Proceedings of the
XIV Symposium Neuroradiologicum

AF877567

George du Boulay · Andrew Molyneux · Ivan Moseley (Eds.)

Proceedings of the XIV Symposium Neuroradiologicum

London, 17–23 June 1990

With 696 Figures (1273 Separate Illustrations) and 183 Tables

Springer-Verlag Berlin Heidelberg New York
London Paris Tokyo Hong Kong Barcelona

Professor George du Boulay, CBE
Old Manor House
Brington
Huntington
Cambridgeshire PEI8 0PX
United Kingdom

Dr. Andrew Molyneux
Neuroradiology Department
Radcliffe Infirmary
Oxford OX2 6HE
United Kingdom

Dr. Ivan Moseley
Lysholm Department of Radiology
The National Hospital
Queen Square
London WC1N 3BG
United Kingdom

This book appears as a supplement to the journal **Neuroradiology** Volume 33/1991

ISBN 978-3-642-49331-7 ISBN 978-3-642-49329-4 (eBook)
DOI 10.1007/978-3-642-49329-4

This work is subject to copyright. All rights are reserved, whether the whole or part of the material is concerned, specifically the rights of translations, reprinting, reuse of illustrations, recitation, broadcasting, reproduction on microfilms or in other ways, and storage in data banks. Duplication of this publication or parts thereof is only permitted under the provisions of the German Copyright Law of September 9, 1965, in its current version, and a copyright fee must always be paid. Violations fall under the prosecution act of the German Copyright Law.

© Springer Verlag, Berlin Heidelberg 1991
Softcover reprint of the hardcover 1st edition 1991

Product Liability: The publisher can give no guarantee for information about drug dosage and application thereof contained in this book. In every individual case the respective user must check its accuracy by consulting other pharmaceutical literature.
The use of registered names, trademarks, etc. in this publication does not imply, even in the absence of a specific statement, that such names are exempt from the relevant protective laws and regulations and therefore free for general use.

2127/3335-543210 – Printed on acid free paper

Foreword

The scope of neuroradiology is now so wide that no one can be master or mistress of it all. Nevertheless the brains of all neuroradiologists still need, and mostly hold, those basic matrices on which neuroanatomy, physiology and pathology are encoded. A chance to grasp and use what's new in the whole field should be available to all because it might be useful outside its primary application, which is why, even in 1990, it was still appropriate to hold our Symposium in plenary sessions.

There are many national and continental meetings at which training in presentation is almost as much a part of the programme as the reports of scientific advance. In my view the Symposia Neuroradiologica are for discussion of the hot topics, by experts, in the full glare of a critical audience able to take part in discussion and dispute.

At such a meeting same subjects are best dealt with orally: others, where copious pictorial detail or numerical analysis needs to be displayed are better as posters.

These are the main explanations for the material in this volume. The editors and the publisher have worked hard to bring it out while its contents are still valuable to the worldwide community of neuroradiological science.

We are also very grateful to our colleagues Drs Vic McAllister and Keith Hall for their editorial help.

Professor George du Boulay
President, XIV Symposium Neuroradiologicum
London, June 1990

Contents

Session 1: Neuroradiological Controversies 1990

Session 2: Neuro-Ophthalmology 11

Session 3: Cerebral Tumours 1

Session 4: Cerebral Tumours 2

Session 5: Cerebrovascular Disease - Diagnosis

Session 6: Cerebrovascular Disease - Treatment

Session 7: Degenerative Diseases of the Spine

Session 8: Inflammatory Diseases of the Spine

Session 9: Demyelinating Disease

Session 10: Treatment of Cerebral Aneurysms

Session 11: Spine: Including Interventional

Session 12: Spine: Trauma and CSF Flow

Session 13: Intracranial A-V Malformations

Session 14: A-V Malformations and Interventional

Session 15: Intracranial Infections

Session 16: Brain Diseases

Session 17: Paediatrics

Session 18: Cerebrovascular Disease, Funtional

Session 19: Paediatrics

Session 20: Magnetic Resonance: Technical Aspects

Poster Session 1

Poster Session 2

Scientific Exhibits

List of Authors

___ Manuscript not received

SESSION 1
NEUroradiological CONTROVERSIES 1990

Neuroradiology (1991) 33 [Suppl]: 2–4

Neuroradiology
© Springer-Verlag 1991

A data base library as a diagnostic aid in neuroimaging

T. Greitz[1], S. Holte[3], C. Bohm[5], L. Eriksson[1,2], R. Seitz[2], K. Ericson[1], H. Nybäck[3], and S. Stone-Elander[4]

Departments of [1] Neuroradiology, [2] Clinical Neurophysiology and [3] Psychiatry, Karolinska Hospital, Stockholm, Sweden
[4] Karolinska Pharmacy, Karolinska Hospital, Stockholm, Sweden, [5] Department of Physics, Stockholm University, Stockholm, Sweden

Summary. This report describes a method for comparing the data obtained from CT, MRI, SPECT and PET in an individual case with the "mean image" of normal patients. This comparison is analogous to the clinical situation which concerns the state of one individual as compared to a normal population. The mean image is obtained after reformatting the image data of the reference group into a standardised anatomy by using transformations that are inverse to those applied to adapt a computerised brain atlas to the individual case. This allows the image data to be averaged and displayed as a mean image. By subtracting the mean image of a normal group, stored in a data base, from that of the individual patient, deviations from the normal can be displayed in a "subtraction image". Using this method significant deviations from the "normal" could be observed in MRI examinations of cases with brain tumours or hydrocephalus as well as in PET studies using various tracers.

Key words: Computerised brain atlas – Positron emission tomography – Image standardisation – Data processing – Data base library

Neuroradiology may be said to have two main objectives: imaging of the anatomy of the central nervous system and imaging of its function. The main role of the neuroradiologist in imaging of brain function has traditionally been to supply anatomical information that serves two purposes: to identify structures of interest in the functional image and to make a conceptual "normalisation" of the anatomy, thus reducing the bias introduced by the anatomical variations. We have shown in earlier work [1–5] that the first of these tasks can be taken over by computerised, individually adjustable brain atlas (CBA). The purpose of this paper is to discuss the extent to which such an atlas may fulfil the second role of the radiologist.

The construction, anatomical content, accuracy and applications of this atlas have been discussed in earlier publications [1–7]. The atlas may be adapted to the anatomy of any individual as it appears in a set of CT, MR, PET or SPECT images (Fig. 1). The atlas may be said to have two main applications in imaging brain function: to serve as a guide in selecting anatomical regions of interest and to serve as a vehicle to compare results from different individuals. By applying the inverse atlas transformation to the image data volume, it is possible to relate the patient's anatomy as it is presented in the tomographic images to the anatomy of the reference atlas instead of to the patient's individual anatomy. All brains will then have the same anatomical appearance.

It has been shown that this method allows data from different individuals to be averaged and averages from different categories of patients to be compared [4]. Similarly, differences between two functional *states* in group of individuals may be demonstrated [5]. These differences may be displayed and identified in a "subtraction image" or a "significance image".

The clinical situation, however, is different from that of the physiological experiment in that it concerns the state of one individual as compared to a normal population. This comparison can be made by subtracting the reformatted mean image of a normal group from that of the individual patient.

Results

Using the method of subtracting the reformatted mean image of normal reference material from that of the patient (or the converse) significant deviations from the "normal" mean can be observed in MRI examinations of cases of brain tumours or hydrocephalus (Fig. 2) and in

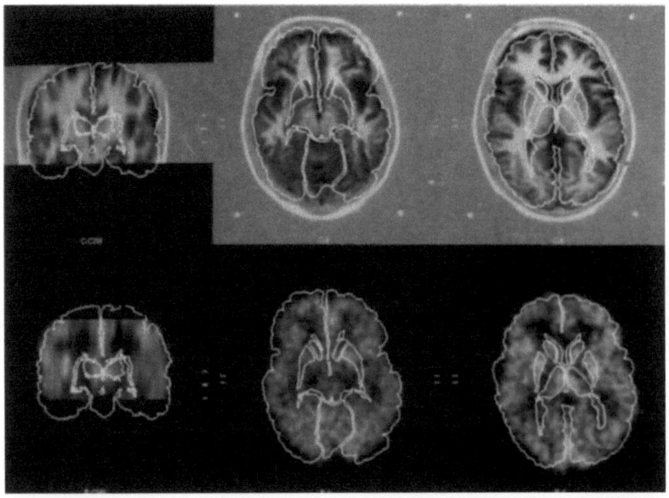

Fig. 1. The computerised atlas has been adapted to a set of MR images (*upper row*) and the reformatted atlas has been transferred to the patient's PET images (*lower row*). The structures displayed include the brain surface, the striatum and the thalamus

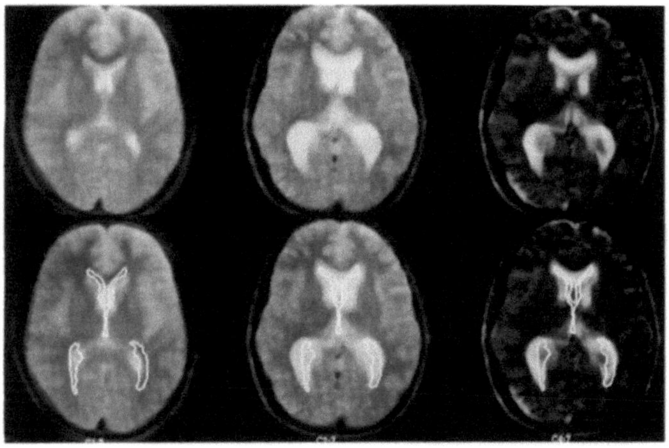

Fig. 2. The image *(right)* obtained by the proposed method, i. e. subtracting the "mean images" of the normal population *(left)* from the patient's MR image *(middle)*, shows the degree of dilatation of the lateral ventricles in this case of hydrocephalus. The ventricular system of the atlas brain is outlined in the lower row

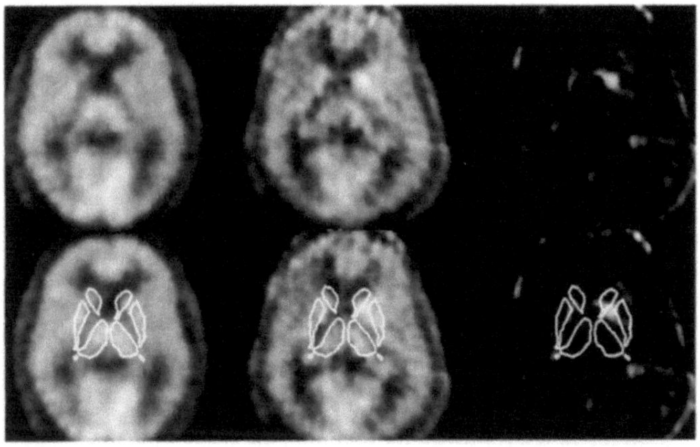

Fig. 3. This PET study using ^{11}C-methionine was considered to reveal "no obvious pathological changes". However, subtracting the "mean image" of a normal population *(left)* from the patient's image *(middle)*, an increased uptake of methionine becomes apparent in the area of the left internal capsule *(right)*. The basal ganglia are outlined in the lower row

PET studies (Fig. 3–5) using various tracers. These include ^{11}C-L-methionine in cases of brain tumors [8], ^{11}C-deoxyglucose in patients with dementia [9] and a benzodiazepine antagonist (^{11}C-RO 15-1788) in cases of epilepsy [10]. One example to show the principle is given in Fig. 2. The mean MR image of the normal individuals is subtracted from the image of a patient with hydrocephalus. The subtraction image shows the degree of dilatation of the ventricular system as compared to the normal group. In tumour cases, the same technique shows in addition to the tumour, the displacement of the brain and ventricular system.

The effect of a physiological stimulation in one individual can be compared with the mean finding at rest in the reference group. The result in the case of a somatosensory activation is shown in Fig. 5.

Alternatively, the response of one individual can be compared with that of the whole reference group. The subtraction image then shows in what respect the response of the individual is different from that of the others.

Discussion

The method of adapting the anatomy of the mean images to the individual case rather than the reverse has certain advantages. The reconstruction of new sections is made by interpolation. The mean image data volume can be stored with better sampling than the ordinary patient study. Therefore, interpolation from the mean images means access to more data than is the case when the individual patient data are used. The formation of new slices would be particularly jeopardised when the individual data set does not cover the entire brain and, at the same time, the slice direction deviates significantly from that of the mean image. In this case it would be impossible to obtain complete data for a correct interpolation at the extreme ends of the stack of slices.

When discussing the extent to which a data base containing a series of CT, MRI, SPECT or PET images, including functional images using various tracers, could take over the role of the radiologist, it is necessary to bear in mind the advances in instrumentation and computer science. It seems very likely that data collection, as well as methods of data handling, will be quite different in the future. The three-dimensional recording of data, already a reality in MRI, combined with computerised methods to recognise and retrieve any plane in the image, will make reproducible alignment and reproducible fixation unnecessary. A step in this direction would be the implementation of an automatic adaption of the CBA. These advances will free not only the radiologist but also the technicians from part of their responsibility.

Computers will undoubtly play an increasing role in radiological diagnostic work. Some kind of a computerised brain atlas (cf. [1–13]) is likely be used by every neuroradiologist. Computers will serve as advisers in the

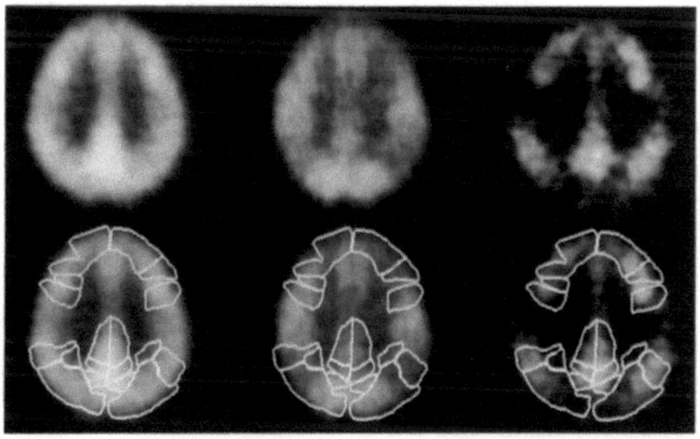

Fig. 4. The metabolic rate of glucose as measured with PET using ^{11}C-deoxyglucose is significantly decreased in several areas of the cortex in this patient suffering from dementia. This is perhaps best seen in the image *(right)* produced by subtracting the patient's data *(middle)* from the mean data obtained in a reference group of seven age-matched normal controls *(left)*. The atlas identifies the most affected regions *(lower row)* at this level as the following Brodmann areas: 6, 7, 8, 9, 19 (lateral part), 23, 34, and 39, all bilaterally

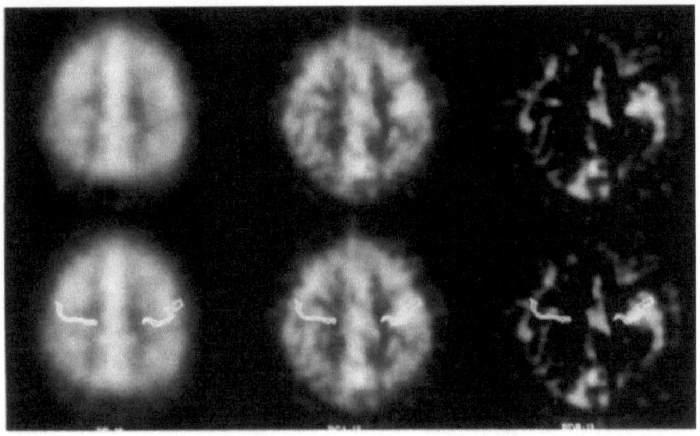

Fig. 5. Using the method of subtracting a reference "mean image" *(left)* from the finding in the individual case *(middle),* the effect of a physiological stimulation in one individual may be compared with the mean finding at rest in the reference group. The effect on regional cerebral blood flow (measured with ^{11}C-fluoromethane) by exposing the right hand of a volunteer to vibrations is shown in the subtraction views *(right).* The central sulcus is outlined in the lower row

interpretation of images [14]. The radiologist will look at a variety of new images and work interactively with a data base that gives access to these new images, including mean images of various reference groups. The data base will allow a rapid and automatic reconstruction of diagnostic images such as subtraction images and significance images. However, the radiologist will still be the expert interpreter of the radiological image, with the knowledge to choose between available methods, providing of course he (or she) is prepared to deal with them all.

Acknowledgment. Supported by a grant from the Swedish Medical Research Council

References

1. Bohm C, Greitz T, Kingsley D, Berggren BM, Olsson L (1983) Adjustable computerized stereotaxic brain atlas for transmission and emission tomography. AJNR 4: 731–733
2. Bohm C, Greitz T, Kingsley D, Berggren BM, Olsson L (1985) A computerized individually variable stereotaxic brain atlas. In: Greitz T (ed) The metabolism of the human brain studied with positron emission tomography. Raven Press, New York, pp 85–91
3. Bohm C, Greitz T, Berggren BM (1985) Selection of PET ROIs from a computerized brain atlas. J Cereb Blood Flow Metab 5 [Suppl 1]: S613–S614
4. Bohm C, Greitz T, Blomqvist G, Farde L, Forsgren PO, Kingsley D, Sjögren I, Wiesel FA, Wik G (1986) Applications of a computerized adjustable brain atlas in positron emission tomography. Acta Radiol [Suppl] 369: 449–452
5. Greitz T, Bohm C, Eriksson L, Mogard J, Roland P, Seitz R, Wiesel FA (1989) The construction of a functional brain atlas: elimination of bias from anatomical variations at PET by reformatting three-dimensional data into a standardized anatomy. In: Ottosson D, Rostène W (eds) Wenner-Gren International Symposium Series, vol 53. MacMillan, pp 137–140
6. Greitz T, Bohm C, Holte S, Eriksson, L (1990) A computerized brain atlas – construction, anatomical content and some applications. J Comput Assist Tomogr (in press)
7. Seitz RJ, Bohm C, Greitz T, Roland PE, Eriksson L, Blomqvist G, Rosenkvist G, Nordell B (1990) Accuracy and precision of the computerized brain atlas program for localization and quantification in positron emission tomography. J Cereb Blood Flow Metab (in press)
8. Ericson K, Lilja A, Bergström M, Blomqvist G, Collins VP, Eriksson L, Ehrin E, Holst H von, Lundquist H, Långström B, Mosskin M (1985) Positron emission tomography with ^{11}C-methyl-l-methionine, ^{11}C-d-glucose and ^{68}Ga-EDTA in the examination of supratentorial tumours. J Comput Assist Tomogr 9: 683–689
9. Nybäck H, Nyman H, Blomqvist S, Sjögren I, Stone-Elander S (1990) Brain metabolism in Alzheimer's dementia: studies of ^{11}C-deoxyglucose accumulation, CSF monoaminee metabolites and neuropsychological test performance in patients and healthy volunteers. J Neurol Neurosurg Psychiatry (in press)
10. Savic I, Roland P, Sedvall G, Persson A, Pauli S, Widén L (1988) In-vivo demonstration of reduced benzodiazepine receptor binding in human epileptic foci. Lancet 8616
11. Evans AC, Beil C, Marett S, Thompson C, Hakim A (1988) Anatomical-functional correlation using an adjustable MRI-based region of interest atlas with positron emission tomography. J Cereb Blood Flow Metab 8: 513–530
12. Fox PT, Perlmutter JS, Raichle ME (1985) A stereotactic method of localization for positron emission tomography. J Comput Assist Tomogr 9: 141–153
13. Mazziotta JC, Koslow SH (1987) Assessment of goals and obstacles in data acquisition and analysis from emission tomography. Report of a series of international Workshops. J Cereb Blood Flow Metab 7: S1–S31
14. Teather D, Teather BA, Wills KM, du Boulay GH, Plummer D, Isherwood I, Gholkar A (1988) Evaluation of computer advisor in the interpretation of CT images of the head. Neuroradiology 30: 511–517

Prof. Torgny Greitz
Department of Neuroradiology
Karolinska Hospital
10401 Stockholm
Sweden

Neuroradiology (1991) 33 [Suppl]: 5–7

Neuro-radiology
© Springer-Verlag 1991

MR discography: a comparison with CT discography and cryomicrotome

II. Clinical applications: work in progress

A. E. Rosenbaum[1], S. Yu[1], N. Szeverenyi[1], H. A. Yuan[2], R. G. Donelson[2], C. M. Mills[3], and B. Fredrickson[2]

[1] Department of Radiology, MR Research Laboratory, and
[2] Department of Orthopedic Surgery, SUNY Health Science Center at Syracuse, New York, USA
[3] San Francisco Neuroskeletal Imaging, San Francisco, California, USA

Summary. The emotional issues concerning discography have been addressed briefly here and some of the many distinguished players in this controversy are cited. Discography remains a very important diagnostic technique in spinal centers for determining the indication for and type of spine operation to be performed to treat symptomatic intervertebral disc disease. Herniation with nerve compression can be readily detected by MRI and CT. When clinical manifestations do not correlate precisely and when symptoms are disabling while equivocal or normal imaging studies obtain, discography may demonstrate the pathologic basis. CT has become the definitive imaging mode for discography while MR has evolved as the optimal spinal imaging technique currently. Should discography by MR not also be included in the armamentarium? Animal toxicology and clinical trials are needed to support these CT-MR-cryomicrotome studies showing MRI to be superior to CT. Perhaps the most likely secondary spin-off of MR discography would be its use for better interpreting routine MRI.

Key words: Magnetic resonance imaging – Discography – Contrast enhancement – Intervertebral disc – Spinal surgery

No radiologically related procedure concerning intervertebral discs (or any other technique) has provoked greater opposing views than discography [1–7]. Despite the elegant clinical science in its conception [8, 9] and early, enthusiastic large follow-up series [10, 11], a solitary, misleading communication by Holt [12] clouded the value of the procedure and rapidly reversed its usage. Moreover, that study [12] performed on 21-to-41 year-old (mean 26) imprisoned "volunteers" uncovered one degenerate and eight herniated intervertebral discs at L4–5 ($n = 24$) and four degenerate and six herniated discs at L5–S1 ($n = 20$). Holt concluded that since there had been no history of back pain or sciatica, that the degenerated and herniated discs found on discography were spurious. Previous anatomic studies and now later CT and MR detect degenerate and herniated discs at a similar frequency in asymptomatic or unrelatedly symptomatic, similar younger age patients. Direct refutation of all aspects of Holt's paper has been advanced [13].

Nonetheless, over the two decades since that report, the emotionally charged positions of distinguished radiologists, orthopedic and neurosurgeons have been discounted so that centers specializing in research on and surgery of intervertebral disc disease [14], could further serve their patients. These centers have reported the procedure to be meaningful and the most pertinent imaging-functional test in their armamentarium when low back and neurologic signs and symptoms do not correlate well with the routine, often noninvasive, imaging studies [14, 15].

CT discography has largely supplanted film-screen discography for demonstrating tears [14, 15]. Since the inception of discography [8, 9], the immediate response of pain, whether similar, dissimilar or precisely reproductive of symptoms following an intradiscal injection, remains a crucial component of the procedure [14].

In the MR era, is the use of discography redundant and remarkably morbid? Certainly the patient with normal MRI would seem very unlikely to have pain of disc origin. Unfortunately, normal MRI does not exclude intrinsic disc disease demonstrable by discography [16]. Our experience agrees with this. Radial tears of the annulus may be detected on T2-weighted images by their hyperintensity within the annulus [17]. In cadavers, T2-weighted MRI shows fewer (10/15) radial tears than CT discography; this was affirmed by cryomicrotome sectioning [17]. Gadolinium (Gd)-DTPA-enhanced MRI has also been reported to visualize radial tears [18]; what percentage of those present is unknown. The resounding question remains as to whether degenerate or herniated disc disease is the cause of that particular patient's symptoms; discography can be of benefit in deciding operability to reduce "failed back" syndrome.

Our experimentation (part I) has shown that a Gd-containing contrast medium can be imaged intradiscally after it is markedly diluted (e.g., 1:1000). Cryomicrotome sectioning was used to judge between the CT and MR intradiscal observations. MR more closely approximated the anatomic findings (Figs. 1–3). The intrinsic disordered architecture of the intervertebral disc and how abnormal

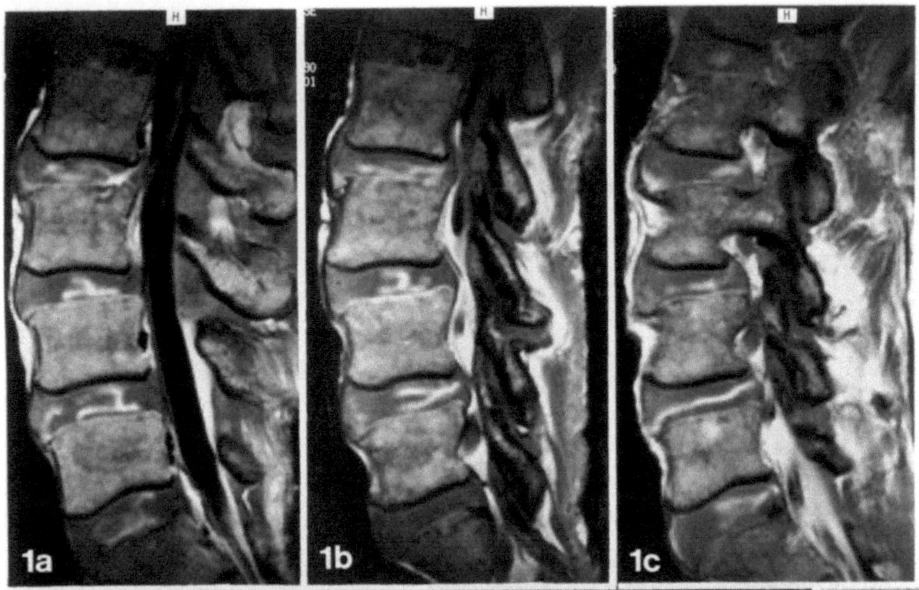

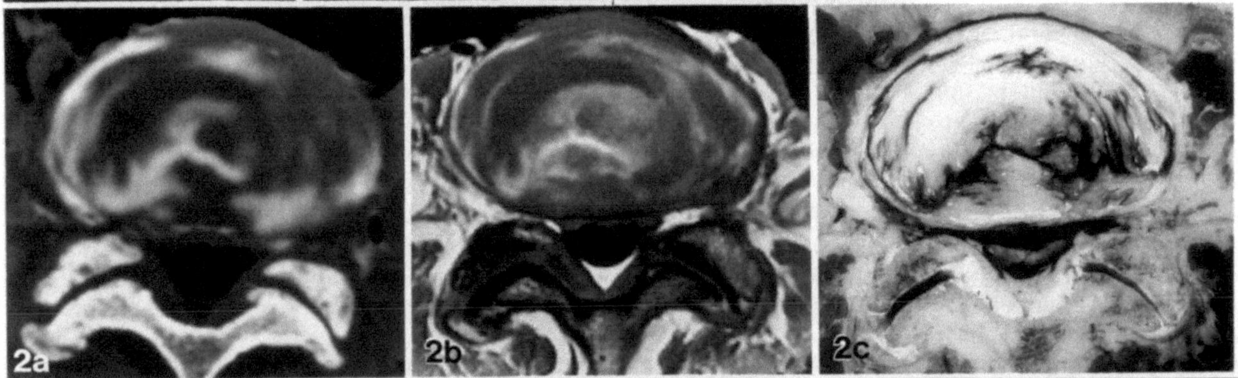

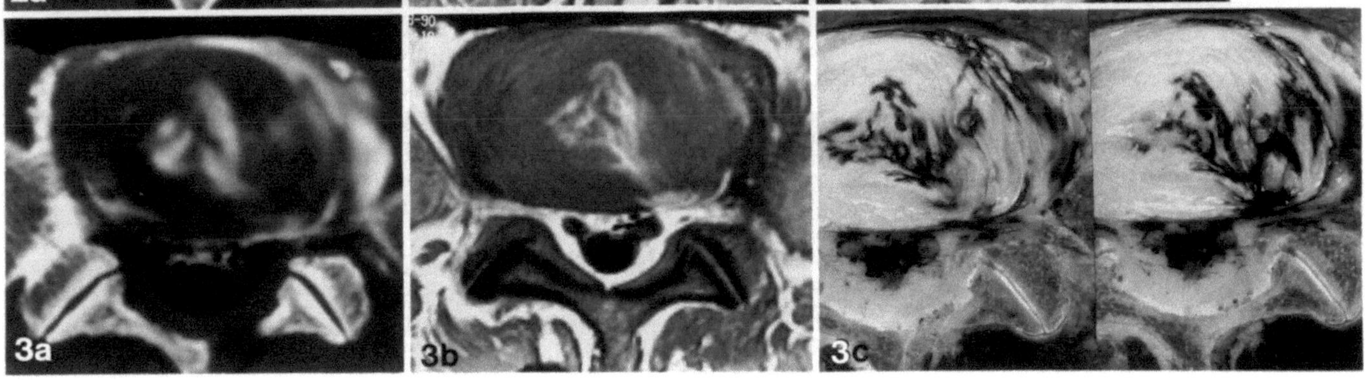

Fig. 1 a–c. Sagittal sections of MR discography of the lumbar discs; T1-weighted spin echo. **a** Mid sagittal section. All five discs are well opacified. L1–2 and L3–4 contain discrete central collections, i. e., show a nucleogram. The L2–3 contrast medium is broader antero-posteriorly denoting contrast material in the annulus; also that disc is mildly narrowed and bulges principally anteriorly. L4–5 is also bulged anteriorly and contrast material is seen in the annulus anteriorly. L5–S1 shows no thinning and the central agglomeration of the contrast material. **b** Right parasagittal section. The L4–5 posterior linear collection representing a radial tear is now seen. **c** Left parasagittal section demonstrates a remarkable single linear fissure visualized from antero-inferiorly to postero-superiorly. L5–S1 shows a posterior radial tear

Fig. 2 a–c. CT-MR-cryomicrotome correlation of L4–5 disc (same specimen as Fig. 1). **a** CT, there is a radial tear on the right which courses from the nucleus to the periphery of the annulus. The tear is broader posteriorly than anteriorly. Circumferential annular tears are seen bilaterally. **b** MR, the beginning of the radial tear within the nucleus is more discrete and better defined its sharper edges despite it appearing narrower. The tightly twisted right posterolateral portion of the tear is more discretely defined by MR and correlates well with the cryomicrotome section. The circumferential annular tears are better defined. **c** Cryomicrotome, the fast green dye allows for readily tracking the tears. Morphologic correlation is closer to MR than CT

Fig. 3 a–c. CT-MR-cryomicrotome correlation of L5–S1 disc. **a** CT, the nucleogram funnels into the postero-lateral radial tear. Circumferential tears are also seen. **b** MR, the delicate breadth and sideward tracking of the radial tear is more distinct than on CT. The intrinsic nuclear disturbance and disrupted annular architecture is displayed better on MR than CT. **c** Cryomicrotome, the deranged morphology better parallels that seen on MR. The radial tear more precisely parallels the imaging of it by MR contrast medium and fast green dye tracked through radial and circumferential tears were well portrayed by MR discography. Although it is doubtful that MR discography would become widespread, another advantage of its use would be to use its superior delineation of intradiscal architecture so that "plain" and intravenously enhanced MR spinal images could be even more skillfully interpreted.

The future direction for its use in man would require toxicologic studies to confirm that an intradiscal injection is safe and that it confers the same disease diagnostic distinguishing features as previous agents, e.g., nonionic iodinated contrast media.

The dilution of gadopentatate dimeglumine with iohexol (and fast green dye) was used so that CT and MR could be more precisely compared from the same injection. However, for MR discography to be performed in man, a similar Gd-iodide mixture would be necessary to allow for "fluoroscopy" of the gadopentatate complex as it is injected into the disc. Moreover, were there the need to do CT rather than MR of the dual contrast medium injected disc(s), this would be possible. The safety of Gd-based contrast media would appear even better as nonionic media are released.

References

1. Peterson HO (1958) Discography. Postgrad Med 23: 512–17
2. Taveras J (1967) Is discography a useful diagnostic procedure? J Assoc Can Radiol 19: 294–295
3. Butt WP, Wortzman G, Simmons EH (1968) Letters to the editor. J Assoc Can Radiol 19: 2–3
4. Shapiro R (1986) Current status of lumbar diskography. Radiology 159: 815
5. Scullin DR (1987) Letters to the editor: lumbar diskography. Radiology 162: 284
6. Bernard TN (1987) Letters to the editor: don't discard diskography. Radiology 162: 285
7. Errico TJ Letters to the editor: the role of diskography in the 1980s. Radiology 162: 285
8. Lindblom K (1948) Diagnostic puncture of intervertebral discs in sciatica. Acta Orthop Scand 17: 231–239
9. Hirsch C (1948) An attempt to diagnose the level of a disc lesion clinically by disc puncture. Acta Orthop Scand 18: 132–139
10. Collis JS Jr, Gardner WJ (1962) Lumbar discography – an analysis of one thousand cases. J Neurosurg 19: 452–459
11. Cloward RB (1962) Discussion – lumbar discography. J Neurosurg 19: 459–460
12. Holt EP (1968) The question of lumbar discography. J Bone Joint Surg 50 A: 720–726
13. Simmons JW, Aprill CN, Dwyer AP, Brodsky AE (1988) A reassessment of Holt's data on "the question of lumbar discography". Clin Orthop 237: 120–123
14. Vanharanta H, Guyer RD, Ohnmeiss DD, Stith WJ, Sachs BL, Aprill C, Spivey M, Rashbaum RF, Hochschuler SH, Videman T, Selby DK, Terry A, Mooney V (1988) Disc deterioration in low-back syndromes. A prospective, multi-center CT/discography study. Spine 13: 1349–1351
15. Jackson RP, Cain JE Jr, Jacobs RR, Cooper BR, McManus GE (1989) The neuroradiologic diagnosis of lumbar herniated nucleus pulposus. I. A comparison of computed tomography (CT), myelography, CT-myelography, discography, and CT-discography. Spine 14: 1356–1361
16. Kornberg M (1989) Discography and magnetic resonance imaging in the diagnosis of lumbar disc disruption. Spine 14: 1368–1372
17. Yu S, Haughton VM, Sether LA, Wagner M (1989) Comparison of MR and discography in detecting radial tears of the annulus: a postmortem study. AJNR 10: 1077–1081
18. Ross JS, Modic MT, Masaryk TJ (1989) Tears of the annulus fibrosus: assessment with Gd-DTPA-enhanced MR imaging. AJNR 10: 1251–1254

Dr. A. E. Rosenbaum
Suny Health Science Center at Syracuse,
750 East Adams Street
Syracuse, New York, USA

Neuroradiology (1991) 33 [Suppl]: 8–10

Neuro radiology
© Springer-Verlag 1991

Applications of computer simulated MRI

G. J. Sivewright[1], X. P. Zhu[2], I. Isherwood[2], and C. J. Taylor[1]

Departments of [1] Medical Biophysics and [2] Diagnostic Radiology, University of Manchester, Manchester, UK

Summary. A large-scale simulation of MRI was developed on vector processing supercomputers. The model has been applied to produce simulated images of normal and abnormal neuroanatomy with and without artefacts. Models of the cervical spinal cord have been produced and the effects of chemical shift, flow and errors in signal processing demonstrated.

Key words: Magnetic resonance imaging – Computer simulation – Artefacts – Anatomical models

---

This article describes applications of a large-scale simulation of MRI [1–3]. MRI is a complex procedure involving interactions between nuclear spin populations and magnetic fields. The underlying physical processes are well understood [4] and suitable for accurate computer simulation [1]. The imaging process is computed over arrays of vectors representing the magnetisation in a polarised object. Values of proton density and T1 and T2 relaxation parameters are associated with each position. Other parameters, such as chemical shift and flow velocity, may be introduced where appropriate. Effects of magnetic gradients, RF pulses and relaxation processes are calculated by numerical integration of the Bloch equations. Raw data acquisition is modelled by periodically summing the transverse components of magnetisation from the whole object array in the presence of phase and frequency encoding gradients. Images are reconstructed by applying two-dimensional Fourier transforms (2DFT) to the simulated raw data.

Large-scale simulation of MRI demands intensive computer processing. The simulation was developed on CDC Cyber 205 and Amdahl VP1200 vector processing supercomputers at Manchester Computer Centre [2]. The peak processing speed of the VP1200 is 571 Mflops (millions of floating point operations per second). This high performance allowed results to be calculated for large object arrays (e.g. $256 \times 256 \times 32$).

In this article a number of phenomena relevant to neuroradiological imaging are examined. Anatomical models were constructed by assigning appropriate MR parameters to an object array. Numerical methods, including cubic spline interpolation and matrix rotation, were used to define the boundaries of the different tissue types. Effects of chemical shift were simulated for a demyelinating lesion in the spinal cord. The principle of flow velocity encoding has also been demonstrated. Several artefacts arising from signal processing errors were examined and their effects demonstrated on a model of the cervical spine.

Chemical shift artefacts

Considerable current interest is directed at monitoring the process of demyelination and plaque formation in patients with multiple sclerosis (MS) [5]. A model of the spinal cord which consisted of grey and white matter surrounded by a layer of cerebrospinal fluid (CSF) was constructed. A small demyelinating plaque in the white matter of the cord was assigned resonant frequency values representing both inflammatory and lipid tissue components. A chemical shift difference of 3.5 ppm was assigned between the lipid and water components.

The chemical shift phenomenon is illustrated in T_1-weighted images generated using a simulated spin echo sequence (SE 200/15) (Fig. 1). Display resolution is approximately 0.15×0.15 mm. As the field strength is increased, the lipid component of the MS plaque is shifted relative to the water component, due to its different resonance frequency. Complete spatial separation of the water and lipid components is evident at 1.5 T, whilst no chemical shift effect is visible at 0.02 T. This model can be used to estimate the effects of chemical shift artefacts on the appearance of MR images under different circumstances, ranging from variations in gradient strength and resonance frequencies to the composition of the lesion itself etc. Such simulations can also be of value in the development of techniques for separation of lipid and water in specific circumstances.

Flow encoding

Techniques for measuring flow information have important applications in the study of central nervous system disorders. Here, we use the MRI simulation simply to demonstrate the principle of flow encoding. An object was defined to consist of a circular region with proton density and relaxation times different from the background. The model assumed laminar flow in a direction perpendicular to the slice. The velocity information was encoded by applying a pair of short gradient pulses in the slice-select direction, either side of a 180° pulse in a spin echo pulse se-

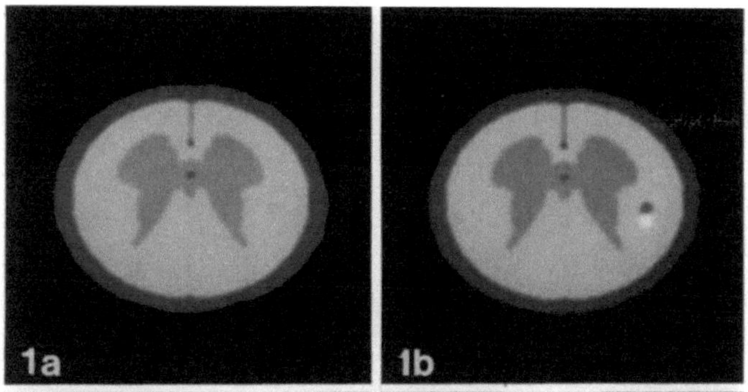

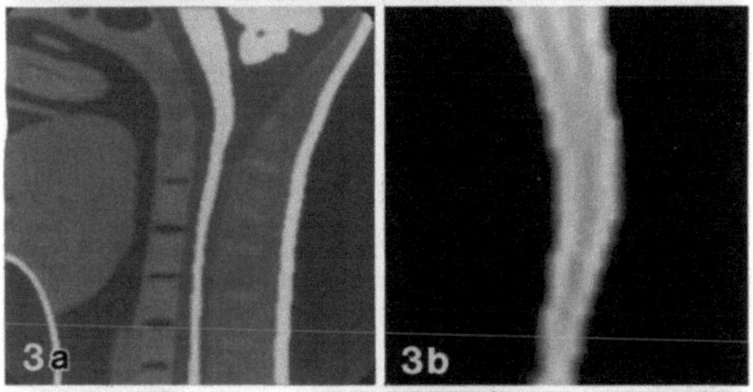

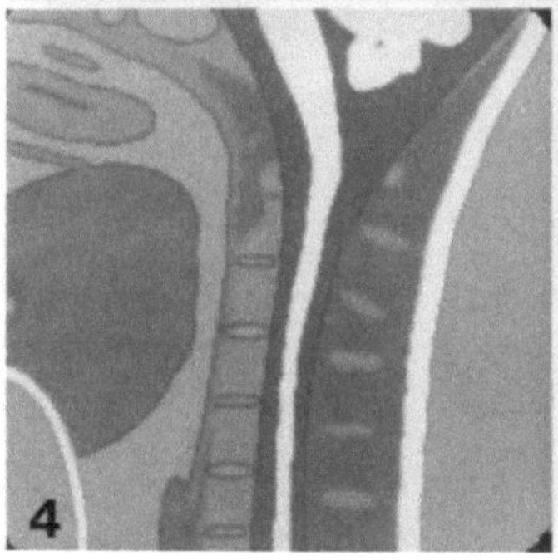

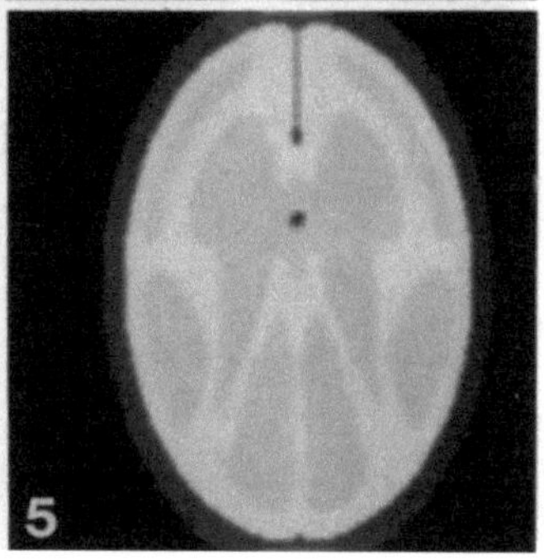

Fig. 1. Simulated spin echo MR images of the spinal cord in transverse section at 0.02 T (**a**) and 1.5 T (**b**). At high field, the lipid component of a modelled multiple sclerosis lesion is shifted relative to the water component, due to its different resonance frequency

Fig. 3 a–b. Simulated spin echo MR images of the cervical spine. **a** An apparent linear low-intensity abnormality in the cervical spinal cord was produced by attenuating the magnitude of high-order phase-encoding gradients. **b** The artefact is more evident in an enlarged and windowed view of the spinal cord

Fig. 4. Simulated spin echo MR images of the cervical spine. Truncation of the MR signal peak reduces low spatial frequencies and produces "outlining" artefacts at the edges of tissue structures

Fig. 5. Simulated spin echo MR images of the spinal cord in transverse section. Incorrect setting of gradients can produce spatial distortion and image wrap-around

quence [6]. Stationary spins were completely rephased by the 180° pulse whilst moving spins retained a degree of phase encoding that was a function of both the gradient and the flow velocity. The phase information was maintained during 2DFT reconstruction. Figure 2a and b shows reconstructed real and imaginary image data that combine the phase and magnitude information. Figure 2c is a reconstructed phase map that contains the flow velocity information. The surface plot in Fig. 2d displays the signal magnitude distribution, which is not affected by the flow.

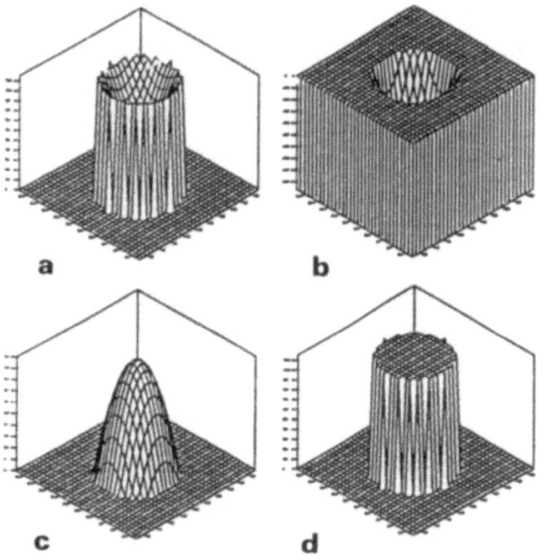

Fig. 2. a–d. Application of a flow mapping sequence to a model of laminar flow in a direction perpendicular to the slice. Reconstructed real (**a**) and imaginary (**b**) images. The velocity and signal intensity distributions can be resolved in phase (**c**) and magnitude (**d**) computed maps.

Reconstruction artefacts

Here we use the simulation to illustrate how a number of common artefacts can affect the appearance of clinical MR images. A model was produced of the cervical spine, comprising bone, intervertebral discs, muscle, fat, CSF and air. The different tissue structures were assigned appropriate values of MR parameters. Simulated spin echo sequences were used to collect signals from the model. Scan parameters were set up to simulate SE2000/150, SE200/15 and SE740/40 sequences.

A commonly encountered artefact consists of a linear, low-signal abnormality in the cervical spinal cord. This artefact may be confused with a syrinx or other intramedullary lesion (Fig. 3). We have produced the artefact by attenuating the magnitude of high-order phase-encoding gradients thus mimicking the effects of gradient saturation. Other causes of such an artefact might include Gibb's phenomenon [7] or pulsatile flow in the CSF.

Another type of artefact results from insufficient attenuation of the received signal before data collection, resulting in a truncation of the signal peak. The resulting image shows loss of low spatial frequencies and relative highlighting of high frequencies. Figure 4 illustrates such a situation with spurious edges at tissue boundaries and reduced contrast between air and surrounding tissues.

Incorrect adjustment of imaging gradients [7] can cause spatial distortion as shown in Fig. 5. Wrap-around artefacts are also apparent in this image. Regions of the object lying outside the field of view possess frequencies outside the imaging bandwidth. The signals are therefore undersampled and become aliased back into the image.

Conclusion

We have demonstrated clinically relevant applications of a large-scale computer simulation of MRI. The simulation was developed in order to provide a means of theoretical assessment of clinical MRI techniques. Implementing the software on high-performance computers has provided the capability to model MR processes with high accuracy and resolution.

References

1. Machin M, Hickey DS, Isherwood I (1989) Supercomputers and magnetic resonance imaging. In: Feig E (ed) Advances in magnetic resonance imaging. Ablex, New Jersey, pp 225–254
2. Machin M, Hickey DS, Sivewright GJ, Robinson EM, Isherwood I (1989) Large scale simulation of magnetic resonance imaging. In: Supercomputing at Manchester Computing Centre 1987–89. MCC, Manchester, p 109
3. Sivewright GJ, Machin M, Hickey DS (1990) Supercomputer simulation of magnetic resonance imaging. Comput Methods Programs Biomed (in press)
4. Mansfield P, Morris PG (1982) NMR imaging in biomedicine. Academic Press, London
5. Thompson AJ, Kermonde AG, MacManus DG, Kendall BE, Kingsley DPE, Moseley IF, McDonald WI (1990) Patterns of disease activity in multiple sclerosis: clinical and magnetic resonance imaging study. Br Med J 300: 631–634
6. Bryant DJ, Payne JA, Firmin DN, Longmore DB (1984) Measurement of flow with NMR imaging using a gradient pulse and phase difference technique. J Comput Assist Tomogr 8: 588–593
7. Henkelman RM, Brouskill MJ (1987) Artifacts in magnetic resonance imaging. Review of MR in medicine, vol 2. Pergamon, New York

Prof. I. Isherwood
University of Manchester
Department of Diagnostic Radiology
Stopford Building
Oxford Road
Manchester M13 9PT, UK

SESSION 2
NEURO-OPHTHALMOLOGY

Neuroradiology (1991) 33 [Suppl]: 12–14

Neuro radiology
© Springer-Verlag 1991

The transdiaphragmatic (transhypophyseal foramen) suprasellar pituitary gland: a normal variant

B. Kaufman[1], W. R. Selman[2], and S. C. Amartur[1]

[1] Department of Radiology, [2] Division of Neurosurgery, University Hospitals of Cleveland/Case Western Reserve University, Cleveland, Ohio, USA

Summary. A normal transdiaphragmatic and suprasellar location of the superior surface of the normal pituitary gland (PG) may result when the diaphragma sellae is incomplete (hypophyseal foramen) in association with a small pituitary fossa. The shape of the glandular extension may be one of a spectrum ranging from minimal to pronounced, the larger having a pyramidal and/or "head and shoulders" configuration. The height of the gland can be greater than the currently utilized normal linear measurements. Glandular contact with the optic chiasm has not been associated with visual field defects. The location and status of the diaphragma sellae can be determined by MRI. Abnormal PG enlargement may also present an identical suprasellar pyramidal appearance, but abnormal tissue characterization and gadolinium enhancement will differentiate between normal and abnormal glands.

Key words: Transhypophyseal foramen – Pituitary gland – Suprasellar – Physiological hypertrophy

We have observed on coronal MRI studies of normal pituitary glands (PGs) a spectrum of transdiaphragmatic suprasellar glandular extensions ranging from a minimal focal convexity to a large focal convex glandular extension which may be in contact with the optic chiasm (OC). The height of the glandular extension, convex configuration of the superior surface and apparent increase in glandular size would be considered abnormal by existing standards which, however, are now being challenged [1–5].

We present case material supporting the proposition that these transdiaphragmatic suprasellar glandular extensions are normal PG variants and probably are the result of a congenitally incomplete diaphragma sellae in association with a normal gland in a small sella turcica (ST) or a physiological hypertrophied gland in a normal or small ST.

Patients and methods

A highly selected group of 22 cases with a suprasellar extension of the PG exhibiting a minimal to large focal convexity and a suspected increased gland height on coronal sections was examined. Only cases with normal STs and visual fields were included.

Age distribution was (1) birth to 10 years: 2 infants (1 week, 6 weeks); (2) 11–20 years: 5 females (13–19 years), 2 males (18 years); and (3) 21 years and older: 13 females [21–46 years (mean, 31 years; median, 28 years)].

The reasons for the MRI studies were as follows. Six patients had suprasellar hyperdensities on CT, 4 had hypothalamic dysfunction, and 12 were investigated for entities other than endocrine abnormalities or visual field defects.

Volume estimation of the PG was done in 1 case (Fig. 1). The steps in the volume estimation algorithm for the PG are as follows:
1. The 3D data set was resampled in all the three axes to provide isotropic 1 mm^3 voxels.
2. A contour enclosing the gland was drawn on a graphics console (Vicom image processor) for each slice of the resampled data set. Number of voxels enclosed by the contour was determined.
3. Sum total of the number of voxels in the resampled data set represents the volume of the gland.

The ST size and configuration were subjectively assessed on the MRI studies. Transphenoidal surgery followed on one 14-year-old female suspected of having a non-functioning adenoma. Initial MR examination was for headaches.

MR examinations were with either 1.0 T or 1.5 T units at multiple institutions. All cases had T1-weighted images in sagittal and coronal planes, 8 had gadolinium (Gd) enhancement, and 3 had spin density and T2-weighted images.

Results

As the result of our case selections, all had a superior gland surface which classically would be considered as probably abnormal in configuration and height [1–4].

Endocrine studies were normal in 15 patients. Seven (including 2 infants) were considered clinically as endocrinologically normal.

Transphenoidal surgery for a suspected non-functioning pituitary adenoma in the 14-year-old female revealed normal histology (Fig. 1).

Eight cases had a small sella (shallow or narrow in width). A small normal sella is illustrated in Fig. 1, and a very small shallow sella is seen in Fig. 2.

The PG touched the OC in 9 cases without visual field defects (Figs. 1, 2). All PGs were above the planum sphenoidale (PS) and a chiasmatic sulcus was not present.

The PG did not touch the OC in 11 cases. In 8, the pituitary was above the PS without a chiasmatic sulcus. In 3 with a chiasmatic sulcus the PG was below the PS.

Both infants had a pyramidal suprasellar PG extension which almost touched the OC (Fig. 3).

A moderate supradiaphragmatic extension was seen with a suspected partially incomplete diaphragma (Fig. 4).

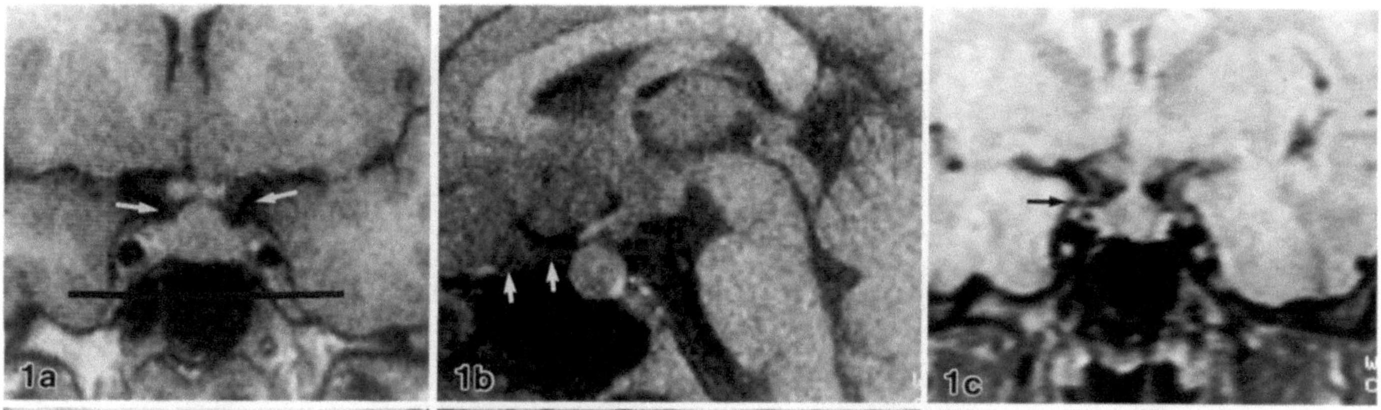

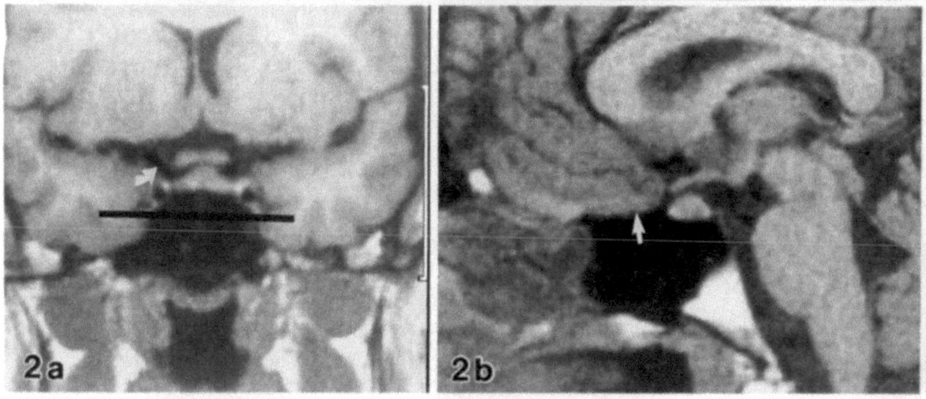

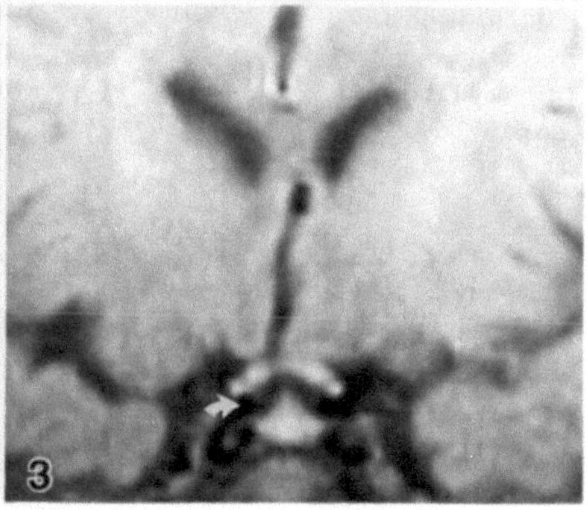

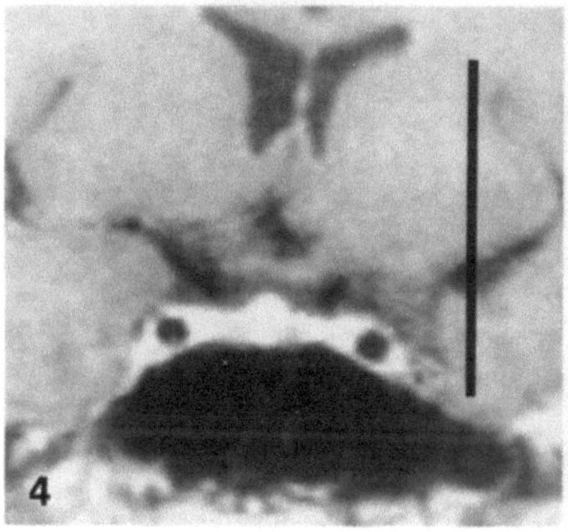

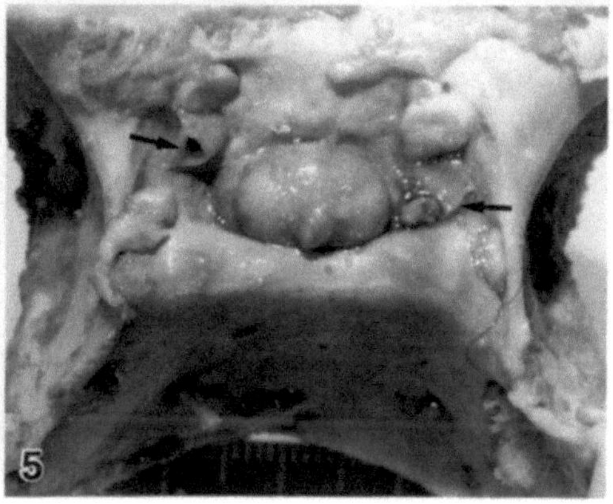

Fig. 1a–c. Transdiaphragmatic suprasellar pituitary gland (PG) in an endocrinologically normal 14-year-old female with menstrual irregularities. Surgery for a non-functioning adenoma revealed normal histology. **a** The PG extends through a suspected incompetent diaphragma sellae and is in contact with the optic chiasm (OC). The transdiaphragmatic glandular extension results in a "head and shoulders" configuration. The edge of the diaphragma sellae is located immediately below the supradiaphragmatic part of the internal carotid arteries *(arrows)*. Gland height is 11.4 mm (scale = 50 mm). Coronal SE 400/17. **b** The central portion of the PG is round, extends above the planum sphenoidale *(arrows)* and is in contact with the OC. Sella turcica dimensions on films; height = 6 mm, length = 11 mm, and width = 12 mm. Calculated volume of the pituitary = 850 mm^3. Sagittal SE 400/17. **c** The peripheral rim of the diaphragma sella is seen as a horizontal linear hypointensity *(arrow)* immediately below and in contact with the supradiaphragmatic portion of the internal carotid artery. The PG has a pyramidal configuration in this plane. Coronal spin density 2000/35

Fig. 2a, b. This case illustrates a small sella turcica and a suprasellar PG in a 26-year-old female with seizures, normal pituitary function and no visual field defects. CT showed a suprasellar enhancing mass. **a** The PG (height = 7.5 mm) is in contact with the OC. The supradiaphragmatic internal carotid artery *(arrow)* indicates the level of the diaphragma sellae. Coronal SE 500/17. Scale = 50 mm. **b** Sella turcica is shallow and small (film measurements where length = 10 mm, height = 4 mm, and width = 14 mm). On this section the PG is above the planum *(arrow)* and triangular but was round on a more medial section through the hypophyseal stalk. Sagittal SE 500/17

Fig. 3. Coronal T1-weighted image in a 6-week-old infant studied for an occipital meningocele. The PG almost touches the OC. The supradiaphragmatic internal carotid artery *(arrow)* indicates the plane of the diaphragma sellae

Fig. 4. This case illustrates a part of the spectrum of transdiaphragmatic PG extension associated with a shallow sella turcica and a partially incompetent diaphragma sellae. The gland extends above the diaphragma sellae but is not in contact with the optic chiasm. Height of gland = 7.7 mm. Coronal SE 760/20 with Gd enhancement. (Scale = 50 mm)

Fig. 5. Dorsal en bloc view of the sphenoid bone of a 15-year-old primigravida postpartum female who died with eclampsia. This case illustrates a congenitally incompetent diaphragma sellae and the post partum edematous and hypertrophied PG extending to a supradiaphragmatic position. The width of the diaphragma sellae opening is 13 mm. Gland is greater than 13 mm and, therefore, when viewed in a coronal plane there would be a central elevation of the gland. The supradiaphragmatic intradural internal carotid arteries (*arrows,* one artery with a thrombus in lumen) can be used to define the plane of the diaphragma sellae. (Scale in mm)

The diaphragma sellae could be identified on coronal spin density or T2-weighted images (Fig. 1) [6]. The plane of the diaphragma sellae could be identified by locating the supradiaphragmatic (intradural) portion of the internal carotid artery (ICA) (Figs. 1–4) which is immediately above the diaphragma sellae. Thus, a supradiaphragmatic location of the PG could be defined. An en bloc sphenoid bone specimen illustrates these artery and diaphragma relationships and shows a postpartum edematous and hypertrophied PG extending through a congenitally incompetent diaphragma sellae (Fig. 5).

Volume estimation of the PG in the surgically treated patient (Fig. 1) yielded a volume of 850 mm^3. Even considering the fact that volume is not exactly equivalent to mass or weight measurements the result was at the upper range of published normal values of weight of adult female PGs [7, 8]. The volume of the sella was 396 mm^3.

Discussion

We suggest that a transdiaphragmatic suprasellar PG is the result of the relationships of the volume of the PG, the volume and configuration of the ST, and the intactness of the diaphragma sellae, and is a normal variant. At autopsy about 80% of the sella diaphragms have varying degrees of incompleteness ranging from a small central opening, the hypophyseal foramen, to near absence with a small remaining peripheral rim (Fig. 5) [7, 9, 10]. The diaphragma sellae can be visualized directly on MRI utilizing appropriate techniques [6] or the location of the diaphragma sellae can be determined by identifying the intradural (supradiaphragmatic) portion of the ICA (Figs. 1–4), in contact with the diaphragma sellae inferiorly.

With a large central opening and a rigid peripheral rim of the diaphragm, the expected gland configuration would be that seen in Figs. 1 and 2. A small diaphragmatic defect probably would result in an extension as seen in Fig. 4.

We have postulated a deficient diaphragmatic sellae in these cases but do not have anatomical proof. A thin but intact diaphragma sella or dilatation of the variable hypophyseal foramen may permit the same glandular configurations to occur.

A shallow ST is accepted as a normal variation [11] and predisposes to an extrasellar PG location.

We have no explanation at this time as to why visual field defects were not present in the nine adult cases in which the gland touched the chiasm. Seventeen cases had the PG above the PS in sagittal views. The gland in this location is seen on CT, axial and coronal views, as a suprasellar mass.

Elster et al. [12] have shown statistically physiological hypertrophy of the PG in adolescence (ages 11–20 years) confirming previous impressions [2–4, 13]. The coronal and sagittal configurations of the PG in Fig. 4 of Elster et al. [12] are comparable to our Fig. 1, and were their demonstration of a normal appearance representing physiological hypertrophy seen in 25% of female teenagers.

Our case material and the highly selective method used do not lend themselves to statistical analysis and comparison with the study of Elster et al. [12]. In addition, their study was based on the appearance of the gland on sagittal MR views. Our case (Fig. 1) is in all likelihood an example of physiological hypertrophy of the PG. We have seen four females (ages 24, 26, 27, and 45 years) who had glands touching the OC, thus suggesting that the occurrence is not rare. The two infant cases show that the transdiaphragmatic glandular extension is probably associated with a congenitally incompetent diaphragma sellae. At autopsy in infants, the PG has been observed projecting through a deficient diaphragma sellae [14].

While the morphological aspects of the described transdiaphragmatic suprasellar PG and pituitary adenomas may have identical images, endocrinological studies and tissue characterization utilizing the basic MR sequences and Gd enhancement can differentiate abnormal PG enlargement from the normal PG variant described.

In summary, when the normal or physiological hypertrophied PG exceeds the volume of the small or normal small ST and there is an incomplete diaphragma sellae the gland will protude. This normal variant is not rare and occurs in all age groups.

References

1. Syverstsen AL (1979) The computed tomographic appearance of the normal pituitary gland and pituitary microadenomas. Radiology 133: 385–391
2. Swartz JD, Russell KB, Basile BA (1983) High-resolution computed tomographic appearance of the intrasellar contents in women of child bearing age. Radiology 147: 115–117
3. Wolpert SM, Molitch ME, Goldman JA, Wood JB (1984) Size, shape, and appearance of the normal female pituitary gland. AJR 143: 377–381
4. Peyster RG, Hoover ED, Viscarello RR (1983) CT appearance of the adolescent and preadolescent pituitary gland. AJNR 4: 411–414
5. Cattin F, Bonneville JF, Tang YS (1990) The convex pituitary gland. Diagn Intervent Radiol 2 (in press)
6. Daniels DL, Pojunas KW, Kilgore DP (1989) MRI of the diaphragma sellae. AJNR 7: 765–767
7. Bergland RM, Ray BS, Torack RM (1968) Anatomical variations in the pituitary gland and adjacent structures in 225 human autopsy cases. J Neurosurg 28: 93–99
8. Rasmussen AT (1934) The weight of the principal components of the normal hypophysis cerebri of the adult human female. Am J Anat 55: 253–275
9. Busch W (1951) Die Morphologie der Sella turcica und ihre Beziehungen zur Hypophyse. Virchows Arch [A] 320: 437–458
10. Kaufman B, Chamberlin WB (1972) The ubiquitous "empty" sella turcica. Acta Radiol Diagn 13: 413–425
11. Matsui T, Teramoto A, Fukushima T, Manaka S, Sano K (1981) Clinical and roentgenological measurement of normal sella turcica statistical research of 1000 cases. Brain Nerve 33: 187–194
12. Elster AD, Chen MYM, Williams DW, Key LL (1990) Pituitary gland: MR imaging of physiologic hypertrophy in adolescence. Radiology 174: 681–685
13. Hayakawa K, Konishi Y, Matsuda T (1989) Development and aging of brain midline structures: assessment with MR imaging. Radiology 172: 171–177
14. Sunderland S (1945) The meningeal relations of the human hypophysis cerebri. J Anat 79: 33–37

Dr. Benjamin Kaufman
Department of Radiology
University Hospitals of Cleveland/
Case Western Reserve University
2074 Abington Road
Cleveland, OH 44106, USA

Neuroradiology (1991) 33 [Suppl]: 15–17

Neuro-radiology
© Springer-Verlag 1991

Emergency decompression of the optic nerve in patients who lose vision with craniofacial fractures: the role of radiological examination

K. J. Momose and M. Joseph

Department of Radiology and Otolaryngology, Massachusetts General Hospital and Massachusetts Eye and Ear Infirmary, Boston, Massachusetts, USA

Summary. The traumatic force to the optic nerve and optic canal was quantified by analyzing CT findings to predict the degree of damage to the optic nerve. Sixty-four patients thought to have traumatic optic neuropathy were studied, of whom 24 were chosen for decompressive surgery. The results in the operated and nonoperated cases are discussed.

Key words: Computed tomography – Traumatic optic neuropathy – Decompressive surgery

A small but significant number of patients sustaining craniofacial fractures develop sudden blindness at the time of the accident or shortly afterwards, due to traumatic swelling of the optic nerve from torsion injury [1]. With immediate decompression of the optic nerve by external ethmoidectomy and sphenoidectomy, the blind eye can be restored to normal vision in a significant number of cases [2, 3].

Difficulty arises in case selection, as some patients may recover their vision spontaneously and some will never recover in spite of decompressive surgery. The benefit of decompressive surgery depends on the severity and site of the lesion in the optic nerve; an immediate decision to operate is essential when surgery is indicated.

This paper is an attempt to use radiological findings (mainly CT) to quantitate the destructive force reaching the optic canal and absorbed by the optic nerve. The three factors which determine the destructive external force in a specific area of the facial skeleton are the causative agent, the direction of the force and the amount of the force. The last of these is the most important factor. The cause of the external force is usually grouped under motor vehicle accidents, assault, and accidental falls. The amount of external force impinging on a specific area of the head and face is expressed by comminution or the number of fracture lines and their extent. Noting the width of the fracture line and the amount of displacement of the bony fragments is important as in case 1; Fig. 1 a, b. The depth of the destructive force is expressed by the presence and type of canalicular and paracanalicular fractures as in case 2; Fig. 2 a, b. The traumatic force on the optic nerve is expressed indirectly by the amount of brain contusion, swelling, and hematoma; free blood and air in the intracranial space also indicate the degree of force applied to the optic nerve and optic canal.

The most frequent site of traumatic optic neuropathy is around the intracanalicular segment of the nerve. This is explained by relative fixity of the intracanalicular portion of the optic nerve which leads to excessive movement of the portion of the optic nerve immediately beyond either end of the canal. It is also due to the limited size of the optic canal, which gives little or no space for a traumatized, swollen optic nerve to expand. The types of optic nerve lesion encountered in traumatic optic neuropathy are dural or interstitial hemorrhage resulting from torsion injuries and infarction due to vascular damage [4, 5]. With sufficient force, the optic nerve can be partially or completely transected. There are many types of decompressive surgical procedure [2, 3]; external ethmoidectomy and sphenoidectomy were chosen as the quickest and safest decompressive procedures when performed by an otolaryngologist with a special interest in optic neuropathy [6].

Quantitation of the traumatic force to the orbital apex was attempted in 64 patients thought to have traumatic optic neuropathy. Most were studied by CT in the coronal and axial planes. Twenty-four were treated by decompressive surgery: 8 had no light perception before surgery; 4 made no improvement after surgery, but there was a variable degree of improvement in the remaining 4. One patient had complete recovery of her vision, 2 had slight improvement and 1 could count fingers at 15 cm. Three patients who could see only finger movements preoperatively experienced a significant improvement in visual acuity after surgery. Two patients whose visual acuity was 20/200 prior to surgery made no improvement postoperatively, but lack of improvement in 1 of these could be related to a significant delay before decompressive surgery. Eleven other patients experienced slight to moderate improvement in their vision after decompression. The remaining 40 cases were not treated surgically because of: (1) the severity of damage to the eye or brain, or both; (2) excessive delay in the decision to operate; (3) inaccessibility of surgical help at the time of accident; and (4) refusal by the patient or consultant for decompressive surgery.

Discussion

All patients with traumatic optic neuropathy from craniofacial fractures should be studied by CT [6–8] to facilitate selection of those who will benefit from decompressive

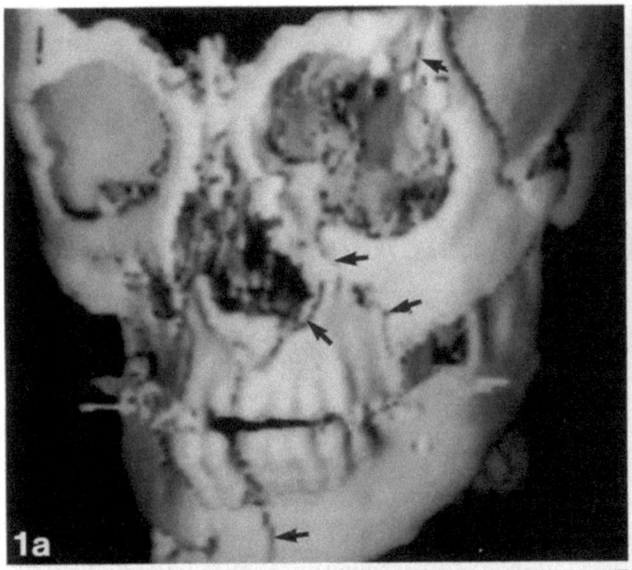

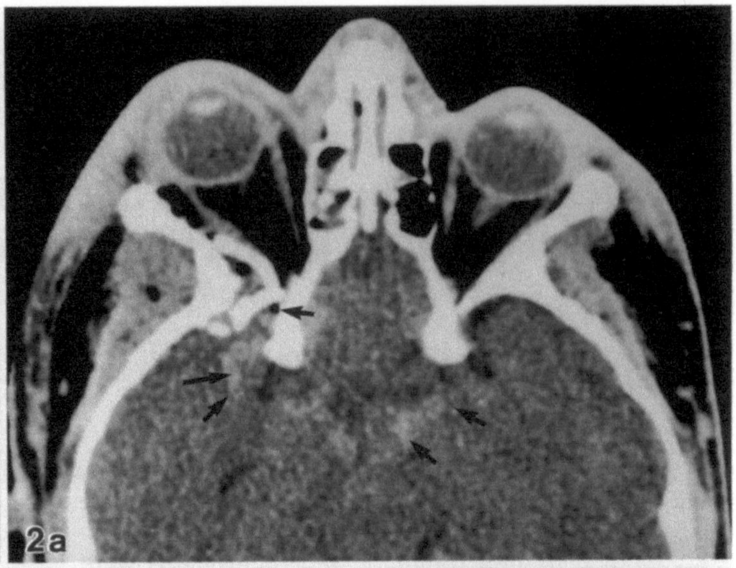

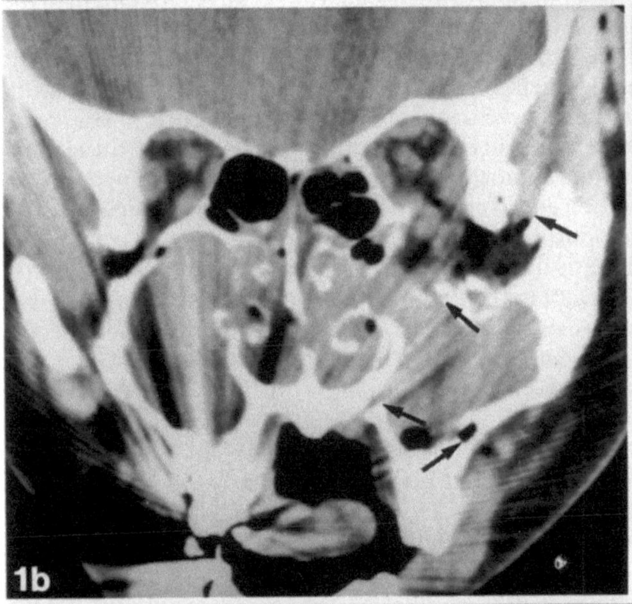

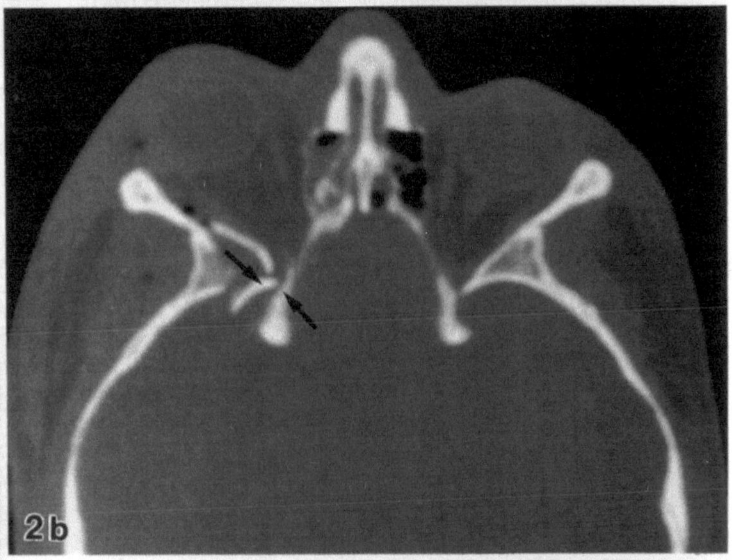

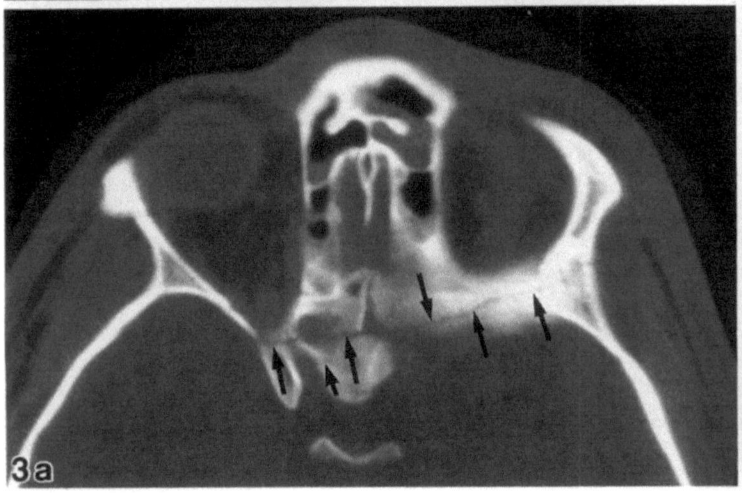

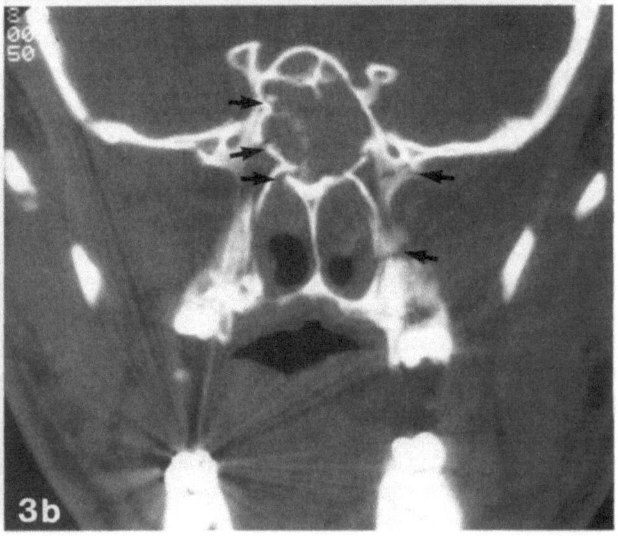

surgery. CT should be obtained in coronal and axial planes; frontal or sagittal reconstructions can be made. All CT images should be studied with separate windows for the brain, eye and osseous structures. At present, CT is the best single available radiological procedure for demonstration of fractures, acute hematomas, and traumatic changes in the orbit and brain. The amount of trauma to the optic nerve can be predicted by quantitating the direct force to the optic nerve. The indirect force to the optic nerve can be quantitated by the types of optic canal frac-

Fig. 1. **a** Three-dimensional CT frontal reconstruction of the facial skeleton to demonstrate the fracture lines *(arrows)* extending into the orbital apex with displacement of the bony fragments. **b** Coronal CT in the same patient to demonstrate comminution *(lower arrows)*, and displacement *(upper arrows)* of the bony fragments from considerable external force applied to the anterolateral aspect of the face

Fig. 2. **a** Soft tissue window for the brain and eye to demonstrate severe internal force on the optic canal and the surrounding structures. Note free blood *(arrows)* and air *(upper arrow)* in the basal cisterns. **b** Bone window in the same patient shows fracture fragments *(arrow)* deforming and compromising the optic canal. There was no recovery of vision after surgery

Fig. 3. **a** Bone window CT at the level of the optic canals shows a long oblique fracture line *(arrows)* extending from anterior to the optic canal on the left into the optic canal on the right, the result of a blow centered about the anterior portion of the left zygomatic arch. **b** Coronal section through the optic canal shows slight deformity in the outline of the sphenoid sinus with multiple fracture lines in its wall and base *(arrows on left)* and fractures of the pterygoid plates *(arrows on right)*. The optic canals are not deformed, which explains complete recovery of the left optic nerve without surgery

◄

ture and recording the presence or absence of contusion and hemorrhage in the frontal and temporal lobes. In most instances, correlation of CT and neuro-ophthalmological findings enables prediction as to whether the optic nerve should be decompressed. However, there were cases in this series in which CT findings led to overestimation of the traumatic force to the optic nerve, as in case 3; Fig. 3 a, b, where there were bilateral intra- and paracanalicular fractures. Although decompressive surgery was recommended for the left eye, the patient refused, and 1 month later had 20/20 vision in the left eye. CT can also lead to underestimation of the traumatic force to the eye by showing little or no change in or near the optic canal or in the frontal or temporal lobes, in patients with classical clinical findings of optic neuropathy. Unless these patients undergo immediate decompressive surgery, permanent damage to the optic nerve may result. Three such patients in this series had bicycle accidents.

CT is the most practical modality for assessment of the craniofacial structures in patients with traumatic optic neuropathy. The amount of external and internal traumatic force to the optic nerve can be predicted by analyzing craniofacial fractures demonstrated by CT in axial and coronal planes with special soft tissue and bone windows. Although quantification of the external and internal forces to the optic nerve will allow identification of most patients who should or should not have decompressive surgery, there are cases in which the CT findings do not correlate with the clinical findings. For proper assessment of any case of traumatic optic neuropathy, neuro-ophthalmological findings should be integrated with CT findings.

References

1. Kline L, Morawetz RB, Swaid SN (1984) Indirect injury of the optic nerve. Neurosurgery 14: 756–764
2. Sofferman R (1981) Sphenoethmoid approach to the optic nerve. Laryngoscope 91: 184–196
3. Fukuda Y (1975) Results in 400 cases of surgical decompression of the optic nerve. Mod Probl Ophthalmol 14: 474
4. Walsh FB (1966) Pathologic clinical correlations. Indirect trauma to the optic nerves and chiasm. II. Certain cerebral involvements associated with defective blood supply. Invest Ophthalmol 5: 433–449
5. Lindenberg R, Walsh FB, Sacks GJ (1973) Neuropathology of vision. An atlas. Lea and Febiger, Philadelphia, pp 92–102
6. Joseph M, Lessell, Rizzo J, Momose KJ (1990) Extracranial decompression of optic nerve for indirect optic neuropathy. Arch Ophthalmol (in press)
7. Manfredi SJ, Raji MR, Sprinkle PM, Weinstein GW, Minardi LM, Swanson T (1981) Computerized tomographic scan findings in facial fractures associated with blindness. Plast Reconstr Surg 68: 479–491
8. Seiff SR, Berger MS, Guyon J, Pitts LH (1984) Computed tomographic evaluation of the optic canal in sudden traumatic blindness. Am J Ophthalmol 98: 751–755

Dr. K. Jack Momose
Department of Radiology and Otolaryngology
Massachusetts General Hospital
Boston, MA 02114, USA

SESSION 3
CEREBRAL TUMOURS 1

Neuroradiology (1991) 33 [Suppl]: 20–21

Neuro radiology
© Springer-Verlag 1991

Grading of oligodendrogliomas: correlation of neuroradiology and proliferation index

J. Berkefeld[1], C. Lang[2], H. Hacker[1], and W. Schlote[2]

Departments of [1] Neuroradiology and [2] Neuropathology, University of Frankfurt, Frankfurt, Federal Republic of Germany

Summary. The results of neuroradiological grading of 30 oligodendrogliomas were correlated to conventional histology and a proliferation index, which was determined by the monoclonal antibody Ki-67. A good correspondence of neuroradiological criteria and the proliferation index was given in 90% of the cases and demonstrates the value of the radiological method, to detect early stages of malignant transformation. Disagreement between neuroradiology and conventional histology could be observed more frequently than differences from the grading made by Ki-67-values.

Key words: Brain tumours, grading – Oligodendrogliomas

Materials and methods

Neuroradiological grading of 30 oligodendrogliomas in 23 patients (7 recurrences) was done before operation to determine the degree of malignancy. All patients had CT and angiography; 8 cases were studied by MRI. Contrast enhancement in CT or MRI and angiographic findings (tumour blush, pathological vessels, early venous drainage) were used as parameters to distinguish three categories of tumours: low-grade malignancy, high-grade malignancy and the high-grade subgroup of tumours behaving like glioblastomas.

The occurrence of enhancement and tumour blush is considered to be a sign of vascular proliferation or disturbance of the blood-brain barrier indicating malignant tumour growth. Analogous to histological grading we used grade II for low-grade processes and grade III and IV for high-grade malignant tumours, which were treated by radiotherapy after operation. Table 1 shows the expression of radiological signs in the different tumour groups.

The results of neuroradiological grading were correlated to the findings of conventional histology and to the percentage of cells reacting with the proliferation marker Ki-67. Ki-67 is a monoclonal antibody, recognizing proliferating cells in all phases of the cell-cyclus except G 0 [1, 2]. Conventional histology can only detect the mitosis itself. The percentage of positive cells was counted in 40 fields of view for each tumour. High median values of Ki-67 (more than 5%) were considered to be an indicator for malignant transformation.

Results

With increasing ratios of Ki-67-positive cells radiological findings suggested grade III or IV-malignancy. The number of tumour recurrences also increased. Five of 18 tumours graded as II by histology were radiologically grade III and had Ki-67 values of 5.7% or more. Tumours with less than 5% positive cells showed no histological or radiological signs of high-grade malignancy.

In the grade III group (determined by histology and Ki-67) there were two tumours (same patient), where radiology appeared to be falsely negative (Figs. 1, 2).

Agreement of radiology and histology could be observed in 23 of 30 caes (76%); agreement of radiology and Ki-67 was as much as 90% (27 of 30). Histology and proliferation marker gave identical results in 80% (24) of the cases.

Discussion

The good correspondence of neuroradiological grading and the proliferation marker Ki-67 underlines the importance of the radiological method, which is a valuable diagnostic tool to predict the degree of malignancy before operation. At the borderline between grade II and grade III tumours conventional histology missed the grade III transformation in five cases, which appeared to be high-grade malignant by radiology and Ki-67 values. The proliferation marker can be considered as an additional criterion to show that CT, MRI and angiography are sensitive enough to detect early stages of vascular proliferation or disturbance of the blood-brain barrier, which are important signs of malignancy. The main advantage of neuroradiology is that we gain an impression of the whole tumour in situ. Both histology and immunohistochemistry have to work with parts of the lesion, which may have dif-

Table 1. Radiological grading of oligodendrogliomas

Malignancy	CT/MRI enhancement	Angiography		
		Tumour blush	Pathological vessels	Early venous drainage
I/II low grade	0	0	0	0
III high grade	+/++	+	+	0
IV glioblastoma	++ Irregular necrosis	+	+	+
II/III[a] borderline	MRI: (+)	(+)	0	0

[a] Three cases with weak enhancement or minimal tumour blush were graded II

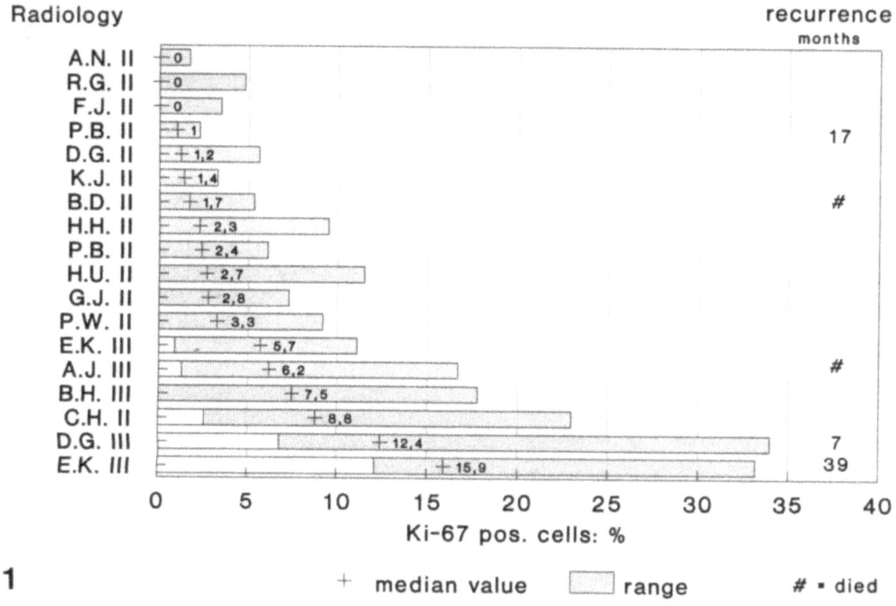

1

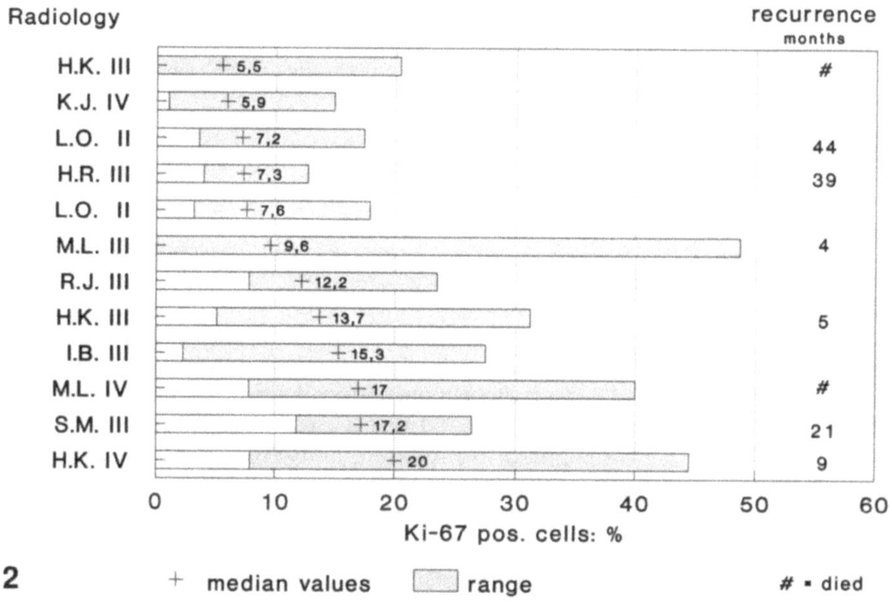

2

Figs. 1, 2. Correspondence of radiological grading and proliferation marker Ki-67 in 30 cases of oligodendrogliomas of histological grade II and III. Note the discrepancies between radiology, Ki-67 and conventional histology at the end of the grade II diagram

ferent degrees of malignant transformation. A few other discrepancies between neuroradiological and neuropathological methods of grading were revealed in a small number of cases and show the need for further collaborating work between the two disciplines concerning the important question of tumour grading.

References

1. Gerdes J, Schwab U, Lemke H, Stein H (1983) Production of a mouse monoclonal antibody reactive with a human nuclear antigen associated with cell-proliferation. Int J Cancer 31: 13–20
2. Gerdes J, Lemke H, Baisch H, Wacker H-H, Schwab U, Stein H (1984) Cell cycle analysis of a cell proliferation-associated human nuclear antigen defined by the monoclonal antibody Ki-67. J Immunol 133: 1710–1715

Dr. Joachim Berkefeld
Department of Radiology
University of Frankfurt
Theodor-Stern-Kai 6–7
W-6000 Frankfurt 70, Federal Republic of Germany

Neuroradiology (1991) 33 [Suppl]: 22–24

Neuro radiology
© Springer-Verlag 1991

Localization of cortical and subcortical lesions with MR brain surface imaging

K. Katada, G. Takesita, H. Anno, Y. Ogura, S. Koga, H. Sano, and T. Kanno

Department of Radiology and Neurosurgery, Fujita Health University Hospital, Toyoake, Japan

Summary. A new MRI technique which permits non-invasive, direct visualization of cerebral sulci and gyri as well as cortical and subcortical lesions as a planar image is introduced. The usefulness of the technique in terms of lesion localization and surgical planning has been evaluated. As this technique, surface anatomy scanning (SAS), can provide excellent images of cortical gyri and sulci, accurate gyral localization was achieved in 87% of the cases. Surgical planning using SAS was performed in ten cases, and was found to be useful in determining the site of skin incision.

Key words: Cerebral cortex – Magnetic resonance imaging – Surgical planning

As the cerebral cortex has a highly specialised functional localization, it is important for neurosurgeons to identify cortical gyri and to know the exact location of the lesion. CT and MRI provide a non-invasive visualization of cortical sulci and gyri; however, it is difficult for these tomographic modalities to identify sulci and gyri as a continuous cortical strip.

The aim of this work is to evaluate the usefulness of the new application of MRI technique which permits non-invasive demonstration of brain surface structures, and to apply this technique to neurosurgical planning.

Materials and methods

The MRI units used in this study were 0.5 T (Toshiba MRT50A) and 1.5 T (Shimazu SMT150) superconducting magnet system. Heavily T2-weighted spin echo sequence (TR/TE = 2000/250 ms) was used to achieve selective enhancement of the signal intensity of the cerebrospinal fluid (CSF). Thus, the CSF within the subarachnoid space on the brain surface was utilized as natural contrast medium, a relief picture of the brain surface being obtained.

Six- to 8-cm-thick slices were used to cover sufficient area of the cerebral cortex to create a planar image of the brain surface. The use of the surface coil was preferable to further enhance the brain surface signal; however, the use of the head coil was required to obtain the parietal view because of the limitation in radiofrequency transmission direction. Image matrix was 256 × 256.

Examination time was 8.5 min for one excitation, and 17 min for two excitations. Post-processing of grey scale reversal and image filtering were applied to achieve better delineation of the sulci.

As a variation of the original spin echo sequence, high-speed brain surface imaging was developed using steady-state gradient echo sequence. The MRI equipment was a 1.5 T superconducting magnet system (SMT-150). The scanning parameters were TR = 60 ms, TE = 34 ms, 60° flip angle, 256 or 512 image matrix, and 4–5 cm slicing gradient. Scanning time with this high-speed imaging varies from 15 s (256 × 256, NEX 1) to 62 s (512 × 512, NEX 2). During the past 3 years, 103 brain surface images were obtained in 88 patients using these techniques, 56 of which were examined for the purpose of lesion localization. These include 26 neoplasms, 12 cerebral infarcts, 6 angiomas and 8 patients with cortical or subcortical brain damages of various aetiologies.

In 10 cases, surface anatomy scanning (SAS) was performed for the purpose of preoperative lesion localization and surgical planning. A water-filled plastic tube was placed on the skin incision line as a marker, which was superimposed onto the SAS image indicating the relative position of the lesion and the skin flap.

Results

Among 56 examinations with cortical and subcortical pathology, good-quality brain surface images were obtained in 49, and the accurate localization of the lesion was achieved in all of these cases (Fig. 1). The remaining 7 cases failed to provide quality images due to technical problems such as motion artefacts. In 10 cases in which surgical planning using SAS was performed, SAS proved to be useful in establishing the plan for craniotomy (Fig. 2). SAS images showed good correlation with actual surgical views in all cases.

It was also useful in correcting skin flap designs in 4 cases (Fig. 3).

High-speed brain surface imaging using steady-state gradient echo technique was performed in 17 cases. Although the image quality was not as good as with the original spin echo technique because of the inhomogeneity due to the magnetic susceptibility effect, major cortical sulci as well as the skin marker were easily identifiable (Fig. 2a), and were considered to be adequate for "test scan" for the surgical planning.

Discussion

The accurate localization of cortical and subcortical lesions on radiological images has special clinical importance because of the highly specialised functional localization of the cerebral cortex [1, 2, 4, 5]. This is especially true in preoperative cases in which the location of the le-

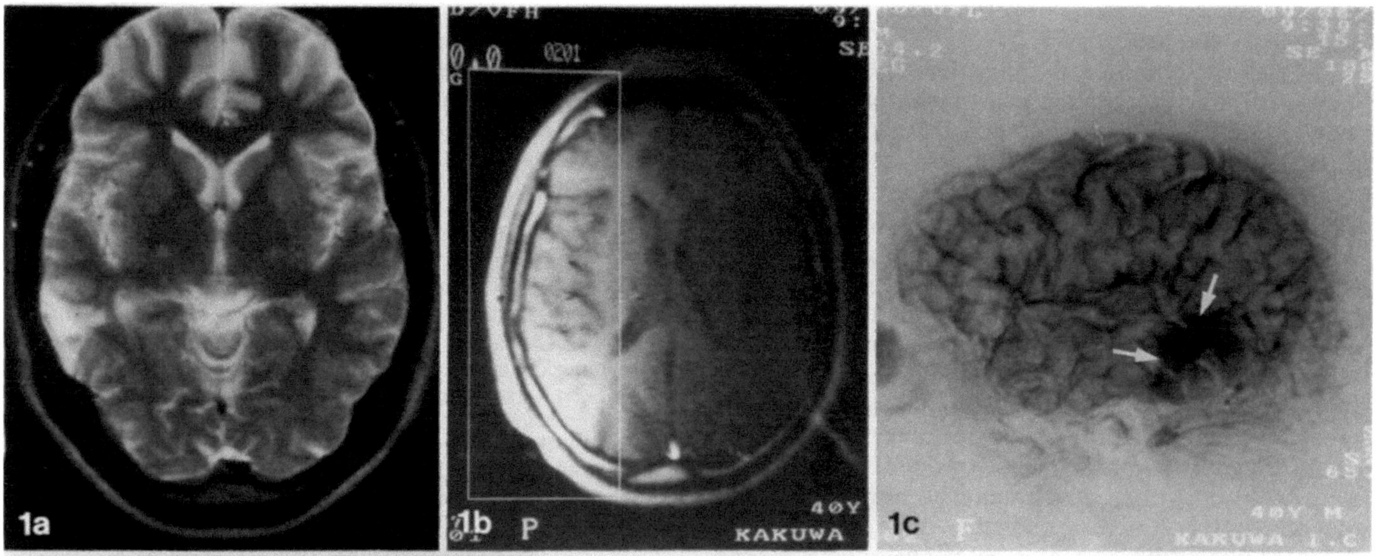

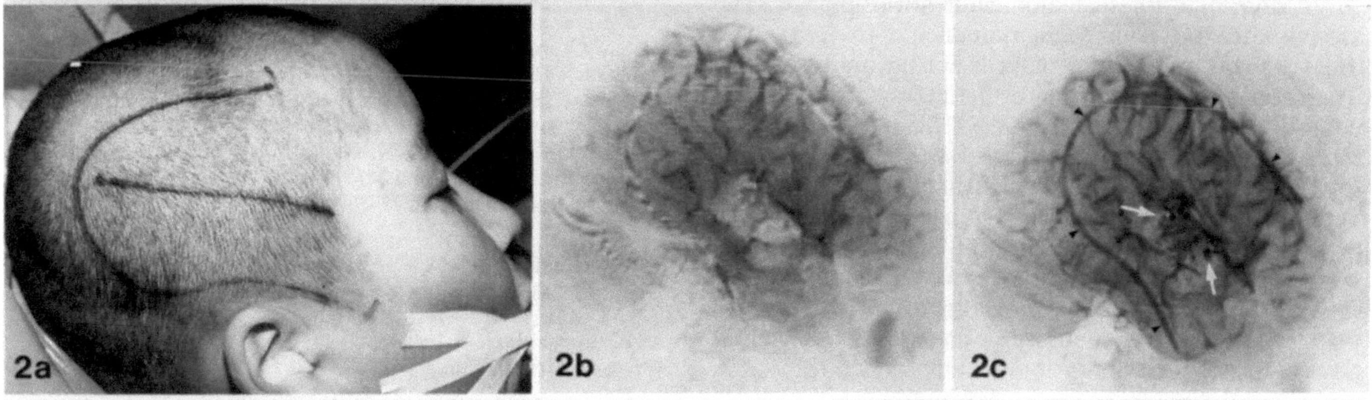

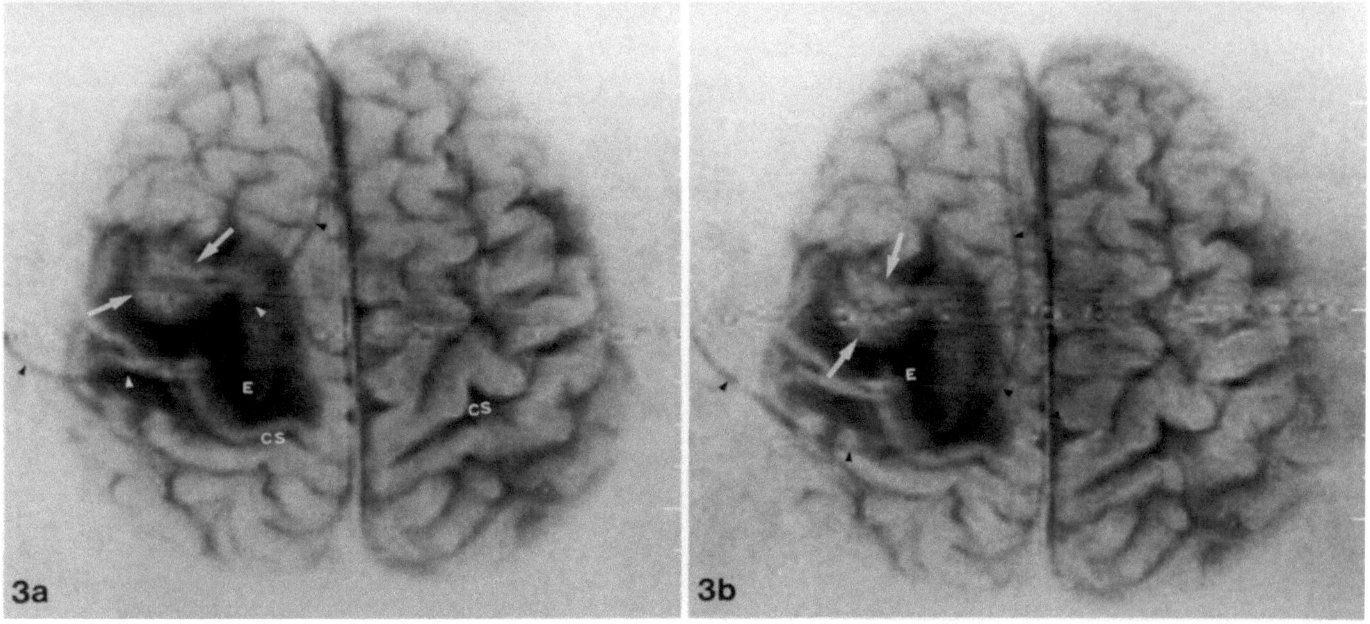

Fig. 1 a–c. Focal epilepsy. **a** Axial T2-weighted image shows focal cortical damage in temporal lobe. **b** Scan plan for lateral surface anatomy scanning (SAS) image. **c** Lateral SAS image demonstrating the lesion located in the middle temporal gyrus *(arrows)*.

Fig. 2 a–c. Surgical planning for right temporal cavernous angioma. **a** Skin flap design. **b** High-speed brain surface imaging with gradient echo sequence. Right lateral view. Inhomogeneous artefact due to magnetic susceptibility is observed. **c** Spin echo SAS image, right lateral view, indicates that the lesion *(arrows)* is located in the superior temporal gyrus. Skin flap plan *(arrowhead)* placed properly

Fig. 3 a, b. Correction of skin flap design by SAS. **a** Initial SAS image, parietal view, indicates that the skin flap *(arrowhead)* is too anteriorly placed against the metastatic tumour in the left frontal lobe *(arrows)*. *E*, Surrounding oedema; CS central sulcus. **b** Second SAS image showing perfect matching of re-designed skin flap plan sion may alter the selection of treatment as well as the prognosis of the patient.

In order to determine the exact location of the lesion, it is essential to identify the gyri to which the lesion belongs. MR SAS can provide excellent visualization of cortical gyri, sulci, fissures and cortical veins. On lateral view, it enabled us to make detailed observation of the sylvian fissure, not only the posterior ramus but also the anterior horizontal ramus, anterior ascending ramus and the ascending part of the posterior ramus. Moreover, the lower part of the precentral sulcus and anterior ascending ramus of the sylvian fissure can easily be differentiated by this technique. These are extremely helpful in identifying the supramarginal gyrus, the angular gyrus, as well as the speech cortex on a lateral SAS image. In the parietal view, precentral sulcus, central sulcus and postcentral sulcus were readily identified, which makes accurate recognition of motor and sensory cortex possible.

In addition to these anatomical features [3], SAS can also visualize the lesion itself as an area of prolonged T2. Thus the exact localization of the lesion becomes possible. The surgical planning is one of the most interesting and clinically useful application of SAS. Skin marks can easily be superimposed onto the brain surface image by applying water-filled plastic tube, which makes simultaneous visualization of the gyri, the lesion and the skin mark possible. Using this capability, the radiologist and the neurosurgeon are able to optimize the size and the site of the skin flap design. Another advantage of SAS in surgical planning is to provide neurosurgeons with good orientations of the surgical view prior to craniotomy. Reasonable scanning time and higher spatial resolution will be significant advantages of SAS against three-dimensional volume rendering technique [6].

For these reasons, we consider that the SAS can be a modality of choice not only for the lesion localization, but also for surgical planning.

References

1. Katada K, Takesita G, Koga S, Asahina M, Kanno T, Asahina K (1987) MR imaging of brain surface structures: surface anatomy scanning (abstract). Radiology [Suppl] 165: 303
2. Salamon G, Lecaque G (1978) Choice of plane of incidence for computed tomography of the cerebral cortex. J Comput Assist Tomogr 2: 93–97
3. Gado M, Hanaway J, Frank R (1979) Functional anatomy of the cerebral cortex by computed tomography. J Comput Assist Tomogr 3: 1–19
4. Hayman LA, Evans RA, Hinck VS (1979) Scalp markers for precise craniotomy siting, using computed tomography. J Comput Assist Tomogr 3: 701–702
5. Naidich TP, Yu RH, King DG, Wholahan JD (1980) Superimposition reformatted CT for preoperative lesion localization and surgical planning. J Comput Assist Tomogr 4: 693–696
6. Levin DN, Hu X, Tan KK, Galhotra BA (1989) Surface of the brain: three-dimensional MR imaging created with volume rendering. Radiology 171: 277–280

Prof. K. Katada
Fujita Health University
School of Hygiene 1–98
Dengakugakubo Kutakake-cho
Toyoake Aichi, Japan

Neuroradiology (1991) 33 [Suppl]: 25–27

Neuro-radiology
© Springer-Verlag 1991

Early postoperative CT and MRI in glioblastoma

M. Forsting[1], F. K. Albert[2], K. Sartor[1], and S. Kunze[2]

Departments of [1] Neuroradiology and [2] Neurosurgery, University of Heidelberg, Heidelberg, Federal Republic of Germany

Summary. Knowledge of the natural history of contrast enhancement after brain tumour resection may help improve postoperative imaging. In a prospective study 42 patients with glioblastomas were evaluated by both CT and MRI before and – at specific intervals – after surgery. Up to the 4th postoperative day areas of enhancement, always better shown by MIR, reflected residual tumour. During the 2nd postoperative week new enhancement occurred along the resection lines. However, increasing protein concentration plus methaemoglobin formation within the resection defect resulted in T1 shortening and made even MRI difficult to interpret. We recommend that postoperative imaging to assess residual enhancing tumour should be performed within the first 4 days after surgery, preferably by MRI. Such a timing minimizes "benign" enhancement due to the surgical trauma. Follow-up of our patients may reveal how the extent of surgical resection influences survival rates.

Key words: Postoperative CT/MRI – Contrast enhancement – Glioblastoma

Malignant brain tumours, specifically glioblastomas, are surgically incurable; optimal therapeutic results require additional measures. To judge tumour response to radiation therapy, chemotherapy or newer types of adjuvant treatment by CT or MRI the contrast–medium–induced tissue enhancement resulting from the surgical trauma must be differentiated from enhancement caused by residual tumour. The extent of tumour resection must also be determined. To improve our postoperative follow-up imaging protocol we wanted first to know what was the natural history of contrast enhancement after brain tumour resection.

Patients and methods

In a prospective study 42 patients with glioblastoma were studied by CT and MRI before and – at specific intervals – after surgery. All CT studies were performed before and after contrast enhancement with 100 ml iohexol 300 (Omnipaque) on a Picker 1200 SX scanner. MRI was performed on a 1.0 T Picker Vista unit. Pre- and postcontrast (0.1 mmol/kg gadolinium-DPTA i. v.) T1-weighted images were obtained with a TR of 600 ms and an echo time (TE) of 20 ms. The slice thickness was 8 mm (CT and MRI).

The first postoperative scan was obtained as soon as possible after surgery, usually between the 1st and 4th postoperative days. Follow-up scans were obtained 1–2 weeks, 4 weeks, 2 months, and 6 months after surgery.

Results

In 40% of patients the first postoperative CT study showed areas of contrast enhancement that corresponded to areas seen on the preoperative scan and thus reflected residual enhancing tumour. There was no enhancement visible in 20% of patients, and in 40% findings were equivocal. The main tissue alteration confounding the interpretation of these early CT studies was haemorrhage at the operative site and enhancement of the adjacent parenchyma (Fig. 1 b).

The first postoperative MRI showed contrast enhancement reflecting residual enhancing tumour in 71% of the patients (Fig. 1 c). Findings were equivocal in only 12% of patients, and in 17% there was no apparent enhancement. Because of the characteristic signal changes due to haemoglobin degradation we had no difficulty in differentiating enhancement from postoperative haemorrhage during the first 4 days after surgery, and we also saw no contrast enhancement related to the surgical trauma during this period. After about 2 weeks widespread enhancement occurred along the resection lines, and this was always more apparent on MRI (Fig. 1 d). Simultaneously, increasing protein content plus formation of methaemoglobin resulted in marked T1 shortening within the resection defect. This made even MRI difficult to interpret (Fig. 2). After 2 months this "benign" enhancement had almost completely resolved. The remaining, surgically induced, dural enhancement was easy to differentiate from enhancing tumour, which appeared more irregular, lobulated or mass-like (Fig. 3).

Discussion

The mechanisms underlying postoperative enhancement are not fully understood. Several hypotheses have been advanced to explain both the presence and time course of contrast enhancement at the operative site [1, 2]. The development of granulation tissue and of neovasculature, as observed experimentally in a canine model, seem best to parallel the enhancement patterns seen on CT [3, 4]. Hyperaemia of the injured area secondary to dysautoregulation may also play a role [5]. Results of animal experiments and of sequential CT after brain tumour resec-

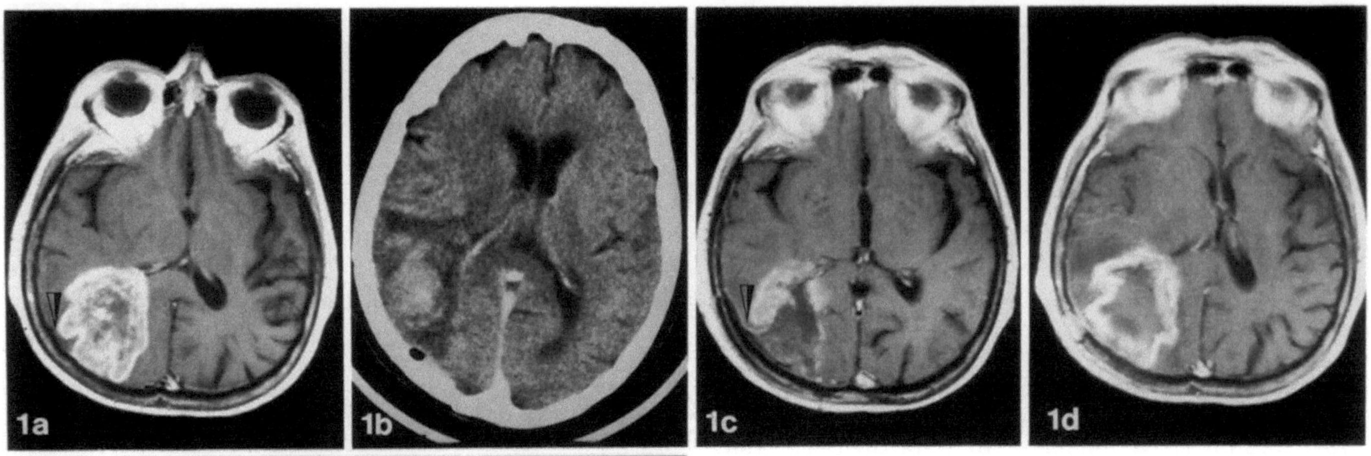

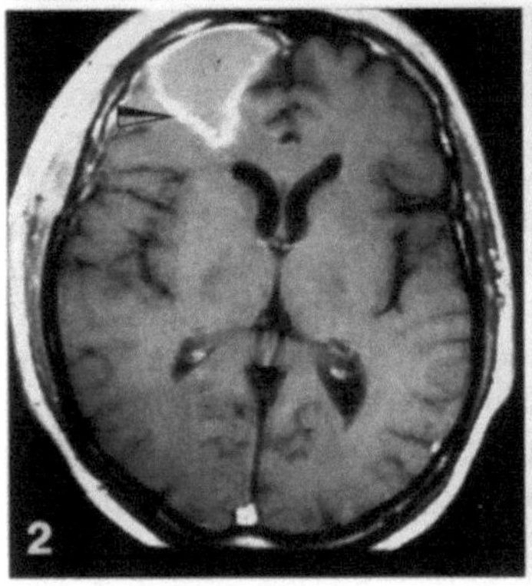

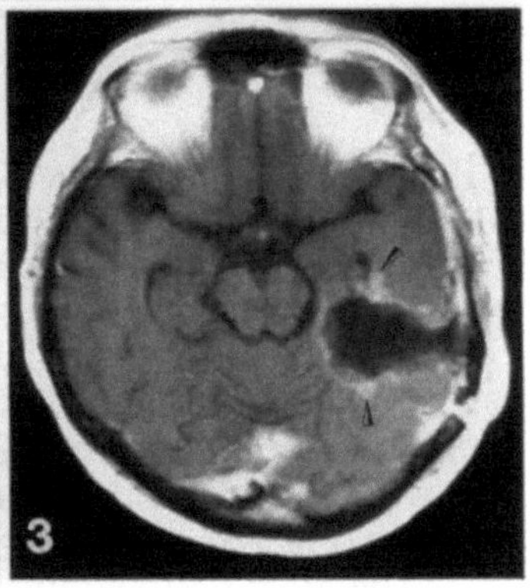

Fig. 1. a T1-weighted contrast-enhanced MRI of a right hemispheric glioblastoma that did not reach brain surface at site marked by *arrowhead.* **b** Contrast-enhanced CT scan obtained 2 days after surgery. It is impossible to differentiate between surgically induced haemorrhage and contrast enhancement. **c** MRI scan obtained on same day as CT in **b.** The enhancing mass corresponds to that part of the tumour that did not reach the brain surface (compare areas marked by *arrowheads* in **a** and **c**). **d** Two weeks after surgery widespread enhancement occurred along the resection lines

Fig. 2. Contrast-enhanced MRI of a patient with a frontal glioblastoma obtained 2 weeks after surgery. "Benign", linear enhancement along the resection lines *(arrowhead)* and T1 shortening due to increasing protein concentration plus formation of methaemoglobin within the resection defect

Fig. 3. Contrast-enhanced MRI of a patient with a left temporal glioblastoma obtained 4 weeks after surgery. Moderate "benign" linear enhancement along resection lines and irregular, lobulated enhancement reflecting residual tumour *(arrowheads)*

tion have shown a delay of enhancement along the operative margins of up to 5 days after surgery [3, 6]. In our study early postoperative CT revealed residual enhancing tumour in 40% of the patients. Unavoidable haemorrhage into the surgical defect and the aforementioned enhancement due to hyperaemia of the adjacent parenchyma made early CT difficult to interpret in 40%.

Theoretically, MRI has advantages in this early postoperative phase. The characteristic signal changes that accompany early haemoglobin degradation should allow easy differentiation of contrast enhancement from surgically induced haemorrhage. Furthermore, the contrast mechanism of Gd-DPTA – as a paramagnetic agent it is visualized not directly but by causing local alterations of the magnetic environment – should minimize the enhancement effect from hypervascularity seen with iodinated contrast media. Even minute amounts of enhancing residual tumour should be visible on MRI, as this modality is about 20 times as sensitive to Gd-DPTA as is CT to iodinated media, based on a mole per kilogram dose of administered contrast medium [7].

Corresponding to these potential advantages of MRI we encountered diagnostic difficulties on the early postoperative MR images in only 12% of patients; in 71% of patients the residual enhancing tumour was easily recognizable. However, neuroradiologically one cannot precisely define the margins of residual neoplasm, and even clear differentiation of tumour from oedema is not feasible. In fact, what one calls "oedema" should be better described as "tumour plus oedema", since pathologically tumour cells may extend beyond abnormal enhancing tissue as seen on MRI [8–10].

It may be reasonably assumed that brain tumour surgery improves the efficacy of postoperative adjuvant treatment. Surgical debulking removes poorly oxygenated cells known to be relatively resistant to radiation, as well as cells in poorly vascularized regions considered to be sequestered from systemic therapy. The data from the ACS-JTS survey show more than a doubling of 5-year survival rates with progressively greater extent of glioblastoma resection [11]. However, more effective ways of adjuvant therapy must be developed to treat these tumours. Quantitative data from tumour response curves based on the amount of residual tumour are probably more accurate than clinical observation in measuring the effect of new therapeutic regimens. We recommend that postoperative imaging to assess residual enhancing tumour should be performed within the first 4 days after surgery, preferably by MRI. Such timing minimizes diagnostic problems associated with "benign" enhancement due to the surgical trauma. Long-term follow-up of our patients may reveal how the extent of tumour resection influences survival rates.

References

1. Bird RC, Drayer BP, Medina M, Rekate HL, Flom RA, Hodak JA (1988) Gd-DPTA- enhanced MR imaging in pediatric patients after brain tumor resection. Radiology 169: 123–126
2. Cairncross JG, Pexman JHW, Rathbone MP, DelMaestro RF (1985) Postoperative contrast enhancement in patients with brain tumor. Ann Neurol 17: 570–572

3. Earnest F, Kelly PJ, Scheithauer BW, Kall BA, Cascino TL, Ehman RL, Forbes GS, Axley PL (1988) Cerebral astrocytomas: histopathologic correlation of MR and CT contrast enhancement with stereotactic biopsy. Radiology 166: 823–827
4. Elster AD, DiPersio DA (1990) Cranial postoperative site: assessment with contrast-enhanced MR imaging. Radiology 174: 93–98
5. Jeffries BF, Kishore PRS, Singh KS, Ghatak NR, Krempa J (1980) Postoperative computed tomographic changes in brain: an experimental study. Radiology 135: 751–753
6. Jeffries BF, Kishore PRS, Singh KS, Ghatak NR, Krempa J (1981) Contrast enhancement in the postoperative brain: Radiology 139: 409–413
7. Johnson PC, Hunt SJ, Drayer BP (1989) Human cerebral gliomas: correlation of postmortem MR imaging and neuropathologic findings. Radiology 170: 211–217
8. Mahaley MS, Mettlin C, Nachimuthu N, Laws ER (1990) Analysis of patterns of care of brain tumor patients in the United States: a study of the brain tumor section of the American Association of Neurological Surgeons and the CNS and Commission on Cancer of the American College of Surgeons. Clin Neurosurg 36: 347–357
9. Penn RD, Walser R, Kurtz D (1976) Tumor volume, luxury perfusion, and regional blood volume changes in man visualized by subtraction computed tomography. J Neurosurg 44: 449–457
10. Runge VM, Clanton JA, Price AC (1985) Evaluation of contrast enhanced MR imaging in a brain-abscess model. AJNR 6: 137–147
11. Zagzag D, Goldenberg M, Brem S (1989) Angiogenesis and blood-brain barrier breakdown modulate CT contrast enhancement: an experimental study in a rabbit brain-tumor model. AJNR 10: 529–534

Dr. M. Forsting
Department of Neuroradiology
Kopfklinikum der Universität
Im Neuenheimer Feld 400
D-6900 Heidelberg
Federal Republic of Germany

Neuroradiology (1991) 33 [Suppl]: 28–30

Neuro radiology
© Springer-Verlag 1991

Brain stem tumours: a clinical and radiological study of 112 patients

R. L. Prevo[1, 3], G. J. Vielvoye[1], and E. A. van der Velde[2]

Departments of [1] Neuroradiology and [2] Medical Statistics, University of Leiden, Leiden, The Netherlands
[3] Department of Radiology, Medisch Spectrum Twente, Hospital Enschede, Enschede, The Netherlands

Summary. Clinical, radiological and histological data of 112 patients with the clinical diagnosis of a brain stem tumour on admission were reviewed. In 75 patients a pontine glioma was suspected and in 37 patients a secondary or extra-axial tumour was found. Histological verification was obtained in 62 patients. In all, 99 CT studies, 56 vertebral angiograms and 34 ventriculograms were compared with clinical data in a statistical evaluation.

Key words: Brain stem tumour – Angiography – Computed tomography – Magnetic resonance imaging

Between 1979 and 1985 the average number of patients, suspected of a brain stem tumour on first admission and the number of people who died from a brain stem tumour were more or less constant. In these years the number of patients who died from a malignant supratentorial tumour of the brain showed a definite increase.

Materials and methods

All major Dutch hospitals were requested to send clinical and radiological records of patients admitted on suspicion of a brain stem tumour in the period January 1978 to January 1984. In all, 75 patients with a primary brain-stem tumour and 37 patients with a secondary or extra-axial tumour were included. Clinical and radiological data were compared. The following clinical information from 112 patients was analysed: age at diagnosis, sex, duration of symptoms before diagnosis, histology, pyramidal tract signs, cerebellar lesions, deficit in sensation, presence of increased intracranial pressure, presence of cranial nerve palsies at the time of diagnosis and at the end of the observation time. Ninety-nine CT studies, 56 vertebral angiograms and 34 ventriculograms were available. The following CT variables were reviewed: tumour density, tumour localization, enhancement and presence of ventriculomegaly. On angiography the position of the basilar artery, posterior inferior cerebellar artery (PICA), anterior inferior cerebellar artery (AICA) and precentral cerebellar vein were noted. It was possible to make seven subdivisions: pontine glioma with and without radiotherapy, metastases, lymphoma, medulloblastoma, ependymoma and miscellaneous. The computer software program SSPS-X 2.1 was used for statistical analysis. Standard statistical methods, like the chi-square test, etc, were performed. Survival distributions were compared with the Lee-Desu test.

Results

A slight male predominance, caused by patients in the groups lymphoma, medulloblastoma and ependymoma, was found. In the other subdivisions, including the gliomas, the sex ratio was equal, agreeing with the series of other authors [1, 2]. Almost half of the patients (51) were below 15 years of age while 41 were older than 35 years of age. A slight increase in the fourth and fifth decades was seen [3–6].

The duration of symptoms and observation time were respectively 9–12 weeks and 25–52 weeks. Pyramidal tract disorders on admission were noted in 84 patients (75.0%), while no statistical association was found between right-and left-sided lesions. Eighty-nine patients (79.5%) demonstrated cerebellar signs. In 52 patients only the medial cerebellar compartment was affected. Sensation disorders were found in 11 patients (9.8%).

Histology was obtained in 62 patients [7, 8]. The incidence of ventriculomegaly was rather high (47.3%), in patients with pontine glioma it was only 33.8%. In this material, palsies of the sixth (56.3%) and seventh (59.8%) cranial nerves occurred most frequently. No significant difference between clinical manifestations on admission and at the end of the observation time could be found. Statistically significant associations were encountered between tumour density and tumour localization, tumour density and cerebellar lesions, and lesions in the combinations of the cranial nerves III–V, VI–VIII, V–VII and VIII–XII. Significant associations were also found between tumour localization and hydrocephalus and cerebellar lesions.

Median survival time of all patients was 42 weeks (Fig. 1). After 1, 2, 3 and 5 years survival times were respectively 46%, 32%, 27% and 22%. One-year survival of untreated patients with a pontine glioma was 30% against 50% for treated patients (Fig. 2). The curves are significantly different ($P = 0.03$).

If the material is subdivided into gliomatous brain stem tumours and tumours of other kinds, the patterns of survival of both groups do not differ significantly ($P = 0.40$, Fig. 3).

Of all CT variables no significant association with length of survival could be found. Histology was obtained by means of biopsy, surgery or autopsy in 62 patients, in whom the diagnosis of an astrocytoma of the brain stem was confirmed in 26 patients. The histology (pathological

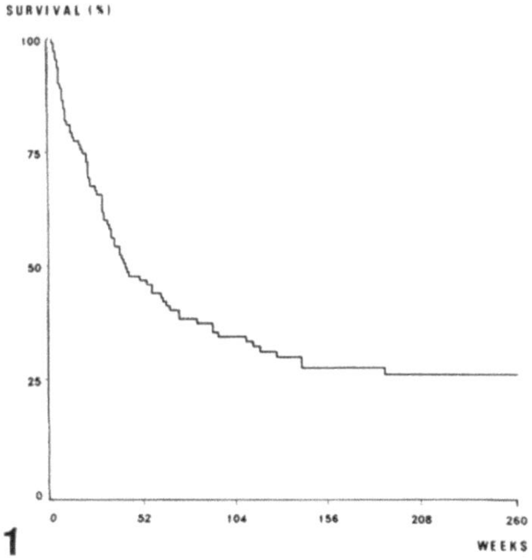

1

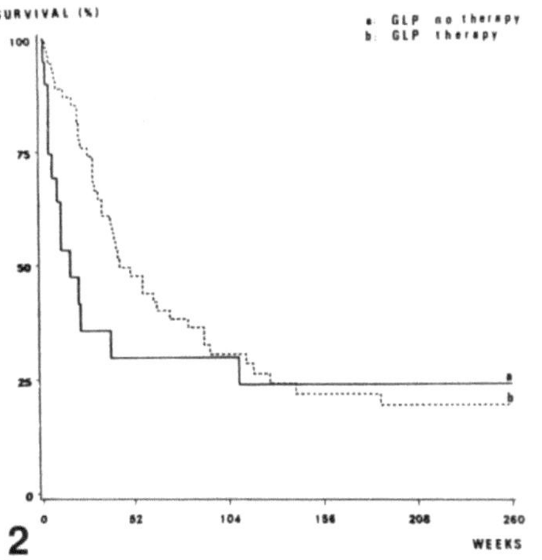

2

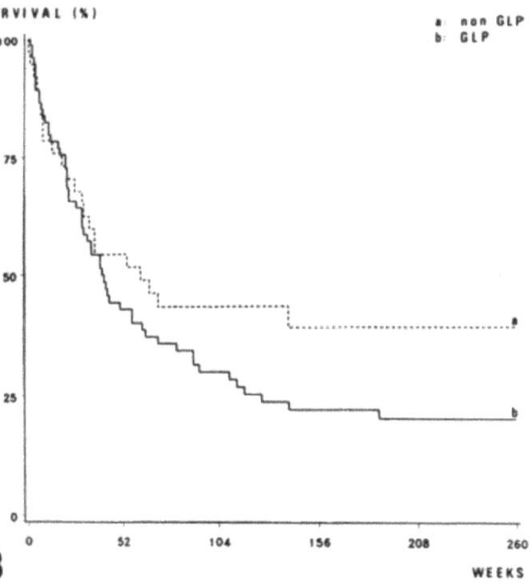

3

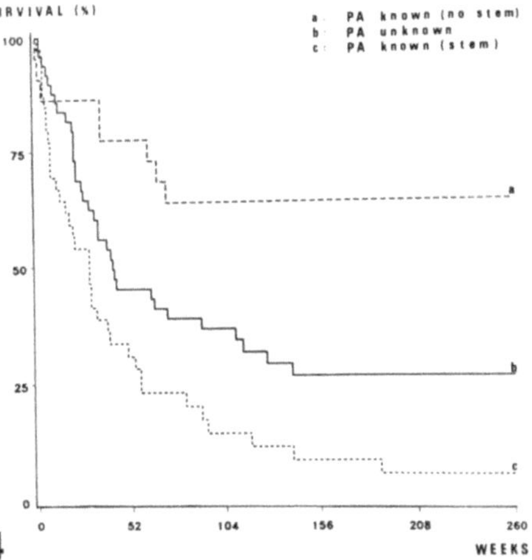

4

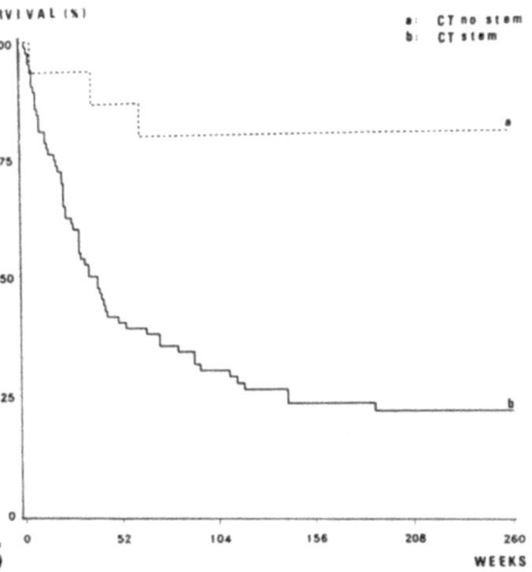

5

Fig. 1. Actuarial life table for all patients with a diagnosis of a brain-stem tumour on admission

Fig. 2. Actuarial life table for 75 patients with a pontine glioma *(GLP)*. Group a: Pontine glioma without therapy; group b: Pontine glioma with therapy

Fig. 3. Actuarial life table for 75 patients with a pontine glioma *(GLP)* and 37 patients with tumours of other kinds (non-GLP)

Fig. 4. Actuarial life table for all patients, subdivided according to the histology of the tumor (PA). Group a: PA known (no stem); group b: PA unknown; group c: PA known (stem)

Fig. 5. Actuarial life table for 99 patients examined with CT scanning. This radiological selection is based on the localization of the tumour with CT scanning. Group a: CT-demonstrated extra-axial tumour (no stem); group b: CT-proven intra-axial tumor (stem)

appearance, PA) was subdivided into: (1) histology unknown (PA unknown) and (2) histology known (PA known). The latter subdivided into PA stem and PA no stem (See below for definition). The curves, also in comparison in pairs, differ significantly in the length of survival ($P < 0.01$, Fig. 4).

According to the appearance of the tumour on CT, a radiological selection was made, which did not confirm the clinical diagnosis in every way. In this selection two subdivisions were made: (1) CT-proven intra-axial tumour (stem) and (2) CT-demonstrated extra-axial tumour (no stem). The variables were significantly associated with the length of survival (Fig. 5).

Discussion

Prognosis of patients, mainly children, with a brain stem glioma is still worse than in patients with a supratentorial glioma, as indicated by these results. In contradiction to the series of Albright et al. [9] we could find no association of CT variables with the length of survival. Treatment should not be homogeneous [10], because in patients with brain stem glioma a broad range in survival and clinical presentation may be seen.

No significant association was found between gliomatous brain stem tumours and tumours of other kinds, because the most important selection criterion for this study was: "suspicion of a space-occupying lesion in the brain stem. At the end of this study only 33 patients were still alive."

Retrospectively we were able to recognize the underlying lesion in about 80%. No additional information was obtained from angiography and ventriculography. Yet angiography can still be used in selected cases, particularly if enhancement is present in CT [11]. In the another 20% of patients with clinical suspicion of a brain stem lesion and an unexpanded brain stem on CT, MRI is required [7, 8, 11, 12]. In case of positive CT, MRI should be performed for radiotherapy planning, especially to show extension of the tumour to the cervicomedullary region, as already mentioned in various recent reports [13].

References

1. Bray PF, Carter S, Taveras JM (1930) Pontine gliomas, a pathologic study and classification of 25 cases. Arch Pathol 9: 799–810
2. Panitch HC, Berg BO (1970) Brainstem tumors of childhood and adolescence. Am J Dis Child 119: 465–472
3. White HH (1963) Brainstem tumors occurring in adults. Neurology 13: 292–300
4. Lassiter KRL, Alexander E, Davis CH, Kelly DL (1971) Surgical treatment of brainstem gliomas. J Neurosurg 34: 719–725
5. Kim TH, Chin Hong W, Pollan S, Hazel JH, Webster JH (1981) Radiotherapy of primary brainstem tumours. J Rad Oncol Biol Phys 6: 51–57

6. Tokuriki Y, Handa H, Yamashita J, Okamura T, Paine JT (1986) Brainstem glioma: an analysis of 85 cases. Acta Neurochir (Wien) 79: 67–73
7. Peterman SB, Steiner RE, Bydder GM, Thomas DJ, Tobias JS, Young IR (1985) Nuclear magnetic resonance imaging (NMR), (MRI), of brain stem tumours. Neuroradiology 27: 202–207
8. Byrne JV, Kendall BE, Kingsley DPE, Moseley IF (1989) Lesions of the brain stem: assessment by magnetic resonance imaging. Neuroradiology 31: 129–133
9. Albright AL, Guthkelch AN, Packer RJ, Price RA, Rourke LB (1986) Prognostic factors in pediatric brainstem gliomas. J Neurosurg 65: 751–755
10. Cohen ME, Duffner PK, Heffner RR, Lacey DJ, Brecher M (1986) Prognostic factors in brainstem gliomas. Neurology 36: 602–605
11. Bradac GB, Schorner W, Bender A, Felix R (1985) MRI (NMR) in the diagnosis of brain-stem tumors. Neuroradiology 27: 208–213
12. Packer RJ, Zimmerman RA, Luerssen TG, Sutton LN, Bilaniuk LT, Bruce DA, Schut L (1989) Brainstem gliomas of childhood: magnetic resonance imaging. Neurology 35: 397–401
13. Stroink AR, Hoffman HJ, Hendrick EB, Humphreys RP (1986) Diagnosis and management of pediatric brain-stem gliomas. J Neurosurg 65: 745–750

Dr. R. L. Prevo
Department of Radiology
Medisch Spectrum Twente
Hospital Enschede
Ariensplein 1
7511 JX Enschede, The Netherlands

Neuroradiology (1991) 33 [Suppl]: 31–32

Neuro radiology
© Springer-Verlag 1991

Meningeal and ependymal abnormalities associated with cranial neoplasms: MR findings

G. Krol, B. Simons, and A. Haimes

Memorial Sloan-Kettering Cancer Center, New York, USA

Summary. Cranial MR studies of patients with histologically proven neoplasms and intracranial enhancing lesions or involvement of cranial vault were assessed for abnormalities of leptomeninges. Segmental or generalized thickening of the membranes, and intraventricular nodules were most frequently observed. Meningeal involvement occurred adjacent to existing parenchymal or vault tumor, or distantly, without anatomical contiguity.

Key words: Cranial neoplasm – Magnetic resonance imaging – Meningeal abnormalities

One hundred and sixteen cases with known neoplasms and MR findings consistent with intracranial involvement were reviewed. Abnormal meningeal enhancement was identified in 19 (Table 1).

Materials and methods

Meningeal changes were categorized according to location and appearance. In consideration of clinical diagnosis, the patients were assigned to three groups: (1) primary brain tumor, (2) brain metastases, (3) cranial vault neoplasm, primary or secondary.

MR studies were performed on a 1.5 T GE Signa Imager. T1- and T2-weighted images were obtained routinely, using spin echo sequences 400/20 and 2000/80/40, respectively. Gadolinium DTPA (Magnevist), 0.2 mml/kg body weight was used as a contrast medium. CT was performed on a GE 9800 scanner. Axial sections were obtained without and with contrast medium (150 cc Renografin 60 or equivalent).

Interpretation of CT and MR examinations was carried out by two neuroradiologists with expertise in imaging of central nervous system neoplasms. The patients included in the study had either brain lesions, undoubtedly interpreted as parenchymal neoplasms or unequivocal neoplastic involvement of cranial vault or skull base, metastatic or direct. Abnormal meningeal enhancement was considered to be present if membrane thickness and segmental length exceeded 1 mm and 2 cm, respectively.

Results

Of 19 patients, 6 had primary brain neoplasms. Metastatic involvement of the brain and vault was present in 10 and 3 cases, respectively. The location of meningeal changes was as follows: convexity, 14; ventricles, 6; basal cisterns, 3; interhemispheric fissure, 2; Sylvian fissures, 2; tentorium, 1. The configuration of the enhancement could be defined as follows: longitudinal thickening (localized or generalized), 16; nodular deposits, ventricles or subarachnoid space (single or multiple), 5; patchy, poorly defined, 3.

Six patients underwent concomitant CT examination without and with contrast medium. Meningeal changes

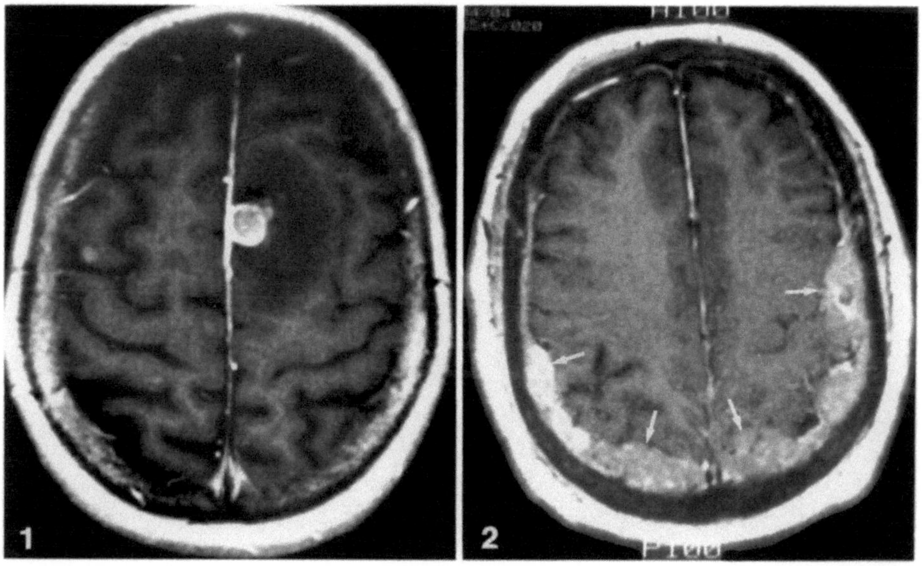

Fig. 1. Focal enhancement of falx cerebri adjacent to interhemispheric (cortical) metastases

Fig. 2. Abnormal enhancement of the convexity membranes secondary to metastatic prostate carcinoma of the calvarium *(arrows)*

Table 1. Histological diagnosis of primary tumors in 19 patients with cranial lesions and coexistent abnormal meningeal or ependymal enhancement

Tumor type	*n*
Glioma	6
Breast carcinoma	3
Lung carcinoma	3
Neuroblastoma	1
Medulloblastoma	1
Prostate carcinoma	1
Head and neck	1
Other	3

appeared to be better defined and could be diagnosed with more confidence on MR in 4 patients. Two studies yielded comparative information. Follow-up MR studies after radiotherapy (RT) were obtained in 3 patients and showed diminution of meningeal enhancement.

Discussion

Meningeal carcinomatosis is a well-recognized although rare form of central nervous system metastasis. The diagnosis is established clinically in conjunction with cerebrospinal fluid (CSF) cytology and biochemical tumor markers. The tumor spread occurs usually as a late complication of malignant intraaxial neoplasms. Less commonly, meningeal infiltration results from metastases from anatomically distant cancers [1–5].

Abnormal enhancement of membranes on contrast-enhanced MR indicates that accumulation of paramagnetic agent takes place, probably via alteration of intravascular–extravascular exchange. Meningeal thickening or enhancement is nonspecific for neoplasm and may be seen in other conditions, particularly inflammatory in nature. Present investigation suggests that involvement of intracranial meninges occurs not only secondar to CSF seeding originating from intracranial (parenchymal) neoplasm but also from direct extension into adjacent membranes, either from superficial parenchymal lesion or from extra-axial tumor, abutting the membranes (Figs. 1, 2). However, there are no data sufficient to classify these meningeal changes as tumoral. Although some cases may represent meningeal extension of the neoplasm, some may actually represent reactive change to the presence of the irritant. Meningeal enhancement associated with benign meningiomas have been described and proven to contain no tumor material. Since only a few patients in the series were treated surgically, the sufficient direct proof is not available. However, positive CSF cytology was present in 5 cases. The regression of meningeal changes after RT paralleling the behavior of the parent lesion suggest that both may be of the same histology.

References

1. Lee Y, Tien RD, Bruner JM (1989) Loculated intracranial leptomeningeal metastases: CT and MR characteristics. AJNR 10: 1171–1179
2. Hwee-Yong Yap, Boh-Seng Yap, Tashima CK (1978) Meningeal carcinoma in breast cancer. Cancer 42: 283–286
3. Redman BG, Tapazoglou E, Al-sarraf M (1986) Meningeal carcinomatosis in head and neck cancer: report of six cases and review of the literature. Cancer 58: 2657–2661
4. Weaver DD, Cross DL, Winn RH, Jane JA (1984) Computed tomographic findings in metastatic dural carcinomatosis. Surg Neurol 21: 190–194
5. Tokumaru A, O'Uchi T, Eguchi T (1990) Prominent meningeal enhancement adjacent to meningioma on gadolinium-DTPA enhanced MR images: histological relation. Radiology 175: 431–433

Dr. George Krol
Memorial Sloan-Kettering Cancer Center
1275 York Avenue
New York, NY 10021, USA

SESSION 4
CEREBRAL TUMOURS 2

Neuroradiology (1991) 33 [Suppl]: 34

Neuro-radiology
© Springer-Verlag 1991

Gadolinium enhancement of the internal auditory canal in posterior fossa meningiomas

P. M. Parizel[1], D. Balériaux[2], M. Van Vyve[3], E. Offeciers[4], G. Forton[4, 5], P. Van de Heyning[5], J. Brotchi[6], and A. M. De Schepper[1]

Departments of [1] Radiology, [3] Neurosurgery and [5] ENT, Antwerp University Hospital, Edegem, Belgium
[4] ENT Department, medical Institute St. Augustinus, Antwerp, Belgium
Departments of [2] Radiology and [6] Neurosurgery, Hôpital Erasme, University of Brussels, Brussels, Belgium

Summary. Gadolinium Gd enhancement within the internal auditory canal (IAC) can occur in meningiomas of the cerebellopontine angle (CPA). In three surgically confirmed cases this enhancement was found to reflect tumour extension into the IAC. The pattern of IAC Gd enhancement was compared with 42 acoustic neuromas (in 38 patients). The most reliable differential diagnostic criteria on MRI in separating CPA meningiomas from acoustic neuromas include the peritumoral dural enhancement, the presence of calcifications, the broad base of attachment to the petrous bone and the lesser T1 increment after Gd injection in meningiomas.

Key words: Gadolinium – Meningioma – Acoustic neuroma – Cerebellopontine angle, neoplasms – Magnetic resonance imaging

Although acoustic neuromas are by far the most common cause of an enhancing lesion in the internal auditory meatus, this finding may also be encountered in posterior fossa meningiomas. The purpose of this communication is to illustrate MRI patterns and to establish differential diagnostic criteria for unenhanced and gadolinium (Gd) enhanced MR examinations of the posterior fossa.

Patients and methods

The MR examinations of 38 patients (14 male, 15 female; age range: 22–78 years; mean age: 56.3 ± 15.4 years) with acoustic nerve tumours (42 lesions; 4 patients had bilateral acoustic neuromas) and 8 patients (2 male, 6 female; age range: 37–80 years; mean age: 63.2 ± 15.2 years) with posterior fossa meningiomas were retrospectively reviewed. In these patient groups, a total of 52 Gd-enhanced MR examinations were performed. Gd-DTPA was used in 38 examinations, Gd-DOTA in 14. Both paramagnetic contrast media were administered intravenously in a dose of 0.1 mmol/kg body weight.

All examinations were performed on a 0.5 T superconducting MR unit (Siemens Magnetom), using a standard 30-cm field of view receiver head coil. The precontrast studies included T1 (short TR), as well as proton density and T2-weighted spin echo images (long TR); the postcontrast MR examination included T1-weighted scans in two or three imaging planes. Additional postcontrast gradient echo (FLASH) sequences were obtained in some cases.

Results and discussion

Gd enhancement within the internal auditory meatus was found in 36 patients with acoustic neuromas and in 3 patients women with large (> 3 cm diameter) meningiomas originating on the posterior surface of the petrous bone. Differential diagnostic criteria for meningiomas include the broad base of attachment to the petrous bone, dural enhancement, the somewhat eccentric location from the internal auditory meatus, the presence of calcifications, the lesser T1 relaxation increment as compared to neuromas.

Conclusion

Enhancement within the internal auditory canal, mimicking an acoustic neuroma, can be encountered in posterior fossa meningiomas. Theoretically, this finding may be caused by direct tumour extension, meningeal hyperaemia, or both. In 3 surgically confirmed cases, this enhancement was found to reflect tumour extension into the internal auditory canal.

Dr. Paul M. Parizel
Department of Radiology
Antwerp University Hospital
Wilrijkstraat 10
B-2520 Edegem, Belgium

Neuroradiology (1991) 33 [Suppl]: 35–36

Neuroradiology

© Springer-Verlag 1991

Cerebrospinal fluid flow measurements in patients with normal pressure hydrocephalus

D. Ott[1], J. Hennig[1], H. Neumann[1], and R. Scheremet[2]

[1] Department of Diagnostic Radiology, [2] Neurosurgical Clinic, University of Freiburg, Freiburg, Federal Republic of Germany

Summary. The diagnostic value of cerebrospinal fluid (CSF) flow measurements in patients with normal pressure hydrocephalus (NPH) was studied using two MRI [double phase encoded (DOPE) and fast Fourier flow (FFF)] techniques. Of 40 patients with the clinical symptoms of NPH, 19 were considered to require a ventricular shunt. Fourteen of these showed abnormal DOPE findings with a reflux pattern at the level of the foramina of Monro with velocities between 0.8 mm and 4 cm/s and increased velocities within the third and fourth ventricle. The FFF results with increased aqueductal flow velocities and hence pulsatility found in all patients examined did not differ from the findings in atrophic hydrocephalus ($n = 2$). The flow studies seem to improve the prediction of the therapeutic response and should be combined with the diagnostic removal of CSF and epidural or intraventricular pressure measurements.

Key words: Normal pressure hydrocephalus – Magnetic resonance imaging – Brain – Cerebrospinal fluid hydrodynamics – Shunt

Fig. 1. DOPE (double phase encoded) findings in normal pressure hydrocephalus: cephalic flow through the foramina of Monro with maximum velocity 4 cm/s *(arrows)* and also upwardly directed flow in the third ventricle *(arrowhead)*

Fig. 2. DOPE findings in atrophic hydrocephalus: no upwards or sideways flow within the lateral ventricles

Fig. 3. Profile-time diagram of aqueductal flow in atrophic hydrocephalus

Although the clinical features of normal pressure hydrocephalus (NPH) are potentially reversible by a shunt operation, some patients do not improve postoperatively. Many diagnostic tests have been introduced in order to improve the prediction of the therapeutic response (CSF tap test [1], CT cisternography, radionuclide studies, epidural or intraventricular pressure measurements, and MRI [2]). The pathophysiological understanding of communicating hydrocephalus is based on disturbed cerebrospinal fluid (CSF) hydrodynamics probably reflected in an alteration of CSF flow which can be measured by MRI [3, 4].

Patients and methods

A total of 40 patients with clinical features of NPH (5 after a subarachnoid haemorrhage (SAH), 1 after tuberculous meningitis), 28 with atrophic and occlusive hydrocephalus were examined by MRI including a T2-weighted image sequence and DOPE (double phase encoded). A reference group consisted of over 50 patients with normal-sized ventricles.

In 6 patients with hydrocephalus and in 5 healthy volunteers the aqueductal flow was measured using the fast Fourier flow (FFF) technique [5]. All MRI studies were performed on a 0.23 or 2 T whole-body system (Bruker, Karlsruhe, FRG). Ten patients each additionally underwent CT cisternography and intraventricular pressure measurements.

Results

After the diagnostic tests 5 patients were classified as atrophic hydrocephalus and 3 were found to have aqueductal stenosis. In 21 patients a shunt operation was con-

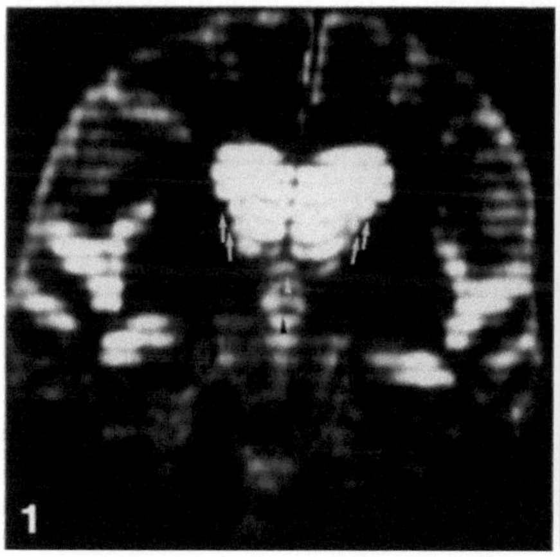

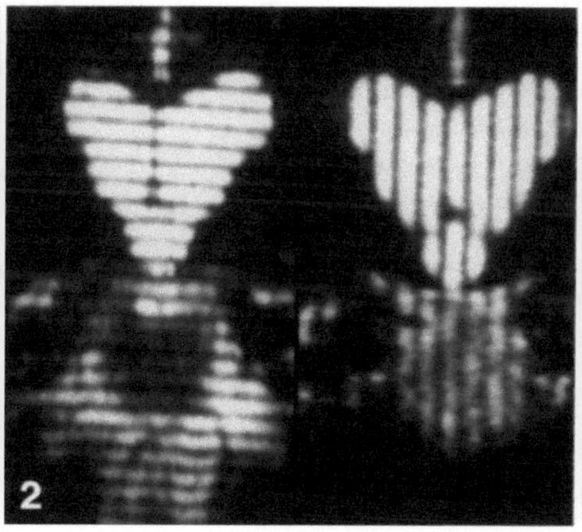

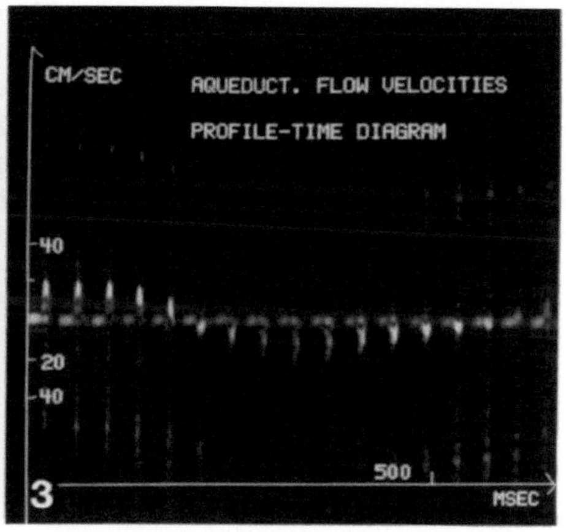

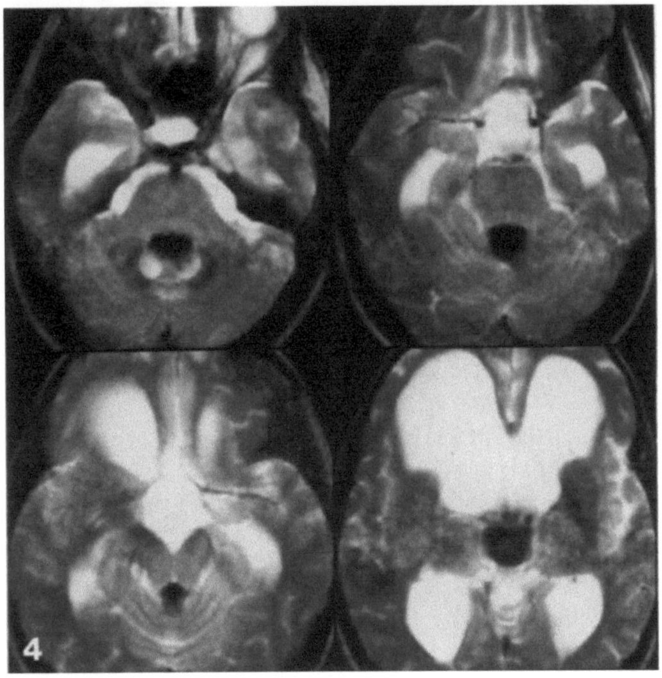

Fig. 4. Extensive signal void in atrophic hydrocephalus (same patient as Fig. 3)

sidered necessary and 12 patients underwent CSF diversion.

Pathological DOPE findings consist of increased flow velocities in the third, fourth and lateral ventricles. The most typical sign of NPH seems to be a "reflux" pattern at the level of the foramina of Monro [6] with marked upward bulging of the interferographic stripes (Fig. 1). In normal-sized ventricles and in atrophic hydrocephalus no upward motion can be detected by DOPE (Fig. 2). 14 of 18 patients with NPH and a clinical shunt indication displayed this sign with varying cephalic (upward) velocities from 0.8 to 40 mm/s. Only 11 of these demonstrated a pathological signal void and 9 patients had increased ependymal hyperintensity on T2-weighted images; white matter lesions were associated in 10 cases.

The pathological DOPE findings correlated better with CT cisternography than with pressure measurements. On the basis of only short-term postoperative results DOPE did not falsely predict positive outcome and falsely predicted negative in 2 patients. The prediction was true (negative and positive combined) in 8 patients.

The aqueductal flow measurements showed a 2- to 5-fold increase of systolic (max. cephalic velocity +20 cm/s) and diastolic (max. caudad velocity −18 cm/s) flow velocities compared with normals. The aqueductal flow velocity in the 2 patients with atrophic hydrocephalus, however, was also markedly increased (Fig. 3). The temporal pattern of flow reversal was always normal. The increased flow velocities correlated well with the extent of signal void (Fig. 4).

Discussion

DOPE and the FFF technique proved to allow accurate measurements of both the slow and fast pulsatile component of CSF circulation. A rather typical pattern with detectable reflux through the foramina of Monro and increased amplitudes was found using DOPE. The hyperdynamic aqueductal flow with marked increase of pulsatility, however, is not specific for NPH, since similar flow dynamics can be proven in atrophic hydrocephalus using the FFF technique. The good correlation of DOPE findings with CT cisternography supports their interpretation as an increased reflux component of the CSF circulation leading to an increased cephalic CSF exchange. The noted divergences from the pressure measurements may be due to the fact that the MRI flow studies do not provide any information about diurnal changes. Compensation mechanisms in malabsorptive hydrocephalus, however, lead to an increased pressure difference at the site of CSF resorption and finally to a normalisation of CSF flow. Whether or not patients with pathological intraventricular pressure and normal CSF flow represent a compensated state that does not respond to a shunt operation can only be decided on long-term results in a larger patient group.

References

1. Wikkelsö C, Andersson H, Blomstrand C, Lindqvist G, Svendsen P (1986) Normal pressure hydrocephalus. Predictive value of the cerebrospinal fluid tap-test. Acta Neurol Scand 73: 566–573
2. Jack CR, Mokri B, Laws ER, Houser OW, Baker HL, Petersen RC (1987) MR findings in normal-pressure hydrocephalus: significance and comparison with other forms of dementia. J Comput Assist Tomogr 11: 923–931
3. Feinberg DA, Mark AS (1987) Human brain motion and cerebrospinal fluid circulation demonstrated with MR velocity imaging. Radiology 163: 793–799
4. Hennig J, Ott D, Friedburg H (1990) Quantification of CSF-flow using a fast MR-technique. Magn Res Med (in press)
5. Hennig J, Mueri M, Brunner P, Friedberg H (1988) Quantitative flow measurements with the fast Fourier flow technique. Radiology 166: 237–240
6. Ott D, Hennig J (1989) DOPE-A fast method to measure CSF motion. Proceedings of the XVth Congress of ESNR. Springer, Berlin Heidelberg New York, pp 63–68

Dr. D. Ott
Department of Diagnostic Radiology
Hugstetterstrasse 55
W-7800 Freiburg
Federal Republic of Germany

Neuroradiology (1991) 33 [Suppl]: 37–39

Neuro-radiology

© Springer-Verlag 1991

Gadolinium-DTPA-enhanced MRI and positron emission tomography of stereotactic laser-induced interstitial thermal therapy in cerebral gliomas

M. Bettag[1], F. Ulrich[1], G. Fürst[2], K.-J. Langen[3], N. Roosen[1], J. C. W. Kiwit[1], S. Hessel[4], U. Mödder[2], and W. J. Bock[1]

Departments of [1] Neurosurgery and [2] Diagnostic Radiology, Heinrich Heine University, Düsseldorf, Federal Republic of Germany
[3] Institute of Medicine, Nuclear Research Centre, Jülich, Federal Republic of Germany
[4] MBB-Medizintechnik GmbH, Application Research, Munich, Federal Republic of Germany

Summary. Stereotactic laser-induced interstitial thermal therapy (SLIITT) is a new method for inducing local hyperthermia in cerebral tumours. As pre- and early post-therapeutic evaluations in five patients with cerebral gliomas WHO grade II and III treated by SLIITT we performed gadolinium-DTPA-enhanced MRI and positron emission tomography (PET). We found that MRI is a sensitive tool for mapping the spatial and temporal distribution of laser-tissue interactions. PET studies using 2-(^{18}F)fluoro-2-D-deoxyglucose showed typical changes in glucose metabolism of the glioma. Both investigations seem to reveal irreversible laser effects in the centre of the tumour probably due to a coagulative necrosis and reversible effects at the tumour margin probably caused by reparative processes after SLIITT. It could be demonstrated that laser-tissue interactions progress with time, depending on laser energy and exposure time.

Key words: Brain tumours – Lasers – Local hyperthermia – Magnetic resonance imaging – Positron emission tomography

The treatment of malignant tumours continues to be a subject of investigation. Several new methods and systems have been introduced into the local therapy of malignancies, among them induced local hyperthermia. The neodymium:yttrium-aluminium-garnet (Nd:YAG) laser with its wavelength of 1.06 m is an excellent source of local hyperthermia because of its low absorption in brain tissue and transmission by an optical fibre. We studied the potential of gadolinium-DTPA (Gd-DTPA) enhanced magnetic resonance imaging (MRI) for visualizing specific effects of stereotactic laser-induced interstitial thermal therapy (SLIITT) in cerebral gliomas in the early postoperative period. Positron emission tomography (PET) was used to reveal changes in glucose metabolism of cerebral gliomas after SLIITT.

Patients and methods

Up to the present, five patients aged between 28 and 70 years were treated by computer-guided SLIITT. All these patients had cerebral gliomas WHO grade II or III confirmed by diagnostic serial stereotactic biopsy. There were two astrocytomas WHO grade II, one mixed glioma WHO grade II–III and 2 anaplastic gliomas WHO grade III. Two gliomas were located in the central motor cortex (Fig. 1 a), one tumour was in the thalamus and two were in the mediobasal temporal lobe. The diameter of the tumours ranged from 1 cm to 3.5 cm. SLIITT was performed by use of a Nd:YAG laser with a wavelength of 1.06 m and its new fiberoptic delivery system, the interstitial thermal therapy (ITT) laser fibre (MBB-Medizintechnik, Munich, FRG). The spatial profile of the ITT fibre is characterised by a circumferential laser beam that extends 2–7 mm proximal to the fibre tip. The tip is flexible and has a biocompatible Teflon sheath that does not cause any tissue adhesion phenomena. A cooling system is not necessary. The ITT laser fibre has an outer diameter of 1.1 mm so that laser treatment can be applied stereotactically. Laser shots are emitted as a continuous wave with an output power of 3–4 W in single or multiple foci depending on the size of the tumour. The exposure time per focus ranges from 5 to 10 min. As pre- and early post-therapeutic investigations we performed contrast enhanced CT and Gd-DTPA-enhanced MRI in all patients. PET studies were obtained in two patients. All MR studies were performed on a Diasonics 0.35 T superconducting magnet system. All images were produced by using spin echo (SE) pulse sequences. Prior to the injection of Gd-DTPA we obtained T1- and T2-weighted images. Following injection of 0.1 mmol/kg Gd-DTPA we performed T1-weighted SE sequences with a short repetition time (TR) of 500 ms and a short echo time (TE) of 30 ms. At least two imaging planes were obtained at each examination. Slice thickness was 5 mm.

In PET we used 2-(^{18}F)fluoro-2-D-deoxyglucose (FDG) for measuring the cerebral metabolic rate for glucose. PET studies were performed pre- and postoperatively (1–3 days and 7–9 days after SLIITT) using the high-resolution Scanditronix PET scanner PC-4096-15WB, which provides 15 brain slices simultaneously. FDG was injected intravenously and a dynamic PET study was acquired over 60 min.

Results

Early postoperative Gd-DTPA-enhanced MR images obtained 1–3 days after SLIITT showed a specific laser-tissue interaction in three of our five patients. There was a marked decrease or complete absence of Gd accumulation in the centre of the glioma and a small, annular, highly increased Gd uptake at the tumour margin (Fig. 1 b). Two patients showed no obvious effect in comparison to the preoperative MR images. Gd-DTPA-enhanced MR images obtained 7–9 days after SLIITT revealed a slight increase in the extent of the central zone of diminished or

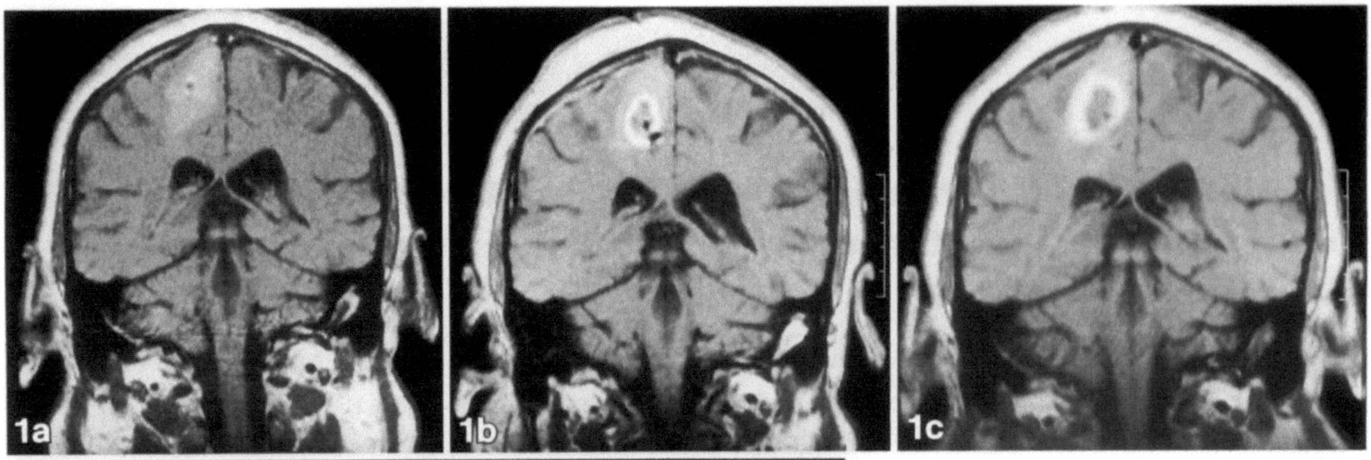

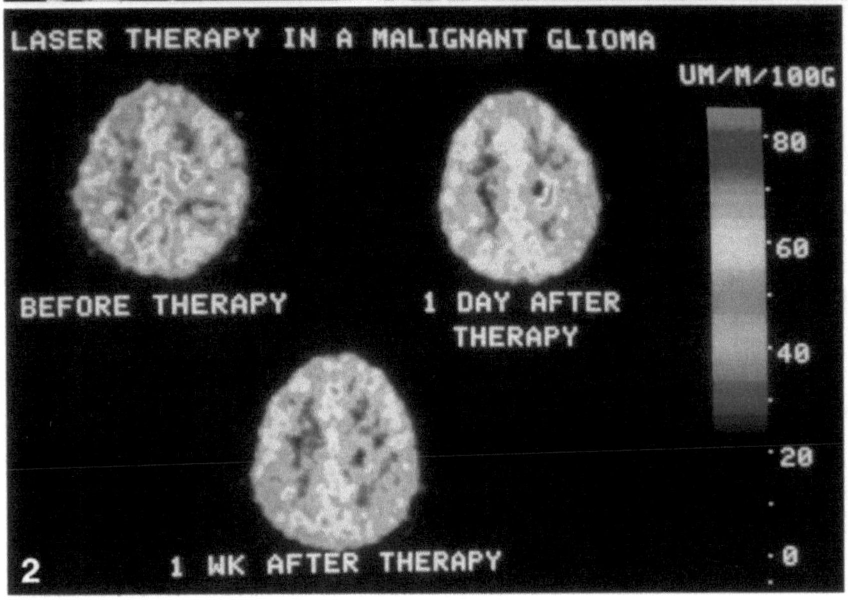

Fig. 1 a–c. Astrocytoma WHO grade II. Post-gadolinium(Gd)-DTPA T1-weighted coronal SE (500/30) images. **a** Pretherapeutic scan demonstrating homogeneous enhancement of the tumour. Relatively sharp demarcation from the adjacent brain tissue. The dot inside the tumour is due to a lesion after diagnostic stereotactic biopsy. **b** Twenty-four hours after stereotactic laser-induced interstitial thermal therapy (SLIITT) a marked decrease of Gd accumulation in the centre of the tumour is seen. Ring- shaped increased enhancement at the tumour margin. **c** One week after SLIITT MR image demonstrating laser-tissue effects have become larger. Signal intensity in the periphery of the tumour is slightly decreased

Fig. 2. Mixed glioma WHO grade II–III. Pretherapeutic PET using FDG revealed a hypermetabolic tumour in the right cortical area. One day after SLIITT PET shows a loss of glucose uptake in the tumour centre and a hypermetabolic rim in the tumour periphery. One week after SLIITT the zone of absent glucose uptake is larger. The previous hypermetabolism at the tumour margin is no longer seen

absent Gd accumulation. The zone of increased Gd uptake at the tumour margin was larger although the signal intensity was slightly diminished (Fig. 1 c).

PET studies using FDG in a patient with a mixed glioma WHO grade II–III 1 day after SLIITT demonstrated a loss of glucose uptake in the centre of the tumour. In contrast, a strong increase in glucose uptake was seen at the tumour margin.

One week later PET revealed the zone of absent central glucose uptake to be larger. Glucose uptake at the tumour margin was in the normal range, the early postoperative hypermetabolism was no longer seen (Fig. 2).

PET studies in a patient with an astrocytoma WHO grade II showed no effects, consistent with MR studies demonstrating no obvious laser-tissue interactions.

Discussion

Heat has been used to treat tumours for at least 100 years [1] by various invasive and noninvasive techniques, e.g. external electromagnetic or ultrasound therapy [2]. There is also the possibility to use lasers for producing hyperthermia in malignancies [3]. The advantages of lasers are the very precise delivery of energy to tissue and the good instrumental control of total energy deposited [4]. Particularly the Nd: YAG laser with its wavelength of 1.06 m involves considerable volumes of laser-tissue interactions by deep penetration into and only slight absorption by living tissue. The property of the Nd: YAG laser that light in the near infrared range can pass down a flexible optical fibre makes it a convenient means of inducing local hyperthermia. The new fibre system of Nd: YAG laser, the ITT fibre, is an excellent tool for interstitial treatment of cerebral tumours. Thermal effects are maximized by use of low power densities and long exposure times [5].

Until now, specific laser effects on brain tissue were mainly analysed by histological studies and by use of thermocouples for measurement of heat diffusion [6]. We used Gd-DTPA-enhanced MRI as a noninvasive and sensitive method of visualizing the qualitative and spatial extent of laser-tissue interactions in cerebral gliomas. Laser irradiation induces changes not only in the thermal motions of the hydrogen photons but also in the distribution and mobility of water and lipids [7]. These alterations result in changed relaxation times. The strong temperature dependence of MR relaxation has been shown in several investigations [7, 8]. The main changes in tissue parameters seem to occur in T1-weighted images, whereas in T2-weighted sequences relatively few alterations are noticed. In our studies early postoperative Gd-enhanced T1-weighted sequences as well as control images 1 week later demonstrate a reduction or loss of Gd accumulation in the centre of the tumour. There is much evidence to suggest that this phenomenon is irreversible, probably due to a coagulative necrosis. The characteristics of Gd uptake at the periphery of the tumour were quite different. In early postoperative images a small zone of highly increased Gd accumulation could be observed. One week later Gd uptake was comparatively diminished, although this zone became larger.

We think this effect could be consistent with a disturbance of the blood-brain barrier at the border of tumour tissue and adjacent normal brain. Because of the alteration with time this seems to be a reversible effect. The fact that tissue changes became more extensive after 7 days may indicate that laser effects do not appear only at the time of application but progress for a certain period. Long-term follow-up studies are necessary to confirm these hypotheses. However, Gd-DTPA-enhanced MRI has proved to be a sensitive tool for mapping the spatial and temporal distribution of laser-tissue interactions in cerebral tumours [9]. In two of five patients typical laser effects could not be demonstrated because of technical problems in SLIITT. There is still the problem of exact volumetric determination of laser energy deposition. Improved control may be possible by using real-time high-speed MR sequences so that imaging can keep pace with the time scale of laser-induced thermal changes. PET of regional cerebral metabolic rate for glucose is a powerful diagnostic and prognostic tool in malignant brain tumours. Strong correlation of increase in glucose uptake and grade of malignancy has been suggested by some research groups [10]. In our studies PET findings gave interesting information additional to the results of MRI.

Early postoperative PET shows a loss of glucose uptake in the tumour centre and an increase in glucose uptake at the tumour margin. Repeated studies 1 week later reveal the zone of absent glucose uptake to be larger. Glucose uptake at the tumour margin was normal. These results underline our suggestion that the effects in the tumour centre are consistent with an irreversible necrotic process and that these alterations progress with time. Changes in glucose uptake at the tumour margin may represent an activation of reparative processes after reversible tissue damage.

However, laser effects in gliomas WHO grade II are difficult to interpret on PET because of only slight glucose hypermetabolism of the tumour. Moreover, very small brain tumours that are especially suitable for stereotactic laser-induced interstitial thermal therapy are often not visible on PET because of its relatively low resolution.

References

1. Busch W (1866) Über den Einfluß welchen heftigere Erysipeln zuweilen auf organisierte Neubildungen ausüben. Verh Naturh Preuss Rhein, Westphal 23: 28–30
2. Cheung AY, Neyzari A (1984) Deep local hyperthermia for cancer therapy: external electromagnetic and ultrasound techniques. Cancer Res [Suppl] 44: 4736–4744
3. Mang TS, Dougherty TJ (1986) Use of the Nd-YAG laser for hyperthermia induction as an adjunct to photodynamic therapy. Laser Surg Med 6: 237
4. Cummins L, Nauenberg M (1983) Thermal effects of laser radiation in biologial tissue. Biophys J 42: 99–102
5. Welch AJ (1984) The thermal response of laser irradiated tissue. IEEE J Quantum Electronics 20: 1471–1481
6. Lajat Y, Patrice T, Nomballais F, Nogues B, Resche F (1987) Effects of 1.06 m wavelength laser radiation applied stereotactically to brain tissue. Laser Surg Med 3: 45–51
7. Bottomley PA, Foster TH, Argersinger RE, Pfeifer LM (1984) A review of normal tissue hydrogen NMR relaxation times and relaxation mechanisms from 1–100 MHz: dependency on tissue type, NMR frequency, temperature, species, excision, and age. Med Phys 11: 425–448
8. Parker DL, Smith V, Sheldon P, Crooks LE, Fussel L (1983) Temperature distribution measurements in two-dimensional NMR imaging. Med Phys 10: 321–325
9. Jolesz FA, Bleier AR, Jakob P, Ruenzel PW, Huttl K, Jako GJ (1988) MR imaging of laser-tissue interactions. Radiology 168: 249–253
10. DiChiro G, DeLaPaz RL, Brooks RA, Sokoloff L, Kornblith PL, Smith BH, Patronas NJ, Kufta CV, Kessler RM, Johnston GS, Manning RG, Wolf AP (1982) Glucose utilization of cerebral gliomas measured by (^{18}F)fluorodeoxyglucose and positron emission tomography. Neurology 32: 1323–1329

Dr. M. Bettag
Department of Neurosurgery
Heinrich-Heine University
Moorenstrasse 5
W-4000 Düsseldorf 1
Federal Republic of Germany

SESSION 5
CEREBROVASCULAR DISEASE – DIAGNOSIS

Neuroradiology (1991) 33 [Suppl]: 42–44

Neuro radiology
© Springer-Verlag 1991

The value of early CT hypodensity in predicting middle cerebral artery haemorrhagic infarction

L. Bozzao[1], U. Angeloni[1], S. Bastianello[1], L. M. Fantozzi[1], A. Pierallini[1], and C. Fieschi[2]

[1] Neuroradiological Section and
[2] III Neurological Clinic, Department of Neurological Sciences, University of Rome "La Sapienza", Rome, Italy

Summary. CT hypodensity is often observed during the first hours of the ischaemic stroke. The value of this sign in predicting possible later development of haemorrhagic infarction (HI) in the injured vascular territories was defined. CT performed within 4 h of 36 supratentorial ischaemic events, showed hypodensity in 25; out of these, 18 developed HI. Angiography performed in the acute phase, showed in all the patients a middle cerebral artery (MCA) or an internal carotid artery embolic occlusion at different sites and defined the state and the efficiency of collateral circulation. Recanalization of the MCA and/or development of a late collateral blood supply through pial arteries after decreased oedema are the two possible mechanisms for secondary bleeding in the ischaemic area. Our data suggest that early hypodensity seen on CT within 4 h of the stroke is a strong predictor of secondary HI in embolic ischaemic stroke.

Key words: Haemorrhagic infarction – Ischaemic stroke – Cerebral angiography – Computed tomography

Haemorrhagic infarction (HI) of ischaemic brain is more common in patients with embolic stroke and large infarcts [1–3]. Restoration of blood flow to an area of embolic infarction is frequently followed by haemorrhage. Experimental studies identified two mechanisms for HI: fragmentation of the embolus within a few days and recanalization of major vessels first occluded; development of a late collateral blood supply through pial arteries after decreased oedema (about 1 week).

Early CT detection of parenchymal ischaemic damage, in patients with middle cerebral artery (MCA) embolic occlusion documented within a few hours by angiography, is predictive of the site of arterial occlusion and the development of chronic brain damage.

Therefore, we studied by sequential CT performed from the acute phase, a consecutive series of 36 patients with supratentorial ischaemic stroke to determine if early CT hypodensity might be predictive for development of HI.

Angiography defined the state of the collateral circulation during the first hours of the developing oedema.

Patients and methods

We have studied 36 patients with supratentorial ischaemic stroke in the territory of the MCA. We performed in all plain CT in the very acute phase of the stroke (4 h) and 1 week from the acute event. Angiography was also performed in the very acute phase (6 h). Four-hour CT allowed us to recognise early changes due to ischaemic brain damage in the MCA territory.

Changes were classified as: lentiform nucleus (LN) hypodensity, cortical hypodensity, LN and cortical hypodensity.

One-week CT showed us the frequency and location of HI. It was classified as: (A) HI involving the LN; (B) HI partially involving the MCA cortical-subcortical regions; (C) HI diffusely involving the MCA cortical-subcortical regions; (D) HI involving the whole MCA territory. The presence on CT of a hyperdense spot along MCA course (HMCAS) was also noted.

Angiography within 6 h showed the frequency and site of vascular occlusions which were classified as: internal carotid artery (ICA) occlusions (cervical, siphon, bifurcation); MCA occlusions (type I: stem-trunk MCA occlusion proximal to the internal lenticulostriate arteries; type II: MCA stem occlusion distal to the lenticulostriate arteries; type III: MCA occlusion at the bifurcation; type IV: MCA peripheral branches occlusion) [4]. Collateral blood circulation was displayed too [5–7].

Results

The CT and angiographic findings are summarized in Table 1. In the 36 patients with brain damage localized to the MCA vascular territory, early CT was normal in 11 and abnormal in 25 [8]. In these 25 patients, slight hypodensity was seen in the LN in 14, in the LN and subcortical-cortical regions in 5, involving only the cortex in the remaining 6 patients.

In the group of 14 patients with early hypodensity localized in the LN (Fig. 1 a), HI was present in 7 of 14 patients. We observed in 4 of them a type A HI (Fig. 1 b); angiography showed a type I MCA occlusion in 1 case, a

Table 1. CT and angiographic findings associated with haemorrhagic infarction

Early hypodensity	HI	Type of arterial occlusion
LN 14	7	4 type I; 1 type II; 2 type III
LN + C 5	5	3 type I; 1 type II; 1 carotid syphon
C 6	6	1 type II; 3 type III; 2 type IV

LN, Lenticular nucleus; C, cortex

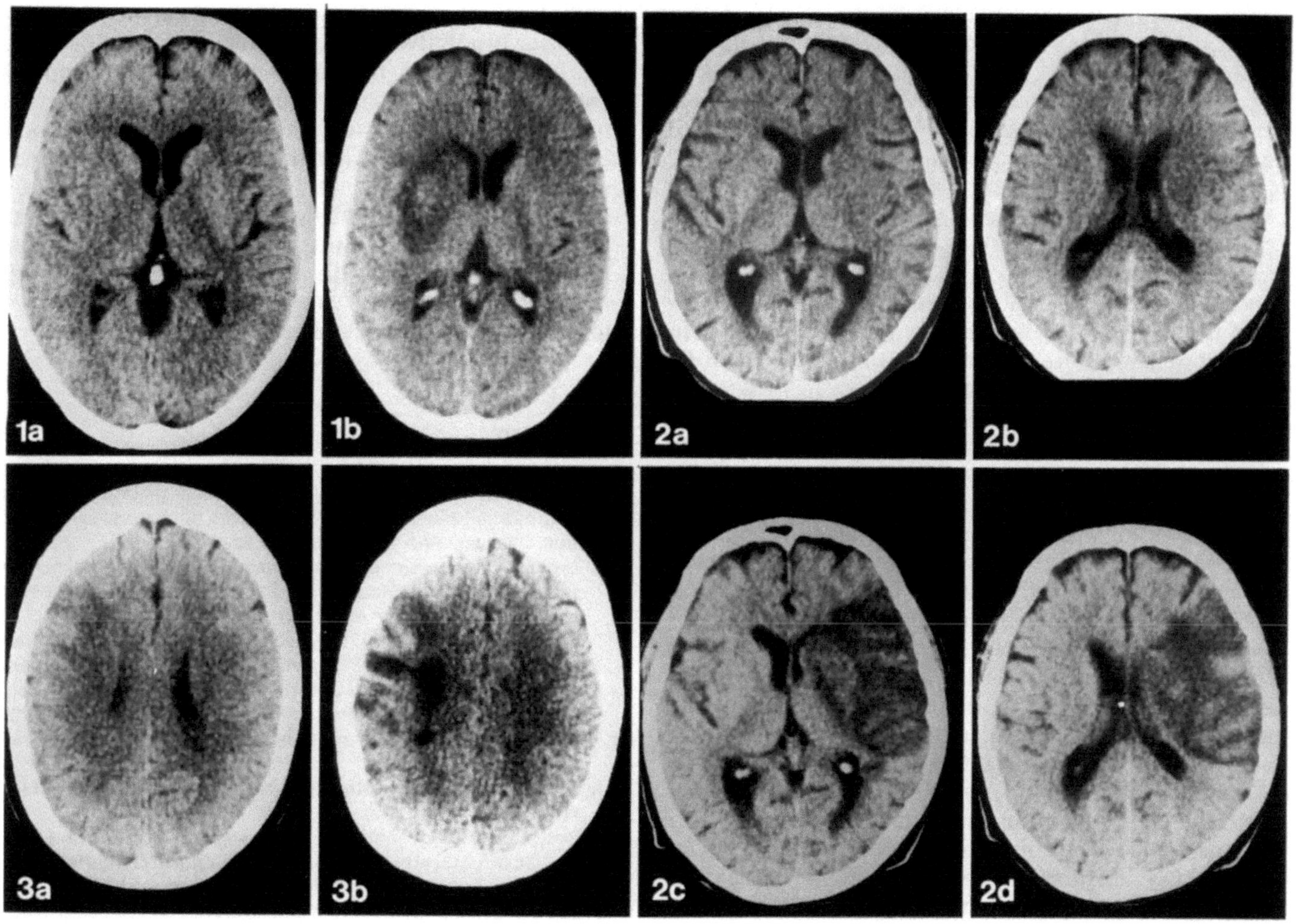

Fig. 1. a Early hypodensity of left lentiform nucleus. **b** Haemorrhagic infarction developed, circumscribed to the left lentiform nucleus

Fig. 2. a Early hypodensity in the right lentiform nucleus and **b** ipsilateral cortical-subcortical regions. **c, d** Development of diffuse haemorrhagic infarction involving right deep and superficial middle cerebral artery (MCA) territory

Fig. 3. a Early hypodensity in left cortical MCA territory. **b** Development of a circumscribed haemorrhagic infarct in the same area

type II in 1, a type III in the remaining 2 patients. Collateral blood supply (CBS) was present in all.

We observed in the other three patients a type D HI; angiography showed a type I MCA occlusion in all with no evidence of CBS in 2.

Seven patients did not show any evidence of HI on 7-day CT; angiography showed an ICA occlusion in 3 of them (cervical, siphon, bifurcation) with good CBS, a type I MCA occlusion in 2 with evidence of CBS in 1 of 2, a type III in the remaining 2 with good CBS in both.

An HMCAS was present in 9 out of these 14 patients. In the group of 5 patients with an early hypodensity localized to the LN and MCA cortical-subcortical regions (Fig. 2a, b) HI was present in all. We oberved a type D HI (Fig. 2c, d) in 4 patients; angiography showed a type I MCA occlusion in 2, a type II MCA in 1 and an ICA occlusion (siphon) in the remaining one. CBS was absent from all. A type C HI was found in the remaining patient: angiography revealed in this case a type I MCA occlusion with no evidence of CBS.

An HMCAS was present in 4 out of these 5 patients. In the group of 6 patients with an isolated early hypodensity in MCA cortical-subcortical regions (Fig. 3a), HI was present in all. We observed in 4 patients a type B HI (Fig. 3b); angiography showed a type III MCA occlusion in 3 with no evidence of CBS in 2 of 3 cases and a type IV in the remaining one with evidence of CBS. We observed in the other 2 patients a type C HI; angiography showed a type II MCA in 1 and a type IV in the other. CBS was absent in both. An HMCAS was present in 3 out of those 6 patients. In the group of patients who did not show any parenchymal hypodensity on early CT we did not find any HI on follow-up controls. In 5 patients angiography revealed a MCA occlusion. We found in 4 of them a type IV and in the remaining one a type III occlusion with good CBS.

Finally in 6 patients angiography did not show arterial occlusions.

Discussion

The frequency of haemorrhagic transformation of a bland infarct is variously reported in previous CT and autopsy studies [1, 9–12]. We detected on CT performed after

7 days from the acute event the presence of an HI in 18 of our 36 patients (50%). Angiography performed within 6 h had shown that an MCA or an ICA occlusion at different sites was present in all. Four-hour CT had also shown an early parenchymal hypodensity in all, making this combination strongly predictive for the haemorrhagic transformation of embolic ischaemic stroke. Haemorrhagic transformation of a bland infarct may be preceded by two pathophysiological steps: there must first be an ischaemic insult of sufficient degree to give rise to disruption of the endothelial vascular wall, then restoration of blood flow into the injured vascular territory must occur. Reperfusion of ischaemic brain is possible within 2 weeks of the stroke either through reopening of the major vessels first occluded or through a late development of leptomeningeal anastomoses. Development of a satisfactorily functioning CBS from cortical anastomoses during the first hours after the stroke may on the contrary be helpful in quickly limiting cortical ischaemic damage [8] and in preventing later haemorrhagic transformation. Development of circumscribed HI in the deep nuclei in patients with early hypodensity of the LN due to main stem MCA occlusion, may be explained only by the reopening of the artery. In all these patients this fact is proved by the disappearance after 7 days of the "hyperdense MCA sign" first detected on early CT, a sign of presence of an embolus in the vessel lumen. The early development of a good CBS through cortical anastomoses preserved cortical regions from the development of early damage and from HI. In three patients of the same group a diffuse HI involving the whole MCA territory developed. In two of these cases early cortical hypodensity was not evident despite the absence of CBS through cortical anastomoses; in these patients a reopening of the MCA could be postulated. The late reperfusion of the injured vascular bed through leptomeningeal anastomoses could be a possible adjunctive mechanism. In the patient with evidence of early CBS, the development of a diffuse HI is probably explained only by an hyper-reperfusion through a reopened MCA. This fact is proved by the absence of "hyperdense MCA sign" present initially on follow-up CT. Development of HI throughout the whole MCA territory in those patients who showed on early CT a hypodensity localized to the LN and in the cortical MCA territories may be explained either by the reopening of main stem MCA first occluded or by this mechanism in association with a late cortical reperfusion through leptomeningeal anastomoses. In these patients, reopening of the MCA first occluded was documented again by the disappearance of the HMCAS on 7-day CT. In the only patient of this group who developed HI diffusely in the cortical MCA territory with no evidence of an early functioning CBS, we found a persistence of HMCAS at follow-up CT. In this case, a late CBS had to be developed for HI. Finally, regarding the development of HI in patients with cortical early hypodensity suffering distal MCA occlusion, this is likely to be due to late reperfusion of the cortex through leptomeningeal anastomoses. Our data confirm that haemorrhagic transformation is a rather common occurrence in embolic ischaemic stroke; in these patients, early CT hypodensity due to artery occlusion is strongly predictive of the development of HI. When the HI is localized to only the basal ganglia reperfusion of these structure may happen only through reopening of the occluded artery. If the HI involves the cortex too, late reperfusion through leptomeningeal anastomoses is likely.

References

1. Fisher CM, Adams RD (1951) Observations on brain embolism with special reference to the mechanism of hemorrhagic infarction. J Neuropathol Exp Neurol 10: 92–94
2. Lodder J, Krijne-Kubat B, Broekman J (1986) Cerebral hemorrhagic infarctions at autopsy: cardiac embolic cause and the relationship to the cause of death. Stroke 17: 626–629
3. Jorgensen L, Torvik A (1969) Ischemic cerebrovascular disease in an autopsy series. 2. Prevalence, location, pathogenesis, and clinical course of cerebral infarcts. J Neurol Sci 9: 285–320
4. Bozzao L, Fantozzi LM, Bastianello S (1989) Angiographic findings in the very early phase (6 hours) of acute ischemic stroke. J Neurol 236: 340–342
5. Osborn AG (1980) Introduction to cerebral angiography. Harper and Row, New York
6. Saito I, Segawa H, Shiokawa Y, Taniguchi M, Tsutsumi K (1987) Middle cerebral artery occlusion: correlation of computed tomography and angiography with clinical outcome. Stroke 18: 863–868
7. Bozzao L, Fantozzi LM, Bastianello S, Bozzao A, Fieschi C (1989) Early collateral blood supply and late parenchymal brain damage in patients with evolving middle cerebral artery distribution cerebral infarction. Stroke 20: 735–740
8. Bozzao L, Bastianello S, Fantozzi LM, Angeloni U, Argentino C, Fieschi C (1989) Correlation of angiographic and sequential CT findings in patients with evolving cerebral infarction. AJNR 10: 1215–1222
9. Yamaguchi T, Minematsu K, Choki J, Sawada T, Ikeda M (1984) Clinical and neuroradiological analysis of thrombotic and embolic cerebral infarction. Jpn Circ J 48: 50–58
10. Hornig CR, Dorndorf W, Agnoli AL (1986) Hemorrhagic infarction – a prospective study. Stroke 17: 179–185
11. Okada Y, Yamaguchi T, Minematsu K, Miyashita T, Sawada T (1989) Hemorrhagic transformation in brain embolism. Stroke 20: 598–603
12. Jorgensen L, Torvik A (1969) Ischemic cerebrovascular disease in an autopsy series. II. J Neurol Sci 1969: 285–320

Dr. L. Bozzao
Department of Neurological Sciences
Neuroradiological Section
University of Rome "La Sapienza"
Viole dell'Università 30
I-00185 Rome, Italy

Neuroradiology (1991) 33 [Suppl]: 45–47

Neuro-radiology
© Springer-Verlag 1991

Dynamic computed tomography in patients with oculomotor palsy: multiplanar and three-dimensional reformations

E. Teasdale, B. Condon, J. Straiton, and P. Macpherson

Department of Neuroradiology, Institute of Neurological Sciences, Southern General Hospital, Govan, Glasgow, UK

Summary. Two-dimensional (2D) multiplanar reformation from dynamic computed tomography (CT) has been shown to be effective in screening for non-subarachnoid haemorrhage aneurysmal third nerve palsy. We describe a method of three-dimensional (3D) analysis of the vessels of the circle of Willis and compare the accuracy of these results with 2D analysis and angiography in 23 patients with third nerve palsy. With 3D analysis there were no false-positive results, but three aneurysms were missed. The 3D technique may be useful in doubtfully abnormal 2D dynamic CT studies.

Key words: Oculomotor palsy – Aneurysm – Dynamic computed tomography – Three-dimensional analysis.

We have previously reported a technique for analysis of the vessels of the circle of Willis by dynamic computed tomography (CT) which will allow accurate noninvasive assessment for use in patients presenting with nonhaemorrhagic oculomotor nerve palsy [1]. This technique was accurate in the diagnosis of vascular abnormalities to a minimum of 2 mm. We have developed a method of three-dimensional (3D) analysis of the same data sets and have analysed this and compared it with the results of both two-dimensional (2D) analysis and angiography.

Patients and methods

In this study 32 patients had dynamic CT carried out by the method previously described [1]. 3D analysis was carried out on all those patients without subarachnoid haemorrhage and in whom the original CT data could be retrieved from tape storage. This resulted in 23 patients' data being available for 3D analysis. All these patients had had prior 2D analysis and angiography.

3D Reformation of CT images. Typically 12 CT slices are acquired which show parts of the vessels under investigation. These vessels initially appear faint because of the high signal from surrounding bone. The procedure for producing pseudo-3D data sets from these data goes through three stages:

1. Thresholding to remove bone signal: Using the interactive thresholding available on the Kontron MIPRON image processing workstation (Kontron, Eching, FRG), any pixels greater than or equal to a typical bone value are set to zero. Any pixels less than or equal to an interactively chosen background level are also set to zero. In this way the contrast between the vessels and surrounding tissues is greatly enhanced.

2. Manual elimination of residual bone signal: Stage 1 does not totally remove the bone signal. At the skull edges partial volume effects may reduce the bone signal to below the upper threshold cut off. Similarly some thin bone in the base of the skull may remain. To remove the bone signal in the skull an observer controlled "mouse" is used to draw a closed line around the brain to exclude the skull. Pixels outside this region of interest (ROI) are set to zero. Similarly ROIs are drawn to enclose the basal bone segments, but this time pixels within this latter ROI are equated to zero. It should be noted that at this stage some operator error may be introduced. Partial volume effects can make it difficult to distinguish between thin bone and vessel. We are now left with only vessels and some slight residual background in the treated images.

3. Construction of pseudo-3D data sets: The 12 treated images are combined to produce a computer generated pseudo-3D construct which can be viewed from a number of angles. Reconstruction is achieved using a maximum extraction algorithm. A series of rays are traced through the stacked slices and only the depth and intensity of the highest voxel value along each ray is retained (this overcomes the summing effect of background which could swamp out the signal from the vessels). The data set is rotated and the procedure is repeated. Two sets of 15 views are obtained. In the first set the view point can be considered to swing laterally across the top of the head

Table 1. Predicted aneurysms causing oculomotor palsy

	2D	3D	Angiography
Ipsilateral PCAA	7	6	7
Basilar AA	1	1	1

PCAA, Posterior communicating artery aneurysm

Table 2. Possible aneurysms

	n	Angiography
2D	4	1 normal 2 loop dominant PCA 1 infundibulum
3D	1	loop dominant PCA

Table 3. Aneurysms at other sites

	2D	3D	Angiography
Ophthalmic AA	1	1	1
Ant. comm. AA	2	2	2
Int. car. bifurcation	0	0	1
Contralateral PCAA	2	0	2

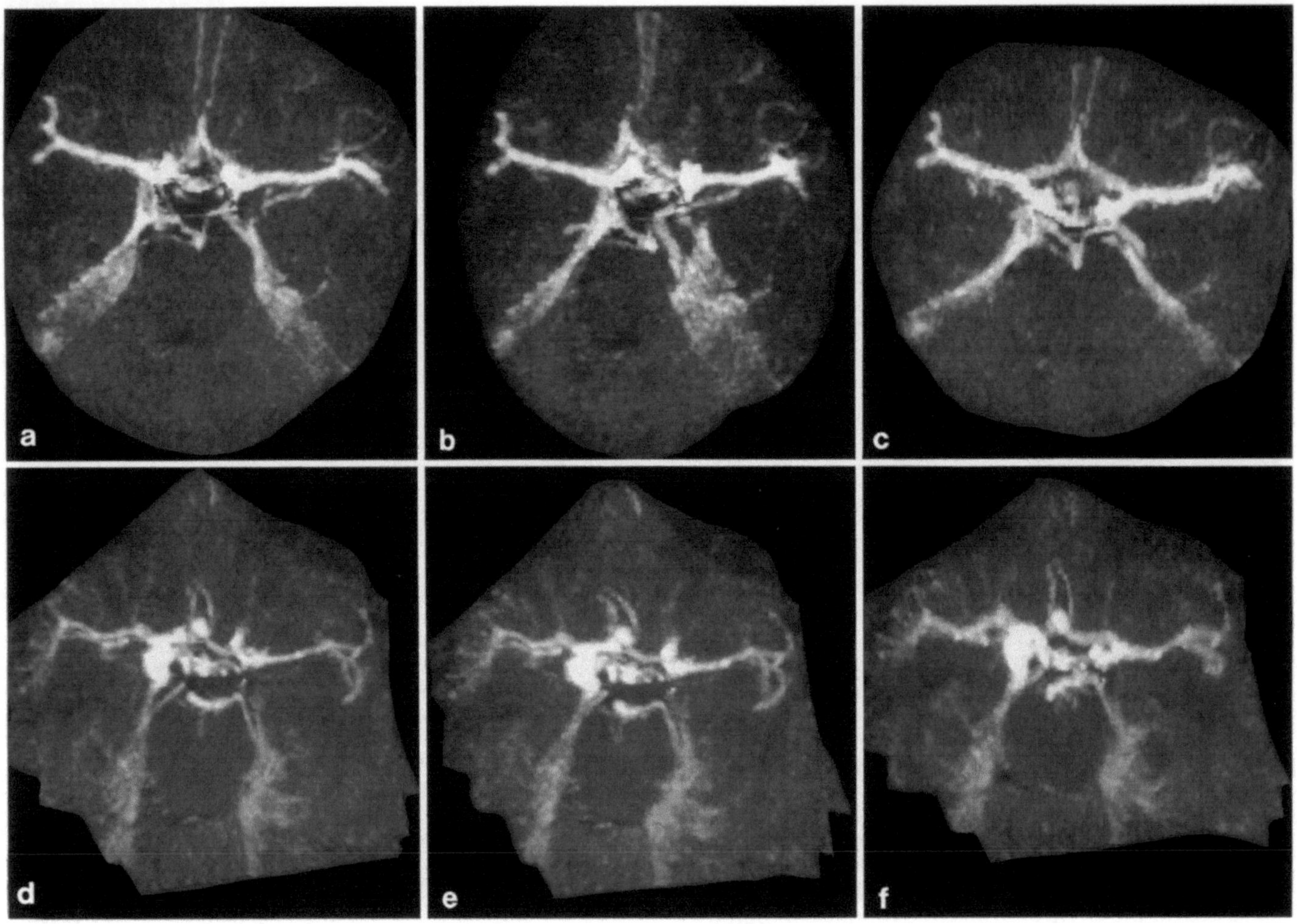

Fig. 1. **a–c** A normal 3D examination; **d–f** a left-sided posterior communicating artery aneurysm and an anterior communicating artery aneurysm. **a** and **d** are viewed from directly above; in **b** and **e** the images have been rotated to the right; in **c** and **f** there is a 24 ° tilt towards the back of the head

from −40 ° to +50 ° (0 ° is the perpendicular to the original slices) in 6 ° increments. In the second the view point swings posterior to anterior along the midline from −40 ° to +50 ° in 6 ° increments. These changing view points can then be viewed in cine mode to show the arterial tree rotating in pseudo-3D and can be zoomed interactively by the operator.

Results

The 3D studies were examined by two neuroradiologists ignorant of the previous 2D or angiographic results. The results are summarised in Tables 1–3 and illustrated in Figs. 1.

Causative ipsilateral posterior communicating artery aneurysms were diagnosed in 7 patients with 2D analysis and in 6 patients with 3D analysis: angiography confirmed 7 aneurysms. The one mainly thrombosed giant basilar aneurysm causing third nerve palsy was correctly identified by both types of CT analysis. Possible but not predicted aneurysms were identified in 4 patients with 2D analysis: angiography showed 1 to be normal, 1 to be a 2-mm infundibulum, and 2 to have large fetal-type posterior communicating arteries. 3D analysis showed only one possible abnormality which was the loop of a fetal posterior communicating artery.

Six aneurysms were present at sites other than the ipsilateral posterior communicating artery origin or the basilar tip. All but one small (< 2 mm) aneurysm at the bifurcation of the internal carotid artery were identified by 2D analysis. 3D analysis identified only three, and in particular did not identify two contralateral posterior communicating artery aneurysms.

Discussion

Our previous publication has shown the value and accuracy of 2D analysis of dynamic CT for non-haemorrhagic oculomotor palsy [1]. We wished to assess the impact of 3D analysis to see if the ability to rotate the image and concentrate only on the blood vessels would add additional information. The results indicate that the 3D technique is less sensitive than the 2D technique and because of this, results in fewer false-positives. However, aneurysms can be missed and 3D analysis failed to demonstrate one causative aneurysm of a size readily detectable on 2D analysis. There is no evidence that aneurysms smaller than 5 mm in their largest diameter are responsible for oculomotor palsy in the absence of subarachnoid haemorrhage [1, 2] and we have shown that lesions of 2 mm can be accurately detected by 2D analysis. It is this sensitivity which is responsible for the greater number of possible abnormalities (false-positives) with the 2D analysis as compared to 3D. Since such small lesions cannot cause oculumotor palsy, perhaps any lesion of this size should be discounted as a insignificant vascular variant. In these cases, additional 3D analysis may result in a greater confidence in excluding pathology and therefore reduce further the need for invasive angiography.

References

1. Teasdale E, Statham P, Straiton J, Macpherson P (1990) Non-invasive radiological investigation of oculomotor palsy. J Neurol Neurosurg Psychiatry (in press)
2. Soni S (1974) Aneurysms of the posterior communicating artery and oculomotor paresis. J Neurol Neurosurg Psychiatry 29: 152–159

E. Teasdale
Institute of Neurological Sciences
Southern General Hospital
1345 Govan Road
Glasgow G51 4TF, UK

Neuroradiology (1991) 33 [Suppl]: 48–49

Neuro
radiology
© Springer-Verlag 1991

Predicting delayed ischaemic deficit in subarachnoid haemorrhage

D. G. Grosset, J. Straiton, I. McDonald, M. Cockburn, M. duTrevou, I. Bone, D. Wyper, and R. Bullock

Institute of Neurological Sciences, Southern General Hospital, Glasgow, UK

Summary. Fifty-nine patients with subarachnoid haemorrhage (SAH) were investigated noninvasively to identify those at risk of delayed cerebral ischaemia. Sixteen patients developed ischaemic deficit but there was no clear relationship with computed tomography blood load and distribution. Serial transcranial Doppler ultrasound (TCD) revealed significantly higher middle cerebral artery flow velocities in those with ischaemic deficit but highest values were often not seen until clinical deterioration had occurred. A rapid rise in flow velocity was observed in advance of clinical signs of ischaemia. Regional blood flow on HM-PAO single photon emission computed tomography (SPECT) in 10 patients with this rapid rise showed focal reduced perfusion in 8, 5 progressing to clinical deficit. A further patient developed infarction before SPECT was performed. Sequential TCD offers potential for identification of patients at risk of delayed ischaemic complications of SAH.

Key words: Subarachnoid haemorrhage – Cerebral ischaemia – Transcranial Doppler ultrasound

Many patients who are initially well after subarachnoid haemorrhage (SAH) and who tolerate early surgical treatment suffer from secondary complications, including delayed ischaemic deficit (DID). The underlying vasospasm and disturbance of autoregulation of cerebral blood flow are poorly understood: treatment is suboptimal and patients most at risk are difficult to identify.

In this prospective study, we examined the use of non-invasive techniques of investigation in an attempt to establish their value in predicting DID after SAH.

Patients and methods

Fifty-nine patients with SAH were examined prospectively. All had cranial computed tomography (CT) on admission, repeated as indicated. Initial CT was graded for blood load after Fisher et al. [1]: grade 1/2, no blood/thin layers; grade 3/4, thick layers. Transcranial Doppler ultrasound (TCD) (EME TC264B, Überlingen, FRG) was performed daily by a standard transtemporal technique, or every 2nd day in those with a more stable clinical course. Arteriography and surgery for aneurysm were carried out within 5 days of haemorrhage when the patient's condition was satisfactory. In selected cases, regional cerebral perfusion was mapped using HM-PAO SPECT (Novo multidetector system).

DID was diagnosed clinically if focal neurological signs and/or reduced conscious level persisted for more than 72 h, in the absence of any other cause for deterioration such as rebleeding, hydrocephalus, or electrolyte imbalance.

Results

Of the 59 patients studied, 53 were fit for early arteriography and aneurysm was confirmed as the source of haemorrhage in 48. DID developed in 16 patients, all with angiographically confirmed aneurysmal SAH. Two of 13 patients with CT blood load grade 1/2 developed DID in comparison to 14 of 46 with greater amounts of subarachnoid blood.

The highest observed middle cerebral artery flow velocities (MCA FVs) were significantly greater in the 16 patients with DID (mean velocities 203.9 ± 15.7 cm/s vs 150.0 ± 8.0, $P = 0.005$, Mann Whitney test). No significant differences in anterior cerebral velocities were seen between the two groups.

For the group of 16 patients developing DID, the MCA FVs plotted in relation to the day of onset of clinical signs showed a rapid rise in velocities in advance of deficit. However, the highest values were not seen until after the onset of deficit (Fig. 1). Ten patients with a rapid rise of FV were selected for further investigation of regional cerebral perfusion by SPECT. Focal reduced perfusion (Fig. 2) was present in 8, with subsequent DID in 5. In those cases with DID, the signs observed corresponded with the site of perfusion abnormality on SPECT and the territory of supply of the vessel with raised FVs (Figs. 2, 3). One further patient developed infarction before SPECT, which showed a focus of hyperperfusion at the site of infarct on

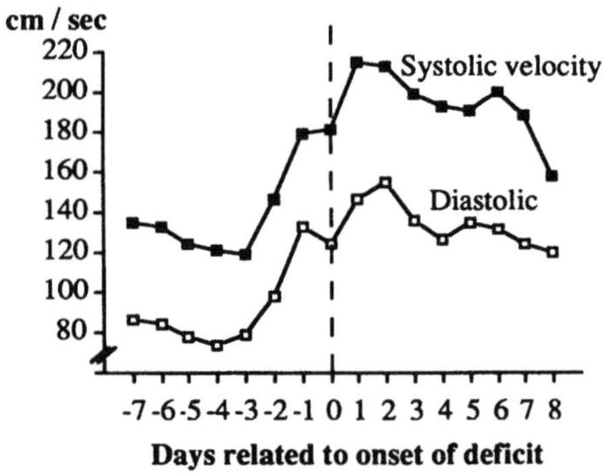

Fig. 1. Middle cerebral artery (MCA) velocity in relation to onset of deficit in 16 patients developing delayed ischaemia. There is a rise in flow velocities from 3 days before the onset of deficit, and a further rise occurs after the onset of deficit

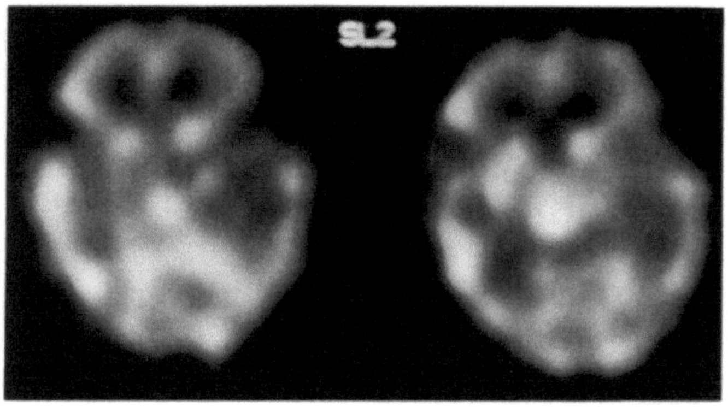

Fig. 2. SPECT cerebral blood flow pattern in a patient with a left MCA aneurysm, and rapidly rising Doppler flow velocities on this artery, showing reduced perfusion in the territory of MCA supply (on reader's right). The patient subsequently developed a right hemiparesis with partial recovery after 1 week

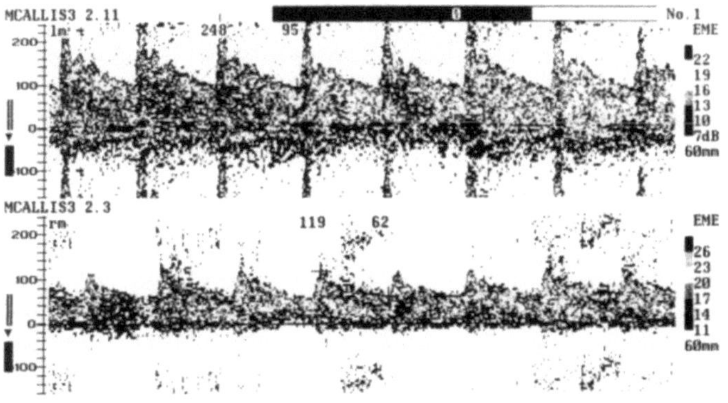

Fig. 3. Transcranial Doppler readings from case in Fig. 2. *Top trace* from left MCA shows elevated velocities (systolic 248, diastolic 95 cm/s); compare to right MCA reading taken on same day *(lower trace)*, with normal reading of 119/62 cm/s

CT. In one case, no SPECT abnormality was found and there was no subsequent ischaemia.

Discussion

The association between subarachnoid blood load on CT and subsequent development of DID has been assessed by several authors [1–3]. Although a greater blood load or substantial localised haematoma predispose to ischaemia, CT data have not proven sufficiently reliable to influence treatment. Our results show that although a greater proportion of those with heavier blood load developed ischaemia, less than one-third of patients with heavier blood load suffered this complication.

Increases in blood flow velocity following SAH have also been described [3–5]. Higher flow velocities are seen in those with ischaemic complications [3, 5], but changes in FVs which precede clinical ischaemia and predict its occurrence have not been described.

We have found rapidly rising MCA FVs in advance of clinical signs of ischaemia. In 10 patients with a rapid rise in FVs, 6 developed ischaemic complications, and 3 had evidence provided by SPECT of subclinical flow reduction. Other authors using SPECT, xenon, and PET [6–9] have demonstrated focal perfusion reduction in association with clinical deficit following SAH, but these techniques are unsuited for frequent repeat examinations. Our findings indicate the sensitivity of TCD, which is eminently suitable for repeat studies and bedside use, in the detection of those at risk of clinical and subclinical cerebral ischaemia.

Serial TCD studies validated against SPECT cerebral blood flow and clinical data on a larger number of patients are needed to quantify the risk of delayed ischaemic complications after SAH. TCD may thus identify patients who require prophylactic treatment.

Acknowledgements. The transcranial Doppler was provided by the Cheast Heart and Stroke Association, Scotland. The Novo scanner was provided by the Wellcome Research Institute. The work was supported in part by Bayer UK.

References

1. Fisher CM, Kistler JP, Davis JM (1980) Relation of cerebral vasospasm to subarachnoid haemorrhage visualized by computerized tomographic scanning. Neurosurgery 6: 1–9
2. Gurusinghe NT, Richardson AE (1984) The value of computed tomography in aneurysmal subarachnoid hemorrhage. The concept of the CT score. J Neurosurg 60: 763–770
3. Seiler RW, Grolimund P, Aaslid R, Huber P, Nornes H (1986) Cerebral vasospasm evaluated by transcranial ultrasound correlated with clinical grade and CT-visualized subarachnoid haemorrhage. J Neurosurg 64: 594–600
4. Compton JS, Redmond S, Symon L (1983) Cerebral blood velocity in subarachnoid haemorrhage: a transcranial Doppler study. J Neurol Neurosurg Psychiatry 50: 1499–1503
5. Sekhar LM, Wechsler LR, Yonas H, Luyckx K, Obrist W (1988) Value of transcranial Doppler examination in the diagnosis of cerebral vasospasm after subarachnoid haemorrhage. Neurosurgery 22: 813–821
6. Nakagawara JP, Nakamura J, Matsuzaki T, Takeda R, Wada K, Toshima M, Suematsu K (1987) Assessment of hemodynamic changes due to delayed cerebral vasospasm in subarachnoid hemorrhage using SPECT and ^{123}I-IMP. In: Wilkins RH (ed) Cerebral vasospasm. Raven Press, New York, pp 79–85
7. Davis S, Andrews J, Lichtenstein M, Kaye K, Tress B, Rossiter S, Salehi N, Binns D (1990) A single-photon emission computed tomography study of hypoperfusion after subarachnoid hemorrhage. Stroke 21: 252–259
8. Yonas H, Sekhard L, Johnson DW, Gur D (1989) Determination of irreversible ischaemia by xenon-enhanced computed tomographic monitoring of cerebral blood flow in patients with symptomatic vasospasm. Neurosurgery 24: 368–372
9. Powers WJ, Grubb RL, Baker RP, Mintun MA, Raichle ME (1985) Regional cerebral blood flow and metabolism in reversible ischaemia due to vasospasm. Determination by positron emission tomography. J Neurosurg 62: 539–546

Dr. D. G. Grosset
Department of Neurology
Institute of Neurological Sciences
Southern General Hospital
Glasgow, UK

Neuroradiology (1991) 33 [Suppl]: 50–52

Neuro
radiology
© Springer-Verlag 1991

Moyamoya disease: MRI and MR angiography

P. Demaerel[1], G. Wilms[1], P. Casaer[2], M. Casteels-Van Daele[2], H. Bosmans[1], G. Marchal[1], and A. L. Baert[1]

Departments of [1] Radiology and [2] Paediatrics, University Hospitals K. U. Leuven, Leuven, Belgium

Summary. MRI is discussed in three children with the Moyamoya syndrome. MR angiography (MRA) was obtained in two of them. The superiority of MRI over CT is well known, as it detects the vascular anomalies (stenosis of major cerbral arteries as well as the hypertrophic collateral circulation) in addition to the ischaemic pathological changes. MRA, although not as detailed as conventional angiography, is very useful for diagnosis and follow-up of this syndrome. Conventional angiography should remain indicated only as preoperative examination.

Key words: Arteries – Occlusive disease – Cerebral blood vessels – Stenosis

The Moyamoya syndrome, first reported by Takeuchi and Shimizu [1], is a rare disease, characterized by a progressive bilateral stenosis of the supraclinoid portions of the internal carotid arteries (ICA) and the proximal parts of the anterior (ACA) and middle cerebral arteries (MCA). This is followed by the development of a hypertrophic collateral circulation from the meningeal branches of the internal and external carotid arteries through the basal ganglia (thalamoperforate and lenticulostriate arteries and (lepto)meningeal anastomoses).

The aetiology is still unknown. Suzuki and Takaku [2] suggested a cerebral type of systemic vascular disease. The autonomic nervous system might also play a role as a pathogenetic factor [3]. The diagnosis is based on radiological examinations, demonstrating the typical misty or smoke-like (moyamoya in Japanese) look of the abnormal vascular network. Adequate medical and/or surgical treatment is not available and remains symptomatic.

Histologically the intima of the stenotic vessel is thickened with fibrous tissue and lipid deposition and is characterized by the absence of inflammatory signs.

Patients and methods

Two boys and one girl, presenting with different but atypical symptoms, were examined by contrast-enhanced (CE) CT, MRI and cerebral angiography. The MR studies were performed with a 1.5 T superconducting magnet (Siemens, Erlangen, FRG). Spin echo axial T2-weighted (TR 2500 ms, TE 15/90 ms) and frontal T1-weighted images (TR 600 ms, TE 15 ms) were obtained with a respective slice thickness of 7 and 5 mm and a slice gap of 1.4 and 1 mm. Gadolinium(Gd)-DTPA (0.1 mmol/kg) was administered in one child. Three dimensional Fourier transform time-of-flight MR angiography (MRA), using a TR of 40 ms, a TE of 10 or 7 ms, a flip angle of 20 °, a volume of 50 ml and a slice thickness of 1 or 1.3 mm as parameters, was obtained in two patients. The method was based on the 3D free induction steady state progression (FISP) sequence with first order flow refocussing gradients. 2D angiographic projections can then be reconstructed by maximum intensity projections along any axis. A set of such projections was displayed on a viewing station (KONTRON-MIPMR workstation) for 3D visualization of the vascular structures.

Discussion

The advent of MRI and MRA has considerably changed the diagnostic approach in moyamoya disease. Radiology has always played a major role in the diagnosis of this syndrome, as clinical presentation remains atypical. Four clinical types are distinguished: the transient ischaemic attack type, the epileptic type, the haemorrhagic type and the infarction type [4]. In this study, the first type was seen in two children and the second type in one. CE CT usually demonstrates only the ischaemic changes: periventricular infarcts, (sub)cortical white matter infarction predominantly in the watershed regions, widening of the sulci and dilatation of the ventricular system. Three types of CT picture have been defined by Yoshii: the normal, the cortical and the wedge type [4]. High resolution CE CT may sometimes demonstrate the collateral circuation.

In addition to these pathological changes, MRI is also capable of visualizing the vascular anomalies, as the major intracranial arteries are imaged due to their rapid blood flow (Fig. 1). A severe stenosis or occlusion is seen as an absence of flow void and the hypertrophic basal ganglionic collaterals are seen as multiple round or tortuous low intensity areas [5, 6].

Stenosis or occlusion of the MCA is best visualized on proton density and T2-weighted images (Fig. 1). ACA stenosis is less easily seen. Occlusion of the intracavernous portion of the ICA is sometimes observed. However, attention has to be paid to fast poststenotic flow which can also produce a flow void. Reports have also proved that sometimes a flow void can be seen in angiographically occluded arteries [7].

The collateral circulation in the basal ganglia, as well as in the thalamus and the parieto-occipital area was clearly depicted in all three patients. An inversion of the signal intensities from grey and white matter in one hemisphere

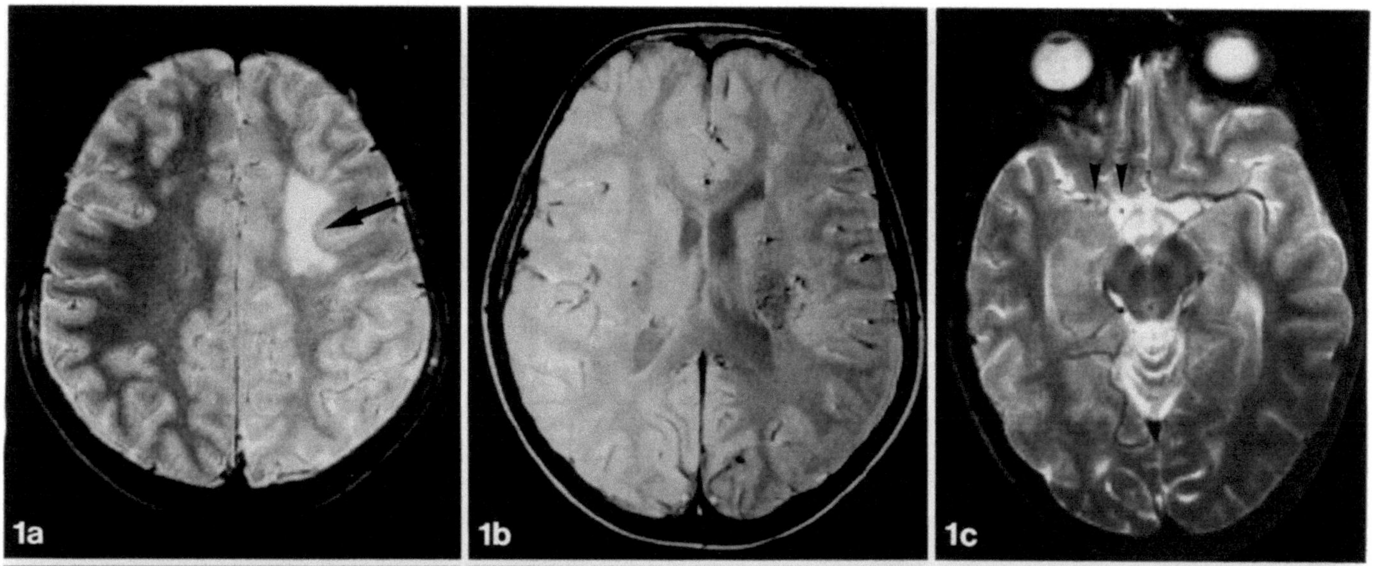

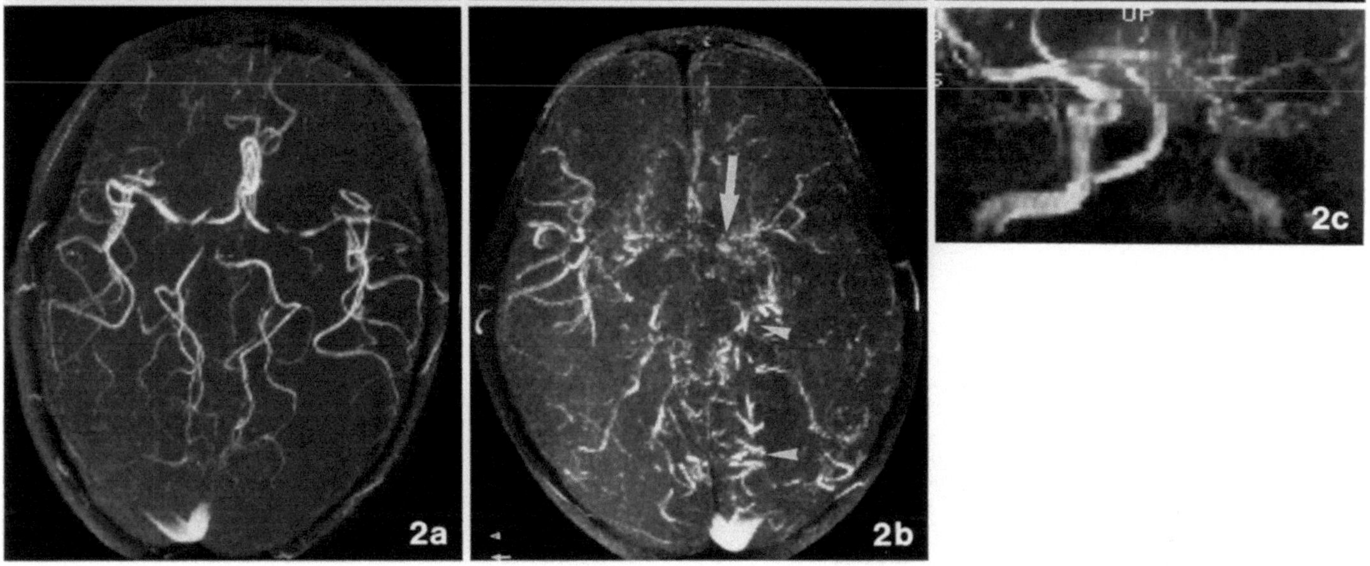

Fig. 1. a Axial SE 2500/90 image demonstrates a watershed infarction in the left hemisphere (♦) and a clear difference in signal intensity between the left and the right hemisphere. **b** Axial SE 2500/15 image visualizes the collateral circulation in the basal ganglia at the left side. **c** Axial SE 2500/90 image shows the absence of flow void in the right middle cerebral artery (MCA) (▶)

Fig. 2. a Normal MR angiography (MRA) in the base of the skull. **b** MRA in a patient demonstrates the stenosis in the left MCA (♦) and the hypertrophic collateral circulation (▶). **c** Rotation of an axial reconstructed image in the frontal direction clearly shows the stenosis of the supraclinoid portion of the left internal carotid artery and of the left MCA

was seen in one patient. This may suggest blood flow asymmetry or abnormal vascularity (Fig. 1). Gd-DTPA meningeal enhancement was observed in that hemisphere.

As already demonstrated, MRA is very promising and may replace conventional angiography in the future [8]. Until now, conventional angiography was the examination of choice in the diagnosis of moyamoya disease [9]. MRA enables us to visualise all vascular abnormalities mentioned above (Fig. 2). The intracavernous portion of the ICA is even better visualized on MRA than on MRI. Moreover, using a viewing station, 3D visualization of the blood vessels become possible (Fig. 2). While the resolution of this technique is not yet equal to that of conventional angiography, it appears probable that MRA will replace angiography with further technical improvements.

MRI's superiority over CT in the diagnosis of the moyamoya syndrome is obvious. An additional MRA, being noninvasive, seems the only necessary investigation in diagnosis and follow-up of moyamoya disease. Today conventional angiography seems indicated only if surgery is planned.

References

1. Takeuchi K, Shimizu K (1957) Hypoplasia of the bilateral internal carotid arteries. Brain Nerve 9: 37–43
2. Suzuki T, Takaku A (1968) The disease showing the abnormal vascular network at the base of the brain particularly found in Japan. Our opinion of dynamic change of this vascular network. Brain Nerve 20: 35–40

3. Welch WC, McBride M, Hido DK, Nelson CN (1988) Moyamoya disease in an infant with autonomic dysfunction: angiographic and MRI findings. J Child Neurol 3: 110–113
4. Maki Y, Enomoto T (1988) Moyamoya disease. Childs Nerv Syst 4: 204–212
5. Fujisawa I, Asato R, Nishimura K, Togashi H, Itoh K, Noma S, Sagoh T, Minami S, Nakano Y, Yonekawa Y, Tarizuka K (1987) moyamoya disease: MR imaging. Radiology 164: 103–105
6. Bruno A, Yuh WTC, Biller J, Adams HP, Cornell SH (1988) Magnetic resonance imaging in young adults with cerebral infarction due to moyamoya disease. Arch Neurol 45: 303–306
7. Rolak LE (1989) MRI in moyamoya disease. Arch Neurol 46: 14
8. Demaerel P, Wilms G, Casteels-Van Daele M, Marchal G, Van Fraeyenhoven L, Bosmans H, Casaer P, Baert AL (1990) Moya-Moya: diagnostic par IRM et angiographie RMN. J Radiol 71: 119–123
9. Maki Y, Horie T, Nakada Y (1968) Angiographical studies on the cases of obstructive disease with abnormal vascular network. J Child Med Soc 45: 272–277

Prof. G. Wilms
Department of Radiology
University Hospitals K. U. Leuven
Herestraat 49
B-3000 Leuven, Belgium

Neuroradiology (1991) 33 [Suppl]: 53–55

Neuroradiology
© Springer-Verlag 1991

MRI of cerebral hypoxia

G. Birbamer[2], F. Aichner[1, 2], S. Felber[2], A. Kampfl[2], K. Berek[1], E. Schmutzhard[1], and F. Gerstenbrand[1]

Departments of [1]Neurology and [2]Magnetic Resonance, University of Innsbruck, Innsbruck, Austria

Summary. MRI findings are described in 24 cases of hypoxic coma. In this study hypoxic damage has occurred as a consequence of diverse conditions such as cardiac arrest, anaesthetic accidents, carbon monoxide poisoning, high altitude brain oedema, drowning, suicidal hanging, hypoglycaemia and shock. The main forms of cerebral damage were watershed infarction and bilateral selective neuronal necrosis within the globus pallidus, putamen, nucleus caudatus, thalamus, parahippocampal gyrus, hippocampus, cerebellum and brainstem nuclei. Whereas watershed infarction indicated failure of circulation, the pattern of damage within the basal ganglia, thalami, temporal lobe and brain stem could not be related to any of the underlying pathogenetic processes. No typical pattern of lesion could be found in regard to the cause of the disease. However, arterial boundary zone involvement indicates the underlying pathogenetic mechanism. The sensitivity of MRI in the detection of hypoxic lesions was greatly superior to that of CT, while specificity based on signal behaviour allowed differentiation of acute and chronic alterations. Based on serial MRI studies prediction of prognostic outcome will be improved.

Key words: Hypoxic coma – Apallic syndrome – Cardiac and circulatory arrest – Oxygenation failure – Magnetic resonance imaging

Disturbance in oxygen supply to the brain can be divided into anoxic or hypoxic anoxia, anaemic anoxia and ischaemia. Though caused by different conditions and diseases, all three categories share equally the potential for depriving brain tissue of its oxygen supply. Until now only a few neuropathological and neuroradiological studies have been reported. The aim of this retrospective study was to analyse MRI findings and their evolution in hypoxic comatose patients and to describe vulnerable areas of brain and the distribution of hypoxic lesions in vivo.

Materials and methods

The median age of the patients was 34 years, ranging from 1 to 78 years, male/female ratio being 1 : 1. The study was performed during a 16-month period, from February 1989 to May 1990. MRI was performed on a 1.5 T Magnetom (Siemens). The current protocol includes sagittal and axial T1-weighted images (550/15) as well as proton density and T2-weighted spin echo images (2400/40/90).

The patients' blood pressure and ECG were continuously monitored and pulsoxymetry and capnography were performed. Nine patients were investigated under general anaesthesia.

Results

The causes and aetiological factors of hypoxia in the 24 comatose patients examined are listed in Table 1. Four patients were investigated in the acute stage, presenting with the clinical signs of decortication, and in 5 the diagnosis of organic brain syndrome was made, whereas the majority were investigated in the chronic stage with an apallic syndrome corresponding to a chronic vegetative state [1].

MRI examinations in all patients revealed multiple, symmetrical and bilateral, focal damage; in 6 the lesions were haemorrhagic (Fig. 1). In order to delineate a distinct pattern of lesions related to aetiology six main regions were defined (cortical border zone, deep white matter, basal ganglia and thalamus, temporal lobe, brain stem, cerebellum and corpus callosum) and correlated with the aetiology. In regard to the aetiology the distribution of lesions was quite various and unspecific, but cortical boundary zones involvement was found only in the cardiovascular group (Fig. 2). There was no significant difference in the number of involved regions in the acute and chronic phases. Patients in the chronic state, however, tend to have more regions involved. Based on signal behaviour, oedema, ischaemia and haemorrhage could be differentiated from cysts, gliosis and necrosis. Occurrence and degree of brain shrinkage increased with the duration of the apallic syndrome.

Discussion

Only recently has MRI been introduced for the assessment of intensive care unit patients. The most important prerequisite is the capability to monitor continuously blood pressure and ECG, to perform oxymetry and capnography. This study documents the applicability of MRI in severely ill patients.

Table 1. Aetiology of hypoxic coma

Drowning accident	4	failure of oxygenation
Carbon monoxide poisoning	2	
Inhalation of inert gases	2	
High altitude brain oedema	1	
Cardiac arrest	4	cardiac and circulation arrest
Hanging	2	
Anaphylaxis	1	
Hypoglycaemia	1	various
Septicaemia	1	
Drug intoxication	2	
Anaesthesia accident	2	

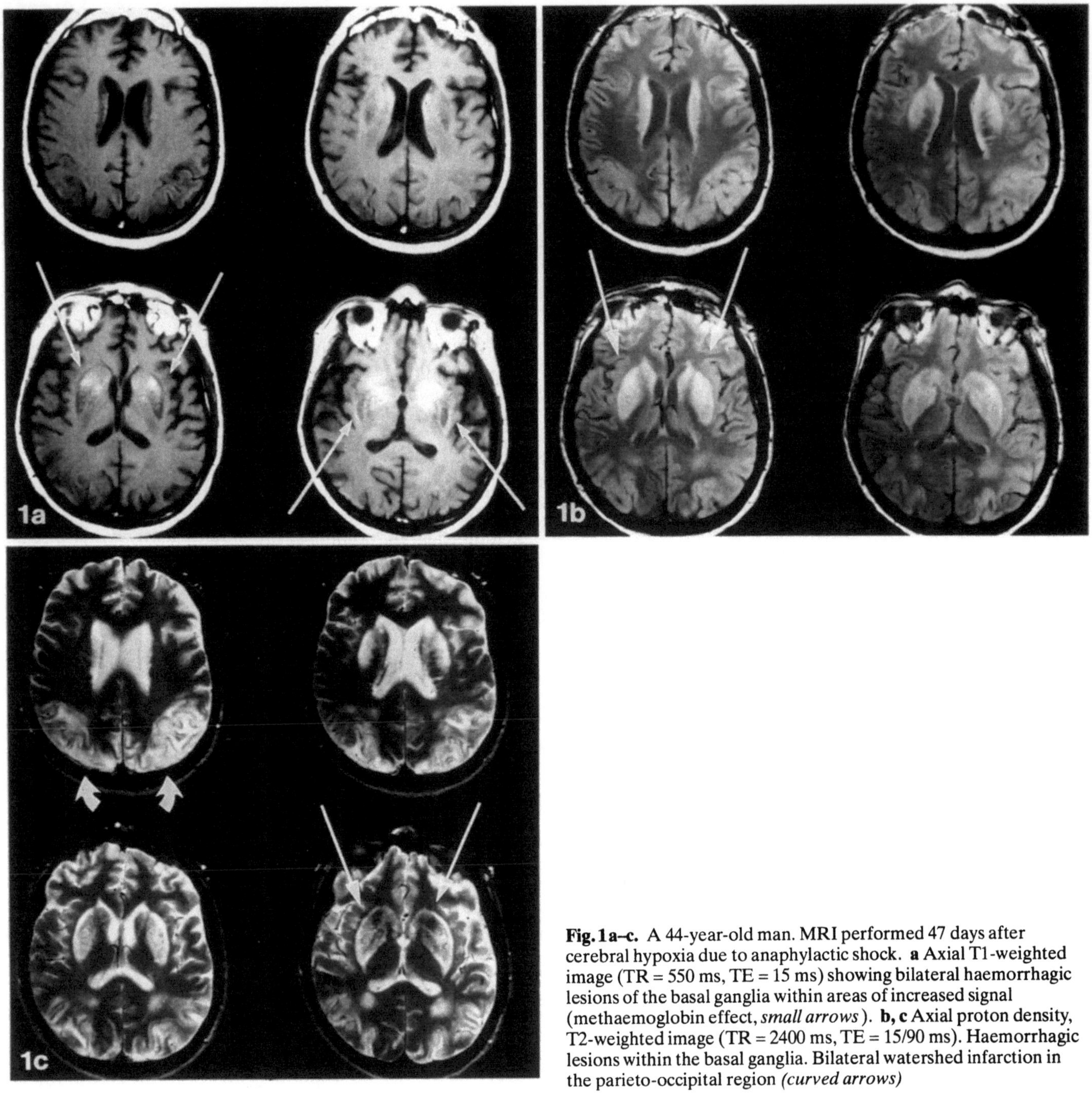

Fig. 1a–c. A 44-year-old man. MRI performed 47 days after cerebral hypoxia due to anaphylactic shock. **a** Axial T1-weighted image (TR = 550 ms, TE = 15 ms) showing bilateral haemorrhagic lesions of the basal ganglia within areas of increased signal (methaemoglobin effect, *small arrows*). **b, c** Axial proton density, T2-weighted image (TR = 2400 ms, TE = 15/90 ms). Haemorrhagic lesions within the basal ganglia. Bilateral watershed infarction in the parieto-occipital region *(curved arrows)*

Multiple focal, symmetrical, bilateral damage was found in most of the patients; 6 cases demonstrated haemorrhagic lesions. Shrinking of the brain was another prominent finding in this study. Based on the clinical data and signal behaviour acute changes like oedema, watershed infarction and haemorrhage could be differentiated from cyst, gliosis and necrosis. The appearance and the degrees of brain shrinkage indicate a trans-synaptical degeneration due to decreased input [2].

In acute anoxic coma, CT usually fails to show any abnormality. Some time later focal infarcts and diffuse and focal atrophy may be evident [3, 4]. The sensitivity of MRI in detecting acute and chronic hypoxic lesions is superior to that of CT [5]. Additional serial MRI studies allow differentiation of acute and chronic alterations of the brain and increase specificity by monitoring the disease.

No typical pattern of lesions could be found in relation to the determining factors of the various conditions causing hypoxic coma. However, arterial boundary zone involvement indicates an underlying pathogenetic mechanism. The reasons behind areas of differential damage and the distribution of hypoxic injury are phylogenetic factors, immaturity and selective vulnerability [6, 7]. Beside these intrinsic factors different levels of toxic metabolites and neurotransmitters may also determine the pattern of hypoxic lesions. In addition, factors such as the degree and duration of circulatory arrest, cerebral energy requirements and pre-existing cerebrovascular morbidity also

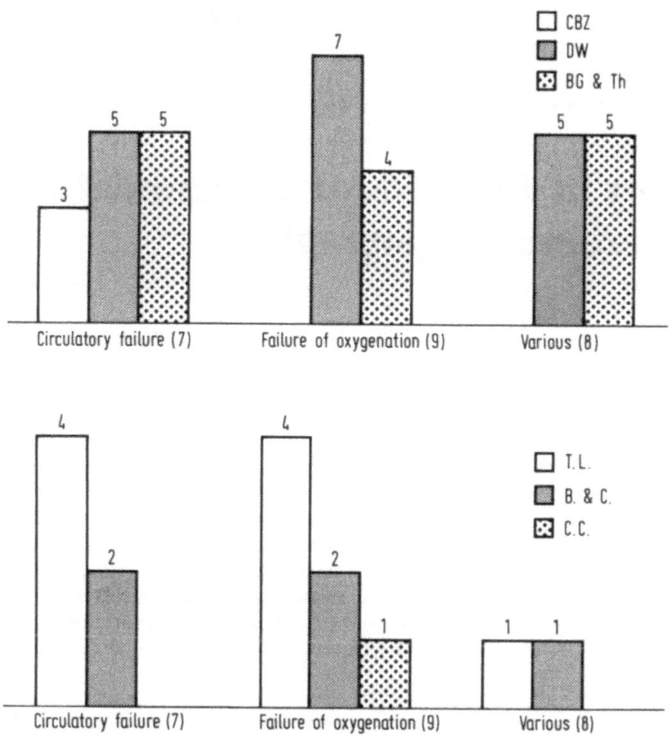

Fig. 2. Anatomical distribution of lesions with regard to aetiology. *GBZ*, Cortical border zone; *DW*, deep white matter; *BG & Th*, basal ganglia and thalamus; *TL*, temporal lobe; *B & C*, brain stem and cerebellum; *C. C.*, corpus callosum

affect the distribution and severity of anoxic cerebral damage.

Neuropathological studies show that the following groups of neurons are vulnerable to even moderate degrees of anoxia: pyramidal cells in Sommer's sector of the hippocampus, Purkinje cells of the cerebellum and the third and fifth layers of the cerebral cortex. More severe degrees of anoxia affect neurons in the amygdala, putamen, caudate nucleus, thalamus and substantia nigra. Profound anoxia affects even brain stem nuclei. The pattern of lesions could be observed in this in vivo MRI study.

References

1. Dalle Ore G, Gerstenbrand F, Lücking CH, Peters G, Peters UH (1977) The apallic syndrome. Springer, Berlin Heidelberg New York
2. Plum F, Posner JB, Hain RF (1962) Delayed neurological deterioration after anoxia. Arch Intern Med 110: 18–25
3. Aichner F, Gerstenbrand F (1989) Computed tomography in cerebrovascular disease. In: Toole JF (ed) Handbook of clinical neurology, vol 10. Vascular diseases. II. Elsevier, Amsterdam, pp 477–480
4. Yagnik P, Gonzalez C (1980) White matter involvement in anoxic encephalopathy in adults. J Comput Assist Tomogr 4: 788–790
5. Horowitz AL, Kaplan R, Sarpel G (1987) Carbon monoxide toxicity: MR imaging in the brain. Radiology 162: 787–788
6. Brierly JB, Graham DI (1984) Hypoxia and vascular disorders of the central nervous system. In: Adams JH, Corsellis JAN, Duchen LW (eds) Greenfield's neuropathology, pp 126–155
7. Cervos-Navarro J, Schneider H (1980) Pathologie des Nervensystems I. Durchblutungsstörungen und Gefäßerkrankungen des Nervensystems. Springer, Berlin Heidelberg New York, pp 67–84

Dr. G. Birbamer
Department of Magnetic Resonance
University of Innsbruck
Anichstrasse 35
A-6020 Innsbruck, Austria

Neuroradiology (1991) 33 [Suppl]: 56–57

Neuro radiology
© Springer-Verlag 1991

High-resolution computed tomography in diagnosis of intracranial aneurysm not well demonstrated on cerebral angiography

P. S. P. Ho[1], C. Y. Chen[1], C. C. Lee[1], M. J. Sun[2], and Y. C. Wang[2]

Departments of [1] Diagnostic Radiology, [2] Neurosurgery, National Defense Medical Center and Tri-Service General Hospital, Taipei, Taiwan, Republic of China

Summary. A 52-year-old female underwent computed tomography (CT) due to a sudden loss of consciousness. The brain CT showed subarachnoid haemorrhage and intracerebral haematoma with ventricular extension. The cerebral angiography was performed 4 weeks later. A berry aneurysm of the left internal carotid artery near the origin of the posterior communicating artery was suspected. The aneurysm neck was not demonstrated on multiple different projections of the left internal carotid angiography. High-resolution CT showed the aneurysm clearly arising from the left internal carotid artery. The aneurysm was then clipped by the neurosurgeon based on our high-resolution CT findings. CT provides a means of investigating cerebral aneurysm especially when cerebral angiography is doubtful.

Key words: Cerebral aneurysm – Computed tomography – Cerebral angiography

Computed tomography (CT) and cerebral angiography are the two main procedures for the neuroradiological investigation of symptomatic intracerebral aneurysms [1]. Although high-resolution CT has high accuracy (97.4%) in the diagnosis of intracerebral aneurysms, determining size and main direction of the aneurysm still depends on cerebral angiography [1–3]. Since high-resolution CT has potential for the visualization of aneurysms, it can be utilized as an alternative method to localize the aneurysm if cerebral angiography does not clearly characterize it effectively.

Case report

A 52-year-old female was admitted because of sudden loss of consciousness. The non-contrast brain CT showed subarachnoid haemorrhage, and intracerebral haematoma with left lateral ventricle extension (Fig. 1). Rupture of an intracerebral aneurysm was highly suspected clinically. A cerebral angiography series including frontal, lateral, transorbital oblique and basal projections was performed 4 weeks after admission.

A berry aneurysm of the left internal carotid artery near the origin of the posterior communicating artery was suspected; however, the aneurysm neck was difficult to separate from the posterior communicating artery (Fig. 2). High-resolution CT technique (Somatom DRH) with 550 mAs, 125 kV, 512 Matrix, 7 s scan time, centered on the circle of Willis, in 1 mm slice thickness following rapid intravenous bolus contrast medium (Angiografin 65% 100 ml) injection with coronal reformation images, clearly showed the aneurysm arising from the supraclinoid portion of the left internal carotid artery (Fig. 3). The patient then underwent a craniotomy based on our high-resolution CT findings. An aneurysm was found arising from the supraclinoid portion of the left internal carotid artery, slightly above and lateral to the origin of the posterior communicating artery. The aneurysm neck was clipped without difficulty (Fig. 4).

Discussion

Although high-resolution CT has been used in the diagnosis of cerebral aneurysm and with a high accuracy rate (97.4%), cerebral angiography is still the definitive procedure in demonstration of the size and location of cerebral aneurysms before surgical treatment [1, 3]. Regarding carotid artery studies, high-resolution CT with image reformation has been used in the study of carotid bifurcation with good results [4]. In this case, high-resolution CT of the head, performed in a rapid series of thin slices during an intravenous bolus injection of contrast medium demonstrated the arteries of the circle of Willis. In addition, the coronal and sagittal reformed imagings clearly showed the aneurysm and surrounding structures. High-resolution CT provides a means of investigating cerebral aneurysm especially when cerebral angiography is doubtful.

References

1. Sarwar M (1983) Intracranial aneurysms. In: Sarwar M, Azar-Kia B, Batnitzky S (eds) Basic neuroradiology. Green, St. Louis, pp 459–485
2. Davis KR, Kistler JP, Heros RC, Davis JM (1982) A neuroradiological approach to the patient with a diagnosis of subarachnoid hemorrhage. Radiol Clin North Am 20: 87–94
3. Schmid UD, Steiger HJ, Huber P (1987) Accuracy of high resolution computed tomography in direct diagnosis of cerebral aneurysms. Neuroradiology 29: 152–159
4. Brant-Zawadzki M, Jeffrey RB Jr (1982) CT with image reformation for noninvasive screening of the carotid bifurcation: early experience. AJNR 3: 395–400

Dr. P. S. P. Ho
Department of Diagnostic Radiology
Tri-Service General Hospital
622, Ting-Chow Road
Taipei, Taiwan 10713, Republic of China

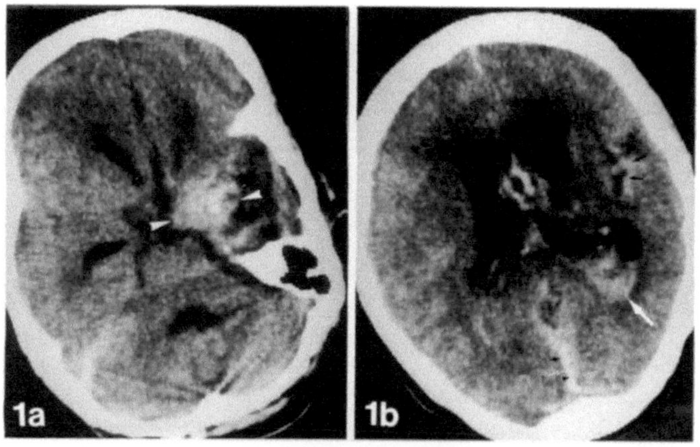

Fig. 1. Non-contrast brain CT showed **a** intracerebral haematoma *(white arrowhead)* in left medial temporal region; **b** intraventricular haematoma *(big white arrow)* and subarachnoid haemorrhage *(small black arrows)*

Fig. 2. Left carotid angiography in (**a**) frontal, (**b**) lateral, (**c**) right oblique, (**d**) left oblique views partially demonstrated the suspicious aneurysm *(small black arrow)* of left internal carotid artery. The basal projection (**e**) did not illustrate the aneurysm

Fig. 3. High-resolution CT imaging with coronal reformation (**a**) showed the aneurysm *(white arrowhead)* and its magnified image (**b**) clearly demonstrated the aneurysm *(white arrowhead)* and internal carotid artery *(I)*

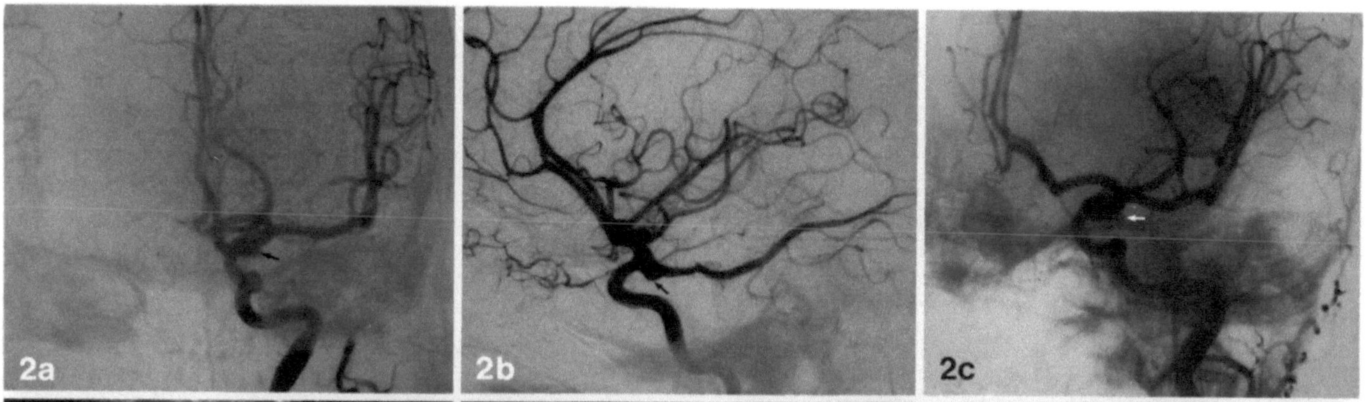

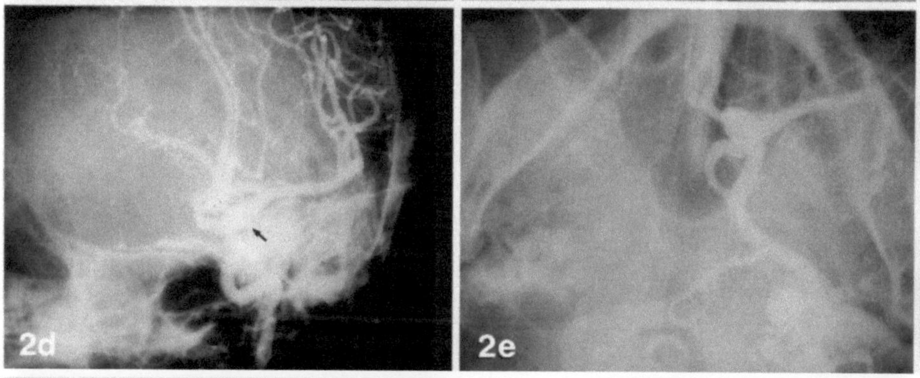

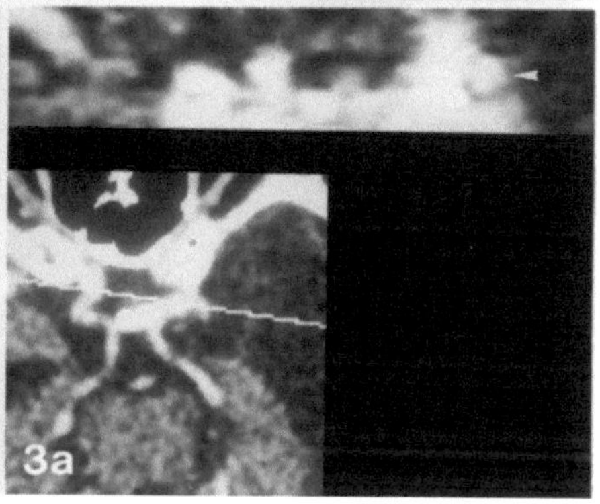

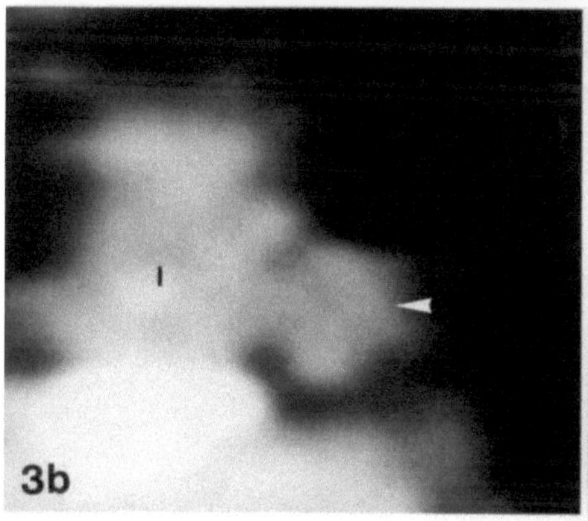

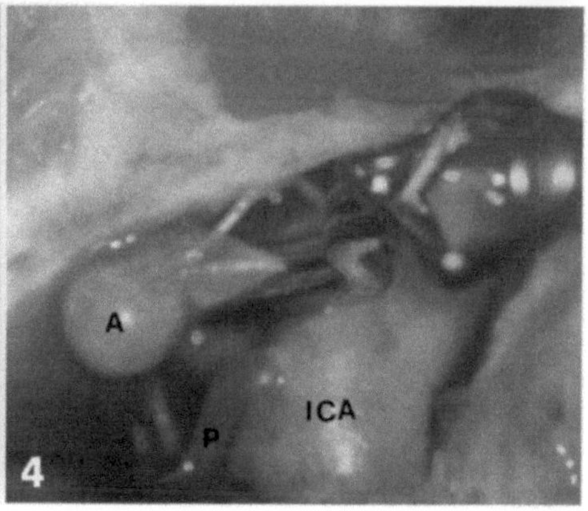

Fig. 4. Photography during operation. The aneurysm *(A)* was clipped. The left internal carotid artery *(ICA)* and posterior communicating artery *(P)* were well illustrated

SESSION 6
CEREBROVASCULAR DISEASE – TREATMENT

Neuroradiology (1991) 33 [Suppl]: 60–62

Neuroradiology
© Springer-Verlag 1991

MRI of experimental cerebral ischemia: response to NMDA antagonist therapy

R. L. DeLaPaz[1], G. K. Steinberg[2], A. Poljack[1], D. Kunis[2], and S. M. Rocklage[3]

[1] Department of Radiology and [2] Division of Neurosurgery, Stanford University Medical Center, Stanford, California, USA
[3] Salutar Corporation, Sunnyvale, California, USA

Summary. MRI was used to assess the efficacy of the *N*-methyl-D-aspartate (NMDA) antagonists dextromethorphan and dextrorphan, for the treatment of cerebral ischemia in an animal model. Marked protective effects of treatment were seen by MRI and histologic measures (67% to 83% reduction in the lesion size, compared to controls). Relaxation time measurements showed that treatment reduced the prolongation of T1 and T2 in lesions. A close correlation was seen between high signal on T2-weighted images, histologic measures of ischemic neuronal damage, and reduced lesion blood flow. Megnetic susceptibility effects of intravascular dysprosium-DTPA-BMA were seen on dynamic gradient recalled acquisition in the steady state (GRASS) images and T2-weighted spin-echo images. This contrast agent enhanced the early detection of ischemia on T2-weighted spin-echo images.

Key words: Magnetic resonance imaging – Experimental cerebral ischemia – *N*-Methyl-D-aspartate antagonist

The rationale for treatment of cerebral ischemia with *N*-methyl-D-aspartate (NMDA) antagonists is the "excitatory hypothesis" which, simply stated, is that overstimulation of neuronal membrane NMDA receptors by excitatory amino acids (e.g. L-glutamate) can cause neuronal cell death [1, 2]. The mechanism for this toxicity appears to be the opening of ion channels that allow rapid influx of extracellular Na^+ and a delayed, slower influx of Ca^{2+} which, together, induce cell swelling (cytotoxic edema), adenosine triphospate depletion, a fall in pH, and activation of intracellular lipases and proteases, leading to cell dissolution and death. In vitro tissue culture studies demonstrate reversal of glutamate toxicity for up to 20 min after exposure by removing extracellular Ca^{2+}, suggesting that a "window of opportunity" after the onset of ischemia exists for treatment with NMDA antagonists [2].This study was undertaken to test this hypothesis in vivo and to assess the utility of MRI for monitoring this therapy.

Materials and methods

Forty-four New Zealand male white rabbits underwent 1 h transorbital internal carotid-middle cerebral-anterior cerebral artery (ICA-MCA-ACA) occlusion and pretreatment or immediate post-treatment with systemic dextromethorphan (D-3-methoxy-*N*-methylmorphinan, DM, 20 mg/kg loading, 10 mg/kg per hour infusion, $n = 14$), dextrorphan (the *O*-demethylated DM metabolite, DX, 15 mg/kg loading, 15 mg/kg per hour infusion, $n = 14$) or normal saline (NS, $n = 16$). Halothane anesthesia was used with monitoring of mean arterial blood pressure heart rate, temperature, pH, expired CO_2, and P_aO_2 as previously described [3].

MR images were obtained at 6 h after onset of occlusion using a GE Signa 1.5 T system with a 15-cm-diameter RF coil, 12 cm field of vision, 3-mm-thick/1-mm gap slices 256 × 256 matrix, coronal plane T1-weighted (600/25) and T2-weighted (2500/25, 50, 75, 100) SE

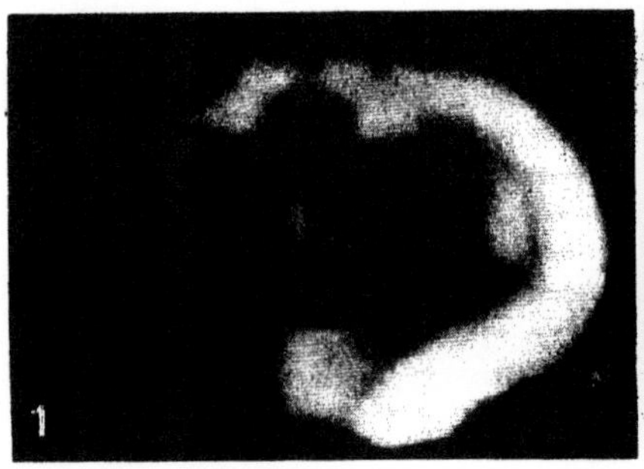

Fig. 1. T2-weighted (SE 2500/100) coronal image shows the typical high signal of an ischemic lesion in the temporal and parietal cortex and white matter *(arrow)*

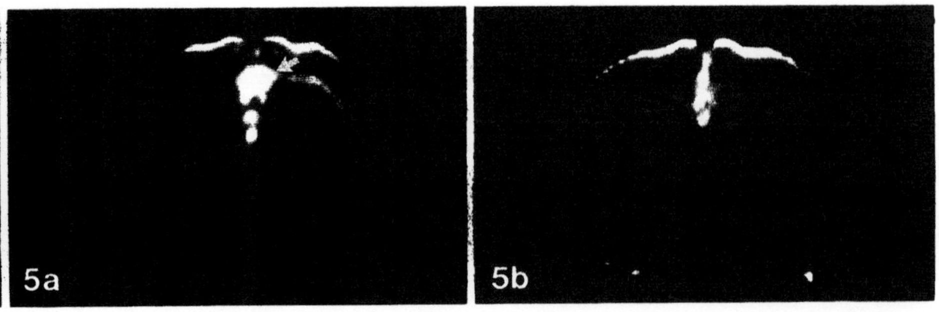

Fig. 5. **a** T2-weighted (SE 2500/100) image at 3 h after onset of ischemia and 10 min after Dy-DTPA infusion shows a medial cortical ischemic lesion *(arrow)* with high signal relative to the rest of the normally perfused brain. **b** On the same pulse sequence 55 min later the lesion area appears nearly isointense with the rest of the brain, probably resulting from washout of intravascular Dy-DTPA-BMA

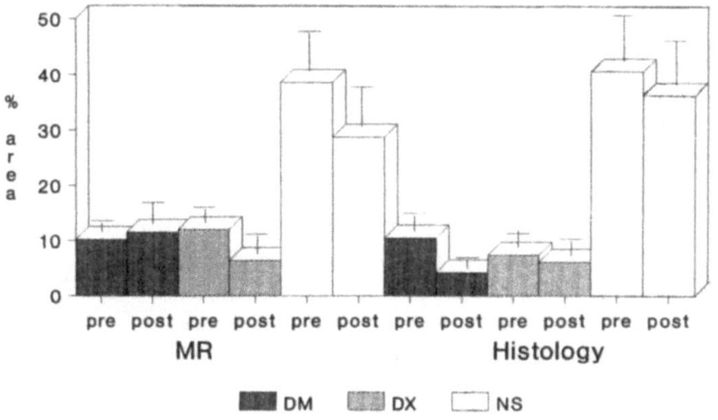

Fig. 2. Bar graph summarizes the marked reduction in lesion size on MRI and histology with *N*-methyl-D-aspartate antagonist therapy

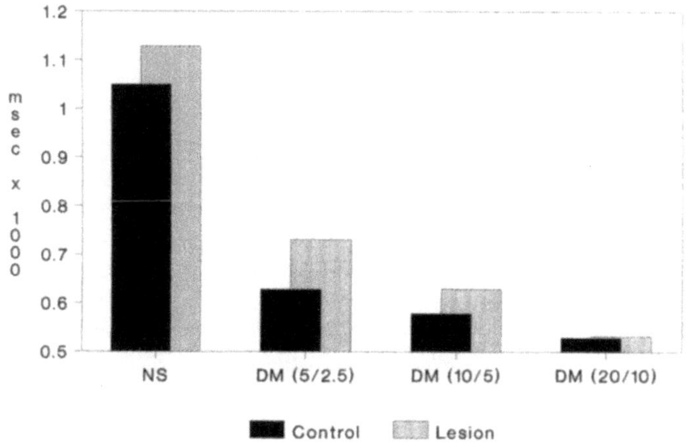

Fig. 3. Bar graph demonstrates the trend toward shorter T1 relaxation times and smaller lesion-to-contralateral hemisphere differences with larger doses of dextromethorphan

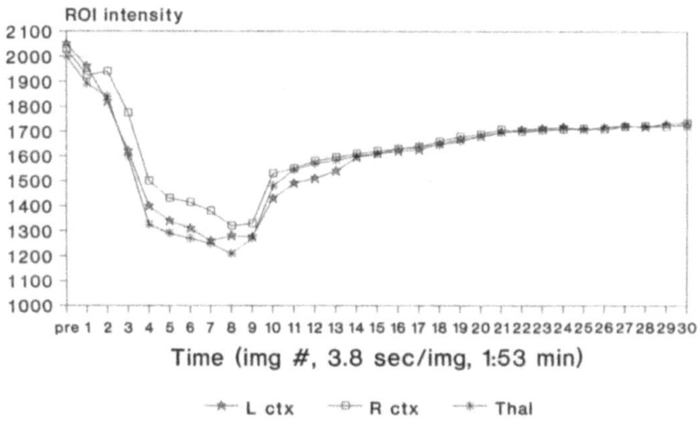

Fig. 4. Plot of image intensity vs time shows a marked drop in signal on serial GRASS images with the "first pass" bolus of intravascular dysprosium (Dy)-DTPA-BMA

pulse sequences (Fig. 1). Lesion size was measured as the area of high signal on T2-weighted images (normalized to the percent of hemisphere area per slice) and correlated directly with the area of ischemic neuronal damage (IND) on H&E histologic sections. T1 and T2 relaxation times were calculated for the central lesion and comparable contralateral hemisphere using an iterative curve-fitting technique (GE product software) in a subgroup of 8 DM and 8 NS animals. Relaxation times were also calculated in two additional groups of 8 animals each, treated with lower doses of DM (10/5 and 5/2.5). Regional cerebral blood flow (rCBF) was measured using standard techniques with 15-μm-diameter [57] Co-labeled microspheres in 1 additional DM and 1 NS animal.

A separate group of 6 animals (5 controls, 1 lesioned) was studied with IV dysprosium (Dy)-DTPA-BMA (Salutar) using gradient echo (GRASS TR 35, TE 25, flip 30, 3.8 s/image rapid sequence) and T2-weighted SE (2500/100) images.

Results

The normalized lesion area on T2-weighted SE images of treated animals was significantly smaller than in untreated animals and corresponded closely to the areas of IND seen on histologic examination (Table 1, Fig. 2). The protective effects of treatment (% reduction in lesion size vs untreated controls) were similar on MRI and histology (Table 1). Significant differences were not seen between DM and DX or between pre- and posttreatment groups. Lesion T1 and T2 were significantly prolonged compared to the contralateral hemisphere in the untreated animals (Table 2). DM (20/10) treated animals showed no increase in T1 and less prolongation of T2 than untreated animals (Table 2). A trend was noted toward shorter T1 relaxation times and smaller differences between lesion and control regions with higher doses of DM (Fig. 3). Although treatment appeared to reduce the T2 lesion- control difference, no clear trend of T2 with increasing DM doses could be identified. Approximately equal reductions in rCBF occurred in the treated and untreated animals (rCBF ml/100 g/min: lesion 1–7, contralateral hemisphere 40–120).

The infusion of Dy-DTPA-BMA produced a marked drop in signal on the rapid sequence GRASS images, initially as a "first pass" bolus effect at 30 s followed by a less

Table 1. Normalized lesion areas

	DM	DX	NS
MRI			
Pretreatment	10.2%*	12.0%*	38.6%
Posttreatment	11.5%	6.4%	28.8%
Protective effect	66.9%	73.4%	
Histology:			
Pretreatment	10.5%	7.4%*	40.6%
Posttreatment	4.2%*	6.1%*	36.2%
Protective effect	81.3%	82.5%	

DM, Dextromethorphan; DX, dextrorphan; NS, normal saline
$*P < 0.05$

Table 2. Relaxation times

	ROI	DM (post)	NS
T1:			
	Contralateral	529 (±40)	1050 (±45)
	Lesion	532 (±42)	1128 (±40)**
	% Increase	0.6%	7.4%
T2:			
	Contralateral	57 (±2)	55 (±2)
	Lesion	62 (±2)*	71 (±2)*
	% Increase	8.7%	29.1%

$**P < 0.05$, $*P < 0.001$
ROI, Region of interest

profound, stabilizing effect at approximately 2 min (Fig. 4). The qualitative effect of this intravascular contrast medium on the T2-weighted SE images is shown in Fig. 5 where the ischemic lesion is seen as high signal relative to the rest of the brain at 3 h following lesion onset and 10 min after contrast medium infusion but appears isointense on the follow-up images at 55 min after contrast medium infusion.

Discussion

The marked reduction in size and the close correlation with histologic change suggest that T2-weighted SE images are a useful tool for monitoring the effects of NMDA antagonist therapy of cerebral ischemia. The tissue parameter identified by high signal on these images is probably primarily cytotoxic edema in these relatively early ischemic lesions. The close correlation of these changes to histologic IND supports this hypothesis, although discrepancies were seen between MRI and histology. These occurred most commonly in the deep striatal structures and marginal "penumbra" zones where low-grade neuronal injury could be seen without substantial edema. These areas of injury may be caused primarily by metabolic/hypoxic mechanisms rather than excitotoxic mechanisms (the striatum is known to have relatively low concentrations of NMDA receptors), or insufficient collateral flow may have inhibited the delivery of NMDA antagonists and the formation of edema, especially vasogenic edema.

The effects of treatment on lesion relaxation times suggest that NMDA antagonists produce substantial changes in intracellular water content and probably also in factors affecting proton relaxation, such as solute concentrations and prevention of protein and membrane breakdown. A tendency for this therapy to reduce lesion T1 and T2 relaxation times toward normal values is clearly seen in the data. The marked shortening of T1 in normal tissue as well as ischemic tissue appears to be DM dose related and, therefore, probably mediated through the NMDA receptor mechanism and it effect on the intracellular environment.

Dy-DTPA-BMA is a contrast agent with a very high magnetic moment (10.6 Bohr magnetons) which induces tissue magnetic susceptibility changes (proportional to the square of the magnetic moment) [4]. The effect of intrasvascular Dy-DTPA-BMA is to enhance magnetic susceptibility markedly within capillaries, creating microscopic magnetic gradients across the capillary walls. These gradients produce T2-dependent signal loss on gradient echo images and diffusion-dependent signal loss on T2-weighted SE images [4, 5].

These relationships are best understood by the equation: $1/T2^* = 1/T2 + 1/T2'$ [5]. Figures 4 and 5 illustrate these effects clearly with marked loss of signal on GRASS images, which are very sensitive to T2*, and a suppression of signal in the normally perfused brain relative to the ischemic lesion on the T2-weighted SE image. The isointensity of the lesion on the delayed T2-weighted SE image is most likely to be due to systemic clearance of Dy-DTPA-BMA as the timing coincides well with the known $t_{1/2}$ of 3–8 min for the rapid phase of intravascular clearance. Isointensity caused by leakage of the contrast agent across the blood-brain barrier into the lesion seems a less likely explanation, but cannot be completely excluded. Quantitative assessment of cerebral blood volume is possible using this effect and this approach may be used for functional brain imaging with MRI in the future [6].

Conclusion

T2-weighted MRI provides a consistent and reliable means of studying cerebral ischemia and is useful for monitoring the effects of experimental NMDA-antagonist therapy. Use of an intravascular contrast medium with strong transverse magnetization effects such as Dy-DTPA-BMA enhances early detection of cerebral ischemia and appears to provide a basis for measurement of cerebral blood volume and a qualitative assessment of tissue perfusion.

References

1. Buchan A (1990) Do NMDA antagonists protect against cerebral ischemia: are clinical trials warranted? Cerebrovasc Brain Metab Rev 2: 1–26
2. Choi D (1990) Methods for antagonizing glutamate neurotoxicity. Cerebrovasc Brain Metab Rev 2: 105–147
3. Steinberg GK, Saleh J, Kunis D, DeLaPaz RL, Zarnegar SR (1988) Protective effect of post-ischemic treatment with the NMDA antagonists, dextromethorphan and dextrorphan after focal cerebral ischemia in rabbits. Stroke 19: 1112–1118
4. Villringer A, Rosen BR, Belliveau JW (1988) Dynamic imaging with lanthanide chelates in normal brain: contrast due to magnetic suceptibility effects. Magn Reson Med 6: 164–174
5. Brown FF (1983) The effect of compartmental location on the proton T2* of small molecules in cell suspension: a cellular field gradient model. J Magn Reson 54: 385–399
6. Belliveau JW, Rosen BR, Kantor HL (1990) Functional cerebral imaging by susceptibility-contrast NMR. Magn Reson Med 14: 538-546

Dr. Robert DeLaPaz
Department of Radiology, Rm. S072
Stanford University Medical Center
Stanford, CA 94305, USA

Neuroradiology (1991) 33 [Suppl]: 63–65

Neuro radiology
© Springer-Verlag 1991

IVT atherectomy with suction for treatment of carotid stenosis: experimental study

F. Y. Tsai, H. Nakashima, D. Wadley, T. V. Myers, and J.-Y. Huang

University of Missouri-Kansas City and Truman Medical Center, School of Medicine, Kansas City, Missouri, USA

Summary. Stroke is the third leading cause of death in the western world. One of the most common causes of stroke is atherosclerotic cerebrovascular disease. The treatment of choice has traditionally been surgical endarterectomy or bybass to restore the cerebral circulation. Those patients at high surgical risk or with surgically inaccessible lesions require an alternative procedure. Over the past several years, percutaneous angioplasty methods have been attempted; however, the potential for dislodging the thrombus and plaque to the distal cerebral circulation has blocked the progress of this nonsurgical intervention. Recently, an IVT atherectomy catheter with a suction device for removal of debris during the cutting of the atheroma, has been developed. We produced and treated an animal model with carotid stenosis with the atherectomy device to determine the safety and feasibility of using it in the treatment of carotid stenosis.

Key words: Carotid artery – Stenosis – Atherectomy

Materials and methods

Mature adult Flemish rabbits weighing approximately 15–20 lb were selected for this study. After the animals arrived from the breeder, they were prepared in the animal laboratory by feeding them a 2% cholesterol diet with peanut oil mixed with a regular rabbit chow for a period of 1 week. The animals were brought to the angiography suite after being carefully anesthetized. The right common carotid artery was selectively catheterized through a femoral approach using a direct femoral cut-down procedure. To induce stenosis, the right carotid artery was dilated using a 4 mm × 2 cm angioplastic balloon (Advanced Cardiac Systems, Mountainview, Calif.). The balloon was inflated for a 1-min period a total of 15 times. The animals were returned to the animal laboratory and continued on the 2% cholesterol and peanut oil diet. At the end of 8 weeks the animals were brought back to the angiography suite to document the presence of stenosis. Selective catheterization of the right common carotid artery was accomplished from the opposite femoral artery (Fig. 1).

After the atherosclerosis had been established, a 5 F IVF atherectomy device (Interventional Technologies, San Diego, Calif.) was advanced to the right common carotid artery through a guiding catheter (Fig. 2). The cutter of the atherectomy catheter with suction device was then passed through the stenotic area under fluoroscopy. Repeat angiography was performed to assess the results (Fig. 3). The procedure was terminated and the brain removed to look for the presence of acute stroke by direct pathologic examination.

Discussion

The rabbit is an excellent animal model to produce atherosclerotic stenosis. The Flemish rabbit has additional advantages for this study because it is larger than regular or New Zealand rabbits. The femoral and carotid arteries are also larger and more suitable for the angioplasty balloon catheter and the atherectomy catheter [1, 2]. A total of 30 Flemish rabbits were included in the study; however, during the early part of our experiment, many animals died from different causes. Flemish rabbits are prone to die with rough handling and the animals must be gently cared for to prevent premature death. A total of 14 rabbits died due to different causes: 3 due to paralysis of hind feet from rough handling; 1 due to abcess at surgical site of femoral arterial cut down; 1 due to total occlusion of both carotid arteries; 2 due to loss of airway; 2 due to perforation of carotid artery during atherectomy procedure; and 5 due to unknown causes during preparation of the animals for angiography.

Twelve of these 14 animals died prior to the second angiographic procedure. Eighteen of 30 rabbits survived to undergo a second angiographic procedure. Two animals died during the atherectomy procedure. Fifteen rabbits developed significant stenosis and survived both procedures. All 15 rabbits had good results with restoration of the carotid artery to normal caliber following treatment with the IVT atherectomy catheter. We have found that one pass with the IVT atherectomy catheter is sufficient to remove the atheroma and restore the vessel to normal caliber.

We have concluded that angioplastic dilatation performed 12–15 times is optimal for producing carotid stenosis. Early in our experiment, angioplastic dilatation was performed only 10 times in 1 animal and the animal failed to develop carotid stenosis. Angioplastic dilatation was performed 20 times in a second animal, and this lead to total occlusion of the carotid artery and death. Subsequently, angioplastic dilatation was performed 15 times, and this produced sufficient carotid stenosis in all animals that survived for a second angiographic procedure.

Arterial spasm was another complication we encountered during the study. Seven of 18 rabbits developed spasm after atherectomy treatment with the IVT atherectomy device, including two of our first rabbits. These ani-

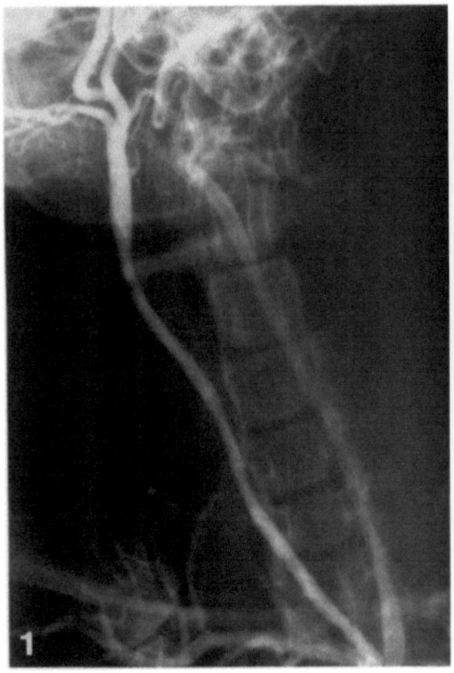

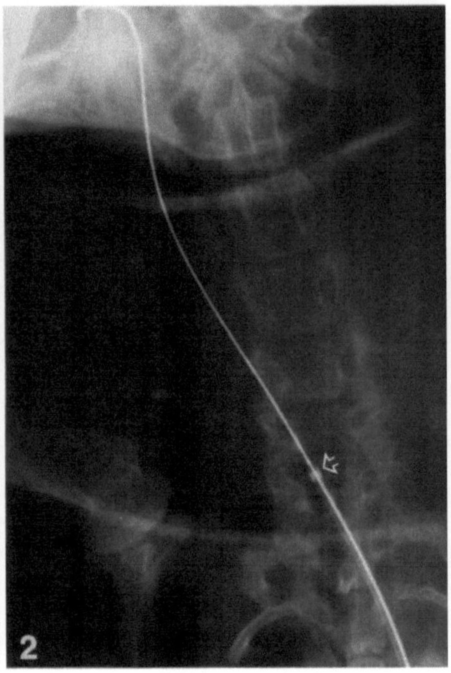

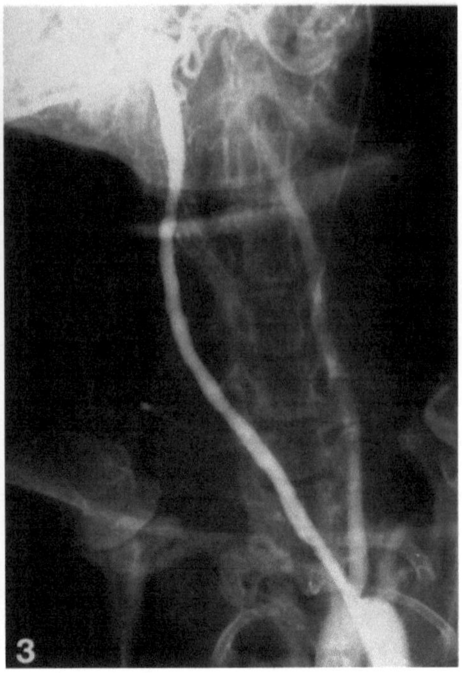

Fig. 1. Moderate degree of stenosis is demonstrated in the proximal half of the right common carotid artery

Fig. 2. Atherectomy device is placed in the right common carotid artery with a small guide wire through a guiding catheter. The cutter *(arrow)* appears as a ring-like structure at the end of atherectomy catheter

Fig. 3. Repeat angiography after atherectomy treatment showed smooth and normal caliber of right common carotid artery. No spasm or vascular injury is noted

mals were not treated with intra-arterial nitroglycerin prior to the second pass of the atherectomy catheters, and this led to perforation of the right common carotid artery. When treated with intra-arterial nitroglycerin, the spasm was relieved and the vessel returned to normal caliber. Three animals developed spasm and were not given intra-arterial nitroglycerin. The carotid artery returned to normal caliber after a period of approximately 30 min without any therapy.

We have seen spasm rather frequently after treatment with the IVT atherectomy device in the carotid. This may also be a problem in humans. However, it does not occur as frequently in treatment of humans with peripheral vascular disease. We believe intra-arterial nitroglycerin may be used routinely to avoid this complication.

Two of 15 animals had an MRI study of the head; however, the brain proved too small for adequate evaluation. Subsequently, 13 of 15 rabbits had removal of the brain for examination by a neuropathologist. No pathologic evidence of acute stroke was detected following treatment with the IVT atherectomy catheter with its suction device, indicating the safety of IVT atherectomy in the treatment of carotid stenosis. The suction device has sufficient suction to remove the debris during excision of atheroma.

Our initial work has been encouraging for several achievements. The Flemish rabbit has proven to be a suitable animal model for the development of atherosclerotic stenosis. Although arteriosclerosis may develop just with a cholesterol diet without mechanical injury to the artery in rabbits, it may take longer to achieve the result. The method which we have used in this study may be open to criticism about the stenosis having neointimal fibrosis in addition to natural arteriosclerosis generated by the cholesterol diet [1, 2]. However, it fulfilled our original intention of testing the safety and ability of the device for the removal of atheroma and debris simultaneously. IVT atherectomy is probably better than other forms because of the attached suction [3–10]. We have been able to use the IVT atherectomy catheter to remove the atheroma without dislodging fragments to the distal intracerebral circulation.

References

1. Constantinides P, Booth J, Carlson G (1960) Production of advanced cholesterol atherosclerosis in the rabbit. Arch Pathol 70: 712–724
2. Wojcicki J, Samochowiec L, Jaworska M (1985) A search for a model of experimental atherosclerosis comparative studies in rabbits, guinea pigs and rats. Pol J Pharmacol Pharm 37: 11–21
3. Simpson JB, Johnson DE, Tha Pliyal HV, Mark DS, Braden LJ (1985) Transluminal atherectomy: a new approach to the treatment of atherosclerotic vascular disease. Circulation 72 [Suppl 3]: 146
4. Kensey K, Nash J, Abrahams C, Zarins CK (1987) Recanalization of obstructive arteries with a flexible rotating tip catheter. Radiology 165: 387–389
5. Schwarten DE, Katzen BT, Simpson JB, Cutcliff WB (1988) Simpson catheter for percutaneous transluminal removal of atheroma. AJR 150: 799–801
6. Snyder SO Jr (1988) The Kensey catheter: preliminary result with a transluminal atherectomy tool. J Vasc Surg 8: 541–543

7. Simpson JB, Selmon MR, Roberts MG, Cipriano PR, Hayden WG, Johnson DE (1988) Transluminal atherectomy for occlusive peripheral vascular disease. Am J Cardiol 61: 966–1016
8. Belli AM, Cumberland DC (1989) Percutaneous atherectomy – early experience in Sheffield. Clin Radiol 40: 122–126
9. Langes K, Schofer J, Bleifield W, Mathey DG (1989) Catheter atherectomy-functional results in peripheral arterial disease. Angiology 40: 830–834
10. Wholey MH, Smith JAM, Godlewski P, Nagurka M (1989) Recanalization of total arterial occlusions with Kensey dynamic angioplasty catheter. Radiology 172: : 95–98

Dr. Fong Y. Tsai
Truman Medical Center
2301 Holmes Road
Kansas City, MO 64108, USA

Neuroradiology (1991) 33 [Suppl]: 66–68

Neuro radiology
© Springer-Verlag 1991

A laboratory and clinical evaluation of laser angioplasty in the treatment of atheromatous disease of the carotid bifurcation

I. W. Turnbull[1] and C. M. Bannister[2]

Departments of [1] Radiology and [2] Neurosurgery, North Manchester General Hospital, Crumpsall, Manchester, UK

Summary. Thirty-nine segments of carotid artery were removed at autopsy; cannulae were sutured into the common carotid artery and internal carotid artery and the system initially perfused with saline and, then, with whole blood. A laser probe was passed up the common carotid artery and across the bifurcation during continuous blood perfusion. Samples of effluent were obtained during and immediately after the laser treatment. It was possible to determine the number of fragments in each sample and, using staining techniques, to assess their likely chemical composition and origin. The results confirm that (1) superficial fatty plaque is vapourised into solution; (2) the surface of fibrous atheroma becomes coagulated, presenting a smooth glazed appearance which is thought to be less thrombogenic, both effects being confirmed histologically; (3) fragments were found even before treatment; (4) there was no change in the number of fragments found before or after treatment; (5) most of the fragments resulted from vessel handling; but some could be traced to the densely adherent fibrous atheroma. Laser angioplasty has now been employed successfully to treat carotid atheroma in four patients.

Key words: Laser angioplasty – Carotid atheroma – particulate matter.

The bifurcations of 39 carotid arteries were removed at autopsy from subjects over the age of 65. The external carotid artery was occluded and cannulae were tied into the common and internal carotid arteries. The vessels were washed out with normal saline to remove postmortem blood clot and debris, and then perfused with normal saline. Once a constant flow was established, samples of fluid were collected from the internal carotid artery cannula. The perfusate was then changed to anticoagulated

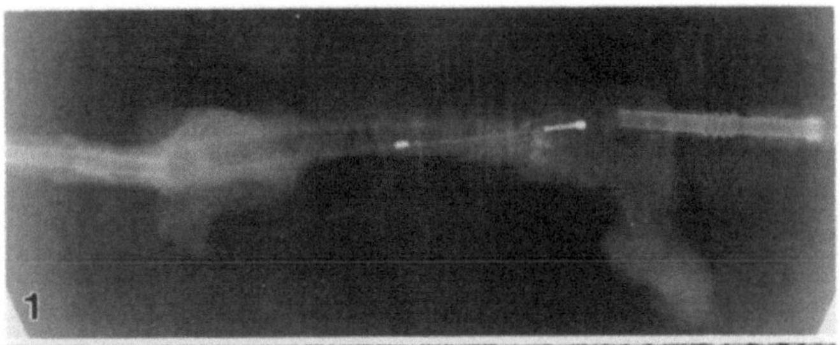

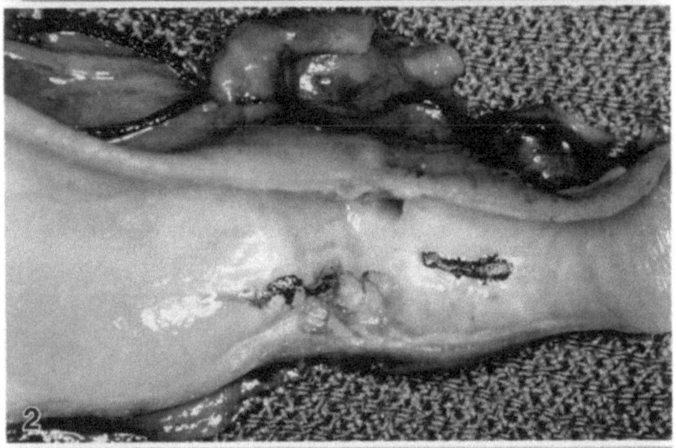

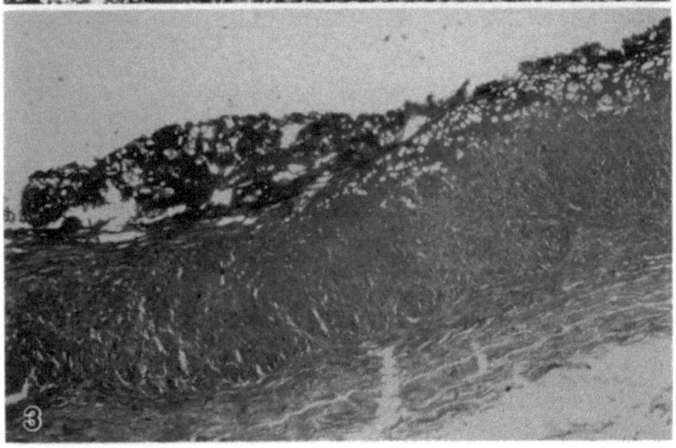

Fig. 1. Cannulae are shown secured within the common carotid and internal carotid arteries. The branches of the external carotid artery have been tied off. The laser probe is seen passing the carotid bifurcation which contains calcified atheromatous plaques

Fig. 2. Naked-eye appearance of opened vessel following laser treatment. Thermal burns on the dependent aspect of the wall are easily recognized as dark char lines. Superficial fatty plaque has been vapourised, leaving a smooth dull patch of the luminal surface, whilst the densely fibrous adherent plaque remaining is glazed and its surface free of any adherent material

Fig. 3. Histological section of an internal carotid artery demonstrates eosinophilic material on luminal surface where superficial fatty plaque has been vapourised. There is some minor disruption of the internal elastic lamina underlying this, but no thermal damage is observed in the outer layers of the media or adventitia. The surface of the remaining fibrous plaque is coagulated to form a smooth, slightly refractile eosinophilic surface. There is no adherent material present

Table 1. Gross morphological appearances of the last 21 carotid arteries examined

Calcification	43%
Ulcerated atheroma	38%
Thrombus ± haemorrhage	19%
Severe stenosis	14%
Visible burn	48%

whole blood and further samples were obtained. An argon laser probe (Trimedyne Argon Laser, Nycomed, UK) was heated with 10 W of energy and passed about 6 times through the common and internal carotid arteries at the same time as blood was perfused through them (Fig. 1). Samples of the outflow from the internal carotid artery were collected during and immediately after laser treatment.

After treatment, the arteries were opened longitudinally and the amount of atheroma and ulceration present was assessed. The presence of any calcification, thrombus and mural haemorrhages was recorded, and any thermal damage noted. The arteries were then fixed in buffered formalin and processed through to paraffin wax for histological examination. Sections of the arteries were stained with haematoxylin and eosin and by Miller's method for optimal visualisation of elastic fibres [1].

Blood samples were treated with lysing agents to rupture the red cells. Two millilitres of each of the fluid samples were centrifuged. The resulting aggregates were resuspended in normal saline and smears of all the samples were made from the same volume of fluid. The smears were stained for DNA, calcium and lipids, and with specific antisera against factor VIII and lectin ulex. Slides were prepared by the Cytospin and the direct smear methods, and the size and number of any fragments present were ascertained. The two methods of slide preparation were chosen in order to verify the counting techniques.

Results

The incidence of calcification, ulceration, adherent thrombus and mural haemorrhage in the last 21 vessels examined are shown in Table 1. Almost half had a visible laser burn on the intimal surface of the vessel (Fig. 2). The burns always occurred on the part of the artery which was dependent when the laser probe was passed through it. In many of the arteries areas were identified where the athermatous material had been vapourised away by the laser to leave behind a smooth, dull patch of the luminal surface (Fig. 2). Where the athermatous plaque was densely fibrous, the laser glazed the lesion to produce a shiny surface free of adherent material (Fig. 2).

Histology showed the presence of eosinophilic material on the luminal surface of the vessels where the atheroma had been burnt away (Fig. 3). In some vessels there was minor disruption of the internal elastic lamina underlying these areas (Fig. 3). More deeply placed tissues had undergone heat coagulation but the damage did not extent beyond the inner part of the media. No damage was seen in the outer layers of the media or in the adventitia in any of the vessels.

In spite of careful handling, a significant number of fragments was seen in the fluid samples collected before laser treatment was begun. Most had a diameter of less than 50 µm, but some measured 50–100 µm, others 100–150 µm, and a few were larger than 150 µm. In the first 18 vessels examined there was an increase in the number of fragments measuring 25–50 µm after laser treatment (Table 2). It was thought the most likely explanation for this was excessive handling of the vessels which took place during cannulation and perfusion. Gentler handling of the remaining 21 arteries resulted in no increase in the numbers of particles of any size after treatment, and in fact, there may even have been a small decrease in their numbers in the post-treatment samples (Table 3). In general, it was noted that the more severely the artery was affected by atheroma, the greater the number of fragments present, both before and after treatment. It was gratifying to note that there was an excellent correlation between the number of fragments counted using the Cytospin and direct smear methods of slide preparation (Table 2). Fragments were classified as either soft or jagged according to their appearance. Some of the soft fragments stained positively for DNA, suggesting that they were nuclear debris produced during red cell lysis. Other soft fragments stained positively with antisera to factor VIII and lectin ulex implying an endothelial or blood cell origin. Jagged fragments only took up collagen stains and were thus probably derived from the atheromatous plaques.

Table 2. Total number and size of all fragments pre/post laser treatment in first 18 cases

	Pre	Post	Pre	Post	Pre	Post	Pre	Post	Pre	Post
	Less than 20 µm		20–50 µm		50–100 µm		100–150 µm		Greater than	150 µm
Cytospin method										
Range	1–21	2–11	5–21	11–23	4–7	2–6	1–6	0–3	1–3	0–2
(Mean)	(6.75)	(7.75)	(13.75)	(16.75)	(5.25)	(4)	(1.75)	(1.5)	(1)	(1)
Direct smear method										
Range	10–14	8–17	11–23	13–41	3–7	2–11	0–1	0–6	1–3	0–4
(Mean)	(11.75)	(12.75)	(15.5)	(21.25)	(4.5)	(5)	(0.75)	(1.75)	(2)	(2)
Mean of both methods	9.25	10.25	14.63	19.0	4.88	4.5	1.25	1.63	1.5	1.5

Table 3. Number and size of soft and jagged fragments pre/post laser treatment in last 18 cases

	"Soft"		"Jagged"	
	< 50 μm	> 50 μm	< 50 μm	> 50 μm
Pre	534.2	86.5	15.2	3.6
Post	459.6	71.9	16.7	3.5

Discussion

This study has shown that laser treatment can remove superficial atheromatous plaques from cadaver carotid arteries, leaving behind a thin layer of coagulated, refractile, eosinophilic material on the treated surface. Larger aggregates of atheromatous material are not completely removed but that which remains is glazed and its surface is free of adherent thrombus. It is to be hoped that the treated areas will not be able to act as a source of emboli and that the glazing will render them permanently antithrombogenic. Since heat damage was restricted to the wall of the artery in the immediate vicinity of the treated area, and the release of fragments into the vessel was not substantially increased by treatment, it would seem that laser angioplasty of atheromatous cervical carotid arteries in patients can be carried out without a significant risk of perforating the vessel, or of causing cerebral ischaemia by particulate propagation.

Encouraged by these results, we have now started a long-term study to assess the clinical efficacy of laser angioplasty. Patients selected for treatment are those who have episodic signs and symptoms of cerebral ischaemia, in whom medical treatment with antiplatelet agents has failed, and in whom angiography has shown an ulcerative lesion of the carotid arteries without a haemodynamically significant stenosis. To date, four patients have been treated without complications. In each case, follow-up over several months has shown complete cessation of their presenting ischaemic symptoms.

Reference

1. Miller PJ (1971) An elastic stain. Med Lab Tech 28: 148–149

J. W. Turnbull
Departments of Radiology and Neurosurgery
North Manchester General Hospital
Delauneys Road
Crumpsall, Manchester, UK

Neuroradiology (1991) 33 [Suppl]: 69–71

Neuro-radiology
© Springer-Verlag 1991

Local intra-arterial fibrinolysis in acute middle cerebral artery occlusion

G. Siepmann[1], M. Müller-Jensen[1], H. Goossens[2], L. Lachenmeyer[2], and H. Zeumer[1]

Departments of [1] Neuroradiology and [2] Neurology, University of Hamburg, Hamburg, Federal Republic of Germany

Summary. The improvement of superselective catheterisation techniques opened the possibility of administering fibrinolytic agents very close to an embolus within the middle cerebral artery (MCA). In patients exhibiting a stroke due to embolic MCA occlusion fibrinolytic recanalisation of the MCA seems to be a rational approach. Up till now 11 treatments have been done. Good results (recanalisation and clinical recovery) could be achieved in 5 cases. An unchanged clinical state was found in 6 cases. Superselective catheterisation allows angiography even distal to the occlusion site in order to show whether peripheral vessels are patent, a possibly important prognostic criterion. It is now possible to put the tip of the catheter between the wall of the MCA and the embolus for fibrinolysis, offering a recanalisation rate of 80%.

Key words: Middle cerebral artery occlusion – Local intra-arterial fibrinolysis – Stroke therapy

We have shown that local intra-arterial fibrinolysis (LIF) is a rational and effective treatment in acute thrombembolic basilar stroke [1, 2]. The results of i.v. tissue plasminogen activator (tPA) fibrinolysis in carotid territory strokes are, according to our and other workers' (personal communication) observations not yet convincingly useful. Since it had been demonstrated that local fibrinolysis may be an effective treatment in acute carotid territory stroke [3, 4], we recently decided to try this method again.

Methods

The technical equipment for performing local fibrinolysis such as digital subtraction angiography, microcatheters and contrast media has been improved significantly in recent years, as has been described elsewhere [2]. New microcatheter systems such as the Tracker catheter offer the opportunity to administer fibrinolytic agents very close to an embolus within the middle cerebral artery (MCA). It was usually also possible to bypass occluding MCA emboli in order to display the downstream vessels. Afterwards the catheter tip has been positioned between the wall of the MCA and the embolus.

Results

Eleven patients with acute hemiplegia due to MCA occlusion have been treated with a maximum dose of 750,000 IU urokinase over a period of 2 h. All patients underwent LIF in the first 6 h after stroke. Using superselective angiography four major types of embolic occlusion within the carotid system could be demonstrated.

Type I shows an occlusion in the internal carotid artery at the level of the anterior choroidal artery leading to hemiplegia.

Type II shows an embolic occlusion proximal to the bi- or trifurcation occluding the lenticulostriatal arteries. The bi- or trifurcational vessels however are not occluded by thromboembolic material.

Type III shows an occlusion not only at the (bi-)trifurcation of the MCA but additionally an occlusion of at least one main branch of the MCA.

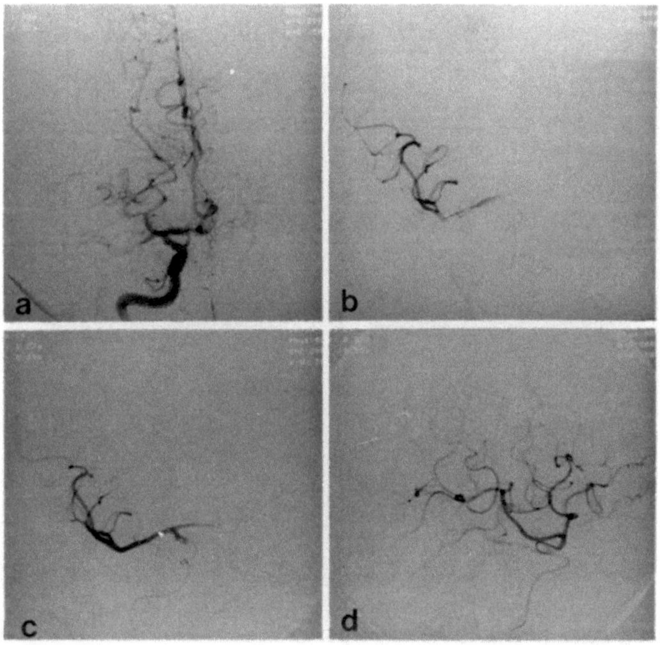

Fig. 1 a–d. Case 1. **a** Selective internal carotid artery (ICA) angiogram demonstrates middle cerebral artery (MCA) occlusion. **b** Microcatheterisation shows type II MCA occlusion. **c** Anteroposterior, **d** lateral superselective angiogram after local intra-arterial fibrinolysis (LIF) demonstrates complete recanalisation

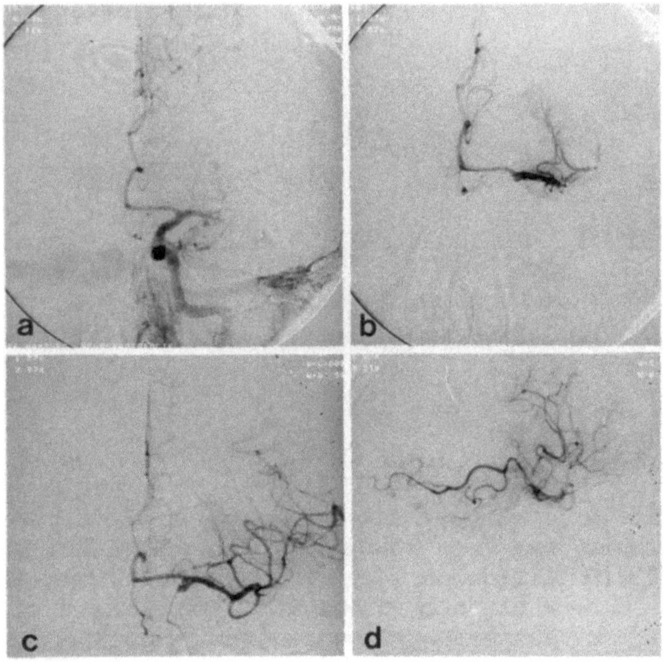

Fig. 2 a–d. Case 2. **a** Selective ICA angiogram shows MCA occlusion. **b** Superselective angiogram at the beginning of LIF. **c** Anteroposterior, **d** lateral superselective angiogram after LIF demonstrating incomplete recanalisation

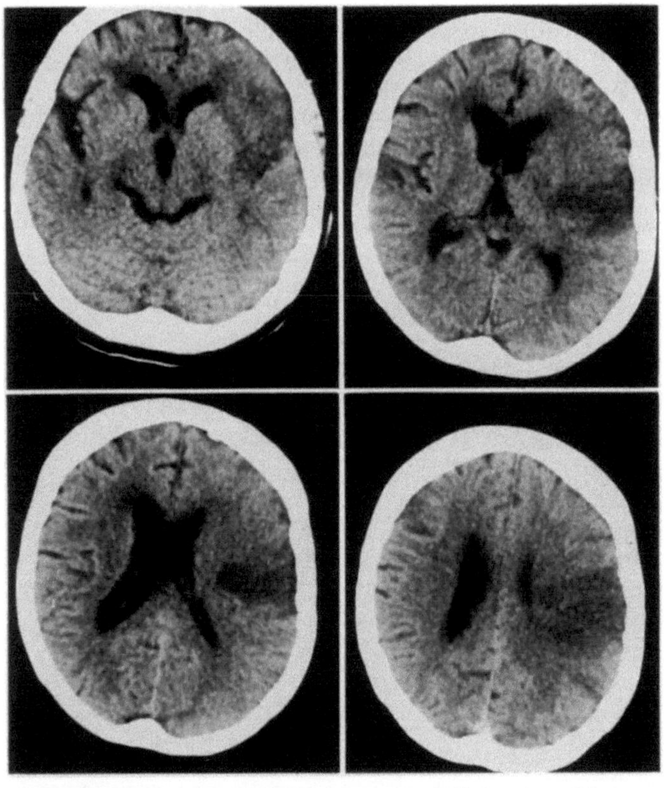

Fig. 3. Postfibrinolysis CT demonstrates partial infarction of the territory of the MCA localised in the central area

Type IV exhibits only a peripheral branch occlusion of the MCA. This type of occlusion never has been treated with our technique.

With the "M" type of carotid territory stroke multiple occlusions within the MCA and the anterior cerebral artery (ACA) territories are demonstrable.

Case reports

Case 1

A 60-year-old female patient suffered from hypertension and atrial fibrillation. She was admitted 4 h after the onset of a left-sided complete hemiplegia. Cerebral angiography showed occlusion of the MCA with collaterals from leptomeningeal anastomoses arising from the ACA. After microcatheterisation had demonstrated a type II MCA occlusion the tip of the microcatheter was positioned at the embolus surface. Only 600,000 units urokinase administered during a period of 1.5 h were necessary to recanalise the vessel. The postfibrinolysis angiogram showed complete revascularisation. Recovery to a normal neurological status was obtained in this patient. Some mild hemiparesis disappeared during the 1st week. Postfibrinolysis CT showed no infarct or haemorrhage (Fig. 1).

Case 2

A 73-year-old female patient exhibited a right-sided complete hemiplegia and aphasia 3 h before admision. The superselective angiogram showed a type III MCA occlusion with an embolus lodging in the middle main branch of the trifurcation of the MCA. After LIF treatment an incomplete recanalisation was seen. Only the M1 segment and two major MCA branches could be visualised. Despite LIF the middle branch of the MCA remained occluded. Postfibrinolysis CT demonstrated an infarcted area in the territory of the MCA localised to the central area. The patient continued to have severe hemiplegia with only minimal improvement (Figs. 2, 3).

Case 3

A 53-year-old male patient suffered from aortic valve stenosis and arterial hypertension. Cerebral angiography was performed 4 h after the onset of complete left-sided hemiplegia and aphasia. Clot was seen in the carotid siphon, the A1 segment of the ACA and the M1 segment of the MCA. Multiple emboli were demonstrated within the peripheral vessels. After fibrinolysis only an incomplete recanalisation was demonstrated in the trifurcational area. Revisualisation of the peripheral vessels was not achieved. CT 1 day later showed infarction of the whole MCA territory and of parts of the ACA territory. The patient died of brain swelling and final herniation.

A summary of the results is shown in Table 1. No space-occupying bleeding occurred in our cases. Minor spotty haemorrhagic transformation of the infarcted areas was seen in three cases.

Discussion

Unlike basilar territory strokes, MCA strokes are not usually lethal. From several studies it is well known that the clinical outcome of MCA occlusion is very variable [5–8]. Early spontaneous fibrinolysis may be one of the reasons for good recovery. However, spontaneous fibrinolysis only rarely occurs very early. Thus LIF offers the opportunity to speed up the recanalisation. Our results show that at least partial recanalisation seems achievable in most of the patients up to the 6th hour after stroke. Excellent outcome was, however, only found in those patients in whom complete recanalisation was demonstrated. Obviously the optimal chance for complete recanalisation was present in those patients who exhibited a type I or a type II occlusion. The outcome of type III occlusions seems to be determined by chance, depending only on which of the trifurcational branches is involved

Table 1. Outcome of 11 patients with different types of MCA occlusions. Local intra-arterial fibrinolysis for carotid territory stroke

Outcome with neurological deficits	No.	Type of occlusion				Recanalisation		
		I	II	III	M	Complete	Incomplete	None
Mild	5	1	4			5		
Moderate	2			1	1		2	
Severe	1			1			1	
Death	3				3		1	2

and which is not recanalisable (case 2). Finally, the existence of collateral pathways plays a major role as demonstrated particularly in the "M" type occlusion, in which not only the MCA but the collateralising ACA is occluded. Having shown that MCA recanalisation (at least partially) is usually possible, without severe complications in our series, we feel it now necessary to test the hypothesis in a larger number of patients. Using LIF it is possible to improve the clinical outcome in certain cases by speeding up MCA recanalisation. The benefit from LIF is the greater the more proximally (type I and II) the embolus is sited.

References

1. Adams HP, Damasio HC, Putman SF, Damasio AR (1983) Middle cerebral artery occlusion as a cause of isolated subcortical infarction. Stroke 14: 948–951
2. Bozzao L, Fantozzi LM, Bastianello S, Bossao A, Fieschi C (1989) Early collateral blood supply and late parenchymal brain damage in patients with middle cerebral artery occlusion. Stroke 20: 735–740
3. Brückmann H, Ferbert A, Zoppo GJ del, Hacke W, Zeumer H (1986) The acute vertebral-basilar thrombosis. Angiological – clinical comparison and therapeutic implications. Acta Radiol [Suppl] 369: 38–42
4. Saito I, Serugawa H, Shiokawa S, Tsutsumi K (1987) Middle cerebral artery occlusion: correlation of computed tomography and angiography with clinical outcome. Stroke 18: 863–868
5. Taneda M, Shimada N, Tsuchiya T (1985) Transient neurological deficits due to embolic occlusion and reopening of the cerebral arteries. Stroke 16: 522–524
6. Theron J, Courtheoux P, Casasco A, Alachkar F, Notari F, Ganem F, Maiza D (1989) Local intraarterial fibrinolysis in carotid territory. AJNR 10: 753–756
7. Zeumer H, Freitag H-J, Grzyska U, Neunzig H-P (1989) Local intra-arterial fibrinolysis in acute vertebrobasilar occlusion. Technical developments and recent results. Neuroradiology 31: 336–340
8. Zeumer H, Hündgen R, Ferbert A, Ringelstein EB (1984) Local intraarterial fibrinolytic therapy in inaccessible internal carotid occlusion. Neuroradiology 26: 315–317

Dr. G. Siepmann
Department of Neuroradiology
University of Hamburg
Martinistrasse 52
W-2000 Hamburg-Eppendorf
Federal Republic of Germany

Neuroradiology (1991) 33 [Suppl]: 72–74

Neuro radiology
© Springer-Verlag 1991

Intraluminal thrombosis associated with carotid bifurcation stenosis is an indication for emergency carotid endarterectomy

J. H. W. Pexman

Departments of Diagnostic Radiology und Clinical Neurological Sciences, Victoria Hospital, The University of Western Ontario, London, Ontario, Canada

Summary. The treatment of intraluminal thrombus at the common carotid bifurcation in patients with an ischemic cerebral event is controversial. Some favour anticoagulation whilst others suggest emergency carotid endarterectomy. A personal series of seven cases is presented. Five patients continued having ischemic events whilst on anticoagulants. Six faired excellently following emergency endarterectomy with no postoperative ischemic events and were well at between 3 and 6 months postoperatively. The operation for one patient was planned for 24 h following the angiogram, but unfortunately she suffered a severe stroke at 18 h whilst on heparin.

Key words: Intraluminal thrombus – Carotid artery – Carotid endarterectomy – Emergency surgery – Anticoagulation

It has recently been suggested that the angiographic demonstration of intraluminal thrombus in association with carotid bifurcation stenosis is associated with an increased risk of subsequent embolic and ischemic complications following carotid endarterectomy [1]. Conventional wisdom has held that one of the strongest indications for urgent carotid endarterectomy is the finding of an intraluminal thrombus associated with an arteriosclerotic plaque at the carotid bifurcation in a patient with ipsilateral ischemic symptoms [2]. A personal collection of seven symptomatic patients with intraluminal thrombus diagnosed angiographically is presented.

Subjects and methods

One hundred consecutive cerebral angiograms which were performed by one neuroradiologist were studied. They met our department's criteria for carotid endarterectomy which are: more than 70% vessel diameter stenosis, an obvious ulcer or an intraluminal thrombus at the internal carotid artery origin or the common carotid artery bifurcation. Eight patients were thought to have a thrombus, and seven charts were available for review. The patients were aged between 64 and 76 years; three were female and four were male. The risk of a stroke from angiography is 0.2% [3] and we are a center in the North American Endarterectomy Trial with a less than 4% surgical morbidity [4].

Results

The charts revealed that two patients had mild strokes: case 5 had a stroke 45 days prior to the angiogram, and case 6 at 24 days prior to the angiogram (Table 1). One patient had a transient ischemic attack (TIA) 90 days prior to the angiogram and four patients had their first TIA 2–13 days prior to the angiogram. Five patients had their last TIA 1–2 days before the angiogram. Four were operated on within 6 h and the other within 2 days and all five had excellent results. Case 5 who had two TIAs and one attack

Table 1. The results of endarterectomy in patients with carotid bifurcation thrombus

Case no.	Sex	Age (years)	Medical treatment	Angiographic findings in addition to thrombus	Timing of symptoms in relationship to procedures: Days to angiogram: First TIA	Last TIA	Operation	Thrombus-confirmed	Clinical results
1	M	71	Aspirin, persantin heparin	Ulcer	2	1	1/4	Yes	Well – 11 years later
2	F	70	Aspirin, persantin heparin	85% stenosis	13 daily →	1	1/4	Yes	Well – 3 months later
3	M	74		90% stenosis	7	2	1/4	Yes	Well – 4 months later
4	M	76	Aspirin, persantin	75% stenosis	8	1	1/4	Yes	Well – 6 months later
5	F	66	Aspirin, persantin heparin	90% stenosis	45 mild stroke 10	4	planned for 1 done at 20	No	Stroked despite heparin 18 h after angiogram
6	F	64		80% stenosis	24 mild stroke		11	Yes	Well 11 months later stroke at 12 months in atrial fibrillation
7	M	69	Aspirin, persantin	50% stenosis ulceration	90 several	2	4	No	Well – 10 weeks later

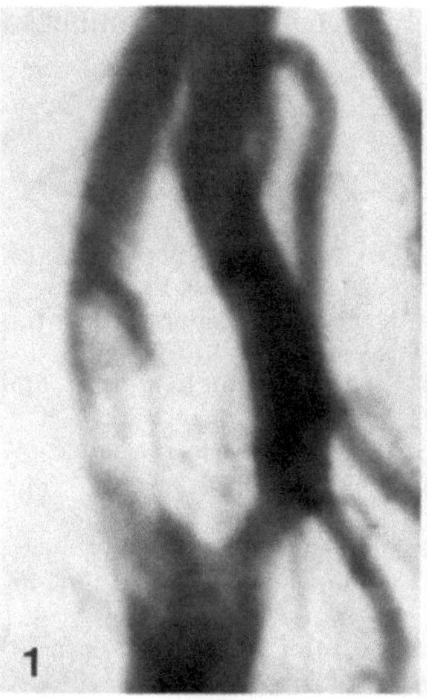

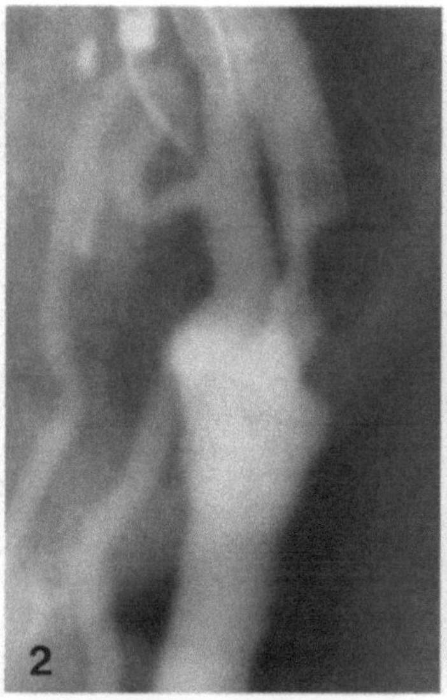

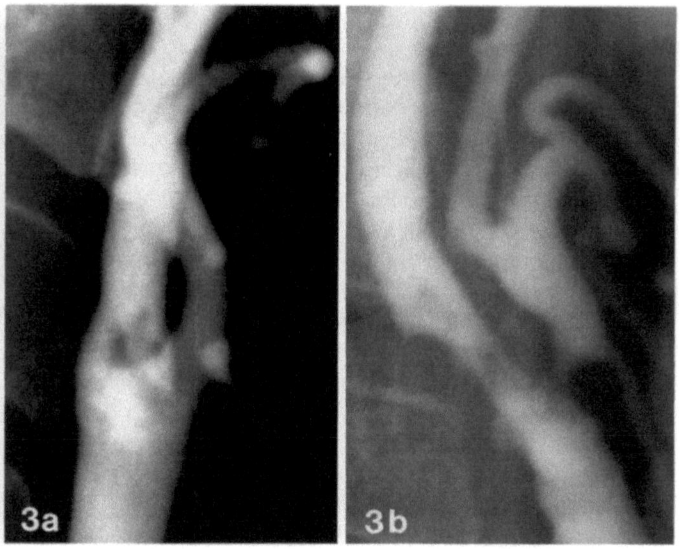

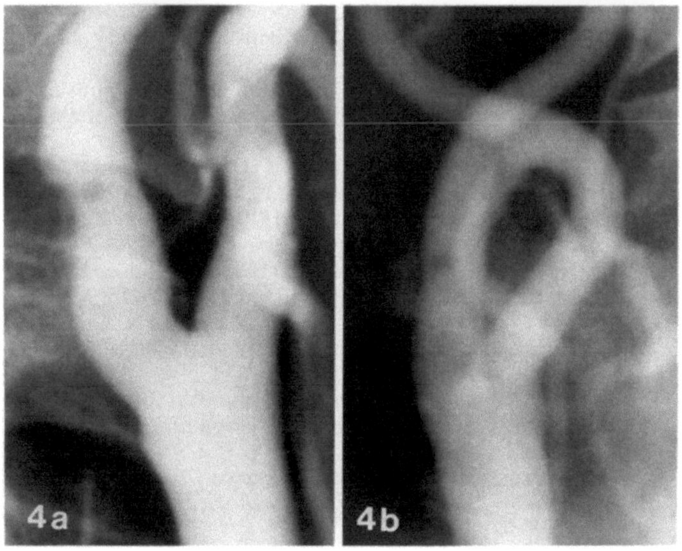

Fig. 1. Case 3. Large elongated clot filling origin of internal carotid artery

Fig. 2. Case 6. Oblong clot above an 80% stenosis

Fig. 3. **a** Case 1. Irregular clot (back) above irregular ulcer (white) at internal carotid artery origin. **b** Case 2. Irregular clot above stenosis in internal carotid artery. Also marked stenosis of external carotid artery origin

Fig. 4 a, b. Case 8. No clinical details. Ball-like clot above 30% stenosis shown on lateral and anteroposterior views

of amaurosis fugax between 10 and 4 days before the angiogram had his operation planned for 24 h following the angiogram, but despite being on heparin had a major stroke at 18 h and his operation was then delayed 20 days. Two other patients had their TIAs whilst on heparin, aspirin and persantin, and two more had them whilst on aspirin and persantin. Case 6 was operated on 11 days after the angiogram and 35 days from the onset of the stroke. Thrombus was found in this patient and in the four patients whose first TIA occurred 1–4 days before the angiogram. In case 5, no thrombus was found and it was presumed to have caused the stroke. Endarterectomy in case 7, whose first TIA occurred 90 days prior to the operation, showed no thrombus, but cholesterol clumps. The degree of atherosclerosis at the carotid bifurcation in each case is indicated in Table 1 and Figs. 1–3.

Discussion

In conventional angiography the most conclusive angiographic feature of intraluminal thrombus is the presence of contrast medium surrounding a smooth elongated filling defect within the vessel in at least two projections perpendicular to each other [5]. Usually a convex margin is seen on at least one projection with the contrast medium extending between the thrombus and the vessel wall. The shape may be variable, being elongated (Fig. 1), cylindrical, or oblong (Fig. 2) and may be irregular (Fig. 3) or ball-like (Fig. 4). In my series there were no cases with the string sign [6]. Dissected flaps or atheromatous projections may sometimes be mistaken for thrombus and laminar flow may be mistaken for thrombus on digital subtraction angiography.

Intraluminal thrombus was found histologically in six patients when the last ischemic event occurred 7 weeks before endarterectomy and no thrombus was found in six patients after 7 weeks [7]. In another series thrombus or other friable material was found in 66% of 24 patients operated upon within the first 4 weeks of a TIA, but in only 21% of 28 patients who were operated upon after a longer interval [8]. My cases fit this pattern. Thrombus was present in all four cases operated upon within 15 days of their first attack and in one case undergoing operation at 5 weeks. The two other patients had their endarterectomies at 35 and 94 days respectively and no thrombus was found. In the former it was thought to have caused the stroke prior to the first scheduled date for endarterectomy.

Thrombus is not often seen during cerebral angiography. I saw it in approximately 1% of patients undergoing angiography for arteriosclerotic cerebral vascular disease and in 7% of patients with severe disease. Others [5, 8, 9] recorded incidences between 0.4% and 1.5%, whilst one series quoted 6.6% [10].

The efficiency of emergency carotid endarterectomy depends upon the skill of the surgeon and our neurosurgeon fulfills the NASCET criteria with a less than 4% morbidity [4]. In 1984, prior to these trials, the overall morbidity and mortality resulting from carotid endarterectomy in the United States were conservatively estimated at 10% [11].

Intraluminal thrombosis has been associated with concurrent disease and coagulation defects [12, 13]. Carotid endarterectomy is not recommended for these.

The merits of carotid endarterectomy versus anticoagulation for intraluminal thrombus associated with arteriosclerotic disease at the carotid bifurcation remain controversial. In a review of the literature [14] 49 patients treated surgically gave 30 good results (67%) and 14 patients treated medically produced 7 good outcomes (50%). The authors recommend surgical therapy if the underlying disease involves an accessible lesion in a patient with transient ischemic attacks, mild neurological deficits, or progressive stroke despite medical therapy. The proponents of anticoagulation [1, 9, 15] had their cases analyzed and to some extent rebutted in an accompanying editorial [2]. These authors [9] treated 14 patients with anticoagulants and 11 (79%) had no new ischemic events. Sixteen different patients were treated surgically, and there were no new events in 10 (63%). Two major and two minor strokes followed surgery. The editor [2] noted that thrombectomy or surgical occlusion of the carotid artery was performed instead of endarterectomy in the two patients that had major strokes, and that one of these patients who underwent thrombectomy on two occasions may have had a hypercoaguable state. All five of my patients who had anticoagulants had ischemic events (0%) whilst all six patients treated with early endarterectomy had no new events (100%). In our hands, emergency carotid endarterectomy is strongly recommended for recurrent transient events caused by intraluminal thrombus at the stenosed carotid bifurcation.

References

1. Pelz D, Buchan AM, White C, Fox AJ (1989) Radiological risk factors in carotid endarterectomy patients. AJNR 10: 873
2. Heros RC (1988) Carotid endarterectomy in patients with intraluminal thrombus (editorial). Stroke 19: 681–687
3. Pexman JHW, Coates RK (1983) Amnesia after femorocerebral angiography. AJNR 4: 979–983
4. North American Symptomatic Carotid Endarterectomy Study Group (1987) Carotid endarterectomy: three critical evaluations. Stroke 19: 987–989
5. Roberson GH, Scott WR, Rosenbaum AE (1973) Thrombi at the site of carotid stenosis: radiographic diagnosis. Radiology 109: 353–356
6. Mehigan JT, Olcott C (1980) The carotid "string" sign differential diagnosis and management. Am J Surg 140: 137–143
7. Gurning AJ, Pickering GW, Robb-Smith AHT, Russel RR (1964) Mural thrombosis of the internal carotid artery and subsequent embolism. Q J Med 33: 155–195
8. Harrison M, Marshall J (1977) The finding of thrombus at carotid endarterectomy and its relationship to the timing of surgery. Br J Surg 64: 511–512
9. Buchan A, Gates P, Pelz D, Barnett HJM (1988) Intraluminal thrombus in the cerebral circulation. Stroke 19: 681–687
10. Kishore PRS, Chase NE, Kricheff II (1971) Carotid stenosis and intracranial emboli. Radiology 100: 351–356
11. Barnett HJM, Plum F, Walton JN (1984) Carotid endarterectomy – an expression of concern (editorial). Stroke 15: 941–943
12. Caplan L, Stein R, Patel D, Amico L, Cashman N, Gewertz B (1986) Intraluminal clot of the carotid artery detected radiographically. Neurology 34: 1175–1181
13. Pessin MS, Abbolt DT, Prager RJ, Batson RA, Scott RM (1986) Clinical and angiographic fractures of carotid circulation thrombus. Neurology 36: 518–523
14. Biller J, Adams HP Jr, Bogrini D, Godersky JC, Smoker WRK, Kongable G (1986) Intraluminal clot of the carotid artery. Surg Neurol 25: 467–477
15. Pelz DM, Buchan A, Fox AJ, Barnett HJM, Vinuela F (1986) Intraluminal thrombus of the internal carotid arteries: angiographic demonstration of resolution with anticoagulant therapy alone. Radiology 160: 369–373

Dr. J. H. Warwick Pexman
Department of Diagnostic Radiology
Victoria Hospital
London, Ontario, N6A 4G5, Canada

Neuroradiology (1991) 33 [Suppl]: 75–78

Neuro
radiology
© Springer-Verlag 1991

Comprehensive experience on intraplaque hemorrhage of the carotid artery

E. D. Cacayorin[1], L. Hochhauser[1], C. J. Hodge[2], C. H. Bredenberg[3], A. Culebras[4], B. H. Guyer[+], S. Sheren*, G. H. Collins[5], and R. A. Schwartz[3]

Departments of [1] Radiology, [2] Neurosurgery,
[3] Surgery, [4] Department of Neurology, Veterans Administration Medical Center, Syracuse, New York, USA

Summary. Gross and histologic analyses of 78 carotid endarterectomy specimens removed from 71 patients showed intraplaque hemorrhage (subintimal hemorrhage) and necrosis in 74 (94.8%); all but 3 were symptomatic. In 66 (95.6%) of 69 carotid arteries with lucent plaques on intravenously enhanced computed tomography (CT), the presence of subintimal hemorrhage and necrosis and the maximal areas of involvement were accurately predicted preoperatively. The pathologic zones were readily identified as areas of circumferential and eccentric focal mural thickening frequently associated with moderate to severe luminal stenosis. Local, expansile areas of intraplaque hemorrhage were consistently observed in 30 (39%) atheromatous plaques causing significant stenosis in marked disparity to the contralateral asymptomatic carotid artery as shown by angiography (including 7 without CT examinations) and CT. There was preponderant involvement of the distal common carotid, carotid bifurcation and proximal internal carotid artery segments. Most patients with hemorrhagic and necrotic plaques had ipsilateral recent (within 6 weeks) neurologic manifestations predominantly in the form of transient ischemic attack, amaurosis fugax and stroke. Our experience reflects the high incidence of intraplaque hemorrhage in carotid related cerebroembolic events. Its presence can be consistently implicated by the demonstration of a markedly lucent plaque on CT and the observation of a symptomatic focal carotid stenosis in marked disparity to the contralateral asymptomatic carotid artery on CT and angiography.

Key words: Intraplaque hemorrhage – Carotid artery – Transient ischemic attack – Computed tomography – Angiography

---

The prevalent finding of intraplaque hemorrhage in endoarterectomy specimens from symptomatic patients in the studies of Imparato et al. [1] and Lusby et al. [2] has generated enormous interest in the atherosclerotic changes of the carotid wall in addition to the vascular surface changes of ulceration and thrombus formation [3, 4] that have been widely implicated in carotid related cerebroembolic events. We are currently confronted with the emergence of a strong and reasonable hypothesis on the interrelated role of the flow limiting expansile mound of intraplaque hemorrhage to stress related intimal disruption and thrombus formation, mechanisms that could lead to the production of cerebral ischemia and infarction [1, 2, 5]. This article explores the effectiveness of CT and angiography in detecting intraplaque hemorrhage.

Patients and methods

Seventy-one patients (54 males, 17 females, from 41 to 89 years of age) who underwent 80 carotid endarterectomies with atheromatous plaques available for gross and histologic examinations (78 specimens available) comprise this series. CT, using the technique we previously described [6], was performed on 64 patients; all had conventional film/screen or digital subtraction angiography. The predominant neurologic manifestations of the patients were noted; signs and symptoms occurring within 6 weeks of the time of evaluation were considered recent, others were entered as old.

On CT, the carotid wall and the luminal diameter were carefully evaluated. The presence of markedly lucent plaque, its extent, and associated luminal narrowing were noted. Carotid stenosis was graded on the size of the lumen relative to the external diameter of the artery. Narrowing was considered mild when 25% or less, moderate 26–50%, moderately severe 51–75%, and severe when greater than 75% of the external diameter.

Stenosis on angiography based on the degree of stenosis relative to the normal higher or lower carotid lumen. When there was discrepancy in the degree of stenosis in two views, the severest narrowing was entered into the data. When there was discrepancy between stenosis on CT and angiography, CT was considered more accurate.

The carotid plaque removed from each patient was carefully examined grossly and/or histologically allowing close segmental and positional correlation with the CT and angiographic findings. In 52 endarterectomy specimens, gross and microscopic analyses were performed (GHC, AC) and in 26 where obvious necrosis and hemorrhage were present, no histologic examinations were undertaken. Grossly, hemorrhage/necrosis was assumed when mural thickening showed a loose, friable mesh of "grumous" material, cavitation and brownish to dark discoloration (CJH, CHB, RAS). Attempts were made to determine the presence of ulcerations grossly and/or histologically.

[+] Former fellow,
* Former medical student of the SUNY Health Science Center at Syracuse, 750 East Adams Street, New York, USA

Results

The presentations in the 78 endarterectomy specimens included ipsilateral recent transient ischemic attack, amaurosis fugax and stroke in 69, chronic or old similar manifestations in 5, none in 3, non-specific in 1. Carotid stenosis was severe in 58 (74%), moderately severe in 11 (14%), moderate in 5, mild in 3 and segmental occlusion with distal patency in 1 patient. Hemorrhagic and necrotic plaques exhibited severe stenosis in 56, moderately severe in 11, moderate in 4, mild in 1, and complete occlusion in 1.

Sixty-nine markedly lucent plaques were observed on CT (Table 1). In 66 (95.6%), the eccentric focal and circumferential mural thickenings (Figs. 1–3) were proved to represent intraplaque hemorrhage and necrosis, grossly (19) and histologically (50). By histology, both subintimal hemorrhage (varying ages and degrees) and necrosis were noted in 41, while necrosis only was noted in 6. Other frequent findings on microscopy included inflammatory cellular infiltrates, cholesterol crystals and lipid deposits, calcification, intimal fibrosis, proteinaceous fluid/precipitate and neovascularity. One lucent plaque associated with mild stenosis yielded only cholesterol deposits with no subintimal hemorrhage or necrosis; another showed inflammatory cells, intimal fibrosis, cholesterol and calcium deposits; and a third, with moderate stenosis, revealed a proteinaceous fluid filled cystic cavity without hemorrhage by histology. Two nonlucent (isodense with muscle) plaques showed on microscopy predominantly fibrolipid collections and intimal fibrosis without subintimal hemorrhage. Grossly and histologically at least 43 (55%) ulcers (Figs. 2, 3) were found; histologic analyses commonly showed inflammatory cellular infiltrates and neovascularity around the ulcers. Endothelial loss and fibrosis along with platelet aggregates and thrombi were also not uncommonly seen.

Significant disparity by at least two grades relative to the contralateral asymptomatic carotid artery was noted in 30 symptomatic carotid stenoses (Fig. 4). All proved histologically and grossly to represent local mounds of subintimal hemorrhage and necrosis.

Discussion

A major site of predilection for atheromatous plaque formation is the carotid bifurcation, which is readily accessible to physical and diagnostic investigation. Despite this apparent advantage, the pathologic changes that lead to carotid artery-related cerebral embolic events have remained incompletely understood. As a consequence, the therapeutic approaches to carotid lesions, such as carotid endarterectomy and thrombolytic therapy, are still controversial. The high incidence of intraplaque hemorrhage and necrosis in symptomatic atheromatous plaques has drawn attention to the carotid wall itself and efforts are being made to correlate these changes with the vascular surface abnormalities.

In radiology, technological trends have shifted to the study of intramural abnormalities which are not demonstrable by angiography, which is restricted to assessing endothelial and intraluminal changes only. Bluth et al. [10] have suggested high resolution sonography for determination of the presence or absence of intraplaque hemorrhage. However, our early involvement with sonography in this area has been significantly limited by plaque calcification and severe luminal stenoses, which are frequently encountered. The potential for MRI of the carotid bifurcation is currently being explored but it is limited by carotid pulsation and flow turbulence in stenotic carotid segments [11].

We have primarily relied on CT in the evaluation of the carotid wall as it accurately depicts both the wall and the lumen, in cross-section, usually being unaffected by plaque calcification. CT may also demonstrate progression of changes in the plaque.

Table 1. Markedly lucent plaques on CT

Histologically and grossly	
Subintimal hemorrhage/necrosis	41
Necrosis only	6
Cholesterol deposit only	1
Proteinaceous fluid cyst	1
Inflammatory cells/intimal/fibrosis/cholesterol	1
Grossly only	
Hemorrhagic/necrotic	19
Total	69

Fig. 1. Intravenously enhanced CT shows circumferential lucent mural thickening *(arrows)* causing mild luminal narrowing *(L)* of the distal left common carotid artery. The lucent plaque reflects the presence of subintimal hemorrhage and necrosis. The right distal common carotid artery also shows mild atherosclerotic subintimal thickening. Normally, the carotid wall is essentially imperceptible on CT. *J*, Jugular vein

Fig. 2. a Lateral view of a left common carotid angiogram demonstrating severe stenosis of the proximal internal carotid *(arrow)* and external carotid arteries. Also evident is a luminal bulging *(arrowheads)* which could represent either ulceration or normal lumen in an eccentric plaque. **b** CT at the level of the luminal bulge showing the direction of the focal luminal outpouching *(white arrow)* towards a markedly lucent moderate carotid wall thickening *(smaller white arrows)*. Smaller luminal protrusions *(curved arrows)* into the lucent plaque are also present. The findings are typical of ulcerations into a hemorrhagic and necrotic plaque. Calcification is evident anteriorly *(black arrows)*

Fig. 3. a CT depicting another ulceration *(dark arrow)* into a milder hemorrhagic and necrotic markedly lucent carotid artery wall *(white arrowheads)*. Note the almost imperceptible wall of the normal left common carotid bifurcation. **b** Gross specimen. Note the correlative ulceration *(curved arrow)* in addition to the marked irregularity of the plaque and evident brownish to darkish discolorations *(arrowheads)* reflecting areas of intraplaque hemorrhage and necrosis. *I*, Internal carotid artery; *E*, external carotid artery

Fig. 4. a Intraplaque hemorrhage can cause severe shelved and irregular segmental stenosis *(arrows)* in marked disparity to the contralateral asymptomatic side. Note also the probable large ulceration at the carotid bifurcation *(arrowheads)*. **b** Endarterectomy specimen *(entire and hemisection)* showing the extensive hemorrhagic and necrotic portions of the common carotid bifurcation and proximal internal carotid artery that caused the severe irregular segmental stenosis. *I*, Internal carotid artery; *E*, external carotid artery

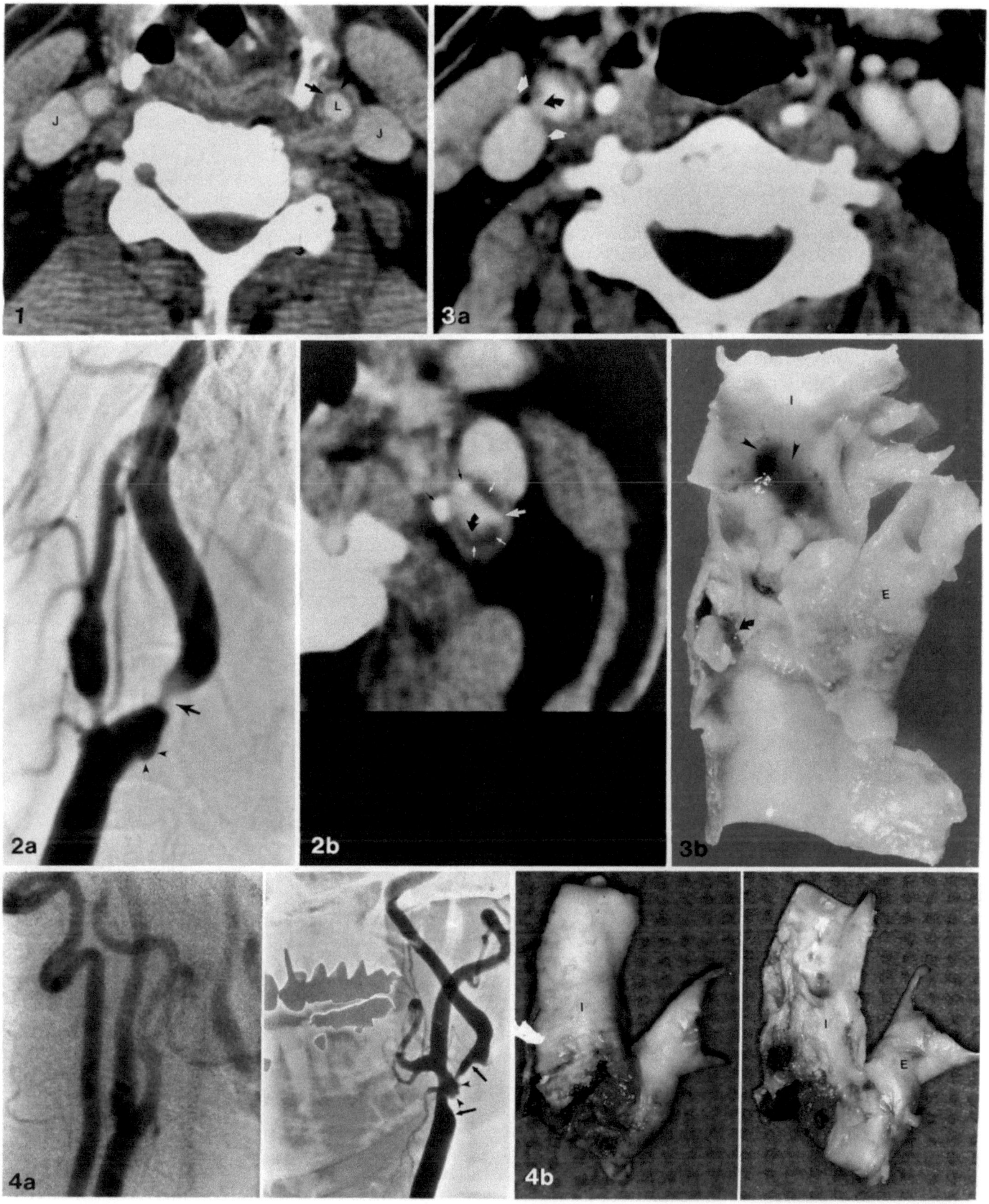

In this series, CT played a major role in predicting preoperatively the existence of intraplaque hemorrhage and necrosis. Thus, 66 of 69 (95.6%) end-arterectomy specimens that were examined demonstrated a close correlation between the hemorrhagic and necrotic areas and markedly lucent mural thickenings seen on CT. In 6 lucent carotid plaques, areas of necrosis only were seen, without subintimal hemorrhage. This observation raises the possibility that necrosis may antedate the development of subintimal hemorrhage. The majority of plaques (41) showed varying degrees and ages of subintimal hemorrhage, necrosis, inflammatory cell infiltrates, cholesterol and calcific deposits, fibrosis and neovascularity. Most (98.6%) of the hemorrhagic and necrotic plaques were moderately to severely stenotic on CT and angiography. Isodense plaques consisting mainly of fibrolipid collections and intimal fibrosis were observed in two cases. Plain cholesterol deposits, without significant inflammatory changes or necrosis, accounted for one lucent plaque, associated with mild stenosis.

The clinical relevance of intraplaque hemorrhage and necrosis is confirmed by the frequent association of ipsilateral, usually recent, manifestations of cerebral ischemia, such as TIA, amaurosis fugax or stroke, in the majority of our patients. We conclude that the observation of a markedly lucent mural thickening on CT, and the finding of significant carotid stenosis that is in great disparity with the contralateral carotid artery, strongly suggests the existence of intraplaque hemorrhage and necrosis, especially when accompanied by ipsilateral neurologic manifestations.

References

1. Imparato AM, Riles TS, Gorstein F (1979) The carotid bifurcation plaque: pathological findings associated with cerebral ischemia. Stroke 10: 238–245
2. Lusby RJ, Ferrell LD, Ehrenfeld WK, Stoney RJ, Wylie EJ (1982) Carotid plaque hemorrhage. Arch Surg 117: 1479–1488
3. Barnett HJM (1979) The pathophysiology of transient cerebral ischemic attacks. Med Clin North Am 63: 649–679
4. Hertzer NR, Beven EG, Benjamin SP (1977) Ultramicroscopic ulcerations and thrombi of carotid bifurcation. Arch Surg 112: 1394–1402
5. Fisher M, Blumenfeld AM, Smith TW (1987) The importance of carotid artery plaque disruption and hemorrhage. Arch Neurol 44: 1086–1089
6. Leeson MD, Cacayorin ED, Iliya AR (1985) Atheromatous extracranial carotid arteries: CT evaluation correlated with arteriography and pathologic examination. Radiology 156: 397–402
7. Winslow CM, Solomon DH, Chassin MR, Kosecoff J (1988) The appropriateness of carotid endarterectomy. N Engl J Med 318: 721–727
8. Caplan LR (1986) Carotid artery disease. N Engl J Med 315: 886–888
9. Imparato AM, Riles TS, Mintzer R (1983) The importance of hemorrhage in the relationship between gross morphologic and cerebral symptoms in 376 carotid artery plaques. Ann Surg 197: 195–203
10. Bluth EI, Kay D, Merritt CRB (1986) Sonographic characterization of carotid plaque: detection of hemorrhage. AJNR 7: 311–315
11. Masaryk TJ, Ross JS, Modic MT, Lenz GW, Haacke EM (1988) Carotid bifurcation: MR imaging. Radiology 166: 461–466

Dr. E. D. Cacayorin
State University of New York of Syracuse
Department of Radiology
750 E. Adams Street
Syracuse, NY 13210, USA

Neuroradiology (1991) 33 [Suppl]: 79–81

Neuro-radiology
© Springer-Verlag 1991

Temporal changes in red blood cell hydration: application to MRI of hemorrhage

H. Y. Chin[1], K. H. Taber[1], L. A. Hayman[1], J. J. Ford[1], and J. B. Kirkpatrick[2]

Departments of [1] Radiology and [2] Pathology, Baylor College of Medicine, Houston, Texas, USA

Summary. It has been established that red blood cell (RBC) dehydration causes significant changes in MRI signal intensity by decreasing both the T1 and T2 relaxation times. This study was conducted to determine if these changes occurred in blood clots maintained at body temperature for times ranging from 15 min to 10 days. Venous blood was used to form clots which were stored at 37°C. The shape and diameter of 20–50 RBCs were measured in the fresh and fixed states. By 12–48 h after clot formation virtually all RBCs lost their biconcave shape and became spherical echinocytes. The volume of these cells decreased by at least 15% over the next 72 h. This change indicates a decrease in the fraction of the cell weight occupied by water of 0.05, which is large enough to alter MR signal intensity significantly. The authors conclude that dehydration of RBCs occurs in vitro within an aging clot. If these changes occur in vivo they should cause a significant decrease in signal intensity on long TR/TE (T2-weighted) images.

Key words: Red blood cells – Brain hemorrhage – Blood, magnetic resonance studies

---

Current theory cannot explain the hypointense appearance of blood which has been observed clinically in acute hemorrhage at field strengths as low at 0.15 T on long TR/TE spin echo MR images [1, 2]. Histological studies of red blood cells (RBCs) within a clot have shown a temporal decrease in RBC size [3]. The purpose of the present study was to quantitate these temporal changes in RBC size and shape and measure the accompanying changes in serum chemistry. It is possible that the changes in RBC size are large enough to affect MR signal intensity of clinical images of hemorrhage. It has been established previously that changes in RBC hydration alter T1 and T2 relaxation times and therefore will affect MR image intensity [4–6].

Methods

Venous blood from three normal male volunteers was used to form 33 blood clots which were then stored at 37°C in a water bath. Sterile procedures were maintained during sample preparation. Over a period of time from 15 min to 10 days individual clots were removed and examined. No evidence of bacterial contamination was noted. The serum, including all cells not adhering to the clot, was aspirated from the clot, then centrifuged to precipitate the cellular debris. The supernatant was aspirated and analyzed for osmolality, glucose, total protein, and hemoglobin concentration.

A wet preparation was made by allowing the clot to touch a glass slide. To obtain a consistent thickness for the wet preparation, two wedges of one cover slip thickness were placed on the ends of the glass slide prior to placing a cover slip over the preparation. This also allowed the RBCs to remain suspended in serum. The shape and diameter of 20–50 RBCs from the surface of each clot were immediately measured under oil immersion on an Axiomat microscope (Zeiss, FRG) utilizing the Nomarski optics and video enhancement.

The remaining clot was promptly fixed in 10% formalin for a minimum of 3 days. The clot was then paraffin–embedded and sectioned for microscopic examination. The shape and diameter of another 20–50 RBCs were measured, and the internal structure of the clot was assessed.

Results

Red blood cells

During the first 4–6 h the RBCs gradually settled and formed a clot. Initially they retained this normal biconcave shape, they showed normal rouleaux formation, and the cells had a pliable, shimmering appearance (Fig. 1a) At 2–4 h spurs appeared on the membrane surface, and many RBCs were flattened disks rather than biconcave. At 6 h approximately 40% of the RBCs were flattened disks, and less rouleaux formation was present. At 24 h approximately 80%of the RBCs became spherical with extensive spur formation. Less than 20% of the cells now showed rouleaux formation (Fig. 1b).

At 2 days many spurs had pinched off from the parent RBC. The volume of the cells decreased by at least 15% over the next 72 h (Fig. 2). There was complete loss of rouleaux formation, and the RBCs no longer shimmered.

At 4 days the serum was tinged by hemoglobin released from lysed RBCs. Approximately 30% of the cells were ghosts. Many of the RBCs still had spurs, but they were less prominent. At 6 days the color of the serum had deepened, and about 60% of the cells were ghosts (Fig. 1c). The serum continued to deepen in color as RBC lysis progressed. There were no further changes in the microscopic appearance of the RBCs through day 10.

Serum

Serum accumulated above the clot during the first 4–6 h of observation. A summary of the serum chemistry changes is given in Table 1. A profound decrease in glucose con-

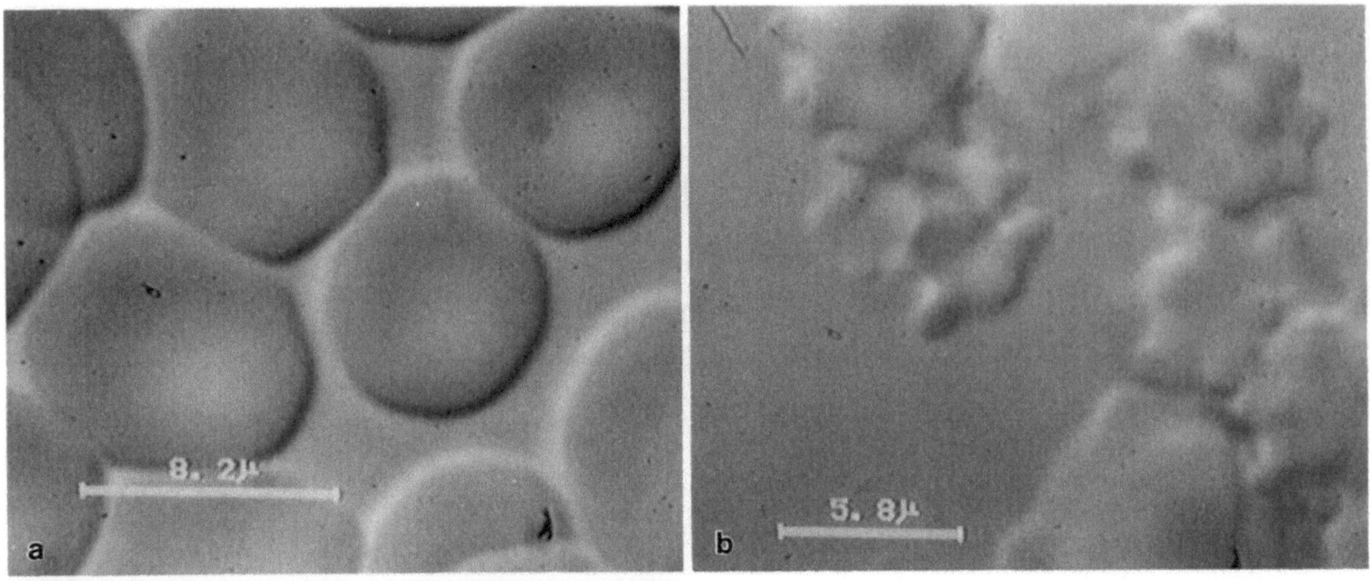

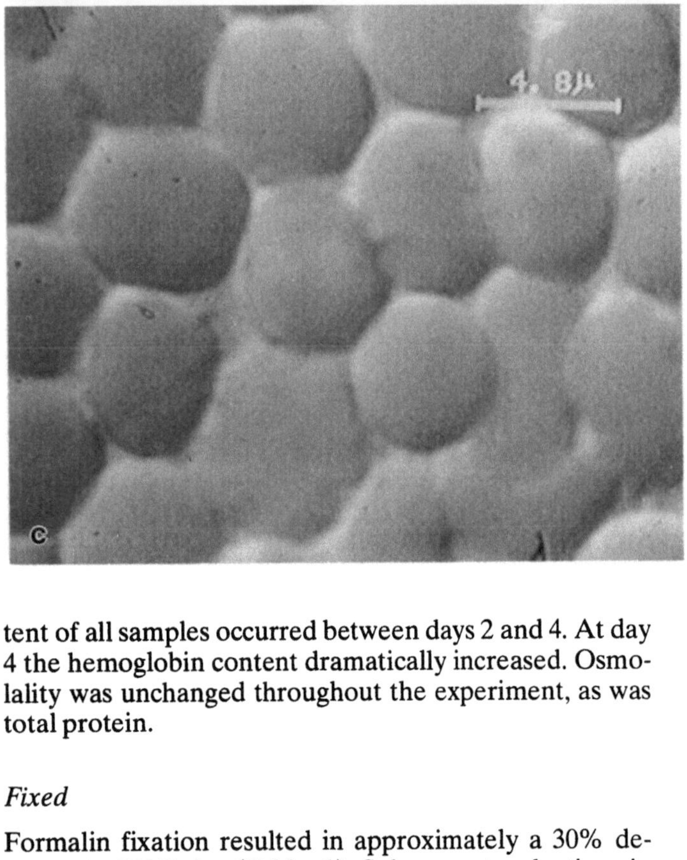

Fig. 1a–c. Appearance of red blood cells (RBCs) from the surface of fresh clot following incubation at 37°C for: **a** 1 h; **b** 2 days ;**c** 6 days. Note the transformation from the normal biconcave disk to echinocyte

tent of all samples occurred between days 2 and 4. At day 4 the hemoglobin content dramatically increased. Osmolality was unchanged throughout the experiment, as was total protein.

Fixed

Formalin fixation resulted in approximately a 30% decrease in RBC size (Table 1). Subsequent reductions in RBC size, which were dramatic in the wet preparations, were partially masked by this fixation shrinkage. A comparison of the size changes in the fresh and fixed clots, as well as the associated changes in serum glucose, is shown in Fig. 2.

A clear internal structure was present in the paraffin-embedded sections of the fixed clots. At the earliest time (15 min) the fibrin was present as swirlings, strands and lakes. The periphery of the clot was formed by a rim of densely packed RBCs. During the first few hours of clot formation the macroscopic inhomogenity of the clot slowly increased as clumps of fibrin and RBCs formed within lakes of serum.

Discussion

Contracted clot formation occurred over about a 6 h period, during which time the RBCs became permanently fixed within the fibrin network and lost their normal biconcave appearance. The conversion to spheres, with spur formation, occurred between 6 and 24 h in most cases, and thereafter the RBCs gradually lost volume as "spurs" of membrane were shed. At 4 days many RBCs broke up, releasing hemoglobin into the serum. This process continued for the remainder of the experiment.

Depletion of serum glucose, the primary energy source of RBC metabolism, caused the expected changes in RBC conformation and size (i. e., echinocyte formation and eventual cell lysis). In addition, the shimmering appearance of the RBCs also disappeared as the glucose level dropped in the serum.

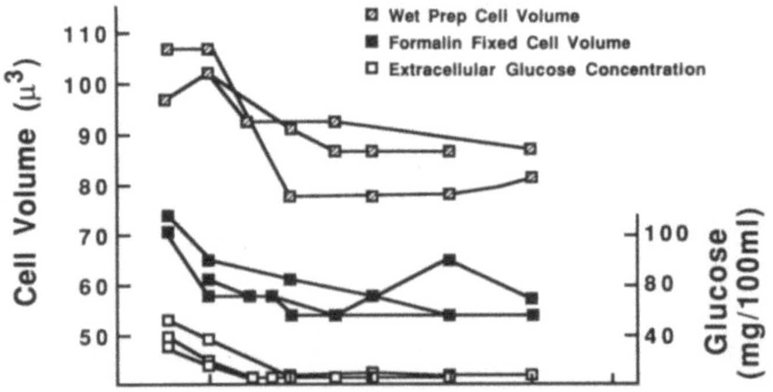

Fig. 2. Temporal changes in RBC size from fresh and formalin–fixed preparations and the parallel changes in serum glucose

Table 1. Serum chemistry analysis

Time	% Diameter change from fresh to fixed	Glucose (mg %)	Osmolality (mosmol)	Hemoglobin (g %)	Protein (g %)
15	29	–	280	21	8.90
min	–	89	–	2	7.50
	29	89	279	31	7.80
1 h	32	–	275	–	8.71
	26	73	–	11	7.50
	34	87	283	7	7.00
2 h	22	66	282	25	8.48
	–	–	–	–	–
	32	72	284	7	6.80
4 h	27	47	280	21	–
	–	–	–	–	–
	–	–	–	–	–
6 h	23	57	281	29	8.46
	27	53	–	18	7.80
	30	50	281	23	7.30
1 day	12	53	284	22	8.84
	11	29	–	25	7.90
	32	36	283	34	7.40
2 day	15	36	289	31	8.60
	17	13	–	36	7.60
	16	19	279	37	6.90
4 day	8	4	282	259	8.49
	14	6	–	334	7.50
	16	1	287	676	7.70
6 day	9	6	281	633	8.53
	16	5	–	1230	8.50
	13	0	294	2030	8.50
8 day	1	1	285	1606	9.67
	–	–	–	–	–
	15	0	300	4244	9.80
10 day	11	1	303	2552	10.13
	15	3	–	4784	12.50
	–	–	–	–	–

Once the RBCs became spherical they underwent a decrease in volume of at least 15%. This indicates a decrease in the fraction of the cell weight occupied by water of a minimum of 0.05. Our previously reported spectroscopic studies, carried out at 0.24T, indicate that this change in RBC volume would cause at least a 25% reduction in T2 relaxation time and a 15% reduction in T1 relaxation time in blood with a hemoglobin concentration of about 30 g%. Others have reported similar MRI effects [4–6].

When the RBC size measurements were compared prior to and following fixation it was clear that the formalin-induced shrinkage masked the decrease in size that accompanied clot aging (Fig. 2). This may explain why changes in RBC size have not been reported in formalin-fixed intracerebral hematomas.

In summary, current theory cannot explain the hypointense appearance of blood which has been observed clinically in acute hemorrhage at field strengths as low as 0.15 T on long TR/TE spin echo MR images [1, 2]. The results of the present in vitro study suggest that dehydration of the RBCs within hemorrhage could be responsible. Although the time frame for these changes does not perfectly match the MR signal changes in vivo, the presence of more rapid energy depletion in vivo could account for the difference.

References

1. Gomori JM, Grossman RI, Goldberg HI, Zimmerman RA, Bilaniuk LT(1985) Intracranial hematomas: imaging by high field MR. Radiology 157: 87–93
2. Bydder GM, Pennock JM, Porteous R, Dubowitz LMS, Gadian DG, Young IR (1988) MRI of intracerebral haematoma at low field (0.15 T) using T2–dependent partial saturation sequences. Neuroradiology 30: 367–371
3. Alanen A, Kormano M (1985) Correlation of the echogenicity and structure of clotted blood. J Ultrasound Med 4: 421–425
4. Kuntz ID, Zipp A (1977) Water in biological systems. N Engl J Med 297: 262–265
5. Fabry ME, Eisenstadt M (1978) Water exchange across red cell membranes. II. Measurement by nuclear magnetic resonance T1, T2 and T12 hybrid relaxation. The effects of osmolarity, cell volume, and medium. J Membr Biol 42: 375–398
6. Sullivan SG, Stern A, Rosenthal JS, Minkoff LA; Winston A (1988) NMR water–proton spin–lattice relaxation time of human red blood cells and red blood cell suspensions. FEBS Lett 234: 349–352

Dr. K. H. Taber
Department of Radiology, Baylor College of Medicine,
One Baylor Plaza
Houston, Texas 77030, USA

SESSION 7
DEGENERATIVE DISEASES OF THE SPINE

Neuroradiology (1991) 33 [Suppl]: 84–85

Neuro radiology
© Springer-Verlag 1991

The natural history of lumbar disc herniations assessed by a CT follow-up study

K. Pardatscher[1], D. L. Fiore[2], and A. Barbiero[3]

[1] Department of Neuroradiology, University of Catanzaro, Catanzaro, Italy
[2] Department of Neuroradiology, Padua Hospital, Padua, Italy
[3] Orthopaedic Clinic, Padua, Italy

Summary. A prospective follow-up CT study was carried out in 98 patients with symptomatic and CT-proven lumbar disc herniation, treated conservatively by a combination of various symptomatic therapy modalities only. The high success rate of this treatment in relieving symptoms and signs (90%), allowed us to follow the natural history of disc herniation. A significant reduction in herniated disc size was seen in 30.4% of this group at 6 months and in 60% of those examined 12 to 24 months after the first CT scan. In a few cases (7.7%), herniation had disappeared completely. These findings are of the utmost importance to all concerned in the diagnosis and treatment, of whatever type, of lumbar disc herniation.

Key words: Lumbar disc herniation – Computed tomography – Follow-up study – Lumbar disc herniation – Conservative treatment

The successful result of a particular kind of conservative, and essentially non-pharmacological, treatment of low back and radicular pain, the latter usually implying nerve root compression by lumbar disc prolapse or bony entrapment, has offered the opportunity to follow up symptomatic lumbar disc herniations. This allows us to gain an insight into the natural history of disc disease and the relationship between structural and functional factors in causing clinical problems. There is, as yet, little agreement on this in the literature.

Teplick [1] reported in 1985 on 15 cases in whom an unequivocal spontaneous regression or disappearance of a herniated lumbar nucleus pulposus was documented on follow-up CT study. He suspected that spontaneous regression of a herniated disc may not be a rare occurrence, though he found no previous reports on this subject, and suggested that a follow-up study on more extended series could be rewarding.

Materials and methods

One hundred and sixty-five patients affected by low back and radicular pain due to spinal degenerative changes, assessed by lumbar CT, were treated with a combination of symptomatic treatment modalities consisting of acupuncture, manipulation and laser applications on trigger points. All patients underwent an initial thorough neurological and orthopaedic examination. Follow-up clinical examinations were performed at 1 month, 3 months, 6 months, 1 year and 2 years, by the same orthopaedic medicine specialist who had performed the pretreatment clinical examination. An improvement in the clinical picture in more than 90% of patients within the first 15–20 days, without any further resort to drugs or surgical procedures, made this group suitable for follow up serial CT, carried out 2 and 62 months after the first examination.

For the purpose of this study, the size of the disc herniations and the clinical signs and symptoms were graded according to criteria reported elsewhere [2, 3]. In brief, based on the CT findings, the size of disc herniations was measured and related to the midsagittal diameter of the spinal canal taken at the nearest interpedicular plane. They were classified as small when measuring 25% or less, medium from 26% to 50%, and large those more than 50% of the spinal canal. Clinical patterns were graded as type A, type B or type C in relation to the increasing severity of low back and radicular pain scored on a scale ranging from 0 to 100, and also on physical signs such as the impairment of spinal mobility in flexion and extension, the degree of impairment of straight leg raising, muscle weakness (quadriceps, extensor hallucis longus and gastrocnemius) and any decrease in lower limb reflexes. At follow-up, each patient was assigned to either a marked improvement (satisfactory outcome) group or to a slight/no improvement (unsatisfactory outcome) group. Results were considered excellent if patients were symptom-free, good if they had least 80% pain relief, and fair with at least 60% pain relief.

Results

In the group of 165 patients consecutively considered, 98 had disc herniation, ten at two levels, giving a total of 108. Minor disc bulges, as well as central and lateral bony canal stenosis, were also present in a large numbers of cases. The size of the disc herniation was assessed as small at 48 levels, medium at 50 and large at 10. There were 17 intraforaminal sites.

At the initial evaluation of the group of 48 small lesions, the clinical pattern was type A in 17%, type B in 55% and type C in 26%. In the group of 50 medium-sized herniations type A was seen in 8%, type B in 52% and type C in 40%. In the 10 large lesions the figures were type A in 20%, type B in 50% and type C in 30%.

Eighty-eight percent of patients were assigned to the marked improvement (satisfactory outcome) group. The remainder, in the unsatisfactory outcome group, went to surgery even though some had achieved at least a 60% relief of pain.

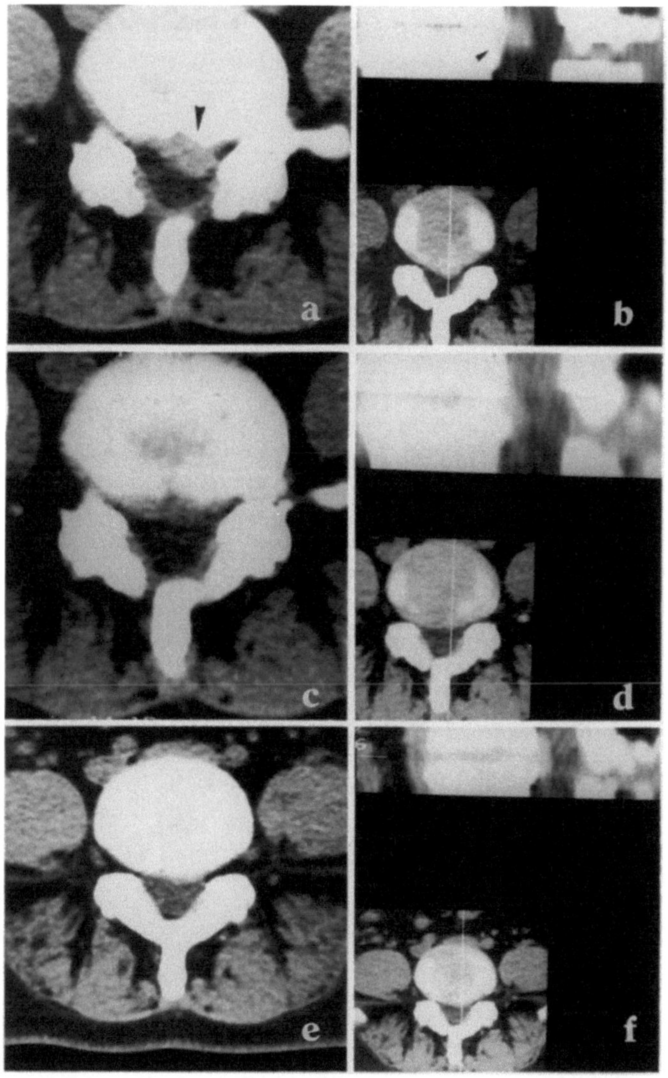

Fig. 1 a–f. A 40-year-old lady with sciatica and muscular weakness in the left leg for 14 days. **a, b** CT at the enrolling stage showing large left disc herniation at L4–L5 level. **c, d** Considerable size reduction at the control performed after 6 months and **e** after 22 months; even though **f** a mild increase is noted in the sagittal reconstruction. S_1 deficit disappeared by one year

Seventy-one patients, with 78 disc herniations, had CT follow-up studies at 2 to 62 months, 48 having 2 CT scans and 23 having 3. A decrease in the size of the herniated nucleus pulposus was seen in 31 discs (39.7%), with disappearance in 6 (7.7%), no change in 35 (44.8%) and an increase in 6 (7.7%). Among the group classified as showing size reduction are two cases showing a definite decrease on the second CT, but with a less prominent increase again on the third (Fig. 1). Among the 'unchanged' group there was one patient showing a 50% decrease on the second CT but a return to the initial appearance on the third.

Discussion

There is, as reported in the literature, a marked lack of consistency between the size of a lumbar disc herniation and the severity of the neurological symptoms and signs it produces. The same applies to the response to treatment, such as chemonucleolysis and disc aspiration [4]. It would be expected that clinical improvement would reflect a structural change in the disc. However, in one study [5], despite a successful clinical response to chemonucleolysis in 17 of 21 patients, changes in the size, location, shape and homogenity of the disc herniation were uncommon at a 6 week CT follow-up; a slight decrease in the size was observed in only 2 (8.3%) herniations.

In our series, the reflex therapy protocol has been as good in the treatment of cases with a small disc prolapse as those with a large herniation and spinal stenosis. The follow-up CT studies show that a decrease in size of a disc herniation happens quite frequently, though not in a linear manner. More infrequently, there can be a complete disappearance or even an increase in size.

Exactly how a disc herniation decreases remains a subject for speculation. Dehydration, shrinkage, retraction of a herniated nucleus pulposus back through the annulus fibrosis, or even fragmentation have been postulated. Other possibilities include decongestion of the epidural venous plexus and remodelling activity by granulation tissue.

References

1. Teplick JG (1985) Spontaneous regression of herniated nucleus pulposus. AJNR 6: 331–335
2. Barbiero A, Pardatscher K (1989) Trattamento riflessoterapico di lombalgie paralizzanti e non paralizzanti. In: Barbiero A, Ceccherrelli F, Giron GP, Pardatscher K (eds) La lombosciatalgia: problemi di etiopatogenesi e terapia. La Garangola, Padua, pp 141–171
3. Postacchini F, Lami R, Massobrio M (1987) Chemonucleolysis versus surgery in lumbar disc herniations: correlation of the results to preoperative clinical pattern and size of the herniation. Spine 12: 87–96
4. Gentry LR, Strother CM, Turski PA, Javid MJ, Sackett JF (1985) Chymopapain chemonucleolysis: correlation of diagnostic radiographic factors and clinical outcome. AJNR 6: 311–320
5. Gentry LR, Turski PA, Strother CM, Javid MJ, Sackett JF (1985) Chymopapain chemonucleolysis: CT changes after treatment. AJNR 6: 311–320

Prof. Kurt Pardatscher
Cattedra di Neuroradiologia
Facoltà di Medicina e Chirurgia
Università degli Studi
I-88100 Catanzaro, Italy

Neuroradiology (1991) 33 [Suppl]: 86–88

Neuro radiology

© Springer-Verlag 1991

Breaches in the blood-brain barrier in head-injured patients shown by gadolinium-enhanced magnetic resonance imaging

D. M. Hadley[1], P. Macpherson[1], D. A. Lang[2], and G. M. Teasdale[2]

Departments of [1] Neuroradiology and [2] Neurosurgery, Institute of Neurological Sciences, Glasgow, UK

Summary. Ten head-injured patients selected to represent a variety of patterns and degrees of brain damage were studied with gadolinium (Gd)-enhanced MRI at various times from 36 h to 6 days following trauma. Clinical and biochemical parameters were closely monitored. T2-weighted and sequential pre- and post-Gd T1-weighted MR images were prospectively assessed for signal change. An index of percentage enhancement was calculated for regions of interest to assess the time course of blood-brain-barrier leakage. No clinically important side-effects were reported. One patient in coma had a normal CT and MR examination and showed no evidence of enhancement. Six patients imaged within 4 days of injury had 27 lesions but no evidence of blood-brain-barrier breakdown despite the presence of marked oedema on the pre-enhancement images. Three patients examined between 4 and 6 days showed marked enhancement of all their lesions. Local dural/meningeal enhancement was noted adjacent to fractures or contusions regardless of the time after injury. This temporal difference in permeability has implications for the biodistribution of intravenous drugs and the pathogenesis of the sequelae of head injury.

Key words: Magnetic resonance imaging – Blood-brain barrier – Head injury – Gadolinium enhancement

---

The endothelial cells of the cerebral capillaries restrict the movement of many molecules from the blood to brain and this has given rise to the concept of the blood-brain barrier (BBB). This is now known to be a complex physiological phenomenon [1] based on the continuous tight junctions between the endothelium of the cerebral capillaries which prevent the passage of protein molecules from the capillary lumen through the endothelium into the extravascular space. Intravenous administration of a paramagnetic magnetic resonance (MR) contrast medium can produce lesion enhancement due to T1 shortening mainly as a result of leakage of the agent from the intravascular space through regions of increased BBB permeability [2, 3]. This shows many intracranial lesions more clearly but has not previously been studied in head-injured patients. We have investigated the permeability of BBB in a series of recently head-injured patients using MRI and gadolinium-DTPA (Gd-DTPA) and have assessed the tolerance of patients to this agent.

Patients and methods

Ten patients (9 male, 1 female) aged between 19 and 60 years (mean 36 years) were selected to represent a variety of patterns and degrees of brain damage. Nine patients had depression of their conscious level and one had developed focal signs. The patients' clinical condition was closely monitored and recorded. MR studies were performed at various times within the 1st week after injury. Serum iron, renal and hepatic function were assessed before and at 4, 24 and 48 h after administration of the contrast medium. The study received approval from the Ethical Comittee of the Institute of Neurological Sciences and informed consent was obtained for each patient, usually from a relative.

MRI was performed with a Picker 0.15 T resistive imager operating at 6.38 MHz. T2- and T1-weighted axial sequences (TR2000/TE80 and TR2000/TI400/TE40 respectively) were ob-

Table 1. Minor biochemical abnormalities noted after single and double doses of gadolinium-DTPA

Gd-DTPA dose	Patient no.	Bilirubin	Creatinine	Iron	AST	AIT	γGT	Other
	1	–	–	↓ 24 h[b]	–	–	–	–
0.1 mmol/kg	2	↑ 24 h[a]	–	↓ 24 h[b]	–	↑ 24 h[a]	–	–
	3	–	–	–	–	–		Diuresis
	4	–	–	↓ 24 h[b]	–	–	–	–
	5	–	–	–	–	↓ 24 h[a]	–	–
	6	–	–	–	–	–	–	–
0.2 mmol/kg	7	–	–	–	–	–	↑[a]	–
	8	–	–	↑ [a]24 h	–	–	↑ C_2H_5OH	–
	9	–	–	–	–	–	–	–
	10	–	–	↑ [a]24 h	–	–	–	

[a] Very minor

[b] Related to primary injuries or operation

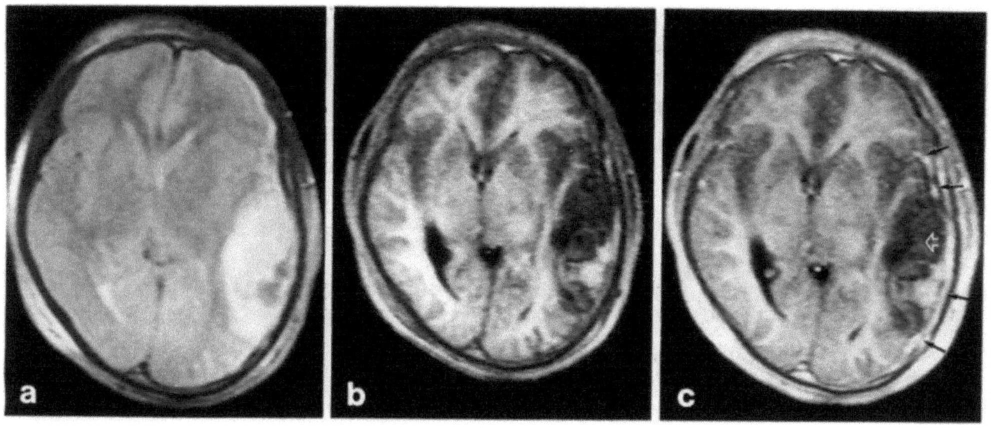

Fig. 1 a–c. A 20-year-old man involved in a road traffic accident imaged on the 4th day. **a** T2-weighted (SE2000/80) and **b** T1-weighted (IR2000/400/40) pre-enhanced sections through a space-occupying cortical and subcortical haemorrhagic contusion with marked oedema and associated with a thin subdural haematoma. Following Gd-DTPA (**c**) the T1-weighted image shows subtle enhancement in the contusion *(open arrow)* but marked meningeal enhancement *(closed arrows)*

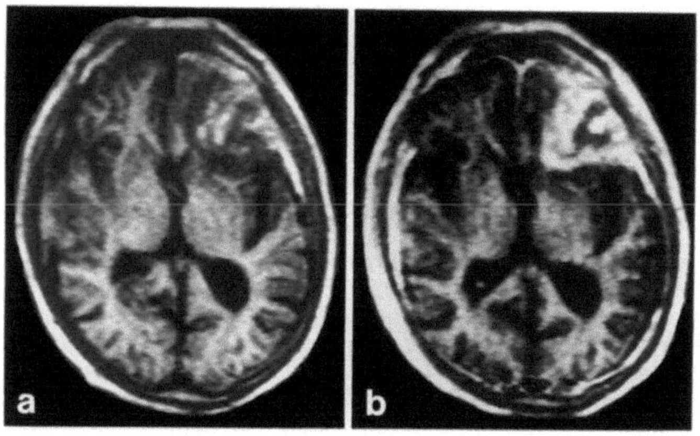

Fig. 2. a, b A 52-yerar-old man who had been assaulted, imaged on day 6. **a** T1-weighted (IR2000/400/40) pre-enhencement section shows frontal haemorrhagic contusion which (**b**) shows marked blood-brain barrier leakage in the area of surrounding oedema and, in addition, superficial meningeal enhancement

tained. Gd-DTPA was given intravenously without altering the patient's position in the imager between the initial and postcontrast examination. The first five patients received 0.1 mmol/kg; the next five received a double dose. T1-weighted imaging was repeatedly performed from 5 min after injection of contrast and up to six sequences were carried out in the 1st hour with a further one between 4 and 6 h. The time interval from injury ranged from 36 h to 6 days.

The images were viewed prospectively by two neuroradiologists blinded to the clinical data. The degree of enhancement was assessed visually and in addition an index of enhancement was calculated for regions of interest by normalising the tissue signal intensities to an area of normal white matter. This has been shown to be unaffected by Gd-DTPA and small differences caused by tuning and attenuation are eliminated [4, 5].

Results

No side-effects were reported by the conscious patients and no adverse reaction to Gd-DTPA was observed in the sedated or ventilated patients. In six patients there were temporary slight elevations of the serum iron, bilirubin or transanimases. One patient had a significant elevation of the glutamyl transferase (GT) which lasted for several weeks; this may have been due to the Gd as his pre-contrast level was normal, but he also had a long history of severe alcohol abuse. One further patient had a minimal elevation of gamma-GT (Table 1). These biochemical changes are not thought to be clinically important and did not influence treatment. Three patients showed reductions of serum iron at 24 h; this was attributed to rehydration after haemorrhage occurring at injury or at operation. The unenhanced images of nine patients showed abnormalities attributable to recent head injury. Seven patients had cortical contusions which extended into the subcortical white matter; one patient had a purely cortical lesion and one patient had a shear lesion in the deep white matter. Small extradural and intracerebral haematomas were shown in eight patients. Only one patient had a normal MR image. Following Gd each patient showed normal enhancement of the nasal mucosa pituitary gland and cavernous sinuses. New intracerebral lesions were not visualised on the post-Gd images. The images from the

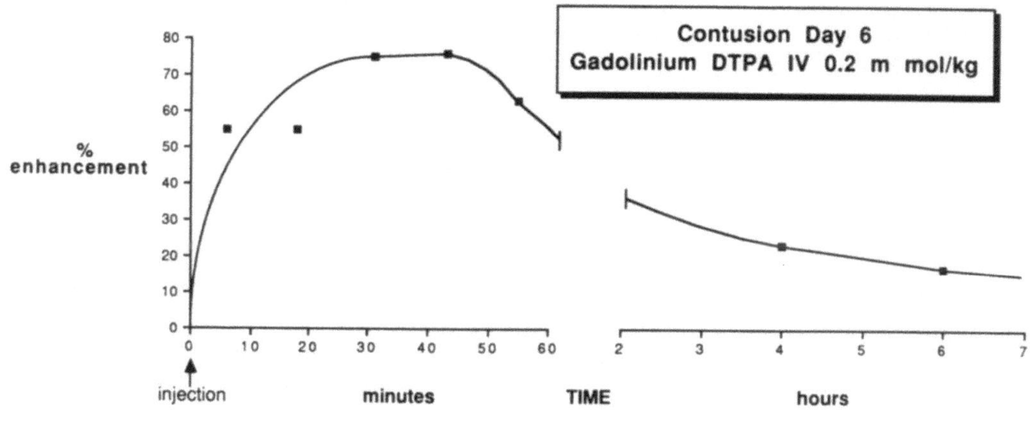

Fig. 3. Percentage enhancement over time

patient with the normal MR study remained normal after high-dose Gd. Six patients with 27 lesions showed no enhancement despite there being marked oedema on the T1- and T2 -weighted images. Each had been studied within 4 days of injury. By contrast, three patients examined between 4 and 6 days of injury showed marked enhancement of all their lesions. This was evident at 6 min, plateaued quickly and lasted for at least 4 h (Fig.3). The shortened T1 signal was noted initially either in the hypointense oedematous brain around the contusion or haematoma or in the periphery of contusions not showing central haemorrhage (Fig.1).

The dura mater around haematomas, burst lobes and associated with fractures showed increasing enhancement up to 40 min after administration (Fig.2). This was observed in six patients. Dural enhancement was not seen in the three patients who did not have a skull fracture.

Discussion

Gd-DTPA has a low molecular weight of 592. It is able to cross from the intravascular to the brain extracellular space only when BBB characteristics are absent. We did not observe intraparenchymal enhancement of any lesion in a patient studied within the first few days of head injury. This shows that the lesions demonstrated by MRI are not accompanied by gross increase in permeability of the BBB at this stage. This pattern is in accord with studies using iodinated contrast media and CT and with preliminary observations using SPECT imaging [6, 7]. By contrast, marked enhancement after Gd-DTPA was noted in each of the patients studied 4–6 days after injury (Fig.2).

These observations indicated that the early increase in water content shown as oedema surrounding a contusion occurs before gross BBB leakage is detectable. It suggests that in the early stages after injury, the oedema noted to have a long T1 and long T2 signal more closely resembles cytotoxic swelling than marked vasogenic transudation, which appears only some days after injury. This suggests that pathophysiological concepts based upon models in which there is an early vasogenic component may not be relevant to the management of acute head injury in man.

The dura mater is supplied by vessels with peripheral characteristics and the relative lack of enhancement of normal dura mater may reflect its extremely low perfusion rate. Our finding of marked meningeal enhancement adjacent to haemorrhage or injured meninges may reflect an enhanced meningeal circulation similar to that recently found at the site previous cranial surgery [8]. Although these focal areas of linear enhancement are unlikely to be important in the pathophysiology of acute brain damage, they do highlight fractures and small areas of traumatised meninges which may confirm a head injury when an intraparenchymal lesion is not noted.

Conclusion

Acutely head-injured patients tolerated Gd-DTPA well. Our results suggest that initally BBB permeability is not grossly increased but focal meningeal enhancement occurred early after injury. Marked enhancement around parenchymal contusions and haematomas was seen only after the 4th day. This temporal difference in permeability has implications for the biodistribution of intravenous drugs and for the pathogenesis of the sequelae of head injury.

References

1. Sage MR (1982) Blood-brain barrier; phenomenon of increasing importance to the imaging clinician. AJR 138: 887–898
2. Caille JM, Lemanceau B, Bonnemain B (1983) Gadolinium as a contrast agent for NMR. AJNR 4: 1041–1042
3. McNamara MT (1987) Paramagnetic contrast media for magnetic resonance imaging of the central nervous system. In: Brant-Zawadzki M, Norman D (eds) Magnetic resonance imaging of the central nervous system. Raven Press, New York, pp 97–107
4. Kilgore DP, Berger RIC, Daniels DL (1986) Cranial tissues – normal MR appearance after intravenous injection of Gd DTPA. Radiology 160: 757–761
5. Macpherson P, Hadley DM, Teasdale E (1989) Pituitary microadenomas. Does gadolinium enhance their demonstration? Neuroradiology 31: 293–298
6. Mauser HW, Van Nieuwenhuizen O, Veiga-Pires JA (1984) Is contrast enhanced CT indicated in acute head injury? Neuroradiology 26: 31–32
7. Bullock R, Statham P, Patterson J (1989) Tomographic mapping of CBF, CBV and blood brain barrier changes in humans after focal head injury by SPECT: mechanisms for late deterioration. In Hoff JT, Betz AI (eds) Intracranial pressure V11. Springer, Berlin Heidelberg New York, pp 637–639
8. Elster AD, Dipersio DA (1990) Cranial post-operative site: assessment with contrast-enhanced MR imaging. Radiology 174: 93–98

Dr. D.M. Hadley
Department of Neuroradiology,
Institute of Neurological Sciences,
1345 Govan Road,
Glasgow G51 4TF, UK

Neuroradiology (1991) 33 [Suppl]: 89–91

Neuro radiology

© Springer-Verlag 1991

Outpatient iohexol lumbar, cervical and total column myelography in 883 patients

R. S. Boulos and T. W. Free

Division of Neuroradiology, Department of Diagnostic Radiology, Henry Ford Hospital, Detroit, Michigan, USA

Summary. Water-soluble non-ionic contrast media have radically changed the practice of myelography. Several reports about outpatient lumbar myelography have already been published. We report our results in 800 lumbar, 66 ccrvical and 17 complete myelograms performed with iohexol on an outpatient basis. Introduction was by lumbar puncture using a 20- or 22-gauge needle. CT scans were obtained in 2–3 h and the patients were discharged in 5–6 h. Each patient was contacted after 24 h. Reactions lasting 24 h or less were considered mild and were not recorded. Reactions lasting 1–3 days were considered moderate, while reactions lasting more than 3 days or requiring hospitalization were considered severe. In the lumbar group, 52 patients had a total of 91 moderate or severe side effects. In the cervical and complete group, 10 patients suffered a total of 18 reactions. Seven patients had to be hospitalized. Our results compare favorably with those published and demonstrate the safety and utility of this approach provided a well-organized and controlled program is instituted. Tremendous reduction in the cost of work-up of patients can thus be achieved.

Key words: Outpatient myelography – Iohexol – Lumbar myelography – Cervical myelography – Total column myelography

The introduction of the water-soluble non-ionic contrast media as substitutes for Pantopaque has radically changed the technique, the post-procedure care and the side effects of myelography. A much smaller needle (20 or 22 gauge) is used for the puncture and there is no need for removal of the contrast medium at the end of the test, thereby curbing the loss of cerebrospinal fluid (CSF). It has been shown that such loss of CSF at the puncture site is a major contributing factor for post-myelography headache [1, 2]. A recent article concludes that the use of still smaller needles, i.e. 25 or 26 gauge, further decreases the incidence of headaches [3]. Patients need not be maintained in the horizontal position following the procedure. On the contrary, a semi-upright position is required in order to minimize the intracranial penetration of the contrast medium in high concentration. It has been demonstrated that patients may walk about after the procedure without a significant increase in the side effects compared to non-ambulatory patients [4, 5]. Based on these facts and coupled with the recent trend toward reducing health care costs, it became feasible to perform myelography on an outpatient basis. Several reports on outpatient lumbar myelography with the non-ionic contrast have already appeared in the English literature [6–10]. An earlier article in 1979 [11] reported the use of the outpatient approach in 30 lumbar myelograms with the ionic contrast media Dimer-X (meglumine iocarmate). However, hospitalization continued to be required for cervical and complete myelograms in most centers. Drawing upon our successful experience with outpatient lumbar myelography, we started in 1989 to systematically perform cervical and complete myelography on outpatients. The purpose of this article is to: (1) describe our program of outpatient myelography; (2) present and analyze its results and side effects in 883 studies; (3) demonstrate its safety, efficacy and cost-effectiveness for lumbar, cervical and total column myelography.

Patients and methods

During the period from 1 July 1987 to 30 September 1989, we performed 800 lumbar, 66 cervical and 17 complete outpatient iohexol myelograms. Of these, 53% were on male patients and 47% on females, whose ages ranged from 12 to 82 years.

The outpatient myelography program at Henry Ford Hospital is tightly organized and controlled. It is supervised by the staff neuroradiologists and is administered by the neuroradiology coordinators. There is close collaboration with the referring departments through their coordinators. The neuroradiology suite has a fully equipped recovery room next to the procedure room for pre- and post-procedure care. Day-care hospital beds are used for holding the patients until they are discharged. The myelography room has biplane fluoroscopic and radiographic capability.

Patient selection

Patients are excluded if they have any of the standard contraindications. Patients with a history of mild or moderate contrast medium reactions are given anti-allergy premedication. Additionally, all candidates must be ambulatory, able to comprehend and follow instructions and have a reliable means of transportation by an escort and a support care system at home.

Flow pattern

The flow pattern is depicted in Table 1. The coordinator meets with the referred patients and their families and gives them a full explanation of the procedure and the pre- and post-procedure instructions.

Table 1. Flow pattern

1
Referring physician schedules appointment for OP myelography for eligible patients

2
Neuroradiology coordinator meets with patient and family and explains and instructs them about procedure and pre- and post-procedure care.

3
Outpatient laboratory tests – PT, PTT, BUN and creatinine obtained in the week preceding the procedure.

4
Pre-myelogram preparation in special studies recovery room. Consent form signed after explanation. IV started and premedication given.

5
Myelography – biplane fluoroscopy and radiography. L2–3 puncture, 22-gauge needle. 10–14 cc iohexol 210.

6
Post-myelogram care in day-care hospital beds. Post-myelogram CT in 2–3 h. Discharge in 5–6 h with escort. Follow-up phone call in 24 h.

Blood coagulation and renal function tests are obtained in the outpatient laboratory in the week preceding the scheduled date of the procedure. Patients are kept hydrated and an intravenous line is routinely started before the procedure. Light premedication is given if necessary. An informed consent is obtained in each case.

All procedures were done via lumbar puncture, mostly at the L2–3 interspace using a 20- or 22-gauge needle. Iohexol 180, 240 or a mixture of the two (210) was used and the volume varied from 10 to 14 cc. Cervical and complete myelography patients received an intravenous injection of 10 mg dexamethasone after the completion of the procedure and each was given three 5-mg doses of prednisone to be taken orally in the first 24 h. Post-myelogram CT was obtained 2–3 h after the test. Patients stayed in the day-care hospital for 5–6 h in the semi-sitting position and were encouraged to drink fluids. They were checked by the neuroradiologist before being discharged in the company of a reliable escort. Each patient was given a phone number to call in case of any reaction or complication. All patients were contacted 24 h after the test by the coordinator and were asked about their reaction both in general and with regard to specific side effects. Mild reactions that resolved within the first 24 h were not recorded. Reactions taking up to 3 days to resolve were considered moderate, while those persisting more than 3 days or requiring hospitalization were considered severe.

Results

All the examinations were completed without technical difficulty or immediate complications. In a small minority (5%), the dilution of the contrast resulted in suboptimal visualization of the cervical area by the conventional radiographs. However, the addition of the post-myelogram CT resulted in a diagnostic study in every case.

With regard to side effects, no seizures, neuropsychiatric disturbances or neurologic deficits occurred. A total of 109 instances of moderate and severe reactions, occurring singly or in combination, was encountered in 62 patients (52 lumbar and 10 cervical or complete myelograms). The overall incidence of side effects was, therefore, 12.4%. The incidence of each of the side effects according to the type of study is shown in Table 2. The most common was headache followed by nausea and vomiting. Seven patients had to be admitted to the hospital for 2–3 days because of severe headache: 5 were in the lumbar group and 2 had cervical myelograms. There was no statistically significant relationship of the side effects to age or sex.

Discussion

To the best of our knowledge, this report is the first to examine in a systematic way the use of the outpatient approach in cervical and total columnar myelography and compare its results with lumbar myelography.

Our results compare very favorably with the published results of outpatient and inpatient lumbar myelography [6–10, 12–14]. We believe this is due, in large measure, to the strict criteria we established for performing the procedure and for the pre- and post-procedural care as well as to the close collaboration with the referring departments.

Our program of outpatient myelography is strictly controlled and organized under the supervision of the staff neuroradiologists and is administered by reliable coordinators who are well-trained and knowledgeable former neuroradiology technologists. All patients are thoroughly screened before inclusion and the necessary blood coagulation and renal function tests are obtained. They receive detailed explanation and instructions at the time of scheduling the test and throughout the procedure and post-procedure period. The availability of a well-equipped recovery room as part of the neuroradiology suite helps in administering the immediate pre- and post-procedure care. Patients are kept well hydrated. During the procedure, every effort is made to reduce the intracra-

Table 2. Results

	Incidence of side effects			
	Lumbar ($n = 800$)		Cx and complete ($n = 83$)	
	No.	%	No.	%
Total	91	11.4	18	21.7
Headache	46	5.8	10	12.0
Nausea	23	2.9	4	4.8
Vomiting	19	2.4	3	3.6
Pain	3	0.4	–	–
General weakness	–	–	1	1.2
Hospitalization	5	0.6	2	2.4

Table 3. Percentage of outpatient myelograms 1987–1989

	Lumbar	Cervical	Complete
1987	22.8%	2%	0%
1988	53.1%	2%	0%
1989	65.6%	45.3%	5.5%

nial passage of the contrast medium. This is facilitated by having available biplane fluoroscopy and radiography. The great majority of the spinal punctures were by 22-gauge needles, although lately we have started experimenting with the 25-gauge needle. Expert nursing care is provided in the day-care hospital beds. We routinely use corticosteroids prophylactically for the first 24 h following the procedure in all cervical and complete myelograms. Patients have ready access to the neuroradiologist and/or the referring physician at any time.

Or patients varied in age from 12 to 82 years. A recent report on outpatient performance of invasive procedures in pediatric patients includes 44 myelograms, some of which were total [15]. The results suggest that pediatric patients tolerate the procedure quite well. Since our results show no effect of higher age on the incidence of side effects, it appears that outpatient myelography is a safe procedure at all ages.

No serious or life-threatening complications were encountered among our patients. Moreover, the vast majority of the side effects could be managed at home with bedrest, hydration and regular medical treatment. Only 0.6% of the lumbar myelogram patients and 2.4% of the cervical and complete group required hospitalization for 2–3 days after their initial discharge because of severe headache. While this clearly demonstrates the safety of this approach, it is essential that all patients have the assurance of easy access to a physician and prompt hospitalization if the need arises.

The cost-savings of outpatient myelography are self-evident when compared with the cost of routine hospitalization. Physicians' and patients' acceptance of this approach is attested by the increasing percentage of myelograms of all kinds performed on an outpatient basis in our institution (Table 3). This trend is expected to continue especially with the use of smaller needles that was shown to result in less side effects [3].

Conclusions

1. Outpatient iohexol, lumbar, cervical and total column myelography is a safe and cost-effective procedure which is well tolerated by patients and accepted by referring physicians with no loss in quality provided the program is tightly organized and controlled.
2. Proper patient selection, pre-procedure instruction and preparation, expert performance of the procedure and reliable post-procedure care and follow-up are essential for assuring the safety and efficacy of outpatient cervical and total columnar myelography.
3. It appears that extremes of age per se are not limiting factors so that the procedure can be safe in both the pediatric and the geriatric age groups.
4. Further reduction in incidence and severity of side effects is to be expected with the use of still smaller needles (25 or 26 gauge).

References

1. Sand T, Stooner LJ, Dale L, Salvesen R (1987) Side effects after diagnostic lumbar puncture and lumbar Iohexol myelography. Neuroradiology 29: 385–388
2. Nestvold K, Sortland O (1988) Lumbar myelography with iohexol. Adverse effects compared with spinal puncture. Acta Radiol 29: 637–640
3. Vezina JL, Fontaine S, Laperrière J (1989) Outpatient myelography with a fine-needle technique: an appraisal. AJNR 10: 615–617
4. Sykes RHD, Wasenaar W, Clark P (1981) Incidence of adverse effects following metrizamide myelography in non-ambulatory and ambulatory patients. Radiology 138: 625–627
5. Macpherson P, Teasdale E, Macpherson PY (1983) Radiculography: is routine bed rest really necessary? Clin Radiol 34: 325–326
6. Kostiner AI, Krook PM (1985) Outpatient lumbar myelography with metrizamide. Radiology 155: 383–385
7. Postacchini F, Massobrio M (1985) Outpatient lumbar myelography. Analysis of complications after myelography comparing outpatients with inpatients. Spine 10: 567–570
8. Badami JP, Baker RA, Scholz FJ, McLaughlin M (1986) Outpatient metrizamide myelography: prospective evaluation of safety and cost-effectiveness. Br Radiology 158: 175–177
9. Choudhri AH, Rowlands PC, Barber CJ, Johnson J, Stevens JM (1989) Outpatient myelography: an acceptable and cost-effective technique. Br J Radiol 62: 253–255
10. Wang H, Binet EF, Gabrielsen TO, Rosenbaum A (1989) Lumbar myelography with iohexol in outpatients: prospective multicenter evaluation of safety. Radiology 173: 239–242
11. Van Niekerk JP (1979) Myelography using water-soluble contrast media as an outpatient procedure. S Afr Med J 55: 550–551
12. Gabrielsen TO, Gebarski SS, Knake IE, Latack IT, Yang PT, Hoff IT (1984) Iohexol vs. metrizamide for lumbar myelography: double blind trial. AJNR 5: 181–183
13. Hindmarsh T (1984) Lumbar myelography with iohexol and metrizamide: a double blind clinical trial. Acta Radiol 25: 365–368
14. Kieffer SA, Binet EF, Davis DO (1984) Lumbar myelography with iohexol and metrizamide: a comparative multicenter prospective study. Radiology 151: 665–670
15. Diament MJ, Bird CR, Stanley P (1988) Outpatient performance of invasive radiologic procedures in pediatric patients. Radiology 166: 401–403

Dr. Roushdy S. Boulos
Department of Diagnostic Radiology
Henry Ford Hospital
2799 W. Grand Boulevard
Detroit, Michigan, USA

Neuroradiology (1991) 33 [Suppl]: 92–94

Neuro
radiology
© Springer-Verlag 1991

Delayed and prolonged side effects of myelography with water soluble media

R. J. V. Bartlett[1] and J. T. Lamb[2]

[1] Department of Radiology, Hull Royal Infirmary, Hull, UK [2] Department of Radiology, Leeds General Infirmary, Leeds, UK

Summary. The occurence of side-effects, especially headache, in the 24 h following myelography has been extensively investigated, though reported results vary widely. Only recently has it become apparent that many patients are debilitated for a much longer period. The results of two separate but related trials are reported. Patients were assessed by questionnaire 2 weeks after myelography. A considerable proportion of patients did not develop symptoms until after they had been discharged from hospital. Females reported more side-effects than males. Many patients consider myelography to be an extremely unpleasant examination.

Key words: Lumbar myelography – Delayed side-effects

Side-effects after water soluble myelography have been well documented, though reported results vary considerably (Table 1) ([1, 2]; Lamb and Bartlett unpublished data). The relevance of post-procedural aftercare and the implications for outpatient studies have received attention [3–6]. Most reports concentrate on the first 24 h after the investigation. Some recent studies have followed patients up for a longer period [7, 8].

Many side-effects are considered to be due to the lumbar puncture and subsequent loss of cerebrospinal fluid [6, 9, 10] (CSF). "Chemical meningitis" may occur as a rare complication of myelography, and this implies to us that the contrast medium still plays a role in the genesis of side-effects.

Patients and methods

Group 1

The 508 patients in this group were recruited in Leeds between 1987 and 1989. All suitable patients undergoing lumbar myelography were given a questionnaire by the radiologist. They were also given a covering letter requesting details of the onset and duration of symptoms which they thought had been caused by the investigation. The wording was intended to reassure, but provided information on how to contact the X-ray department if advice were needed. A stamped, addressed envelope was supplied.

Myelography was performed in a standard manner, with demonstration of the lower end of the spinal cord at the end of the study. Contrast medium was drawn up with a 5 µm filter and injected via a 22-gauge lumbar puncture needle. Generally 3 ml CSF were removed. All studies were performed with iohexol, except in 10 patients given iopamidol or iotrolan, who had experienced side-effects previously after iohexol myelography. Only 2 of these patients remained asymptomatic after the second myelogram. Contrast medium doses varied from 2 to 3 g iodine.

All patients remained in hospital for 24 h. On return to the ward, they were permitted to sit in a chair or in bed, and limited ambulation was permitted (e.g. to the toilet). Fluids were encouraged. Exclusions were emergency studies, children under 15 years, known significant sensitivity to contrast, mentally disturbed or unco-operative patients, and known epileptics. Drugs known to lower the seizure threshold were witheld for 24 h. Because of the way in which surgery for lumbar disc disease is organised in this centre, and the exclusion of acute cases, only 14 patients underwent surgery during the study period, precluding full evaluation of their data.

Group 2

One hundred patients recruited in Hull were part of a blind comparative trial of iohexol and iotrolan. Their consent was obtained for admission into a randomised clinical trial, and this could have generated some anxiety. Myelographic technique exclusions were the same as in group 1. As in that group, 3 ml CSF were removed and contrast medium dose was 10 ml 240 mg/I (per millilitre). Aftercare was for the patient to sit with three pillows in bed for 3 h, and then to be semisupine in bed for 12 h. Ambulation was discouraged. These patients were interviewed in detail 4 and 24 h after myelography and subjected to a neurological examination. This was performed by an investigator who was "blind" to the myelographic details. Prior to being discharged the patients were given a questionnaire. If the questionnaire was not returned after 2 weeks the patient was contacted again by letter and if necessary by telephone.

Results

Group 1

Forty-nine percent of patients were female; hence there is no sex bias in this group. Of the female patients 68.4% were symptomatic, as were 53.5% of the males. Headache was considered moderate if analgesics were required;

Table 1. Lumbar myelography – side-effects in hospital

610 Patients	22-Gauge needle	
% Patients with:	Iohexol	Iopamidol
Headache	19	25
Nausea/vomiting	6	7
Exacerbation of pain	12	14

(Lamb et al. 1985)

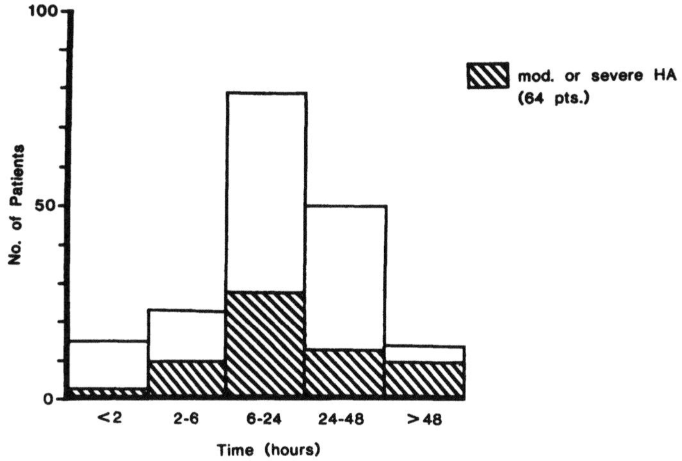

Fig. 1. Time of onset of headache in 181 patients in group 1; ▧, moderate or severe headache (64 patients)

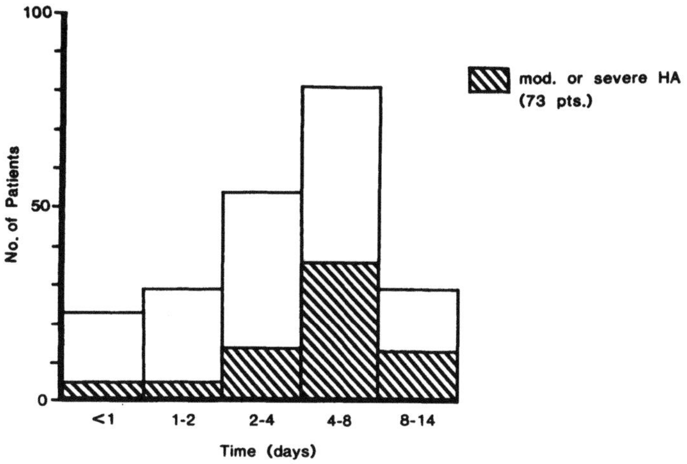

Fig. 2. Duration of headache in 216 patients in group 1; ▧, moderate or severe headache (73 patients)

severe headache caused the patient to return to bed. The subgroups of headaches are mutually exclusive. We cannot assess accurately from our data how many headaches were genuinely postural. Many patients reported exacerbation of back or leg pain which they did not believe was part of their underlying clinical problem. Lassitude, dizziness, faintness, depression, agitation and disturbed sleep have been grouped together as "emotional" symptoms. Side-effects are shown in Table 2, and for males and females separately in Table 3.

Other side-effects reported but not shown in the Tables were photophobia in 4 patients, blurred or distorted vision in 8, altered sense of hearing in 11, a rash in 4, and diarrhoea in 3; muscle jerks or twitches were reported by 20 patients but were relatively short lived.

Symptoms attributed to the myelogram occurred in 309 patients, 75% of whom suffered headache, and of those suffering from headaches 75% also had other symptoms. Of the symptomatic patients, 54% complained of exacerbated back or leg pain. Thirteen patients (2.6%) were severely incapacitated, i. e. they called their general practitioner or the X-ray department to complain of their symptoms.

In the 233 patients suffering from headache, good data on the time of onset were available in 181 and on its duration in 216; the proportions were similar in the subgroups with moderate and severe headaches. These are summarised in Figs. 1 and 2. The duration of exacerbated back or leg pain is summarised in Fig. 3, but we have insufficient data to analyse the onset of that symptom.

Group 2

We obtained 94 questionnaires (6% loss). Four patients had surgery shortly after the study, and 2 could not be traced. Of those in whom results were available, 47 received iotrolan and 47 iohexol. The mean age in the iotrolan group was 43 years (25 male, 22 female) and in the iohexol group 42 years (20 male, 27 female). In the total group of 94 patients 52.1% were female.

Table 2. Group 1 – side effects

		%
Headache:	mild	31.0
	moderate	12.6
	severe	2.4
Mild nausea		8.5
Severe nausea and/or vomiting		8.5
Exacerbation of leg/back pain		32.9
Emotional symptoms		26.2

Table 3. Group 1 – side effects analysed by sex

	% of female patients	% of male patients
Headache mild	32.8	29.1
Headache moderate/severe	17.6	12.4
Nausea/vomiting	22.8	11.2
Back/leg pain	36.8	29.1
Emotional symptoms	32.8	19.8

Table 4. Group 2 – headaches

		Iotrolan (47)	Iohexol (47)
On ward	mild	18	6
	moderate	6	7
	severe	0	2
At home	mild	9	13
	moderate	8	9
	severe	1	1

Table 5. Group 2 – side-effects at home

		%
Headache	mild	22
	moderate	17
	severe	2
Mild nausea		7
Severe nausea/vomiting		12
Exacerbation of back/leg pain		26
Emotional symptoms		33

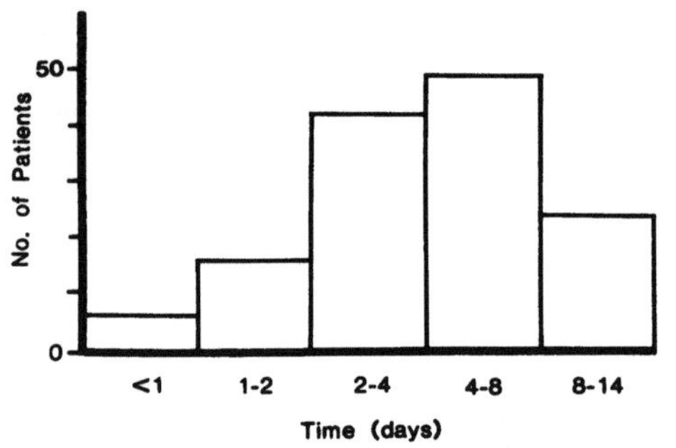

Fig. 3. Duration of back or leg pain in 137 patients in group 1

Headache in this group is shown in Table 4. The only significant difference between the contrast agents is for "mild headaches". The numbers of all other side-effects were very similar, and the results for the combined group of 94 patients are shown in Table 5.

Sixty-one patients (65% of the total) had at least one symptom at home. Of these a small proportion (23%) had been entirely well whilst in hospital. Of these symptomatic patients, 72% were polysymptomatic. Eight patients were considered to be severely distressed at home.

Discussion

Results in group 1 could have been influenced by the fact that not all questionnaires were returned, but group 2 is a tightly controlled group with a high response rate. The incidence of reported side-effects at home is very similar (e.g. group 1 total headaches 46%, group 2 43%).

All symptoms were reported more commonly by women, confirming previous observations. Incapacitating symptoms were equally distributed in group 2, but females predominated in group 1 (8 females, 5 males). The high incidence of incapacitating side-effects reported in group 2 may reflect the close attention given to these patients. It does nevertheless give an accurate indication of the numbers of myelogram patients who need to contact their general practitioner or other medical attendant after they have been discharged home. This result is almost identical to that reported by Davies et al. [8]. Of the patients in group 2 who sought further medical attention after being discharged, 2 had been entirely well for the first 24 h; indeed only half the patients had significant symptoms whilst on the ward.

Patients in group 1 were permitted to be ambulant immediately after the myelogram. Despite this, the onset of headaches was delayed for more than 24 h in 35% of the patients (Table 4 – total headache and moderate/severe headache). Thus many patients did not develop symptoms until they had returned home.

Many patients suffer symptoms which last for a week or even longer, and very similar findings are noted for total headache, moderate/severe headache, and for exacerbation of pain (Figs. 2, 3). The design of these studies does not permit analysis of symptoms lasting more than 2 weeks but there is clearly a small "tail" to the histogram in Figs. 2 and 3).

In conclusion, results based on a questionnaire carry risks of inaccuracy. Any method of assessing symptoms after myelography is subjective and susceptible to bias. We should accept what patients tell us about their investigation. Much patient suffering is occurring at home. Primary care doctors are aware of many of these patients, but the radiologists and hospital specialists are usually sheltered from their protests. We would like to know how frequently complaints would be made by patients undergoing diagnostic lumbar puncture if they were presented with our questionnaire in similar circumstances. One cannot obtain a strictly comparable group but we are pursuing a study of this nature.

Whatever contribution to side-effects originates from the contrast medium and to what extent the lumbar puncture is responsible is irrelevant from the patient's point of view. Myelography remains an unpleasant investigation. Many patients are less than enthusiastic to have myelography repeated. This is important at a time when noninvasive techniques are becoming more widely available.

Acknowledgements. We would like to thank S. Bingham for typing the manuskript.

References

1. Sand T (1989) Which factors affect reported headache incidence after lumbar myelography? Neuroradiology 31: 55–59
2. Maly P (1989) Sex and age related difference in post-myelographic adverse reactions. Neuroradiology 31: 331–335
3. Macpherson P, Teasdale E, Macpherson PY (1983) Radiculography: is routine bed rest really necessary. Clinical Radiol 34: 325–326
4. Kuuliala IK, Göransson HJ (1987) Adverse reactions after iohexol lumbar myelography: influence and postprocedural positioning. AJR 149: 389–390
5. Sykes RHD, Wasenaar W, Clark P (1981) Incidence of adverse effects following metrizamide myelography in nonambulatory and ambulatory patients. Radiology 138: 625–627
6. Sand T, Myhr G, Stovner LJ, Dale LG, Tangerud A (1989) Side effects after ambulatory lumbar iohexol myelography. Neuroradiology 31: 49–54
7. Skalpe IO, Nakstad P (1988) Myelography with iohexol (Omnipaque); a clinical report with special reference to the adverse effects Neuroradiology 30: 169–174
8. Davies AM, Evans N, Chandy J (1989) Outpatient lumbar radiculography: comparison of iopamidol and iohexol and a literature review. Br J Radiol 62: 716–723
9. Tourtellotte WW, Henderson WG, Tucker RP, Gillano O, Walker JE, Kokman E (1972) A randomized double-blind clinical trial comparing the 22 versus 26 gauge needle in the production of the post -lumbar puncture syndrome in normal individuals. Headache 12: 73–78
10. Sand T, Stovner LJ, Dale L, Salvesen R (1987) Side effects after diagnostic lumbar puncture and lumbar iohexol myelography. Neuroradiology 29: 385–388

Dr. R. Bartlett
Department of Radiology
Hull Royal Infirmary, Anlaby Road
Hull, Yorkshire, UK

Neuroradiology (1991) 33 [Suppl]: 95–96

Neuro radiology
© Springer-Verlag 1991

CT of the postoperative lumbar spine: is contrast enhancement necessary?

C. S. McKinstry and K. E. Bell

Department of Neuroradiology, Royal Victoria Hospital, Belfast, UK

Summary. Thirty-eight lumbar disc levels were re-explored following CT in patients with a failed back surgery syndrome. Comparison of the noncontrast CT (NCCT) and contrast-enhanced CT (CECT) with the operative findings showed that in the majority of cases, NCCT was sufficient for diagnosis. CECT was useful in confirming the extent of epidural fibrosis. A major source of error using both techniques was the presence of undetected disc fragments embedded in scar tissue.

Key words: Lumbar disc – Computed tomography – Contrast media

Following the advent of high-resolution CT, interpretation of the findings in patients with a failed back surgery syndrome (FBSS) was based on the known appearances of virgin disc prolapse on noncontrast CT (NCCT) [1]. Subsequently, use of intravenous contrast medium was reported to improve the accuracy of the technique [2–4]. More recently, the need for routine enhancement to distinguish recurrent disc prolapse from fibrosis has been questioned, although as in most such studies the number of re-explorations to confirm the CT prediction was small [5]. Our aim was to assess the accuracy of NCCT and contrast-enhanced CT (CECT) in a series of surgically verified cases.

Table 1. Noncontrast CT and surgical findings

Diagnosis	CT	Surgery
Disc protrusion	13	11
Epidural fibrosis	7	5
Bony stenosis	8	8
Pseudomeningocele	1	1
Bone fragment	1	1
Indeterminate	8	
Total	38	

Table 2. NCCT indeterminate: contrast-enhanced CT and surgical findings

Diagnosis	CT	Surgery
Epidural fibrosis	5	4
Disc protrusion and fibrosis	1	1
Indeterminate	2	Fibrosis and disc fragment

Methods and results

One hundred and two consecutive CT studies were performed on 100 patients at 131 previously explored disc levels, between 6 months and 13 years after surgery. Thirty-eight levels were subsequently re-explored within 7 months of CT, and these form the basis of this report.

Results of NCCT and comparison with the findings at re-exploration are shown in Table 1. Where an extradural soft tissue abnormality was seen at the disc margin with possible compromise of the adjacent nerve root or thecal sac, differentiation between "true" recurrent disc protrusion and epidural fibrosis was made on the basis of the morphology of the tissue and its density. Recurrent disc protrusion indented or displaced neural tissue and had a density of over 65 CT units (Fig. 1): fibrosis retracted or engulfed neural tissue and did not measure over 50 CT units (Fig. 2). Material not fitting these criteria was designated as indeterminate.

All patients with possible disc prolapse or fibrosis were given a bolus of 100 ml intravenous contrast medium (Niopam 300, Merck) and rescanned immediately. Enhancement was confirmed by a rise of at least 10 CT units in density. CECT did not alter a firm NCCT diagnosis (Fig. 1, 2) but was useful in those which were indeterminate on NCCT, mainly in confirming the presence of significant epidural fibrosis. In one case, a large recurrent fragment with a rim of enhancing fibrosis was seen (Fig. 3).

NCCT was incorrect at four levels. In two, recurrent disc prolapse was suspected: at one an epidural vein was found which had not enhanced on CECT. In this patient a significant delay had occurred between contrast injection and repeat scanning. In the second, the surgeon reported a bulging degenerate disc and it is felt that positional factors may have been responsible as CT was always done in the supine position. At two other levels, small fragments were found within the suspected epidural fibrosis.

CECT was incorrect at one level in missing a small disc fragment within fibrosis. Two levels remained indeterminate and small fragments with fibrosis were again found.

Discussion

Infrequent causes of FBSS such as bony stenosis can be diagnosed on NCCT; however, in most cases distinction must be made between recurrent disc protrusion and epidural scar tissue. It is also important to recognise the difference between a "true" recurrent disc protrusion (Fig. 1) and small disc fragment or fragments buried in epidural scar.

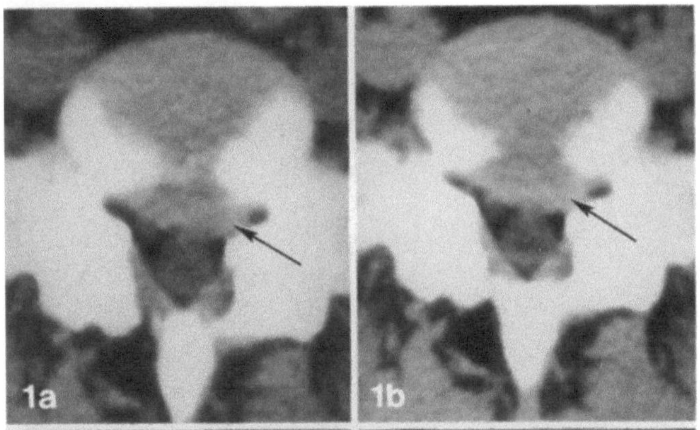

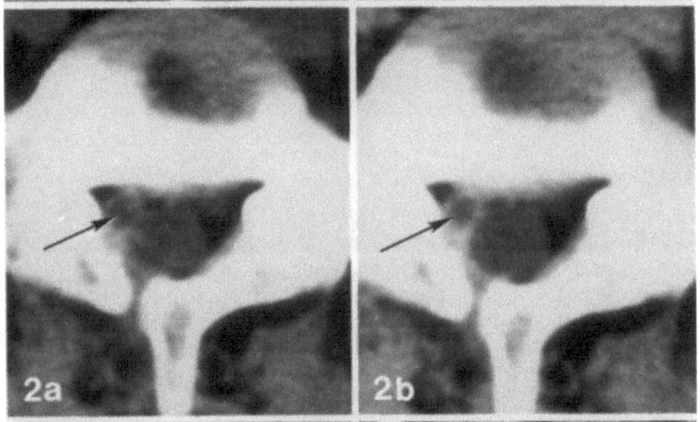

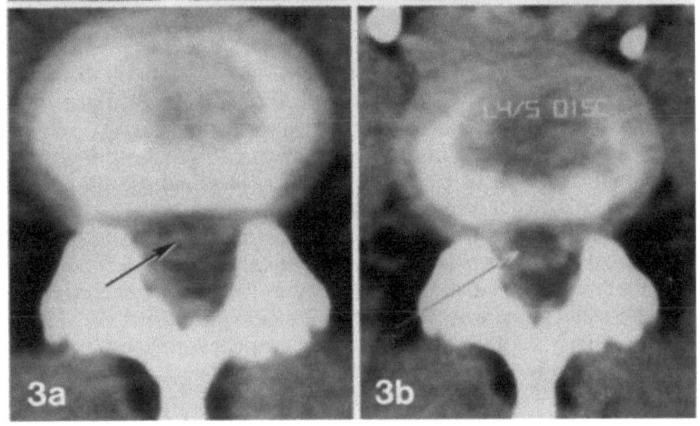

Fig. 1 a, b. A 36-year-old man complaining of back pain and sciatica following a lifting strain. Noncontrast CT (NCCT) (**a**) and contrast-enhanced CT (CECT) (**b**) at level of previous microsurgical discectomy 6 years previously. Dense (> 65 CT units) recurrent disc protrusion *(arrow)* displaces nerve root (compare normal side) on NCCT. Nonenhancement on NECT did not alter diagnosis

Fig. 2 a, b. A 40-year-old man with low back pain following laminectomy and discectomy 4 years previously. NCCT (**a**) shows scarring at laminectomy site and retraction of thecal sac. Note low density nerve root *(arrow)* which is highlighted by enhancing fibrosis on CECT. However, CECT has not altered diagnosis

Fig. 3 a, b. A 30-year-old woman with low back pain radiating to right foot and ankle 2 years after previous discectomy. NCCT (**a**) suggests soft tissue mass at posterior disc margin *(arrow)*, but density is indeterminate and configuration is unclear. CECT (**b**) confirms presence of large nonenhancing disc protrusion with rim of fibrosis, indenting thecal sac *(arrow)*

"Mass-like" scar tissue has been described which may simulate a recurrent disc protrusion [2, 6, 7], and also use of density measurements on NCCT has been questioned [8]. However, in our large series of surgically confirmed cases, true recurrent disc protrusion was reliably diagnosed on NCCT, when technical factors were taken into account. The major problem is to decide whether a small disc fragment is present within epidural scar tissue. Both NCCT and CECT were able to predict the presence of scar, but both had difficulty in excluding the presence of small fragments. Differentiation from engulfed nerve root can sometimes be made [6, 7] but is frequently difficult [3, 8].

A recent study has indicated that differentiation of true recurrent disc protrusion from the presence of significant epidural fibrosis is the main prognostic indicator for re-exploration, whether or not small disc fragments are present within the fibrotic material [9]. Selective use of CECT in FBSS would therefore be even more appropriate under these circumstances.

References

1. Teplick JG, Haskin ME (1983) Computed tomography of the postoperative lumbar spine. AJR 141: 865–884
2. Schubiger O, Valavanis A (1982) CT differentiation between recurrent disc herniation and postoperative scar formation: the value of contrast enhancement. Neuroradiology 22: 251–254
3. Brown BM, Bedell JE, Frank E (1986) Contrast enhanced computed tomography scanning of the postoperative spine. Surg Neurol 25: 351–356
4. Schell GR, Modesti LM, Cacayorin ED (1986) Diagnostic value of computed tomography in recurrent pain after discectomy. Neurosurgery 20: 302–309
5. Dixon AK, Bannon RP (1987) Computed tomography of the postoperative lumbar spine: the need for, and optimal dose of, intravenous contrast medium. Br J Radiol 60: 215–222
6. Schubiger O, Valavanis A (1983) Postoperative lumbar CT: technique, results and indications. AJNR 4: 595–597
7. Teplick JG, Haskin ME (1984) Intravenous contrast-enhanced CT of the lumbar spine. AJR 143: 845–855
8. Braun IF, Hoffmann JC, Davis PC, Landman JA, Tindall GT (1985) Contrast enhancement in CT differentiation between recurrent disc herniation and postoperative scar: prospective study. AJR 145: 785–790
9. Ebeling U, Kalbarcyk H, Reuben HJ (1989) Microsurgical reoperation following lumbar disc surgery. J Neurosurg 70: 397–404

Dr. C. S. McKinstry
Department of Neuroradiology
Royal Victoria Hospital
Grosvenor Road
Belfast BT12 6BA, UK

Neuroradiology (1991) 33 [Suppl]: 97–98

Neuro radiology
© Springer-Verlag 1991

Recurrent herniations following surgery: the significance of MRI in 90 cases

D. Krause, J. L. Drape, P. Boyer, and J. Tongio

Departments of Radiology and Neurosurgery, University Hospital, Strasbourg, France

Summary. The authors present a series of 90 patients investigated using CT and MRI for recurrent lumbosciatic pain following disc surgery. Diagnostic conclusions based on CT sections alone were not apparent; CT was insufficient in one-third of cases. MRI combined with intravenous gadolinium can distinguish between ordinary postoperative scar tissue and a possible recurrent disc fragment. This study underlines the incidence of fibrosis combined with herniation (i.e. 46%).

Key words: Scar tissue – Fibrosis – Recurrent herniation – Magnetic resonance imaging – Gadolinium

Scar formation and recurrent herniation are the most frequent causes of persistent or recurrent pain following disc surgery. Scar formation following surgery is commonplace and cannot be immediately incriminated in the recurrence of symptoms following lumbar surgery.

Clinical and radiological investigations often only permit a tentative diagnosis, especially since a herniation and scar may be associated. Differentiation between the two important, since they determine the therapeutic approach and the prognosis. MRI has already proven its reliability in this particular field; the aim of this study was to demonstrate its capabilities in a series of patients investigated postoperatively [1–4].

Patients and methods

In 1988 and 1989 90 patients previously operated upon for disc herniation were investigated by CT and MRI. In 23, the examinations were performed within 6 months surgery; the interval was greater for the remaining 67 (from 6 months to a few years). There were 37 women and 53 men, with a mean age of 43.7 years. The pain prompting radiological work-up had evolved over several weeks on average, and in 75% of cases was typical L5 or S1 radicular pain. L4 (2); L5 (28); S1 (39); and L5 + S1 (12). Isolated pain was less commonly found (9).

Computed tomography. Millimetric sections (1.5 mm thick) are aimed at detecting a mass effect on the root, which is particularly difficult to do within the fibrosis.

Magnetic resonance imaging [5–10]. After disc surgery, we used the following protocol: 1. Sagittal T1-weighted SE sections, 2. Sagittal T1-weighted sections after the administration of gadolinium-DTPA, 3. Axial T1-weighted SE sections.

Results

Of our 90 patients, 62 had CT interpretations concordant with the MRI results: isolated herniation (11); herniation and fibrosis (27); and isolated fibrosis (24; with bulging in 10). In the 28 other patients (31%), CT was insufficient to reach a conclusion, resulting in a high rate of false positives and false negatives.

1. Fibrosis: In 70 patients fibrosis gave poor contrast; it was hypointense (22) or isointense (40) in comparison to the disc; it was less often hyperintense (8). 2. Enhancement by gadolinium: In 23 patients investigated within 6 months of surgery, fibrosis enhanced in 75% and the operated disc in 43%. In 67 patients explored after an interval of at least 6 months, enhancement rates were lower: fibrosis 53%, and disc 40%. 3. MRI and the diagnosis of fibrosis-herniation: There was a normal appearance in 8% of the patients; isolated herniation in 10%; herniation and fibrosis, which were well differentiated, in 46%; and isolated fibrosis in 36% (with bulging in 18%). 4. Visualization of nerve roots: The nerve roots were well visualized by CT in 60 patients (66%) and by MRI in 81 (90%). The combination of herniation and fibrosis was the most frequent finding (46%). 5. MRI vs CT (Fig. 1): Differences in analysis involved 28 cases considered difficult to evaluate using CT, giving false positives or negatives. The major problem was that of isolated fibrosis, which was better shown with MRI [15]. Fibrosis may conceal a herniation (9 false negatives). However, MRI has certain limitations: 4 unresolved cases, with CT being more informative in 2 of them.

Discussion

In cases of recurrent pain following disc surgery, MRI is a more capable technique than CT for differentiating a herniated fragment from epidural fibrosis. Its sensitivity may reach 96% if sagittal and axial sections are performed early after injection of gadolinium. Investigations using T1-weighted sequences are more rapid; T2-weighted sequences are not indispensable.

The following characterized the operated segment. Scar tissue enhanced strongly early in 80%. The enhancement was heterogeneous during the first few minutes and subsequently became homogeneous. Contiguous disc

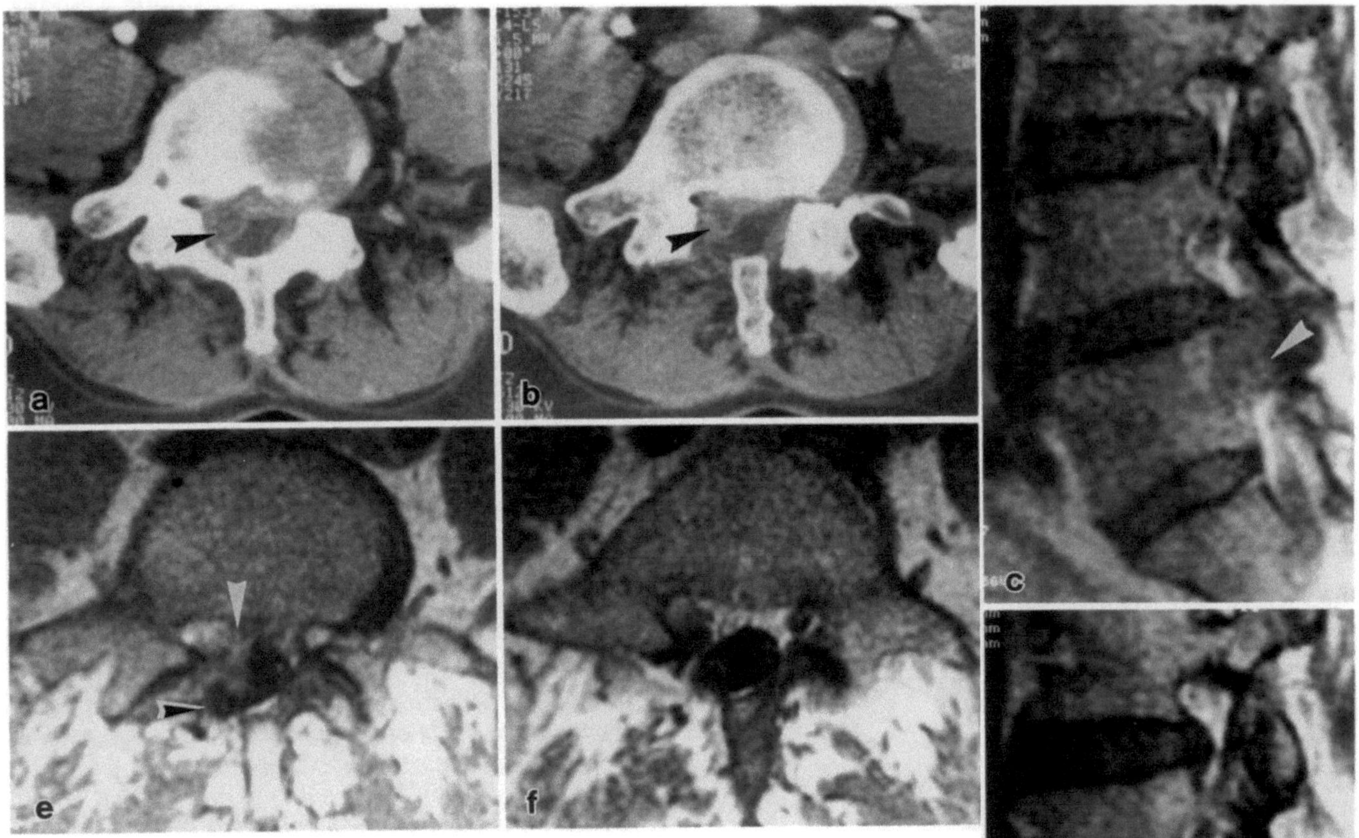

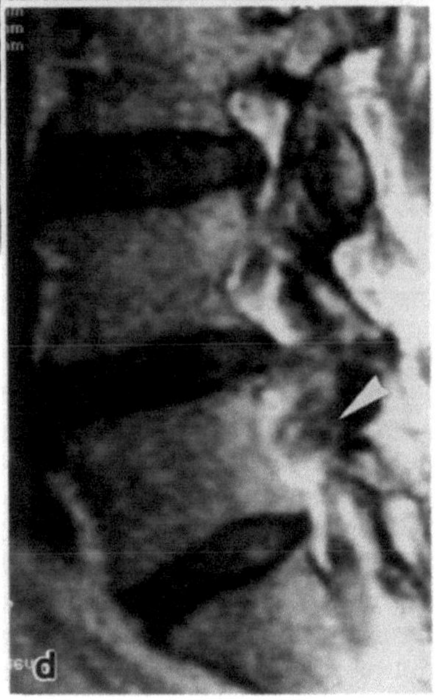

Fig. 1a–f. A 56-year-old patient. Intervention for L4–5 right disc herniation 6 months previously. New recurrence of sciatica with a motor deficit. **a, b** CT with iodinated contrast injection: probably hypodense free fragment within the lateral recess, surrounded by the contrast *(arrowhead)*. L5 root is not clearly distinguished opposite the fenestration (hemi-laminectomy). **c** Right lateral sagittal section (T1-weighted SE): filling in of the pedicular region by low signal material *(arrowhead)*. **d** Same section after gadolinium-DTPA: enhancement of the scar tissue surrounding the nerve root or a large free fragment? *(arrowhead)*. **e, f** Axial sections. All the lateral recess is obscured by a disc fragment. L5 root is still recognizable (hyposignal of the sheath) behind the extruded fragment

fragments were perfectly identified in almost all cases. In half the cases, there was a delayed enhancement of the end-plates and disc beginning at 30 min.

References

1. Bundschuh CV, Modic MT, Ross JS, Masaryk TJ, Bohlmann H (1988) Epidural fibrosis and recurrent disc herniation in the lumbar spine: MR imaging assessment. AJNR 9: 169–178
2. Crouzet G, Bronnier L, Vasdev A, Lebas GF (1990) IRM et hernie discale lombaire. Acquisitions rhumatologiques. La hernie discale lombaire. Masson, Paris, pp 60–72
3. Drape JL, Krause D, Martin JC, Tongio J, Maitrot D, Buchheit F, Vautravers P (1990) Récidives herniaires postchirurgicales. Intérêt de l'IRM. Acquisitions rhumatologiques. La hernie discale lombaire. Masson, Paris, pp 345–351
4. Frocrain L, Duvauferrier R, Charles G, Ramee A, Pawolotsky Y (1987) Intérêt de l'imagerie par résonance magnétique dans le diagnostic des lombosciatiques récidivantes post-operatoires. J Radiol 68: 385–391
5. Hochhauser L, Kieffer SA, Cacayorin ED, Petro GR, Teller WF (1988) Recurrent postdiskectomy low back pain: MR-surgical correlation. AJNR 9: 769–774
6. Hueftle MG, Modic MT, Ross JS (1988) Lumbar spine: postoperative MR imaging with Gd-DTPA. Radiology 167: 817–824
7. Krause D, Drape JL, Woerly B, Kardous N, Tongio J (1988) Hernies discales lombaires: intérêt des coupes obliques en résonance magnétique nucléaire. J Neuroradiol 15: 305–324
8. Krause D, Drape JL, Woerly B, Maitrot D, Tongio J (1990) CT and MRI of disc herniations. Springer, Berlin Heidelberg New York
9. Picard L, Bracard S, Chevrot A, Prere J, Valk J Rachis opéré. Imagerie du rachis et de la moëlle. Vigot, Paris, pp 725–729
10. Ross JS, Delamarter R, Hueftle MG, Masaryk TJ, Aikawa M, Carter J, Vandyke C, Modic MT (1989) Gadolinium DTPA enhanced MR imaging of the post-operative lumbar spine: time course and mechanisms of enhancement. ANR 10: 37–46

Dr. D. Krause
Departments of Radiology and Neurosurgery
University Hospital, Strasbourg, France

Neuroradiology (1991) 33 [Suppl]: 99–100

Neuro
radiology
© Springer-Verlag 1991

Gadolinium-DTPA-enhanced MRI of the asymptomatic postdiscectomy lumbar spine: early postoperative results

N. Roosen[1], T. Kahn[2], M. Messing[1], R. P. Trappe[2], U. Moedder[2], E. Lins[1], and W. J. Bock[1]

Departments of [1] Neurosurgery and [2] Diagnostic Radiology, University Hospital, Heinrich-Heine-University Düsseldorf, Düsseldorf, Federal Republic of Germany

Summary. We studied 30 patients with an uncomplicated clinical course after surgery for lumbar disc herniation, using gadolinium (Gd)-DTPA-enhanced 0.35 T spin-echo MRI within 4–12 days of operation: the goal was to define the normal healing process following this type of surgery. At surgery we found disc protrusion (10%), herniation (57%), or sequestration (33%). Postoperative MRI demonstrated major protrusion in 4% and minor protrusion in 27%. There was strong epidural enhancement in 83% and moderate enhancement in 17%. The enhancing tissue had mass effect in 67% of cases. Delineation of intraspinal structures was excellent after administration of Gd-DTPA. Although Gd-DTPA-enhanced MRI of the postdiscectomy lumbar spine gives good visualization of the intraspinal space, the rather high incidence of abnormalities seen on MRI in asymptomatic patients clearly demonstrates that post-operative assessment still depends strongly upon clinical examination, and that neuroimaging, however sophisticated, has a complementary role in the process of medical decision making.

Key words: Magnetic resonance imaging – Gadolinium-DTPA – Lumbar spine – Intervertebral disc herniation

---

Although surgery for herniated lumbar disc is widely performed, assessment of outcome is not straightforward and depends upon a wide variety of factors [1]. Modern imaging techniques such as CT and MRI promised to facilitate postoperative study of patients, due to their ability to depict soft tissues with great detail. However, with regard to CT, clinical studies were disappointing [2, 3]. MRI has not yet been studied extensively and relatively few reports have been published, usually involving longterm follow-up of symptomatic patients [4]. Therefore, to complement our previous studies on early CT evaluation of asymptomatic postdiscectomy patients [3], we initiated a prospective clinical study using gadolinium (Gd)-DTPA-enhanced MRI to examine the normal course of healing after surgery for herniated lumbar intervertebral disc. Knowledge of normal findings should give base-line information against which to judge MRI results in symptomatic patients.

Patients and methods

We studied 30 patients with an uncomplicated clinical course after lumbar intervertebral disc surgery. Their mean age was 46 years, range 26–70 years. The discs involved were: L5–S1 39%, L4–5 50%, and L3–4 11%.

MRI was performed with a Diasonics 0.35 T superconductive imager. We obtained axial and sagittal slices using T1- and T2-weighted spin-echo pulse sequences (SE 500/30 and SE 2000/40–80). T1-weighted images were acquired before and after i. v. administration of 0.1 mmol/kg body weight Gd-DTPA. MRI examination was carried out within 4–12 days of surgery.

The operative findings were categorized as disc protrusion (bulging), herniation (clear extension and extrusion of disc material through the annulus fibrosus or even through the posterior longitudinal ligament), or sequestration (free sequestrum within the spinal canal).

Postoperative MRI was studied with special attention to persisting protrusion of disc material (major or minor), epidural contrast enhancement (strong, moderate, slight or absent), mass effect, and visibility of normal intraspinal structures (nerve roots, etc...).

Results

At operation we found 10% disc protrusion, 57% herniation, and 33% sequestration. MRI signs of persistent protrusion were seen in 31% of cases: major in 4%, and minor in 27%.

All patients demonstrated epidural enhancement after Gd administration, marked in 83%, and moderate in 17% of cases. The enhancing tissue had mass effect in 67% of patients. Due to this enhancement visibility of intraspinal structures such as nerve roots was tremendously increased. Enhancing tissue was not confined to the intraspinal space, but extended extraspinally along the surgical approach, well into the subcutaneous tissue.

Case report

A 34-year-old man presented with acute pain in the right S1 dermatome, which had occurred during heavy physical work about 4 weeks earlier. During recent years he had episodes of low back pain, but never had radicular pain.

Examination revealed hypaesthesia and hypalgesia in the right S1 dermatome. The ankle jerk was absent on the right. There was no weakness. Straight leg raising was reduced to 45 °. The lumbar spine was immobile and its musculature tender to palpation. CT demonstrated a disc herniation at L5–S1 on the right.

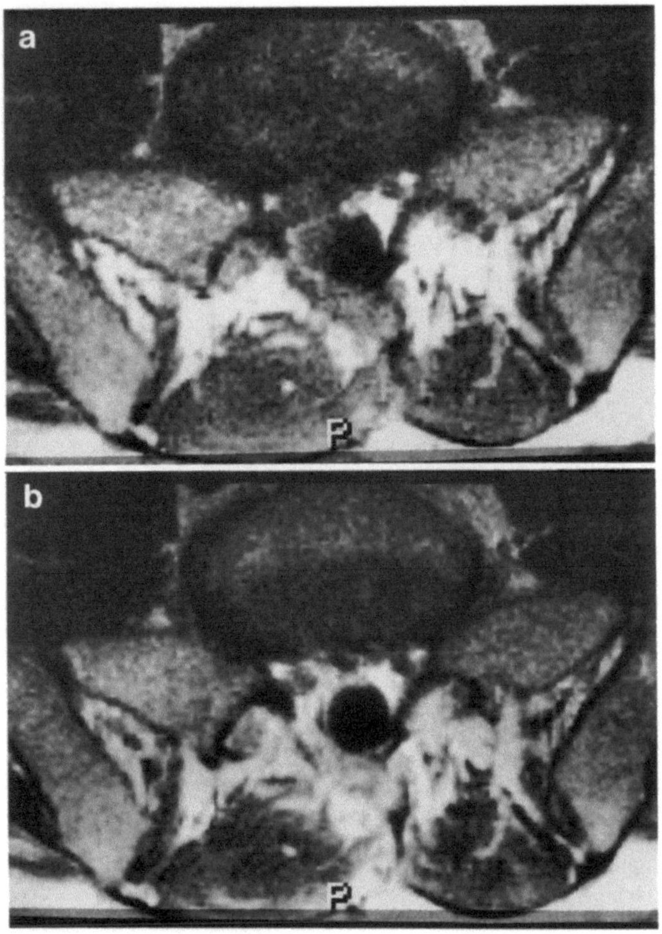

Fig. 1 a, b. Axial T1-weighted image of the L5–S1 disc space at the 9th post-operative day. The non-enhanced image (**a**) is not as informative as the gadolinium (Gd)-DTPA-enhanced scan (**b**). The intraspinal structures such as the nerve root, the border of the disc space, and the anterolateral border of the dural sac, are seen well on the Gd-DTPA-enhanced MR image

At operation a multisequestrated disc herniation was found (17 October 1989). The postoperative course was uneventful. The radicular symptoms disappeared, the patients was discharged after 1 week, and resumed work about 2 months later. At follow-up visit (5 April 1990) he was still doing very well.

Early postoperative MRI was performed on day 9. Axial T1-weighted images before and after Gd-DTPA (Fig. 1). demonstrated extensive epidural contrast enhancement, which resulted in good delineation of the posterior border of the disc space, of the right S1 nerve root, and of the dural sac. The contrast enhancement can be followed extending through the paravertebral muscles into the subcutaneous tissue.

Discussion

A multitude of reports on evaluation of failed back surgery have appeared [5, 6]. None, whether involving myelography, CT, or even MR, has yielded unequivocal criteria for establishing correct diagnoses; a major drawback is that most of these publications do not consider the normal healing process after low back surgery! Only knowledge of this normal healing after lumbar discectomy will allow us to evaluate symptomatic patients correctly.

Reports in the literature as well as our own experience with early postoperative CT in asymptomatic patients suggest that in at least 50% of cases no useful information on the intraspinal situation can be obtained due to "blurry" pictures, and that clear images are seen in at most 10%–15% of cases [3, 7]. A slight improvement might result from i. v. contrast medium; as far as we know, this has not been investigated in asymptomatic patients.

The only published MRI study in asymptomatic early-postdiscectomy patients concerns ten patients [8]: five demonstrated persisting disc protrusion, and Gd-DTPA administration was very helpful in delineating intraspinal structures. Enhancement was found in all cases. The results in our 30 patients confirm the findings of Steiner [8].

Therefore, we think it essential for the clinician and the radiologist to be aware of the relatively high incidence of MRI abnormalities in asymptomatic patients in the early postoperative period. This means that the clinical condition of the patient (i. e., pain? paresis? deterioration? amelioration?) should be the primary criterion for further decision making on the future management of that individual patient!

References

1. Waddell G, Reilly S, Torsney B, Allan DB, Morris EW, Di Paola MP, Birchner M, Finlayson D (1988) Assessment of the outcome of low back surgery. J Bone Joint Surg [Br] 70: 723–727
2. Cervellini P, Curri D, Volpin L, Bernardi L, Pinna V, Benedetti A (1988) Computed tomography of epidural fibrosis after discectomy: a comparison between symptomatic and asymptomatic patients. Neurosurgery 23: 710–713
3. Roosen N, Botzenhard A, Lins E, Bock WJ (1987) Computed tomography (CT) findings during the first two weeks after uncomplicated surgery for lumbar disk herniation. In: Calabro A, Leonardi M (eds) Computer aided neuroradiology. CIC Edizioni Internazionali, Rome, pp 507–510
4. Sotiropoulos S, Chafetz NI, Lang P, Winkler M, Morris JM, Weinstein PR, Genant HK (1989) Differentiation between postoperative scar and recurrent disc herniation: prospective comparison of MR, CT, and contrast-enhanced CT. AJNR 10: 639–643
5. Burton CV, Kirkaldy-Willis WH, Yong-Hing K, Heitthoff KB (1981) Causes of failure of surgery on the lumbar spine. Clin Orthop 157: 191–199
6. Ros JS, Modic MT, Masaryk TJ, Hueftle MG (1988) The postoperative lumbar spine. Semin Roentgenol 13: 125–136
7. Hammer B, Boehm-Jurkovic H, Nedden D zur, Valencak E, Moshenipour I (1986) Der Wert der frühen postoperativen CT-Untersuchung nach lumbaler Bandscheibenoperation. ROEFO 145: 586
8. Steiner H (1989) MR-Tomographie nach lumbalen Bandscheibenoperationen: differentialdiagnostische Möglichkeiten durch Gd-DTPA. ROEFO 151: 179–185

Dr. Norbert Roosen
Brain Tumor Research Center
Department of Neurosurgery
University of California
San Francisco, CA 94143, USA

SESSION 8
INFLAMMATORY DISEASES OF THE SPINE

Neuroradiology (1991) 33 [Suppl]: 102–105

Neuro radiology
© Springer-Verlag 1991

Cord atrophy in late-onset Pott's paraplegia

L. C. Handler and P. C. Corr

Neuroradiology Unit, Groote Schuur Hospital and University of Cape Town, Cape Town, South Africa

Summary. From a group of 171 patients with Pott's paraplegia, 40 with the myelographic feature of cord atrophy were selected for study. Constant associated features were peridural fibrosis and a variable holdup in contrast medium flow which amounted to nothing more than an incomplete block. Thirty-six had clinical evidence of "quiescent" late-onset Pott's paraplegia. Four were ascribed to the "reactivated" late-onset category. It is postulated that cord atrophy develops over a period of years and may be present before clinical features of cord decompensation manifest. It probably results in gradual progressive deterioration in cord function and militates against a successful outcome for anterior spinal fusion.

Key words: Pott's paraplegia, late-onset – Tuberculous spondylitis – Myelography – Spinal cord atrophy

As the disease progresses the clinical manifestations of tuberculous spondylitis change from those of backache and progressive truncal deformity to paraparesis or worse. The incidence of the disease itself and the frequency with which it causes cord compression are in large measure dependent on the socioeconomic status of the geographical region, the availability of adequate treatment and the nature of the referral hospital. Large series have reported incidences of paraplegia in tuberculous spondylitis of 10.6% (Hong Kong 1964) [1], 16.2% Ulster (1970) [2], 20% (Egypt 1967) [3], 47% (South Africa 1987) [4], 60% (Saudi Arabia 1985) [5].

In most patients paraplegia is the result of active tuberculosis (TB); it develops within 2 years of onset of spondylitis and is known as acute-onset Pott's disease. Often this occurs during childhood. Occasionally reactivation of infection is the cause.

In a minority, maybe 20% of those with Pott's disease, paraparesis gradually develops in the absence of reactivation long after the subacute episode may have been forgotten [6]. A number of explanations have been offered [6, 7] and pathological description of the cord atrophy found in late-onset Pott's paraplegia are indeed scanty [6, 8, 9]

This report deals with the myelographic features of the quiescent type of late-onset Pott's paraplegia – a rather uncommon manifestation of burnt out tuberculous spondylitis.

Materials and methods

Over a 20-year period (1970–1989) virtually all cases of Pott's paraplegia had myelography. From amongst the 171 cases so studied 40 were found to have cord atrophy. Their clinical notes were studied to assess the temporal sequence of events, disease activity, operation and follow-up. Plain radiographs, myelograms and CT studies were independently reviewed. Signs of activity, the angle and radius of curvature of the kyphos were assessed on plain radiographs and narrowing of the contrast medium column and the enclosed cord were evaluated on myelography often aided by linear tomography. In 5 instances computed tomography (CT) was done and in 3 of these magnetic resonance imaging (MRI) as well.

Myelographic technique was directed at defining the width of the contrast medium column in the region of the gibbus and the cord diameter in sagittal and coronal planes. Initially iophendylate (Myodil) was used and, following the advent of nonionic agents, iohexol 300 × 15 ml have been used, both with equal success. The kyphotic segment was studied in the supine position and a horizontal X-ray beam was used for the lateral projection. Radiological review took place in the absence of specific clinical information (eg. evidence of reactivation).

Results

Clinical findings

All the patients were from the economically deprived section of the community with an average age of 30 years (range 3–66 years). Lower limb weakness and spasticity were present in 33 and paraplegia in 7. Cord symptoms had been present for periods that ranged from 1 to 16 years. Particular attention was paid to the latent interval since the initial spondylitis. Many patients had no recollection but in 16 the interval ranged between 2 and 49 years with an average of 23 years.

Reactivation of a tuberculous focus was also assessed. An elevated erythrocyte sedimentation rate (ESR) was recorded in 11, 4 of whom also had some backache. Radiological signs of activity were present in 4 of those with a raised ESR. In the other 36 healed tuberculous damage was the radiographic feature.

Myelography

Cord atrophy was a constant feature but its severity varied. Reduction in the coronal diameter of the cord varied between 1 mm and 5 mm (in 6 patients). Only 2 of those with marked atrophy were paraplegic and in 1 of these a myelogram done 8 years earlier (at which time he had

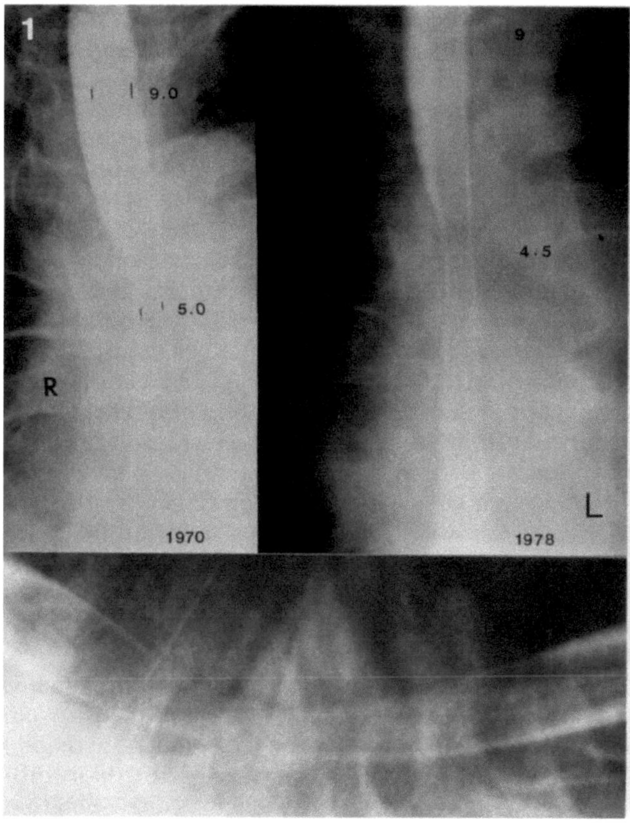

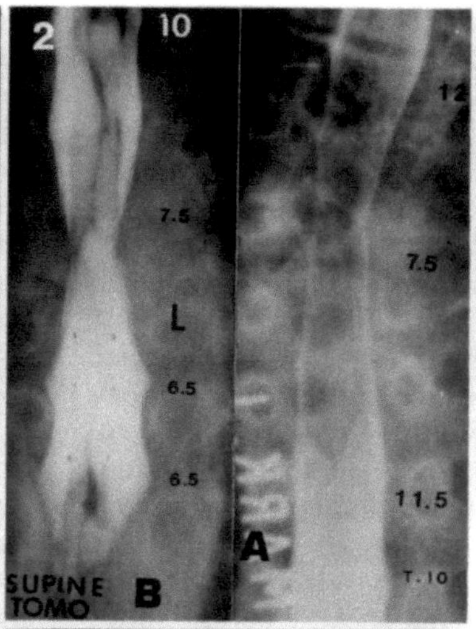

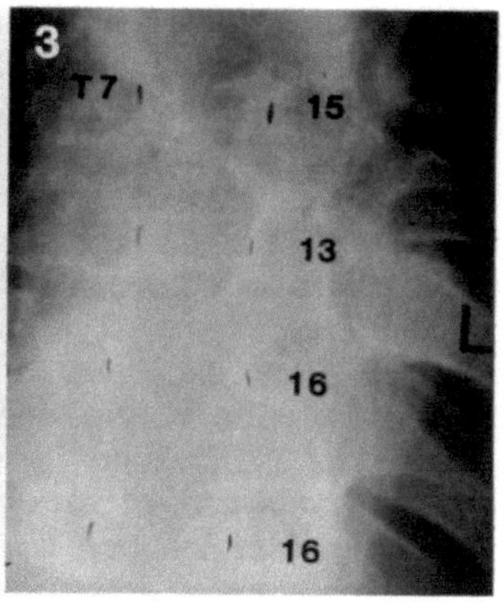

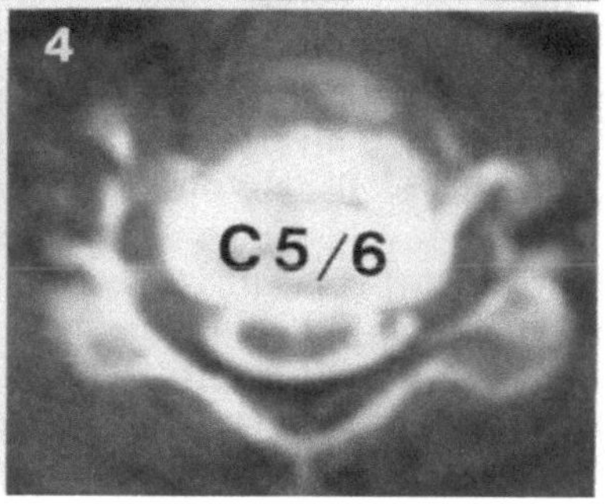

Fig. 1. Cord atrophy: coronal diameter of the cord was reduced from 9 mm to 5 mm and 4.5 mm. Associated loss of reserve resulted in deterioration of clinical function from mildly spastic gait to paraplegia over 8 years. Lateral view with patient supine demonstrated mild gibbus with large radius curvature. Male, 43 years in 1970. Latent interval: 30 years

Fig. 2 a, b. Cord atrophy and peridural fibrosis: **a** cord narrowed from 12 mm to 7.5 mm at apex kyphos. Peridural fibrosis has resulted in widening of the extradural space from T4 to T8. Subarachnoid space has been reduced from 13 to 8 mm.
Female, 8 years; latent interval unknown.
b Cord atrophy extends below the gibbus in another patient. Coronal diameter above the kyphos is 10 mm and below 6.5 mm. Contrast column has been narrowed by bony mass and peridural fibrosis.
Male, 26 years; latent interval: 21 years

Fig. 3. Growth disturbance has caused focal reduction in interpedicular distance at T8.
Male, 32 years with progressive paraparesis of 5 years' duration. Tuberculous spondylitis treated 23 years earlier at age 9 years

Fig. 4. CT: severe atrophy of cervical cord. The contrast-filled subarachnoid excluded a current compressive lesion. Female, years; latent interval: unknown

nothing more than a mildly progressive spastic gait of 5 years' duration), looked no different (Fig. 1).

Reduction of subarachnoid space in the region of the kyphos was a feature in virtually all. Here too the constriction varied and in some instances the space available for the cord was halved (Fig. 2a). This constriction was due to peridural fibrosis when the region was exposed at surgery (anterior spinal fusion).

Interpedicular distances were reduced in some of the diseased vertebrae in 19 patients. The reduction varied between 1 mm and 3 mm (Fig. 3). Posterior extension of the caries from its point of origin in a vertebral body into the pedicles, transverse processes or ribs was reported in 18.

Computed tomography was carried in 5 patients (Fig. 4). The bony destruction was slightly more extensive, especially posteriorly into the pedicles, than on plain films. The paravertebral mass was more readily appreciated but the canal contents were not. Only in children under age 5 years could invasion of the thecal canal by caseous material, but not the status of the cord be recognised. A quadriplegic with a midthoracic gibbus was shown to have a syrinx 6 h after intrathecal contrast medium had been instilled.

Magnetic resonance imaging studies in 4 patients were not of quality sufficient to identify demyelination or infarction in cords distorted and constricted by canals deformed by TB.

Discussion

The clinical features of this series are those of late-onset Pott's paraplegia [6, 9], also called perhaps more appropriately paraplegia of healing [10]. The salient features are those of a slowly progressive paraparesis developing after a latent period measured in years as was the situation in this series. In only 4 cases was it due to reactivation of the tuberculous process. In older series [6, 11] with less effective chemotherapy it was more commonly due to reactivated bone disease. Identification of activity was not an easy task because the disease seemed to grumble on without much clinical evidence – in our case backache was scarcely a prominent feature and although the ESR was raised it did not attain the high values seen during the acute phase of initial spondylitis. The radiological changes of activity, viz., a paravertebral mass and bony destruction with fuzzy ill-defined edges, were likewise muted and difficult to identify amongst the deformity and products of previous repair. Subtle clinical features and radiological signs pointed to reactivation in 4 patients, all of whom were paraplegic when investigated.

Myelographic features of late-onset Pott's disease have not been adequately reported because earlier authors [10] felt that the investigation had nothing to offer, probably because poor technique confused the issue [1, 9]. A recent report [12] included a series of 50 myelograms but no reference was made to the quiescent late-onset group.

The thinned atrophic segment of cord is peculiar to this condition and has not been identified in kyphoscoliotic patients with or without cord decompensation. (Cord diameters were measured in that entity to establish whether stretching was a causative factor). The severity of cord thinning did not correlate closely with the severity of paraparesis because only 1 of the 6 patients with severe atrophy was paraplegic. Another became paraplegic after a 7-year interval between myelograms, which showed minimal change in the interim (Fig. 1). Neither was there any correlation with the angle of the gibbus nor its radius of curvature.

Peridural fibrosis was the only feature that was consistently associated with cord atrophy and here there was a linear relationship (Fig. 1, 2). The concentric constriction of the contrast medium column in the kyphos due to peridural fibrosis resulted in a holdup in the flow of contrast medium, which was never complete and mostly of mild to moderate severity. Frequently it barely constituted much of an obstruction and often the holdup in flow was considered to be due to changes in spinal curvature rather than an extradural blockage.

The distinctive myelographic picture was therefore one of a cord tapering down to a coronal diameter of 5 mm or 6 mm over a distance of 30 mm or 40 mm within a contrast medium column that was also tapered over a similar distance.

CT (5 cases) (Fig. 4) and MRI (3 cases) have not yielded any more information regarding the nature of the cord lesion than a syrinx in one patient.

Pathogenesis

Very little unformation is available on the neuropathology, and that which is deals more with the tuberculous process penetrating the dura [11, 13]. Cord atrophy with a loss of differentiation between the grey and white matter, scanty blood vessels and perivascular fibrosis have been reported [6, 9]. Because of the unavailability of specimens the frequency of their occurrence and association with cord symptoms have not been determined. Much more is known about the peridural fibrosis because current surgical practice calls for complete exposure of the dural canal during anterior spinal fusion [8, 13]. A greyish membrane up to 5 mm thick constricts the dura and has been found even in those without clinical evidence of cord compression [14, 15]. Because peridural fibrosis was constantly associated it has been speculated that it played a causative role in the development of cord atrophy with ischaemia being the immediate cause. Once initiated by ischaemia or pressure the cord atrophy progressed without further stimulus resulting in slowly deteriorating lower limb function. Subtle vascular damage by cord movement over a gibbus during flexion and extension has been proposed and may be a contributory factor [7]. However, a sharp bony gibbus was an infrequent feature, and the cord certainly was not stretched because there was always collapse of more than one vertrebral body.

Bony destruction was obvious in the vertebral bodies but in 21 cases one or more pedicles were also destroyed. The narrowed interpedicular distance noted more readily on tomography than on CT must reflect a growth disturbance because it was observed in when bony disease started in childhood or early adolescence (Fig. 3).

Prognostic significance

What is the significance of cord atrophy? Repeat myelography was done at an interval of 1 year in 3 patients and after 8 years in a fourth. In this last patient both the atrophy and the fibrosis were unchanged but his clinical status had deteriorated from a spastic gait to paraplegia.

Anterior spinal fusion with strut grafting was done after removal of dural fibrosis and any bony spur at the gibbus in 28 patients. Complete recovery was reported in 7 (25%) but all 4 patients with reactivated disease were part of this group. Partial recovery occurred in another 6, making the total with a favourable surgical outcome 13 (46%). Unfortunately postoperative deterioration occurred in 5 (18%). This compares unfavourably with the outcome for the same operation done in those with acute-onset paraplegia without any cord atrophy: 75% made a complete recovery and a further 10% showed improvement [1]. The presence of cord atrophy and peridural fibrosis in our series is associated with a satisfactory surgical outcome only half as frequently (46% vs 86%). A recent report [15] on the outcome of surgical decompression in acute-onset paraplegia makes an interesting comparison with our series especially in that socioeconomic conditions were similar in the two areas. Ninety-five per cent of those with paraplegia of less than 3 months' duration made a complete recovery. If, however, cord compression had been present for longer than 3 months a satisfactory outcome was achieved in 77%.

References

1. Hodgson AR, Yau A, Kwon JS, Kim D (1964) A clinical study of 100 consecutive cases of Pott's paraplegia. Clin Orthop 36: 128–150
2. Martin NS (1970) Tuberculosis of the spine: a study of the results of treatment during the last 25 yrs. J Bone Joint Surg [Br] 52 : 613–628
3. Guirguis AR (1967) Pott's paraplegia. J Bone Joint Surg [Br] 49: 658–667
4. Adendorff JJ, Boeke EJ, Lazarus C (1987) Pott's paraplegia. S Afr Med J 71: 427–428
5. Lifeso RM, Weaver P, Harder EH (1985) Tuberculous spondylitis in adults. J Bone Joint Surg [Am] 67A: 1405–1413
6. Butler RW (1935) Paraplegia in Pott's disease with special reference to the pathology and aetiology. Br J Surg 22: 738–768
7. Jones BS (1972) The management of late onset Pott's paraplegia caused by a bony ridge. S Afr Med J 46: 1664–1670
8. Hodgson AR, Stock FE, Fang HSY, Ong GB (1960) Anterior spinal fusion: the operative approach and pathological findings in 412 patients with Pott's disease of the spine. Br J Surg 48: 172–178
9. Griffiths DL, Seddon HJ, Roaf R (1956) In: Pott's paraplegia. Oxford University Press, London, pp 7–40
10. Hodgson AR, Wong W, Yau A (1969) X ray appearances of tuberculosis of the spine. Thomas, Springfield, pp 110–124
11. Seddon HJ (1946) Discussion on spinal caries with paraplegia. Proc R Med 39: 723–730
12. Weaver P, Lifeso RM (1984) Radilogical diagnosis of tuberculosis of the adult spine. Skeletal Radiol 12: 178–186
13. Hughes JT (1966) In: Pathology of the spinal cord. Lloyd-Luke, London, pp 73–74
14. Hodgson AR, Stock FE (1960) Anterior spine fusion for the treatment of tuberculosis of the spine: the operative findings and results of treatment in the first one hundred cases. J Bone Surg [Am] 42A: 295–310
15. Govender S, Charles RW, Naidoo KS, Goga IE (1988) Results of surgical decompression in chronic tuberculous paraplegia. S Afr Med J 74: 58–59

Prof. L. C. Handler
Neuroradiology C7
Groote Schuur Hospital
Cape Town
7925 South Africa

Neuroradiology (1991) 33 [Suppl]: 106–108

Neuro radiology
© Springer-Verlag 1991

Tuberculous atlanto-axial dislocation

N. Khandelwal[1], V. K. Khosla[2], N. Malik[1], B. D. Radotra[3], V. K. Kak[2], and S. Suri[1]

Departments of [1] Radiodiagnosis, [2] Neurosurgery, and
[3] Pathology, Postgraduate Institute of Medical Education and Research, Chandigarh, India

Summary. Tuberculous atlanto-axial dislocation (AAD) is extremely rare. Of 145 cases of AAD treated at our institute, 15 were due to tuberculosis. Neck pain or restricted neck movements were the predominant presenting features. Based on the radiological findings the disease was staged: stage I, AAD with retropharyngeal mass or abscess (RPAB) and normal bony architecture (5 cases); stage II, AAD with or without RPAB and with minimal bony destruction (4 cases); stage III, AAD with or without RPAB and with gross bony destruction (6 cases). Conservative treatment was effective in stage I and for some patients in stage II, while patients in stage III needed surgery. CT was helpful in early diagnosis, staging, treatment planning and follow-up of these patients.

Key words: Tuberculosis – Atlanto-axial joint – Computed tomography – Staging – Instability

Although tuberculosis is common in India, tuberculous involvement of the craniovertebral region is rare, accounting for less than 1% of all spinal tuberculosis [1]. Tuberculous atlanto-axial dislocation (TB-AAD) is extremely rare, with only a few reports in the English language literature, stressing mainly the management aspects [1–3]. We present the radiological findings in 15 patients with TB-AAD, divided into three stages, and outline the principles of management in relation to the radiological staging.

Patients and methods

Between 1977 and early 1990, 145 patients with AAD were treated at our institute. A diagnosis of tuberculosis was made in 15 of these, 9 males and 6 females between 12 and 55 years of age.

Clinical presentation. A varying degree of nuchal pain was present in all patients, and neck movements were restricted in 9. Other features included torticollis (4 patients), dysphagia (3), neck swelling (2) and low grade fever (5). Examination revealed varying degrees of neurological deficit in 10 patients, with a twelfth cranial nerve palsy in one. Routine haematological examination was normal, except for a raised erythrocyte sedimentation rate in 3 patients. Five patients had evidence of tuberculosis on chest radiography, 3 with active and 2 with healed lesions. Two patients developed AAD while on antituberculous treatment (ATT) and in another 2 patients tuberculous involvement developed in the lungs and skull respectively while they were on ATT for TB-AAD.

Radiological studies. Plain radiography of the upper cervical spine was carried out in all cases. All patients had myelograms (Myodil 4; water-soluble contrast medium 11). Conventional tomograms were obtained in 6 patients, and CT in 9. In 7 patients both plain CT and CT following myelography (CTM) were carried out. Plain CT studies only were obtained in 2 patients.

Diagnosis. Histopathological proof of tuberculosis was obtained in 14 cases. In 1 case, the CT and the clinical findings were highly suggestive of tuberculosis. Seven patients had open surgical biopsy (transoral 2, posterior approach 5). Fine-needle aspiration cytology was obtained from a retropharyngeal mass or abscess (RPAB) (5 patients), a cervical lymph node (1 patient) or a skull lesion (1 patient); in 2 cases acid-fast bacilli were demonstrated in the RPAB.

Table 1. Pathological basis of tuberculous atlanto-axial dislocation (AAD)

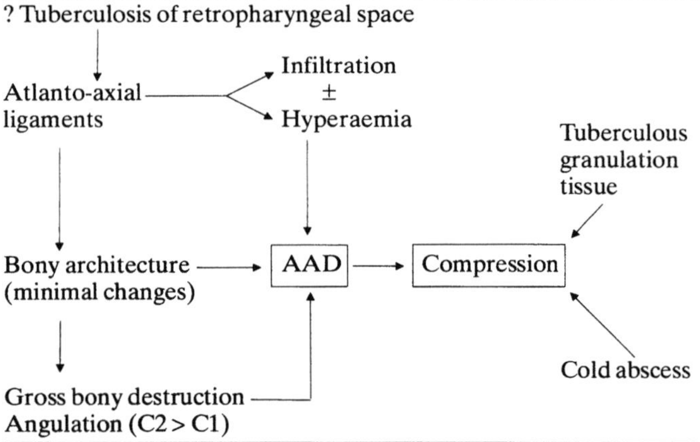

Table 2. Radiological findings

Stage 1 (? Mainly ligamentous involvement)	
[5]	Retropharyngeal mass Atlanto-axial dislocation/subluxation Normal bony architecture
Stage II	
[4]	Retropharyngeal mass ± AAD Mild alteration of bony architecture
Stage III	
[6]	Retropharyngeal mass ± AAD Gross bony destruction/angulation (C2 > C1) ±

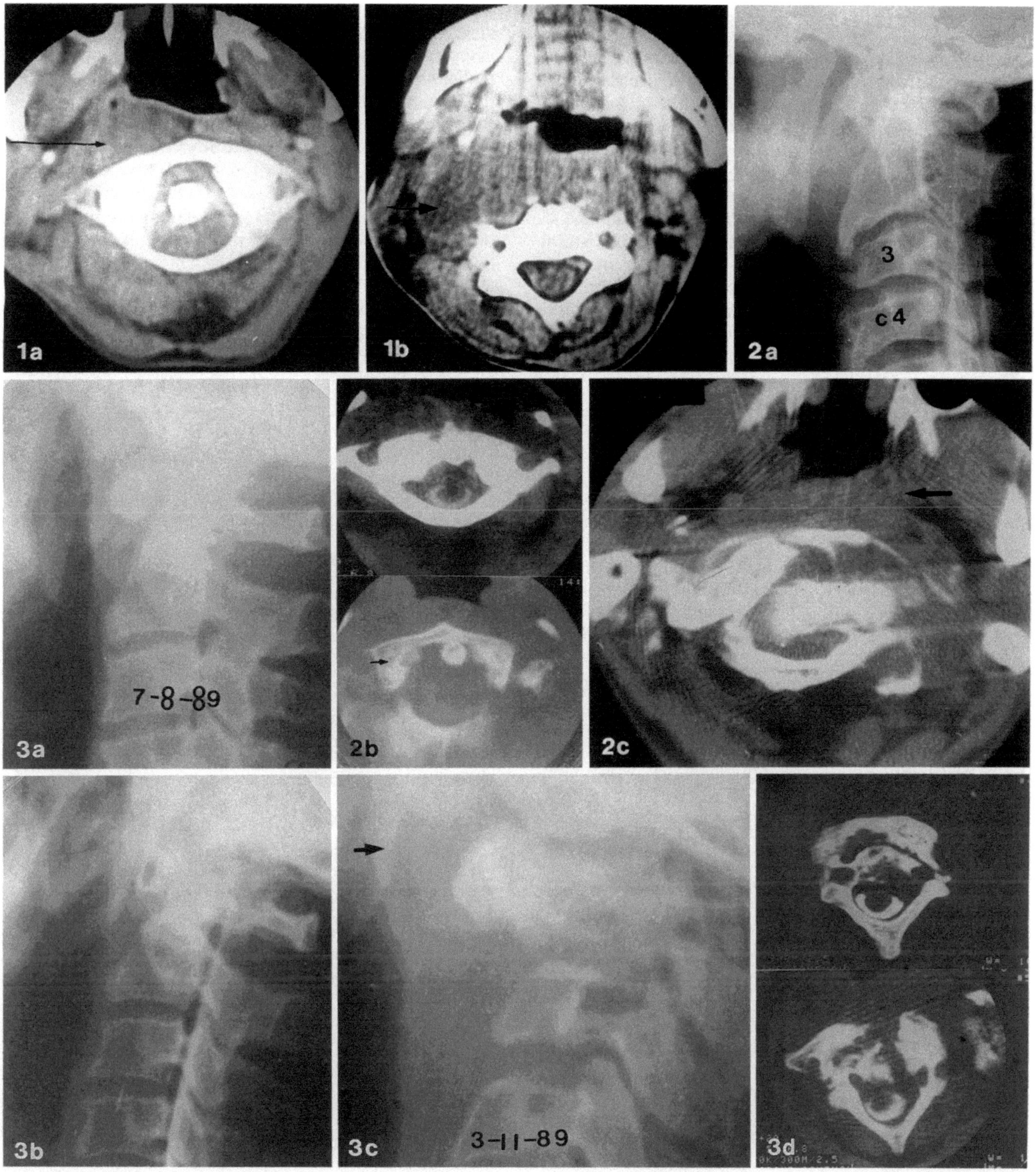

Fig. 1 a, b. Stage I showing atlanto-axial dislocation (AAD) and large retropharyngeal abscess (RPAB) *(arrow)*

Fig. 2 a–c. Stage II: **a** myelogram showing anterior extradural compression from foramen magnum to C3; **b** myelogram (CTM) demonstrating extradural soft tissue (tuberculous granulation tissue) and mild bony destruction *(arrow)*; **c** CT in another case showing destruction of lateral mass of C1 with small RPAB *(arrow)*

Fig. 3 a–d. Stage III: **a, b** plain radiograph and myelogram showing AAD and normal soft tissue; **c** plain radiograph showing gross bony destruction and large RPAB *(arrow)*; **d** CTM confirming the destruction of C1 and C2 and minimal anterior compression

Results

Three radiological groups emerged, indicating one continuous pathological process. The pathological sequence of TB-AAD is summarised in Table 1 while the radiological staging is summarised in Table 2. There were 5 patients in stage I (Fig. 1), 4 in stage II (Fig. 2), and 6 in stage III (Fig. 3).

ATT was started in all cases if the clinical and radiological features favoured TB-ADD. Drainage of the RPAB, cervical traction and external immobilisation was performed immediately in all patients. In the early part of the study surgery was carried out in all patients irrespective of staging of the disease, for spinal instability, but later in the series conservative management in stage I (2 cases) and stage II (2 cases) was found to be effective.

Discussion

The spinal cord at the cervicomedullary junction is compromised in tuberculosis by atlanto-axial instability, tuberculous cold abscess or granulation tissue, or by direct invasion [3]. The mechanism of AAD and the pathological basis of the disease are described adequately in the literature [2]. Early accurate diagnosis with complete radiological evaluation helps in better management of this curable condition [4, 5].

Conservative treatment, i.e. rest, cervical traction, evacuation of abscess and external immobilisation along with ATT, leads to clinical and radiological healing in the early stages [1]. Surgery is indicated when there is gross bony destruction with or without angulation, major compressive neurological deficit, or an unstable spine following conservative treatment [1].

Dynamic plain radiography and tomograms of the cervical spine (lateral flexion/extension and anteroposterior projections) confirm the presence of AAD, demonstrate the RPAB and the extent of bony destruction, and provide the baseline for the follow-up of these patients. Myelography demonstrates the degree and direction of cord compression. CT and CTM have the advantage of early detection and total demonstration of soft tissue and bony involvement, showing the degree and direction of cord compression and thus helping in deciding the surgical approach. CT is also useful for delineation of early signs of healing during follow-up [5, 6].

TB-AAD is thus a definite entity. Being a curable condition, it demands a high index of suspicion for early detection. The suggested radiological staging is of great help in its management.

References

1. Tuli SM (1974) Tuberculosis of craniovertebral region. Clin Orthop 104: 209–212
2. Pandya SK (1971) Tuberculous atlanto-axial dislocation (with remarks on the mechanism of dislocation). Neurology India 19: 116–221
3. Fang D, Leong JCY, Fang HSY (1983) Tuberculosis of upper cervical spine. J Bone Joint Surg 65-B: 47–50
4. Karapurkar AP (1988) Tuberculous atlanto-axial disease including dislocations. NIMHANS J [Suppl]: 89–88
5. Dowd CF (1986) Tuberculous spondylitis resulting in AAD. Skeletal Radiol 15: 65–68
6. Osborne D, Triolo P, Dubois P (1983) Assessment of cranio-vertebral junction and atlanto-axial region using metrizamide enhanced CT in flexion and extension. AJNR 4: 843–845

Dr. V. K. Khosla
Department of Neurosurgery
P. G. I. M. E. R.
Chandigarh-160012, India

Neuroradiology (1991) 33 [Suppl]: 109–110

Neuro-radiology
© Springer-Verlag 1991

Pott's paraplegia and tuberculous spondylitis: evaluation by magnetic resonance

P. Corr[1], L. Handler[1], and H. Davey[2]

[1] Department of Radiology, University of Cape Town/Groote Schuur [2] Red Cross Children's Hospitals, Cape Town, South Africa

Summary. Fifty-five patients with proven tuberculous spondylitis were evaluated by magnetic resonance imaging (MRI). Twenty-nine of these patients had paraparesis of varying severity. Fourteen patients had anterior spinal decompressions and fibula in situ grafts. MRI accurately defined the extent of spondylitis and its spread into the paravertebral soft tissue and spinal canal. The presence and degree of spinal cord compression is well demonstrated by MRI and correlates with the myelographic findings. The presence of a high-intensity cord signal on the T2-weighted scan indicated a poor prognosis for neurological recovery, while the presence of a normal cord signal pointed to a good prognosis for recovery.

Key words: Spine – Magnetic resonsance imaging Tuberculosis – Pott's paraplegia.

Tuberculous spondylitis remains a common disease in the Third World. As many as 30–50% of patients present with paraparesis or paraplegia and an essentially curable disease often results in life-long disability [1].

Paraparesis is most often due to extradural cord compression by tuberculous pus or caseous material. These patients often recover completely after anterior spinal decompression and fibula strut graft insertion [2]. However, a number of patients do not recover after decompression and this is thought to be focal myelopathy.

The aim of this study was to evaluate the MR features of tuberculous spondylitis and to determine its value in the assessment of spinal cord compression and detection of intramedullary lesions. We hoped by using MRI to identify those patients who were unlikely to recover function after spinal decompression.

Patients and methods

Fifty-five patients with biopsy- or culture-proven spinal tuberculosis were studied.

All patients were imaged by using 0.5 T Elscint unit with a spinal surface coil. Spin echo sequences in the sagittal and coronal planes were used (T1-weighted scan: TE 30/TR 500 ms; T2-weighted scan: TE 30, 90, 120/TR 2000 ms. CT scans and plain radiographs were also performed and 14 patients with paraparesis had myelograms.

Results

Thirty-six adults and 19 children were studied, of whom 28 had neurological complications (23 with paraparesis, 4 with paraplegia and 1 with quadraplegia). Fourteen patients had anterior spinal decompressions.

The commonest site of involvement was the thoracolumbar region, followed by the lower thoracic and lumbar spine. Cervical spine involvement was uncommon. Forty-five percent of patients had active pulmonary tuberculosis.

MRI accurately demonstrated both the bony and soft tissue involvement. On the T1-weighted scan there was a focal decreased signal intensity in 90% of patients with a corresponding increased signal intensity on the T2-weighted scan in 85% of patients. Only 26.5% of patients had an increased focal signal in the adjacent vertebral disc on the T2-weighted scan, while the signal was normal in 67%.

The presence and extent of the intraspinal abscess and associated cord compression correlates well with myelographic findings (Figs. 1, 2).

Focal high-intensity cord signals were detected on the T2-weighted images in 9 patients, none of whom made any significant recovery after decompression and anti-TB chemotherapy (Figs. 3, 4). Seven of these lesions were in keeping with focal myelopathy which persisted after repeat imaging 6 months later. Two patients with long-standing neurology had focal syrinx formation.

Discussion

MRI provides critical information for the treatment of Pott's paraplegia that previously was only available by myelography and follow-on CT examination. The ability to accurately detect the presence and assess the degree of cord compression non-invasively allows for early spinal decompression.

MRI is particularly useful in the follow-up of patients with neurology to confirm response to chemotherapy as seen by a diminution in the size of the extra- and intraspinal abscesses (Figs. 5, 6).

The presence of a high-intensity focal cord signal on the T2-weighted scan suggests a poor prognosis for neurological recovery ($P < 0.01$). These lesions probably repre-

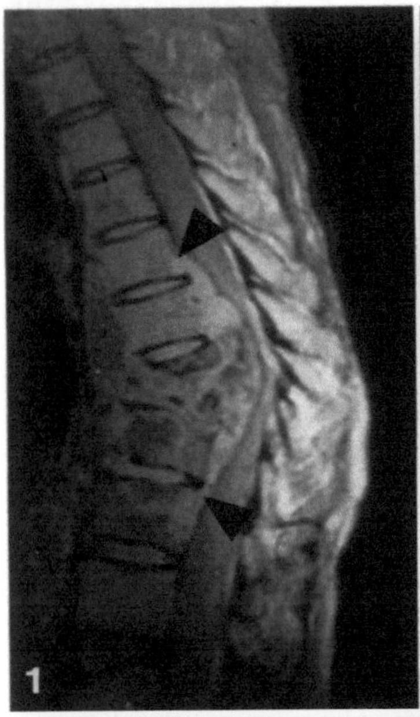
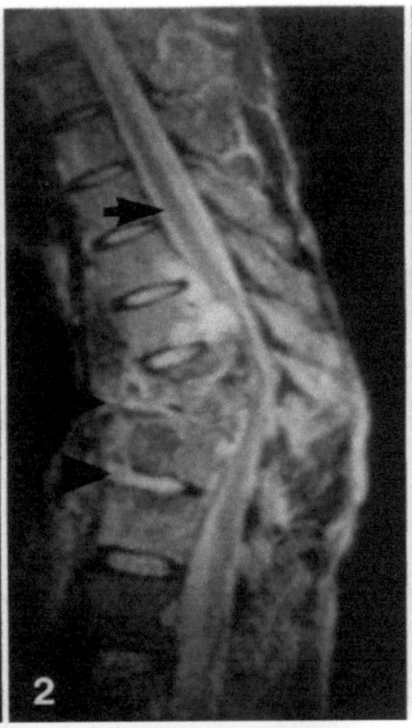
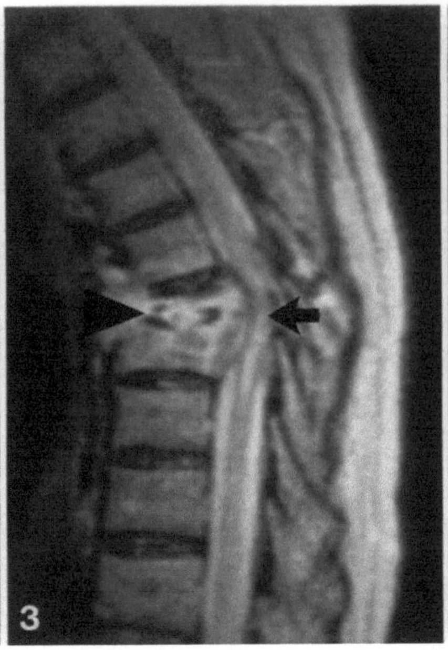
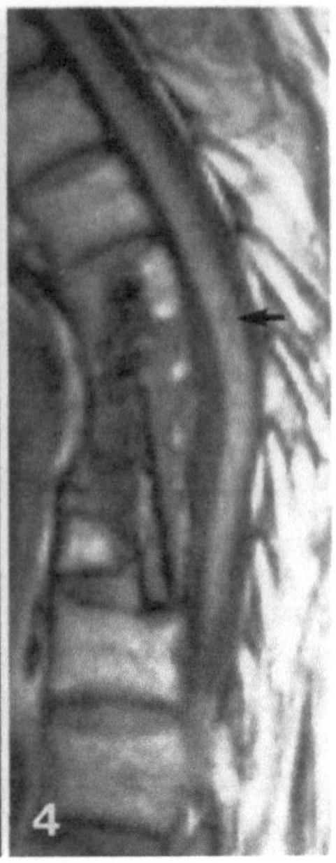
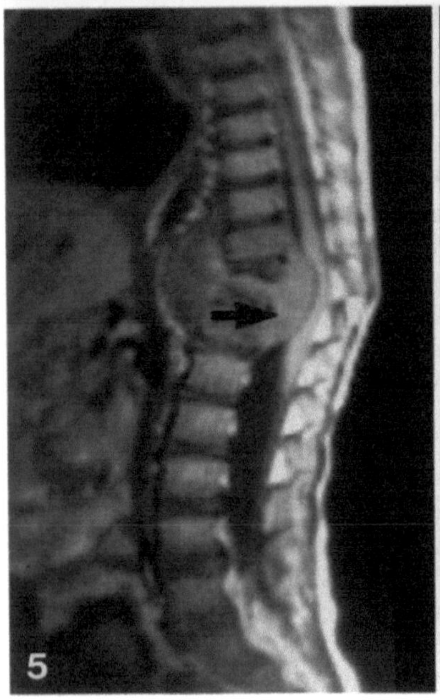
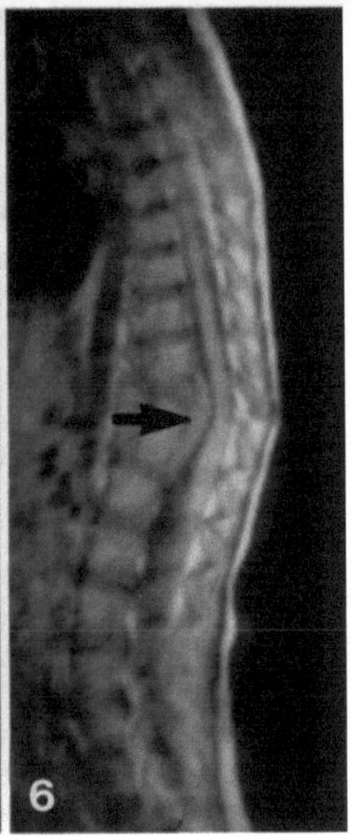

Fig. 1. Proton density sagittal image of a 30-year-old man with Pott's paraplegia. Note the large anterior extradural abscess causing thecal sac compression *(arrowheads)*

Fig. 2. T2-weighted sagittal scan of the same patient demonstrates the spinal cord compression *(arrow)* clearly

Fig. 3. T2-weighted sagittal scan of the mid-thoracic spine of 60-year-old patient with paraplegia. Note the collapsed high-intensity vertebral bodies and the intervening disc *(arrowhead)* and the anterior extradural cord compression. There is a high-intensity cord signal *(arrow)*. This patient did not recover after surgery

Fig. 4. T1 sagittal scan in the same patient 6 months after decompression. Note focal low-intensity lesion in the cord persists. There was no neurological improvement

Fig. 5 T1-weighted sagittal scan of a 3-year-old with paraparesis. Note the intraspinal abscess *(arrow)* causing cord compression

Fig. 6. T1-weighted sagittal scan of the same patient after 6 weeks of chemotherapy with marked clinical improvement. The intraspinal abscess is now much smaller *(arrow)*

sent focal myelopathy on the basis of ischaemia from associated cord compression [3].

The absence of signal changes in the intervertebral disc in two-thirds of patients appears distinct from pyogenic osteitis, where there is invariably a high-intensity signal in the disc and adjacent vertebral end-plates [4]. Tuberculous spondylitis may thus mimic metastatic disease on MRI [5].

This study demonstrates the value of MRI in providing an accurate evaluation of the spine and the spinal cord in tuberculous spondylitis.

References

1. Tuli S (1969) Treatment of neurological complications in tuberculosis of the spine. J Bone Joint Surg [Am] 51: 4
2. Lifeso R, Weaver P, Harder E (1985) Tuberculous spondylitis in adults. J Bone Joint Surg [Am] 67: 1405–1413
3. Takahashi M, Yamashita Y, Sakamoto Y (1989) Chronic cervical cord compression: clinical significance of increased intensity on MR images. Radiology 173: 219–224
4. Modic M, Feiglin D (1985) Vertebral osteomyelitis using MR. Radiology 157: 157–166
5. Smith A, Weinstein M, Mizushima A, Coughlin B (1989) MR imaging characteristics of tuberculous spondylitis vs vertebral osteomyelitis. AJNR 10: 619–625

P. Corr M. B., Ch. B., F. F. Rad (D) S. A.
Department of Radiology
Groote Schuur Hospital, Observatory
7925 Cape Town
South Africa

Neuroradiology (1991) 33 [Suppl]: 111–113

Neuro radiology

© Springer-Verlag 1991

Spinal arachnoiditis: MR appearances

S. B. Desai, V. C. Shah, O. J. Tavri, and P. Rao

Department of Magnetic Resonance Imaging, Breach Candy Hospital and Research Centre, Bombay, India

Summary. A retrospective review of 2012 spinal MRIs was performed to study MR characteristics of spinal arachnoiditis. Confirmation was obtained by myelography. Gadolinium-DTPA studies were also obtained in a few cases.

Key words: Spine – Arachnoiditis – Tuberculosis – Magnetic resonance imaging

Materials and methods

Twenty-five patients with spinal arachnoiditis were studied. Detailed clinical assessments and routine investigations were carried out in all cases. Criteria for diagnosis of arachnoiditis were: (1) clinical suspicion, (2) cerebrospinal fluid (CSF) studies, (3) associated cerebral infective lesion, (4) characteristic myelographic findings, (5) MRI appearances.

Myelograms were done with either 6–9 ml of Myodil or 10 ml of 180–300 mg% water soluble contrast medium. All MRI studies were obtained on Siemens Magnetom operating at 1.0 T. A rectangular surface coil was used. Multislice spin-echo images were obtained with short repetition time (TR) of 0.5–0.75 s and longer TR of 2.5–3.0 s and echo delay time (TE) of 17, 23 and 90 ms. Axial, sagittal and coronal images were obtained. Slice thickness was 4–5 mm with interslice gap of 0.4–0.8 mm. MRI was compared with myelograms.

Results

Controls

None of 10 patients in a control group showed any findings suggestive of arachnoiditis. The normal appearances of lumbar nerve roots on axial MR images varied from a mass of soft tissue signal in the lower portion of the theca at L2 to discrete laterally placed cresents at L5, as observed by Ross et al. [1] and Reicher et al. [2].

Midline sagittal images showed the roots as a single band of intermediate signal intensity along the dorsal aspect of the theca progressively tapering from the conus to L4–5 level. The thoracic subarachnoid space was of even calibre, symmetrical and homogeneously hypointense.

Postoperative patients

Of the 25 patients, 13 had undergone operation for a disc lesion or canal stenosis (Table 1), twelve in the lumbar region and 1 in the cervical spine. Myelograms were obtained in 5 cases prior to MRI and in the rest following MRI, and showed characteristic features of arachnoiditis [1, 3, 4]. MRI features consistent with arachnoiditis, fell into three distinct groups as observed by Ross et al. [1].

Group I (6 patients). The predominant feature was central conglomeration of nerve roots (Fig. 1). Peripheral dura mater was not thickened.

Group II (6 patients). The predominant feature was clumping of the lumbar nerve roots, adherent dorsally to the meninges with focal meningeal thickening, giving an appearance of a theca devoid of nerve roots (Fig. 2).

Group III (3 patients). The predominant feature was altered signal intensity of the CSF, best appreciated on T1-weighted and proton-density MR images (Fig. 3). The lumbar nerve roots were ill defined, with areas of focal "filling defect" within this subarachnoid space.

Post-Myodil myelogram. There was an overlap with the patients who had undergone Myodil study prior to operation [5] and for lumbar disease diagnostic work-up [6]. The MRI appearances of post-Myodil myelogram arachnoiditis were identical with postoperative arachnoiditis [1, 3, 4, 7]. In many patients, sagittal T1-weighted and T2-weighted images revealed a "twisted rope" appearance of nerve roots [3, 7]. Residual Myodil droplets were invariably identified and gave signal intensity compatible with fat (hyperintense on T1-weighted images and progressively hypointense on T2-weighted images).

Postinfective (tuberculous meningitis). The commonest myelographic finding, seen in 5 of 7 patients, was irregular, incomplete or complete block at different thoracic levels (Fig. 4 a, b). The cord contour was usually ill-defined. There were large, irregular, serpiginous, nodular filling defects in the subarachnoid space. The nodular defects were small and focal or long, irregular and scattered throughout the dorsal spine.

CT following myelography was obtained in only 2 cases and showed irregular nodular soft tissue mass-like lesions in the subarachnoid space with compression of the thoracic cord. On T1-weighted MRI the CSF in the involved segment was of altered signal intensity (higher than normal). The thoracic cord was usually irregular in contour. On

Table 1. Significant previous history

Postoperative	13
TBM (AFB + ve = 3; Chest + ve = 1)	7
Myodil myelography	15

TBM, Tuberculosis meningitis; AFB, acid fast bacilli

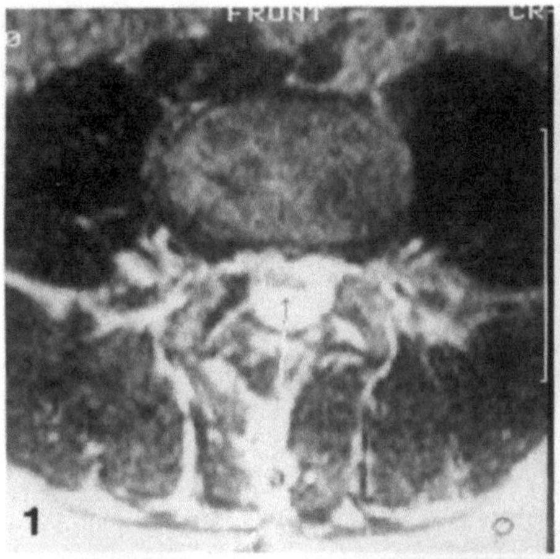

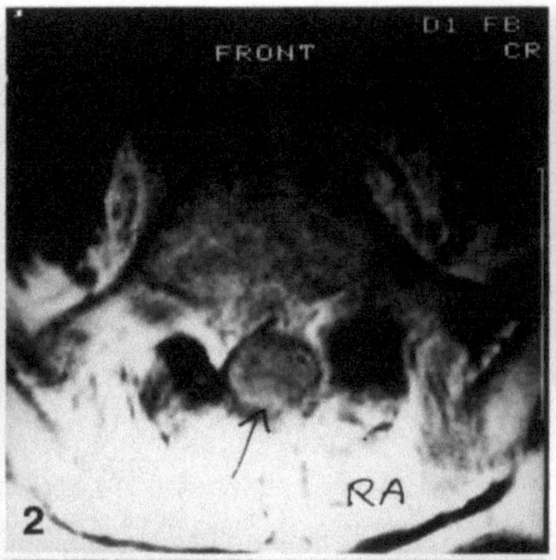

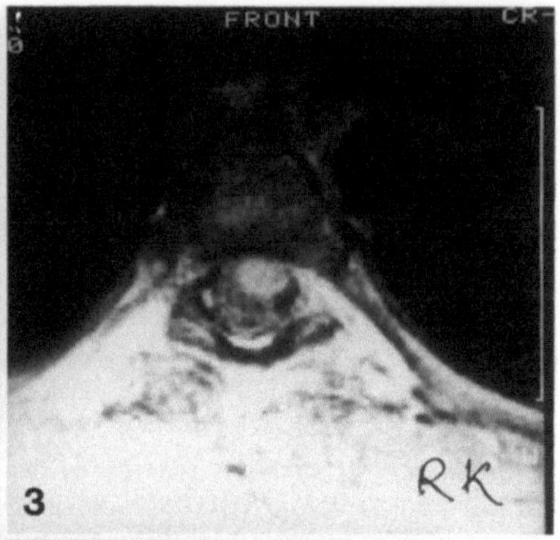

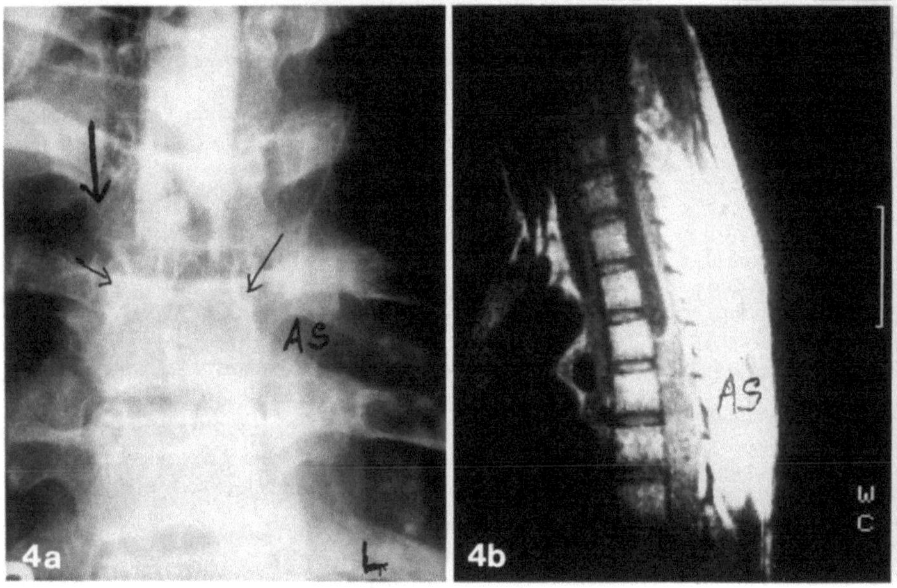

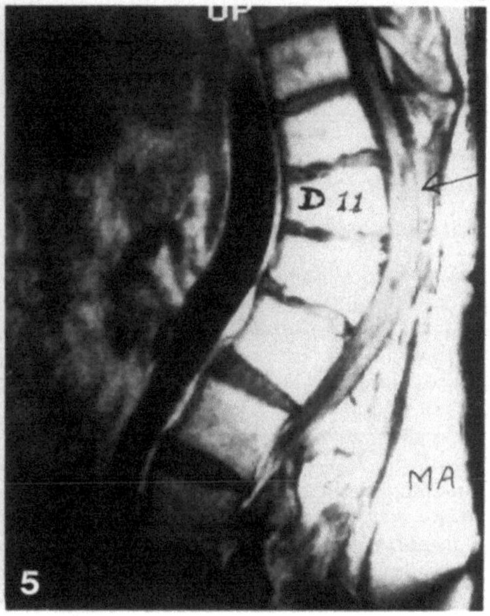

Fig. 1. Group I arachnoiditis. T2-weighted axial image at L3 showing central conglomeration of nerve roots

Fig. 2. Group II arachnoiditis. Proton-density axial image at L5 showing empty thecal sac appearance

Fig. 3. Group III arachnoiditis. Proton-density axial image showing altered cerebrospinal fluid (CSF) intensity and filling defects in subarachnoid space

Fig. 4 a, b. Tuberculous arachnoiditis: **a** complete block on myelogram; **b** T1-weighted sagittal image showing irregular cord contour and altered CSF signal

Fig. 5. With gadolinium-DTPA. T1-weighted sagittal MR image reveals extensive enhancement of dura-arachnoid mater complex

proton density images there was appreciable increase in the signal intensity of the CSF in the involved segment as compared with the rest of the thoracolumbar subarachnoid space with indistinct CSF/cord interface. This could not be appreciated on second-echo images. The thoracic cord, however, revealed focal areas of high signal intensity on T2-weighted images signifying oedema, infarct [4], cord atrophy in 5 cases or focal syrinx in 4 cases [5] (Table 2).

In 7 patients intravenous gadolinium-DTPA was injected in a dose of 0.02 ml/kg body weight. Gd-DTPA-enhanced T1-weighted MRI revealed patchy plaque-like and nodular enhancement along the thoracic subarachnoid space in 6 patients and ring enhancement in 1 patient (Table 3). Extensive enhancement of the dura–arachnoid mater complex was seen in 1 patient (Fig. 5). In 2 patients there was irregular patchy enhancement of the thoracic cord with associated mild cord swelling.

Discussion

Arachnoiditis is the cause of pain in 5%–15% of postoperative patients [1, 3, 4, 8, 9] and is the commonest spinal inflammatory disease [8]. In arachnoiditis, there is prominent fibrinous exudate with negligible inflammatory cellular reaction. The fibrin covered roots have a tendency to adhere to themselves and to the thecal sac. During the reparative stage, dense collagenous adhesions are formed by proliferating fibrocytes. In cases of tuberculous arachnoiditis, tuberculoma or tubercular abscesses may be associated [1, 6, 10, 11].

Tuberculous arachnoiditis is more aptly described as tuberculous radiculomyelitis and can be primary or secondary [10]. Conventional and CT myelography reveal clumping of nerve roots, dural adhesions and multiple filling defects.

Two distinct types of myelographic appearances of arachnoiditis are described by Jorgensen et al. [12]. Of

Table 2. Associated cord lesions

1. Oedema/infarct	4 (16)	25%
2. Atrophy	6 (16)	37.3%
3. Syrinx	4 (16)	25%

Table 3. Post-gadolinium-DTPA MR arachnoiditis

Patchy cord enhancement	2
Extrinsic dura/arachnoid mater complex enhancement	1
Patchy, nodular subarachnoid space enhancement	5
Ring-like subarachnoid space enhancement	1

16 patients with arachnoiditis in the lumbar and dorsolumbar regions, 6 revealed central nerve root clumping (group I). Six showed peripheral adhesions (group II) while 3 showed soft tissue intensity mass-like lesions (group III). We excluded 7 patients with tuberculous arachnoiditis in the dorsal and cervical region and 1 patient with cervical postoperative arachnoiditis from this analysis. However, most tuberculous arachnoiditis falls into group III appearances. In 15 patients there was evidence of residual Myodil, and 6 of 13 postoperative patients had a Myodil myelogram prior to surgery. The majority of these patients showed a long segment of involvement in lumbar and dorsolumbar regions, compared with short segment involvement seen in tuberculous arachnoiditis. The appearance was that of a "twisted rope" of nerve roots [3, 6, 7].

Although typical spinal arachnoiditis is more prevalent in patients aged 30–50 years [6], tuberculous arachnoiditis occurs more commonly in the younger patients [5]. In our series 6 of 7 (99%) were below 30 years of age. Arachnoiditis symptoms occurred a few months to many years following Koch's infection of the chest or brain. The blocks seen on myelograms may be caused by tuberculoma, arachnoid adhesions, epidural granuloma and/or cord swelling. In our series, tuberculous arachnoiditis was predominantly in the thoracic region (6/7, 86%). MRI was superior in evaluating the nature and extent of the block, showing masses consistent with tuberculoma. Multiple fine nodular or coarse defects seen on myelography may represent active granulomas or inactive scar tissue. Differentiation between these is possible with Gd-DTPA-enhanced MRI. Enhancement of the dura-arachnoid mater complex indicates an active meningeal inflammation around the cord. Cord granuloma may reveal ring or homogeneous enhancement. Only MRI can show the cord status. In our of 16 patients with thoracic or cervical involvement, 4 were believed to show cord ischaemia, 7 had cord atrophy and 4 revealed a focal syrinx.

It is not possible to distinguish cord oedema from ischaemia or infarct as all three give high signal intensitity on T2-weighted images. However, the duration of disease is a good indicator and has therapeutic bearing, as the presence of an infarct rules out surgical intervention.

Table 4. Initial clinical impression

Arachnoiditis	9
Cord neoplasm	3
Myelopathy	6
Syrinx	1
Miscellaneous	6
Total	25

The axial T1-weighted and proton-density images are important in diagnosing arachnoiditis. Due to the long T1 of CSF, it is easy to appreciate the higher signal nerve root abnormalities against hypointense CSF. As proteinaceous CSF has shorter T1 and T2 than pure CSF, signal changes are best appreciated on proton-density images, where the exudate appears brighter than normal CSF; it is masked on the T2-weighted images as the exudate merges with CSF. Subtle abnormalities of the cord are appreciated on T2-weighted images.

Gd-DTPA is used to confirm the diagnosis and establish activity of the lesion. MRI features help to exclude canal stenosis or tumours which may mimic arachnoiditis.

In only 9 of our 25 patients (36%) was arachnoiditis suspected clinically (Table 4). MRI was helpful in arriving at the correct diagnosis. As this study is retrospective and some unsuspected/undiagnosed cases of arachnoiditis may not have been included, we cannot exclude false positive or negative MRI in arachnoiditis. However, knowledge of the normal appearances, thin section multiplanar multiecho imaging, use of Gd-DTPA and a greater degree of awareness lead to detection of subtle changes.

References

1. Ross JS, Masaryk TJ, Modic MT, Dalameter R (1987) MR imaging of lumbar arachnoiditis. AJNR 8: 885–892
2. Reicher MA, Gold RH, Hallbach VV, Rauschning W, Wilson G, Lufkin RB (1986) MR imaging of the lumbar spine: anatomic correlations and effects of technical variations. AJR 147: 891–898
3. Pomeranz SJ (1989) Disk disease, spondylosis and related disorders. In: Craniospinal magnetic resonance imaging. Saunders, Philadelphia, pp 541–565
4. Modic MT, Masarck TJ, Ross JS (1989) Inflammatory disease: magnetic resonance imaging of the spine. YBM, Chicago, pp 167–172
5. Arseni G, Samitea DC (1960) Intraspinal tuberculous granuloma. Brain 83: 285–292
6. Chang KH, Han MH, Choi YM, Kim IO (1989) Tuberculous arachnoiditis of the spine: finding on myelography, CT and MR imaging. AJNR 10: 1255–1262
7. Mamourian AC, Briggs RW (1986) Appearances of Pantopaque on MR images. Radiology 158: 457–460
8. Pomeranz SJ (1989) Inflammatory disease of the brain and spine. In: Craniospinal magnetic resonance imaging. Saunders, Philadelphia, pp 436–458
9. Stark DD, Bradley WG (1988) Lumbar spine: magnetic resonance imaging. Mosby, St Louis, pp 678–680
10. Wadia NH, Dastur DK (1969) Spinal meningitides with radiculomyelopathy. I. Clinical and radiological features. J Neurol Sci 8: 239–260
11. Shaw MDM, Sussel JA, Grossart KW (1978) The changing pattern of spinal arachnoiditis. J Neurol Neurosurg Psychiatry 41: 97–107
12. Jorgensen J, Hansen PH, Steenkov V, Quesen N (1975) A clinical and radiological study of chronic lower spinal arachnoiditis. Neuroradiology 9: 139–144

Dr. S. B. Desai
Magnetic Resonance Imaging
Breach Candy Hospital & Research Centre
60-B, Bhulabhai Desai Road, Bombay-400026, India

Neuroradiology (1991) 33 [Suppl]: 114–116

Neuro-radiology
© Springer-Verlag 1991

Differentiation of benign versus metastatic vertebral body compression fractures

S. W. Horowitz, M. Fine, and B. Azar-Kia

Department of Radiology, Loyola University Medical Center, Maywood, Illinois, USA

Summary. Six patients with benign fractures showed a sharply demarcated vertical band of preserved bone marrow along the dorsal one-third of the compressed vertebral body, while the anterior two-thirds showed decreased signal intensity (SI) with a T1-weighted sequence. This "posterior band sign" seen in benign, and not seen in metastatic, fractures correlates well with the biochemical theory of the "three column spine". The latter defines compression fracture by an intact "middle column" which includes the dorsal one-third of the vertebral body, posterior annulus fibrosus, and posterior longitudinal ligament. Metastatic fractures showed either complete or irregular bone marrow replacement of multiple vertebral bodies and of posterior elements. Other benign patterns included a horizontal band of low SI adjacent to the superior or inferior vertebral endplate, isointense or increased SI of the vertebral body in images with a T1-weighted sequence. Two fractures were indeterminate.

Key words: Spine – Magnetic resonance imaging – Secondary neoplasms

A frequent clinical dilemma is to distinguish between benign and pathologic vertebral body compression fractures. Plain spine radiographs, CT, and radionuclide scintigrapy may not distinguish the underlying nature of compression fractures in the absence of diffuse metastases. Other MRI studies [1, 2] have described signal intensity and morphologic criteria to aid in differentiation between these entities. The purpose of this study was to describe another useful sign in their distinction.

Patients and methods

Utilizing a 1.5 T magnet (GE signa), MRI was performed in 30 patients with thoracic of lumbar compression fractures due to metastatic (20 fractures, 11 patients) or benign process (31 fractures, 19 patients), including trauma and osteoporosis. Pathologic proof and/or follow up MR scans were available in a few cases, and the diagnosis in the other cases was substantiated by clinical correlation and follow-up.

Results

A sharply delineated isointense vertical band of preserved bone marrow along the dorsal one-third of the compressed vertebral body, with decreased signal intensity (SI) of the anterior two-thirds, was seen on images made with a T1-weighted sequence in six benign (Figs. 1, 2) fractures and no metastatic fracture. The isointense "posterior band sign" corresponds to the intact middle column of the biomechanical three column spine theory (Fig. 3) [3]. SI characteristics may vary with time while still exhibiting a sharply demarcated band along the dorsal vertebral body (Fig. 4).

Other benign compression patterns on T1-weighted sequence images included homogeneous isointense vertebral body (9 fractures), a horizontal band of decreased SI adjacent to the superior or inferior vertebral endplate (11 fractures), and increased SI of the vertebral body (3 fractures).

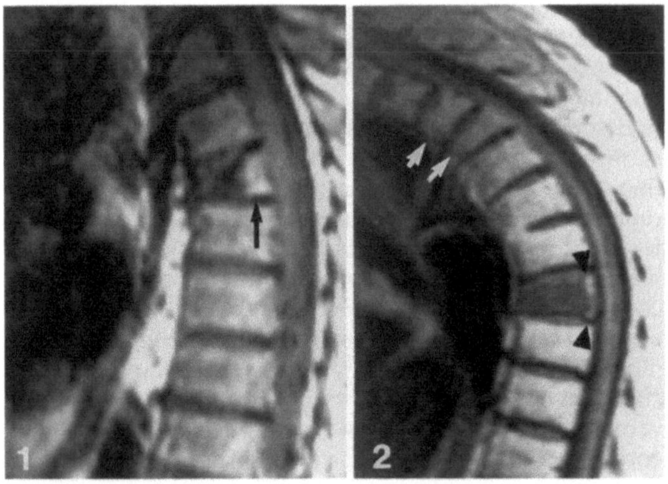

Fig. 1. A 37-year-old male. Trauma 6 years previously had caused T4 anterior wedge fracture. An isointense "posterior band" *(arrow)* is sharply delineated at the dorsal third of the vertebral body, while the anterior two-thirds are hypointense on T1-weighted images

Fig. 2. A 72-year-old female with osteoporosis, kyphosis, and history of breast carcinoma. Isointense anterior wedge fractures of T3 and T4 *(arrows)* are old, due to osteoporosis. Recent compression of T8 shows "posterior band sign" *(arrowheads)* characteristic of benign fracture, not metastatic breast carcinoma. Follow-up MR scan 5 months later (not shown) showed homogeneously isointense T8 vertebral body, confirming the benign nature of the fracture

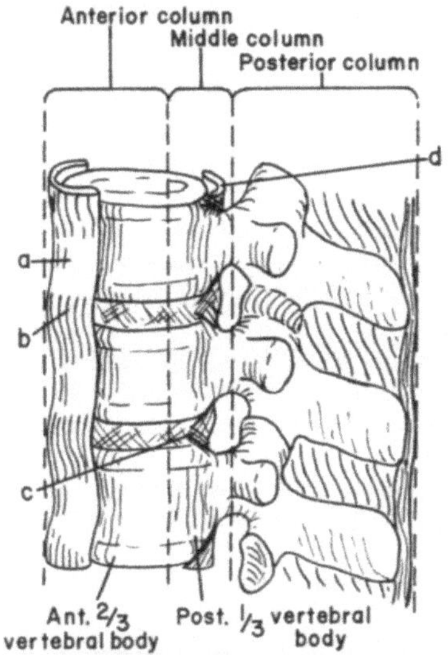

Fig. 3. Biomechanical three column spine theory of Denis.
a, Anterior longitudinal ligament;
b, anterior annulus fibrosus ;
c, posterior annulus fibrosus;
d, posterior longitudinal ligament

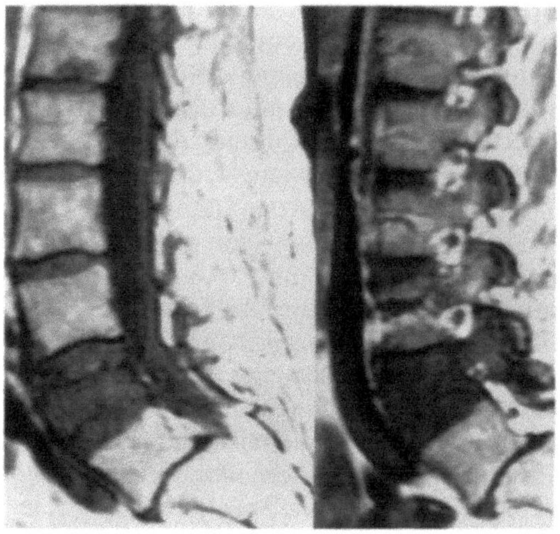

Fig. 5. A 54-year-old female with metastatic breast carcinoma. Hypointense signal of entire compressed vertebral body and posterior elements of L5 on T1-weighted sequence. Smaller metastatic foci of L1 and L4 vertebral bodies

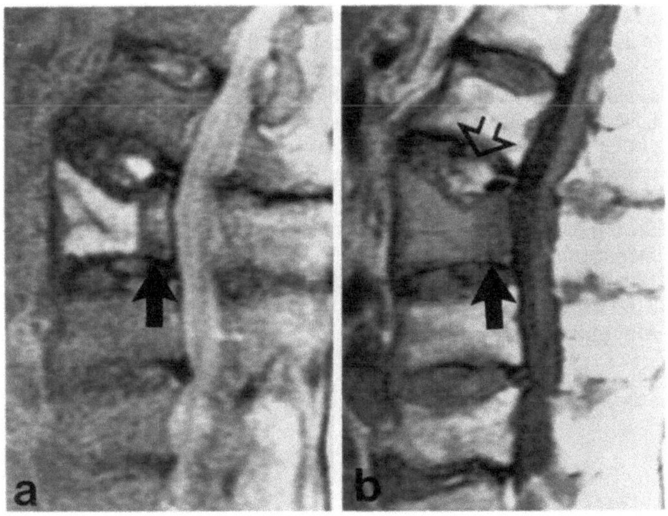

Fig. 4. a, b. A 91-year-old osteoporotic female. Back pain began 4 days prior to MR scan. **a** Decreased height of the L3 vertebral body is greatest centrally with bowing of superior endplate. On T2-weighted sequence, marked hyperintensity of anterior column due to increased fluid. Sharply demarcated, isointense band at dorsalvertebral body *(arrow).* **b** Entire vertebral body is hypointense on T1-weighted sequence, with sharp posterior band *(arrow)* distinguishing this from metastatic pattern. Hyperintensity within L2–3 disc on T1-weighted sequence due to methemoglobin *(open arrow)*

The SI patterns seen in metastatic compression fractures included complete (15 fractures) or irregular (5 fractures) replacemnt of bone marrow by decreased SI on T1-weighted sequence images in multiple vertebral bodies and posterior elements (Fig. 5). Diffusely decreased SI throughout the spine on T1 weighting was noted in 2 of the 20 metastatic patients.

Two fractures were indeterminate by pattern.

Discussion

The biochemical concept of the "three column spine" and its significance in classification of thoracolumbar spine injuries was introduced by Denis in 1983 [3]. The anterior column includes the anterior two-thirds of the vertebral body, anterior longitudinal ligament, and anterior annulus fibrosus. Benign, simple compression fracture is a failure of the anterior column under compression. The middle column consists of the posterior one-third of vertebral body, posterior annulus fibrosus, posterior longitudinal ligament, and anterior aspect of pedicles. It is of major importance that the middle column is intact in benign compression fracture and acts as a hinge which differentiates simple compression fracture from the other categories of post-traumatic fracture (burst, seat-belt, fracture-dislocation). The posterior column includes posterolateral facet capsular ligaments, ligamentum flavum, posterior laminar structures, supraspinous and interspinous ligaments. In severe compression, there may be partial tension failure of the posterior column. Loss of any two of the three structural columns results in instability.

In six of our benign fractures, the sharply delineated "posterior band sign" illustrates and confirms the biomechanical concept of the three column spine. the decreased SI of the anterior two-thirds of the vertebral body corresponds to the compressed anterior column. The isointense posterior one-third of the vertebral body corresponds to the intact middle column of the three column spine. The height of the anterior vertebral body is decreased, the height of the posterior aspect of the body remains unchanged, and the posterior cortex of the body is intact.

The SI characteristics of this biomechanical model may vary with time while still exhibiting a distinct "posterior band sign". Acutely, there may be marked increase in SI on T2-weighted sequence of the anterior column secondary to increased fluid. The latter edema may be seen throughout the vertebral body as decreased SI on T1-weighted sequence, perhaps combined with an element of hemorrhage in the anterior column.

While benign compression fracture follows the biomechanical forces described above, the posterior band sign was not seen in metastatic fracture, the latter collapse due to complete or irregular infiltration of bone marrow by tumor. The high incidence of complete bone marrow replacement and the irregular configuration of incomplete infiltration by metastatic tumor have been previously described [1, 2]. Metastatic disease may invade the vertebral column through the nutrient artery supply to the midportion of each vertebral body and the posterior elements [4] or via Batson's venous plexus [4–6]. Both the mechanism and location of bone marrow involvement differ in metastatic versus benign vertebral fractures.

Other patterns of benign compression fracture, previously described [1, 2, 7] and also noted in this study, included a horizontal band of low SI adjacent to the superior or inferior vertebral endplate. The most frequent type of compression fracture involves failure of the superior endplate anteriorly; however, there are isolated failures of the inferior endplate and sometimes failure of both endplates [3]. Other benign patterns included increased SI on T1-weighted images in either subacute or chronic fractures [7], possibly secondary to subacute hemorrhage, compaction of bone marrow, or chronic conversion of hematopoietic to yellow fatty marrow [8]. Chronic compression fractures commonly exhibit reversal to homogeneously isointense SI throughout the vertebral body as edema resolves. The time frame or the latter has not been completely elucidated, although others have suggested 1–3 months [2].

In conclusion, the posterior band sign is an adjunct to previously described MR criteria to differentiate between benign and malignant vertebral body compression fractures. Such distinction may not always be possible by MR criteria in a small percentage of cases.

Refernces

1. Yuh WT, Zachar CK, Barloon TJ, Sato Y, Sickels WJ, Hawes DR (1989) Vertebral compression fractures: distinction between benign and malignant causes with MR imaging. Radiology 172: 215–218
2. Baker LL, Goodman SB, Perkash I, Lane B, Enzmann DR (1990) Benign versus pathologic compression of vertebral bodies: assessment with conventinal spin-echo, chemical -shift, and STIR MR imaging. Radioligy 174: 495–502
3. Denis F (1983) Three column spine and its significance in the classification of acute thoracolumbar spinal injuries. Spine 8: 817–831
4. Meyer PR (1989) Surgery of spine trauma. Churchill Livingstone, New York, pp 61–106
5. Batson OV (1942) The vertebral vein system as a mechanism for the spread of metastases. Am J Roentgenol 48: 715–718
6. Abrams HL (1957) The vertebral azygous venous systems and some variations in systemic venous return. Radiology 69: 508–525
7. Modic MT, Masaryk T, Paushter D (1986) Magnetic resonance imaging of the spine. Radiol Clin North Am 24: 229–245
8. Modic MT, Steinberg PM, Ross JS, Masaryk TJ, Carter JR (1988) Degenerative disk disease: assessment of changes in vertebral body marrow with MR imaging. Radiology 166: 193–199

Dr. Sandra W. Horowitz
Department of Radiology
Loyola University Medical Center
2160 South First Avenue
Maywood, IL 60153, USA

SESSION 9
DEMYELINATING DISEASE

Neuroradiology (1991) 33 [Suppl]: 118–120

Neuro
radiology
© Springer-Verlag 1991

Value of T2-MRI features in differentiating ischaemic, vascular inflammatory and primary demyelinating diseases

P. A. Lyrer and E. W. Radü

Department of Neuroradiology, Kantonsspital, Basel, Switzerland

Summary. T2-weighted MRI of 69 patients, in three diagnostic groups: multiple sclerosis (MS) (28 patients), vascular ischaemic disease (34 patients) and vascular inflammatory disease (7 patients), were reviewed without clinical data and white matter lesions were analysed. The prominent features are: MS – diffuse, usually round lesions with blurred edges in the periventricular area and white matter; vascular ischaemic diseases – indented sharply edged lesions with prominent atrophy in over 50%; and vascular inflammatory disease lesions: lying at the grey/white border with sharp or blurred edges without cerebral atrophy. A diagnostic score was established which assisted in differentiating the three entities.

Key words: Magnetic resonance imaging – White matter lesions – Multiple sclerosis – Vascular ischaemic disease – Vascular inflammatory disease

Since MRI was first shown to be useful in detecting white matter lesions in T2-weighted images [1, 2] many authors have described multiple diseases with signal-intense spots in brain MRI scans. Lesions in cases of multiple sclerosis (MS) [3, 4], vascular ischaemic diseases [5], neuropsychiatric systemic lupus erythematosus (SLE) [6], CNS sarcoidosis [7], CNS syphilis [8] and vasculitis with involvement of the CNS [9] were described. In infections [10], AIDS [11] and strokes the diagnosis will be made using clinical findings, laboratory tests, CT and MRI. On the other hand, distinguishing similar, slowly progressing diseases like MS, different forms of cerebral vasculitis or subcortical vascular ischaemic degenerative diseases may be difficult in the early stages. In these cases MRI may have higher predictive value in pointing to the aetiology than clinical examination, laboratory tests or CT.

We therefore tried to find typical features of lesions in T2-MRI scans that might distinguish multiple sclerosis, vascular ischaemic diseases (hypertensive and with risk factors such as diabetes mellitus or heavy smoking) and inflammatory diseases (SLE, syphilis, angitis etc.).

Patients and methods

We reviewed brain MRI of 69 neurological patients which showed pathological high signal spots on T2-weighted images. T2 axial images 6–7 mm thick were obtained (TR 2000 ms, TE 90 ms) on a 2T Siemens MR imager working at 1.5 T. The images were analysed blind to the clinical diagnosis by two neuroradiologists. High signal lesions were described referring to criteria [2–4, 9] such as localization: periventricular; separated from ventricles in the white matter; grey/white border; grey matter; one region or multiple regions (hemispheres, mesencephalon, cerebellum, brain stem and medulla oblongata), size 0–0.5 mm, 0.5 mm, more than 20 mm in diameter), number (0–3, 4–10, more than 10) and morphology (round, sharp, round, blurred, irregular or star-shaped with or without atrophy.

Based on all clinical data presented in the final report the population was divided into three diagnostic groups: (1) MS, 28 cases, mean age 44.4 years (range 25–64); (2) vascular ischaemic diseases (multiple transient ischaemic attacks and risk factors), 34 cases, mean age 62.0 years (range 37–81); (3) vascular inflammatory diseases (SLE, CNS syphilis, temporal arteritis), 7 cases, mean age 46.6 years (range 22–76).

The relative incidence of all above-mentioned options was summarized for each diagnostic group and statistical analysis was performed using 2×2 contingency tables [12].

Results

MRI features in the three diagnostic groups are shown in Fig. 1. MS lesions were located predominantly periventricularly 75% (21/28 patients), and separated from ventricles, 89.3% (25/28 patients) in the white matter. Most lesions 85.7% (24/28 patients) were 0.5–2.0 cm in diameter, and numbered four to ten in 50% (14/28 patients) or even more in 42.9% (12/28 patients). The edges were blurred and the lesions usually round, 92.6% (26/28 patients) and atrophy was not present 85.7% (24/28 patients).

Cases of vascular ischaemic disease were characterized by lesions predominantly in white matter, separated from ventricles, 97.1% (33/34 patients) with fewer periventricularly, 70.6% (24/34 patients), mostly only in one region, 61.8% (21/34 patients). Usually there were more than ten lesions, 58.3% (20/34 patients) commonly 0.5–2.0 cm, 73.5% (24/34 patients), or in fewer cases 0–0.5 cm in diameter, 58.9% (20/34 patients). In approximatively half the cases we noted atrophy, 47.1% (16/34 patients). The lesions were characterized by irregular edges, 76.5% (26/34 patients) or round shape with a sharp edge, 47.1% (19/34 patients).

Cases of vascular inflammatory disease revealed lesions located mainly at the grey/white border, 85.7% (6/7 patients) and in white matter, 100% (7/7 patients). Usually they were 0.5–2.0 cm in diameter, 85.7% (6/7 patients). They were round and sharply edged, 71.4% (5/7 patients) and atrophy was present in 2 cases, 28%.

Comparison of the three diagnostic entities

Localization of lesions. Diffusely distributed lesions were commonest in MS, while lesions in one region were found

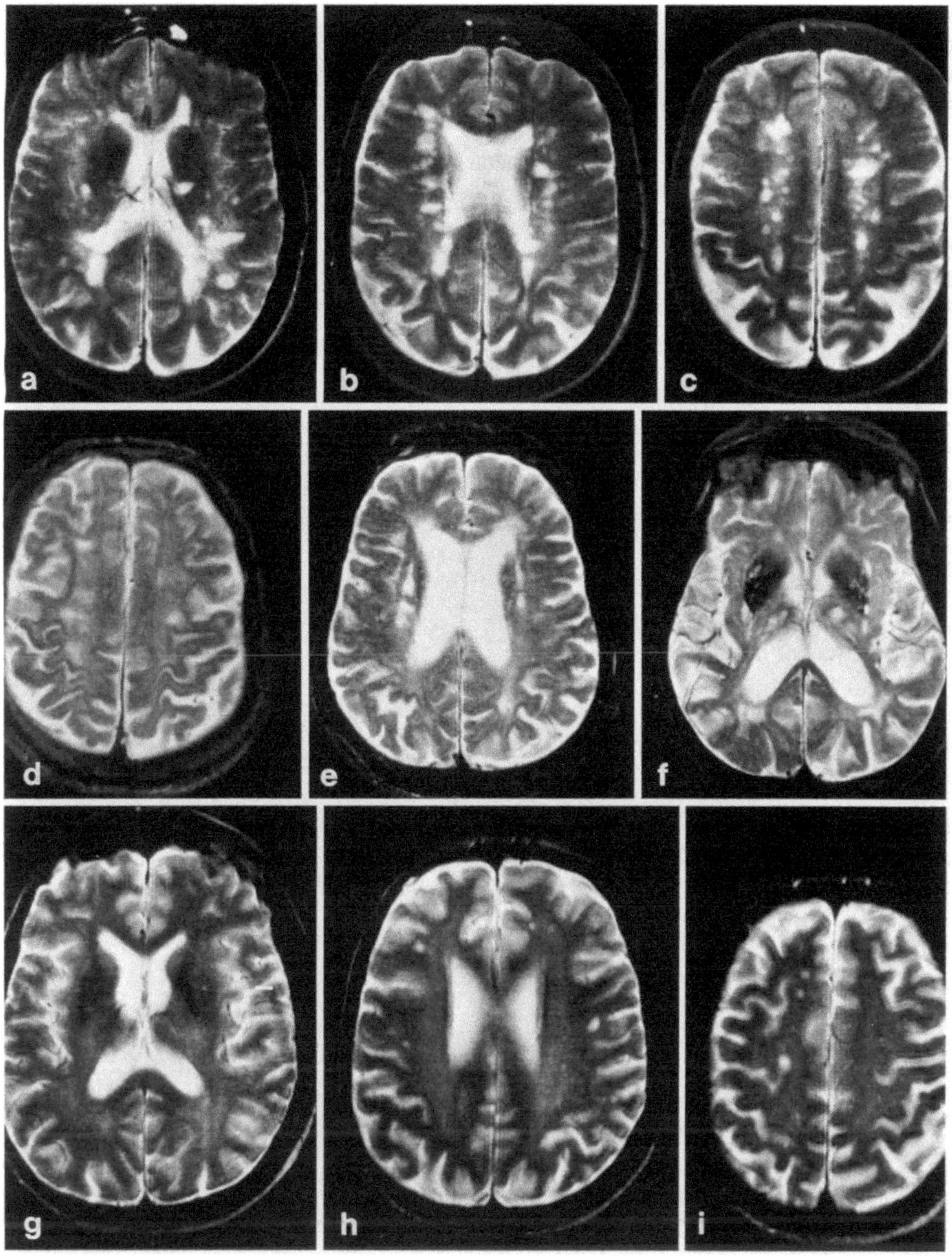

Fig. 1. MRI in: **a–c** multiple sclerosis; **d–f** cerebrovascular ischaemic disease; **g–i** cerebrovascular inflammatory disease

all cases lesions were mostly found in the white matter without contact with ventricles. Lesions in the border zone of white and grey matter are more frequent in vascular ischaemic and vascular inflammatory diseases ($P < 0.05$).

Size of lesions. No significant difference was found in the three groups.

Number of lesions. In most cases of MS we found four to ten lesions, while vascular ischaemic diseases often showed more than ten lesions ($P < 0.1$).

Morphology and atrophy. Lesions of vascular ischaemic origin were usually irregular and sharply edged, while lesions of MS or vascular inflammatory disease were round and blurred, less frequent sharply edged ($P < 0.05$). Atrophy was present in nearly half the cases of vascular ischaemic disease, while it was rare in the other groups ($P < 0.05$).

Discussion

The pathological appearances of MS plaques, vascular ischaemic and inflammatory lesions like those of SLE or polarteritis nodosa differ as a result of their underlying pathological nature. Localization, size and number of lesions may help to distinguish them from each other. With CT it is impossible to detect the differences because density resolution is too low. The lesions are seen well in T2-weighted MRI but all look very similar and it is again difficult to differentiate them.

Looking at localization, all lesions tend to be situated in the white matter, because vascular and inflammatory processes take place here. However MS and vascular ischaemic lesions were situated mostly in the periventricular area and vascular inflammatory lesions were located at the border of the grey and white matter and cortex. These findings fit perfectly with the pathological nature of these diseases.

Distribution: MS lesions were diffuse and often lay in several areas. Vascular inflammatory lesions lay anywhere in the hemisphere but exclusively in one area, mainly subcortically at the border between grey and white matter. This observation is supported by Martin and Noetzel [13], who showed diffuse involvement of vessels but few infarcts in the subcortical and cortical region in cases with cerebral arteritis.

The shapes were also different. In MS most lesions were round with a blurred edge. They seem to coalesce, especially along the ventricles and they could not be separated from one another. By contrast, the vascular lesions were sharply demarcated, irregular and separated from each other. These findings support pathological observations which show MS lesions diffusely around the veins and vascular ischaemic lesions sharply demarcated in the territory of one cerebral artery or its branch.

The size of the lesions was mainly between 0.5 and 2 cm. Smaller lesions were seen in vascular ischaemic diseases and larger ones in vascular inflammatory diseases. In general the size distribution of is very similar and so size itself does not seem useful for discriminating the different pathologies.

Usually over ten separate lesions are seen in vascular ischaemic diseases. MS patients with large numbers of lesions are not as frequent in our series as one might expect. Only MS patients with a short clinical history form part of our study, and if it is true that the longer history of MS are more lesions are seen, this may provide an explanation.

One clinical feature which was not used in our investigation but which seems to be important is the patient's age. The distribution in our cases is quite different. MS patients are much younger (44.4 years) than those with vascular ischaemic diseases (62.0 years).

Although the diagnosis of cerebral atrophy is difficult, we used wide cerebral sulci and large ventricles (Evans index > 0.35) as two criteria. Although those criteria may be questionable the absence or presence of cerebral atrophy thus identified seems to distinguish between MS and vascular inflammatory lesions, in which atrophy was absent, and vascular ischaemic lesions, in which atrophy was present.

No single parameter which can distinguish the three clinical diagnoses by itself, but constellations of parameters are very typical for each group. In MS lesions are round with blurred edges, there is no cortical atrophy and there are only lesions in the white matter and the periventricular area; there are no lesions in the border between grey and white matter. In vascular ischaemic diseases there are usually more than ten lesions with sharp irregular edges and general cerebral atrophy; in vascular inflammatory diseases the lesions lie mainly at the border of grey and white matter, are usually single, have sharp or blurred edges and produce no cerebral atrophy.

Using these seven criteria, MS, vascular ischaemic disease and vascular inflammatory disease lesions can be separated quite usefully and their probabilities can be established. The scoring method is now used prospectively (Table 1).

Table 1. Diagnostic score

Features	Multiple sclerosis	Vascular ischaemic disease	Vascular inflammatory disease
Localization			
grey/white matter	–	+	+
diffuse	+	–	–
Number			
> 10	–	+ (*)	–
Morphology			
irregular	–	+ (*)	–
sharp	–	+ (*)	+
blurred	+ (*)	–	+
atrophy present	– (*)	– (*)	–
Sum/rank	/	/	/

References

1. Young JR, Hall AS, Pallis CA, Legg NJ, Bydder GM, Steiner RE (1981) Nuclear magnetic resonance imaging of the brain in multiple sclerosis. Lancet II: 1063–1066
2. Gerard G, Weisberg LA (1986) MRI periventricular lesions in adults. Neurology 36: 998–1001
3. Fazekas F, Offenbacher H, Fuchs S, Schmidt R, Niederhorn K, Horner S, Lechner H (1988) Criteria for an increased specificity of MRI interpretation in elderly subject with suspected multiple sclerosis. Neurology 38: 1822–1825
4. Reider-Grosswasser I, Kott E, Benmair J, Hubermann M, Machtey Y, Gelernter I (1988) MRI prameters in multiple sclerosis patients. Neuroradiology 30: 219–233
5. Erkinjuntti T, Ketonen L, Sulkava R, Sipponen J, Vuorialho M, Iivanainen M (1987) Do white matter changes on MRI and CT differentiate vascular dementia from Alzheimer's disease? J Neurol Neurosurg Psychiatry 50: 37–42
6. McCune WJ, McGuire A, Aisen A, Gebarski S (1988) Identification of brain lesions in neuropsychiatry systemic lupus erythematosus by magnetic resonance scanning, Arthritis Rheum 31: 159–166
7. Miller DH, Kendall BE, Barter S, Johnson G, McManus DG, Logsdail SJ, Ormerod IEC, McDonald WI (1988) MRI in central nervous system sarcoidosis. Neurology 38: 378–388
8. Holland BA, Perrett LV, Mills CM (1986) Meningovascular syphilis: CT and MR findings. Radiology 158: 439–442
9. Miller DH, Ormerod IEC, Gibson A, Boulay EP du, Rudge P, McDonald WI (1987) MR brain scanning in patients with vasculitis: differentiation from multiple sclerosis, Neuroradiology 29: 226–231
10. Schroth G, Kretschmar K, Gawehn J, Voigt K (1987) Advantage of MRI in the diagnosis of cerebral infections. Neuroradiology 29: 120–126
11. Olsen WL, Longo FM, Mills CM, Norman D (1988) White matter disease in AIDS: findings at MRI. Neuroradiology 169: 445–448
12. Matthew DE, Farewell VT (1988) Using and understanding medical statistics, 2nd edn. Karger, Basle
13. Martin H, Noetzel H (1959) Gehirnbeteiligung bei generalisierter Panarteriitis Nodosa. Beitr Pathol Anat 121: 347

Dr. E. W. Radü
Leiter der Neuroradiologischen Abteilung
Kantonsspital Basel
CH-4031 Basel, Switzerland

Neuroradiology (1991) 33 [Suppl]: 121–122

Neuro radiology
© Springer-Verlag 1991

Multiple sclerosis associated with sinusitis: a case-controlled MRI study

S. Lang[1], M. Brainin[1,2], A. Neuhold[2], and L. Wicke[2]

[1] Department of Neurology, Landesnervenklinik Gugging/Klosterneuburg, Austria
[2] Institute for Diagnostic Imaging, Krankenanstalt Rudolfinerhaus, Vienna, Austria

Summary. A recent revival of the microbial hypothesis suggests that multiple sclerosis (MS) is caused by a direct spread of infection to the central nervous system. According to this hypothesis, oral spirochaetes spread from a submucosal abscess within the paranasal sinuses through thin bone or where the bone is deficient and disseminate in the cerebrospinal fluid producing a perivascular inflammation. The exacerbations of MS have been shown to be associated with exacerbations of mucosal inflammation. This hypothesis accounts for most epidemiological, genetic and clinical characteristics of MS. In order to substantiate this hypothesis a retrospective study of the MRI studies of 100 consecutive clinically definite MS patients was performed and compared to an age- and demographically-matched control group ($n = 100$). In no case were clinical signs or symptoms of acute sinusitis reported. The review of the MRI and the rating of the mucosal pathology of the ethmoid and sphenoid sinuses was performed independently by two neuroradiologists: 0, normal or near-to-normal with hypertrophic mucosa (lining); 1, inflammatory changes with partial obstruction of at least one sinus; 2, opacification without obliteration; 3, opacification with obliteration. Although there was tendency towards a higher prevalence in the MS group, no significant group difference of opacified sinuses (with and without obliteration) was found (MS: 21%; controls: 16%). It is concluded that the prevalence of asymptomatic inflammation of the ethmoid and sphenoid sinuses as seen by means of MRI is similar to the percentage range known from previous CT studies and that immunological long-term effects may also play a role in the remitting and relapsing course of MS.

Key words: Multiple sclerosis – Aetiology – Sinusitis – Magnetic resonance imaging

The aetiology of multiple sclerosis (MS) has remained entirely obscure in spite of a number of hypotheses based on epidemiological, genetic, virological and experimental data. No breakthrough has been achieved in more than 35 years of intensive research. As McDonald summarized in a recent overview [1]: "We do not know the nature of the environmental agent, nor do we understand the sequence of events which follows exposure to it, nor the mechanism of tissue damage. We still have no satisfactory explanation for the apparent cycles of quiescence and activity in the disease and we do not know what determines whether a patient will die within 5 years of the first symptoms or be fit after 50 years". Remarkable recent technical advances such as MRI have to date yielded no data as to elucidate the origin of the disease [2]. In our view, this frustrating and bewildering resumé implies the need for new efforts based on new concepts of the disease.

One such is the "spirochaetal hypothesis" put forward by Gay and Dick in 1986 [3]. They hypothesized a direct spread of infection from a diseased sinus to the central nervous system (CNS) as the primary event in MS. This is based on two facts. Firstly, a statistical and anatomical re-evaluation of the findings of Steiner (1954) and other contemporary workers has shown that the rejection of the spirochaetal hypothesis seemed to be unsubstantiated; secondly, in a retrospective, case-controlled study, Gay et al. [4] were able to find an association between MS and chronic sinusitis. This led to a most intriguing hypothesis which could fully explain the origin of MS. Oral spirochaetes, known to have a predilection for chronically inflamed mucosa, invade the CNS from chronic submucosal microabscesses in the sphenoid sinus through thin bone or where the bone is deficient. The organisms disseminate through the cerebrospinal fluid (CSF) and along tributaries of the cavernous sinus producing a meningovascular inflammation initially involving the Virchow-Robin spaces. The site of entry may account for the localization of the first symptoms. The exacerbations of MS are caused by the intermittent invasion of the CNS by an oral spirochaete associated with exacerbations of mucosal inflammation. The specific age-of-attack curve in MS is explained by the direct association with sinusitis and risk is carried in MS by carrying mucosal damage acquired after the sphenoid sinus is pneumatized in the second decade of life. The geographical distribution of MS is explained by the world distribution of respiratory infections as known from the literature. The apparent rarity of MS among Japanese may be caused by differences in the ossification and anatomy of the sphenoid bone. Other spirochaetal infections, such as Lyme borreliosis, are also known to show chronic relapsing as well as chronic progressive courses in addition to intrathecal immunoglobulin production and oligoclonal bands [5].

Table 1. Prevalence of asymptomatic chronic sinusitis in MS-patients and age-matched controls

	MS ($n = 100$)	Controls ($n = 100$)	Significance
Mean age (SD) in years	46.9 (13.3)	46.1 (14.1)	
Ethmoid sinusitis with partial/complete obstruction (%)	14	12	NS
Sphenoid sinusitis with partial/complete obstruction (%)	7	4	NS

MS, Multiple sclerosis; SD, standard deviation; NS, not significant

The aim of our study was to substantiate this hypothesis by using the sensitivity of MRI to detect mucosal inflammation in the nose and paranasal sinuses.

Patients and methods

One hundred MR studies of patients with clinically definite MS (Poser Committee Criteria) were examined and compared with 100 of age-matched control patients (headache: $n = 17$; epilepsy: $n = 18$; tumour: $n = 21$; vascular: $n = 25$; other: $n = 19$). All patients were residents within the geographical area of Vienna or the surrounding province of Lower Austria. In no case was acute or chronic sinusitis known at the time of the MR examination. The disease duration and the disability status of the MS patients were not considered, as long as the diagnosis had been established on clinical grounds as well as by examination of the CSF (elevated intrathecal immunoglobulin production and oligoclonal bands). All patients considered for this study had had a complete brain MRI examination (0.5 T, Gyroscan) using spin-echo sequences with contiguous transverse slices without injection of contrast media. Only those patients were included in whom at least the upper nasal cavity and paranasal sinuses were visualized, which usually is the case when investigating at the posterior fossa level. The assessment of the MR images was done independently by two neuroradiologists who were not familiar with the object of this study. Interpretation was restricted to the ethmoid or sphenoid sinuses. Three grades of mucosal pathology were used: 0, normal or near-to-normal with discrete lining of the mucosa; 1, inflammatory changes with partial obstruction of at least one sinus; 2, inflammatory changes with complete obstruction of at least one sinus. Statistical evaluation was performed by means of cross-tabulation analyses with Yates's correction.

Results

The mean age in both groups was 46 years (Table 1). Inflammatory changes (grade I or II) of the ethmoid sinus were seen in 14% of MS patients and 12% of the control patients. The difference was not significant (chi square = 0.11, $df = 1$, NS). When considering pathological changes in the sphenoid sinus the MS group showed inflammatory changes in 7% and the control group in 4%, respectively. This difference was also not significant (chi square = 0.49, $df = 1$, NS).

Discussion

MRI has been shown to be a sensitive tool for the detection of mucosal inflammation within the nose and paranasal sinuses. Differentiation between inflammatory changes and other pathological, e.g. tumorous conditions can be achieved more reliably than is the case with CT. The specificity for MRI to differentiate between inflammatory and non-inflammatory changes has been shown in one series with pathologically confirmed cases that inflammation of the mucosa tends to show a bright signal on T2 scans, whereas 95% of all tumours of the nasal cavities have an intermediate T2 signal [6]. This is of diagnostic importance in cases with complete obliteration of a sinus.

We therefore utilized this sensitivity and specificity of MRI to investigate the varying frequency of asymptomatic inflammation of the ethmoid and sphenoid cells in MS patients and age-matched controls residing in the same geographical area. Although there was a tendency for MS patients to show a higher prevalence, the differences did not reach a significant level. To our knowledge there are only CT data on the frequency of asymptomatic ethmoid sinus abnormalities to date. These have been found in 17 of 156 adults, corresponding to 10.9% [7], which compares with the 12% prevalence we found in our control group by means of MRI.

By means of a retrospective, case-controlled MRI study we were not able to substantiate the Gay-Dick hypothesis of a direct association between MS and chronic sinusitis. This does not imply that the hypothesis is not valid. It only shows that MS patients do not show a higher frequency of asymptomatic mucosal inflammation in the ethmoid and sphenoid sinuses at all times, irrespective of illness duration and disease activity. It might also be held that the ability to detect microbial microabscesses of the nasal mucosa by means of MRI is not sufficient. On the other hand, our findings could also imply that a direct spirochaetal invasion of the CNS is not the only pathogenetic factor contributing to the progression of the disease but that some unknown immunological factors triggered by such invasions (e.g. molecular mimicry) also determine the further course of the illness.

References

1. McDonald WI (1986) The mystery of the origin of multiple sclerosis. J Neurol Neurosurg Psychiatry 49: 113–123
2. McDonald WI (1989) Diagnosis of multiple sclerosis remains essentially clinical though silent lesions can now be identified. Br Med J 299: 635–637
3. Gay D, Dick G (1986) Is multiple sclerosis caused by an oral spirochaete? Lancet i: 75–77
4. Gay D, Dick G, Upton G (1986) Multiple sclerosis associated with sinusitis. A case controlled study in general practice. Lancet i: 815–819
5. Omasits M, Seiser A, Brainin M (1989) Zur chronisch rezidivierenden und schubhaft verlaufenden Neuroborreliose. Wien Klin Wochenschr 102: 4–12
6. Som PM, Shapiro MD, Biller HF, Sasaki C, Lawson W (1988) Sinonasal tumors and inflammatory tissues: differentiation with MR imaging. Radiology 167: 803–808
7. Duvoisin B, Agrifoglio A (1989) Prevalence of ethmoid sinus abnormalities on brain CT of asymptomatic adults. AJNR 10: 599–601

Dr. Michael Brainin
Department of Neurology
Landesnervenklinik Gugging
Hauptstrasse 2
A-3400 Maria Gugging/Klosterneuburg, Austria

Neuroradiology (1991) 33 [Suppl]: 123–124

Neuro radiology
© Springer-Verlag 1991

Correlation between structural brain lesions and emotional and cognitive function in patients with multiple sclerosis: an MRI study

C. F. Gonzalez[1], D. R. Mitchell[2], T. Sachetti[2], J. D. Seward[2], R. L. Knobler[3], and F. D. Lublin[3]

Departments of [1] Radiology, [2] Psychiatry, and [3] Neurology, Thomas Jefferson University Hospital, Philadelphia, USA

Summary. Forty-two patients in the acute phase of multiple sclerosis (MS) were studied with MRI and a battery of neuropsychological tests to determine the correlation beween the quantity and distribution of MS plaques in the brain and the emotional and cognitive profile. A semiautomated quantitative system was utilized to measure MRI variables such as focal distribution of the lesions in specific regions of the white matter, total lesion area, size of the corpus callosum, and ventricular brain ratio. Our findings indicate good correlation between cognitive dysfunction and altered emotional status with the total lesion area. The greatest correlation was found with lesions in the parietal and occipital areas. This suggests that white matter damage in this region may result in dementia and affective changes such as euphoria and depression.

Key words: Magnetic resonance imaging – Multiple sclerosis – Dementia – Euphoria – Depression

Numerous studies have attempted to relate both cognitive and emotional dysfunction to lesions identified on MR images in patients with multiple sclerosis (MS) [1–5]. Using MRI analysis of the MS lesion, Rao et al. [1] demonstrated a relationship between the lesion load shown on MRI and the patient's cognitive dysfunction. However, the relationship between the localization of MS lesions in the brain and cognitive performance and emotional disturbance has not as yet been established. In the present study, we have measured both the distribution and the extent of focal lesions in several areas of the brain in MS patients. The purpose of this study was to determine whether focal involvement in specific regions of the white matter, as measured by MRI, had a direct effect upon cognitive performance and mood states. The MRI indices included total lesion area (TLA), area of lesions localized in each of the frontal, temporal, and parieto-occipital regions, size of the corpus callosum, and the ventricular-brain ratio (VBR).

Materials and methods

Forty-two patients with definite MS who met the criteria of Poser et al. [6] were selected from the Multiple Sclerosis Comprehensive Clinical Center of Thomas Jefferson University. Patients were excluded if they had a history of alcohol abuse, drug abuse or a nervous system disorder other than MS. They were studied with MRI and a battery of neuropsychological tests.

The neuropsychological tests administered in this study were used to evaluate a wide range of cognitive functions, including information processing speed, verbal and nonverbal memory, abstract reasoning, visuoperceptual and language skills. Neurological abnormalities were measured using the Kurtzke Expanded Disability Status Scale and Scripps Neurological Rating Scale [7] and the Mini Mental State Examination (MMSE) [8]. Mood states were measured based upon extensive psychiatric interviews, the Hopkins Euphoria Rating Scale [9] and the Minnesota Multiphasic Personality Inventory [10].

MR images were acquired on the GE 1.5 T whole-body Signa unit to estimate the area of cerebral lesions. Sagittal, coronal and axial images of the brain were obtained, with a 5-mm slice thickness, using 2D multi-sclice, T1- and T2-weighted sequences. For T1-weighting, a spin echo sequence was used with single specification of TE = 20 ms and TR = 600 ms. In the T2-weighted spin echo sequence, TR was 2000 ms and the two echoes were acquired at 20 and 80 ms, respectively. On each slice, the lesions were outlined using the MRI console "region of interest" facility. The neuroradiologist who outlined the lesions was blinded to the subject's performance on cognitive, behavioral or neurological testing. The area of the lesion (in cm^2) and the average pixel intensity were recorded. For the correctional analyses, TLA was obtained by summing areas from all cerebral lesions identified on axial slices.

Results

The distribution of quantitative lesion area (cm^2) is presented in Table 1. Lesions were also rated in three categories according to depth from the cortex: subcortical, intermediate, and periventricular. The greatest area of involvement was periventricular (lesion mean area = 7.48 cm^2), followed by the intermediate (mean lesion area = 6.00 cm^2) and subcortical (mean lesion area = 1.18 cm^2) localizations.

Cognitive and disability variables and TLA on MRI, are presented in Table 2. In contrast, neither neurological rating scales (Kurtzke, Scripps) nor the MMSE correlated with TLA. These findings confirm the inadequacy of these tests in assessing the degree of cerebral damage resulting from MS.

The 42 patients examined were categorized into four groups based upon their emotional presentation during psychiatric interview: euphoric ($n = 8$), depressed ($n = 16$), mixed mood state ($n = 5$), and normal function-

Table 1. Distribution of lesion area

Region	Mean area (cm^2)	Range
Left frontal	1.39	0– 7.30
Left temporal	0.94	0– 8.28
Left parieo-occipital	4.68	0–16.08
Right frontal	1.74	0–19.51
Right temporal	1.23	0–15.22
Right parieto-occipital	4.66	0–24.40
Total lesion area	14.06	0–72.9

Table 2. Pearson *r* correlations between total MRI lesion area and cognitive/disability variables

Cognitive/disability variable	*r*	Probability less Than
Abstract reasoning	−0.65	0.0001
Language	−0.43	0.005
Verbal memory	−0.42	0.007
Figural memory information	−0.62	0.0001
Processing speed	−0.62	0.0001
Visuoperceptual	−0.52	0.0007

ing ($n = 13$). Patients in the mixed mood state were euphoric in appearance, but reported a feeling of depression. A discriminant analysis was performed to determine the relative importance of lesion localization upon emotional functioning. Results suggest that lesions in descending order in the right parieto-occipital, left parieto-occipital, and left temporal regions significantly discriminated among the four categories of mood state ($F = 1.87$, $P > 0.03$). The mixed mood state group had the greatest lesion load in these regions. The mixed group also had a significantly greater VBR and a significantly smaller callosal area than the normal group.

Discussion

The right and left parieto-occipital regions of the brain had the highest concentration of lesions in our study population. Lesions were rarely found in the subcortical areas, and were concentrated mainly in the periventricular and intermediate white matter. There was a direct correlation between the number of lesions seen in these areas and the degree of dementia as indicated by the results of cognitive testing and personality changes determined by psychiatric interview of these patients.

Cerebral lesions in MS are by no means clinically silent, but appear to be associated with a "subcortical dementia" characterized by both cognitive and emotional dysfunction. Although the effects of these cerebral lesions were apparent on neuropsychological testing this was not the case with the neurological examination.

Our results are surprising, since it was expected that a greater compromise of both the frontal and the temporal lobes would have been demonstrated, as indicated by our preliminary results and other reports of the organic basis of psychiatric disease. However, the present analysis shows that damage to the subcortical white matter of the parieto-occipital areas can result in dementia associated with affective changes of euphoria and depression [12].

This is of particular interest considering the degree of cortical involvement in the parieto-occipital regions in other dementing diseases and their associated psychological and neurological findings. Further analysis of these findings is now in progress.

References

1. Rao SM, Leo GJ, Haughton VM, St. Aubin-Faubert P, Bernardin BS (1989) Correlation of magnetic resonance imaging with neuropsychological testing in multiple sclerosis. Neurology 39: 161–166
2. Rao SM, Hammeke TA, Speech TJ (1987) Wisconsin card sorting test performance in relapsing-remitting and chronic-progressive multiple sclerosis. J Consult Clin Psychol 55: 263–265
3. Franklin GM, Heaton RK, Nelson LM, Filley CM, Seibert C (1988) Correlation of neuropsychological and MRI findings in chronic/progressive multiple sclerosis. Neurology 38: 1826–1829
4. Huber SJ, Paulson GW, Shuttleworth EC (1987) Magnetic resonance imaging correlates of dementia in multiple sclerosis. Arch Neurol 44: 732–736
5. Peyser JM, Poser CM (1986) Neuropsychological correlates of multiple sclerosis. In: Filskov SB, Boll TJ (eds) Handbook of clinical neuropsychology, vol 2. Wiley, New York, pp 364–397
6. Poser CM, Paty DW, Scheinberg L (1983) New diagnostic criteria for multiple sclerosis: guidelines for research protocols. Ann Neurol 13: 227–231
7. Kurtzke JF (1983) Rating neurologic impairment in multiple sclerosis: an expanded disability status scale (EDSS). Neurology 33: 1444–1452
8. Swirsky-Sacchetti T, Field H, Mitchell D, Seward J, Lublin F, Knobler R, Gonzalez CF. The mini-mental state, neuropsychological testing, and magnetic resonance imaging: clinicopathologic correlations in the white matter dementia of multiple sclerosis. J Neurol Neurosurg Psychiatry (in press)
9. Derogatis LR (1978) Hopkins psychiatric rating scale
10. Davis LJ (1971) MMPI correlates with disability in multiple sclerosis. Psychol Rep 28: 700
11. Hoff AL, Shukla S, Cook BL, Aronson TA, Ollo CL, Pass HL (1988) Cognitive function in maniacs with associated neurologic factors. J Affect Dis 14: 251–255

Dr. Carlos F. Gonzalez
Department of Radiology
Thomas Jefferson University Hospital
1009 Main Building
10th and Sansom Streets
Philadelphia, PA 19107, USA

Neuroradiology (1991) 33 [Suppl]: 125–126

Neuro
radiology
© Springer-Verlag 1991

Onset and duration of blood-brain barrier breakdown in multiple sclerosis

A. J. Thompson, A. G. Kermode, B. D. Youl, P. S. Tofts, D. G. MacManus, B. E. Kendall, D. P. E. Kingsley, I. F. Moseley, and W. I. McDonald

MS NMR Research Group, Instute of Neurology, London, UK

Summary. In a serial gadolinium-enhanced MRI study of secondary progressive multiple sclerosis (MS) enhancement, indicating blood-brain barrier breakdown and inflammation, was seen in the vast majority of new lesions (87%) and in the centre and at the periphery of pre-existing lesions. In four cases enhancement was the first abnormality seen on MRI. The duration of enhancement ranged from 2 weeks to greater than 2 months. The area of enhancement was frequently smaller than the T2-weighted abnormality and the latter usually decreased in size to correspond approximately with the area of enhancement. Gadolinium-enhanced MRI is likely to play an important role in the serial assessment of MS patients in therapeutic trials.

Key words: Multiple sclerosis – Blood-brain barrier breakdown – Gadolinium enhancement

The pathogenesis of the lesion in multiple sclerosis (MS) remains obscure mainly because of the ethical unacceptability of getting tissue sequentially during the course of the disease. The introduction of magnetic resonance imaging (MRI) and particularly the use of gadolinium (Gd) enhancement have given new insight into the natural history of the MS lesion and of the disease process as a whole [1, 2]. Studies of chronic relapsing experimental allergic encephalomyelitis, an experimental model of immune mediated demyelination have demonstrated that Gd enhancement indicates blood-brain barrier breakdown in the presence of inflammation [3]. In MS two patterns of enhancement are seen; solid uniform enhancement shown by serial scanning to occur in entirely new lesions [4] and ring enhancement which is seen in the chronic lesions [4]. This corresponds with the known morphology of inflammation seen at post-mortem. Using Gd-DTPA we have studied the relationship of blood-brain barrier breakdown and inflammation to the evolving lesion [5] and addressed the following questions:

1. When does it occur?
2. How does it relate to the natural history of the lesion?
3. How long does it last?

Materials and methods

Serial enhanced MRI was carried out on 12 patients with clinically definite MS [6] who had passed from the relapsing/remitting phase of the disease into the progressive phase (secondary progressive

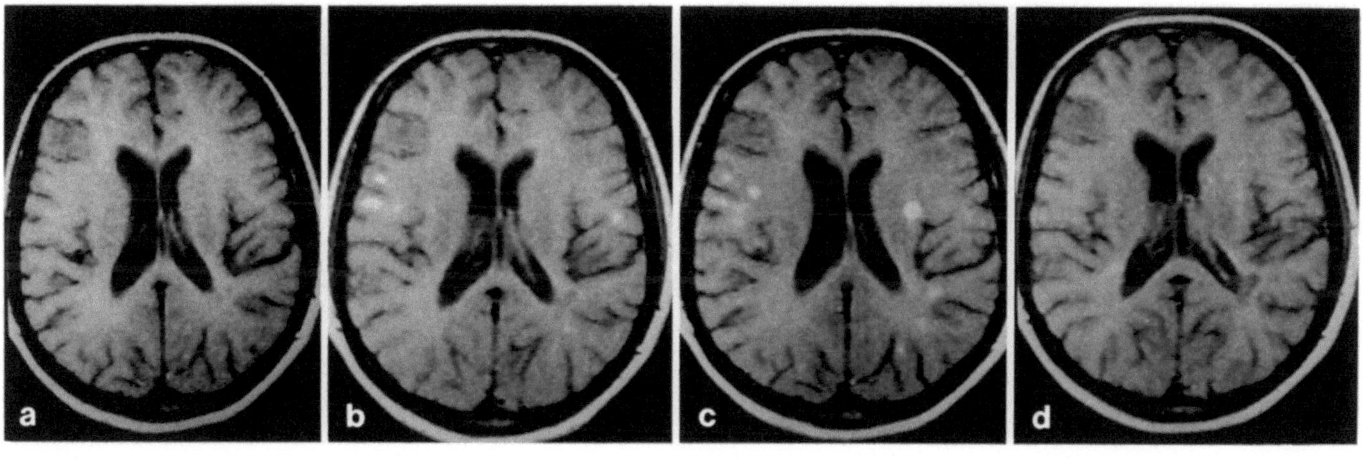

Fig. 1 a–d. Serial enhanced T1-weighted MRI (SE 500/40) from a 25-year-old female with secondary progressive multiple sclerosis. The images were taken at monthly intervals and during the period of follow-up the patient had a single clinical relapse from which she made a good recovery. No enhancement is seen in the first image and in the second image there is a cluster of lesions in the left parietal area with a single lesion on the right. One month later the areas of enhancement in the left parietal lesion have reduced in size and the lesion on the right hand side has disappeared. However, three new lesions have appeared on the right: two in the posterior parietal white matter and one in the centrum semiovale. In the final study the previous lesions are no longer seen and the only area of enhancement is adjacent to the posterior body of the left ventricle

MS). Imaging was carried out on a Picker 0.5 T superconducting machine (SE 2000/60 5-mm contiguous slices). The patients were studied fortnightly for 3 months and then monthly. Gd-DTPA was given monthly in the first 6 patients and in the second 6, at each study and T1-weighted enhanced images were obtained (SE 500/40). The imaging plane was determined by four oblique pilots to achieve consistency of imaging plane throughout the study.

Results

During the study there were four occasions when Gd enhancement preceded any definite MRI abnormality and in one case enhancement occurred not only before the lesion appeared on T2-weighted MRI but before the patient had the relevant symptoms. These findings provide strong support for the view that blood-brain barrier breakdown is an important early event in the development of the new lesion of MS.

The frequency of new lesions far exceeded the number of clinical events. In the 12 patients studied, 109 new lesions were seen (18.3 new lesions/patient per year). During the 6 months 10 patients deteriorated and there were 17 clinical events. Thus new MRI lesions occurred 7 times as frequently as their clinical events.

Enhancement was seen in 87% of new lesions. It also occurred at the edge and in the centre of pre-existing lesions. From their initial presentation new lesions were observed to increase in size for 2–4 weeks. The area of abnormality on T2-weighted MRI was greater than the area of enhancement with Gd-DTPA. When enhancement ceased the T2-weighted abnormality usually diminished to a size corresponding approximately with the initial area of enhancement. The duration of enhancement ranged from 2 weeks to greater than 2 months and was approximately 1 month in the majority of patients (67%) (Fig. 1).

Discussion

In this study we have shown that enhancement, indicating blood-brain barrier breakdown and inflammation, may be the first detectable abnormality seen on MRI, indicating that it is an early and perhaps crucial event in the evolution of the new lesion. As has been previously shown in relapsing/remitting [1, 7] and secondary progressive ([8]; Thompson et al., to be published) MS enhancement was seen in almost all lesions lasting between 2 weeks and 2 months and was significantly more frequent than clinical events.

These findings have important implications for the conducting of clinical trials. If MRI is to be used to monitor disease activity it is clear that simply measuring lesion area or counting new lesions is likely to be misleading. We have shown that Gd enhancement can appear in apparently homogeneous lesions and that the lesion area fluctuates markedly during the natural history of the enhanced lesion. Thus it is likely that serial enhanced imaging will play an important part in assessing future treatments in MS.

References

1. Miller DH, Rudge P, Johnson G, Kendall BE, MacManus DG, Moseley IF, Barnes D, McDonald WI (1988) Serial Gadolinium enhanced magnetic resonance imaging in multiple sclerosis. Brain 111: 927–939
2. Willoughby EW, Grochowski E, Li DKB (1989) Serial magnetic resonance scanning in multiple sclerosis: a second prospective study in relapsing patients. Ann Neurol 25: 43–49
3. Hawkins CP, Munro P, Mackenzie F, Kesselring J, Tofts PS, du Boulay EPGH, Landon DN, McDonald WI (1990) Duration of blood-brain barrier breakdown in chronic relapsing experimental allergic encephalomyelitis studied using Gadolinium-DTPA and protein markers. Brain 113: 365–378
4. Kermode AG, Tofts PS, Thompson AJ, MacManus DG, Rudge P, Kendall BE, Kingsley DPE, Moseley IF, du Boulay EPGH, McDonald WI (1990) Heterogenity of blood-brain barrier changes in multiple sclerosis: an MRI study. Neurology 40: 229–235
5. Kermode AG, Thompson AJ, Tofts PS (1990) Breakdown of the blood-brain barrier precedes symptoms and other MRI signs of new lesions in multiple sclerosis: pathogenic and clinical implications. Brain (in press)
6. Poser CM, Paty DW, Scheinberg L, McDonald WI, Davis FA, Ebers GC, Johnson KP, Sibley WA, Silberberg DH, Tourtellotte WW (1983) New diagnostic criteria for multiple sclerosis: guidelines for research protocols. Ann Neurol 13: 227–231
7. Grossman RI, Braffman BH, Brorson JR (1988) Multiple sclerosis: serial study of gadolinium-enhanced MR imaging. Radiology 169: 117–122
8. Kappos L, Stadt D, Rohrbach E (1988) Gadolinium-DTPA-enhanced magnetic resonance imaging in the evaluation of different disease courses and disease acitivty in MS. Neurology 38 [Suppl 1]: 255

Alan J. Thompson
Multiple Sclerosis NMR Research Group
Institute of Neurology
Queen Square
London WC1N 3BG, UK

Neuroradiology (1991) 33 [Suppl]: 127–128

Neuro radiology

© Springer-Verlag 1991

Gadolinium enhancement of new MRI lesions in progressive multiple sclerosis

A. J. Thompson, C. P. Hawkins, A. G. Kermode, B. Youl, D. G. MacManus, B. E. Kendall, D. P. E. Kingsley, I. F. Moseley, and W. I. McDonald

MS NMR Research Group, Institute of Neurology, Queen Square, London, UK

Summary. Clinical and immunogenetic differences between primary progressive (1 °P) and secondary progressive (2 °P) multiple sclerosis (MS) are well described. A recent magnetic resonance imaging (MRI) study has demonstrated differences in the pattern and extent of abnormality on cerebral MRI between the two groups. In this serial study with gadolinium-enhanced MRI, 24 patients (12 with 1 °P and 12 with 2 °P disease) were studied over a 6-month period. In the 2 °P group, 109 new lesions were seen over the study period and 87% of these showed enhancement. By contrast, in the 1 °P patients only 20 new lesions were seen and only 1 of these enhanced. There was no difference in the degree of clinical deterioration between the two groups during the study. These findings suggest that there may be a less marked inflammatory component in the evolution of new lesions in patients with 1 °P MS when compared to those with 2 °P disease.

Key words: Multiple sclerosis – Magnetic resonance imaging – Gadolinium-DTPA – Enhancement

Multiple sclerosis (MS) is a demyelinating disease, in which inflammation is known to occur. Usually, an initial relapsing and remitting course is followed by the development of progressive disability – secondary progressive (2 °P) disease. In a small group of patients the condition is progressive from onset without clinical relapses or remissions – primary progressive (1 °P) [1]. There is evidence for immunogenetic differences between the two types of MS [2]. It is important to understand the different pathological changes which might explain these different types of progressive disease in order to plan putative treatments. A serial study was thus conducted using magnetic resonance imaging (MRI) with gadolinium (Gd)-DTPA enhancement to elucidate differences in the natural history of the MS lesion.

Patients and methods

Twenty-four patients with definite MS (Poser criteria) [3] were studied – 12 with 1 °P and 12 with 2 °P disease. There was no significant difference in the mean age, duration of illness or degree of disability (as measured by the Extended Kurtzke Disability Status Scale [4]) between the two groups. Patients were studied over a period of 6 months. A 0.5 T Picker International imager was used. Unenhanced T2-weighted images of the brain were performed every 2 weeks for the first 3 months and then monthly in all patients (SE 2000/60, 5 mm slice thickness, 256 phase-encoding increments), and sagittal images of the cervical and thoracic cord in 12 patients (SE 1500/80). Enhanced T1-weighted images following injection of Gd-DTPA 0.1 mmol/kg (SE 500/40, 5 mm slice thickness, 128 phase-encoding increments) were undertaken in all patients, and sagittal images of the spinal cord in 12 patients. In the first 12 patients (6 1 °P and 6 2 °P) studies were performed with Gd-DTPA injection monthly, and in the second 12 patients, every 2 weeks for the first 3 months and then monthly.

Results

On the T2-weighted unenhanced images there were fewer brain lesions, which were smaller and less likely to be confluent in the 1 °P group than in the 2 °P patients ($P = < 0.05$).

In the serial study, there was no difference in the degree of clinical deterioration between the two groups. In the 2 °P group, 109 new brain lesions were observed on MRI over the 6-month period (18.3 lesions/year per patient), 87% of which were Gd-DTPA-enhancing (Fig. 1). In contrast, only 20 new lesions were seen in the 1 °P group (3.3 lesions/year per patient) and only 1 of these enhanced ($P = < 0.05$ and $P = < 0.005$ respectively) (Fig. 2). There was no difference in the number of spinal cord lesions between the two groups.

Discussion

This study has shown that in patients with 1 °P MS there are fewer and smaller MRI lesions in the brain than in patients with 2 °P disease. In the serial study, new brain lesions were observed less frequently in 1 °P (3.3 lesions/year) than in 2 °P patients (18.3 lesions/year). In addition, enhancement of new lesions with Gd-DTPA was a rare occurrence in the 1 °P group, but a very frequent finding (87%) in 2 °P disease. Enhancement with Gd-DTPA reflects blood-brain barrier breakdown associated with inflammation in MS lesions [5, 6] and we thus conclude that there may be less inflammatory disease activity in the brains of 1 °P patients than in patients with 2 °P disease. It could be that the nature of the MS lesion itself is different – a less inflammatory and more demyelinating pathology in 1 °P than in 2 °P disease.

It is important to appreciate that patients with 1 °P MS may have few MRI abnormalities visible in the brain. Since the dynamic behaviour of the individual lesion and of the disease process in 1 °P and 2 °P disease is so differ-

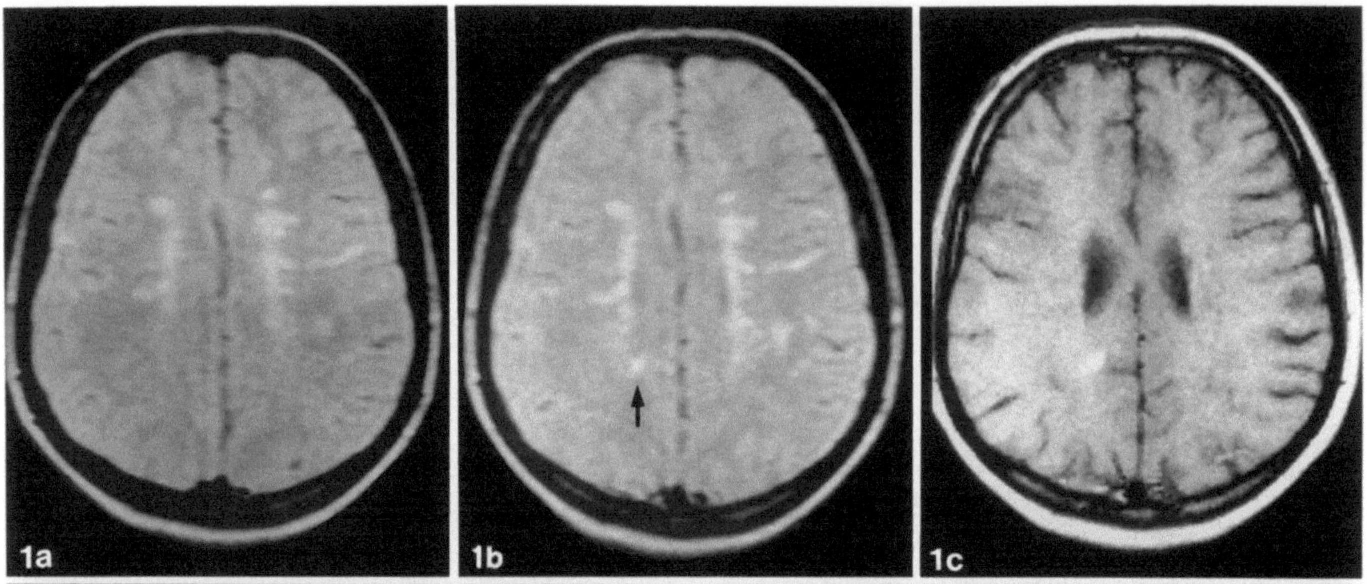

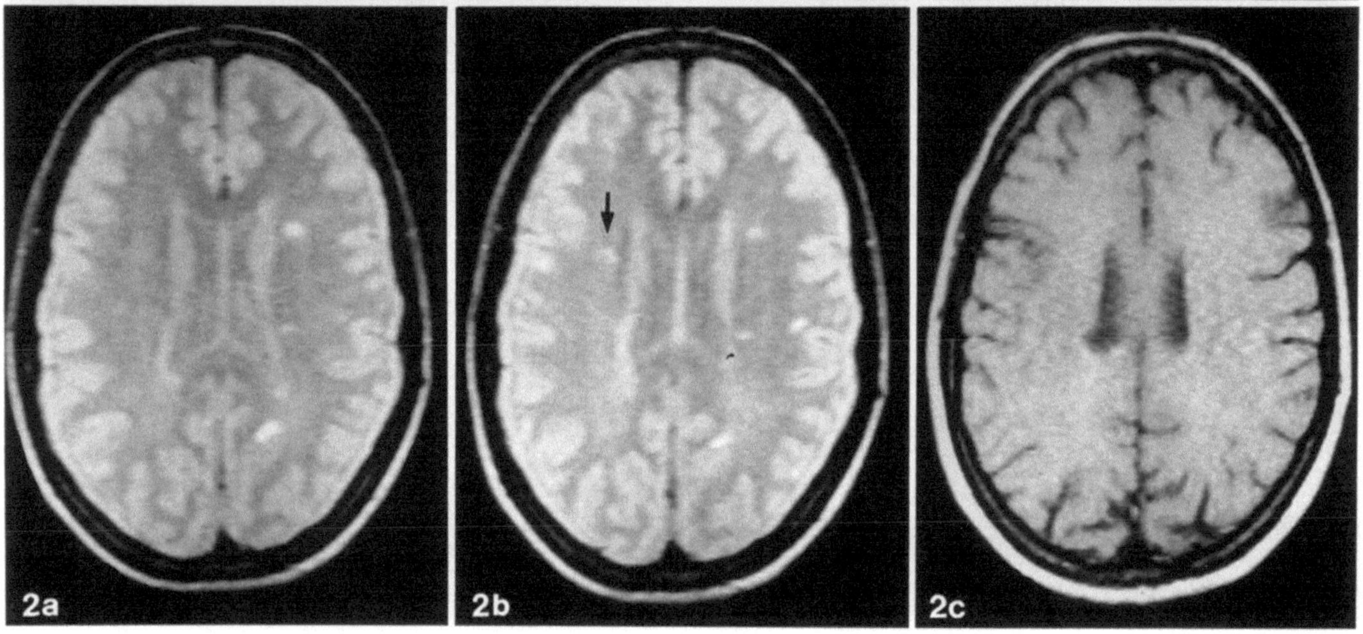

Fig. 1 a–c. MRI from a patient with secondary progressive multiple sclerosis (MS). **a** T2-weighted image (SE 2000/60) showing extensive periventricular abnormalities. **b** On serial studies (SE 2000/60), a new lesion is seen *(arrow)*. **c** The new lesion enhances with Gd-DTPA (0.1 mmol/kg, SE 500/40)

Fig. 2 a–c. MRI from a patient with primary progressive MS. **a** T2-weighted image (SE 2000/60) showing few, small white matter lesions. **b** On serial studies (SE 2000/60), a new lesion is seen *(arrow)*. **c** The new lesion does not enhance with Gd-DTPA (0.1 mmol/kg, SE 500/40)

---

ent, patients with 1 °P MS should be considered as a separate group in studies evaluating putative treatments.

References

1. Thompson AJ, Kermode AG, MacManus DG, Kendall BE, Kingsley DPE, Moseley IF, McDonald WI (1990) Patterns of disease activity in multiple sclerosis: clinical and magnetic resonance imaging study. Br Med J 300: 631–634
2. Olerup O, Hillert J, Fredrikson S, Olsson T, Kam-Hansen S, Moller E, Carlson B, Wallin J (1989) Primarily chronic progressive and relapsing/remitting multiple sclerosis: two immunogenetically distinct disease entities. Proc Natl Acad Sci USA 86: 7113–7117
3. Poser CM, Paty DW, Scheinberg L, McDonald WI, Davis FA, Ebers GC, Johnson KP, Sibley WA, Silberberg DH, Tourtellotte WW (1983) New diagnostic criteria for multiple sclerosis; guidelines for research protocols. Ann Neurol 13: 227–231
4. Kurtzke JF (1983) Rating neurologic impairment in multiple sclerosis: an expanding disability status scale (EDSS). Neurology 33: 1444–1452
5. Kermode AG, Tofts PS, Thompson AJ, MacManus DG, Rudge P, Kendall BE, Kingsley DPE, Moseley IF, du Boulay EPGH, McDonald WI (1990) Heterogeneity of blood-brain barrier changes in multiple sclerosis: an MRI study. Neurology 40: 229–235
6. Hawkins CP, Munro PMG, MacKenzie F, Kesselring J, Tofts PS, du Boulay EPGH, Landon DN, McDonald WI (1990) Duration and selectivity of blood-brain barrier breakdown in chronic relapsing experimental allergic encephalomyelitis using Gd-DTPA and protein markers. Brain 113: 365–378

A. J. Thompson
MS NMR Research Group, Institute of Neurology
Queen Square, London, UK

Neuroradiology (1991) 33 [Suppl]: 129–130

Neuro radiology

© Springer-Verlag 1991

Optic nerves show gadolinium enhancement in early acute optic neuritis

B. D. Youl, D. H. Miller, D. G. MacManus, S. G. Moore, D. Barnes, A. G. Kermode, C. P. Hawkins, B. E. Kendall, I. F. Moseley, P. S. Tofts, A. J. Thompson, and W. I. McDonald

The Multiple Sclerosis NMR Research Group, Institute of Neurology, Queen Square, London, UK

Summary. A technique allowing the demonstration of optic nerve gadolinium enhancement in acute optic neuritis is described. Enhancement is detected as a fall in signal return using a STIR sequence (an inversion recovery sequence with short TI) and a binocular orbital surface coil. An illustrated example is given. The use of the method may further the understanding of the pathophysiology of this and other related conditions, and may assist in the monitoring of treatment.

Key words: Optic neuritis – Magnetic resonance imaging – Gadolinium

Use of the intravenous contrast agent gadolinium(Gd)-DTPA (Schering) has shown that enhancement is a consistent early feature in the lesions of relapsing/remitting and secondary progressive multiple sclerosis [1, 2]. Studies using the chronic relapsing experimental allergic encephalomyelitis model of immune-mediated demyelination have indicated that Gd enhancement occurs in areas of blood-brain barrier breakdown, in the presence of inflammation [3]. We now demonstrate optic nerve enhancement in cases of acute optic neuritis.

Materials and methods

MRI (0.5 T Picker superconducting magnet) was performed before and after the injection of Gd-DTPA (0.2 mmol/kg), with the subject remaining in the imager throughout, to minimise movement. A short TI inversion recovery (STIR) sequence [4] was used (IR 2000/40/150) enabling the suppression of signal from orbital fat. A binocular orbital surface coil was provided by the manufacturer. Five-millimetre contiguous coronal slices from the head of the optic nerve to the optic chiasm were obtained. Signal attenuation was set manually.

Prior to contrast administration, lesions were identified as foci of increased signal within the nerve. Images were then examined for evidence of signal decrement, corresponding to shortening of T1, following contrast injection. This is the equivalent of lesion enhancement using conventional T1-weighted spin echo sequences, as shown in the case of a central white matter lesion, in Fig. 1 a and b.

Results

An example of optic nerve enhancement is shown in Fig. 2. A 31-year-old male had presented with isolated left optic neuritis 6 months prior to the MRI, and had now developed right optic neuritis, of 8 days' duration. On examination, clinical signs consistent with the diagnosis were elicited, including pallor of the left disc and swelling of the right, on fundoscopy. Preinjection STIR sequences demonstrated increased signal return from both optic nerves (Fig. 2 a), consistent with optic neuritis [5]. Following injection, there was decreased signal from the right, but not the left optic nerve, indicating enhancement of the right nerve only. Using an axial T1-weighted spin echo sequence (SE 500/40), with 5-mm slice thickness, enhancement was confirmed in the intracranial portion of the right optic nerve (Fig. 2 c), though signal from orbital fat obscured the intraorbital portion of this structure.

Discussion

This technique provides an effective means of detecting blood-brain barrier breakdown, and by implication, inflammation, in acute optic neuritis. Further studies are being carried out with a view to determining the frequency of enhancement in such patients, its duration, and its correlation with clinical and electrophysiological parameters. The demonstration of this feature may allow further understanding of the pathophysiology of this condition, and assist in the monitoring of treatment in this and other inflammatory and neoplastic disorders of the optic nerve.

Acknowledgement. The multiple Sclerosis NMR Research Group is supported by the Multiple Sclerosis Society of Great Britain and Northern Ireland.

References

1. Kermode AG, Tofts PS, Thompson AJ, MacManus DG, Rudge P, Kendall BE, Kingsley DPE, Moseley IF, du Boulay EPGH, McDonald WI (1990) Heterogeneity of blood-brain barrier changes in multiple sclerosis: an MRI study. Neurology 40: 229–235
2. Thompson AJ, Kermode AG, MacManus DG, Kendall BE, Kingsley DPE, Moseley IF, McDonald WI (1990) Patterns of dis-

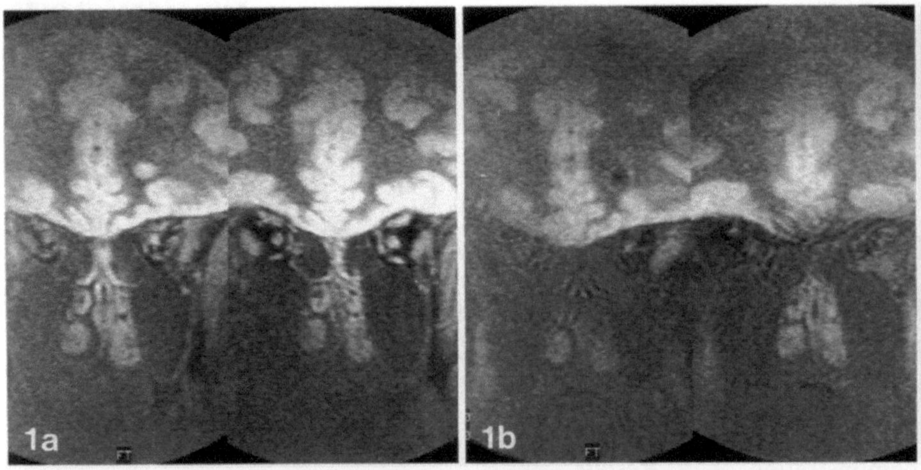

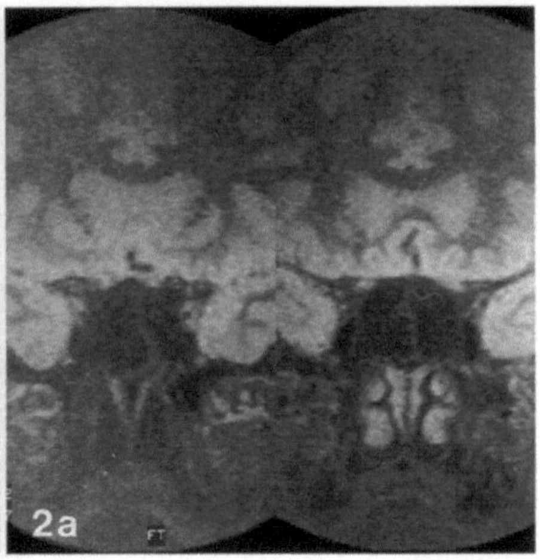

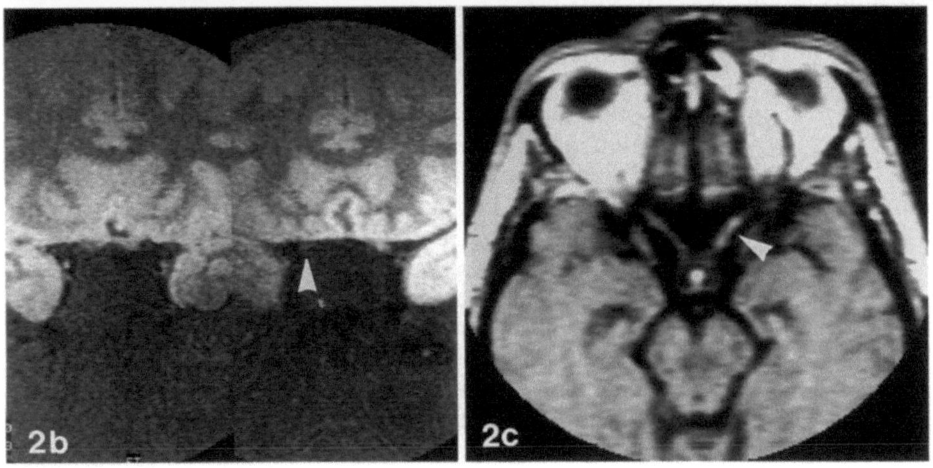

Fig. 1. **a** A 20-year-old female with isolated left optic neuritis. Lesion returning high signal in left frontal white matter. **b** Following contrast medium injection, there is a decrease in signal returned. Axial pre- and post-contrast T1-weighted spin echo sequences using a head coil confirmed lesion enhancement

Fig. 2. **a** Precontrast STIR. Increased signal is returned from both optic nerves, consistent with optic neuritis. **b** Following injection, whilst the left nerve still returns high signal, the right nerve *(arrow)* shows signal decrement, i.e. "enhancement". **c** SE 500/40 sequence showing "conventional" enhancement of the right optic nerve *(arrow)*. This shows increased signal, which had not been present on a precontrast image

ease activity in multiple sclerosis: clinical and magnetic resonance imaging study. Br Med J 300: 631–634

3. Hawkins CP, Munro PMG, MacKenzie F, Kesselring J, Tofts PS, du Boulay EPGH, Landon DN, McDonald WI (1990) Duration and selectivity of blood-brain barrier breakdown in chronic relapsing experimental allergic encephalomyelitis using Gd-DTPA and protein markers. Brain 113: 365–378
4. Johnson G, Miller DH, MacManus D, Tofts PS, Barnes D, du Boulay EPGH, McDonald WI (1987) STIR sequences in NMR imaging of the optic nerve. Neuroradiology 29: 238–245
4. Miller DH, Newton MR, Poel JC van der, du Boulay EPGH, Halliday AM, Kendall BE, Johnson G, MacManus DG, Moseley IF, McDonald WI (1988) Magnetic resonance imaging of the optic nerve in optic neuritis. Neurology 38: 175–179

David Miller
Institute of Neurology
Queen Square, London WC1N, UK

Neuroradiology (1991) 33 [Suppl]: 131–133

Neuro radiology

© Springer-Verlag 1991

Repeated gadolinium MRI in acute experimental allergic encephalomyelitis

S. J. Karlik[1, 2, 3], R. T. Stavraky[2], L. Grant[1], C. Norley[1], D. H. Lee[1, 3], and J. H. Noseworthy[3]

Departments of [1] Diagnostic Radiology and Nuclear Medicine, [2] Physiology and [3] Clinical Neurological Sciences, University of Western Ontario, London, Ontario, Canada

Summary. Serial brain MRI (3–4 day intervals) with gadolinium (Gd)-DTPA have been performed on 18 juvenile Hartley guinea pigs during acute central nervous system (CNS) – induced experimental allergic encephalomyelitis. Opening and closing of the blood-brain barrier (BBB) was observed and correlated with clinical and T2-weighted MR abnormalities. Enhancement by Gd-DTPA was observed at the first signs of clinical disease and prior to T2-weighted changes. Parenchymal Gd was observed in the most severe cases in the presence of subarachnoid or cisternal enhancement. Abnormal T2-weighted MRI continued after the BBB was again impermeable to Gd-DTPA. Sequential MRI provides a useful means to test potential interventions in BBB disease.

Key words: Experimental allergic encephalomyelitis – Gadolinium-DTPA – Multiple sclerosis – Magnetic resonance imaging

Experimental allergic encephalomyelitis (EAE) is a widely employed animal model of multiple sclerosis (MS). This model has been developed in many species [1] and comes primarily in two forms: (1) the acute monophasic form, which is dominated neuropathologically by inflammation and edema with some demyelination and (2) the chronic-relapsing, chronic-progressive or relapsing-remitting forms, which have demyelinated plaques [2, 3]. All animals which proceed to chronic forms initially undergo an acute phase. During this acute phase, the blood-brain barrier (BBB) is disrupted during inflammatory events and edema has been observed by a variety of techniques [4–6] including NMR spectroscopy [7] and MRI [8–10]. By performing gadolinium (Gd) MRI in the chronic model, changes in the BBB as a function of disease can be delineated [9, 10]. The studies reported here demonstrate the ability of repeated cardiac puncture to show BBB opening and closing in the same animal as a function of disease state. This paper illustrates the relationship between clinical findings, MRI abnormalities and BBB permeability.

Materials and methods

Eighteen, 230–250 g Hartley juvenile females (Charles River, Canada) were used for this study. All animals were immunized with homogenized whole isologous central nervous system (CNS) – in complete Freund's adjuvant (CFA) with Mycobacterium tuberculosis. Each animal received a nucal injection of 0.5 ml a 1:1 mixture of CNS and CFA with 7 mg/10 ml of mycobacterium. During pre-acute (day 0–9), acute (day 10–21), and recovery (> 21) phases, MRI was performed with Gd at 3–4 day intervals on either a Bruker 1.9T-MSL 30 system using a specially constructed double-saddle head coil or a GE Signa 1.5T clinical scanner using the extremity coil. After a mid-sagittal localizer, coronal 3-mm contiguous T2-weighted images were obtained using a TR of 2000 and TE of 34, 68, 102, and 136 ms. T1 sequences were TR500; TE34 with 3-mm contiguous coronal slices pre – and post – Gd injection. Magnevist was injected by the intracardiac route. Animals were sedated with i. p. ketamine – xylazine (10:1, 1 ml/kg). Repetitive i.m. injections produced inflammatory reactions at the site of injection.

Clinical assessments were performed daily on a scale included in Fig. 1. T2-weighted MR images were read blind to the clinical status or treatment of the animal and the abnormality was rated on an MRI scale (Fig. 2).

Results

Guinea pigs treated with whole CNS – CFA underwent an acute disease, in which loss of weight was accompanied by varying degrees of spinal neurological signs, including poor righting reflexes, ataxia, incontinence and hind limb paralysis (Fig. 1). Of the 18 animals, 5 reached a clinical assessment of 4 (terminal paralysis). All animals which showed significant clinical signs (> 1) showed enhancement by Gd-DTPA during active disease. There was one animal which showed no clinical signs, had normal T2-weighted MRI and did not enhance with Gd.

On days 10–20, T2-weighted images showed profound white matter edema, particularly in the corpus callosum, cingulum, and external capsules. Extensive parenchymal Gd-DTPA enhancement was accompanied by subarachnoid enhancement. During the recovery phase, on days 20–35, there was residual T2 abnormality observed in the external capsules and near the midline in the cingulum. At this time, there was subarachnoid enhancement. When the animals were in late recovery phase, Gd enhancement disappeared entirely, although the MRI scores remained abnormal (> 1). Figures 3 and 4 are representative animals imaged in the acute phase. Figure 3 illustrates comparative T1-weighted coronal images of guinea pig head showing subarachnoid/cisternal enhancement and Fig. 4 shows the perimesencephalic cisternal enhancement in more detail.

Figure 5 summarizes the typical course of acute events in EAE. After sensitization, the animals' body weight be-

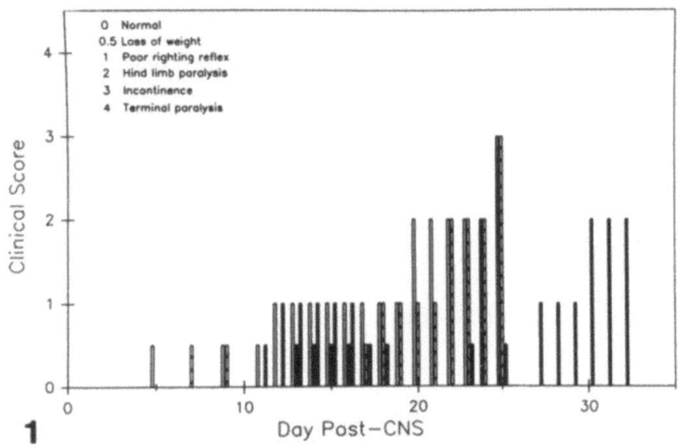

1

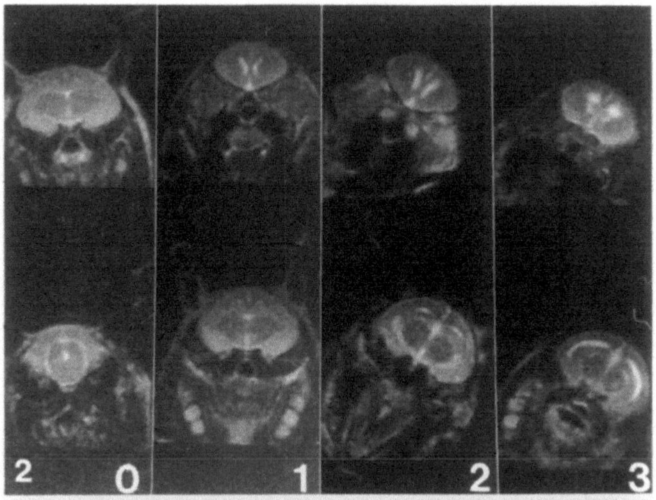

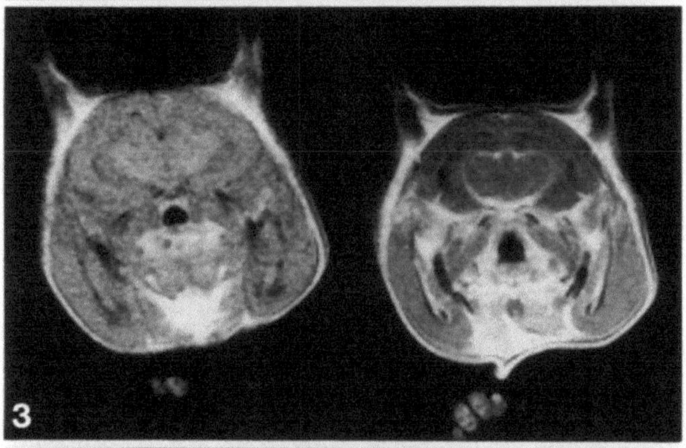

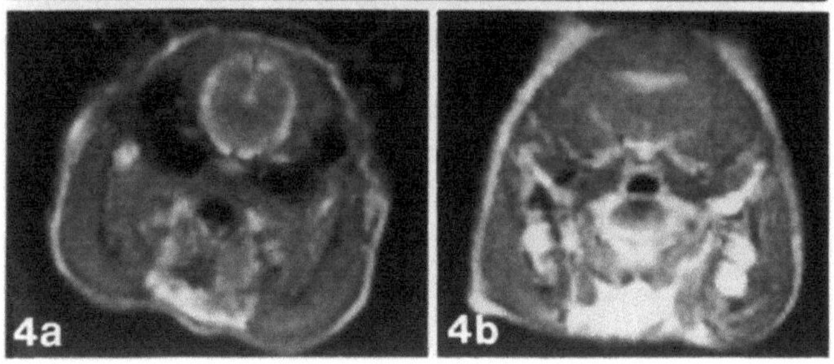

gins to drop around day 10–15. A clinical score of 0.5 indicates loss of weight only. There is a precipitous drop in weight when the animal becomes ataxic. At this time, Gd enhancement is observed before there is abnormal T2-weighted MRI. As the loss of weight proceeds, and addi-

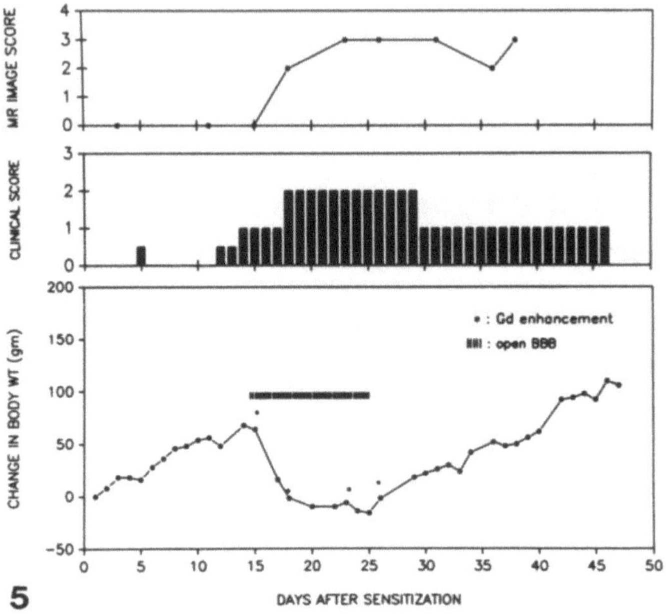

5

Fig. 1. Clinical score (0–4) plotted for three Hartley guinea pigs (□, ⊟, ■) showing typical heterogeneity of clinical progress in acute experimental allergic encephalomyelitis (EAE)

Fig. 2. MRI scoring scale for T2-weighted images: 0, normal; 1, slightly abnormal; 2 moderate and 3, severe

Fig. 3. T1-weighted pre- (left) and post- (right) gadolinium (Gd) for an acute EAE guinea pig (MRI score 3)

Fig. 4. **a** Subarachnoid Gd enhancement in an acute EAE guinea pig (MRI score 2). **b** Cisternal, periventricular and subarachnoid enhancement in an acute EAE guinea pig (MRI score 3)

Fig. 5. Composite overall clinical and MR temporal profile of a representative acute EAE guinea pig. Change in body weight, clinical score and MR score plotted on days after immunization. Gd-DTPA enhancement indicates blood-brain barrier *(BBB)* disruption

tional spinal cord signs arise, Gd enhancement continues and the MRI score worsens. Finally, at approximately day 25–30, Gd enhancement ceases, and the animal begins to improve in clinical signs. However, the MRI score continues to be abnormal.

Discussion

The purpose of this paper was to illustrate alterations in BBB permeability during the acute events associated with EAE. Repeated Gd imaging has allowed the delineation of BBB opening and closing with concomitant comparisons of clinical and MRI status. Repeated cardiac puncture has proved to be an effective means to deliver vascular contrast medium to an animal which has no readily available veins. The clinical progress through the acute phase correlates with the changes in the BBB and T2-weighted MRI abnormalities in white matter and periventricularly. In addition, Gd enhancement precedes the appearance of the T2-weighted abnormalities. Therefore, utilization of repeated MRI imaging with Gd enhancement (utilized for the detection and characterization of abnormalities in MS patients [11–13]) is fruitful in this animal model. This model will provide a mechanism to examine agents or treatments which may affect the BBB in inflammatory disorders.

Acknowledgement. This work was supported by the Multiple Sclerosis Society of Canada and the Upjohn Company.

References

1. Paterson PY (1976) Experimental autoimmune encephalomyelitis: induction, pathogenesis and suppression. In: Meischer PA, Muller-Eberhand HJ (eds) Textbook of neuropathology. Grune and Stratton, New York pp 179–212
2. Lassman H, Wisniewski HM (1979) Chronic – relapsing experimental allergic encephalomyelitis: effect of age at the time of sensitization on clinical course and pathology. Acta Neuropathol (Berl) 47: 111–116
3. Pender MP, Nguyens KB, Willenborg DO (1989) Demyelination and early remyelination in experimental allergic encephalomyelitis possibly transferred with myelin basic protein – sensitized lymphocytes in the Lewis rat. J Neuroimmunol 25: 125–142
4. Bergman RK, Munoz JJ, Portis JL (1978) Vascular permeability changes in the central nervous system of rats with hyperacute experimental allergic encephalomyelitis induced with the aid of a substance from Bordatella pertussis. Infect Immun 21: 627–637
5. Sobel RA, Schneeberger EE, Colvin RB (1988) The immunopathology of acute experimental allergic encephalomyelitis. Am J Pathol 131: 547–558
6. Stewart WA, Alvord EC, Hruby S, Hall LD, Patey DW (1985) Early detection of experimental allergic encephalomyelitis by magnetic resonance imaging. Lancet II: 898
7. O'Brien JT, Noseworthy JH, Gilbert JJ, Karlik SJ (1987) NMR changes in experimental allergic encephalomyelitis: NMR changes precede clinical and pathological events. Magn Reson Med 5: 109–117
8. Grossman RI, Lisak RP, Macchi PJ, Joseph PM (1987) MR of acute experimental allergic encephalomyelitis. AJNR 8: 1045–1048
9. Hawkins CP, Munro PMG, MacKenzie F, Kesselring J, Tofts PS, DuBoulay EPGH, Landon DN, McDonald WI (1990) Duration and selectivity of blood-brain-barrier breakdown in chronic relapsing experimental allergic encephalomyelitis studied with gadolinium-DTPA and protein markers. Brain 113: 365–378
10. Kuharik MA, Edwards MK, Farlow MR, Becker GJ, Azzarelli B, Klatte EC, Augustyn GT, Dreesen RG (1988) Gadolinium-enhanced MR imaging of acute and chronic experimental demyelinating lesions. AJNR 9: 643–648
11. Kermode AG, Tofts PS, Thompson AJ, MacManus DG, Rudge P, Kendall BE, Kingsley DPE, Moseley IF, DuBoulay EPGH, McDonald WI (1990) Heterogeneity of blood-brain-barrier changes in multiple sclerosis: an MRI study with gadolinium-DTPA enhancement. Neurology 40: 229–235
12. Bastianello S, Pozzilli C, Bernardi S, Bozzao L, Fantozzi LM, Buttinelli C, Fieschi C (1990) Serial study of gadolinium-DTPA MRI enhancement in multiple sclerosis. Neurology 40: 581–595
13. Wiebe S, Karlik SJ, Lee D, Hopkins MB, Vandervoort MK, Rice GPA, Ebers GC, Noseworthy JH (1990) Serial cranial and spinal cord quantitative MRI in multiple sclerosis: clinical correlations. Neurology [Suppl] 40: 377

Dr. Stephen J. Karlik
Department of Diagnostic Radiology, 2MR21
University Hospital
P. O. Box 5339, Postal Stn. A
London, Ontario, N6A 5A5
Canada

SESSION 10
TREATMENT OF CEREBRAL ANEURYSMS

Neuroradiology (1991) 33 [Suppl]: 136–138

Neuro radiology
© Springer-Verlag 1991

Interventional neurovascular treatment of intracavernous aneurysms

R. T. Higashida[1], V. V. Halbach[1], C. F. Dowd[1], S. L. Barnwell[1], B. Dormandy[2], J. Bell[2], and G. B. Hieshima[1]

[1] Departments of Radiology and Neurological Surgery, Interventional Neuroradiology Section, University of California at San Francisco, San Francisco, California, USA
[2] Interventional Therapeutics Corporation, South San Francisco, California, USA

Summary. The direct surgical approach to large and giant intracavernous aneurysms is rarely attempted due to the surrounding cavernous sinus. It is now technically feasible to treat these aneurysms by interventional neurovascular techniques in selected cases. For ectatic and broad-based aneurysms, test occlusion, followed by permanent balloon occlusion of the carotid artery and aneurysm can be performed. If a well defined neck to the aneurysm is present, a balloon can be navigated directly into it for occlusion, with preservation of the parent vessel. So far our group has treated 102 patients with an intracavernous aneurysm by this technique. In 77 cases (75.6%), parent vessel occlusion was performed. In the remaining 25 cases (24.5%), direct occlusion of the aneurysm was achieved. Complications included transient cerebral ischemia in 9 cases, stroke in 7 cases, and 1 death. Endovascular therapy can be effective for treatment of intracavernous aneurysms.

Key words: Intracavernous aneurysms – Interventional neuroradiology – Balloon occlusion – Aneurysm therapy – Detachable balloons

Interventional treatment of intracavernous aneurysms was first reported in the early 1970s [1]. The technique involved direct puncture of the cervical internal carotid artery and occlusion with latex balloons (Fig. 1). Improvements in catheter and microballoon technology, along with permanent solidifying materials, have now allowed the interventionalist the capability of directly guiding the balloon into the aneurysm while preserving the parent vessel, if a well-defined neck to the aneurysm can be identified [2] (Fig. 2). This technique is especially useful for intracavernous aneurysms, due to the relative inaccessibility by direct surgical exposure of this segment of the carotid artery [3]. Over the past 10 years, our group has treated 102 patients with an intracavernous aneurysm by endovascular balloon occlusion techniques. Our current technique and therapeutic results are presented.

Materials and methods

Since 1981, our group has treated a total of 215 patients with an intracranial aneurysm by interventional techniques. The largest single group, patients with an intracavernous aneurysm, constituted 102 cases (47.4%). Patients ranged in age from 11 to 83 years of age (mean 47.0). They included 80 females and 22 males. The clinical

1

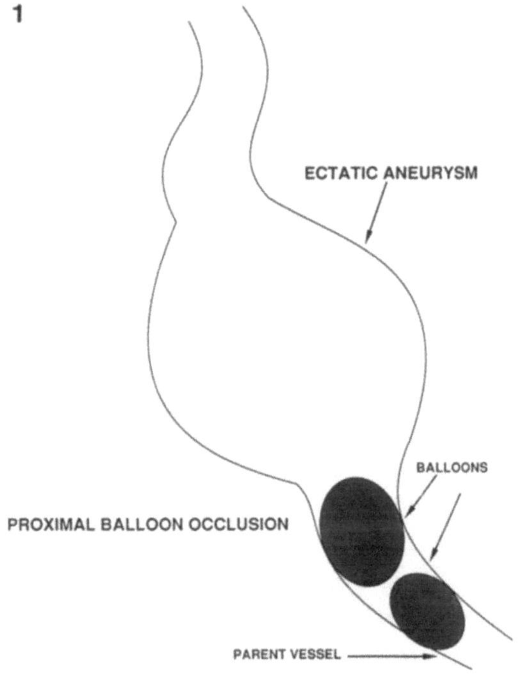

2

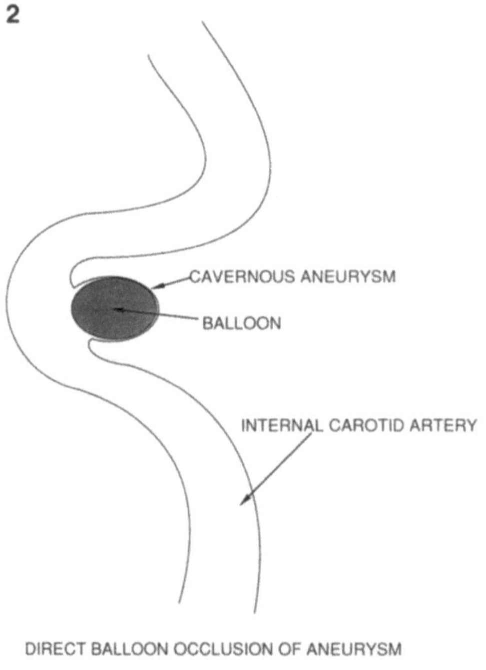

Fig. 1. Proximal occlusion of an ectatic aneurysm using two detachable balloons for occlusion of the aneurysm and parent vessel

Fig. 2. Treatment of an intracavernous aneurysm by placement of the balloon directly into the aneurysm for obliteration, with preservation of the normal internal carotid artery

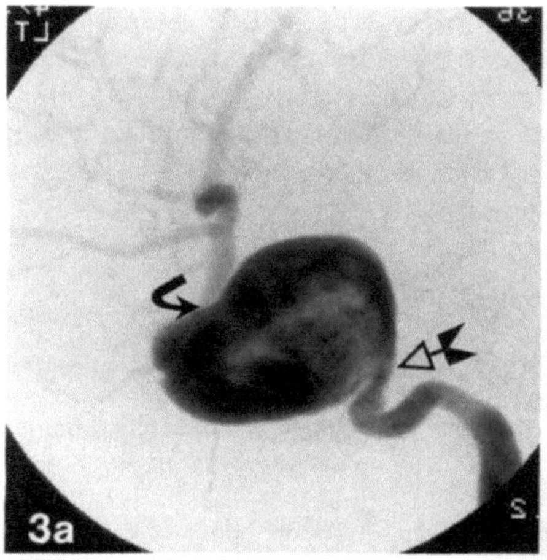
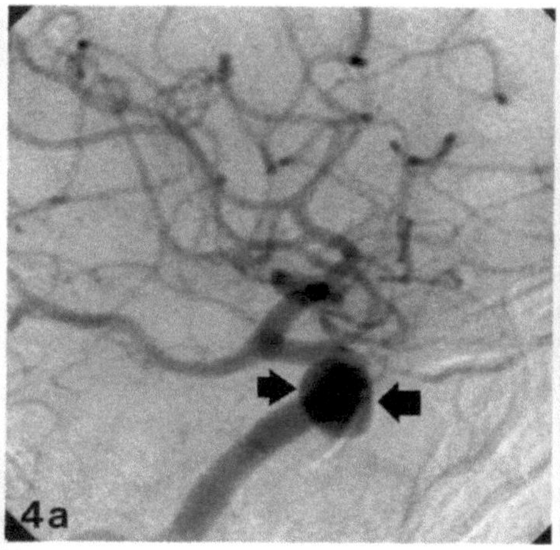
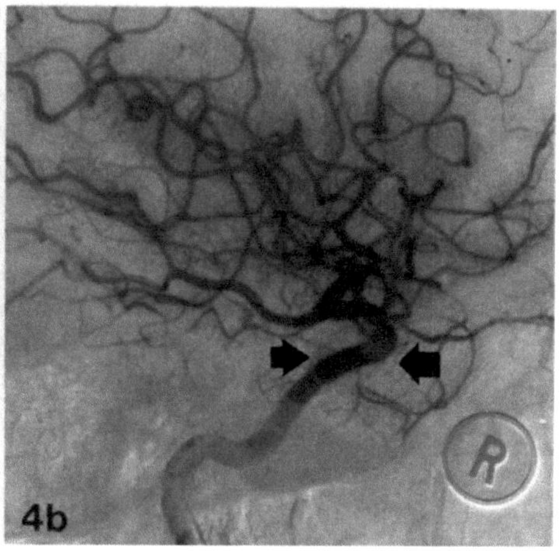
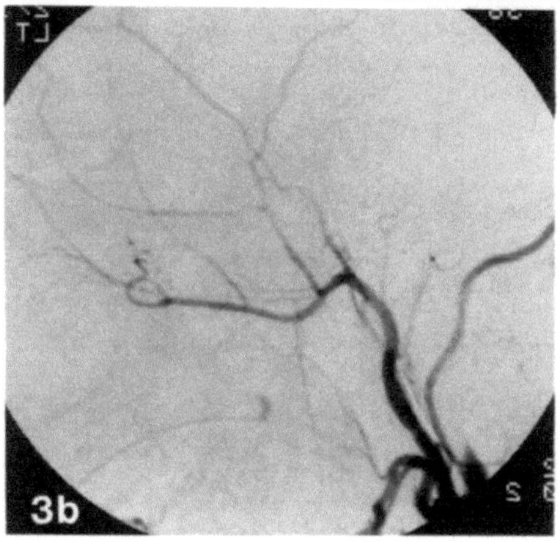

Fig. 3. **a** Internal carotid arteriogram demonstrates a giant intracavernous ectatic aneurysm. Note that the inflow (*large arrow*) and outflow (*curved arrow*) are separate. **b** Following occlusion of the internal carotid artery with two silicone detachable balloons, the common carotid artery injection demonstrates occlusion of the aneurysm and parent vessel

Fig. 4.a Cerebral arteriogram demonstrates a large intracavernous aneurysm (*arrows*) with a well-defined neck. **b** Following placement of a single detachable balloon into the aneurysm (*arrows*), there is complete obliteration of the aneurysm, with preservation of the normal internal carotid artery

presentation included 74 patients with mass effect (72.5%), 10 patients with a traumatic pseudoaneurysm (9.8%), 8 patients with transient cerebral ischemia (7.8%), 7 patients with rupture of an intracavernous aneurysm resulting in a carotid cavernous sinus fistula (6.9%), and 3 patients with an acute subarachnoid hemorrhage (2.9%). In 41 cases the aneurysm was giant, measuring more than 2.5 cm in diameter.

All patients underwent a complete cerebral arteriogram to demonstrate the location, size, and neck of the aneurysm, and to exclude multiple aneurysms in other locations. Collateral circulation was studied by compression of the ipsilateral carotid artery while injecting the contralateral carotid and dominant vertebral artery. External carotid vessels were examined in case an intracranial to extracranial bypass procedure was required in conjunction with carotid occlusion therapy. Correlation with CT and/or MRI was made to study mass effect and intraluminal thrombus within the aneurysm.

All patients underwent a trial of temporary carotid occlusion prior to therapy. Systemic anticoagulation was administered by giving heparin (72 units/kg) IV, and checked by an activated clotting time. From a transfemoral approach under local anesthesia, a 7.0 Fr catheter, with an affixed balloon (Medi-tech, Watertown, Mass.), was then placed into the proximal cervical internal carotid artery. The balloon was then inflated for 30 min to occlude temporarily the carotid artery and neurological testing was performed. Arterial pressures before and after balloon occlusion were measured. For aneurysms with ectatic or broad based necks, carotid occlusion using detachable balloons was then performed if the patient tolerated the test occlusion.

At our institution, we are utilizing the ITC silicone detachable balloon occluder system (Interventional Therapeutics Corporation, South San Francisco, Calif. [4]). The ITC 1.5 DSB balloon measures 1.5 mm × 5.1 mm uninflated, will accept 0.50 ml of fluid, and expand to 7.5 mm × 13.5 mm. The balloon is attached to a 2.0 F catheter. It is detached by simple traction and has an internal miter valve which will self-seal to prevent deflation. The balloon is flow-directed through the intracranial circulation under direct fluoroscopic vizualization. Once in the proper position, it is inflated to produce occlusion of the carotid artery and aneurysm neck, and then detached. A second balloon is then placed proximal to the first balloon and also detached. We routinely use two balloons placed in tandem for carotid artery occlusion (Fig. 3 a, b).

For aneurysms with a well-defined neck, the balloon can be directly guided into the aneurysm. The contrast medium used to opacify the balloon is then aspirated and exchanged with a liquid polymer (2-hydroxyethylmethacrylate), allowed to solidify, and then detached [5]. A final postembolization arteriogram is performed to insure obliteration of the aneurysm, and preservation of the normal internal carotid artery (Fig. 4 a, b).

Patients were observed in the neurological observation unit for 2–4 days, and if stable discharged. Follow-up both clinically and radiographically is performed at 1, 3, and 12 months postembolization. Plain skull radiographs, CT, MRI, and/or angiography are performed to insure continued obliteration and thrombosis of the aneurysm.

Results

In our series of 102 cases, 77 patients (75.5%) shown to have an ectatic or broad based intracavernous aneurysm were treated by parent vessel occlusion therapy. Only 2 patients (2.0%) in this group did not tolerate temporary test occlusion and required an extracranial to intracranial bypass graft procedure prior to balloon occlusion therapy. In 25 patients (24.5%), a well-defined neck to the aneurysm was present and direct balloon occlusion of the aneurysm could therefore be performed.

Permanent complications in this series occurred in 7 patients (6.9%) who developed a stroke during or following treatment. Nine patients (8.8%) developed a transient ischemic event. These patients were treated with volume expansion for cerebral ischemic symptoms, or with antiplatelet and anticoagulant medications if a thromboembolic event was suspected. All patients' symptoms resolved after appropriate medical therapy was instituted. There was 1 death in this series resulting from a delayed stroke following carotid occlusion treatment.

Radiological follow-up has demonstrated aneurysm thrombosis in all cases treated by carotid occlusion therapy. Follow-up has ranged from 6 months to 10 years (mean 63 months). In general, there was alleviation of symptoms by 3–6 months for patients presenting with symptoms of mass effect. For patients treated by direct occlusion, 18 patients had complete aneurysm occlusion on follow-up studies. Seven patients had subtotal occlusion, but remain stable neurologically.

Discussion

Surgical approaches in the past, for patients presenting with an intracavernous aneurysm, have included gradual occlusion of the common or internal carotid artery using an external clamp applied to the exposed cervical vessel or direct ligation by clipping of the supraclinoid carotid artery [6–11]. The incidence of reported complications associated with these techniques varies. Scott reviewed 909 cases and reported a combined operative mortality for carotid ligation of 17% and an additional morbidity rate of 33%. In another series of 21 cases, he reported a 19% rate of fatal delayed subarachnoid hemorrhage from carotid artery ligation [12].

Several large series of patients treated by endovascular techniques for intracranial aneurysms have recently been reported from different centers. Serbinenko [1] reported upon 82 patients successfully treated by occlusion of the carotid siphon using latex balloons in 1974. Debrun et al. [13] in 1981 and Berenstein et al. [14] in 1984 also reported upon the efficacy of this technique for large and giant aneurysms involving the internal carotid artery. In 1987, Fox et al. [15] described 68 patients treated by parent vessel occlusion therapy using detachable balloons. They reported a 13.2% incidence of delayed cerebral ischemia, 1.5% permanent morbidity (1 stroke), and no mortality.

In our current series of 102 patients with an intracavernous aneurysm, we report a permanent morbidity rate of 6.7% and a mortality rate of 0.98%. An additional 8.8% of patients had a transient ischemic event with resolution of symptoms. We conclude that treatment of symptomatic intracavernous aneurysms, utilizing detachable balloons, can be performed with morbidity and mortality acceptable when compared to surgical treatment. Certainly the long-term follow-up of patients treated by proximal balloon occlusion indicates that this can be efficacious, relatively safe and lead to resolution of symptoms. Treatment of patients by direct balloon occlusion of their aneurysm also appears to be feasible; however, the long-term follow-up of these patients is ongoing.

References

1. Serbinenko FA (1974) Balloon catheterization and occlusion of major cerebral vessels. J Neurosurg 41: 125–145
2. Halbach VV, Higashida RT, Hieshima GB (1987) Treatment of intracranial aneurysms by balloon embolization therapy. Semin Intervent Radiol 4: 261–268
3. Higashida RT, Halbach VV, Dowd CF, Barnwell SL, Dormandy B, Bell J, Hieshima GB (1990) Endovascular detachable balloon embolization therapy of cavernous carotid artery aneurysms: results in 87 cases. J Neurosurg 72 (in press)
4. Higashida RT, Halbach VV, Dormandy B, Bell J, Hieshima GB (1990) Endovascular treatment of intracranial aneurysms with a new silicone microballoon device: technical considerations and indications for therapy. Radiology 174: 687–691
5. Goto K, Halbach VV, Hardin CW, Higashida RT, Hieshima GB (1988) Permanent inflation of detachable balloons with a low-viscosity, hydrophilic polymerizing system. Radiology 169: 787–790
6. Galbraith JG, Clark RM (1974) Role of carotid ligation in the management of intracranial carotid aneurysms. Clin Neurosurg 21: 171–181
7. Roski RA, Spetzler RF, Nulsen FE (1981) Late complications of carotid ligation in the treatment of intracranial aneurysms. J Neurosurg 54: 583–587
8. Gurdjian ES, Lindner DW, Thomas LM (1975) Experiences with ligation of the common carotid artery for treatment of aneurysms of the internal carotid artery. J Neurosurg 23: 311–318
9. Brackett CE Jr (1953) The complications of carotid artery ligation in the neck. J Neurosurg 10: 91–106
10. Giannotta SL, McGillicuddy JE, Kindt GW (1979) Gradual carotid artery occlusion in the treatment of inaccessible internal carotid artery aneurysms. Neurosurgery 5: 417–421
11. Kak VK, Taylor AR, Gordon DS (1973) Proximal carotid ligation for internal carotid aneurysms: a long term follow up study. J Neurosurg 39: 503–513
12. Scott M, Skwarok E (1961) The treatment of cerebral aneurysms by ligation of the common carotid artery. Surg Gynecol Obstet 113: 54–61
13. Debrun G, Fox A, Drake C (1981) Giant unclippable aneurysms: treatment with detachable balloons. Am J Neuroradiol 2: 167–173
14. Berenstein A, Ransohoff J, Kuppersmith M (1984) Transvascular treatment of giant aneurysms of the cavernous carotid and vertebral arteries: functional investigation and embolization. Surg Neurol 21: 3–21
15. Fox AJ, Viñuela F, Pelz DM, Peerless SJ, Ferguson G, Drake CG, Debrun G (1987) Use of detachable balloons for proximal artery occlusion in the treatment of unclippable cerebral aneurysms. J Neurosurg 66: 40–46

Dr. Randall T. Higashida
Interventional Neuroradiology Section
University of California at San Francisco Medical Center
505 Parnassus Avenue L-352
San Francisco, California, USA

Neuroradiology (1991) 33 [Suppl]: 139–141

Neuro radiology

© Springer-Verlag 1991

Interventional therapy for intracranial aneurysms by direct balloon occlusion: clinical protocol and therapeutic results

R. T. Higashida[1], V. V. Halbach[1], S. L. Barnwell[1], C. Dowd[1], G. B. Hieshima[1], B. Dormandy[2], and J. Bell[2]

[1] Departments of Radiology and Neurological Surgery, Interventional Neuroradiology Section, San Francisco, California, USA
[2] Interventional Therapeutics Corporation, South San Francisco, California, USA

Summary. Interventional treatment of complex and surgically difficult intracranial aneurysms is now being performed by direct balloon occlusion. From a transfemoral approach under local anesthesia, a silicone microballoon can be flow directed through the intracranial circulation and guided directly into the aneurysm. The balloon is then filled with a polymerizing material, allowed to solidify, and detached. The aneurysm is thus excluded from the circulation with preservation of the parent vessel. Since 1981, our group has treated 215 cases of intracranial aneurysm of which 88 (40.9%) were treated by direct aneurysm occlusion. Patients ranged in age from 15 to 83 years of age. Complications related to therapy included 16 deaths (18.2%) and 9 cases of stroke (10.2%). Interventional techniques utilizing detachable balloons may be a useful therapeutic alternative to surgery in selected cases.

Key words: Aneurysm therapy – Detachable balloons – Intracranial aneurysms – Balloon occlusion – Interventional neuroradiology

Interventional neurovascular techniques utilizing detachable balloons were first described in the early 1970s by Serbinenko [1,2]. Since then, with recent advances in microballoon technology, steerable guidewires and microcatheters, high resolution fluoroscopy with road-mapping capability, and newer polymerizing materials, it has become feasible to guide a balloon directly into the aneurysm for obliteration while preserving the parent vessel [3– 5]. Since 1984, 88 patients have been treated by our group, using this technique for aneurysms involving both the anterior and posterior circulation. Our current clinical indications, technique, and therapeutic results are described.

Materials and methods

Since 1981, we have treated 215 patients with an intracranial aneurysm by intravascular detachable balloon occlusion techniques. In 1984, with the development of 2- hydroxyethyl-methacrylate (HEMA), as a solidification material within silicone balloons, it became possible to place a balloon directly into the aneurysm and preserve the parent vessel [6, 7]. A permanent solidification material within the aneurysm was required in order to insure that the aneurysm continued to remain occluded should the balloon shell deterioriate or the valve leak. In 88 cases (40.9%) this treatment goal has been achieved. Patients ranged in age from 15 to 83 years (mean: 49 years), and included 63 cases involving the anterior and 25 the posterior circulation. Twenty patients (22.7%) were treated for a giant aneurysm larger than 2.5 cm.

Our current indications for balloon occlusion therapy include surgical exploration with inability to clip the aneurysm, ectatic and broad based aneurysms without a well-defined neck, aneurysms in surgically difficult anatomical locations such as the petrous and cavernous internal carotid artery, and intolerance of general anesthesia [8].

All procedures were performed in the interventional neurovascular radiology suite under direct fluoroscopic visualization. Patients are mildly sedated with intravenous diazepam, morphine sulfate, and/or midazalom hydrochloride. A high resolution, rapid sequence, subtraction arteriogram is performed of the aneurysm, to show the size, shape, and relationship of the aneurysm neck to the parent vessel. Careful measurements are made of the aneurysm size and compared with recent CT and/or MRI studies to look for intraluminal thrombus [8, 9]. In the non-acute patient, embolization therapy may be delayed for 6 weeks to allow fresh thrombus to organize or lyse. This is to avoid inadvertently dislodging clot while placing balloons in the aneurysm.

Patients are then given intravenous heparin (5000 units for a 70 kg patient), for systemic anticoagulation. A guiding 7.3 or 8.0 Fr catheter is placed from the femoral artery into the cervical internal carotid or dominant vertrebral artery, depending upon aneurysm location. The correct size and configuration are then selected. At our institution we are utilizing the ITC detachable balloon occluder system (Interventional Therapeutics Corporation, South San Francisco, Calif.) for aneurysm therapy (Fig. 1). The advantages of this balloon, over latex balloons, are that it is biocompatible, non-biodegradable within the intravascular system, and due to the inherent properties of silicone, is softer and more malleable, thereby decreasing stress upon the aneurysm and reducing the risk of inadvertent rupture. Using road-mapping technique, in which the neurovascular architecture is superimposed over the real-time fluoroscopic image, the balloon can be flow – directed or catheter – guided into the aneurysm. Once the balloon is well situated within the aneurysm, the contrast used to visualize the balloon is aspirated and exchanged with HEMA, which is then allowed to solidify over 40-60 min (Fig. 2 a–c). For large and giant aneurysms, more than one balloon may be required for complete aneurysm obliteration. (Fig. 3 a, b)

A post-embolization arteriogram is performed to assess aneurysm exclusion and patency of the parent vessel in all cases. Patients are then observed in the neurosurgical observation unit for 2-4 days and if stable, discharged. Clinical and radiological follow-up is performed at 1, 3 and 12 months post-treatment to insure continued aneurysm obliteration.

Results

In the 88 patients treated by this technique, our mortality rate was 18.2% (16 deaths) [10]. The cause of death in 11 patients was aneurysm rupture due to subtotal occlusion. The other 5 deaths were due to stroke in 2 cases, myocar-

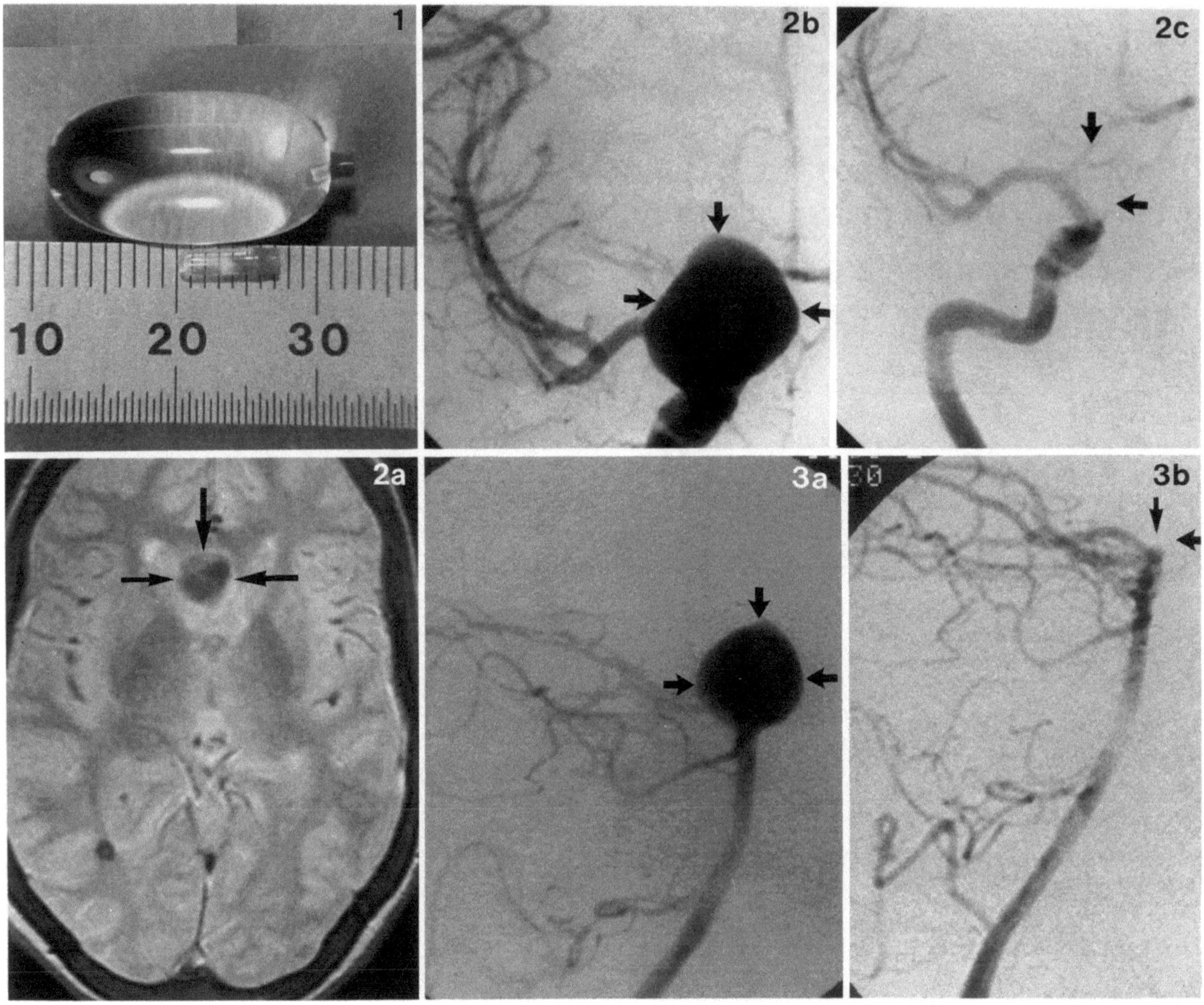

Fig. 1. Picture of ITC detachable silicone balloon system used for direct aneurysm occlusion therapy. The 1.5 DSB balloon measures 1.5 mm × 7.3 mm uninflated (foreground), will accept 0.90 ml of fluid, and expands to 8.5 mm × 21.0 mm (background)

Fig. 2. **a** MRI scan demonstrating a large aneurysm *(arrows)* which was compressing the optic chiasm. **b** Arteriogram confirming the presence of a giant supraclinoid internal carotid artery aneurysm *(arrows)* projecting superiorly and medially. **c** Following placement of a single detachable silicone balloon into the aneurysm *(arrows)*, there is complete obliteration of the aneurysm, with preservation of the normal distal intracranial circulation

Fig. 3. **a** Vertebral arteriogram, lateral view, demonstrates a large distal basilar artery aneurysm *(arrows)*, in a patient presenting with an acute subarachnoid hemorrhage. **b** Following treatment with multiple balloons placed directly into the aneurysm *(arrows)* from a transfemoral approach, there is complete obliteration with preservation of the basilar artery and distal posterior circulation

dial infarction in 2 cases, and pulmonary embolus in 1 patient. In general, these patients were in poor medical condition prior to therapy.

Our permanent morbidity rate was 10.2%: 9 patients that suffered from a stroke. In 5 patients, this was due to a thromboembolic event during the procedure, either from clot forming on the balloon and catheter, or from dislodgement of thrombus from within the aneurysm during balloon placement. This occurred in spite of placing patients on adequate doses of systemic anticoagulants during the procedure. In 2 cases, the balloon shifted after detachment causing occlusion of the parent vessel. In 1 patient, during the polymerization phase of HEMA solidification, the balloon ruptured causing a stroke. In a second patient, a balloon prematurely detached resulting in an embolus to the middle cerebral artery. Long term follow-up in these patients demonstrated that in 7 cases (77.8%) there was improvement in neurological function with only mild to moderate functional impairment. Two patients however continue to have fixed dense deficits. Clinical and radiological follow-up has ranged from 6 months to 6 years (mean 39 months).

Discussion

Direct endovascular balloon occlusion of intracranial aneurysms is now being performed at several major neurological centers. The largest published series is from the

Kiev Neurosurgical Institute by Romodanov and Shcheglov [11]. In 1982, they reported upon the treatment of 119 patients with latex balloons for aneurysm therapy. In 78.2% of cases they were able to successfully occlude the aneurysm and preserved the parent vessel. Only 12.6% of patients required parent vessel occlusion, and in only 9.2% of cases were they unable to successfully treat the aneurysm by endovascular balloon occlusion techniques. They reported a 96.7% good to excellent result following therapy.

Moret et al. [12] in 1990 reported a series of 60 patients with saccular aneurysms treated by direct balloon occlusion. Their reported morbidity rate was 10% neurological complications, 10% failure to treat the aneurysm, 8% partial recanalization requiring retreatment, and 4% mortality.

In our current series of 88 patients treated by direct aneurysm occlusion we report an overall mortality rate of 18.2% and a permanent morbidity rate of 10.2%. The differences in these statistics we believe is due to patient selection criteria. Since we view this as an adjuvant to surgery, we are only accepting patients that are medically unstable and are poor candidates for general anesthesia. A large percentage of our patients also presented with large and giant intracranial aneurysms which were judged difficult to clip surgically, or with acute subarachnoid hemorrhage.

In conclusion, we believe that detachable balloon occlusion therapy of intracranial aneurysms is feasible. However, long term follow-up of these patients both clinically and radiographically is still required. As continued developments in endovascular occlusion techniques utilizing detachable balloons, catheters, and other materials evolve, the safety, efficacy, and usefulness of these techniques will continue to improve.

References

1. Serbinenko FA (1971) Catheterization and occlusion of cerebral major vessels and prospects for the development of vascular neurosurgery. Vopr Neirokhir 35:17–27
2. Serbinenko FA (1974) Ballon catheterization and occlusion of major cerebral vessels, J Neurosurg 41:125–145
3. Higashida RT, Halbach VV, Hieshima GB (1989) Treatment of complex intracranial aneurysms by interventional techniques. In: Margulis AR, Gooding CA (eds) Diagnostic radiology. University of California Printing Services, California, pp 357–360
4. Debrun G, Fox A, Drake C (1981) Giant unclippable aneurysms: treatment with detachable balloons. Am Neuroradiol 2:167–173
5. Halbach VV, Higashida RT, Hieshima GB (1987) Treatment of intracranial aneurysms by balloon embolization therapy. Semin Intervent Radio 4:261–268
6. Goto K, Halbach VV, Hardin CW, Higashida RT, Hieshima GB (1988) Permanent inflation of detachable balloons with a low-viscosity, hydrophilic polymerizing system. Radiology 169: 787–790
7. Taki W, Handa H, Yamagata S (1980) Radio-opaque solidifying liquids for releasable balloon technique: technical note. Surg Neurol 13:140–142
8. Higashida RT, Halbach VV, Dormandy B, Bell J, Hieshima GB (1990) Endovascular treatment of intranial aneurysms with a new silicone microballoon device: technical considerations and indications for therapy. Radiology 174:687–691
9. Tsuruda J, Halbach VV, Higashida RT MR evaluation of large intracranial aneurysms using cine low flip angle gradient-refocused imaging. AJNR 9:415–424
10. Higashida RT, Halbach VV, Barnwell SL, Dowd CF, Dormandy B, Bell J, Hieshima GB (1990) Treatment of intracranial aneurysms with preservation of the parent vessel. AJNR (in press)
11. Romodanov AP, Shcheglov VI (1982) Intravascular occlusion of saccular aneurysms of the cerebral arteries by means of a detachable balloon catheter. In: Krayenbuhl H (ed) Advances and technical standards in neurosurgery, vol 9. Springer Vienna New York, pp 25–49
12. Moret J, Picard L, Mawad M (1990) A critical study on endosaccular treatment of berry aneurysms based on 60 cases (abstract). Proceedings from the 28th Annual Meeting of the American Society of Neuroradiology. Los Angeles, California. Am J Neuroradiol (in press)

Dr. T. Randall
Departments of Radiology and Neurological Surgery
Interventional Neuroradiology Section
University of California
505 Parnassus Avenue L–352
San Francisco, California, USA

Neuroradiology (1991) 33 [Suppl]: 142–143

Neuro
radiology
© Springer-Verlag 1991

Occlusion of the anterior superior ophthalmic vein in carotid-cavernous fistulae acutely aggravating visual symptoms

C. F. Dowd[1], V. V. Halbach[1, 2], R. T. Higashida[1, 2], S. L. Barnwell[1, 2], and G. B. Hieshima[1, 2]

Departments of [1] Radiology and [2] Neurological Surgery, University of California, San Francisco, California, USA

Summary. Acute occlusion of the anterior superior ophthalmic vein in the setting of a carotid-cavernous fistula (CCF) can produce dramatic and dangerous ophthalmological sequelae, including loss of vision and elevation of intraocular pressure. We present our experience with this phenomenon and its proposed mechanism of action in 11 patients. The treatment regimen includes aggressive embolization to close the fistula urgently, and administration of pharmacological agents (beta-blocker, carbonic anhydrase inhibitor) to reduce aqueous humor production. Physicians who treat CCF patients should be familiar with this phenomenon and its therapy.

Key words: Cavernous sinus – Cerebral blood vessels, therapeutic blockade – Carotid cavernous fistula – Superior ophthalmic vein – Ophthalmic veins

Carotid-cavernous fistulae (CCF) are classified as either direct or indirect (dural), based on the anatomy of the arterial feeder(s). A direct CCF consists of a direct communication between the cavernous portion of the internal carotid artery (ICA) and the surrounding cavernous sinus, usually as a result of trauma [1] or rupture of a cavernous carotid aneurysm. An indirect CCF consists of a dural-based arteriovenous fistula in the wall of the cavernous sinus, supplied by small cavernous branches of the ICA and/or branches of the external carotid artery [2], often arising spontaneously in middle-aged women. In either type, the superior ophthalmic vein (SOV), which normally drains the orbit toward the cavernous sinus, responds to the elevated venous pressure by reversing its direction of flow and transmitting elevated venous pressure *to* the orbit, producing proptosis, chemosis, pain, ophthalmoplegia, and bruit [3, 4]. When this venous drainage pathway is obstructed anteriorly *and* the CCF persists, further elevation of venous pressure may aggravate symptoms acutely. Loss of vision and elevation of intraocular pressure (IOP) may occur, necessitating urgent therapy to save vision. We report our experience with this phenomenon in 11 patients.

Patients and methods

Eleven adult patients with a CCF experienced abrupt worsening of ocular symptoms as a result of acute occlusion of the anterior SOV. Patients' ages ranged from 17 to 66 years; 6 patients were female and 5 male. Six CCFs were indirect and 5 direct. Acute anterior SOV occlusion was produced iatrogenically in 9 patients during transvascular embolization procedures, and occured spontaneously in 2 patients known to have an untreated CCF.

Results

All 11 patients experienced rapid proptosis as a result of acute SOV occlusion. Six patients suffered acute loss of visual acuity. Documented elevation of IOP occurred in 5 patients. In 10 of 11 patients, aggressive embolization was undertaken to close the remaining fistula and to reduce the pressure in the arterialized SOV; this was successful in 8 patients (Fig. 1). In the 3 remaining patients, symptoms abated when the CCF underwent spontaneous thrombosis.

Discussion

Sanders and Hoyt [5] proposed that hypoxia was the major etiologic factor in producing visual loss in CCF patients. Given that retinal perfusion is proportional to the arteriovenous pressure gradient in the orbit, perfusion will diminish when the venous pressure is raised, a condition which exists in a CCF. Although *acute* elevation of IOP will not embarass visual function by itself, it can contribute to visual failure by elevating venous pressure within the globe even further. In response to this reduced arteriovenous pressure gradient, the retinal vascular bed compensates by dilating venules and opening precapillary shunts. When this compensatory mechanism is exhausted, retinal perfusion falls below the level needed to meet local metabolic requirements, retinal tissue becomes hypoxic, and visual failure ensues.

Abrupt occlusion of the anterior SOV would dramatically and acutely elevate venous pressure above the level already produced by the presence of a CCF, because there would by one less route of drainage for the pressurized cavernous sinus. This further elevation in venous pressure would be transmitted to the eye and could produce visual loss and elevated IOP, a condition which necessitates urgent therapy to save vision [6].

The first goal of treatment is closure of the CCF by aggressive embolization techniques. This would eliminate the factor which produces elevated venous pressure, and retinal perfusion would improve as venous pressure decreased.

IOP can be reduced by lowering production of aqueous humor. Agents which can be used for this pur-

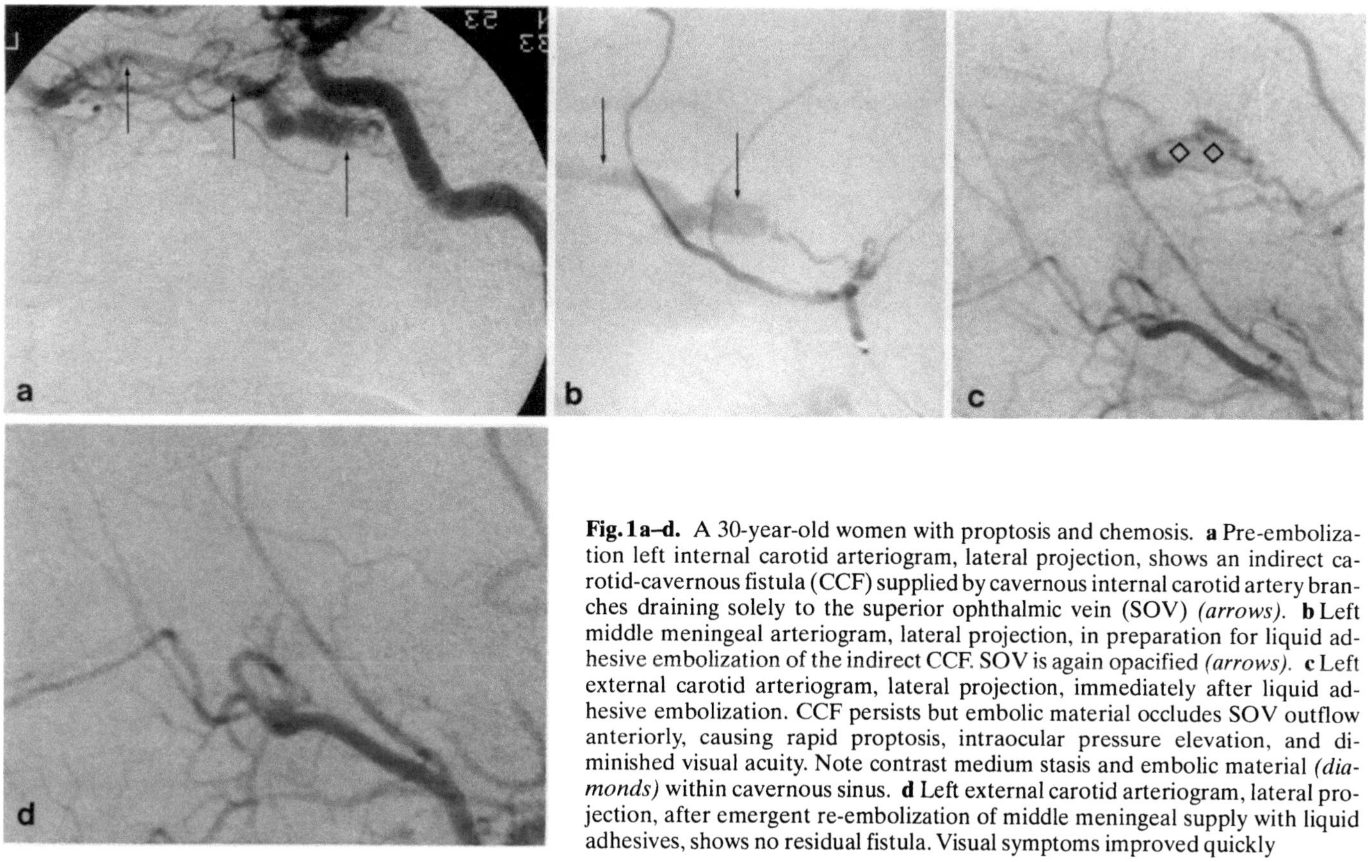

Fig. 1a–d. A 30-year-old women with proptosis and chemosis. **a** Pre-embolization left internal carotid arteriogram, lateral projection, shows an indirect carotid-cavernous fistula (CCF) supplied by cavernous internal carotid artery branches draining solely to the superior ophthalmic vein (SOV) *(arrows)*. **b** Left middle meningeal arteriogram, lateral projection, in preparation for liquid adhesive embolization of the indirect CCF. SOV is again opacified *(arrows)*. **c** Left external carotid arteriogram, lateral projection, immediately after liquid adhesive embolization. CCF persists but embolic material occludes SOV outflow anteriorly, causing rapid proptosis, intraocular pressure elevation, and diminished visual acuity. Note contrast medium stasis and embolic material *(diamonds)* within cavernous sinus. **d** Left external carotid arteriogram, lateral projection, after emergent re-embolization of middle meningeal supply with liquid adhesives, shows no residual fistula. Visual symptoms improved quickly

pose include beta-blockers (such as timolol maleate) and carbonic anhydrase inhibitors (such as acetazolamide).

Finally, performance of a canthotomy will reduce IOP and venous pressure temporarily by allowing more space into which the contents of the orbit may expand. Nevertheless, unless the CCF is closed either spontaneously or iatrogenically, elevation of venous pressure produced by the combination of patent CCF and anterior SOV occlusion will persist, aggravating visual symptoms.

Acute occlusion of the anterior SOV in a patient with a CCF can produce abrupt worsening of visual symptoms. One must be able to recognize and treat this phenomenon to avoid permanent loss of vision.

References

1. Debrun G, Lacour P, Viñuela F, Fox A, Drake CG, Caron JP (1981) Treatment of 54 traumatic carotid-cavernous fistulas. J Neurosurg 55: 678–692
2. Viñuela F, Fox AJ, Debrun GM, Peerless SJ, Drake CG (1984) Spontaneous carotid-cavernous fistulas: clinical, radiological, and therapeutic considerations. J Neurosurg 60: 976–984
3. Kupersmith MJ, Berenstein A, Flamm E, Ransohoff J (1986) Neuroophthalmologic abnormalities and intravascular therapy of traumatic carotid cavernous fistulas. Ophthalmology 93: 906–912
4. Grove AS (1984) The dural shunt syndrome: pathophysiology and clinical course. Ophthalmology 91: 31–43
5. Sanders MD, Hoyt WF (1969) Hypoxic ocular sequelae of carotid cavernous fistulas. Br J Ophthalmol 53: 82–97
6. Halbach VV, Hieshima GB, Higashida RT, Reicher M (1987) Carotid cavernous fistulae: indications for urgent treatment. AJNR 8: 627–633

Dr. C. F. Dowd
Neuroradiology L-352
University of California Medical Center
San Francisco, CA 94143-0628, USA

SESSION 11
SPINE: INCLUDING INTERVENTIONAL

Neuroradiology (1991) 33 [Suppl]: 146–148

Neuro
radiology
© Springer-Verlag 1991

Cervical chemonucleolysis: a study of 130 cases

D. Krause[1], J. Tongio[1], J. L. Drape[1], and D. Maitrot[2]

Departments of [1] Radiology and [2] Neurosurgery, University Hospital, Strasbourg-Hautepierre, France

Summary. The authors present a series of 130 patients who have undergone cervical chemonucleolysis. All had experienced cervicobrachial neuralgia resistant to medical treatment, due to a posterolateral or foraminal disc herniation. In terms of the root pain, good results were obtained: 48 patients showed resolution within 24 h following Chymodiactin injection, and 64 others did so within the 1st week. This overall success rate of 86% allows one to consider cervical nucleolysis as a viable alternative to disc microsurgery.

Key words: Root pain – Root pain – Chymodiactin – Cervical disc herniation – Cervicobrachial neuralgia

Cervicobrachial neuralgia (CBN) in young patients usually affects subjects without a radicular history and involves incapacitating hyperalgesia of sudden onset which is accentuated by coughing and at night. The condition renders daily activity difficult. The physical examination often reveals a motor, reflex, or sensory deficit; dysaesthesia or a pins-and-needles sensation are less often cited by patients.

Medical treatment usually leads to resolution of the root pain. However, a certain number of cases are refractory; one may then consider percutaneous disc injection techniques like those practised at the lumbar level.

Cervical chemonucleolysis is a recent therapeutic procedure. Only certain medical teams perform it [1–3].

Some use chymopapain, whereas others resort to Iniprol, Aprotinine [4, 5] or the intradiscal injection of corticosteroids (i.e. Triamcinolone Retard, [6]).

Over the past 3 years we have developed cervical chemonucleolysis as a treatment for CBN, although this application is classically cited as a contraindication by the product manufacturer.

The aims of this study were to analyse the results obtained in 130 treated patients (January 1987–March 1990) and to elucidate by means of routine postdiscography CT (following nucleolysis) the mechanism of nucleus pulposus extrusion through the peripheral annulus fibrosus.

Patients and methods

Mean age and sex. One hundred and thirty patients were treated for typical CBN refractory to medical treatment for several weeks. The mean age was 42.4 years; there were 90 men and 40 women.

Clinical picture. All patients had constant and significant root pain which was often aggravated at night (i.e. 40%–50% of cases). Deficits were frequently observed: motor deficit (63 patients); reflex deficit (52); sensory deficit (45); and dysaesthesiae (30).

Interval between CBN onset and nucleolysis. This interval concerned the widely varying duration of medical treatment. The mean interval for the 130 patients was 2.5 months.

Levels involved. In the major part of our series, there was almost always a monoradicular distribution whose course suggested C7 or C6 involvement. Pathological levels: C4–5, 3 cases; C5–6, 32 cases; C6–7, 90 cases; C7–T1, 5 cases.

Technique. Chemonucleolysis was performed in a radiology department. The disc was located by fluoroscopy, using a mobile gantry permitting anteroposterior and lateral views. Patients were in a strictly supine position, with the head erect and facing forward. All were treated by neuroleptanalgesia combining Fentanyl and Hyponovel.

Disc injection. This is achieved using a 22-gauge needle whose extremity has been rounded, in order to attain the central portion of the nucleus. One first pushes the patient's right jugular and carotid vessels downward (with the operator's left hand), leaving the sternocleidomastoid laterally and the airways and digestive pathways medially. The approach is anterolateral, passing along the trachea and with the needle tip orientated inward. One perceives a slight resistance when the needle enters the disc.

Discography. It is always performed. One injects 0.3–0.4 ml of nonionic contrast medium (i.e. Iopamiron 300); this may revive the patient's pain (i.e. 23/130). Anteroposterior and lateral plain films confirm the nucleography and often reveal a "foliated" or lamellar anteroposterior appearance as well as the passage of contrast medium towards the foramen; this is not a contraindication to enzyme injection. The herniation is not often opacified on lateral projections, given the small quantities injected.

Nucleolysis. Its practice obviously entails the observance of the classic contraindications, especially that of spinal cord compression due to a large herniation. The injection is performed slowly over a period of about 10 min. Starting 10 months ago (August 1989) we reduced the amount of Chymodiactin injected from 2000 to 1500 units (i.e. 0.7–0.8 ml).

Postdiscography CT. Because of the small amounts of contrast medium injected into the intervertebral space prior to chemonucleolysis, discography was not capable of accurately showing contrast medium dispersal outside the disc. In cases involving foraminal herniations we consider it important to verify their attainment by the contrast medium and, thus, by the enzyme. Postdiscography CT was thus performed 30 min after nucleolysis. The following appearances were observed (i.e. 126/130).

1. At the level of the herniated disc one observed the opacification of a medially located, linear extrusion channel passing through the annulus fibrosus. The fragment itself was more lateral and close to the intervertebral foramen. This was observed in 56 of 130 patients (Fig. 1).
2. The size of the herniation: large fragments were outlined by the contrast medium, whereas smaller ones appeared "drowned" and directly opacified.

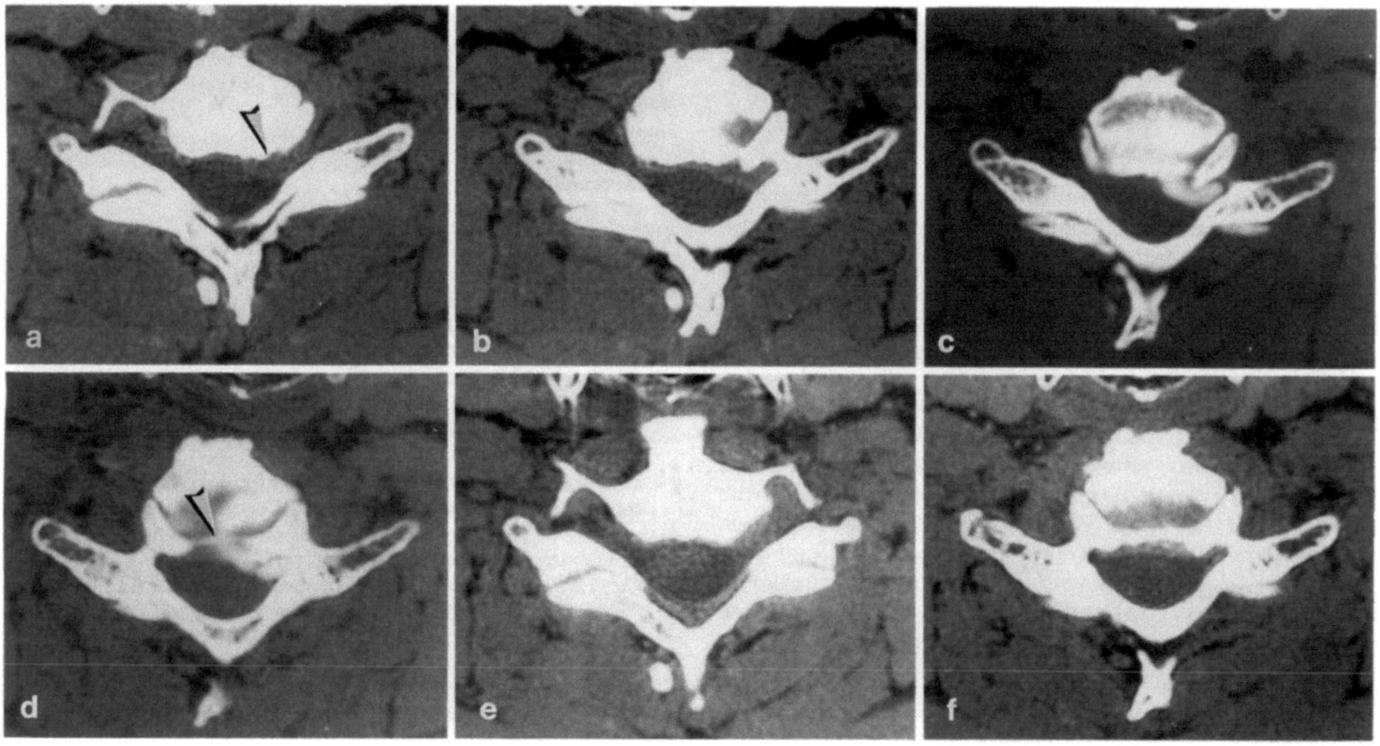

Fig. 1 a–f. A 51-year-old patient; acute neuralgia (C7), resistant to medical treatment, of 2 months duration. **a, b** Left lateral herniation at the foramen entrance *(arrowhead)*. **c, d** Postdiscography CT 30 min after cervical chemonucleolysis (0.8 ml Chymodiactin injected). The tear of the annulus is directly seen, in the middle part of the disc: the fragment is laterally opacified. **e, f** CT 3 months later (the patient is definitively healed). Disappearance of the foraminal herniation at C6–C7. After cervical chemonucleolysis, 87% of patients are cured of their neuralgia within the 1st week

3. The location of herniations: certain herniation fragments were very lateral or within the foramen, especially if they were small. The extrusion channel was laterally located (i.e. next to the uncinate process) and less distinct (i.e. 25/130).

4. Unopacified or poorly opacified fragments: 13/130.

5. Herniations and cervical rheumatoid arthritis: the herniation involved predisposed subjects (i.e. foraminal uncarthrosis). Postdiscography CT irrefutably showed the fragments which had decompensated these subjects (i.e. 17/130).

6. Disc degeneration: in certain cases, postdiscography CT showed a lack of differentiation between the annulus and the nucleus. The herniation image may correspond to a posterolateral bulging in the annulus. These infrequent cases were found in an older patient subgroup (i.e. 15/130).

Results

Clinical picture

Clinical follow-up after chemonucleolysis is simple; after the procedure, the patient is confined to bed for 24 h. The hospital stay is a short one, usually lasting 3 days. Normal activity is eventually resumed 4–6 weeks after chemonucleolysis.

Pain. Regression of the root pain following the intradiscal injection of Chymodiactin is both rapid and constant. The pain decreases or disappears within hours after nucleolysis:

clear reduction of the CBN within 24 h	(48/130);
very significant decrease after 8 days	(64/130);
uncertain improvement after 15 days	(7/130);
unmodified after 4 weeks	(9/130).

Deficits. In most patients, follow-up examinations during the first few weeks following chemonucleolysis showed segmental muscle power to be back to normal. The same was true for the sensory and reflex deficits:

motor deficit – regression after 4 weeks	(55/63);
reflex deficit – improvement (4th week)	(43/52);
sensory disorders – regression (4th week)	(38/45).

Dysaesthesiae. These may persist several days after chemonucleolysis (i.e. 11/130), despite the resolution of root pain.

Neck pain. At present, the smaller doses injected considerably reduce postchemonucleolysis neck pain. In certain cases (i.e. 20 ×), it was recommended that a Schanz neck brace be worn.

Failures

In 9 patients, the CBN seemed to be unchanged after 6 weeks (9/130). In 4 patients with associated pathological conditions (i.e. scapulohumeral periarthritis; carpal tunnel syndrome), the presenting clinical picture did not allow one a priori to rule out the disc herniation as the cause of the arm or shoulder pain. Five other patients were operated upon between the 3rd and 4th weeks. In 3 of these instances, a hard herniated fragment resulting in compression was found; these may have been annulus fibrosus fragments from an older degenerated disc. The remaining 2 patients were operated upon for a severe foraminal uncarthrosis existing in combination with the herniation.

Complications

We can cite here two complications encountered early in our study (i.e. in the 12th and 14th patients, respectively): spondylodiscitis and subarachnoid haemorrhage, both of which had favourable outcomes.

Long-term CT follow-up after chemonucleolysis

Thirty-nine patients were investigated between 2 and 5 months after chemonucleolysis (39/130). The treated disc almost always showed a reduced height. In all cases, follow-up CT showed a resolution of the venous stasis due to the herniation (i.e. 39/130). A minor posteromedian bulging (i.e. 9/130) or intradiscal gas (i.e. 8/39) may persist. The images indicative of rapid resolution of the herniated fragment which are observed at the cervical level are in complete contrast with those at the lumbar level a few months following nucleolysis. (Fig. 1)

Discussion

Because of the rapid resolution of root pain and the brief hospital stay (i.e. 3 days), cervical chemonucleolysis appears to be gaining ground on disc microsurgery. In our experience, we have not observed recurrences at the treated segment or those above or below it. By virtue of its therapeutic efficacy, cervical chemonucleolysis represents an alternative to surgery capable of long-term preservation of the intervertebral space.

References

1. Bonafé A (1986) Chymopapaîn cervical chemonucleolysis. Preliminary results in 15 cases. In: Bonneville JF (ed) Focus on chemonucleolysis. Springer, Berlin Heidelberg New York
2. Krause D, Tongio J, Drape JL, Woerly B, Maitrot D, Boyer P, Buchheit F (1989) Chémonucléolyse cervicale (70 cas). 2e Congrès Interrachis, Marseille
3. Krause D, Tongio J, Maitrot D, Vautravers P, Drape JL, Martin JC, Lecocq J (1990) Chémonucléolyse cervicale (100 cas). Rev Med Orthop 21: 13–16
4. Lazorthes Y, Verdie JC, Richard J, Théron J, Houteville JP, Courtheaux P (1985) Chemonucleolysis of cervical discs: preliminary results in 15 cases of root compression. In: Sutton IC (ed) Current concepts in chemonucleolysis, pp 217–223
5. Théron J, Courtheaux F, Hazebroucq V, Delorme CL, Loyau G (1989) Traitement des névralgies cervico-brachiales par injection intra-discale d'Hexacetonide de Triamcinolone. Rachis 1: 351–358
6. Lesoin F, Viaud C, Dipaola F, Villette L, Autricque A, Clarisse J, Jomin M (1986) Traitement des hernies cervicales molles par injection intradiscale percutanée d'Aprotinine. Neurochirurgie 32: 272–275

Dr. D. Krause
Department of Radiology
University Hospital Strasbourg-Hautepierre
France

Neuroradiology (1991) 33 [Suppl]: 149–152

Neuro-radiology
© Springer-Verlag 1991

Percutaneous vertebroplasty with acrylic cement in the treatment of osteoporotic vertebral crush fracture syndrome

C. Debussche-Depriester[1], H. Deramond[1], P. Fardellone[2], A. Heleg[1], J. L. Sebert[2], L. Cartz[3], and P. Galibert[4]

[1] Service de Radiologie A, [2] Service de Rheumatologie, [3] Service de Neurologie, [4] Service de Neurochirurgie, CHU Amiens, Amiens, France

Summary. Vertebral fractures, spontaneous or due to minor trauma are classical complications of osteoporosis. Fractures are often painful, requiring analgesia and immobilisation for some weeks; immobilisation, however, has a negative effect on mineralisation. In order to consolidate the collapsed vertebra and relieve symptoms, the authors have developed a new therapy, percutaneous intrasomatic injection of acrylic cement, which was initially proposed for the cure of aggressive spinal angiomas. After percutaneous biopsy of the vertebra, a 10-gauge needle is inserted in its body and a mixture of tantalum powder and methyl-methacrylate (3–5 cc) paste is injected. Five patients with severe pain due to osteoporotic vertebral crush fracture syndrome were successfully treated by this method. The technique and results are detailed.

Key words: Vertebroplasty – Osteoporosis – Crush fracture syndrome

Vertebral fractures are classic complications of osteoporosis and are the result of mechanical failure of demineralised vertebrae.

This state induces invalidating clinical manifestations. Until recently analgesic drugs were administered and the patient immobilised; however this increases demineralisation [1–3]. Recently it has been shown that the administration of calcitonin reduces pain [4, 5]. It is important to act quickly to reduce pain thereby reducing immobilisation.

In order to alleviate fracture-induced pain, we used a method for consolidating the pathological vertebrae: percutaneous vertebroplasty with acrylic cement, described initially for treatment of aggressive spinal angiomas [6, 7]. A previous in vitro study showed that intrasomatic acrylic cement injection was followed by increased resistance to external compression [6].

Patients suffering from painful vertebral fracture without neurological complications were treated using this method. In the present study we will consider only the first five patients for whom we have at least 1 year's follow-up.

This paper describes the techniques and the results obtained.

Patients and methods

First, percutaneous biopsy of the pathological vertebra is performed; then a 10-gauge needle is inserted in the vertebral body by a posterolateral approach. After that, a phlebogram is performed, by injection of 3–5 cc of contrast medium through the needle. The transosseous phlebogram shows the vertebral veins, the epidural plexus and the perivertebral veins. It is important in assessing the risk of perivertebral cement.

The third stage consists of injection of acrylic cement whatever the results of the phlebography because the cement's viscosity is different from that of the contrast medium and it may therefore spread differently. A 6 cc mixture is obtained by mixing 4 vol. methyl-methacrylate powder to 1 vol. liquid methyl-polymethacrylate and adding 1 g tantalum powder. In a few minutes the viscosity of this liquid increases. When the mixture has obtained the viscosity of toothpaste it is injected through the needle using 2.5 ml syringes.

The injection is monitored fluoroscopically: at the slightest suspicion of epidural or perivertebral overflow the injection is stopped. In all cases unilateral puncture only permitted the injection of half the vertebra. It was therefore necessary to carry out a contralateral puncture under the same conditions.

Vertebroplasty was carried out in to five patients (two males, three females, aged 45–86 years). The clinical characteristics of these patients are shown in Table 1. All had spinal osteoporosis with radiological evidence of vertebral fractures (cases 1, 2, 5), or reduced bone density measured by lumbar dual photon absorptiometry. The diagnosis of simple osteoporosis was confirmed in all cases by negative laboratory investigations and the absence of neoplastic cells in biopsy immediately before vertebroplasty.

For all patients pain was the principal cause of medical consultation and hospitalisation. The vertebroplasty was carried out 3 weeks to 5 months after the initial symptoms. All patients had previously been treated by analgesic drugs, calcium and immobilisation. Vertebroplasty was undertaken because of persistent of pain.

Results

Patients 1, 2 and 5 were all old (76, 86, and 84 years). They suffered from intense mechanically-induced pain which immobilised them. All were capable of standing and walking 48 h after the vertebroplasty. None showed any sign of spinal or radicular complications. In each case the vertebroplasty achieved its objective: suppression of pain.

In one case (no. 3), after T7 vertebroplasty and immediate suppression of pain, the pain reappeared 1 month later but in attenuated form and localised to the right paravertebral region. After infiltration of the posterior articular processes, the pain disappeared, In another case (no. 4) 6 weeks after treatment the patient felt some discomfort after prolonged physical effort but his work was not hampered.

Postvertebroplasty clinical surveillance at intervals of 12, 15 and 18 months has shown excellent results in all

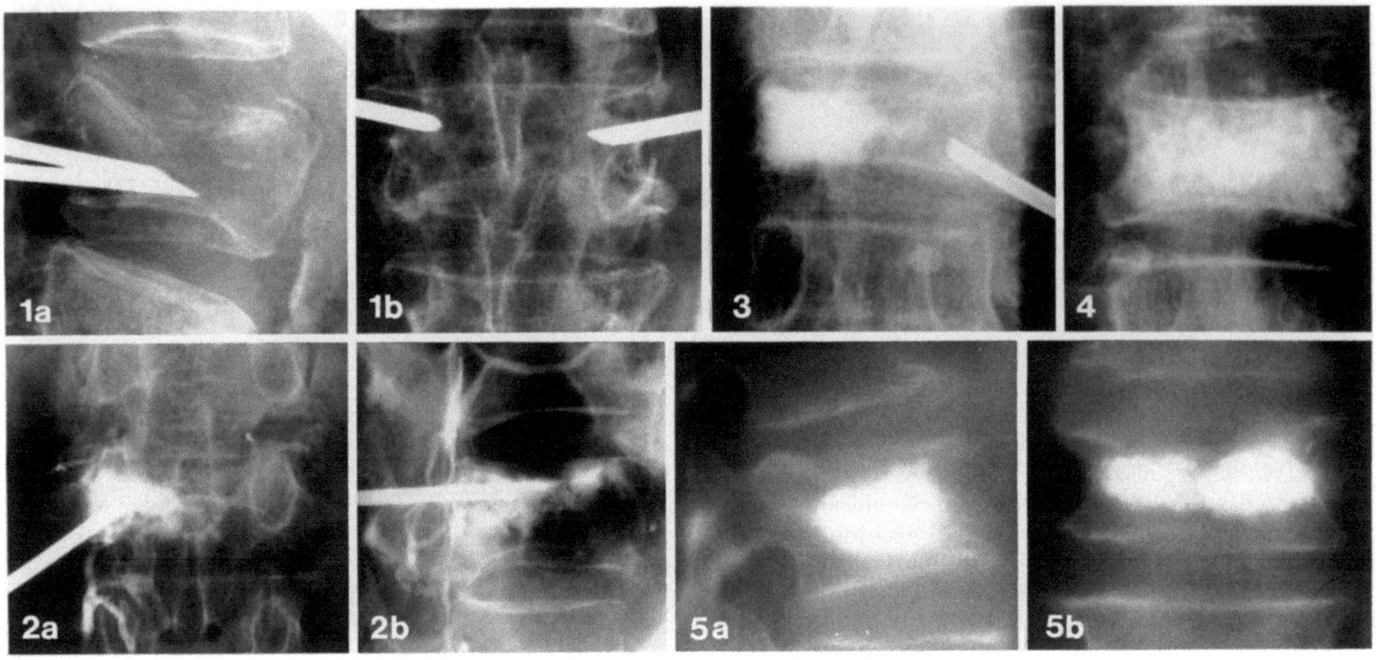

Fig. 1 a, b. Case 5. Two 10 gauge needles are inserted in L3; sagittal and frontal views

Fig. 2 a, b. Case 1. Phlebography (frontal and sagittal views); the epidural plexus and perivertebral veins were injected

Fig. 3. Case 4. After cement injection of the right T9 hemivertebra, we inserted a second needle by left postero-lateral approach

Fig. 4. Case 3. Control after T7 vertebroplasty; homogeneous cement injection

Fig. 5 a, b. Case 3. Radiotomographies (frontal and sagittal views) after L3 vertebroplasty

cases. X-rays showed perfect stability of acrylic cement injections in both form and localisation. Moreover, we have not noted any change in height of the treated vertebra nor to those above and below.

Discussion

The spectacular effect on pain in a case of a vertebral angioma after peroperative acrylic cement treatment encouraged us to develop this percutaneous method [6]. Our objective was to suppress, using vertebral consolidation, the sometimes extremely incapacitating root pain present in association with vertebral angiomas.

Simultaneously in vitro studies confirmed the vertebral consolidation effect obtained by cement injection [6].

The excellent, long-lasting (up to 5 years) clinical results in vertebral angiomas prompted us to extend this method to severe osteoporotic vertebral crush fractures.

Osteoporosis is a metabolic bone disease characterised by reduction of bone mass leading to diminished bone strength and fractures. It is now recognised as a major public health problem because of its high cost and increasing incidence linked to progressive aging of the population and other age-unrelated and not well-known factors [1, 2]. The commonest sites of osteoporotic fractures are the hip, the distal radius and the vertebrae. Hip fractures in the elderly represent the major consequence of osteoporosis and are associated with increased mortality. Vertebral compression fractures occur most frequently in post-menopausal women aged 60 years or older, after minimal trauma or spontaneously.

Vertebral fractures usually cause acute symptoms with pain of variable intensity localised at the fracture site. These symptoms tend to subside after 4–6 weeks, but severe back pain may persist for many weeks. Repetition of fracture episodes is usual and can cause serious morbidity [3]. Later consequences of vertebral fractures include less of height, kyphosis and chronic pain due to distortion of the normal anatomy of the spine.

Medical treatment of osteoporosis is aimed at prevention of vertebral fracture and uses antiresorptive (oestrogen, calcitonin) or bone formation stimulating drugs (fluoride) [2, 11]. Treatment of the vertebral crush fracture syndrome is usually limited to bed-rest and analgesic drugs. However, immobilisation is potentially harmful leading to classical decubitus complications and to increased bone resorption, which can worsen bone demineralisation [9].

Recently calcitonin has been proposed for treatment of acute vertebral fractures for its antiresorptive activity and specific central analgesic effect [4, 5].

Our patients had persistent severe pain despite prolonged medical treatment. Acrylic cement vertebroplasty was proposed to alleviate symptoms and reduce duration of immobilisation. Immediate results were excellent in all cases, with complete relief of pain and the patients were capable of standing and walking 24–48 h after the procedure.

Why were these results achieved? Mechanically induced pain was suppressed due to vertebral consolidation which in turn suppressed vertebral plasticity.

Table 1. Clinical characteristics of the five patients and results

Patient no.	Age/sex	Localisation	Clinical characteristics	Previous treatments	Evolution after vertebroplasty
1	76 F	L1	Severe lumbago, bedridden, one other collapsed vertebra	Immobilisation, analgesic drugs, for 6 weeks	Complete disappearance of pain; 48 h after injection she was able to ride again; 18 months follow-up
2	86 F	T12 + L1	Fall, fracture T12 + L1, severe lumbago, bedridden, one other collapsed vertebra	Immobilisation, analgesics, for 2 months	Complete disappearance of pain; 15 months follow-up
3	54 M	17	Heaving effort, back pain	Immobilisation, analgesic drugs, calcium, for 2 months	Immediate complete disappearance of pain; 1 month later: minimal right paravertebral pain eased by infiltration; 12 months follow-up
4	45 M	19	Fall, mechanical pain	Immobilisation, analgesic drugs, calcium, during 5 months	Immediate complete disappearance of pain; at 3 months: discomfort after prolonged physical effort; 12 months follow-up
5	84 F	L3	Severe lumbago, bedridden, two other collapsed vertebrae	Immobilisation, analgesic drugs, calcium, for 3 weeks	Complcte disappearance of pain; 48 h after she rides again; 12 months follow-up

The use of large needles is indispensable due to the viscosity of the cement. Injection is facilitated by the use of a small syringe (2.5 ml). An opacifier must be added to the cement to ensure effective monitoring of the mixture and immediate abandonment of injection in the case of perivertebral or epidural injection. Tantalum powder is recommended because it is particularly radio-opaque and increases the solidity of the cement [7].

What are the risk of the method? No accident happened during the treatments. In four cases, general anaesthesia was used and in the fifth neuroleptanalgesia. General anaesthesia is not obligatory, it does assure greater comfort for both the patient and the operator. All our vertebroplasties are now carried out under neuroleptanalgesia.

Because the quantities of acrylic cement used in vertebroplasty are far less than those used in orthopaedic surgery, the risk of allergic accidents, hypotension and pulmonary emboli is only theoretical. None of these complications were observed [10, 11]. No carcinogenic effect has as yet been attributed to acrylic cement [12].

During phlebography the distribution of the contrast medium differs from that of the cement. In the case of perivertebral injection of cement, the injection is abandoned and a new puncture is effected. Injection of anterior or lateral veins is without consequences, but injection of epidural veins can be a source of complications. This underlines the importance of fluoroscopic monitoring during injection of cement. Injection of insufficient cement due to an advanced state of solidification is also a problem. One must then undertake a new puncture of the part of the vertebra not yet injected and recommence the procedure.

Conclusion

These preliminary results show that acrylic cement vertebroplasty can be used successfully in the treatment of osteoporotic vertebral crush fracture syndrome. This procedure seems particularly useful when conventional medical treatment has been insufficient it is simple and safe but has to be rigorously performed.

Acknowledgement: We wish to thank Simon Stone for his assistance in this study.

References

1. Obrant KJ, Bengner U, Johnell O, Nilsson BE, Sernbo I (1989) Increasing age-adjusted risk of fragility fractures: a sign of increasing osteoporosis in successive generations? Calcif Tissue Int 44: 157–167
2. Riggs BL, Melton LJ III (1988) Osteoporosis, Etiology, Diagnosis and management. Raven Press, New York
3. Adams PH (1983) The clinical spectrum of osteoporosis. In: Dixon AStJ, Russell RGG, Stamp TCB (eds) Osteoporosis, a multi-disciplinary problem. Academic Press and Royal Society of Medicine, London, pp 127–132
4. Gennary C (1989) Salmon calcitonin (Miacalcic) nasal spray in prevention and treatment of osteoporosis. Clin Rheumatol 8 [Suppl 2]: 61–65
5. Levernieux J, Julien D, Caulin F (1986) The effect of calcitonin on bone pain and acute resorption related to recent osteoporotic crush fractures. Result of a double blind and an open study. In: Cecchettin M, Segre G (eds) Calciotropic hormones and calcium metabolism. Elsevier, Amsterdam, pp 171–178
6. Galibert P, Deramond H, Rosat P, Le Gards D (1987) Note préliminaire sur le traitement des angiomes vertébraux par vertébroplastie acrylique percutanée. Neuro-Chirurgie 33: 166–168
7. Deramond H, Darrasson R, Galibert P (1989) Percutaneous vertebroplasty with acrylic cement in the treatment of aggressive spinal angiomas. Rachis 2: 143–153

8. Nagat de Deuxchaisnes C (1983) The pathogenesis and treatment of involutional osteoporosis. In: Dixon AStJ, Russel RGG, Stamp TCB (eds) Osteoporosis, a multi-disciplinary problem. Academic Press and Royal Society of Medicine, London, pp 291–333
9. Minaire P (1989) Immobilisation osteoporosis: a review. Clin Rheumatol 8 [Suppl 2]: 95–103
10. Schlag G, Schliep HJ, Dingeldein E, Grieben A, Ringsdore W (1976) Does methylmethacrylate induce cardiovascular complications during alloarthroplasty surgery of the hip joint? Anaesthesist 25: 60–67
11. Svartling N, Pfaffli P, Tarkkanen L (1985) Methylmetacrylate blood levels in patients with femoral neck fracture. Arch Orthop Trauma Surg 104: 242–246
12. Feith R (1975) Side effects of acrylic cement implanted into bone. Acta Orthop Scand [Suppl] 1975: 161

Dr. Claude Debussche-Depriester
Service de Radiologie A
F-80054 Amiens cedex, France

Neuroradiology (1991) 33 [Suppl]: 153–155

Neuroradiology
© Springer-Verlag 1991

Vein of Galen malformation: clinical relevance of angiographic classification, and utility of MRI in treatment planning

D. Seidenwurm and A. Berenstein

New York University Medical School, New York, USA

Summary. Vein of Galen malformations may be divided angiographically into two groups: patients with fistulae alone and patients with an arteriovenous malformation nidus. The age and symptoms at presentation differ between the two groups. Fistula patients present earlier in life and are more likely to have heart failure and hydrocephalus than the nidus group. Venous outflow obstruction, thought to be etiologically important, is identified in 31 of 34 patients in our series. MRI proved superior to CT in noninvasive evaluation. Lesion category, vascular supply and venous drainage were reliably identified by MRI.

Key words: Vein of Galen malformation – Arteriovenous malformation – Magnetic resonance imaging – Surgical neuroangiography

Vein of Galen malformation (VOGM) is a uncommon congenital anomaly of the cerebral circulation in which enlarged deep venous structures of the Galenic system are fed by abnormal arteriovenous communications in the midline [1–4]. These may be single or multiple arteriovenous fistulae, or they may be a more complex pial arteriovenous malformation. In virtually all of these cases, some type of venous outflow restriction is present [5].

Recent advances in endovascular therapy have produced a resurgence of interest in this lesion [6–9]. Developments in noninvasive imaging techniques have prompted a reassessment of the optimum methods for diagnostic investigation of these patients [10].

Materials and methods

Thirty-four consecutive patients with VOGM were reviewed. Angiograms, CT and MR were reviewed for the presence of arteriovenous malformation (AVM) nidus or direct fistulae, presence of venous outflow constraint, and the identity of feeding arteries and draining veins. Clinical records were reviewed primarily for the age and symptoms at presentation.

Results

Patients were divided angiographically into two groups, those in whom an AVM nidus was present (Fig. 1), and those in whom AV fistulization alone was present (Fig. 2). There were 17 patients in each group. The AVM nidus was thalamic in 16 of 17 patients.

Angiographic differentiation of these groups had clinical relevance (Fig. 3). The presenting symptoms and age of onset differed between the groups ($P = 0.01$). In the fistula group the age of onset was skewed heavily to the newborn period with mean age 4.2 months, median 1 month. In the nidus group the ages averaged 15.3 months at presentation, median 9 months. The presenting symptoms differed between the two groups.

Venous outflow constraint was identified angiographically in 31 of the 34 patients in our series (Fig. 4). Fifteen of the 17 nidus and 16 of 17 fistula patients exhibited this finding. The straight sinus was absent in 16 cases.

The comparative ability of CT and MRI to categorize patients as nidus or fistula patients, to identify arterial feeders and venous drainage, and to identify venous out-

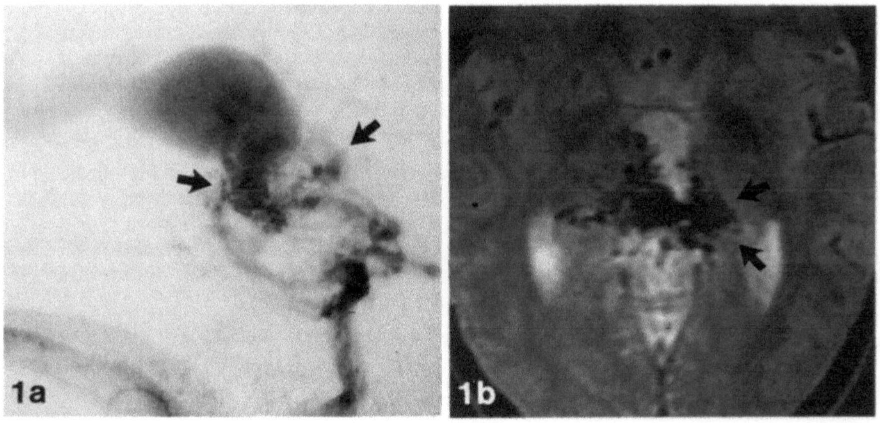

Fig. 1a, b. Nidus group. **a** Vertebral arteriogram demonstrates arteriovenous malformation nidus *(arrows)*, enlarged vein of Galen and anomalous falcine sinus. Lateral projection, anterior on reader's right. **b** Axial T2-weighted spin echo MRI demonstrates tangles of thalamic vessels representing the nidus *(arrows)*

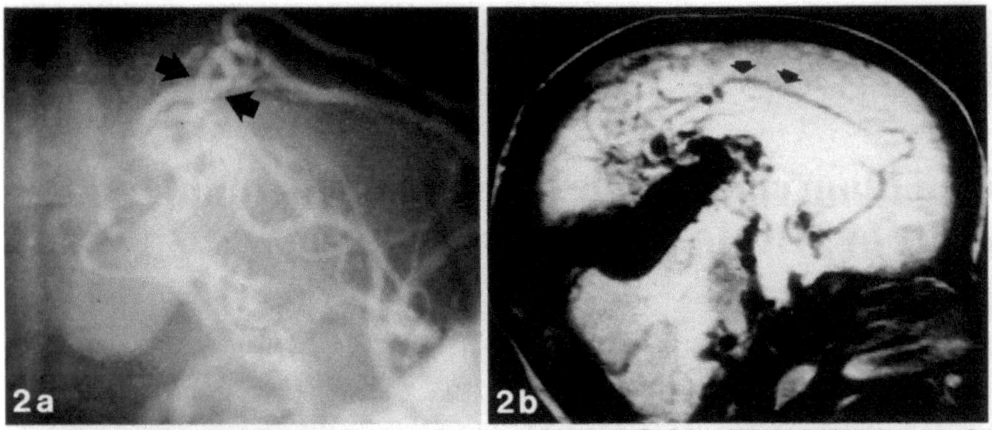

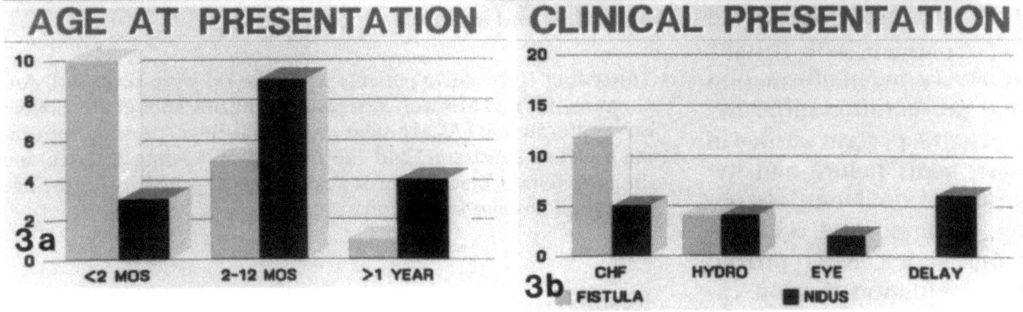

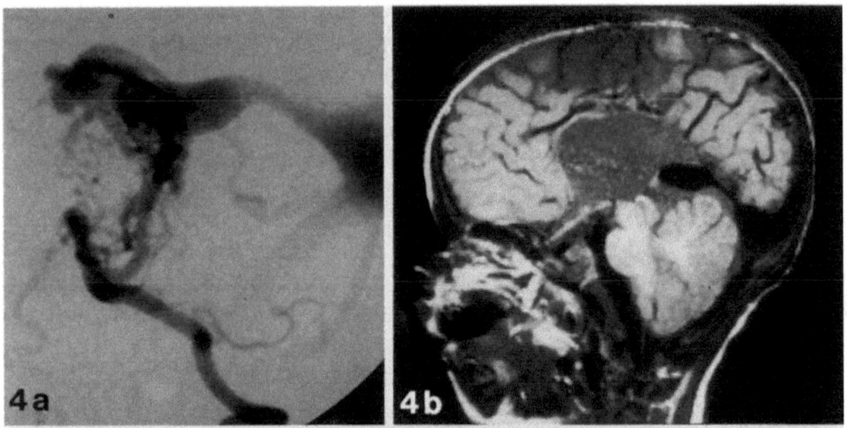

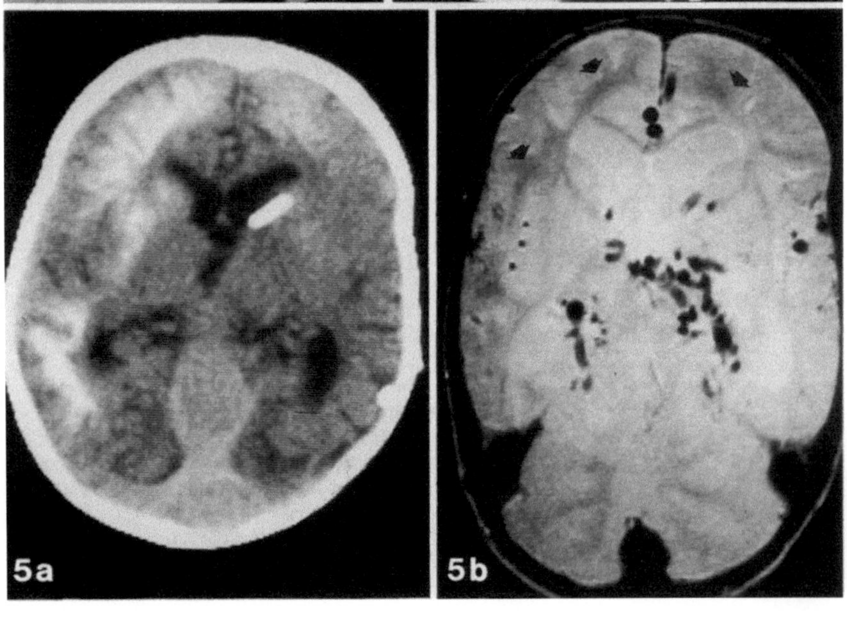

Fig. 2 a, b. Fistula group. **a** Carotid arteriogram demonstrates anterior cerebral artery fistula *(arrows)* to enlarged vein of Galen. Lateral projection, anterior on reader's right. **b** Sagittal T2-weighted gradient echo MRI demonstrated enlarged anterior cerebral artery *(arrows)* and vein of Galen; no nidus is recognized, but direct fistula is not demonstrated. Anterior on reader's right

Fig. 3 a, b. Population characteristics. **a** Distribution of age of onset of symptoms for fistula and nidus patients. Note the skew toward the newborn period in the fistula group. **b** Distribution of symptoms at presentation of the two groups. Note that fistula patients presented with congestive heart failure *(CHF)* or hydrocephalus, while developmental delay and ocular symptoms were present in the nidus group

Fig. 4 a, b. Venous constraint. **a** Vertebral arteriogram demonstrates narrowing of straight sinus. Lateral projection, anterior on reader's left. **b** Sagittal T1-weighted spin echo MRI demonstrates the same finding. Anterior on reader's left

Fig. 5 a, b. Cerebral calcification. **a** CT demonstrates diffuse cerebral calcification. **b** T2-weighted spin echo MRI findings are extremely subtle *(arrows)*

flow constraint, was evaluated. Sixteen patients had MRI; of these 14 had CT.

No cross-sectional imaging study identified a direct arteriovenous fistula, and no false nidus was diagnosed. The nidus was correctly identified by MRI in 8 of 8 cases and by CT in 3 of 6 cases. Therefore, MRI categorized 16 of 16 cases correctly while CT correctly categorized 11 of 16.

Major arterial trunks were identified correctly in 14 of 16 cases with MRI and by CT in 8 of 14. Primary branch vessels were identified correctly in 15 of 16 by MRI and in 5 of 14 cases by CT. Secondary branches were identified correctly in 11 of 16 cases by MRI and in no case by CT. MRI was superior to CT in the identification of arterial feeders in 11 and equal to CT in 3 of 14 cases in which both studies were available.

Significant features of venous anatomy included identification of draining veins, venous anomalies and venous constraints. MRI identified these features of venous anatomy in 15 of 16 cases, and CT in 7 of 14 cases. Overall, MRI was superior to CT in 8 and equal to CT in 6 of 14 cases in which both studies were performed.

A single patient exhibited cerebral calcification on CT (Fig. 5).

Discussion

Our data demonstrate the relevance of a simple classification of VOGM. The ability of MRI to demonstrate vascular anatomy in a manner superior to CT is important because the precarious clinical condition of these patients requires expeditious evaluation. If the primary feeding arteries can be predicted prior to angiography, a limited diagnostic and therapeutic procedure can be performed in one sitting. Noninvasive identification of the venous drainage, particularly when anomalies or stenoses are present, may be useful when venous approaches to endovascular therapy are employed.

References

1. Litvak J, Yahr MD, Ransohoff J (1960) Aneurysms of the great vein of Galen and midline cerebral arteriovenous anomalies. J Neurosurg 17: 945–954
2. Gold AP, Ransohoff J, Carter S (1964) Vein of Galen malformation. Acta Neurol Scand [Suppl] 40: 5–31
3. Amacher AL, Shillito J (1973) The syndromes and surgical treatment of aneurysms of the great vein of Galen. J Neurosurg 39: 89–98
4. Hoffman HJ, Chuang S, Hendrick EB, Humphreys RP (1982) Aneurysms of the vein of Galen. J Neurosurg 57: 316–322
5. Lasjaunias P, TerBrugge K, Lopez Ibor L (1987) The role of dural anomalies in vein of Galen aneurysms: report of six cases and review of the literature. AJNR 8: 185–192
6. Epstein F, Berenstein A (1981) Pediatric vascular anomalies: combined neurosurgical and neuroradiologic intervention. In: American Society of Pediatric Neurosurgery (eds) Concepts in Pediatric Neurosurgery I. Karger, New York, pp 49–68
7. Berenstein A, Epstein F (1982) Vein of Galen malformations: Combined neurosurgical and neuroradiological intervention. In: American Association of Neurolocial Surgeons (eds) Pediatric neurosurgery, surgery of the developing nervous system. Grune and Stratton, New York, pp 637–657
8. Lasjaunias P, TerBrugge K, Lopez Ibor L (1987) Vein of Galen dilatation, anatamo-clinical forms and endovascular treatment, 14 cases. Neurochirurgie 33: 315–333
9. Mickele JP, Quisling RG (1987) The transtorcular embolization of vein of Galen aneurysms. J Neurosurg 64: 731–735
10. Martelli A, Scotti G, Harwood-Nash DC, Fitz CR, Chuang S (1980) Aneurysms of the vein of Galen in children: CT and angiographic correlation. Neuroradiology 20: 123–133

Dr. David Seidenwurm
Department of Radiology
Peninsula Hospital
Burlingame, CA 94010, USA

SESSION 12
SPINE: TRAUMA AND CSF FLOW

Neuroradiology (1991) 33 [Suppl]: 158–160

Neuroradiology

© Springer-Verlag 1991

MRI evaluation of sequential changes of the injured spinal cord

J. Shinzato[1], K. Yoshizumi[1], Y. Sakamoto[1], Y. Yamashita[1], Y. Korogi[1], H. Bussaka[1], T. Sakae[2], and M. Takahashi[1]

[1] Department of Radiology, Kumamoto University School of Medicine, Kumamoto, Japan
[2] Department of Orthopedics, Kumamoto Orthopedic Hospital, Kumamoto, Japan

Summary. Thirty-seven cases of acute spinal cord injury were studied with MRI and correlated with the neurological findings. Nineteen out of 37 cases were followed by sequential MRI for 10 days to 1 year. Cord abnormalities, including cord compression, cord swelling, and abnormal signal intensities were observed on the initial MR images, followed by various changes, depending on the nature of the initial damage on the subsequent MR images. The most frequent initial changes within the cord included isointensity on both T1- and T2-weighted images or isointensity on T1-weighted images and hyperintensity on T2-weighted images, followed at 2 months by persistence of isointensity on T1-weighted images and hyperintensity on T2-weighted images. The most common final MR appearance was hypointensity on T1-weighted images and hyperintensity on T2-weighted images. The size of the hyperintense area on T2-weighted images was the most important finding in predicting the prognosis of spinal cord injuries.

Key words: Spinal cord injury – Sequential magnetic resonance imaging – Neurological changes of cord trauma

Spinal cord injury is not an uncommon occurrence and the major imaging techniques recently applied have been conventional radiography with tomography, CT, myelography and CT myelography. Although these imaging modalities can provide useful diagnostics information, direct information about the spinal cord can not be obtained. With the recent introduction of MRI for spinal cord trauma, it has been shown that direct information about the cord itself can now be obtained [1–3].

The purpose of this report is to study evolution of sequential MR findings of the injured spinal cord with special attention to prognosis.

Materials and methods

Patients. Thirty-seven cases (32 males, 5 females; 14–78 years of age, mean 47.0 years) of acute spinal cord injury were studied with MRI between April 1988 and March 1990 at the Kumamoto University and its affiliated hospitals. MRI was performed in 10 cases within 6 h of the injury, in 13 cases within 24 h and in another 14 patients within 7 days. Follow-up MRI was performed in 19 patients.
Treatment. Patients were observed from 3 to 26 months after injuries. Surgical decompression was performed in 24 patients. Thirteen patients were treated conservatively. Traction for a dislocated vertebrae was performed immediately in 4 patients.
MRI technique. MRI was performed with two 0.5 T superconductive MR units (Philips Gyroscan, T5 and S5) with a surface coil. Spin-echo images were obtained with 400450/30/4 (TR/TE/excitations) sequence as T1-weighted images, 1600–1800/50/2 sequence as proton-density-weighted images and 1600–1800/100/2 sequence as T2-weighted images. The slice thickness was 5–7 mm. Patients in poor condition were examined with reduced averaging. Images were acquired using a field of view of 6×15 square cm and a 256×256 matrix.
Analysis. The neurological function of the spinal cord at the initial time of MRI and final clinical outcome was classified according to the classification of Frankel et al. [4].

Spinal cord injuries were classified into five patterns by signal intensity within the spinal cord: type 0, isointensity on both T1- and T2-weighted images; type I, isointensity on T1-weighted images and hyperintensity on T2-weighted images; type II, hypointensity on T1-weighted images and hyperintensity on T2-weighted images; type III, hyperintensity on T1- and T2-weighted images; type IV, spinal cord atrophy or syringomyelia.

Results

Extramedullary abnormalities

In 37 patients, various abnormalities were observed in the extramedullary structures: fracture in 26 cases, subluxation in 17, ligamentous injury in 15 and paravertebral

Table 1. Sequential changes of MRI patterns (no. cases)

Type (T1WI, T2WI)	Interval from injury		
	Less than 1 week	Less than 2 months	More than 2 months
Type 0 (Iso, Iso)	0 (5) →	0 (1) I (3) →	I (1) II (1) II (1)
Type I (Iso, Hyper)	I (12) →	I (9) → II (1)	0 (1) II (4) II (1) II (2)
Type II (Hypo, Hyper)	II (1) →	I (1) →	II (1)
Type III (Hyper, Hyper)	III (1) →	I (1)	
	19	16	13

T1WI, T1-weighted image; T2WI, T2-weighted image

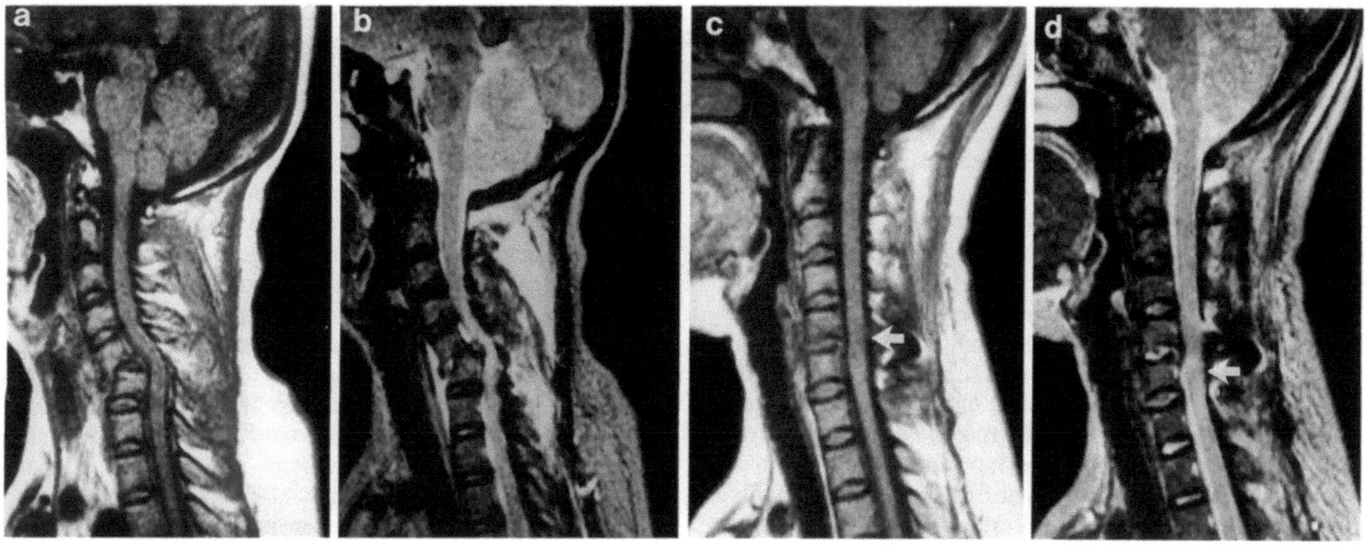

Fig. 1 a–d. A 47-year-old female who had cervical spinal cord injury by diving into the pool: **a** T1-weighted image (TR 400/TE 30), 24 h after injury, shows subluxation of C5–6, ligament injury and prevertebral haematoma. The spinal cord is compressed but isointense; **b** on T2-weighted image (TR 1600/TE 100), hyperintense area of the spinal cord extends from C4 to C6; **c** T1-weighted image (TR 400/TE 30), 2 months after injury, shows hypointense area at the level of C5–6; **d** on T2-weighted image (TR 1600/TE 100), hyperintense area of the spinal cord has diminished. She had a quadriplegia initially, but later she recovered (Frankel A–D) and was able to resume her daily life

Table 2. Relationship of initial MRI patterns to neurological function

MR patterns (T1WI, T2WI)	No. of cases	Neurological function		
		Complete recovery	Improvement	No improvement
Type 0 (Iso, Iso)	8	3	5	0
Type I (Iso, Hyper)	25	6	8	11
Type II (Hypo, Hyper)	1	0	0	1
Type III (Hyper, Hyper)	3	0	0	3
Total	37	9	13	15

Table 3. Relationship of extent of high signal intensity area on subsequent T2-weighted images to neurological recovery

Extent of high signal intensity	No. of cases	Neurological function		
		Complete recovery	Improvement	No improvement
Less than 1 vertebral body	9	1	8	0
Between 1 and 2 vertebral bodies	3	1	2	0
More than 2 vertebral bodies	5	0	0	5
Total	17	2	10	5

Two cases showed isointensity with complete recovery

haematoma in 26. Traumatic disc herniation was found in 2 patients.

Intramedullary abnormalities

Spinal cord abnormalities demonstrated on MRI were: swelling in 22, compression in 32 and abnormal signal intensity on T2-weighted images in 29 patients.

Severe cord compression was observed in 11 cases, moderate compression in 18 and minimal compression in 3. The causes of cord compression included subluxation of the vertebral body in 14 and burst fracture of the vertebral body in 9, ossification of the posterior longitudinal ligament, disc hernia or spinal canal stenosis in 3 each, and osteophyte in 1.

MR pattern of initial and sequential MR images

On the initial MRI study, types I and 0 were most frequently observed, however, on sequential MRI study, types I and II were frequent. Sequential patterns most often observed were from types 0 or I to type I in less than 2 months and then type I to type II with elapse of more than 2 months (Table 1).

Relationship of MR patterns to neurological function

Patients with type 0 at the initial examination showed relatively good recovery (Table 2). Approximately half of the patients with type I showed complete recovery or improvement. Patients with types II or III did not show significant improvement.

Patients with small areas of hyperintensity on subsequent T2-weighted images showed neurological improvement (Fig. 1), while patients with larger areas of hyperintensity extending more than two vertebral bodies showed no neurological recovery (Table 3). Patients with isointensity on T2-weighted images all had neurological improvement.

Discussion

A variety of pathological changes can be detected on MRI, including intramedullary and extramedullary lesions [1, 5]. The most important advantage of MRI is the ability to demonstrate changes within the cord accurately by signal intensity changes.

Contusion, ischaemia, haemorrhage and associated oedema develop at an early stage after cord trauma [5]. In the subacute stage, various pathological changes take place including myelomalacia, gliosis, demyelination, fibrosis and necrosis within the spinal cord. In the chronic stage, these changes turn into cyst formation, atrophy and syringomyelia. These sequential changes of spinal cord trauma can be imaged with MRI to good advantage. However, there is considerable overlap in the signal intensity patterns and it is sometimes difficult to suggest which pathological processes are taking place within the traumatised cord.

We have classified spinal cord abnormalities due to trauma into five patterns. Type 0 indicates small areas of contusion, oedema, and ischaemia or gliosis and myelomalacia which can not be demonstrated by MRI. When haemorrhage and contusion, or gliosis and myelomalacia are more prominent, then the MRI patterns may appear as type I. Type II indicates more marked changes since there is definite hypointensity on T1-weighted images. That is, haemorrhage or oedema in the acute stage and extensive myelomalacia or cyst formation in the chronic stage. In type III, more extensive haemorrhage is likely which is manifest as high signal intensity on both T1-and T2-weighted images. Type IV indicates chronic changes including cyst formation, myelomalacia, atrophy and syrinx formation.

The MRI patterns overlap considerably and depend upon the degree of pathological changes and superimposed haemorrhage. MRI patterns have been proposed and explained on the basis of pathological changes. Kulkarni et al. [2] classified their findings into three patterns on T2-weighted images. Most lesions were attributed to haemorrhage, cord oedema and contusion. Mirvis et al. [3] also attempted to classify MR signal characteristics and explained the findings on the basis of focal oedema and haemorrhage. In any event, patterns at the time of initial trauma is isointensity on T1- and T2-weighted images and isointensity on both T1-weighted images and hyperintensity on T2-weighted images. MRI less than 2 months after the initial trauma most commonly reveals type I with isointensity on T1-weighted images and hyperintensity on T2-weighted images. This indicates that the early changes of oedema, ischaemia and contusion have subsided and demyelination, myelomalacia, gliosis, and other necrotic changes are taking place. On MRI of trauma more than 2 months old, type II develops as the most frequent pattern, indicating cyst formation or necrosis within the spinal cord. Syringomyelia and spinal cord atrophy may follow these changes.

Various authors have attempted to correlate MRI patterns with clinical outcome or prognosis [1–3]. In particular, Kulkarni et al. [2] reported that spinal cord haemorrhage indicated the most severe anatomical and physiological injury to the spinal cord, whereas focal areas of petechial haemorrhage and oedema indicated the possibility of significant improvement in neurological function. We have also correlated various aspects of the MRI patterns with the neurological recovery. The most important prognostic indicator was the extent of high signal intensity area on subsequent T2-weighted images. Cord compression on the initial MRI was also important. Patients with marked cord compression tended to show no significant improvement compared with patients having moderate and minimal compression. Initial MRI pattern was important; type 0 showed a better prognosis than type I.

Because of the numerous advantages of MRI over other diagnostic modalities in the investigation of acute and chronic spinal cord trauma, MRI is the most important diagnostic modality together with plain radiography. CT may be performed for assessment of bony fragments and subtle fractures [1]. Myelography, CT myelography and angiography will not be used widely in the investigation of spinal cord trauma.

References

1. Kalfas I, Wilberger J, Goldberg A, Prostko ER (1988) Magnetic resonance imaging in acute spinal cord trauma. Neurosurgery 23: 295–299
2. Kulkarni MV, McArdle CB, Kopanicky D, Miner M, Cotler HB, Lee KF, Harris JH (1987) Acute spinal cord injury: MR imaging at 1.5 T. Radiology 164: 837–843
3. Mirvis SE, Geisler FH, Jelinek JJ, Joslyn JN, Gellad F (1988) Acute cervical spine trauma: evaluation with 1.5-T MR imaging. Radiology 166: 807–816
4. Frankel HL, Hancock DO, Hyslop G (1969) The value of postural reduction in initial management of closed injuries of the spine with paraplegia and tetraplegia. Paraplegia 7: 179–192
5. Enzmann DR, DeLePaz RL, Rubin JB (1990) Magnetic resonance imaging of the spine. Mosby, St. Louis, pp 237–259

Dr. J. Shinzato
Department of Radiology
Kumamoto University School of Medicine
Kumamoto, Japan

Neuroradiology (1991) 33 [Suppl]: 161–163

Neuro radiology

© Springer-Verlag 1991

MRI evaluation of whiplash injuries

R. W. Parrish, D. P. E. Kingsley, B. E. Kendall, and I. F. Moseley

Queen Square Imaging Centre, The National Hospital for Neurology and Neurosurgery, London, UK

Summary. Abnormalities of cervical spinal posture or of disc disruption were significantly more common in a group of 60 patients with whiplash syndrome than in a non-injured control population and, as anticipated, had a higher incidence with advancing age. Disc abnormality, if present, was usually at a single level, most commonly C5–6. Alteration of cervical curve is an important finding, and may reflect associated soft-tissue injury, muscular or ligamentous.

Key words: Cervical spine, trauma – Whiplash injury – Magnetic resonance imaging

Traumatic hyperextension injury to the neck, the so-called whiplash injury, is a common consequence of rear-end motor vehicle collisions. Its clinical course may be subacute or chronic, and is frequently a cause of prolonged disability.This report deals with the magnetic resonance imaging (MRI) findings in a series of 60 patients who had experienced whiplash injuries and makes comparison with a group of 98 non-injured controls.

Patients and methods

Sixty patients who had experienced whiplash injury to the neck were examined by MRI.

Imaging was performed on a Picker 0.26T system, the standard protocol being moderately T1-weighted (TR440, TE26) sagittal and axial sequences with a section thickness of 5 mm; this was usually supplemented by sagittal T2-weighted (TR1500,TE80) imaging without motion suppression, using a section thickness of 10 mm.

Patients with more severe injuries, such as vertebral fractures or dislocations were excluded from the analysis, as were patients who had undergone surgery. Ninety-eight age-matched patients with a clinical diagnosis of multiple sclerosis and no history of significant trauma, examined using the same imaging sequences, formed a control group. Plain radiographs of the cervical spine performed at or near the time of injury were also examined so that correlation could be made with the MR images.

Patients were grouped according to the time interval between injury and MRI: less than 6 months, 6–24 months and longer than 24 months.

Results

The whiplash patient group's ages ranged from 20 to 69 years, with 1 patient aged 81 years (mean 38.6); the control group ages ranged from 21 to 60 years, with 1 patient aged 14 years (mean 38.9).

Patients and controls were grouped into ages by decades for analysis – no significant difference existing between the mean ages of patients and controls in any decade group.

Overall, 62% of patients and 32% of controls had abnormal MRI findings, with an increasing frequency in both groups with age (Table 1). There was a significant increase in spinal or intervertebral disc disease in patients as compared to controls for the two decades 20–29 years ($p < 0.05$) and 30–39 years ($p < 0.001$) with a non-significant trend in the same direction in the next two decade groups (Fig. 1). The proportion of normal to abnormal patients did not vary significantly when analysed in respect of interval between injury and the MRI study, i.e. the patients with symptoms of greater duration were not more likely to have abnormal images.

In both patient and control groups disc abnormality was more often at a single level (C5–6) than at multiple levels; the groups did not differ significantly in this respect. There was no difference in the location or distribution of disc abnormality by decade in either group.

Reversal of the normal cervical lordosis was observed in 9 patients (15%) without demonstrable disc disruption, and in 4 with an abnormality at a single level only (7%) (Fig. 2). None of the abnormal control subjects showed reversal of the cervical curve. There were 18 patients with abnormal neurological physical signs (30%), of whom 12 had abnormal MRI findings. The severity of changes did not correlate with the presence of physical signs.

Marked asymmetry of bulk of the sternocleidomastoid muscles was noted in two patients (Fig. 3), and generalised muscle wasting with increased intermuscular fat was a notable feature in a further patient (Fig. 4).

Table 1. Percentage abnormal

Decade group	Patients	Controls
10–19		0 (n = 1)
20–29	41.7 (n = 12)	5.6 (n = 18)
30–39	64.0 (n = 25)	17.1 (n = 35)
40–49	61.5 (n = 13)	46.7 (n = 30)
50–59	85.7 (n = 7)	69.2 (n = 13)
60–69	50 (n = 2)	100 (n = 1)
70 +	100 (n = 1)	
Total	61.6 (n = 60)	31.7 (n = 98)

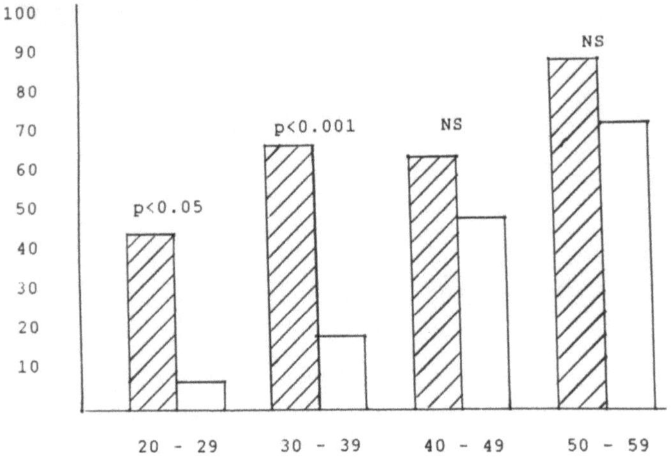

Fig. 1. Percentage abnormality by decade for patients *(hatched columns)* and controls *(open columns)*

Discussion

Despite the frequency of whiplash injury of the neck there is no general agreement about the exact pathological nature of the injury and the significance of accompanying symptoms and signs.

The symptom-complex known as the whiplash syndrome probably results from a variety of traumatic disruptions, of which the majority may be ligamentous or muscular, and therefore not associated with neurological signs. Superimposed on this is a variable component of disc derangement or herniation which can give rise to neurological symptoms and signs. One group [1] exclude disc herniation as part of the whiplash syndrome, confining their definition to a musculoligamentous sprain or strain of the cervical region.

Another series [2] of 50 cases of whiplash injury records symptoms of cervical radiculopathy in 70%, usually accompanied by muscle spasm but less frequently by physical signs. An identical percentage of our patients (42 patients) had reported symptoms suggesting cervical radiculopathy, and in 37 (62%) localised neck pain was a prominent feature.

Eighteen (30%) of our patients had physical signs, usually in the form of loss or reduction of arm reflexes, and 12 (20%) of these had abnormal MRI findings. This is comparable to the incidence of abnormality seen in the patient group as a whole: thus the presence of neurological signs did not have any predictive value for demonstrable MRI abnormality.This could be explained by the relative difficulty of demonstrating cervical nerve root compression with a low field (0.26 T) system. A more likely explanation is that many symptoms arise from ligamentous or muscle injury which is anatomically subtle, and may remain undetected on the images. Since 70% of our patients had symptoms but no neurological signs a large proportion may have had pain arising from soft tissue structures such as muscles and ligaments, suggesting that soft tissue injuries may be present even when all imaging studies are negative. Animal experiments [3] showed that tearing of the anterior longitudinal ligament and separation of the disc from the associated vertebra never occurred without damage to the anterior cervical muscles.

Plain cervical radiographs were infrequently performed at the time of injury, possibly because many hours or even days may elapse before symptoms reach sufficient severity for medical advice to be sought. We were able to examine so few (5 cases) that no conclusions can be drawn about pre-existing degenerative changes acting as a risk factor for whiplash injury. Other work [4, 5] suggests that prior degenerative changes are a strong indicator of an unfavourable outcome following a hyperextension injury, but conversely, one report described 146 patients with a whiplash syndrome, none of whom had degenerative changes on plain films at the time of injury [6].

Loss or even reversal of the cervical curve, noted in 13 patients with no demonstrable disc abnormality or abnormality at a single level, was not seen in any of the control group. An analysis of plain radiographs after whiplash injury noted increasing frequency of this finding in patients with more severe symptoms and physical signs [4]. The authors stated that abnormal curves in the cervical spine, presumably reflecting spasm of the neck muscles,

Fig. 2. Reversal of cervical lordosis

Fig. 3. Asymmetry of sternocleidomastoid muscles

Fig. 4. Generalised wasting of nuchal muscles

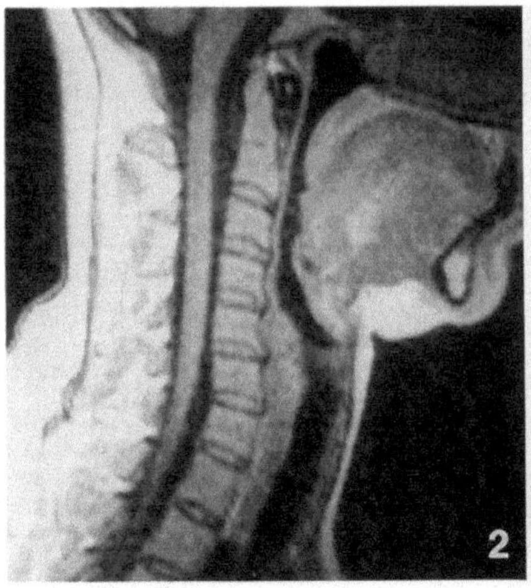

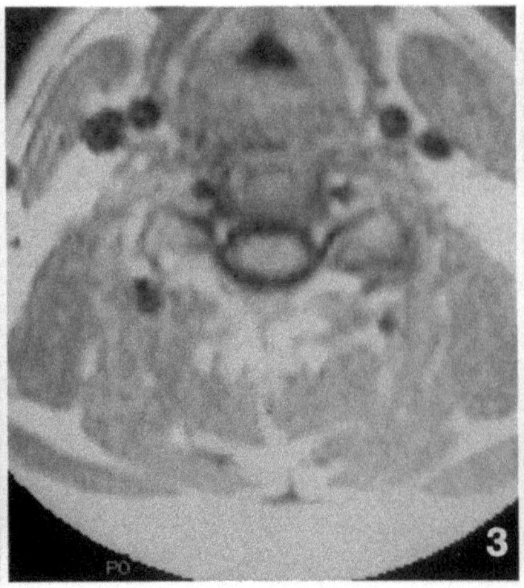

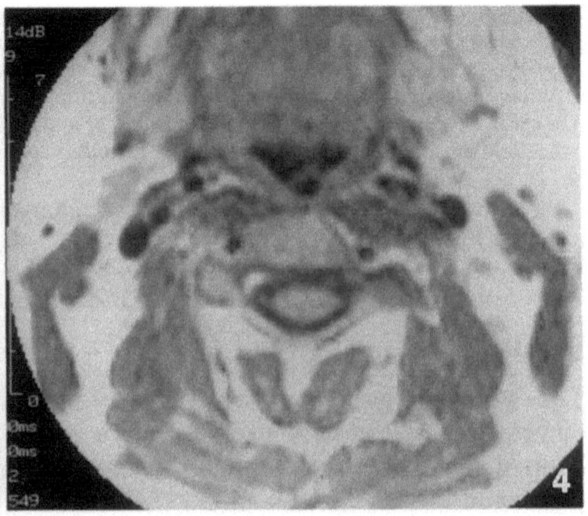

were more common in patients with a poor outcome, a conclusion also reached by other authors [1].

The 3 patients in our series with muscle asymmetry or wasting may have lost muscle bulk secondarily to disuse due to pain. However, it has been claimed [7] that whiplash injury is more common in subjects with slight muscular development and that this was due to insufficient muscular strength available to resist the injuring forces. Several authors have suggested that this may explain the reported female predominance in the whiplash syndrome.

References

1. Hirsch SA, Hirsch PJ, Hiramoto H, Weiss A (1988) Whiplash syndrome – fact or fiction? Orthop Clin North Am 19: 791–795
2. Gay JR, Abbott KH (1953) Common whiplash injuries of the neck. JAMA 152: 1698–1704
3. Macnab I (1973) The whiplash syndrome. Clin Neurosurg 20: 232–241
4. Norris SH, Watt I (1983) The prognosis of neck injuries resulting from rear-end vehicle collisions. J Bone Joint Surg [Br] 65: 608–611
5. Miles KA, Maimaris C, Finlay D, Barnes MR (1988) The incidence and prognostic significance of radiological abnormalities in soft tissue injuries to the cervical spine. Skeletal Radiol 17: 493–496
6. Hohl M (1974) Soft-tissue injuries of the neck in automobile accidents. J Bone Joint Surg [Am] 56: 1675–1682
7. La Rocca H (1978) Acceleration injuries of the neck. Clin neurosurg 25: 209–217

R. W. Parrish
Queen Square Imaging Centre
The National Hospital for Neurology and Neurosurgery
Queen Square
London WC1N 3BG, UK

Neuroradiology (1991) 33 [Suppl]: 164–166

Neuro-radiology
© Springer-Verlag 1991

The MRI appearances of subacute and chronic spinal trauma

R. W. Kerslake, T. Jaspan, and B. S. Worthington

Department of Radiology, Queens Medical Centre, University Hospital, Nottingham, UK

Summary. The MR images of 69 patients who had sustained previous spinal trauma were retrospectively reviewed. Abnormalities of the vertebral column were present in 79% and of the spinal cord in 51%. Cord atrophy was present in 13 cases (17%), syringohydromyelia in 10 (13%) and changes consistent with cystic myelomalacia in 8 (11%). In all but 1 case where syringohydromyelia was present, focal canal stenosis of at least 40% was present. Differing patterns of syringohydromyelia above and below the level of injury were the rule. MRI has the unique capability of displaying noninvasively the late sequelae of spinal trauma. The extraspinal soft tissues, vertebral column and spinal cord may be evaluated simultaneously.

Key words: Spinal cord injuries – Magnetic resonance imaging – Syringomyelia

MRI is ideally suited to the evaluation of the previously injured spinal cord. Assessment of the vertebral column, intervertebral discs and changes in spinal cord morphology and signal characteristics may be simultaneously and noninvasively carried out. The information obtained may be of value in determining patient management.

Materials and methods

Seventy-four MRI examinations of 69 patients who had sustained spinal trauma from 3 weeks to 40 years previously were retrospectively analysed. The age range of the patients was 18–75 years. There were 45 males and 24 females. Injuries involved the cervical region in 33 cases, upper thoracic (T1–6) in 7, lower thoracic (T7–10) in 6, thoracolumbar (T11–L2) in 21 and low lumbar (L3–5) in 4; two or more levels were involved in 4 cases.

MRI was performed at 0.15 T using dedicated surface coils and 7 mm section thickness in all cases. Short TR/short TE spin-echo (TR 500/TE 40) sagittal images were obtained in all cases, supplemented by sagittal plane long TR/long TE (TR 1600/TE 80) or short tau inversion recovery (STIR) sequences and axial plane TR 500/TE 40 sequences in most instances. A consensus report for each set of images was produced by two radiologists experienced in MRI.

Results

Eleven (15%) of the examinations were entirely normal. Changes in the extraspinal soft tissues, comprising regions of high signal intensity in the posterior ligamentous complex, were shown in 2 cases. These studies were obtained within 6 weeks of injury and the abnormalities were best appreciated using the STIR sequence. The vertebral column was normal in 15 cases; of these, spinal cord lesions were shown in 5 (atrophy 2, cystic myelomalacia 2, syrinx 1, the latter occurring following a stab wound).

Abnormalities of the vertebral column or intervertebral discs were present in 59 cases (79%). The changes demonstrated included fractures of the vertebral body (49 cases), focal bony canal stenosis (21 cases), vertical vertebral body cleft (6 cases) and altered vertebral body signal intensity (6 cases). Disc protrusions were present, either as isolated features or in association with bony changes, in 16 cases. These were associated with cord changes in 11 cases (compression 6, atrophy 2, syrinx 2, contusion 1).

Intraspinal abnormalities were shown in 38 cases (51%). Spinal cord compression or displacement was present in 17 cases, due to bony narrowing in 11 and disc protrusion in 6. Atrophy of the spinal cord was shown in 13 cases but was not seen earlier than 4 months following trauma. The changes were maximal at the site of injury and involved between 3 and 11 spinal segments, mean 5.7. Myelomalacic changes were present in 4 of these and syringohydromyelia in 2. The features of cystic myelomalacia (focal moderately well-defined high signal

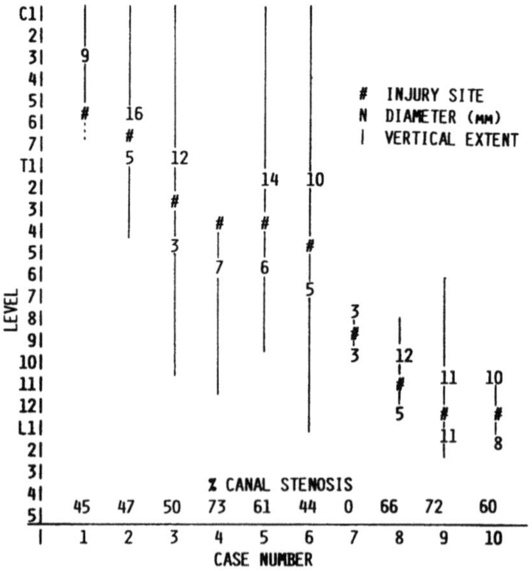

Fig. 1. Post-traumatic syringohydromyelia: location and diameter related to original injury site and degree of canal stenosis

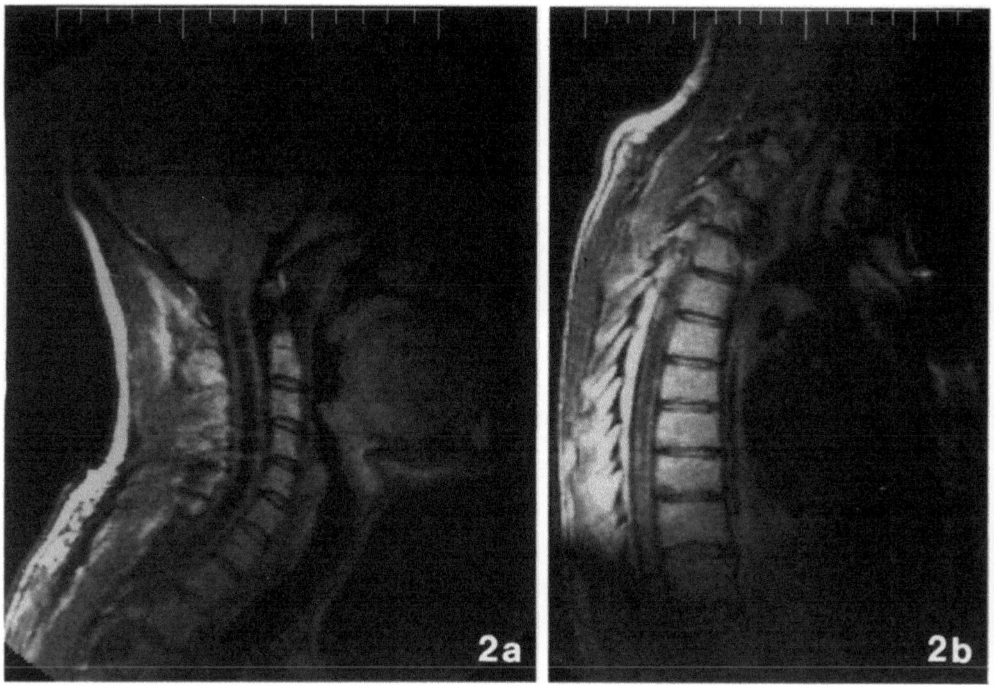

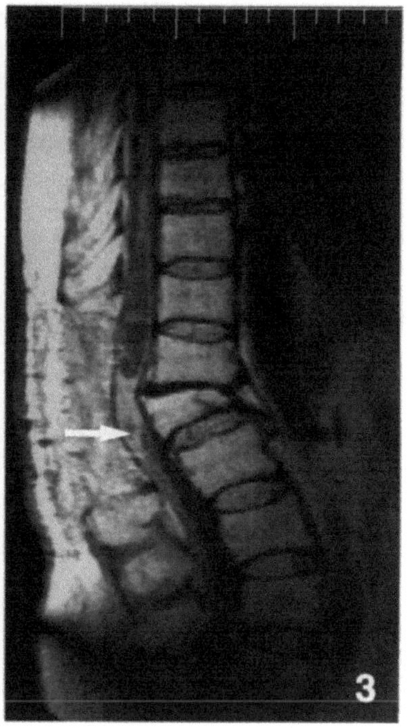

Fig. 2a, b. Sagittal SE 500/40 images showing: **a** expanded cervical cord with large syrinx containing multiple fibroglial septations; **b** in the thoracic region the syrinx is unilocular and the cord is only slightly expanded

Fig. 3. Sagittal SE 500/40 sequence demonstrates distended lower thoracic cord containing a septated syrinx. Note previous laminectomy: the spinal cord occupies the entire canal at the level of the previous burst fracture, below which there is a very small syrinx *(arrow)*

intensity on T2-weighted images with or without small punctate regions of low signal intensity on T1-weighted images) were present in 8 cases. This pattern was not seen in any patient examined within 6 months of trauma and was usually, but not invariably, accompanied by other intraspinal abnormalities (cord compression or atrophy).

Syringohydromyelic cavities (syrinxes) were present in 10 patients, but were not seen earlier than 6 months following trauma. The were well-defined regions of low signal intensity within the cord substance on T1-weighted images and involved between 3 and 20 spinal segments. In 4 of 6 cervical or upper thoracic injuries the size of the cavity above the level of injury was considerably greater than that below the level of injury (Fig. 1). Focal canal stenosis of 44–60% was present in these cases and the cord was noted to occupy the entire width of the spinal canal at the level of injury. Typically, the cord was enlarged and the syrinx contained multiple fibroglial bands or septations above the level of injury (Fig. 2a), whilst below, the cavity was smooth walled and the cord only minimally expanded (Fig. 2b). A similar but less marked pattern of abnormalities was seen in thoracolumbar injuries following which a syrinx had developed (Fig. 3).

Discussion

The late sequelae of spinal trauma include spinal cord atrophy, tethering, myelomalacia and syringohydromyelia. These may be localised to the injury site or *extensively* involve untraumatised regions of the spinal cord. Abnormalities of the vertebral column and intervertebral discs may occur due to the original injury or as a result of instability associated with decompressive surgery; they may in turn cause further cord injury.

Clinicopathological studies have resulted in the concept of a spectrum of post-traumatic spinal cord pathology from arachnoiditis through microcystic degeneration to syringohydromyelia [1–3]. Delayed CT following water-soluble myelography may show contrast medium accumulation within the spinal cord in both cystic and non-cystic myelopathy [2]. MRI appears to be more reliable in predicting the presence of surgically drainable cord cysts [4, 5] but microcystic degeneration may mimic these appearances [1]. Intraoperative ultrasound should permit an accurate distinction to be made before myelotomy is undertaken [1, 5].

Syringohydromyelia may occur as a consequence of extramedullary compressive lesions, possibly due to ischaemia of the cord with secondary degeneration of the grey matter, to filling of the central canal by extra-choroidally produced cerebrospinal fluid (CSF) [6], or to neuroglial damage with enlargement of extracellular perivascular spaces [7]. The formation of arachnoid adhesions either as a result of the initial injury or due to later surgery may alter CSF dynamics such that abnormal entry of CSF into the cord via the enlarged Virchow–Robin spaces may result in the formation of a cord cyst [6] which enlarges and propagates due to a water-hammer effect [7]. If there is a high-grade subarachnoid block with focal compression of the cord cyst by a fracture and/or dislocation, locally altered CSF dynamics may result in turbulence of CSF within the cyst above the block and stagnation below, contributing to a variable appearance of the cyst in there two locations [5]. MRI is of value in defining the morphological appearances of post–traumatic cord cysts prior to consideration of surgical drainage.

References

1. MacDonald RL, Findlay JM,Tator CH (1988) Microcystic spinal cord degeneration causing posttraumatic myelopathy. J Neurosurg 68: 466–471
2. Stevens JM, Olney JS, Kendall BE (1985) Post–traumatic cystic and non–cystic myelopathy. Neuroradiology 27: 48–56
3. Yamashita M, Takahashi M, Matsuno Y, Sakamoto Y, Oguni T, Sakae T (1989) MR imaging of chronic spinal cord injuries. Radiology 173: 83
4. Quencer RM, Sheldon JJ, Post MJD, Diaz RD, Montalvo BM, Green BA, Eismont FJ (1986) Magnetic resonance imaging of the chronically injured cervical spinal cord. AJNR 7: 457–464
5. Quencer RM (1988) The injured spinal cord. Evaluation with magnetic resonance and intraoperative ultrasonography. Radiol Clin North Am 26: 1025–1045
6. Castillo M, Quencer RM, Green BA, Montalvo BM (1988) Syringomyelia as a consequence of compressive extramedullary lesions: postoperative clinical and radiological manifestations. AJR 150: 391–396
7. Sherman JL, Barkovich AJ, Citrin CM (1986) The MR appearances of syringomyelia: new observations. AJNR 7: 985–995

R. W. Kerslake
MRI Unit
Queens Medical Centre
Nottingham NG7 2UH, UK

Neuroradiology (1991) 33 [Suppl]: 167–169

Neuro-radiology
© Springer-Verlag 1991

Idiopathic and Chiari-associated syringomyelia in adults: observations on cerebrospinal fluid pathways at the foramen magnum using static MRI

A. G. Clifton, J. M. Stevens, and B. E. Kendall

The National Hospitals for Nervous Diseases, Queen Square, London, UK

Summary. Forty patients with idiopathic and Chiari-associated syringomyelia were evaluated for the level of tonsillar and medullary descent and size and flow in cerebrospinal fluid (CSF) spaces across the foramen magnum (FM), with which the cranial extent and degree of distension of the syrinxes were compared. There was no significant association with or even trend towards patients with increasing tonsillar descent or narrow or obstructed CSF pathways having more extensive or more distended syrinxes. Reduction of distension of syrinxes occurred in 66% of operated cases, regardless of whether FM decompression or only shunting of the syrinx had been performed. These trends were unexpected in the light of current hypotheses of syrinx formation in which intermittent obstruction of CSF pathways at the FM is central.

Key words: Syringomyelia – Magnetic resonance – Foramen magnum – Cerebrospinal fluid pathways

The concept of impedance of cerebrospinal fluid (CSF) movement in the cisterns traversing the foramen magnum (FM) is central to several hypotheses about syrinx formation, and many current therapeutic strategies [1, 2]. MRI has contributed new data about syringomyelia and its response to treatment [3, 4], but relatively little attention has been paid to how the varying appearances at the FM relate to the cranial extent and degree of distension of the intramedullary cavities and their response to operative treatment. This study was designed to address these questions within the limitations of the available material.

Materials and methods

Patients in the study were examined on a Vista MR Unit (Picker International Corp) operating at 0.26 Tesla. MR images from all patients diagnosed as having syringomyelia between 1985 and 1990 were reviewed, and cases with known or suspected spinal cord trauma or intraspinal tumours were excluded. This yielded 40 patients. All had sagittal T1-weighted spin echo images (TR 500/TE 26) of adequate quality, but less than half had sagittal T2-weighted images (TR 2000/TE 80–120), of which only 8 were of adequate quality. Only 4 had axial images.

The following observations were made at the FM: (1) level of the cerebellar tonsils and obex for the fourth ventricle with respect to the FM, atlas and axis; (2) evidence of medullary compression; (3) evidence of medullary spur or kink; (4) width of the subarachnoid space across the FM anterior and posterior to the neuraxis. The space was regarded as obliterated if it was invisible, narrowed if it was visible but less than 2 mm in width (not measurable), and normal if it was visible and greater than 2 mm in width (and therefore measurable). When T2-weighted images were available, the presence or absence of CSF flow void in the subarachnoid space and along the floor of the fourth ventricle was recorded. It was also noted whether a communication between the fourth ventricle and syrinx cavity was visible.

These features were correlated with the appearance of the intramedullary cavity. The particular features noted were: (1) whether the cavity was distended, resulting in overall enlargement of the spinal cord, or not distended, so that the cord was normal in size or small; (2) the cranial extent of the cavity.

Pre- and postoperative MRI was available for 6 patients. The above features were compared before and after operation, which consisted of FM decompression in 4 and syringostomy in 2.

Results

In 29 patients the cerebellar tonsils lay below the FM, and these cases were designated as having Chiari-associated syringomyelia. In 23 of these (79%) the tonsils lay between the FM and the C1 arch, and in 8 (21%) they lay below C1. A medullary spur or kink was identified in the cervical canal in 9 (22.5%) and in a further 3 cases the obex lay in the cervical canal. There was evidence of medullary compression in 13 (32.5%). Eleven patients were considered to have idiopathic syringomyelia, and because they may have represented an aetiologically heterogeneous group they were analysed both separately and with the whole material.

The spinal cord was distended in 25 (62.5%) and normal or small in 15 (37.5%). The syrinx was not shown to extend above the axis body in 28 (72%), reached the atlas ring in 18 and extended into the medulla oblongata in 4 (10%). There were no significant differences in these distributions between the Chiari-associated and idiopathic types of syringomyelia.

The correlations obtained are given in Tables 1–4. The outcome of surgery is given in Table 5. No correlation was found between the presence or absence of medullary compression and the appearances of the syrinxes.

Discussion

The hydrodynamics of CSF in syringomyelia are still poorly understood [1, 5–7]. Current therapeutic strategies are influenced by hypotheses of syrinx formation in Chiari

Table 1. Extent of syrinx relative to level of tonsils

Level of tonsils	Upper limit of syrinx		
	Below C2	C1	Medulla
Above FM	4	5	2
FM-C1	2	6	0
At C1	7	6	2
Below C1 arch	5	1	0

FM, Foramen magnum

Table 2. Distension of syrinx relative to level of tonsils

Level of tonsils	Distension of syrinx		
	Distended	Normal	Collapsed
Above FM	7	3	1
FM-C1	6	0	2
At C1	9	3	3
Below C1 arch	3	0	3

Table 3. Distension of syrinx related to size of cerebrospinal fluid (CSF) pathways across FM

		Distension of syrinx (All)		
		Distended	Normal	Collapsed
Anterior	Normal/large	13	4	4
	Small/obliterated	12	2	5
Posterior	Normal/large	10	3	2
	Small/obliterated	15	3	7
		Distension of syrinx (Chiari)		
		Distended	Normal	Collapsed
Anterior	Normal/large	6	1	4
	Small/obliterated	12	2	4
Posterior	Normal/large	3	0	2
	Small/obliterated	15	3	6

malformations to which impedance of CSF flow in the cisterns at the FM is central, especially partial or complete obstruction of the foramen of Magendie, vallecula and cisterna magna by the ectopic cerebellar tonsils and arachnoiditis [1, 5–9]. In a previous study of 93 water soluble myelograms and computed cisternograms in adults with Chiari malformations, 46% of whom had associated syringomyelia, no correlation was found between the size of the vallecula or cisterna magna and the incidence of clinical or radiological syringomyelia, nor was there definite evidence of arachnoiditis; moreover, contrast medium entered the fourth ventricle as often in cases with syrinx as those without [10]. These data provided little support for current hypotheses, or for some aspects of current therapeutic strategies.

Chiari-associated syringomyelia is often classified as communicating syringomyelia or syringohydromyelia [1]. In the hypotheses of Gardner and Angel [5] and Williams [1] cranial CSF is rerouted into the spinal cord via a communication between the fourth ventricle and central canal of the spinal cord; CSF pulsation and intermittently *low* intraspinal pressure due to ball-valve occlusion of the FM by the cerebellar tonsils result in progressive distension of the syrinx. The alternative theory of Aboulker [6] and Ball and Dyan [7] postulates that CSF enters the spinal cord along its length from the spinal subarachnoid space via the Virchow-Robin spaces, driven by a relatively *high* intraspinal pressure caused by obstruction of cisternal CSF flow across the entire FM.

Craniospinal pressure dysjunction has been measured, and has indicated a relatively low intraspinal pressures in some studies [1] and a relatively high intraspinal pressure in others [11].

In a study of MRI examinations and computed cisternograms of 93 adults with Chiari malformations and normal controls the relative lengths of the midbrain, pons and medulla were measured, and the position of the obex and the presence of medullary spurs and kinks were charted [12]. It was found that the medulla was elongated in 71% of patients with Chiari malformation, and that the obex lay in the cervical canal and usually below the ectopic tonsils in 53% of these. The dorsal hump caused by the gracile tubercles frequently protruded by more than 2 mm in such cases, and on computed cisternography similar humps were usually shown to represent medullary kinks, although actual kinking was shown by MRI, where resolution was relatively low, in only 13%.

In the present material it was concluded that the obex lay in the cervical canal and below the level of anatomical obstruction at the FM in 12 cases, constituting 40% of patients with Chiari-associated syringomyelia. Moreover, in 9 of these, the hump caused by the gracile tubercle was large enough to suggest a kink, and in such cases the obex probably was overhung by the herniated distal medulla oblongata. These anatomical features are usually ignored in discussions about syrinx formation, despite being well documented at operation [9].

In patients with Chiari malformations syringomyelia has been found most often when there was arachnoiditis at the FM [9]. The development of CSF pulsations, thought

Table 4. CSF flow void (CSFV) characteristics in the 8 cases with T2-weighted sequences

Case	Extent syrinx cranially	Syrinx distended +/−	CSFV in syrinx +/−	High signal in cord	CSFV at FM		FM narrow or not		CSFV at floor of IV	Level tonsils
					A	P	A	P		
1	C2	+	+	+	+	+	+	+	+	C1/2
2	C2	+	+	+	+	+	+	+	+	C2
3	C3	+	+	+	+	+	+	+	+	C1
4	C2	+/−	+	+	+	−	+	−	+	Arch C1
5	C2	+	+	−	+	+	+	+	+	Arch C1
6	C1	+	+	−	+	+	+	+	+	C1
7	C2	+	+	+	+	+	+	+	−	Arch C1
8	C1	+	+	−	+	+	−	−	−	Below FM

A, Anterior; P, posterior

Table 5. Distension of syrinx pre- and postoperatively and type of surgery in operated patients

Case	Syrinx distended Preop	Type of surgery		Syrinx distended Postop
		FM Decompression	Shunt	
1	+	+	–	–
2	+	+	–	–
3	+	–	+	–
4	+	–	+	+
5	+	+	+	+
6	–	+	–	–

to predispose to syringomyelia after chemically induced arachnoiditis at the FM, has been shown in experimental animals [13] and, unfortunately, MRI may fail to detect even moderate degrees of spinal arachnoiditis [14]. For this study it was considered that MRI could reasonably be expected to detect major degress of impedance of CSF flow on non-gated T2-weighted images, and that the presence of wide subarachnoid cisterns on T1-weighted images could reasonably be expected to indicate free CSF flow in most cases. If obstruction to craniospinal CSF flow across the FM was central to syrinx formation, distension and propagation, some correlation between narrow or obliterated CSF pathways and more extensive and more distended intramedullary cavities would be expected. That there was not even a trend towards such a correlation in the groups as a whole, or in the Chiari-associated cases considered separately, does not support any of the hypotheses cited above. This view was reinforced by the 11 patients with idiopathic syringomyelia in whom the intramedullary cavity was distended in 75%, all of whom had wide craniospinal subarachnoid spaces. However, it is conceded that it may not be correct to consider this group in the same context as Chiari-associated syringomyelia.

The commonest operation to be performed on patients with Chiari-associated syringomyelia is a posterior FM and upper cervical decompression with duroplasty, designed to widen the craniospinal subarachnoid spaces. This is often combined with a syringotomy and some form of shunt; sometimes only syringotomy and shunting procedures are performed. Whatever the operation, the syrinx has been shown to diminish in size in between 60% and 80% of patients [11]. Indeed, it has been asserted that merely performing a subarachnoid lumboperitoneal shunt will often collapse a distended syrinx [11], and we have seen a case with a grossly distended Chiari-associated syrinx on myelography and CT, which despite no surgical intervention, appeared as an atrophic cord in an expanded spinal canal on MRI a week later. Given this variability of response it is difficult to draw definitive conclusions about the precise mechanisms which result in diminution in the size of the syrinx. In this material 4 of the 6 cases for which pre- and postoperative MRI was available indicated a satisfactory radiological result from operation, which was independent of the size of either the anterior or posterior craniospinal subarachnoid spaces preoperatively.

It is probable that the mechanisms of syrinx formation are not the same as those determining subsequent propagation and maintenance of distension. Moreover, static imaging with the patient in a relaxed supine position should not perhaps be expected to indicate the presence of obstruction of the cranio-spinal subarachnoid pathways which is intermittent. The particular MRI equipment at our disposal may well not be sensitive in detecting localised arachnoid adhesions. Nevertheless, that these data, such as they are, do not even hint at the expected trends is a cause for concern. These negative findings are not sufficient to reject current hypotheses totally, nor are they a suitable basis for an alternative formulation.

However, we speculate that both the genesis and propagation of intramedullary cavities are multifactorial processes, some cases being a true communicating hydromyelia, some a syringohydromyelia in which the communication has become obliterated, whereas in others, which may be the majority, an entirely different mechanism may obtain. Perhaps this is the appearance of circumscribed central necrosis within the spinal cord of traumatic and/or ischaemic origin, which subsequently liquefies, as has been documented in cases of post-traumatic and tumour-associated syringomyelia.

References

1. Williams B (1980) On the pathogenesis of syringomyelia: a review. Proc R Soc of Med 73: 798–806
2. Barnett HJM (1973) The epilogue. In: Barnett HJM, Foster JB, Hudgson P (eds) Syringomyelia. Saunders, London, pp 302–313
3. Sherman JL, Barkovich AJ, Citrin CM (1987) The MR appearance of syringomyelia: new observations. AJR 148: 381–391
4. Batzdorf U (1988) Chiari I malformation with syringomyelia: evaluation of surgical therapy by magnetic resonance imaging. J Neurosurg 68: 726–730
5. Gardner WJ, Angel J (1975) The mechanism of syringomyelia and its surgical correction. Clin Neurosurg 6: 131–140
6. Aboulker J (1979) La syringomyelie et les liquides intra-rachidiens. Neurochirurgie 25: [Suppl 1]: 9–144
7. Ball MJ, Dyan AD (1972) Pathogenesis of syringomyelia. Lancet II: 799–801
8. Mohr PD, Strang FA, Sambrook MA, Boddie HG (1977) The clinical and surgical features in 40 patients with primary cerebellar ectopia (adult Chiari malformation). Q J Med 46: 85–96
9. Rhoton AL Jr (1976) Microsurgery of Arnold-Chiari malformation in adults with and without hydromyelia. J Neurosurg 45: 473–483
10. Serva WAD (1985) Chiari malformation in adults: therapeutic and prognostic aspects. Thesis, University of London
11. Park TS, Cail WS, Broaddus WS, Walker MG (1989) Lumboperitoneal shunt combined with myelotomy for treatment of syringohydromyelia. J Neurosurg 70: 721–727
12. Shah V, Martin N, Stevens J, Kendall B (1987) Observations on abnormalities of the cerebellum and medulla in Chiari malformation. Dupont, UK
13. duBoulay G, Shah SH, Currie JC, Logue V (1974) The mechanism of hydromyelia in Chiari type I malformations. Br J Radiol 47: 579–587
14. Norman D (1987) In: Brant-Zawadzki M, Norman D (eds) Magnetic resonance imaging of the central nervous system. Raven Press, New York, p 316

A. G. Clifton
X-Ray Department
Maida Vale Hospital
London, W9 1TL, UK

Neuroradiology (1991) 33 [Suppl]: 170–172

Neuro
radiology
© Springer-Verlag 1991

Three types of syringomyelia in MRI: clinical and experimental results

M. Hermes and E. Donauer

Institute for Neuroradiology and Department of Neurosurgery, Saarland University Hospital, Homburg–Saar, Federal Republic of Germany

Summary. Most cases of syringomyelia are caused by congenital malformations, and these form the basis of our clinical and experimental study. The findings from MRI and clinical examination reveal three types of intramedullary cavities in congenital syringomyelia. We could mimic them by several experimental situations and were able to characterise them. The so–called hydromyelia corresponds to our type of experimental closure of the foramina of Luschka with continuous dilation of the cavity into the cervicomedullary region. The syringomyelia associated with the Chiari II malformation with a very narrow canal at C1 and a balloon–like dilatation of the syrinx corresponds to our experimental type produced by a broad kaolin cuff in the cervicomedullary region. The syringomyelia as seen in Chiari I malformation or in connection with arachnoid adhesions and a narrow canal at C1 has a more discrete intramedullary cavity; this is mimicked by experimental kaolin injection into the cisterna magna. The three experimental types are correlated to clinical findings in our patients.

Key words: Syringomyelia – Hydromyelia – Experimental hydrocephalus – Syringoarachnoidal shunting – Chiari malformation

The present terminology for syringomyelia is not consistent. Ballantine et al. [1] noted a semantic confusion concerning intramedullary cavities. However, good correlation between experimental data and MRI may enable a better classification of syringomyelia.

In this paper we use the term "syringomyelia" only for dysraphic cavities in the spinal cord, usually combined with other malformations of the neural crest such as the Chiari malformation (CM), the Dandy Walker cyst, basilar impression, spina bifida and meningocoele or myelomeningocoele.

With MRI it is now possible to show intramedullary cavities noninvasively. In the absence of other dysraphic signs the diagnosis of syringomyelia has to be checked carefully, at least by gadolinium–enhanced MR images to exdlude other causes such as traumatic or neoplastic intramedullary cavities.

There are also many hypotheses as to the development of syringomyelia [2]. The most widely accepted theory is that of Gardner [3] and Gardner and Angel [4], supplemented by Williams [5, 6]. According to Gardner's hydrodynamic theory, the CSF pressure widens the central canal in case of CSF circulation block. The pulsatile changes of the CSF pressure (Gardner) or the breath–dependent venous pressure changes (Williams) are the cause of the progressive dilatation of the central canal. This can result in syringomyelia that develops from the CSF pressure gradients or pulsations. The form and size of such cavities depend on developmental or CSF dynamics [7].

By injection of kaolin into the cisterna magna we could induce a CSF circulation block from the fourth ventricle similar to the CM in cats ($n = 52$). The dilation of the central canal leads to progressive syringomyelia. Our experimental and clinical follow–up studies over up to 2 years show a similar course to human syringomyelia [8–12]. After the acute phase associated with intracranial pressure increase the central canal widens. With subsequent flow of fluid from the filum terminale into the spinal subarachnoid space the disease seems to stabilise with good clinical condition and balanced CSF pressure. After this "silent phase" there is progression with an increase in the number of cavities and clinical signs of destruction of dorsal columns. With ventriculography we could show that the cavities, predominantly cervical and lumbar, are connected by the narrow cervical central canal to the ventricular system. This narrow connection lies under the kaolin cuff. This is comparable to the narrowing by the descent of the cerebellum in CM. Such cases were mistaken for "non–communicating" syringomyelia.

Depending on the kaolin cuff we find two types of kaolin–induced syringomyelia in cats:
1. A complete block by the kaolin cuff is comparable to the human CM II with a very narrow central canal in this segment and a considerable dilation below like the shape of a claret glass.
2. Incomplete block by the kaolin cuff (10% kaolin) leads to a more discrete cavity like a champagne glass. This corresponds to the human CM I or arachnoid adhesions.

In another experiment with selective block of the foramina of Luschka with cotton wool ($n = 16$) a different type of syringomyelia develops. We find free CSF communication between cerebral and spinal subarachnoid spaces and a wide central canal. This corresponds to "communicating" syringomyelia or hydromyelia [9].

These three experimental forms of syringomyelia show a surprisingly good correlation to clinical and MRI

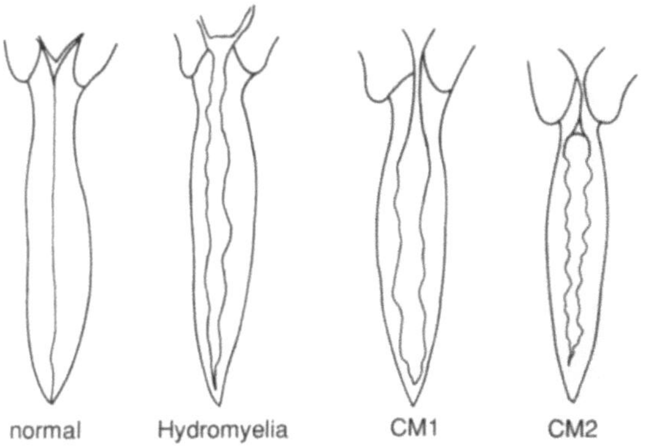

Fig. 1. Patterns of congenital syringomyelia. Different shapes of intramedullary cavities related to hydromyelia, Chiari I *(CM1)* and Chiari II *(CM2)*

findings in human syringomyelia. They confirm observations that show three types of syringomyelia in patients depending on the type of CSF circulation block.

We think that the partial pressure compensation between inner and outer spinal and cerebral CSF spaces is responsible for the dilation of the full length of the central canal. This and the CSF outflow from the filum terminale can compensate for the increased basal pressure of the CSF. But acute pressure changes such as occur in breathing, coughing or venous pressure changes cannot be compensated sufficiently.

Dye or contrast agent injected into the ventricles diffuses to the filum terminale and into the spinal subarachnoid space; however, morphologically there are no channels. The experiments show that neither the reduction of CSF resorption capacity nor the separation of the dilated central canal are responsible for the progression of syringomyelia. The important point is the loss of the ability to compensate for pressure changes caused by the blocking of the outflow of the fourth ventricle. These are the physiological pathways of pressure compensation, and their closure directs the pressure changes into the central canal. Even after the implantation of a shunt, once it has developed a syringomyelic cavity may keep growing.

These ideas only partially explain the pathophysiology of syringomyelia; they do not take the plasticity and biological properties of nervous tissue into account. Ultrastructural investigations, in cats, show typical and reproducible morphological changes with cavities always in the dorsal columns. In the acute phase the ependymal layer is destroyed and is replaced in the chronic state by an astroglial layer so that there is a CSF–parenchymal threshold again.

Even after treatment there is a further progression of the dorsal cavities. These cavities may become very large and communicate only in small areas with the central canal. Outside these areas there appears to be no communication on microscopic sections.

The experimental results on form and size of the cavities suggest not only the hydrodynamic theory of Gardner and Williams, but also the neuroschisis theory of Padget [13, 14] to be of importance. Cavities always develop along weak parts of the neural raphe. In experimentally induced obstructive hydrocephalus the central canal becomes the main CSF drainage pathway but this is inadequate and is considerably elongated with increased resistance. In the filum terminale there is outflow of CSF but no open end of the canal. Increased CSF pressure can only be partially compensated for, and then only after a delay. The onset of reparative mechanisms reduces the elasticity of the tissue. The progression of the syringomyelic cavity

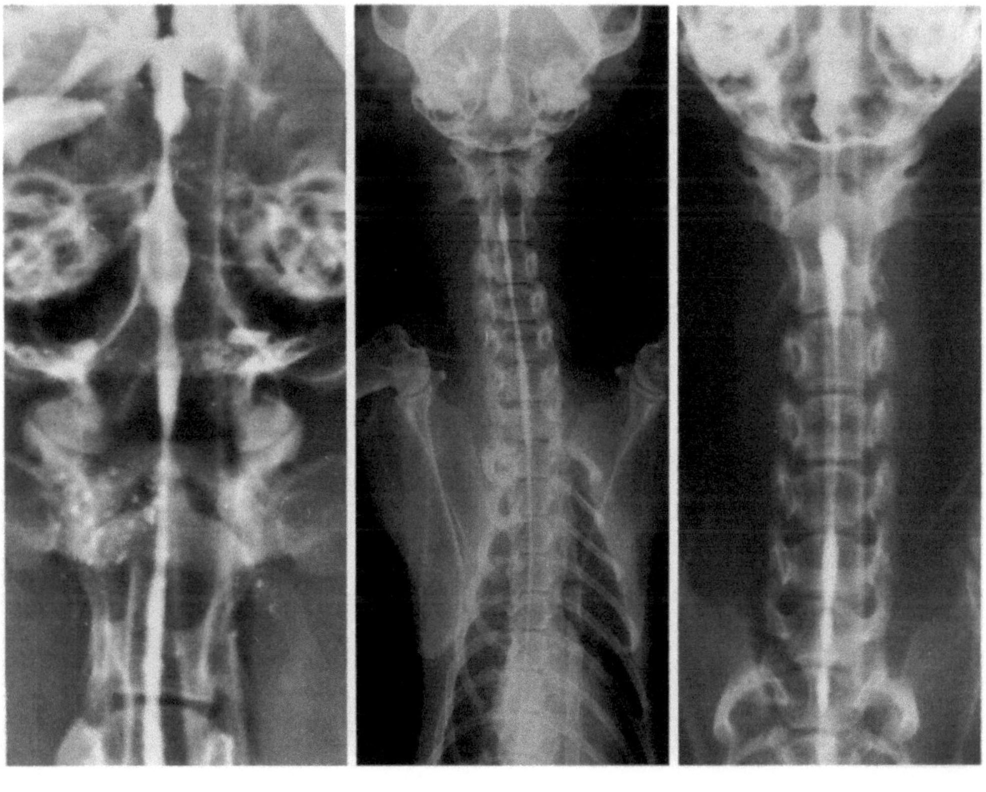

Fig. 2. Intramedullary cavities in experimental syringomyelia. *Left,* Hydromyelia; *middle,* CM1 type; *right,* CM2 type

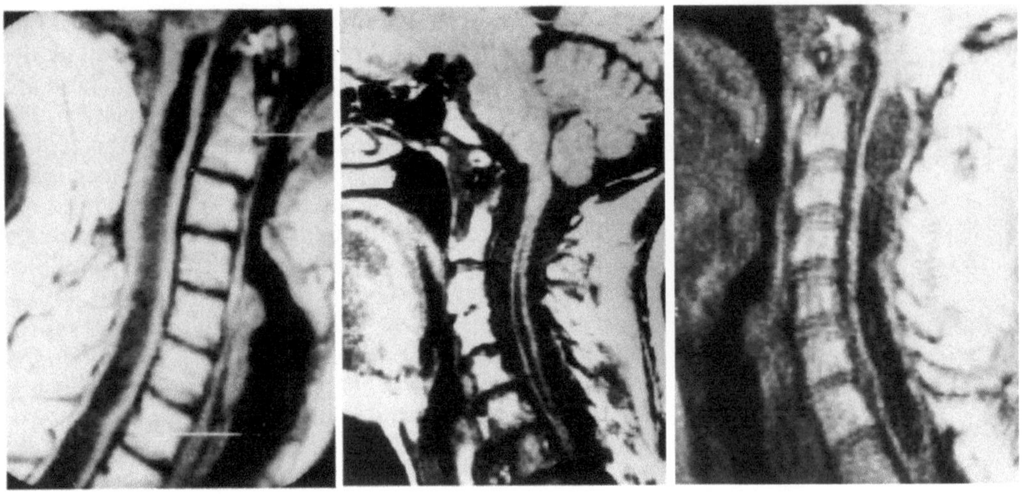

Fig. 3. Sagittal MR images of clinical syringomyelia. *Left,* Hydromyelia; *middle,* CM1 type; *right,* CM2 type

stops only when there is no further tissue elasticity. This underlines the importance of early surgical therapy in congenital syringomyelia.

References

1. Ballantine HT, Ojemann RG, Drew JH (1971) Syringohydromyelia. Prog Neurol Surg 4: 227–245
2. Barnett HJM, Foster JB, Hudgson P (1973) Syringomyelia. In: Walton JN (ed) Major problems in neurology, vol 1. Saunders, Philadelphia
3. Gardner WJ (1965) Hydrodynamic mechanism of syringomyelia: its relationship to myelocoele. J Neurol Neurosurg Psychiatry 28: 247–259
4. Gardner WJ, Angel J (1958) The mechanism of syringomyelia and its surgical correction. Clin Neurosurg 6: 131–140
5. Williams B (1986) Progress in syringomyelia. Neurol Res 8: 130–145
6. Williams B (1972) Combined cisternal and lumbar pressure recordings in the sitting position using differential manometry. J Neurol Neurosurg Psychiatry 35: 142–143
7. Greenfield JG, Blackwood W, McMenemy WH, Meyer A, Norman RM, Russell DS (1963) Neuropathology, vol 2. Arnold, London, p 331
8. Donauer E (1990) Syringomyelia: experimental and clinical studies. Habilitationsschrift, Universität des Saarlandes, Homburg–Saar
9. Faulhauer K, Donauer E (1985) Experimental hydrocephalus and hydrosyringomyelia in the cat. Acta Neurochir (Wien) 74: 72–80
10. Rascher K, Booz KH, Donauer E, Nacimiento AC (1987) Structural alterations in the spinal cord during progressive communicating syringomyelia. An experimental study in the cat. Acta Neuropathol (Berl) 72: 248–255
11. Rascher K, Booz KH, Sonauer G, Donauer E (1988) The filum terminale. A morphological study in the cat. Z Mikrosk Anat Forsch 102: 1–17
12. Booz KH, Faulhauer K, Donauer E, Nieland F (1979) Morphologische Veränderungen an Zentralkanal der Katze nach Kaolin–Injektion in die Zisterna magna. Z Mikrosk Anat Forsch 93
13. Padget DH (1972) Development of so-called dysraphism; with embryonic evidence of clinical Arnold–Chiari and Dandy–Walker malformations. Johns Hopkins Med J 130: 127–165
14. Padget DH (1970) Neuroschisis and human embryonic maldevelopment: new evidence on anencephaly, spina bifida and diverse mammalian defects. J Neuropathol Exp Neurol 29: 192–216

Dr. M. Hermes
Institut für Neuroradiologie
Universitätskliniken
W-6650 Homburg–Saar
Federal Republic of Germany

Neuroradiology (1991) 33 [Suppl]: 173–175

Neuro-radiology
© Springer-Verlag 1991

Magnetic resonance cineflow imaging of cerebrospinal fluid in syringomyelia

T. Abe[1], N. Nakamura[1], R. Watanabe[2], T. Suzuki[1], K. Tashibu[1], H. Onoue[1], and M. Ida[3]

Departments of [1] Neurosurgery, [2] Internal Medicine and [3] Radiology, The Jikei University School of Medicine, Tokyo, Japan

Summary. The cerebrospinal fluid (CSF) hydrodynamics of 17 patients with syringomyelia were analysed using a Toshiba MRT-200 superconducting system (1.5 T) in 3 normal subjects. The turbulent flow of CSF in the cisterna magna which was seen in normal subjects could not be detected before operation in patients with the syringomyelia Chiari malformation complex. Moreover, the CSF in the syrinx moved actively in synchrony with pulsation in the lateral ventricles. After obstruction of the central canal by Gardner's operation, the syrinx decreased in size and pulsatile movements of CSF within it were absent even in patients with a remaining cavity. This suggests that the pulsatile flow inside the syrinx is transmitted from the fourth ventricle through the patent central canal. The pathogenesis of syringomyelia associated with a Chiari malformation is discussed.

Key words: Syringomyelia – Magnetic resonance imaging – Chiari malformation – Cerebrospinal fluid dynamics

The pathogenesis of syringomyelia remains controversial [1, 2]. However, the disturbance of cerebrospinal fluid (CSF) flow at the craniovertebral junction produced by the Chiari malformation or basal arachnoiditis may play an important role in syrinx formation [3].

The hydrodynamics of CSF were analysed in normal subjects or patients with syringomyelia associated with a Chiari malformation using a superconducting MR unit.

Patients and methods

We analysed the flow of CSF in 17 patients with syringomyelia associated with a Chiari malformation, using a Toshiba MRT-200 superconducting system (1.5 T).

Magnetic resonance (MR) cineflow imaging was obtained using the single-slice multiphase imaging method, employing gradient field echoes with a low flip angle of 30°, synchronisation with the R-wave of the electrocardiogram (ECG), an echo time (TE) of 14 ms, a repetition time (TR) of 50 ms and 16 phases. In each case, a midline sagittal image from the aqueduct to the cervical spinal cord was obtained. Axial images at the level of the upper cervical spine in control subjects and at the site of the syrinx in patients with syringomyelia were also obtained.

Results

MR cineflow imaging showed to-and-fro active movements of CSF from the third ventricle to the fourth ventricle, becoming turbulent in the cisterna magna of normal subjects. The CSF around the spinal cord and in the pontine cistern moved actively in synchrony with pulsations in the lateral ventricles. Moreover, in all patients with syringomyelia associated with a Chiari malformation, the cisterna magna was occupied by the descending cerebellar tonsils and the CSF movements in the region of the craniovertebral junction were absent.

The subarachnoid space around the spinal cord was narrowed by the enlarged spinal cord and active CSF movements in that space were not observed as in normal subjects. The most striking finding was that the CSF in the syrinx moved actively in synchrony with pulsations in the ventricles.

Figure 1 A shows a frame from MR cineflow imaging in the midline in a patient with syringomyelia associated with a Chiari malformation. The syrinx shows a mixture of high signal intensity areas and low signal intensity areas. Figure 1 B shows a frame from MR cineflow imaging in the horizontal plane at the level of C3. A high signal intensity area is recognisable in the syrinx. This indicates rapid flow, different from other regions in the syrinx.

Figure 1 C shows a frame from an axial sequence at the level of C7 at the same stage as Fig. 1 B, the high-intensity spot being diffuse and the intensity itself being lowered.

It was considered that local flow in the syrinx observed at C3 slowed at C7 and diffused throughout the cavity.

In case 2, a high signal intensity area inside the syrinx at systole (Fig. 2 A) was decreased in size and intensity during diastole (Fig. 2 B), indicating pulsatile CSF movements inside the syrinx.

After obstruction of the central canal by Gardner's operation, the syrinx decreased in size and pulsatile movements of CSF in the syrinx disappeared (Fig. 2 C). In this patient it was confirmed that the central canal at the obex was patent at surgery.

Discussion

Syringomyelia is not regarded as a single entity, and there are different pathophysiological mechanisms [4]. We have focussed on the hydrodynamics of CSF in patients with

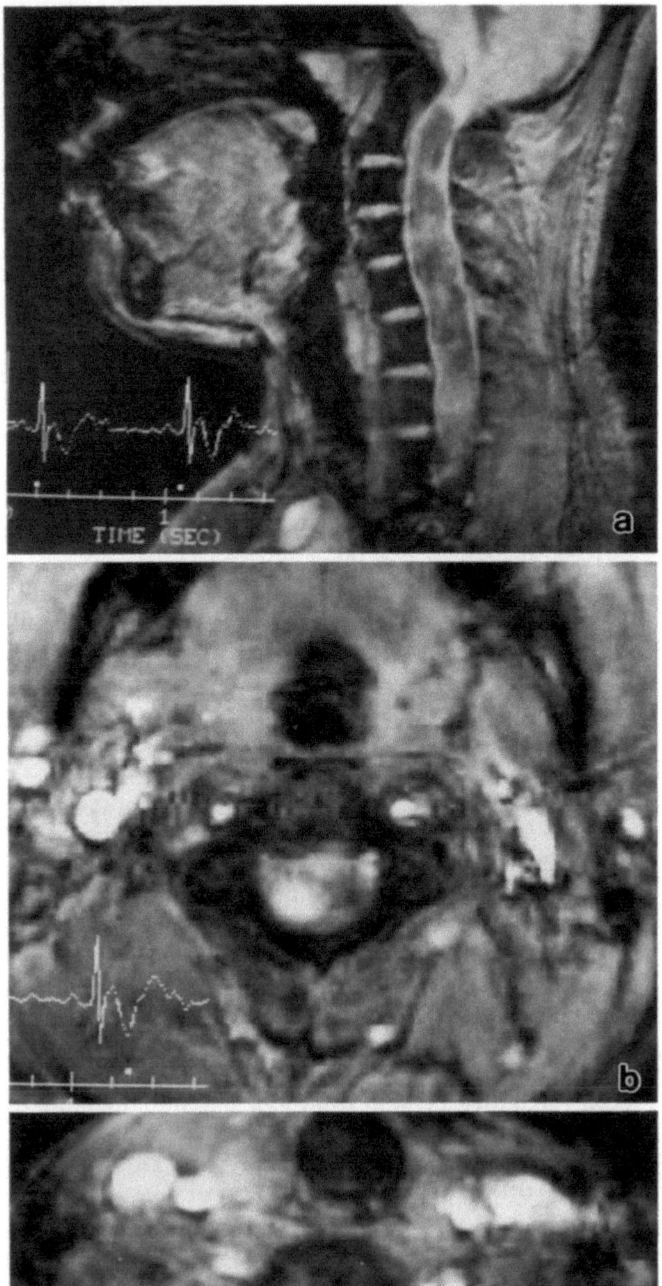

Fig. 1 a–c. Case 1. Frames from MR cineflow imaging of cerebrospinal fluid (CSF) in patient with syringomyelia Chiari malformation complex. **a** Midsagittal plane scan; the syrinx has mixed high and low signal intensity areas. **b** An axial scan at C3: a high signal intensity area recognisable in the syrinx. **c** An axial scan at C7: the high signal intensity area is more diffuse and the signal intensity itself is reduced

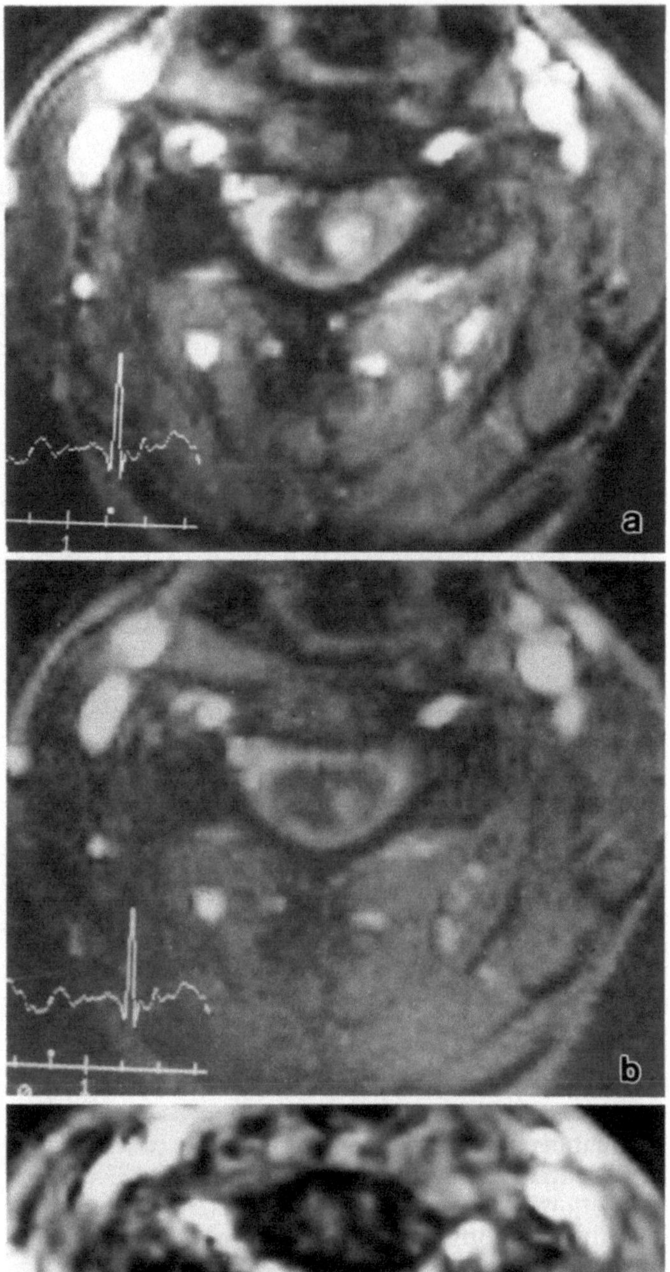

Fig. 2 a–c. Case 2. Frames from an axial scan at the level of C5 in a patient with syringomyelia Chiari malformation complex. **a** Preoperative study during systole: a high signal intensity area is recognisable in the syrinx. **b** Preoperative study during diastole: the high signal intensity area is decreased in size and intensity. **c** Postoperative study during systole: the high signal intensity area can no longer be seen syringomyelia associated with the Chiari malformation and discuss the pathophysiology of this type. Common abnormalities of CSF hydrodynamics in these patients were disturbance of CSF flow around the craniovertebral junction and pulsatile CSF movement in the syrinx. The former was considered to be due to plugging of the foramen magnum by descending cerebellar tonsils. The latter was considered to be transmitted from the fourth ventricle through the patent central canal, for the following reasons:

1. MR cineflow imaging of the upper cervical cord in the horizontal plane revealed locally recognisable pulsatile flow in the syrinx like a jet from the patent central canal into the syrinx. This flow lost its speed in the lower cervical cord and spread throughout the syrinx.

2. In all patients showing pulsations in the syrinx, patency of the central canal was confirmed surgically and the movements were absent, even in patients with a remaining cavity after its obstruction by surgery.

Gardner [5] proposed that the persistence and expansion of the syrinx were promoted directly by the force of pulsatile CSF from the fourth ventricle into a patent central canal via the obex.

Williams [6] also proposed that the pressure difference between the intracranial and spinal compartments produced by the hindbrain malformation impacted into the foramen magnum acted as a ball valve to promote the entry of CSF into the central canal by suction.

The common feature of both theories was that the syrinx was formed by CSF pressure, transmitted from the fourth ventricle via a patent central canal on the basis of CSF flow disturbance around the craniovertebral junction [7].

In our present studies on the hydrodynamics of CSF, we have obtained results that are consistent with both theories.

It is likely that both theories maybe explain the pathogenesis of syringomyelia associated with Chiari malformation.

References

1. Cahan LD, Bentson JR (1982) Considerations in the diagnosis and treatment of syringomyelia and the Chiari malformation. J Neurosurg 57: 24–31
2. Oakes WJ (1985) Chiari malformations, hydromyelia, syringomyelia. In: Wilkins RH, Rengachary SS (eds) Neurosurgery, vol 3, McGraw-Hill, New York, pp 2102–2124
3. Hall P, Turner M, Aichinger S, Bendick P, Campbell R (1980) Experimental syringomyelia. The relationship between intraventricular and intrasyrinx pressures. J Neurosurg 52: 812–817
4. Peerless SJ, Durward QJ (1983) Management of syringomyelia; a pathophysiological approach. Clin Neurosurg 30: 531–576
5. Gardner WJ (1965) Hydrodynamic mechanism of syringomyelia; its relationship to myelocele. J Neurol Neurosurg Psychiatry 28: 247–259
6. Williams B (1969) The distending force in the production of "communicating syringomyelia". Lancet I: 189–193
7. Abe T, Tashibu K, Onoue H, Suzuki T, Nakamua N, Ida M (1990) The evaluation of Gardner's operation for syringomyelia. Spinal Surg 4: 47–53

Dr. T. Abe
Department of Neurosurgery
The Jikei University Aoto Hospital
6-41-2, Aoto, Karsushika-ku
Tokyo, Japan, 125

Neuroradiology (1991) 33 [Suppl]: 176–177

Neuro radiology
© Springer-Verlag 1991

Assessment of aqueductal cerebrospinal fluid flow using the fast field echo technique in MRI

E. Hofmann[1], T. Becker[1], M. Warmuth-Metz[1], J. Meixensberger[2], and R. Schindler[3]

[1] Abteilung für Neuroradiologie in der Kopfklinik, Würzburg, Federal Republic of Germany
[2] Neurochirurgische Universitätsklinik, Würzburg, Federal Republic of Germany
[3] Institut für Röntgendiagnostik, Würzburg, Federal Republic of Germany

Summary. The "fast field echo" sequence, a gradient echo sequence, was used to investigate flow-related changes of signal intensity in the mesencephalic aqueduct. In cardiac-gated T2-weighted midsagittal images the periodically changing signal intensity was described mathematically by a Fourier anlaysis. Using the Fourier coefficients a continuous graph depicting time-dependent signal void could be derived and plotted. Fifteen healthy volunteers were compared with 92 patients in whom a disorder of cerebrospinal fluid (CSF) flow was suspected. Patient subgroups with aqueduct stenosis, communicating and normal pressure hydrocephalus and craniocervical malformations showed a distinctly pathological flow pattern. Compared to invasive techniques our results were sufficiently sensitive to predict CSF flow pathology.

Key words: Aqueduct – Cerebrospinal fluid flow – Hydrocephalus – Magnetic resonance imaging

The pulsatile nature of cerebrospinal fluid (CSF) flow is well known to neurosurgeons. du Boulay [1] described the to-and-fro movement of intraventricular contrast medium which he observed in neuroradiological examinations. With the advent of MRI, CSF pulsations were show to cause signal void in the mesencephalic aqueduct [2]. In cardiac-gated fast imaging sequences the oscillations of CSF flow could for the first time be visualised noninvasively [3].

To our knowledge, little effort has been made to arrive at a mathematical description of the periodic alterations in aqueductal CSF flow. So far, little experience has been reported on the correlation between pathological MRI flow patterns and invasive testing methods.

Materials and methods

A gradient echo sequence, the "fast field echo" (FFE) sequence, was applied to obtain sagittally orientated cardiac-gated images of the mesencephalic aqueduct. This sequence is routinely installed on our Philips Gyroscan S15 scanner. A flip angle of 10° and a TE of 35 ms resulted in T2-weighted images. Slice thickness was 6 mm. The number of phases per cardiac cycle was limited to the default minimum of 8. This corresponds to a time resolution of approximately 100 ms.

From the images obtained a line was drawn perpendicular to the centre of the mesencephalic aqueduct. A profile of intensities along this line was generated by the imager's software. The signal intensity of the aqueduct was represented by a point on the profile and could be measured in every phase of the cardiac cycle (Fig. 1).

Phase shifts and phase dispersion of the moving protons resulted in a decrease of aqueductal signal intensity dependent on the velocity of CSF flow. These periodic signal oscillations were described by a Fourier analysis which in turn enabled us to derive a continuous signal intensity graph from the Fourier coefficients. For each individual patient or volunteer eight coefficients (A_0 to A_4 and B_1 to B_3) were calculated. Fifteen healthy volunteers were examined to establish the normal values. They were compared with 92 patients who were referred with a suspected disorder of CSF dynamics. In 34 patients invasive testing methods (spinal infusion testing, epidural pressure monitoring) were performed; we compared these results with our measurements.

Results

The graph calculated from the coefficients of our control group is shown in Fig. 2. The typical to-and-fro pulsations of aqueductal flow are expressed as oscillations of the signal intensity. There is an initial flow maximum at peak systolic and a late diastolic CSF backwash into the third ventricle, followed by third ventricular outflow beginning about 100–200 ms after the R wave.

Calculation of Fourier coefficients enabled us to perform statistical analysis. Results were assessed by the t-test and Wilcoxon test.

Based on clinical and morphological findings, four patient groups were distinguished: aqueduct stenosis, communicating hydrocephalus, normal pressure hydrocephalus and Chiari I malformation. All had significantly pathological coefficients. In aqueduct stenosis signal oscillations were negligible; the three latter groups showed increased aqueductal CSF pulsations. Their pathological flow patterns are shown in Fig. 3.

Two major patient groups were distinguished: those with aqueductal flow-related signal void ($n = 78$) and those without ("aqueduct stenosis", $n = 15$). Seven of 8 patients classified as aqueduct stenosis showed pathological results in invasive testing, an increase of B-wave frequency being the most consistent finding.

In the remainder of patients pathology in the pressure-volume index (PVI) did not have a significant impact on the Fourier coefficients, whereas changes of mean pressure and outflow resistance were associated with signifi-

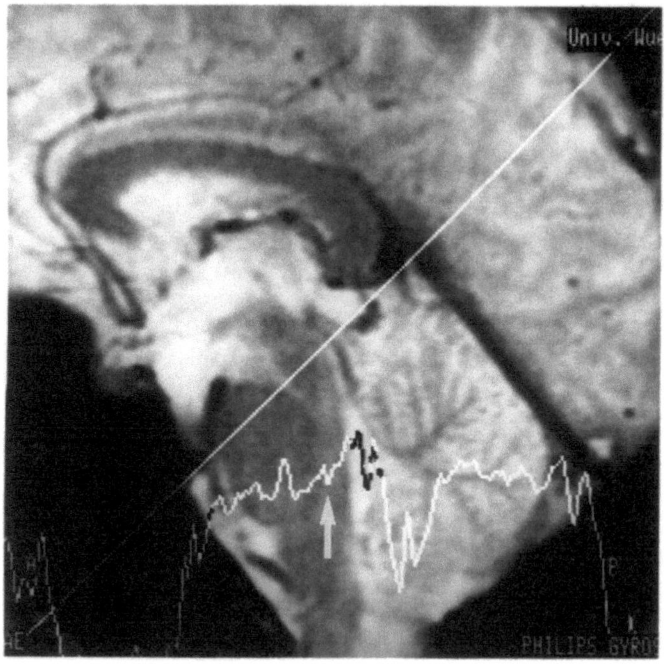

Fig. 1. Intensity profile intersecting centre of aqueduct *(arrow)*. Peak representing reduced signal intensity of the aqueduct ("signal void")

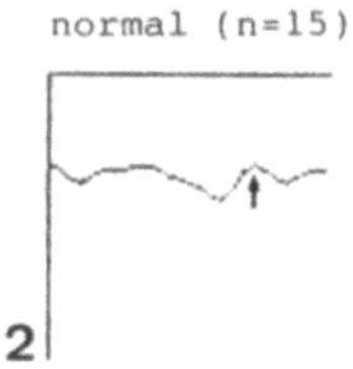

2

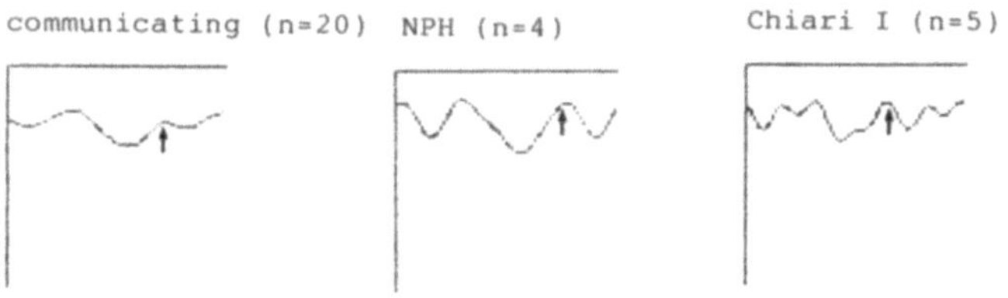

3

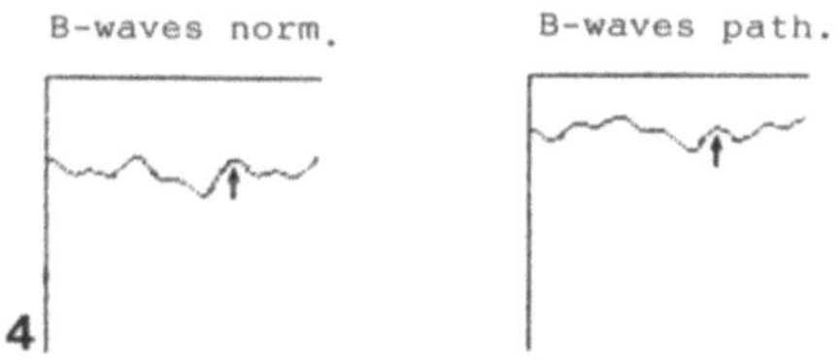

4

Fig. 2. Aqueductal signal intensity plotted over time. Mean value calculated from 15 normal volunteers. *Horizontal axis,* 1000 ms; *vertical axis,* relative units. *Top,* Fast aqueductal flow; *bottom,* slow aqueductal flow. *Arrow,* R wave

Fig. 3. Time-flow velocity graph in communicating hydrocephalus, normal pressure hydrocephalus *(NPH)* and Chiari I malformation. *Arrow,* R wave. Note accelerated flow and increased amplitude of pulsations

Fig. 4. Time-flow velocity graph in patients with normal *(left)* and increased *(right)* frequency of B-waves. *Arrow,* R wave. Note significantly increased flow in pathological group

cantly pathological coefficients, mostly a decrease of A_0. The most significant difference, however, was observed between patients with a pathological increase of B-wave frequency and those without (Fig. 4).

The number of patients with increased CSF secretion and elevated venous sinus pressure was too small to yield statistically significant results.

To assess the sensitivity of our method, we plotted the coefficients of all patients with abnormal invasive testing and compared them with our normal group (data not shown). There was little overlap in the coefficients A_0, indicating high sensitivity. However, some overlap was noted in the coefficients of a higher order. Specificity was difficult to assess as the number of patients with inconclusive results on invasive measuring methods was too small to warrant analysis.

Discussion

The method described above proved useful for non-invasive assessment of aqueductal CSF flow. The Fourier analyis was employed to obtain coefficients comparable among individuals and patient groups, thus making statistical evaluation possible.

We found high flow in patients with communicating hydrocephalus, Chiari I malformations and in patients with the clinical triad of normal pressure hydrocephalus; high flow has hitherto been described only for the latter patient group [4].

In patients in whom invasive testing methods had been performed, there was a good correlation with our noninvasive results. We could not confirm, however, a correlation between changes in intracranial pressure and the time of maximum aqueductal flow [5].

Absence of flow void has to be considered with caution. Threshold velocity causing changes in signal intensity is of the order of 1 cm/s. Flow induced by CSF production alone, if not combined with to-and-fro pulsations, may not be sufficient to cause signal void. Therefore, the finding of aqueduct stenosis as assessed by the FFE sequence is not *per se* pathological as some compensatory slow CSF flow may pass unnoticed on MRI.

References

1. du Boulay GH (1966) Pulsatile movements in the CSF pathways. Br J Radiol 39: 255–262
2. Sherman JL, Citrin CM (1986) Magnetic resonance demonstration of normal CSF flow. AJNR 7: 3–6
3. Klose U, Requardt H, Schroth G, Deimling M (1987) MR-tomographische Darstellung von Liquorpulsationen. Fortschr Röntgenstr 147: 313–319
4. Schroth G, Klose U (1989) MRI of CSF flow in normal pressure hydrocephalus. Psychiatry Res 29: 289–290
5. Ohara S, Nagai H, Ueda Y (1989) CSF pulsatile flow on MRI and its relation to intracranial pressure. In: Hoff JT, Betz AL (eds) Intracranial pressure VII. Springer, Berlin Heidelberg New York

Dr. Erich Hofmann
Abteilung für Neuroradiologie
in der Kopfklinik
Josef-Schneider-Strasse 11
W-8700 Würzburg
Federal Republic of Germany

Neuroradiology (1991) 33 [Suppl]: 178–181

Neuro-radiology
© Springer-Verlag 1991

Notes on the driving forces of the CSF circulation with special emphasis on the piston action of the brain

D. Greitz[1], B. Nordell[2], A. Ericsson[3], F. Ståhlberg[4], and C. Thomsen[5]

Departments of [1] Neuroradiology and [2] Hospital Physics, Karolinska Hospital, Stockholm, Sweden
[3] Department of Hospital Physics, University Hospital, Uppsala, Sweden
[4] Department of Radiation Physics, University of Lund, Sweden
[5] MRI Section, Hvidore Hospital, Copenhagen, Denmark

Summary. The cerebrospinal fluid (CSF) flow at the foramen magnum, in the aqueduct and in the pontine cistern was studied in five volunteers using phase images. The adjacent brain motion was also studied. In one volunteer the motion of the cerebrum was studied using phase images of an SE sequence sensitive to flow below 1 mm. The large pulsations at the foramen magnum, starting before the pulsations in the aqueduct and the pontine cistern, are not consistent with the assumption that the ventricular pulsations or mere brain expansion are the driving force of the CSF circulation. The systolic expansion of the brain, combined with its systolic downward movement, propels the extraventricular CSF, the entire brain acting as a piston. The bulk flow in the anterior and posterior part of the spinal canal, if any, is small and the impression of an "active" spinal circulation may be caused by increased mixing elicited by the pumping brain. When a CSF tracer is present there will be an increased diffusion due to shearing forces in the fluid causing increased area of exchange and gradient of concentration.

Key words: Magnetic resonance imaging – Brain – Movements – Cerebrospinal fluid

Methods

The CSF flow at the foramen magnum, in the aqueduct and in the pontine cistern were studied in five volunteers using phase images obtained with a 0.5 T MRI unit. An axial ECG-gated standard SE sequence with a TE of 30 ms and an effective TR of 1.5–2.5 s was used. The pronounced systolic motion of the cord, brain stem, cerebellum and the basal ganglia could also be observed. To study motion of the cerebral hemispheres velocities below 1 mm/s have to be measured. This was made possible by placing two large flow-encoding slice-selective gradients symmetrically around the 180° pulse in an SE sequence. In one volunteer the brain motion was studied in two additional planes, one at the level of the foramen of Monro and the other above the lateral ventricles. As a model of the spinal CSF circulation a flow phantom with pulsatile flow in plastic tubing was used with a blue colour (methyl-thionine-chloride) as a tracer.

Results

The movements of the brain stem and the cerebellum were larger than those measured supratentorially and decreased in amplitude at more cephalad levels. During systole, they amounted to 2 mm/s in the brain stem and the cerebellum (Fig. 1) and to a mean of 0.5 (0.3–1.3) mm/s in the cerebrum at the level of the basal ganglia (Fig. 2) where the greatest movements were observed in the central parts of the brain (Fig. 3).

The to-and-fro flow at the foramen magnum was 1.0 ml/heart beat in each direction, i.e. about 50 times

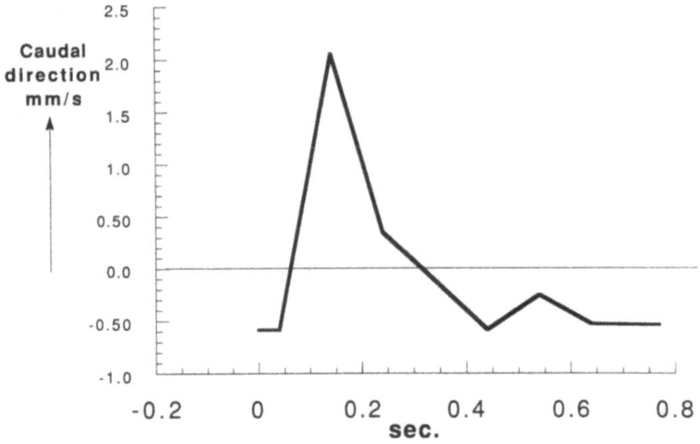

Fig. 1. Brain stem and vermis motion (mm/s) studied with a gated MRI using a standard SE sequence. The peak velocity occurs about 0.18 s after R-wave in the ECG complex and is directed caudally

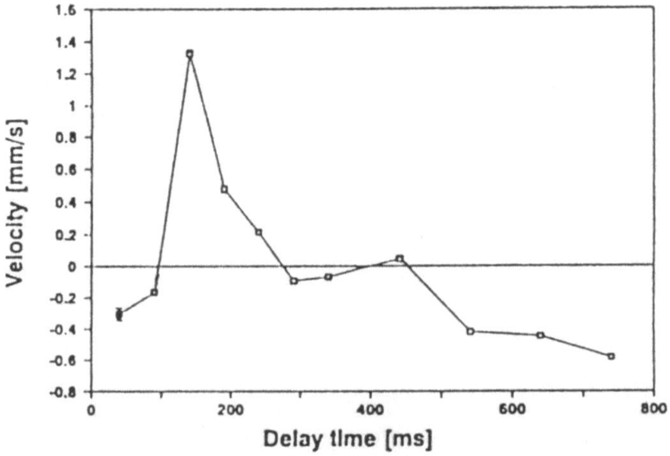

Fig. 2. Brain motion at the basal ganglia studied with a flow enhanced SE sequence. Note the similarity to the brain stem movements in Fig. 1. However, the peak is smaller

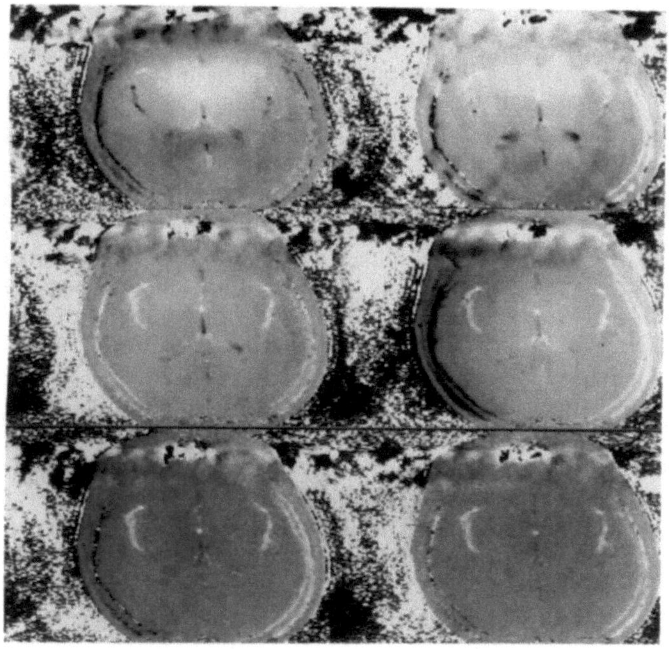

Fig. 3. Phase images illustrating brain movements at the basal ganglia obtained with a flow enhanced technique. The upper two images are in the early systole, the lower two in diastole. The lighter areas represent greater movements downwards. The greatest movements can be observed in the basal ganglia an insular regions as demonstrated in Fig. 2

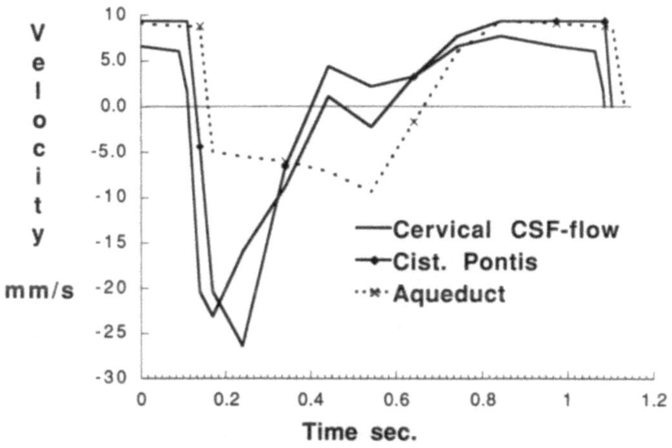

Fig. 4. Pulsatile cerebrospinal fluid (CSF) flow velocities in mm/s measured with a standard SE sequence. The systolic flow in the cervical canal is greater and earlier than in the aqueduct and earlier than in pontine cistern.

greater than in the aqueduct (0.017 ml/beat). Its systolic phase started 50–60 ms earlier than in the aqueduct and earlier than in the pontine cistern (Fig. 4). The CSF displacement in the pontine cistern was 0.32 ml/beat. The displacement of the upper brain stem and the vermis was 0.28 ml/beat. The last two figures represent the supratentorial systolic expansion and the CSF displacement is of the same magnitude as the brain displacement.

The bulk flow measured in the anterior and posterior parts of the spinal canal was 1–3% of the pulsatile flow and within the error of the method (Fig. 5). In four of five cases

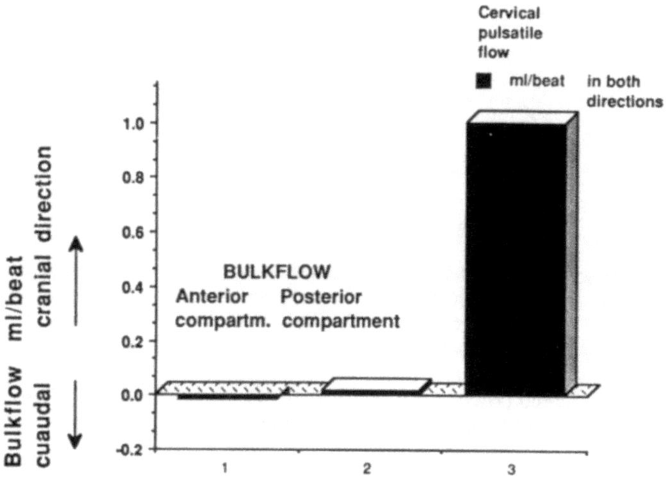

Fig. 5. Bulk flows in the anterior and posterior cervical compartments compared with total pulsatile flow. The bulkflows are only 1–3% of the pulsatile flow and are within error of method

its direction was the reverse of that commonly postulated, i.e. it was directed upwards posteriorly and downwards anteriorly. The pulsatile flow velocities in the anterior compartment were more than 50% greater than in the posterior compartment.

In the phantom study mere diffusion and pulsatile diffusion without and with an artificial cord were compared. In 17 h the tracer moved about 5 cm with simple diffusion, and with pulsatile diffusion 50 cm. When the cord was put into the tubing the tracer moved 80 cm in 30 min with pulsatile diffusion.

In the narrow space between the cord and the spinal canal shearing forces in the fluid will cause the fluid to pulsate with a parabolic flow profile. This will increase the area of diffusion and the gradient of concentration between the CSF and the tracer. If a "cord" is put in to the tubing the effective radius (r) will be about halved. An equation calculated at the Royal Institute of Technology, Stockholm shows that the effective diffusion coefficient will be 32 $[(1/r)^5 = (1/0.5)^5]$ times larger than without the cord, if the volumetric displacement is kept constant. Turbulence may occur behind the nerve roots in the spinal canal because the Reynold number may be exceeded and this will also increase the mixing of the CSF.

Discussion

The existence of an active CSF circulation has been proven mainly by observations of fluid movement at intracranial operations [1] as well as on isotope cisternography [2]. There seems to be a general consensus that the arterial pulsations are the driving force of this circulation.

However, the mechanism by which the arterial pulsations are acting as the driving force is still very much under debate. Many investigators consider the "pump" to be located within the ventricular system. Bering [3] postulated in 1955 that pulsations originated from the choroid plexus. It has, however, been questioned whether the plexus pul-

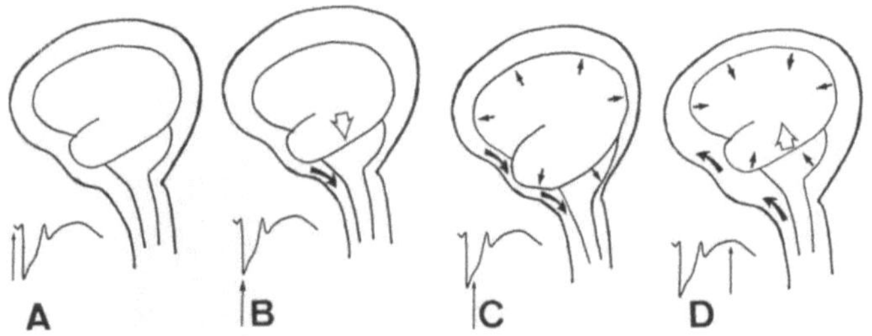

Fig. 6 A–D. Motions of the brain and CSF according to the proposed model. **A** Presystolic phase. **B** In early systole the increased arterial volume causes a rise in the CSF pressure and downward displacement of the brain, its lower surface acting as a piston. **C** Further expansion and downward movement later in systole causes more fluid to be expelled down to the spinal canal. **D** The relatively high pressure in the spinal canal moves the brain upwards as it retracts

sations are large enough to expel the amount of fluid that leaves the ventricles.

O'Connell [1] in 1943 postulated the existence of a third ventricular pump and in 1966 du Boulay [4] was able to demonstrate radiologically that such a pump-like action did actually exist in the closed head in man and he also found another larger pump at the basal cisterns also due to brain expansion [5, 6]. The third ventricular pump is considered to provide effective mixing between the CSF in the third ventricle and the basal cisterns. Using air or contrast ventriculography and cisternography, du Boulay demonstrated large pulse-synchronous pulsations in the upper cervical region as well as in the third ventricle, but very small or absent pulsations in the lateral ventricles. This, he thought, was contradictory to Bering's hypothesis but supported the view held by O'Connell of the third ventricle pump. du Boulay observed systolic antegrade and diastolic retrograde flow in the aqueduct as well as in the cervical region and found the pulsations in the cervical region (1 ml/beat) to be 10 times as large as in the aqueduct (0.1 ml/beat). In our study the cervical pulsations were more than 50 times large. One reason for this discrepancy may be the fact that du Boulay's figures were based on observations of volume variations of the third ventricle and not on direct measurements of the aqueductal flow. Feinberg and Mark [7] [10] using ECG-gated MRI [8, 9], found a systolic compression from above of the lateral ventricles, which they claimed moved CSF downwards in systole and a systolic caudal motion of the diencephalon and the brainstem producing a wave of CSF in the cerebellomedullary cisterns that propagates through the spinal canal.

Finally, Levy and co-workers [11], using gated MRI, found small, pulse-synchronous volume changes of the lateral and third ventricles.

Common to all these authors is the idea that CSF fluid is expelled through the aqueduct by compression of the fluid in the ventricular system in the lateral ventricles, the third ventricle or both, and that this compression is the driving force of the intraventricular CSF circulation. du Boulay and Feinberg also discribed a larger to-and-fro pump in the basal cisterns.

These driving force of the intracranial circulation has also been considered to act on the CSF circulation in the spinal canal, the bulk flow of CSF through the foramen of Magendie continuing posterior to the cord and the dentate ligament, as opposed to the flow in the compartment anterior to the cord, which is thought to be cephalad.

The to-and-fro flow in the aqueduct is small (0.017 ml) as compared to that in the upper cervical region, which is 1.0 ml/beat in each direction. The systole of this large regional to-and-fro flow at the foramen magnum starts after a constant time interval (110 ms) following the beginning of the cardiac cycle, and – what is important – always earlier than the systole in the aqueduct which starts 50–60 ms later. These findings are not compatible with the pulsating ventricles as the driving force of the whole CSF system.

The systolic flow at the foramen magnum starts earlier than in the pontine cistern, making it difficult to explain why the origin of the start of the arterial expansion is within the CSF itself rather than dependent on the downward systolic movement the brain that has been observed by us and others [7, 12]. Unlike Feinberg and Mark [7], we additionally attribute the pulsatile volume changes of the brain a significant role in explaining its pumping action. We consider the downward movements of the central parts of the brain due to CSF and brain being easily vented through the tentorial notch and the foramen magnum rather than due to conservation of momentum.

We postulate (Fig. 6) that the large cervical pulsations are caused by the brain acting as an expanding and retracting piston. It is important to distinguish pulsatile flow and bulk flow when a pumping action is described. A pump without valves is a mixer and causes pulsatile flow but no bulk flow. A pump with valves can cause a bulk flow and is able to contribute to the active CSF circulation. The piston-like action certainly causes effective mixing in the extraventricular CSF spaces, possibly including the spinal canal. It is postulated that the pulsations, in combination with the Pacchionian valves also contribute to the bulk flow, i. e. the active CSF circulation.

The mechanisms behind the active spinal CSF circulation have always been puzzling, as this circulation seems to be two-directional. Thus tracers injected in the lumbar area are transported cephalad and those injected in the ventricles are carried in the caudal direction and both occur at a speed significantly higher than that of simple diffusion. These observations have given rise to the suggestion of a "two-way traffic" in the spinal canal, upwards anterior to the cord and downwards posterior to it. This theory seems, however, to be challenged by the present study as no two-way circulation could be seen in the spinal canal and in addition no consistent and significant bulk flow in any direction could be measured in the spinal canal. It should, however, be emphasised that the bulk flows measured are within the error of the method. Furthermore, large to-and-fro movements could be observed in the cervical region and they were synchronous in the anterior and posterior spinal CSF compartments, the anterior pulsations being greater. This and the results in the phantom study raise the question as to whether the spinal "CSF flow" is in fact a rapid mixture elicited by the pumping brain.

The authors have tried to find a model for the CSF circulation which could fit these observations. This model has the following characteristics. It postulates that the CSF circulation is mainly driven by the compression and remoulding of the intracranial extracerebral CSF spaces by the moving and pulsating brain. It acts by alternating volume increases and decreases and in addition, by moving up and down as a piston. The pulsations caused in combinations with the Pacchionian valves may result in a bulk flow, i.e. an active CSF circulation.

The intraventricular pulsatile flow is undoubtedly driven by compression of the ventricles and serves as a mixing device between the ventricles and the cisterna magna.

The spinal CSF flow is most likely a rapid mixture of the fluid at various levels caused by shearing forces in the fluid causing increased diffusion and elicited by the pumping brain. No consistent and significant bulk flow in any direction could be measured in the cervical canal.

This model will be validated by further studies.

References

1. O'Connell JEA (1943) The vascular factor in intracranial pressure and the maintenance of the cerebrospinal fluid circulation. Brain 73: 165–172
2. Di Chiro G (1966) Observations on the circulation of the cerebrospinal fluid. Acta Radiol Diagn 5: 988–1002
3. Bering EA (1955) Choroid plexus and arterial pulsation of the choroid plexuses as a cerebrospinal fluid pump. Arch Neurol Psychiatry 73: 165–172
4. du Boulay GH (1966) Pulsatile movements in the CSF pathways. Br J Radiol 39: 255–262
5. du Boulay G, O'Connell J, Currie J, Bostick T, Verity P (1972) Further investigations on pulsatile movements in the cerebrospinal fluid pathways. Acta Radiol Diagn 13: 496–523
6. du Boulay GH (1972) Specialisation broadens the view. The significance of a CSF pulse. 2nd Glyn Evans Memorial Lecture. Clin Radiol 23: 401–409
7. Feinberg DA, Mark AS (1986) Human brain motion and cerebrospinal fluid circulation demonstrated with MR velocity imaging. Radiology 16: 527–31
8. Bergstrand G, Bergström M, Nordell B, Ståhlberg F, Ericsson A, Hemmingson A, Sperber G, Thuomas KÅ, Jung B (1985) Cardiac gated MR imaging of cerebrospinal fluid flow. J Comput Assist Tomogr 9: 1003–1006
9. Bergstrand G, Nordell B, Ståhlberg F, Ericsson A, Bergstöm M, Hemmingsson A, Sperber G, Thuomas KÅ, Jung B (1986) Cerebrospinal fluid flow studied with gated magnetic resonance imaging during the various parts of the cardiac cycle. Acta Radiol (Stockh) [Suppl] 369: 490–491
10. Mark AS, Feinberg DA, Sze GK, Brant-Zawadski MN (1986) Gated magnetic resonance imaging of the intracranical cerebrospinal fluid spaces. Acta Radiol (Stockh) [Suppl] 369: 296–299
11. Levy LM, Di Chiro G, Brooks RA, Dwyer AJ, Dietz MJ (1986) Changes in cerebral ventricular dimensions related to the cardiac cycle as seen with gated magnetic resonance imaging. Acta Radiol (Stockh) [Suppl] 369: 300–301
12. Levy LM, Di Chiro G, McCullough DC, Dwyer AJ, Johnson DL, Yang SSL (1988) Fixed spinal cord: diagnosis with MR imaging. Radiology 169: 773–778

Dr. Dan Greitz
Department of Neuroradiology
Karolinska Hospital
S–104 01 Stockholm
Sweden

SESSION 13
INTRACRANIAL A-V MALFORMATIONS

Neuroradiology (1991) 33 [Suppl]: 184–186

Neuro radiology

© Springer-Verlag 1991

Vascular characteristics of intracranial arteriovenous malformations which correlate with symptoms of hemorrhage and steal

M. P. Marks[1], B. Lane[1], G. Steinberg[2], and P. Chang[1]

[1] Departments of Diagnostic Radiology and Nuclear Medicine and [2] Department of Neurosurgery, Stanford University School of Medicine, Stanford, California, USA

Summary. Fifteen vascular characteristics of intracranial arteriovenous malformations (AVMs) were reviewed in 65 patients to identify those correlating with hemorrhage or clinical steal. For hemorrhage a strong positive correlation was found with central venous drainage ($P < 0.0001$), periventricular or intraventricular AVM location ($P = 0.0002$), and intranidus aneurysm ($P = 0.028$). A strong negative correlation was found with angiomatous change ($P = 0.0005$), cortical venous drainage ($P = 0.005$), and mixed venous drainage ($P = 0.021$). Three characteristics correlated highly with steal: angiomatous change ($P < 0.0001$), size ($P < 0.0001$), and peripheral venous drainage ($P = 0.045$). These data should prove useful in identifying patients at higher risk for developing hemorrhage and clinical steal.

Key words: Arteriovenous malformation – Cerebral hemorrhage – Cerebral vascular disorders – Cerebral arteriovenous malformations

Cerebral arteriovenous malformations (AVMs) often present in early adult life, typically by the third decade [1]. Approximately 50% of AVM patients will suffer hemorrhage with significant mortality [2]. Those surviving are often left with debilitating neurological deficits. Others suffer gradually progressive neurological deficits and intellectual deterioration attributable to cerebral steal [3]. This study was undertaken to identify vascular characteristics of AVMs that may predispose to development of hemorrhage or clinical steal.

Subjects and methods

Fifteen vascular characteristics were reviewed in 65 patients utilizing angiography supplement by MRI (46 cases) and CT (19 cases). Patients ranged from 9–69 years (mean 33 years). Of the 65 patients, 45 (69%) had a history of hemorrhage and 9 of 65 (9%) clinical steal. The characteristics studied are listed in the first column of Table 1. Size was determined by a previously described method [4]. Using CT or MRI relationship of the nidus to the ventricle was judged as peri-

Table 1. Vascular characteristics correlating with hemorrhage

Vascular characteristic studied	Number (% of total study group, $n = 65$)	Number with characteristic that bled/number with characteristic (%)	Number with characteristic that bled/total patients that bled, $n = 45$ (%)
1. Size	No correlation with hemorrhage		
2. Lobar location			
3. Periventricular/ Intravent location	24 (37%)	23/24 (96%)	23/45 (51%)
4. Arterial aneurysm	5 (8%)	4/ 5 (80%)	4/45 (9%)
5. Arterial stenoses	3 (5%)	1/ 3 (33%)	2/45 (2%)
6. Angiomatous change	6 (9%)	0/ 6 (0%)	0/45 (0%)
7. Intranidus aneurysm	9 (12%)	9/ 9 (100%)	9/45 (20%)
8. Arteriovenous fistula	0 –	– –	– –
Venous drainage			
9. central	34 (52%)	32/34 (94%)	32/45 (71%)
10. cortical	19 (29%)	7/19 (37%)	7/45 (16%)
11. mixed	12 (19%)	6/12 (50%)	6/45 (13%)
12. Venous stenosis	23 (36%)	19/23 (83%)	19/45 (42%)
13. Delayed drainage	4 (6%)	4/ 4 (100%)	4/45 (9%)
14. Venous ectasia	22 (34%)	15/22 (68%)	15/45 (33%)
15. Venous variation	19 (29%)	14/19 (74%)	14/45 (31%)

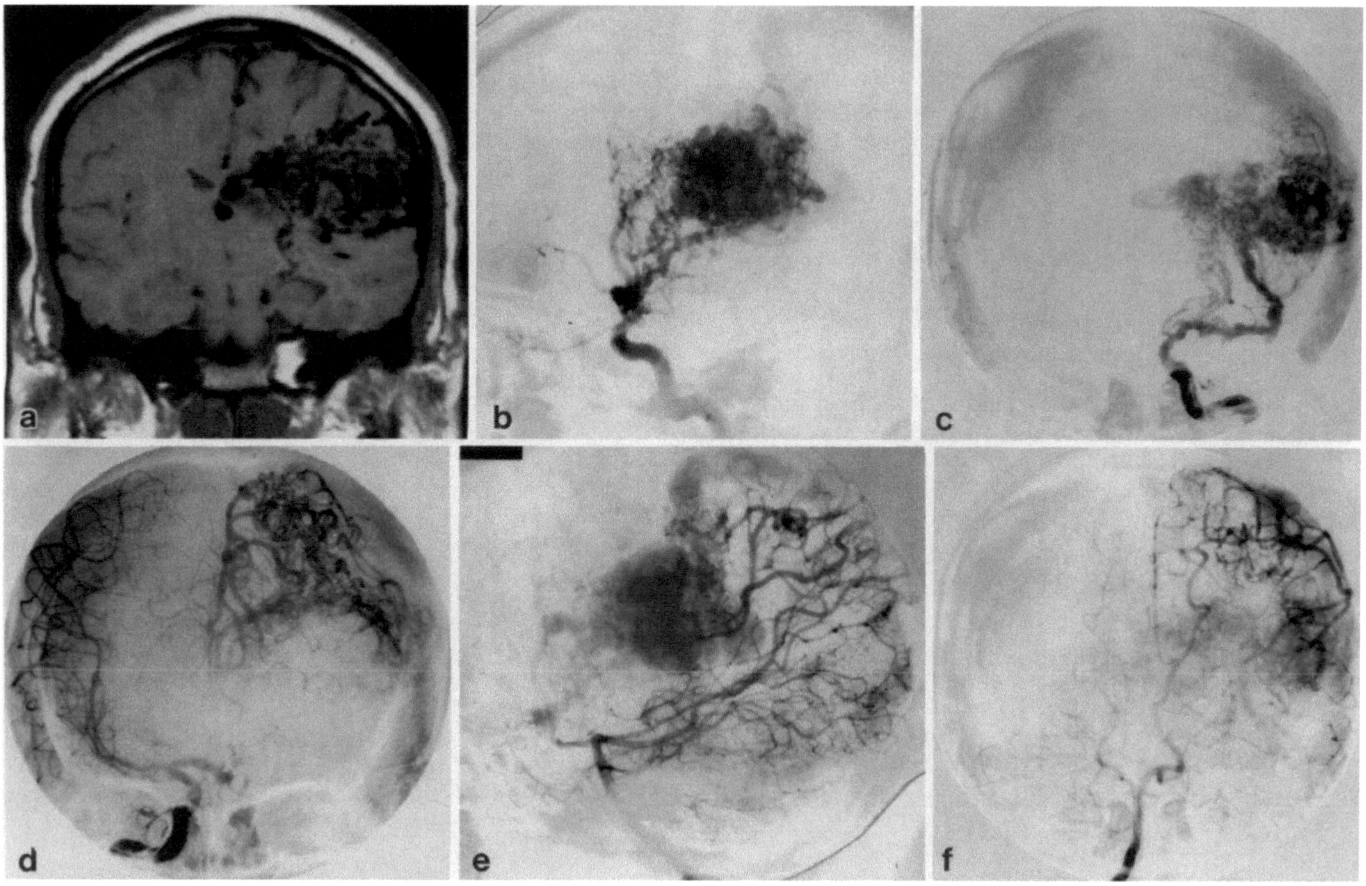

Fig. 1 a–f. Left parietal arteriovenous malformation (AVM) in a patient with gradually progressive right sided weakness, no history of hemorrhage. **a** Coronal T1-weighted MRI demonstrates wedge shaped AVM. **b, c** Lateral and frontal views from left internal carotid angiogram show direct supply to the nidus via lenticulostriate and opercular branches of the middle cerebral artery. **d** Frontal view right internal carotid angiogram; note dilated tangle of vessels from the left anterior cerebral artery which extend over the cortex (angiomatous change). These collateral vessels supplied the superior portion of the AVM nidus in a retrograde fashion. **e, f** Lateral and frontal views from right vertebral angiogram. AVM nidus was noted to fill via the posterior communicating artery; note dilated cortical vessels in the posterior parieto-occipital cortex (angiomatous change). These vessels provided collateral supply to the AVM via retrograde flow through distal branches of the angular and posterior parietal arteries

(occupying a wall) or intra-(partially within) ventricular in location. Arterial or venous stenosis was present when a vessel was narrowed by more than 50%. Arteriovenous (AV) fistulae were noted when there was a large early AV Shunt. Angiomatous change was defined as collateral arterial supply to the nidus from dilated transcortical vessels derived from arteries not usually expected to supply the AVM territory. Venous variation indicated unexpected or anomalous drainage.

Characteristics were analyzed using the Fisher-Irwin exact test (for nominal qualitative characteristics) and the two sample, two-sided t-test (for continuous quantitative characteristics such as size). A multivariate stepwise linear discriminant analysis was performed to identify characteristics which best predicted hemorrhage, as more fully described in an additional publication [5].

Results

Size and lobar location were not found to significantly correlate with hemorrhage. Table 1 lists the other characteristics studied. Central venous drainage ($P < 0.0001$), peri/intraventricular location ($P = 0.0002$), intranidus aneurysm ($P = 0.028$) strongly correlated. Others negatively correlated with hemorrhage: angiomatous change ($P = 0.0005$), cortical venous drainage ($P = 0.005$), and mixed venous drainage ($P = 0.021$). Venous stenosis was the most frequently observed venous characteristic. Of 23 patients, 19 (83%) with venous stenosis also had a history of hemorrhage but this was not statistically significant ($P = 0.09$).

Multivariate discriminant analysis demonstrated three characteristics most predictive of hemorrhage: central venous drainage, angiomatous change (negatively predictive), and intranidus aneurysm. They correctly predicted 35 of 45 cases in which hemorrhage occurred and gave a false negative rate of 15% (10 of 65 patients). All 20 patients without hemorrhage were correctly predicted (0% false positive).

Characteristics strongly correlating with clinical steal were angiomatous change ($P < 0.0001$), size ($P < 0.0001$), and peripheral venous drainage ($P = 0.045$). Mean AVM nidus size for the study group was 31.3 cm^3. Patients with steal had a mean size of 105 cm^3 compared with 19.5 cm^3 in those without steal. Of 45 patients, 6 (9%) had angiomatous change and all 6 had clinical steal. A patient with angiomatous change is shown in Fig. 1. Of 9 patients with clinical steal, 5 had peripheral venous drainage (56%).

Discussion

The three characteristics most predictive of hemorrhage were central venous drainage, intranidus aneurysm, and angiomatous change (negatively predictive). The strong correlation between central venous drainage and hemorrhage may be due to multiple factors. Prior studies have suggested that central or deep lesions are more likely to bleed [6]. Central drainage includes at its final pathway the vein of Galen, implicated as the most common site of venous stenosis [7]. While there may be a trend to hemorrhage with venous stenosis it was not found to be statistically significant in our study. A more important consideration may be the arterial side of the AVM. According to the Hagen-Poiseulle equation flow is proportional to the pressure drop along the length of a tube and change in pressure is directly related to the length of the tube [8]. Therefore if two AVMs have comparable flow rates and similar arterial feeder diameters the variable affecting change in pressure will be the length of the arterial pedicle. Thus the shorter feeding pedicle of a central lesions will undergo less pressure change along its course and the AVM nidus of the deeper central lesion will experience higher arterial pressures.

Angiomatous change represents collateral arterial supply to the AVM nidus from dilated transcortical vessels. These collaterals derive from arterial territories not directly supplying the nidus. This complex network of dilated cortical vessels often has an appearance similar to that of the AVM and we have termed it "angiomatous change"; however the angiogram does not show early venous drainage from regions of angiomatous change. This characteristic positively correlated with steal and negatively correlated with hemorrhage. We believe these dilated vessels are recruited to meet the demands of the AVM shunt. Autoregulation in AVM vessels has been lost making it a passive vascular system where the rate of blood flow is pressure dependent [9]. Lesions with low perfusion pressures will have lower flow rates. Local arterial supply to the nidus will prove adequate when the perfusion pressure is high. In other AVMs the perfusion pressure remains low despite maximal dilatation of the local arterial supply and the AVM recruits supply from outside its local distribution. These recruited collateral vessels include those seen with angiomatous change. Collateral supply beyond the circle of Willis has been well documented in adults in response to proximal occlusions [10]. Stenosis of larger feeding vessels was seen in 2 of 6 cases with angiomatous change and has been reported previously in AVM patients [11]. This would contribute to lower perfusion pressures. Angiomatous change exists when there is lower perfusion pressure to the AVM which confers a protective effect against hemorrhage but reflects an environment in which clinical steal occurs.

References

1. Luessenhop AJ (1984) Natural history of cerebral arteriovenous malformations. In: Wilson CB, Stein BM (eds) Intracranial arteriovenous malformations, 1st edn. Williams and Wilkins, Baltimore, pp 12–23
2. Wilkins RH (1985) Natural history of intracranial vascular malformations: a review. Neurosurgery 16: 421–430
3. Mohr JP (1984) Neurological manifestations and factors related to therapeutic decisions. In: Wilson CB, Stein BM (eds) Intracranial arteriovenous malformations, 1st edn. Williams and Wilkins, Baltimore, pp 1–11
4. Marks MP, DeLaPaz RL, Fabrikant JI, Frankel KA, Phillips MH, Levy RP, Enzmann DR (1988) Intracranial vascular malformations: imaging of charged-particle radiosurgery. I. Results of therapy. Radiology 168: 447–455
5. Marks MP, Lane B, Steinberg G, Chang P (1990) Angiographic determinants of hemorrhage in intracerebral arteriovenous malformations. Radiology (in press)
6. Willinsky R, Lasjaunias P, Terbrugge K, Pruvost P (1988) Brain arteriovenous malformations: Analysis of the angio architecture in relationship to hemorrhage (based on 152 patients explored and/or treated at the hospital de Bicêtre between 1981 and 1986). J Neuroradiol 15: 225–237
7. Viñuela F, Nombela L, Roach MR, Fox AJ, Pelz DM (1985) Stenotic and occlusive disease of the venous drainage system of deep brain AVM's. J Neurosurg 63: 180–184
8. Nornes H, Grip A (1980) Hemodynamic aspects of cerebral arteriovenous malformations. J Neurosurg 53: 456–464
9. Hassler W (1986) Hemodynamic aspects of cerebral angiomas. Acta Neurochir [Suppl] (Wien) 37: 1–136
10. Hawkins TD (1966) The collateral anastomoses in cerebrovascular occlusion. Clin Radiol 17: 203–219
11. Mawad ME, Hilal SK, Michelsen WJ, Stein B, Ganti SR (1984) Occlusive vascular disease associated with cerebral arteriovenous malformations. Radiology 153: 401–440

Dr. Michael P. Marks
Department of Diagnostic Radiology and Nuclear Medicine
Stanford University School of Medicine
Stanford, CA 94305, USA

Neuroradiology (1991) 33 [Suppl]: 187–189

Neuro radiology
© Springer-Verlag 1991

Brain AVM embolization: influence of amytal test and transient deficit on surgical management

A. J. Fox, D. M. Pelz, and D. H. Lee

University Hospital, University of Western Ontario, London, Ontario, Canada

Summary. Utilizing advances in embolization materials and delivery systems, 43 patients with brain arteriovenous malformations (AVMs) have been embolized over the past 4 years. The cases were predominantly treated prior to surgical resection for complex AVMs in surgically difficult locations; 84% had surgery after embolization and 70% were completely resected. Embolization caused permanent deficit in 5 (11.6%) cases: 3 quadrantanopia, 1 mutism, and 1 cerebellar ataxia. Amytal testing during embolization influenced surgical management in 2 cases. Two other cases were not resected because following embolization transient deficit caused the patient to realize that the risk of surgical resection was unacceptable. In this series embolization enabled the complete resection of large, complex AVMs in the majority of cases.

Key words: Arteriovenous malformation – Cerebral arteries – Therapeutic blockade

Although some small arteriovenous malformations (AVMs) can be completely occluded using acrylic glue [1–3], large, complex AVMs are not successfully obliterated by embolization alone. The cases we currently embolize [4, 5] are mostly presurgical cases in which difficulty in resection is anticipated. The introduction of new embolic materials and delivery systems, and a change in our embolization team during the past 4 years has given the opportunity to present a reassessment of the value of embolizing brain AVMs.

Materials and methods

Forty-three patients with brain AVMs were embolized from August 1986 to May 1990. Wire-dirigible microcatheters were used to access the arterial feeding pedicles in most cases. A mixture of avitene, polyvinyl alcohol and ethanol [6], acrylic glue or both were used as the embolic material [4, 5]. Amytal was injected into feeding arteries before and between embolizations, with clinical monitoring. Outcome was recorded by proportion of AVM embolized, permanent deficit caused by embolization, success of surgical resection, and eventual clinical outcome.

Results

Seventy-six embolization procedures were carried out in 43 patients with brain AVMs. A total of 120 feeders were embolized. Due to a positive amytal test 1 patient (Fig. 1) had no embolic material injected. This patient did not have resection of the AVM because he would not accept the risk of this deficit. In another patient (Fig. 2) endovascular therapy was stopped when a positive amytal test was produced after embolization of most of the AVM. The AVM was resected very carefully and there was no deficit. Amytal testing influenced both the embolization and the surgery in 2 (5%) cases.

Embolization produced permanent deficits in 5 (11.6%) patients. Four were ischemic complications of embolization, 3 were quadrantanopias and 1 was ataxia due to cerebellar infarction. One patient had an intracerebral hemorrhage during the embolization after two feeders had been injected. He immediately underwent surgical removal of the hematoma and partial resection of the AVM in the left frontal lobe. He remained akinetic and mute following the surgery.

Seven patients did not undergo surgery and 2 patients were explored without resected. It was decided not to resect the AVM in 3 patients based on the functional neurological information gained by the embolization procedure, one the positive amytal test mentioned above (Fig. 1). In another two patients (Figs. 3 and 4), temporary deficit caused by partial embolization led to cancellation of further treatment because of the unacceptability of probable deficit.

Total surgical removal was performed after embolization in 30 (70%) of the 43 patients. Twenty-three patients had no deficit after embolization with or without surgery and 5 patients had a deficit which was the same as the one they had before surgery. After surgery 3 patients were left with a deficit which was worse than the original one, 2 patients had new weakness, 5 patients had visual field defects, 2 patients had speech disorders, and 1 patient was ataxic. Two patients (4.6%) died following surgical resection, 1 a week later of complications and the other of uncontrolled bleeding at surgery. Only a minority of the nidus had been blocked in these patients.

Discussion

The goal of therapy of AVMs is their complete obliteration or removal. Embolization at our institution and others has evolved in most instances into a preoperative adjunctive treatment for AVMs which are difficult to excise surgically [4, 5, 7–9].

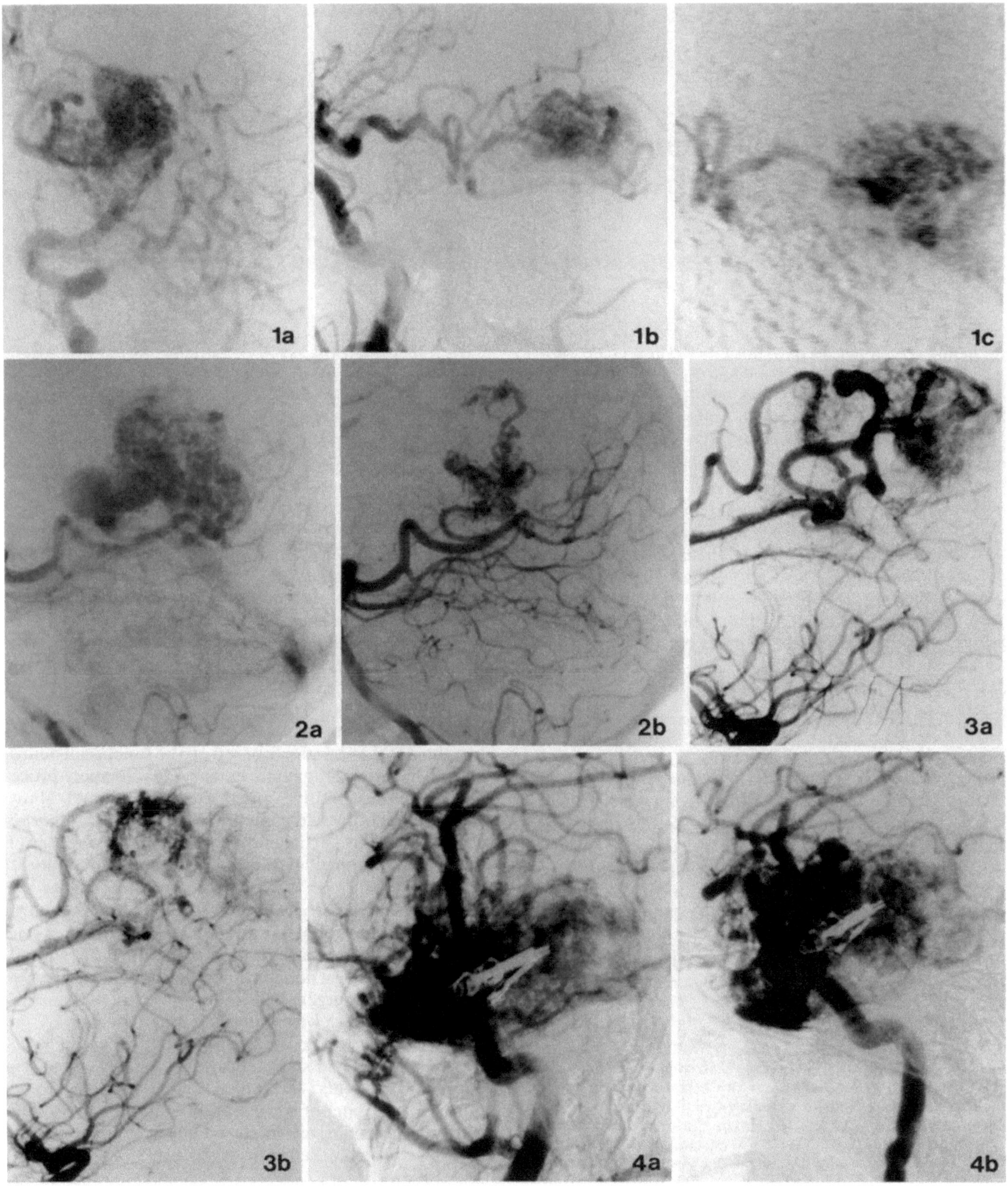

We attempt to occlude as much of the AVM as safely as possible prior to surgical resection, to reduce operative time and potential bleeding and, whenever possible, to block feeders which are difficult for the surgeon to access. This recent series produced a permanent deficit from embolization in 5 (11.6%) of 43 cases, 2 (4.6%) of which were serious. There were no deaths following embolization.

It is difficult to place a relative value on the embolization as it relates to the surgical resection and patient outcome. On postoperative angiography 70% of these surgically difficult AVMs had been completely resected. Two

(4.6%) patients died following surgery, and 13 patients (30%) were made clinically worse. Three (7%) of the 13 were much worse after the surgical resection. Five patients had serious complications of treatment, 2 of which were directly caused by the embolization. No more than one-third of the AVM was occluded by embolization in the 2 patients who subsequently died after surgery. It is possible that more extensive embolization might have produced a different result in one of these fatal cases where the embolization had been stopped because of the high risk of causing a deficit.

Although the goal of embolization in these complex AVMs is to enable surgical resection and reduce blood loss, embolization with amytal testing yields neurological information which can be useful when making decisions about therapy. Amytal injected into an AVM feeder can give a false-negative result because most of the amytal will be preferentially sucked through the AVM and not necessarily predict the effect of embolization on the brain. Indeed, deficits produced by embolization generally occur where the amytal test has been negative. A positive amytal test however is very important information which influences patient management. The same situation can occur when embolization produces a neurological deficit and the patient is given an immediate understanding of the permanent risks of the treatment. In a sense, these patients end up with the ultimate form of informed consent.

Fig. 1 a–c. A 52-year-old man with left occipital temporal arteriovenous malformation (AVM). Anteroposterior **(a)** and lateral **(b)** views of left carotid angiogram show the AVM fed primarily by a posterior cerebral branch feeder. Superselective angiogram **(c)** shows filling only of the nidus and venous drainage. Injection of 40 mg sodium amytal produced transient hemianopsia, and therefore embolization was not performed. As a result of this experience, the patient refused surgical resection

Fig. 2 a, b. This 52 year-old woman with previous hemorrhage was treated for right medial parieto-occipital AVM prior to surgical resection. Embolization eliminated the pericallosal feeding to anterior superior aspects not shown. Lateral vertebral angiogram prior to embolization **(a)** shows the posterior cerebral part. Lateral vertebral angiogram following embolization **(b)** shows a small amount of AVM continuing to fill by a parieto-occipital branch. Because of the acute angle of origin of that branch, the catheter was just within the branch origin, and amytal testing produced hemianopsia. Further embolization was not carried out. Complete surgical excision was performed without deficit. [Reproduced from Radiology with permission: Fox AJ, Pelz DM, Lee DH (1990) Endovascular therapy of brain AVMs: recent results. Radiology (in press)]

Fig. 3 a, b. This 40 year-old woman with a right medial rolandic AVM presented with progressive spastic hemiparesis. Lateral left carotid angiogram prior to embolization **(a)** shows the anterior cerebral part. Lateral left carotid angiogram following embolization of two feeders **(b)** shows significant reduction in the anterior cerebral component. Amytal tests were negative prior to and in between embolizations. Overnight the patient developed some temporary worsening of the hemiparesis, presumably from edema. This led the patient to refuse embolization of the middle cerebral component, and insist that resection be done only if it appeared that permanent worsening would not occur. The patient was explored with awake cortical mapping and resection was not done because of functional brain within the region of the AVM

Fig. 4 a, b. 41 year-old woman, who had presented with hemorrhage from a basilar aneurysm that was clipped, also had right temporal AVM. Lateral right carotid angiogram prior to embolization **(a)** shows the middle cerebral part. Embolization of only one anterior temporal branch was done, and embolization stopped for technical reasons. Lateral right carotid angiogram after embolization **(b)** does not show much change. However, a serious temporary memory disorder resulted, suggesting that memory function was centred within the right temporal lobe. This precluded further treatment at this time

Conclusion

Patients with large, generally complex AVMs at very high risk for surgical resection can be embolized with complete operative removal of the AVM in most instances. There is a modest risk of producing a permanent deficit from the embolization. These patients are still subject to risk from surgical resection. The neurological information occasionally afforded by amytal and transient deficits caused by embolization can influence subsequent surgical management.

References

1. Berenstein A, Choi IS (1988) Surgical neuroangiography of intracranial lesions. Radiol Clin North Am 26: 1143–1152
2. Debrun G, Viñuela F, Fox AJ (1982) Embolization of cerebral arteriovenous malformations with bucrylate: experience in 46 cases. J Neurosurg 56: 615–627
3. Viñuela F, Fox AJ (1983) Interventional neuroradiology in the management of arteriovenous malformations and fistulas. Neurol Clin 1: 131–154
4. Fox AJ, Pelz DM, Lee DH (1990) Endovascular therapy of brain AVMs: recent results. Radiology (in press)
5. Pelz DM, Fox AJ, Viñuela F, Drake CG, Ferguson GG (1988) Preoperative embolization of brain AVMs with isobutyl-2 cyanoacrylate. AJNR 9: 757–764
6. Fox AJ, Lee DH, Pelz DM, Brothers M, Deveikis J (1988) A thrombotic mixture as a "polymerizing" agent. AJNR 9: 1029
7. Luessenhop AJ, Rosa L (1984) Cerebral arteriovenous malformations: indications for and results of surgery, and the role of intravascular techniques. J Neurosurg 60: 14–22
8. Purdy PD, Samson D, Batjer HH, Risser RC (1990) Preoperative embolization of cerebral arteriovenous malformations with polyvinyl alcohol particles: experience in 51 adults. AJNR 11: 501–510
9. Spetzler RF, Martin NA, Carter LP, Flom RA, Raudzens PA, Wilkinson E (1987) Surgical management of large AVMs by staged embolization and operative excision. J Neurosurg 67: 17–28

Dr. Allan J. Fox
Radiology Department
University Hospital
339 Windermere Rd.
London, Ontario
N6A 5A5, Canada

Neuroradiology (1991) 33 [Suppl]: 190–192

Neuro radiology
© Springer-Verlag 1991

New liquid embolization method for brain arteriovenous malformations: combined infusion of oestrogen-alcohol and polyvinyl acetate

A. Takahashi[1], T. Yoshimoto[2], and T. Sugawara[1]

[1] Department of Neurosurgery, Kohnan Hospital, Sendai, Japan
[2] Division of Neurosurgery, Institute of Brain Diseases, Tohoku University School of Medicine, Sendai, Japan

Summary. A new liquid embolization method using oestrogen-alcohol and polyvinyl acetate was utilized in the treatment of brain arteriovenous malformations (AVMs). Oestrogen dissolved in 25% ethanol (oestrogen-alcohol) causes diffuse capillary and arteriolar obliteration, while ethanol soluble polymer, polyvinyl acetate (PVac solution) causes larger vessel occlusion without catheter glueing, or unwanted tissue reactions. Thirty-six cases of surgically inaccessible or difficult AVM were embolized by the infusion of oestrogen-alcohol followed by PVac solution in 73 sessions. Angiographic cure was achieved in 3 cases, and more than 90% obliteration in 16 cases without any difficulties related to embolic materials. Successful surgical resection was carried out in 8 cases. Adjunct radiation therapy was used in 9 cases which led to progressive diminution of the nidus. This newly developed method may be more effective and safer than the conventional one in the treatment of inoperable brain AVMs and make surgical excision or radiation therapy possible in surgically difficult AVMs.

Key words: Arteriovenous malformation – Embolization – Oestrogen – Polyvinyl acetate – Intravascular neurosurgery

In spite of the recent technical improvements in vascular access for intravascular neurosurgery, the method of embolization becomes more critical for optimum embolization therapy of arteriovenous malformations (AVMs) in brain. We have developed a new liquid embolization method combining a chemical embolization material, oestrogen-alcohol, and water insoluble polymer, polyvinyl acetate (PVac). In this communication, our experience of embolization of 36 cases of surgically inaccessible or difficult brain AVMs is reported.

Materials and methods

From October 1986 to June 1990, we treated 36 patients with brain AVM. Twenty-three were male and 13 were female with an age range from 3 to 57 years old (average age 26.3 years). Initial symptoms were as follows; haemorrhage in 21, seizures in 11, headache in 3 and progressive neurological deficit in 1. They were divided into small and large lesions according to the size of the nidus. Seventeen were large lesions, with a nidus greater than 5 cm in maximum diameter: 7 were located in the cortex, 8 were deeply situated and 2 were in the cerebellum. Of nineteen small lesions, less than 5 cm, 4 were situated in the cortex, 13 were deep and 2 were in the brain stem.

These patients were treated by transfemoral superselective embolization in 73 sessions. The embolization procedures were carried out in an operating room where a high-quality digital subtraction angiography (DSA) unit was installed. Patients were awake with neuroleptic anaesthesia and local anaesthesia with monitoring of neurology, somatosensory evoked potentials, brain stem auditory evoked potentials. General anaesthesia with monitoring of motor evoked potentials was used for a 3-year-old boy who had a choroidal AVM. After femoral puncture, a 5–6 F thin-walled heparinized introducing catheter (Anthron, Toray) was introduced into the vertebral or internal/external carotid artery. Under systemic heparinization, superselective catheterization using a minicatheter with or without leak balloon was performed. To avoid mechanical arterial spasm, an intra-arterial calcium antagonist was usually used (0.2–0.5 mg nicardipine).

After angiographic confirmation of the position of the catheter, a functional test using sodium amytal (50 mg) was carried out. If the amytal test was negative, a further provocation test using lidocaine (30–50 mg) was performed. Then, oestrogen-alcohol (20 mg/1 ml of 25% ethanol) was perfused for 10–20 min with an electrical pump. Oestrogen-alcohol was administered in a volume of 3–10 ml per feeder depending on the size and flow. PVac is a polymer which is insoluble in water but soluble in ethanol. The composition of polymer containing the material (PVac solution) is varied depending on the degree of A-V shunting. Standard compositions are shown in Table 1. Solution A is used for the finest vascular network, while solution D is suitable for fistulous components. The reaction of PVac solution with water, which is considered as reprecipitation, takes place immediately resulting in a gelatinous material which does not adhere to the catheter. PVac solution was injected intermittently under real-time DSA monitoring until adequate obliteration of the lesion was achieved.

To maximize nidus penetration with these embolizing agents, and to minimize damage to normal brain tissue, additional embolization with silk suture or mini-coils was occasionally used for accessory feeders which had other main feeder(s) entering the same compartment. In such cases, care was taken to embolize via the main feeder(s) with oestrogen-alcohol and PVac after the additional embolization.

Results

Total obliteration of the nidus was achieved in 3 cases (8%) (Figs. 1, 2). Clinically, there were no complications after embolization with a follow-up period of 32, 14 and 3 months, respectively. One case showed progressive reduction in the size of the lesion at follow-up angiography 1 and 2 years after embolization. Of the cases of incom-

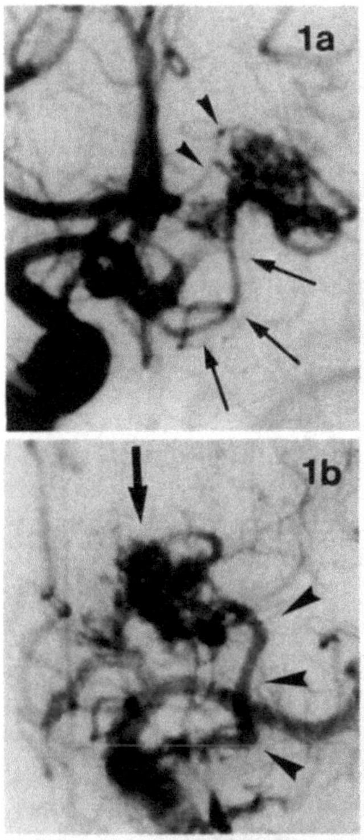

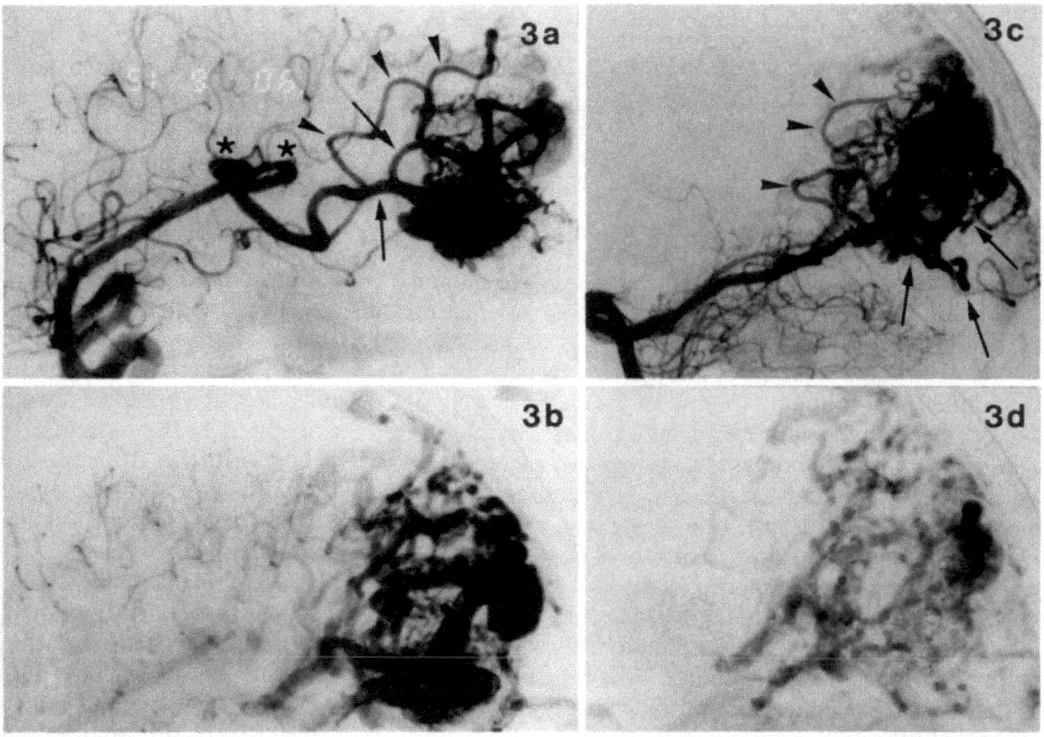

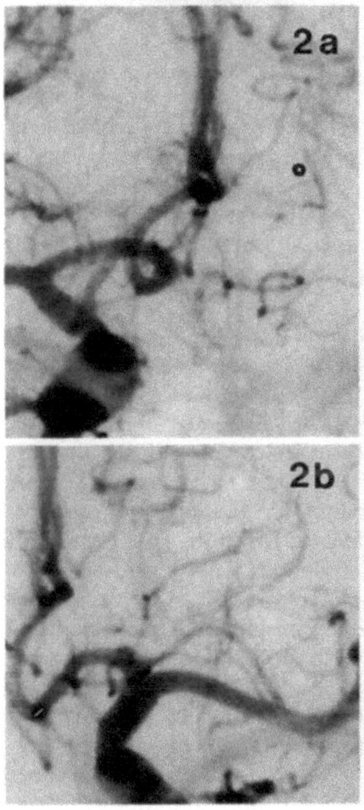

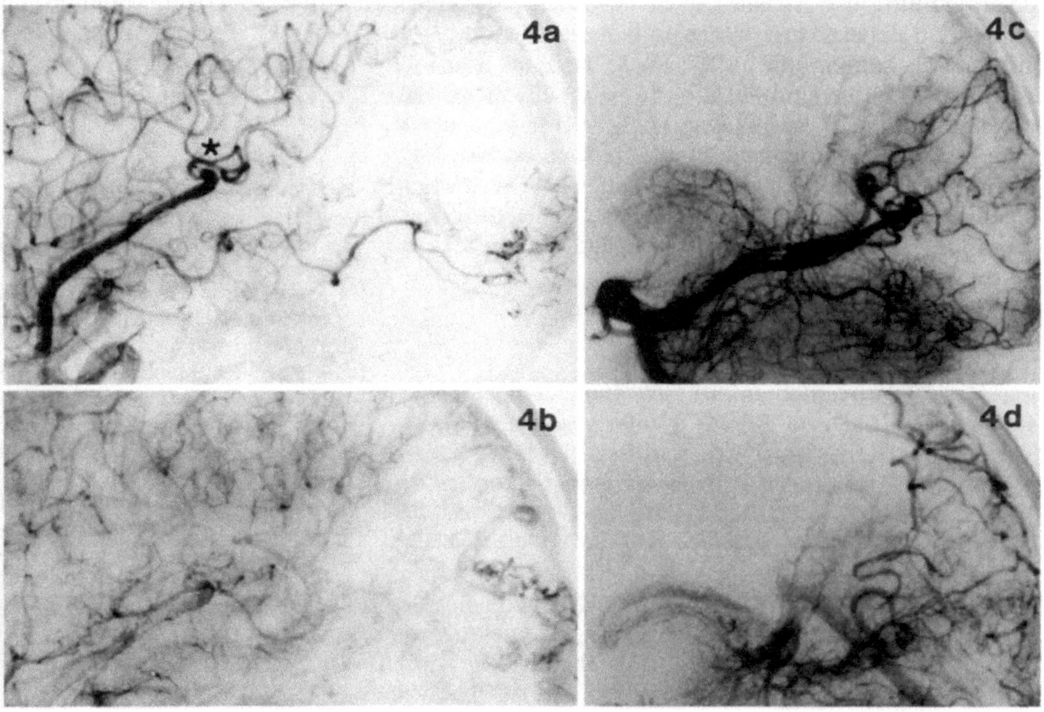

Fig. 1a, b. Pre-embolization angiograms of left deep-seated arteriovenous malformation (AVM) in a 21-year-old male who had bled once. **a** Right internal carotid angiogram showing two feeders derived from left A_1 segment *(arrows* and *arrowheads)*. **b** Left internal carotid angiogram showing nidus *(arrow)* and venous drainage *(arrowhead)*.

Fig. 2a, b. Angiogram 3 weeks after two sessions of embolization. Embolization through each feeder was performed in different sessions. Complete disappearance of nidus is noted. **a** Right internal carotid angiogram. **b** Left internal carotid angiogram

Fig. 3a–d. Pre-embolization angiograms of (large) left occipital AVM in a 57-year-old presenting with a seizure and right upper quadrantanopia. **a** Left internal carotid angiogram, arterial phase, showing two middle cerebral artery (MCA) feeders *(arrows* and *arrowheads)* and nidus. Note two aneurysms on MCA *(asterisks)*. **b** Left internal carotid angiogram, capillary phase, showing drainage with extensive cortical reflux. **c** Right vertebral angiogram, arterial phase, showing two major feeders from posterior cerebral artery (PCA) *(arrows* and *arrowheads)*. **d** Right vertebral angiogram, capillary phase

Fig. 4a–d. Angiogram 3 weeks after two sessions of embolization. Feeders from MCA were embolized in the first session and those from PCA in the second session. Almost all of nidus was obliterated. **a** Left internal carotid angiogram, arterial phase, showing accessory feeders from MCA. Note disappearance of distal MCA aneurysm and marked reduction in another *(asterisk)*. **b** Left internal carotid angiogram, capillary phase, showing disappearance of cortical reflux. **c** Right vertebral angiogram, arterial phase, showing no filling of the lesion. **d** Right vertebral angiogram, capillary phase

Table 1. Composition of polyvinyl acetate solution

Type of solution	A	B	C	D
PVac (ml)	1.00	1.25	1.65	1.00[a]
Ethanol (ml)	2.50	2.45	2.75	2.50
Distilled water (ml)	2.00	1.80	1.10	2.00
Metrizamide (g)	1.25	1.25	1.25	1.25

[a] Higher molecular weight polymer

plete embolization, 16 (44%) showed 90–99% obliteration (Figs. 3, 4), 6 (17%) 70–89%, 6 (17%) 50–69%, and 5 (14%) less than 49% occlusion. Of the 33 cases of incomplete embolization, 8 had subsequent surgical resection, 9 had conventional irradiation (30 Gy in 3 weeks) and the remainder are still being treated or are being closely observed. Among the surgically treated cases, complete resection without difficulty was achieved in 6 cases. During the surgery, the embolized nidus was soft enough to allow easy retraction and transection of the embolized portion with minimal blood loss. Among 4 radiation-treated cases, followed over 24 months, subtotal obliteration was observed in 2 and reduction of the size of the nidus 2.

In the early stages, we had 3 complications related to technical aspects of the catheter. Transient neurological deficits occurred in 7 cases and mild hemiparesis lasting several months in 3. Because of the location of the nidus, visual field defects were observed in 8 cases (quadrantanopia in 5, hemianopia in 3). There were no cases of haemorrhage after embolization in patients with no history of bleeding (15 cases). Among the cases whose initial symptom was haemorrhage, 2 had symptomatic bleeding, with 1 death. Both had large basal ganglia AVMs and rebleeding occurred 3 weeks after staged embolization. Two cases had small haemorrhages 1 week and 3 days after embolization.

Discussion

In spite of improvement in catheters and techniques, it remains difficult to treat AVMs by intravascular methods. Some of the factors causing these difficulties are selection of embolic materials and delivery methods. Although cyanoacrylates have been used extensively over the past decade, these materials may not be considered optimal. The major disadvantage of cyanoacrylates is that they are difficult to manipulate, and may result in complications such as vascular rupture or catheter glueing [1]. They can cause strong tissue reactions and may allow recanalization [2–5].

After experimental and clinical experience of oestrogen as a potent chemical embolizing agent [6–8], we have developed a more effective chemical combination, oestrogen-alcohol, which has the same embolization potential as absolute ethanol with fewer adverse effects in experimental renal artery studies in dogs [9]. Nevertheless, despite its potent embolizing property at the capillary and arteriolar level, larger vessels remains unembolized. It is thought that diffuse intimal damage with preserved blood flow may cause some adverse effects in clinical situations. In fact, initial results with oestrogen-alcohol caused oedema and petechial haemorrhage [9]. For larger vessel occlusion, we have developed another liquid material, PVac solution. PVac was first reported as an experimental embolization agent in 1984 [10]. We have modified it in vivo and in vitro and developed a better composition with more dilute ethanol; because it is ethanol soluble, metrizamide was added instead of lipiodol to make a homogeneous material. In clinical applications, four standard compositions were prepared to adjust the degree of penetration depending on the size of the shunts.

This newly developed combined embolization material fulfils many of the properties required of the ideal agent for intravascular treatment of AVMs, which should be

1. a liquid which can be introduced through a tiny catheter.
2. easy to control, radiopaque and with an infusion time long enough to control the embolization volume; it should not adhere to the catheter.
3. able to diffuse from artery to capillary without propagation into veins, without allowing recanalization.
4. non-toxic, biologically inert, and unreactive with brain parenchyma.
5. resectable in embolized tissue.

This method may be beneficial in a small inoperable AVM as a definitive treatment or in a large AVM as an adjunct to surgical resection or radiation therapy. Long follow-up is necessary before any conclusion about AVMs partially embolized by this method can be reached.

References

1. Deruty R, Lapras CI, Patet JD (1986) Intraoperative embolization of cerebral arteriovenous malformations by means of isobutyl cyanoacrylates (experience in 20 cases). Neurol Res 8: 109–113
2. Brothers MF, Kaufmann JCE, Fox AJ, Deveikis JP (1989) *N*-butyl 2-cyanoacrylate – substitute for IBCA in interventional neuroradiology: histopathologic and polymerization time studies. AJNR 10: 777–786
3. Klara PM, George ED, McDonnell DE, Pevsner PH (1985) Morphological studies of human arteriovenous malformation. J Neurosurg 63: 421–425
4. Rao VPK, Mandalam KR, Gupta AK (1989) Dissolution of isobutyl 2-cyanoacrylate on long-term follow-up. AJNR 10: 135–141
5. Vinters HV, Lundie MJ, Kaufmann JCE (1986) Long term pathological follow-up of cerebral arteriovenous malformations treated by embolization with bucrylate. N Engl J Med 314: 477–483
6. Suzuki J, Komatsu S (1981) New embolization method using estrogen for dural arteriovenous malformation and meningiomas. Surg Neurol 16: 438–442
7. Nagamine Y, Komatsu S, Suzuki J (1983) New embolization method using estrogen on microcirculation. Surg Neurol 20: 269–275
8. Shimizu Y, Nagamine Y, Fujiwara S, Suzuki J, Yamamoto T, Iwasaki Y (1987) An experimental study of vascular damage in oestrogen-induced embolization. Surg Neurol 28: 23–30
9. Takahashi A, Suzuki J (1988) Nonsurgical treatment of AVM: development of new liquid embolization method. In: Suzuki J (ed) Advances in surgery for cerebral stroke. Springer, Tokyo Berlin Heidelberg, pp 215–224
10. Peregrin JH, Jaspar M, Vanecek R, Belan A (1984) New occlusive agent for therapeutic embolization tested in dogs. Cardiovasc Intervent Radiol 7: 97–101

Dr. Akira Takahashi
Department of Neurosurgery
Kohnan Hospital
4-20-1, Nagamachi-minami
Taihaku-ku, Sendai, 982, Japan

Neuroradiology (1991) 33 [Suppl]: 193–194

Neuro-radiology
© Springer-Verlag 1991

A new technique for embolization of cerebral arteriovenous malformations and dural arteriovenous fistulae

K. Goto[1], W. Taki[2], and H. Iwata[3]

[1] Department of Interventional Neuroradiology, Iizuka Hospital, Iizuka, Japan
[2] Department of Neurosurgery, Kyoto University, Kyoto, Japan
[3] Department of Surgical Research, National Cardiovascular Center, Osaka, Japan

Summary. The main features of our system are: a new embolic material (EVAL; ethylene vinyl alcohol copolymer) which solved many of the problems of widely used liquid emboli, and a hydrophilic polymer-coated guide wire which is characterized by low friction and high torque control. This system was proved more effective for embolizing inoperable high flow vascular lesions of the brain and craniofacial regions. We report our experience in cerebral arteriovenous malformations 15 and 11 dural arteriovenous fistulae.

Key words: Embolization – Dural arteriovenous fistula – EVAL (ethylene vinyl alcohol copolymer) – Arteriovenous malformation

Since microcatheters became available, catheterization of deep cerebral arteries has become possible without the use of complex calibrated leak balloon systems. Nevertheless, it is still a time-consuming procedure and with potentially serious clinical complications due mainly to the friction between the catheter and the guide wire, and several undesirable features of liquid emboli. This is a report on our efforts to develop a new technique for safer and faster embolization of various central nervous and craniofacial vascular lesions.

Materials and methods

The main features of the authors' system are as follows: (1) a 0.016 inch Radiofocus plastic guide wire M (Terumo) with a hydrophilic polymer coating and a core made of superelastic alloy [1]; (2) a microcatheter (Tracker 18; Target); (3) a new liquid embolic material EVAL (ethylene vinyl alcohol copolymer) [2] which is made of ethylene vinyl alcohol copolymer dissolved in dimethyl sulphoxide (DMSO); upon contact with circulating blood, DMSO diffuses out immediately and EVAL becomes solid; (4) a Silastic nondetachable balloon catheter (Daw-Corning, Japan) used for flow restriction during EVAL injection in order to prevent escape of embolic material into the venous circulation.

Analysis was made of 39 embolizations performed using this system, in 15 inoperable high flow cerebral arteriovenous malformations (AVMs) and 11 dural arteriovenous fistulae (AVFs) over 1 year.

Case report

A 30-year-old male with a massive AVM in the right cerebellar hemisphere presented with a massive subarachnoid haemorrhage 2 months prior to embolization. Angiography revealed all three right cerebellar arteries to be markedly enlarged and to contribute to the blood supply of the AVM nidus (Fig. 1 a). Microcatheters were placed deep into these arteries with the aid of the hydrophilic polymer-coated guide wire and they were embolized using 0.7–1.0 ml EVAL (Fig. 1 b, c). Four sessions of embolization resulted in obliteration of a large part of the nidus (Fig. 1 d) and disappearance of the venous engorgement.

Results and discussion

With the combination of good torque control and the very low friction properties of the guide wire, the tip of the microcatheter was selectively placed much closer to the nidus, in a more controlled fashion than with conventional guide wire systems. The authors consider optimal flow restriction is mandatory during injection of EVAL, to prevent escape of EVAL into the venous system before solidification. Better flow control could be obtained by the placment of a non-detachable balloon slightly proximal to the tip of the microcatheter than a calibrated leak balloon. As EVAL lacks adhesive properties, sufficient EVAL could be injected in a relatively relaxed atmosphere, and repeat injection of EVAL through the same catheter was possible if required.

Of 15 cerebral AVM cases, complete obliteration of the nidus was obtained in 4 cases, more than 80% obliteration of the nidus in 7, 50–70% in 1 and treatment is still continuing the remaining 3 cases. Total obliteration of the fistula was obtained in 9 of the 11 cases with dural AVF. Inflammatory reaction around the vessels embolized by EVAL, examined in 6 operated cases, was much milder than in patients embolised with cyanoacrylate.

Complications

Two massive haemorrhages occurred during the procedure after the major part of the nidus was obliterated. Neurological deficits were not predicted by sodium amytal testing.

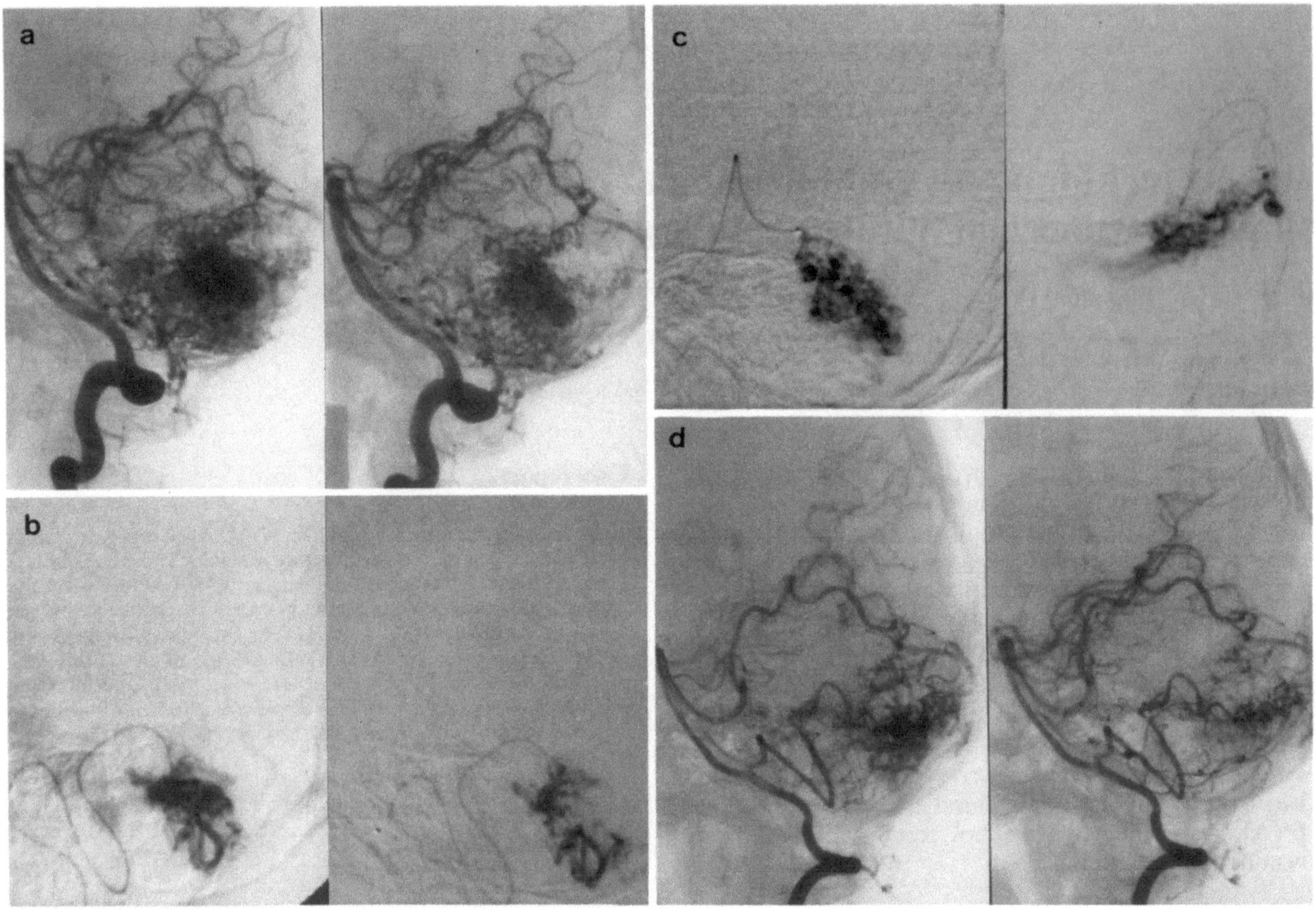

Fig. 1. **a** Vertebral angiography showing arteriovenous malformation (AVM) fed by all cerebellar arteries on the right (stereo). **b** Superselective cannulation of the right posterior inferior cerebellar artery (*left:* test injection using contrast medium; *right:* embolization using 1 ml EVAL). **c** Superselective opacification of the precentral cerebellar artery shows a pseudoaneurysm (*left:* lateral; *right:* AP). **d** Control angiogram showing marked reduction in size of the nidus (stereo). Remaining nidus was excised by surgery without need for blood transfusion

Conclusion

Based upon our experience in 26 cases with AVM and AVF, we feel that our system has considerable advantages over the conventional systems. For further reduction in the procedure time and increase in safety the development of a microcatheter with less friction is desirable.

References

1. Goto K (1991) Low friction high torque guide wire: a new way for superselective catheterization. Technical exhibit no. 442. Neuroradiology 33 (Suppl). Springer, Berlin Heidelberg New York
2. Taki W, Yonekawa Y, Iwata H, Uno A, Yamashita K, Amemiya H (1990) A new liquid material for embolization of arteriovenous malformations. AJNR 11: 163–168

Dr. K. Goto
Department of Interventional Neuroradiology
The Center for the Central Nervous Diseases
Iizuka Hospital
3-83 Yoshio-machi
Iizuka 820, Japan

Neuroradiology (1991) 33 [Suppl]: 195–196

Neuro radiology
© Springer-Verlag 1991

Embolization of arteriovenous malformations using EVAL mixture (a new liquid embolization material)

W. Taki[1], H. Kikuchi[1], H. Iwata[2], S. Nishi[1], K. Yamashita[1], and I. Nakahara[3]

[1] Department of Neurosurgery, Kyoto University Medical School, Kyoto, Japan
[2] Department of Experimental Medicine, National Cardiovascular Center, Osaka, Japan
[3] Department of Neurosurgery, Hamamatsu Rosai Hospital, Hamamatsu, Japan

Summary. For controllable embolization of arteriovenous malformations (AVMs) EVAL mixture, a new liquid material, was developed for use instead of cyanoacrylate derivatives such as isobutyl cyanoacrylate (IBCA) and *N*-butyl cyanoacrylate (NBCA). When the mixture is injected into blood, EVAL (ethylene vinyl alcohol copolymer) instantly forms sponge and occludes the pedicle and nidus. This new liquid material was used in 38 cerebral AVMs. Twenty cases were cured by embolization and the subsequent surgery. The remaining 18 cases was treated by embolization alone. Total embolization was achieved in 1 case. Between 70% and 90% embolization was achieved in 3 cases; 50–70% embolization was achieved in 10 cases. Less than 50% embolization was achieved in 4 cases. Complications were observed in 11 cases. Nine cases were minor or transient. Two cases were moderate. Rebleeding from the AVM was observed in 3 cases at follow-up examinations.

Key words: Cerebral arteriovenous malformation – Embolization – EVAL (ethylene vinyl alcohol copolymer) – Interventional radiology

---

Some cerebral or dural arteriovenous malformations (AVMs) are difficult or impossible to remove surgically because of their size and location. For these AVMs, embolization may be the primary treatment or as an adjunct to surgery or radiotherapy is usually performed using a cyanoacrylate derivatives such as isobutyl cyanoacrylate (IBCA). However, IBCA may glue the balloon to the artery or polymerize within the catheter, leading to an incomplete injection [1, 2]. In addition, polymerized cyanoacylate forms a very hard mass, which is difficult to remove. To overcome these disadvantages, we have developed a radiopaque liquid material for embolization. The material was applied clinically in 38 cerebral AVMs.

Subjects and methods

The embolization liquid that we have developed is a mixture of ethylene vinyl alcohol copolymer (EVAL) and metrizamide dissolved in dimethyl sulphoxide (DMSO). The precise preparation of the mixture has already been reported[3]. In in-vitro experiments, EVAL was injected into water through an 18-gauge needle, in about 3 s, a white gel-like droplet had formed; it had a sponge-like consistency within 15 s. In dogs, injection of EVAL into a renal artery occluded vessels as small as 80 μm in diameter, and histological examination revealed no inflammatory reaction. Since the sponge is elastic and soft, it is easy to cut and handle the nidus packed with an EVAL sponge during surgery.

Since the introduction of EVAL for clinical embolization of AVMs, we have been consulted about patients with 42 cerebral AVMs. Thirty-eight of those were treated using EVAL mixture. The symptoms were intracranial bleeding such as subarachnoid haemorrhage, intraventricular haemorrhage in 24 cases and convulsive or migraneous attack in 14 cases.

Percutaneous transfemoral catheterization was performed and the introducing catheter was guided into the internal carotid artery or the vertebral artery. Through this introducing catheter, a calibrated leak balloon catheter or microcatheter with guide wire was introduced and positioned within the feeding pedicle. By superselective angiography, we ascertained whether the catheter tip was in satis factory position. After the injection of the contrast an amytal test was performed by injecting 1 ml thiopentone sodium or amobarbital (50 mg/ml) through the microcatheter into the feeding pedicle. Immediately after the injection, the neurological status was determined. After confirming that there was no neurological deficit, 2 ml DMSO was injected to irrigate the catheter lumen, and this was followed by injection of the EVAL mixture under fluoroscopic control. The injection was continued and repeated until the feeding pedicle and the nidus were completely occluded. Since the material is not adhesive, multiple repeated injections could be performed. As many feeders as possible were catheterized and embolized.

Results

The results of the embolization of the cerebral AVMs with EVAL mixture were analysed using the grading proposed by Spetzler and Martin [4]. Grade 6 is inoperable because of the life-threatening location of the AVMs. Grades I–5 are determined by adding the each score in three aspects namely the size of the nidus, the location adjacent to the eloquent brain and the pattern of the venous drainage. The higher the grade, the more difficult the surgical removal becomes. The results are shown in Table 1. Twenty cases were cured by the combination of embolization and surgical removal. In these cured cases, one grade 1 case, one grade 2 case, eight grade 3 cases, seven grade 4 cases and three grade 5 cases were included. The surgical removal after EVAL embolization was faulitated with little blood loss. Even in the small

Table 1. Cerebral arteriovenous malformations (AVMs)[a] embolized with EVAL between 22 March 1988 and 31 May 1990

Embolization and surgical removal (20 cases)			
	Grade 1–1		
	Grade 2–1		
	Grade 3–8		
	Grade 4–7		
	Grade 5–3		
Embolization only		18 cases	
	100% embolization	1 case	grade 4–1
	90%	2 cases	grade 4–1 grade 5–1
	70%	1 case	grade 4–1
	50%	10 cases	grade 4–2 grade 5–6 grade 6–2
	30%	3 cases	grade 4–1 grade 5–2
	Feeder ligation effect		
		1 case	grade 3–1

[a] Spetzler's grading of cerebral AVMs was used [4]

Table 2. Complications

Motor weakness	4
Hemianopsia (1 visual agnosia)	2
Quadrantanopsia	3
Cerebellar signs (RIND)	1
Subarachnoid haemorrhage	1
Total	11/38
Re-rupture (embolization only)	3/18

AVM such as grade 1, the embolization was very helpful. The remaining 18 cases were treated by embolization only. One case was embolized 100%. Three cases were resulted in more than 70% embolization. Ten cases resulted in 50–70% embolization. Three cases resulted in less than 50% embolization, mainly 30–50% embolization.

The complications were mainly due to the false-negative result of the barbiturate injection test and are listed in Table 2. Two had moderate worsening of the hemiparesis. One had a visual agnosia; in the remaining eight cases there were minor complications. Rebleeding from the embolized AVM occurred in three cases.

Discussion

EVAL is a copolymer of polyethylene and polyvinyl alcohol (PVA). Both polyethylene and PVA has been used for permanent implantation material and biocompatible. In addition, histological examination of AVMs embolized with EVAL showed no associated inflammatory reaction. DMSO was chosen as a solvent of EVAL because it has been used in humans and its physiological properties have been well documented [5].

The use of EVAL mixture, and subsequent surgical removal was very easy. The EVAL forms a spongy mass in the AVMs and is easy to cut and compress during the surgical removal. This is more favourable than IBCA which forms a relatively hard mass. Because of its non-adhesive character, the catheter manipulation becomes easier and safer. Although the EVAL mixture is useful for embolization, it may not be suitable for some lesions such as a single arteriovenous fistula or an AVM that contains a large arteriovenous fistula, as it is possible that EVAL may pass through the nidus to the venous drainage. This did not occur in our series. EVAL is not biodegradable and recanalization of the embolized AVM appears to be comparable to IBCA. Although almost the entire nidus can be occluded by EVAL, any residual nidus may gradually enlarge. Surgical resection after embolization is necessary when early venous drainage is still observed by postoperative angiography.

References

1. Berenstein A, Kricheff II (1979) Catheter and material selection for transarterial embolization: technical considerations. II. Materials. Radiology 132: 631–639
2. Debrun G, Vinuela F, Fox A (1982) Embolization of cerebral arteriovenous malformations with bucrylate. Experiences in 46 cases. J Neurosurg 56: 615–627
3. Taki W, Yonekawa Y, Iwata H (1990) A new liquid material for embolization of arteriovenous malformations. AJNR 11: 163–168
4. Spetzler RF, Martin NA (1986) A proposed grading system for arateriovenous malformations. J Neurosurg 65: 476–483
5. Mullan S, Torre JC de la, Kajihara K (1973) Use of dimethyl sulfoxide in experimental head and spinal cord injuries. J Neurol Neurosurg Psychiatry 36: 153–154

Dr. W. Taki
Department of Neurosurgery, Kyoto University
Medical School, Kyoto, Japan

SESSION 14
A-V MALFORMATIONS AND INTERVENTIONAL

Neuroradiology (1991) 33 [Suppl]: 198–200

Neuro-radiology
© Springer-Verlag 1991

Vascular perforations resulting from neurointerventional procedures

V. V. Halbach[1, 2], R. T. Higashida[1, 2], C. F. Dowd[1], S. L. Barnwell[2], and G. B. Hieshima[1, 2]

Departments of [1] Radiology, Neurointerventional Section and [2] Neurological Surgery, University of California, San Francisco Medical Center, San Francisco, California, USA

Summary. During the past 5 years, 1,420 neurointerventional endovascular procedures have been performed, resulting in 15 vascular perforations. In 7 patients the suspected mechanism of perforation included a mechanical perforation of a normal vessel, mechanical disruption of a dysplastic vessel in 5 patients, and fluid overinjection in the remaining 4 patients. Treatments for the perforations included reversal of anticoagulants (10 patients), direct closure of the perforation site with coils (5 patients), and particles (2 patients). Closure of the adjacent intravascular compartment was performed in 6 patients with coils and in 4 patients with liquid adhesives, and balloons (2 patients). Immediate consequences of the perforation included headaches (9 patients), seizures (2 patients), hydrocephalus (1 patient), right upper extremity dysmetria (1 patient), diabetes insipidus (2 patients) and 2 deaths. Long-term sequelae in the remaining 13 patients included diabetes insipidus in 1 patient and hydrocephalus treated effectively with shunting. No documented episodes of rehemorrhage have occurred in patients followed for an average of 26 months.

Key words: Neurointerventional procedures – Perforation – Seizures – Hemorrhage – Coils

Vascular perforations have been reported following diagnostic and therapeutic procedures outside the central nervous system; the majority of these perforations are repaired surgically. Only a few scattered reports have dealt with this potentially devastating complication occurring within the central nervous system following diagnostic procedures [1–3] and most recently during intracranial navigation with steerable microcatheters [4]. We report the first series listing the incidence and possible etiologies of these complications, their management, and outcome.

Results

The specific diseases in which vascular perforations occurred included 6 arteriovenous malformations (AVM), 2 spinal AVMs, 3 dural fistulas, 1 vasospasm, 1 carotid cavernous fistula, 1 vein of Galen malformation, and 1 ruptured basilar aneurysm. All 15 patients had CT following the perforation: contrast medium and/or blood were present in 14. The presumed mechanism causing the perforation was fluid overinjection in 4, mechanical disruption of a normal vessel in 6, and mechanical tearing of an aneurysm or dysplastic vessel in 5. Treatments in-

Table 1. Summary of vascular perforations

Case no.	Age/sex	Pathology	Vessel catheterized	Result of perforation	Immediate outcome	Long-term outcome	Follow up (months)
1	50/F	AVM	Ant ch	IVH	HA	O	26
2	8 days/M	Vein of Galen	Vein of Galen	IVH	Hydrocephalus	Hydrocephalus	13
3	34/F	AVM	PCA	SAH, IVH	Mild HA	O	26
4	55/M	AVM	Ant ch	IVH	Mild HA	O	18
5	62/F	TS DAVF	TS	Small subdural	O	O	28
6	72/F	CS DAVF	CS	O	DI	DI	13
7	71/F	Direct CCF	IPS	SAH	HA	O	54
8	33/F	AVM	Ant ch	IVH	HA	O	16
9	45/F	Vasospasm	PCA	Massive SAH	Death		
10	41/F	AVM/aneurysm	PCA	SAH	HA	O	24[a]
11	20/M	Spinal AVM	Ant spinal	SAH	Paraplegia	Recovered	14
12	26/F	Spinal AVM	Ant spinal	SAH	Seizure HA	0	68
13	48/F	CS DAVF	IPS	Cerebellar bleed	Dysmetria	Recovered	20
14	30/M	AVM	MCA branch	SAH	DI seizure	O	11
15	68/M	AVM	PCA	Massive SAH	Death		

AVM, Arteriovenous malformations; HA, headaches; TS, transverse sinus; DAVF, dural arteriovenous fistula; M, male; F, female; IBCA, isobutyl cyanoacrylate; NBCA, normal butylcyanoacrylate; IVH, intraventricular hemorrhage; IPS, inferior petrosal sinus; DI, diabetes insipitus; Ant ch, ant choroidal; CS, cavernous sinus, O, neurologically intact without symptoms

[a] Died; unrelated causes

Table 2. Summary of treatment

Case no.	Reverse heparin	Anticon- vulsants	Coil across perforation	Adjacent intravascular compartment closed: coils	IBCA/ NBCA	particles	balloon	Continued bleeding	Rehemorrhage
1	Yes	Yes	No	No	Yes	No	No	No	No
2	Yes	Yes	Yes	Yes	No	No	No	No	No
3	Yes	No	Yes	No	No	No	Transient	No	No
4	Yes	No	No	No	No	No	Transient	No	No
5	Yes	No	Yes	Yes	Yes	No	No	No	No
6	DNA	No	No	Yes	Yes	No	No	No	No
7	DNA	No	Yes	Yes	No	No	No	No	No
8	Yes	Yes	No	No	No	Yes	No	No	No
9	Yes	No	No	No	No	No	No	Yes	Died
10	Yes	No	No	No	No	No	Permanent	No	No
11	Yes	No	No	No	No	No	Permanent	No	No
12	Yes	Yes	No	No	Yes	No	No	No	No
13	DNA	No	No	Yes	No	No	No	No	No
14	Yes	Yes	Yes	Yes	No	Yes	No	No	No
15	Yes	No	No	No	No	No	No	Yes	Died

cluded reversal of anticoagulation with protamine sulfate in all 12 patients on heparin. Anticonvulsants were administered to 5 patients, 2 following the onset of a seizure related to the extravasation of blood or contrast. Five patients had coils placed at the perforation site and the adjacent intravascular compartment was occluded with coils in 6 patients, liquid adhesives in 4, particles in 2, temporary balloons in 2, and permanent balloons in 2. In 2 patients with massive subarachnoid hemorrhage secondary to a large vessel perforation, death occurred before definitive treatment could be instituted. The immediate outcome of the perforation in the surviving 13 patients included headaches in 7, diabetes insipidus in 2, seizures in 2, dysmetria in 1, paraplegia in 1, hydrocephalus in 1, and death in 2 patients. The long-term sequelae (more than 2 weeks) resulting from the perforation included stable hydrocephalus requiring shunting in 1 vein of Galen malformation; and diabetes insipidus in 1 patient. One patient died from unrelated causes 2 years after treatment. The remaining 12 patients are alive and well and have completely recovered all neurological deficits related to the perforation; they have been followed for 26 months without evidence of rehemorrhage. The patients' age, sex, vascular pathology, location of hemorrhage, outcome and follow up are summarized in Table 1. The various treatments are summarized in Table 2.

Case report

Case 2 is a newborn who presented with severe intractable congestive heart failure. Arteriography disclosed a large vein of Galen malformation (Fig. 1 a). During a transfemoral, transtorcular venous approach, the guidewire was noted to leave the confines of the vein of Galen. The catheter was immediately advanced over the wire across the perforation site and systemic anticoagulation reversed. A contrast medium injection revealed extravasation into the lateral ventricle. A steel Gianturco coil was placed with the tip of the coil in the lateral ventricle, and the remainder of the coil bridging the perforation site and into the vein of Galen. Forty-two additional coils were then rapidly deposited in the vein of Galen to promote thrombosis (Fig. 1 b, c). Postembolization CT demonstrated contrast medium concentrated in the right lateral ventricle (Fig. 1 d). A postembolization arteriogram confirmed thrombosis and occlusion around the perforation site without evidence of pseudoaneurysm formation (Fig. 1 e). The patient developed moderate hydrocephalus following the procedure and was shunted with improvement but has had complete alleviation of his heart failure and 9 months later is neurologically normal and without bruit.

Discussion

The vast majority of vascular perforations occurring outside the central nervous system are repaired surgically. Surgical repair of a perforation occurring during an interventional procedure within the central nervous system is frequently not practical nor possible. The central nervous system is exquisitely sensitive to even small amounts of extravasated blood, therefore immediate elimination of the hemorrhage site is essential for a good outcome. Emergency neurologic surgery may take hours before a bleeding site is approached and in many instances the site of the bleeding is in areas that are difficult or impossible to reach surgically. Therefore the most effective treatment is occlusion of the perforation site by the offending catheter or balloon performed immediately upon recognition of this potentially disastrous occurrence. Roadmapping is essential for safe intracranial navigation and allows immediate recognition should the guidewire or catheter leave the confines of the vascular space as well as permitting detection of even small amounts of extraluminal contrast medium. In many instances the catheter or guidewire is tamponading the perforation site and therefore should not be withdrawn immediately. A small injection of nonionic contrast medium can confirm the extraluminal location but should be aspirated if possible to reduce the risk of seizures. Immediate reversal of anticoagulation is essential and the patient's return to baseline coagulation should be confirmed by laboratory tests. Extravasated contrast medium and blood can produce severe headaches and pain medication should be administered appropriately. Phenothiazines should be avoided as they may lower the

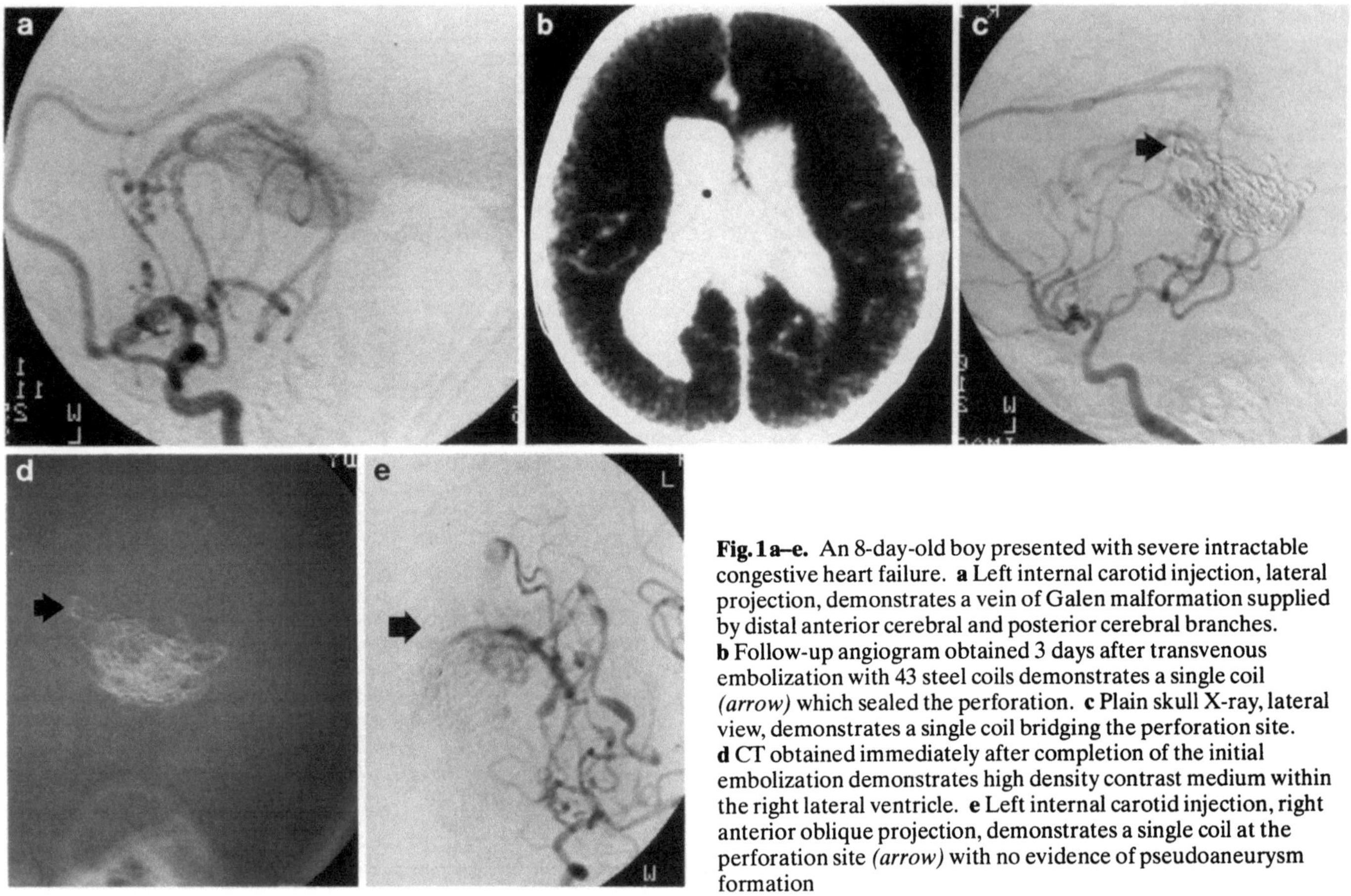

Fig. 1 a–e. An 8-day-old boy presented with severe intractable congestive heart failure. **a** Left internal carotid injection, lateral projection, demonstrates a vein of Galen malformation supplied by distal anterior cerebral and posterior cerebral branches. **b** Follow-up angiogram obtained 3 days after transvenous embolization with 43 steel coils demonstrates a single coil *(arrow)* which sealed the perforation. **c** Plain skull X-ray, lateral view, demonstrates a single coil bridging the perforation site. **d** CT obtained immediately after completion of the initial embolization demonstrates high density contrast medium within the right lateral ventricle. **e** Left internal carotid injection, right anterior oblique projection, demonstrates a single coil at the perforation site *(arrow)* with no evidence of pseudoaneurysm formation

seizure threshold. When technically possible the perforation site and the adjacent intravascular compartment should be closed with embolic material, particularly if rupture of an aneurysm or dysplastic vessel has occurred. A normal vessel can constrict and seal a small perforation. However, a dysplastic vessel or aneurysm lacks the muscular wall and continued extravasation will enlarge and extend the perforation, often resulting an a fatal outcome. Therefore, prompt recognition and closure of the perforation is essential for a good outcome. Anticonvulsant medication should be considered when a large amount of contrast medium and/or blood are pooled extravascularly. While two of our patients developed seizures related to extravasated contrast medium and/or blood, none have had long-term seizures now off medication.

Due to the recent advances in the field of interventional neuroradiology with high resolution fluoroscopy, roadmapping techniques, and advanced embolic materials, it is now possible to access the distal intracerebral vasculature for the treatment of vascular malformations and aneurysms. Despite the development of these newer materials, vascular perforations can rarely occur during endovascular procedures involving the brain and spinal cord. Prompt recognition and closure of the perforations is essential for a good outcome.

References

1. Tsementzis SA, Kennett RP, Hitchcock ER (1984) Rupture of intracranial vascular lesions during arteriography. J Neurol Neurosurg Psychiatry 47: 795–798
2. Dublin AB, French DN (1980) Cerebral aneurysm rupture during angiography with confirmation by computer tomography. A review of intra aneurysmal rupture. Surg Neurol 13: 19–27
3. Shiu PC, Hanafee WN, Wilson GH, Rand RW (1968) Cavernous sinus venography. Radiology 104: 57–62
4. Purdy PD, Sampson D, Batjor HH, Rissen RC (1990) Preoperative embolization of cerebral arteriovenous malformations with polyvinyl alcohol particles: experience in 51 adults. AJNR 11: 501–510

Dr. Van V. Halbach
Department of Radiology
Neurointerventional Section
Box 0628
UCSF Medical Center
San Francisco, CA 94143, USA

Neuroradiology (1991) 33 [Suppl]: 201–202

Neuro radiology
© Springer-Verlag 1991

Contrast medium extravasation during embolization of intracranial arteriovenous malformation without associated intracranial hematoma

B. Azar-Kia, J. T. Barron, S. W. Horowitz, and M. Fine

Loyola University Medical Center, Maywood, Illinois, USA

Summary. We describe the radiographic findings in two patients who underwent intracranial embolization for arteriovenous malformation in whom, during the course of the embolization, extravasation of contrast medium without concomitant hemorrhage was identified on subsequent angiography and confirmed surgically.

Key words: Embolization – Cerebral hemorrhage – Intracranial arteriovenous malformation

Case reports

Case 1

A 25-year-old male was transferred to our facility after a single episode of generalized seizure. CT performed at an outside hospital revealed findings consistent with a right temporoparietal arteriovenous malformation (AVM).

Staged angiography and selective right external and internal carotid artery embolization was performed with sequential occlusion of multiple feeding vessels [1].

During the final session, right carotid angiography was performed (Fig. 1 a), followed by embolization of the anterior choroidal artery. Under fluoroscopy, test injection into the anterior choroidal artery prior to embolization showed contrast medium in the right lateral ventricle. There was no clinical deterioration of the patient's status. Embolization was completed using a mixture of Ivalon particles, 50% dextrose, albumin and contrast material. Postembolization angiography demonstrated the presence of contrast medium within the right lateral ventricle (Fig. 1 b). Overt extravasation was not demonstrated on sequentially filmed injection but was present throughout the examination. CT performed within 6 h of the last embolization revealed complete clearance of the contrast medium from the right ventricle, and no evidence of intraventricular hemorrhage or rupture of the AVM. Definitive surgery was performed within 24 h of the CT, and the neurosurgeon reported finding no evidence of blood in the right lateral ventricle. Complete surgical removal of the AVM was performed without neurological sequelae, and the postoperative course was uneventful.

Case 2

A 21-year-old male was transferred to our institution partially comatose with acute onset of change of mental status and right hemiparesis. Outside CT and repeat CT performed upon admission identified a large left parietal lobe intracerebral hemorrhage (Fig. 2 a). Digital subtraction angiography at the outlying hospital was suggestive of a left parietal AVM. Emergency carotid angiography was performed, confirming the left parietal lobe AVM with feeding vessels from the posterior parietal branches of the left middle cerebral artery (Fig. 2 a).

Selective embolization of the left parietal AVM was performed with injection of Ivalon, 50% dextrose, albumin and contrast. Following embolization, repeat injection of the left middle cerebral artery revealed marked decrease in the size of the AVM. On the postembolization angiography films, there was an intraparenchymal collection of contrast medium (Fig. 3 b) not seen on the pre-embolization study. CT was performed immediately following the angiogram, which demonstrated new areas of increased density in the subarachnoid space and anterior aspect of the left parietal lobe parenchyma not present on the previous CT (Fig. 2 b). A repeat CT examination performed the following day demonstrated complete resolution of these areas of increased density in the subarachnoid space, consistent with reabsorption of contrast medium rather than subarachnoid hemorrhage. An external shunt tube revealed no blood in the cerebrospinal fluid drainage from the time of embolization to the preoperative evaluation. No subarachnoid hemorrhage was found during the subsequent surgical excision of the AVM.

Discussion

Both cases outlined above demonstrate the leakage of contrast medium into the extravascular space of the brain (ventricular system, brain parenchyma and subarachnoid space) without concomitant hemorrhage or blood extravasation. At no time was there evidence of blood within the intracranial extravascular spaces when contrast medium leakage occurred. Our literature search found no previous case reports of contrast medium extravasation following intracranial AVM embolization [2, 3]. The absence of blood within the extravascular spaces as confirmed by the surgeons during the definitive exploratory and AVM removal procedure would speak against the contrast pooling as a result of postembolotherapy reperfusion rupture and hemorrhage which has been widely reported in the literature.

The exact cause of contrast egress into the ventricular system, brain parenchyma and subarachnoid space in our two patients is unclear but it may be related to hemodynamic alterations of the parenchymal AVM [4]. It is our belief that these reports are the first of extravasation of

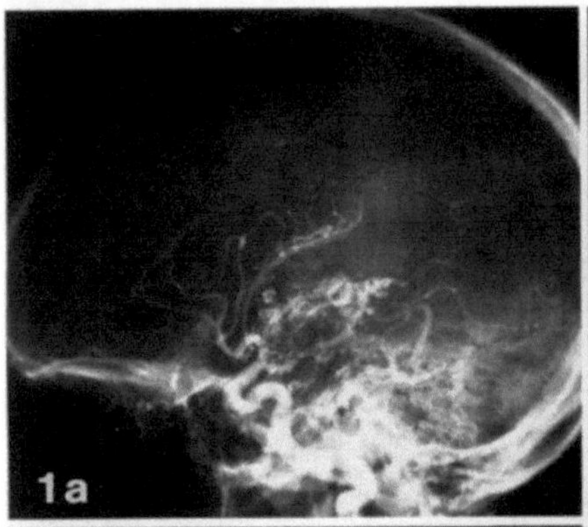

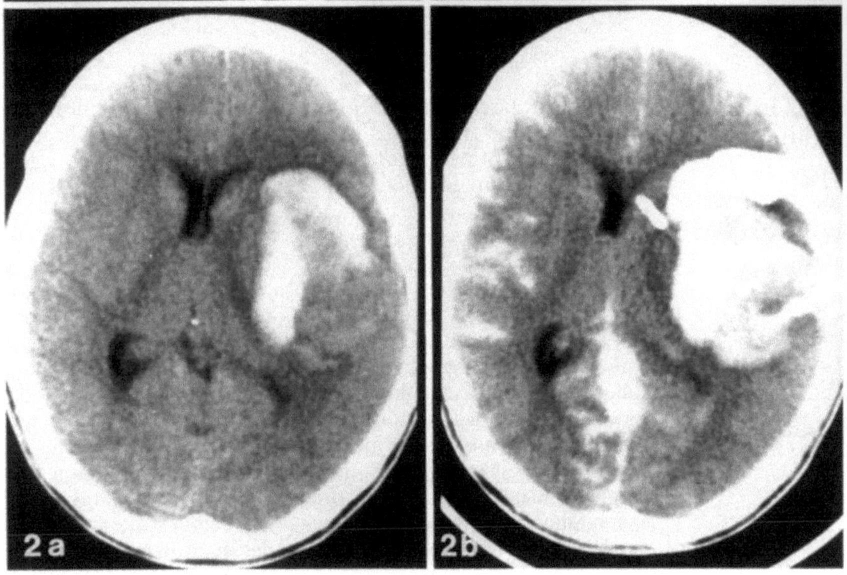

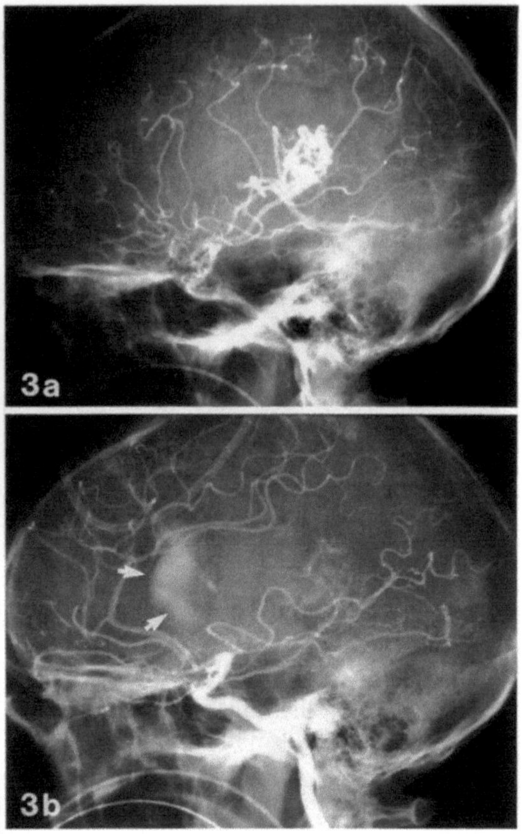

Fig. 1. **a** Arteriovenous malformation (AVM) in the Sylvian fissure before embolization. **b** After embolization, note contrast medium in the body and trigone of the lateral ventricle *(arrow)*

Fig. 2. **a** CT on admission shows intracerebral hematoma in the left temporal region. **b** Postembolization CT showing density of collection of contrast medium anterior and in the hematoma. Also note contrast medium in the subarachnoid space

Fig. 3. **a** Angiogram before embolization showing AVM in the posterior aspect of the Sylvian fissure. **b** Postembolization angiogram shows collection of contrast medium *(arrows)*

contrast medium during embolization procedures for intracranial AVM without antecedent rupture and hemorrhage.

References

1. Andrews BT, Wilson CB (1987) Staged treatment of arteriovenous malformations of the brain. Neurosurgery 21: 314–323
2. Vinters HV, Lundie MJ, Kaufmann JC (1986) Long term pathological follow up of cerebral arteriovenous malformations treated by embolization with bucrylate. N Engl J Med 314: 477–483
3. Jones FD, Boone SC, Whaley RA (1982) Intracranial hemorrhage following attempted embolization and removal of large arteriovenous malformations. Surg Neurol 18: 278–283
4. Halbach VV, Higashida RT, Hieshima GB, Norman D (1987) Normal perfusion pressure breakthrough occurring during treatment of carotid and vertebral fistulas. AJNR 8: 751–756

Dr. Behrooz Azar-Kia
Department of Radiology
Loyola University Medical Center
2160 South First Avenue
Maywood, IL 60153, USA

Neuroradiology (1991) 33 [Suppl]: 203–205

Neuroradiology

© Springer-Verlag 1991

Cost implications of different policies for the treatment of arteriovenous malformations of the brain

M. Nelson[1], G. Bonsor[2], and J. T. Lamb[1]

[1] Section of Neuroradiology, General Infirmary, Leeds, UK
[2] Pinderfields Hospital, Wakefield, UK

Summary. Arteriovenous malformations (AVMs) of the brain may be treated with conventional surgery, gamma-knife or linear accelerator radiosurgery and embolisation. Estimates for the costs of these treatments have been obtained from centres in the United Kingdom and have been used to calculate the costs of three policies for treating brain AVMs. Policies that approximate to present clinical practice are relatively cost-effective. For a single treatment session embolisation costs less than other therapies. Used preoperatively embolisation adds 30–40% to policy costs and when used as the only therapy multiple treatment sessions make embolisation the most costly therapy. Detailed cost-benefit analysis is required for embolisation in the treatment of brain AVMs.

Key words: Arteriovenous malformation – Brain – Costs – Embolisation – Radiosurgery

Clinical policies for treating arteriovenous malformations (AVMs) of the brain vary between neurosurgical centres depending on the availability of surgical expertise and of facilities for radiosurgery and embolisation. Little is known of the effects on health care costs of different treatment policies. The objective of this paper was to assess the costs of three hypothetical treatment policies by applying them to a series of patients referred to our neurosurgical centre using treatment costs from centres in the United Kingdom.

Patients, methods and definitions

New cases of brain AVM were identified by a retrospective review of clinical and radiographic records at our hospitals. As part of a larger survey all clinical notes, CT studies and angiograms were reviewed by one of us (MN). The AVMs were assessed for surgical risk using an established classification, the Spetzler-Martin grade [1]. Demographic data for the population served by our hospitals were obtained from publication of the Government Statistical Service [2, 3].

Information on treatment costs was obtained from finance administration in our hospitals or by personal communication with clinical colleagues in other centres. Costs were calculated for each treatment on an item-cost basis for all activities included in the treatment process. Average durations of inpatient stay and procedure time were assumed. For each treatment modality the calculated cost includes the following elements (a) hotel services; (b) personnel – medical, nursing, technical; (c) disposable items – equipment, contrast agents, drugs; (d) capital depreciation, amortised over 10 years – buildings, equipment. (The cost for gamma-knife radiosurgery at Sheffield is the hospital charge for members of the European Community and is believed to contain other elements).

Three hypothetical treatment policies have been modelled (Figs. 1–3). Treatment decisions in all three policies depend on the morphology of the AVM (size of nidus and Spetzler-Martin grade) and in policies II and III on the clinical presentation of the patient (presence of bleeding or flow-related symptoms).

Policy I allocates AVMs of low and intermediate grade to surgery while high grade lesions have gamma-knife radiosurgery or embolisation depending on the size of the nidus. This type of policy applied before stereotactic linear accelerator radiosurgery was adopted and before it was appreciated that AVM embolisation is often incomplete and does not eliminate the risk of bleeding.

Policy II also allocates AVMs of low and intermediate grade to surgery but adds a single session of preoperative embolisation to eliminate deep feeders and facilitate surgical mobilisation of the nidus. For high grade lesions embolisation is used to control flow-related symptoms and all patients have stereotactic radiosurgery, using the gamma-knife or linear accelerator depending on the size of the nidus. Policy II corresponds to present practise in some UK centres.

In modelling policy III it is noted that surgery for a grade III AVM carries a risk of neurological deficit (16%) which is much higher than that associated with radiosurgery [1, 4, 5]. This risk is acceptable for grade III patients who present with bleeding but not for grade III patients who have not bled; the latter are allocated to the other arm of the policy. In other respects policy III is similar to policy II.

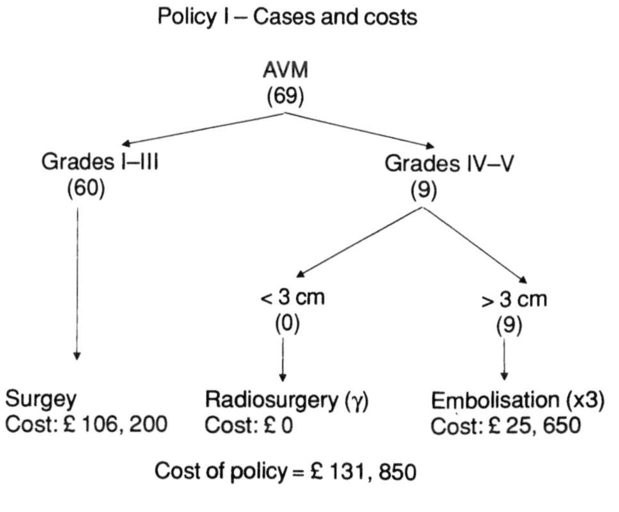

Fig. 1. Policy I: treatment algorithm, patient numbers and costs (patient numbers in parentheses)

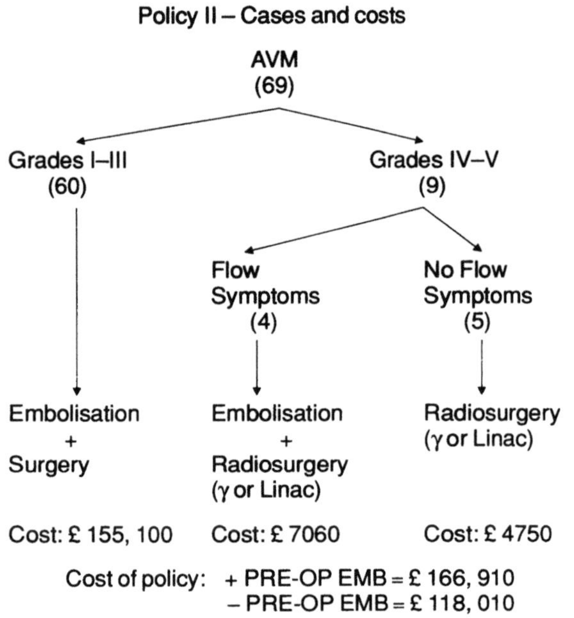

Fig. 2. Policy II: treatment algorithm, patient numbers and costs (patient numbers in parentheses)

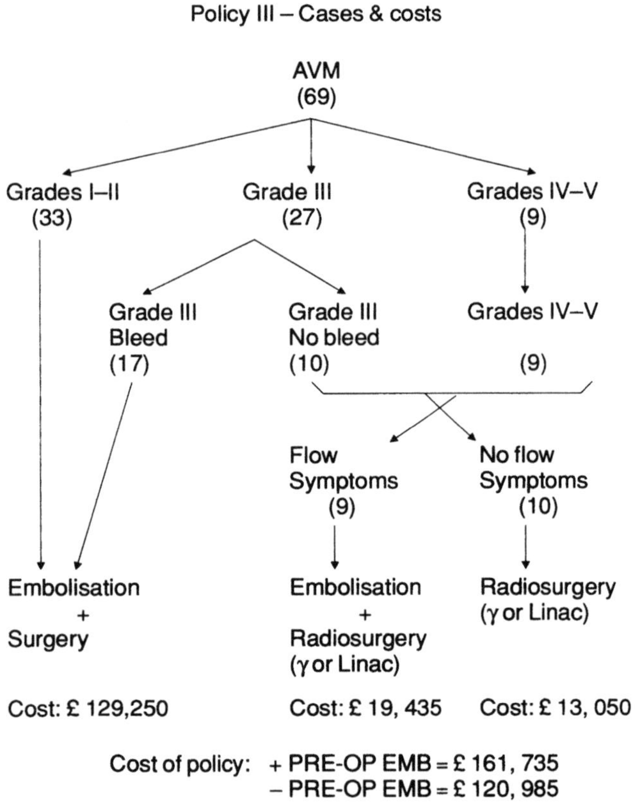

Fig. 3. Policy III: treatment algorithm, patient numbers and costs. (patient numbers in parentheses)

No policy was modelled using embolisation to attempt definitive treatment of any grade of AVM considering the low rate of nidus obliteration with embolisation and the higher risks of neurological deficit, bleeding and death compared to radiosurgery ([4, 5]; A. J. Molyneux, personal communication).

Table 1. Treatment costs for arteriovenous malformations of the brain

Treatment	Centre, year	Cost
Embolisation	Edinburgh, 1989	£ 815
Radiosurgery (linear accelerator)	Birmingham, 1990	£ 950
Surgery	Leeds and Wakefield, 1990	£ 1770
Radiosurgery (gamma-knife)	Sheffield, 1990	(£ 4500)

Results

The population served by our hospitals numbered 2.65 million in 1988. The population is demographically stable, having increased by less than 0.4% since 1984. Population change due to migration in 1988 was 0.11%, well below the national average.

Between July 1983 and December 1988 there were 69 new cases of brain AVM in 68 patients, aged between 6 and 68 years. The clinical presentation was bleeding in 44, symptoms of haemodynamic origin in 12, seizure in 11 and a fixed neurological deficit in 1. On angiography the nidus measured less than 3 cm in 49, 3–6 cm in 13 and greater than 6 cm in 7. The nidus involved evocative brain in 34 and had a deep venous drainage in 42. The Spetzler-Martin grades were: I 17; II 16; III 27; IV 3; V 6.

Treatment costs are given in Table 1. The relatively low costs of embolisation (£ 815) and linear accelerator radiosurgery (£ 950) reflect their low capital depreciation cost. Since embolisation often requires multiple treatment sessions case-costs can be much higher. The high cost of surgery (£ 1770) reflects the high capital depreciation and running costs of operating theatres. The high cost of gamma-knife radiosurgery (£ 4500) reflects a high capital depreciation cost and additional factors that are not costed for the other treatments.

Policy costs are given in Fig. 1–3. Policy I is the simplest policy but is not the cheapest because of the high cost of multiple embolisations for the larger AVMs. Policy II without preoperative embolisation is the cheapest because the number of embolisations is reduced and most of the nonsurgical AVMs are large and receive the cheaper linear accelerator radiosurgery. Policy II with preoperative embolisation is the most costly of all the policies. Policy III costs are similar to those of policy II though preoperative embolisation adds less to costs because fewer AVMs are treated surgically.

Discussion

The incidence of new brain AVMs in this series was 3.4 per million population per year. Most (87%) were low risk for surgery which remains their treatment of choice. The relatively high cost of surgery must be accepted for the benefits of rapidly eliminating an AVM which has bled.

We did not attempt to cost all aspects of AVM management. Diagnostic costs prior to treatment are likely to be similar for all the treatment policies. Costs after treatment are likely to depend on the incidence of adverse effects such as bleeding, neurological deficit and death. These will vary with the type of treatment. If costs after treatment are considered, for surgery the 16% risk of new neurological deficit in grade III patients who have not bled seems unacceptably high. This risk would be reduced by adopting policy III. Comparison of the costs of policies II and III shows that the reduced neurological deficits would be achieved without increased treatment costs.

The low cost of embolisation for a single treatment session is not reflected in its impact on policy costs. Preoperative embolisation adds 30–40% to costs. Attempts to eliminate high grade AVMs with embolisation usually require multiple embolisations and result in case-costs that are higher than those of surgery or radiosurgery. Critical cost-benefit analyses are required for embolisation in both treatment contexts.

References

1. Spetzler RF, Martin NA (1986) A proposed grading system for arteriovenous malformations. J Neurosurg 65: 476–483
2. Office of Population Censuses and Surveys (1984) Population and vital statistics. Local and Health Authority Summary. England and Wales. HMSO, London
3. Office of Population Censuses and Surveys (1988) Key population and vital statistics. Local and Health Authority Areas. England and Wales. HMSO, London
4. Forster DMC, Sutcliffe JC (1990) Unwanted effects after stereotactic radiosurgery for cerebral arteriovenous malformations. Proceedings of the Society of British Neurological Surgeons. J Neurol Neurosurg Psychiatry (in press)
5. Steiner L, Greitz T, Lindqvist C, Lindqvist M, Arndt J (1986) Radiosurgery in intracranial arteriovenous malformations. Acta Radiol (Stockh) [Suppl 369]: 769

M. Nelson
Section of Neuroradiology
General Infirmary
Great George Street
Leeds LS1 3EX, UK

Neuroradiology (1991) 33 [Suppl]: 206–208

Neuro radiology
© Springer-Verlag 1991

Radiosurgical treatment of intracranial arteriovenous malformations with gamma knife

H. Bunge, A. Chinela, L. Lemme-Plaghos, J. Antico, J. Guevara, and L. Steiner

Buenos Aires Gamma Knife Centre, Clínica del Sol, Buenos Aires, Argentina

Summary. Long-term follow-up of 194 patients with intracranial arteriovenous malformations (AVMs) treated with gamma knife radiosurgery is reported. One hundred and twenty-seven had more than 2 years of clinical and CT follow-up. Eighty-six underwent control angiograms more than 2 years after irradiation, showing complete obliteration in 71 cases (81.4%); partial in 13 (15%) and no changes in 3 (3.5%). Five patients (2.6%) suffered rebleeding before complete obliteration, and 6 (3.1%) showed definite neurological deficit of probable radiation aetiology. Gamma knife radiosurgery can be considered as an alternative in AVM treatment.

Key words: Arteriovenous malformation – Radiosurgery – Gamma knife

Brain arteriovenous malformations (AVMs) are congenital vascular abnormalities which present clinically with bleeding, seizures, progressive neurological deficit or other symptoms. The treatment of choice is the complete resection of the lesion, traditionally achieved by surgery. Nevertheless, the development of procedures such as endovascular embolization and stereotactic radiosurgery has provided new therapeutic alternatives that can be used alone or in combination with surgery. Radiosurgery with gamma knife can be a successful and safe approach to those AVMs whose size and location make their surgical removal difficult. It is the purpose of this report to describe the experience gained in the Buenos Aires Gamma Knife Centre, in patients treated with the Leksell stereotactic radiosurgical technique.

Patients and methods

One hundred and ninety-four patients harbouring intracranial AVMs were treated from August 1984 up to March 1988 (32 months). One hundred and forty-five were referred because of spontaneous bleeding, 33 (17%) because of seizures and 16 (8.2%) because of other symptoms. Thirty-seven had had previous surgery and/or endovascular techniques with partial or subtotal resection or occlusion. Ninety-eight were male and 94 were female with an average age of 25.6 years.

The radiosurgical procedure was carried out following the same principles as open stereotactic surgery [1]. A stereotactic frame was fixed to the skull under local anaesthesia, with the exception of children in whom general anaesthesia was performed. Four vessel angiograms were performed by femoral catheterization to identify the AVM's nidus and feeders and determine the stereotactic target. Once the data were available, the coordinates of the single or multiple targets were computerized in order to obtain isodose curves of the three planes (sagittal, coronal and axial) at different levels. Isodose curve diagrams were superimposed on the angiogram films to determine the amount of irradiation to be received by the target and adjacent areas. After this check the coordinates were transferred to the stereotactic frame and the head of the patient was positioned in the collimator helmet for stereotactic irradiation. This procedure was repeated for each treatment in those cases where more than one target was used.

Results

All of the 194 patients have had more than a 2-year follow-up, a period of time considered to be the shortest to assess criteria of definite or partial occlusion of the AVM. Eighty-six have undergone follow-up angiograms which showed complete obliteration in 70 patients (81.4%, Fig. 1), partial in 13 (15%) and no changes in 3 (3.5%, Table 1). In 1 case the angiographic follow-up was carried

Table 1. Results of follow-up angiography (in 194 cases with a 2-year follow-up, about 365 treated)

Type	No.	%
Total obliteration	70	81.4%
Subtotal obliteration	13	15.0%
No changes	3	3.5%
Angiograms	86	100.0%

Table 2. Rebleeding before obliteration (194 cases with a 2-year follow-up)

Outcome	No.	%
No neurological signs	2	1.0%
Death	3	1.5%
Rebleeding	5	2.5%

Table 3. Radiation damage (194 cases with a 2-year follow-up)

Neurological deficit	Cases	%
Transient	6	3.1%
Permanent	6	3.1%
Total	12	6.2%

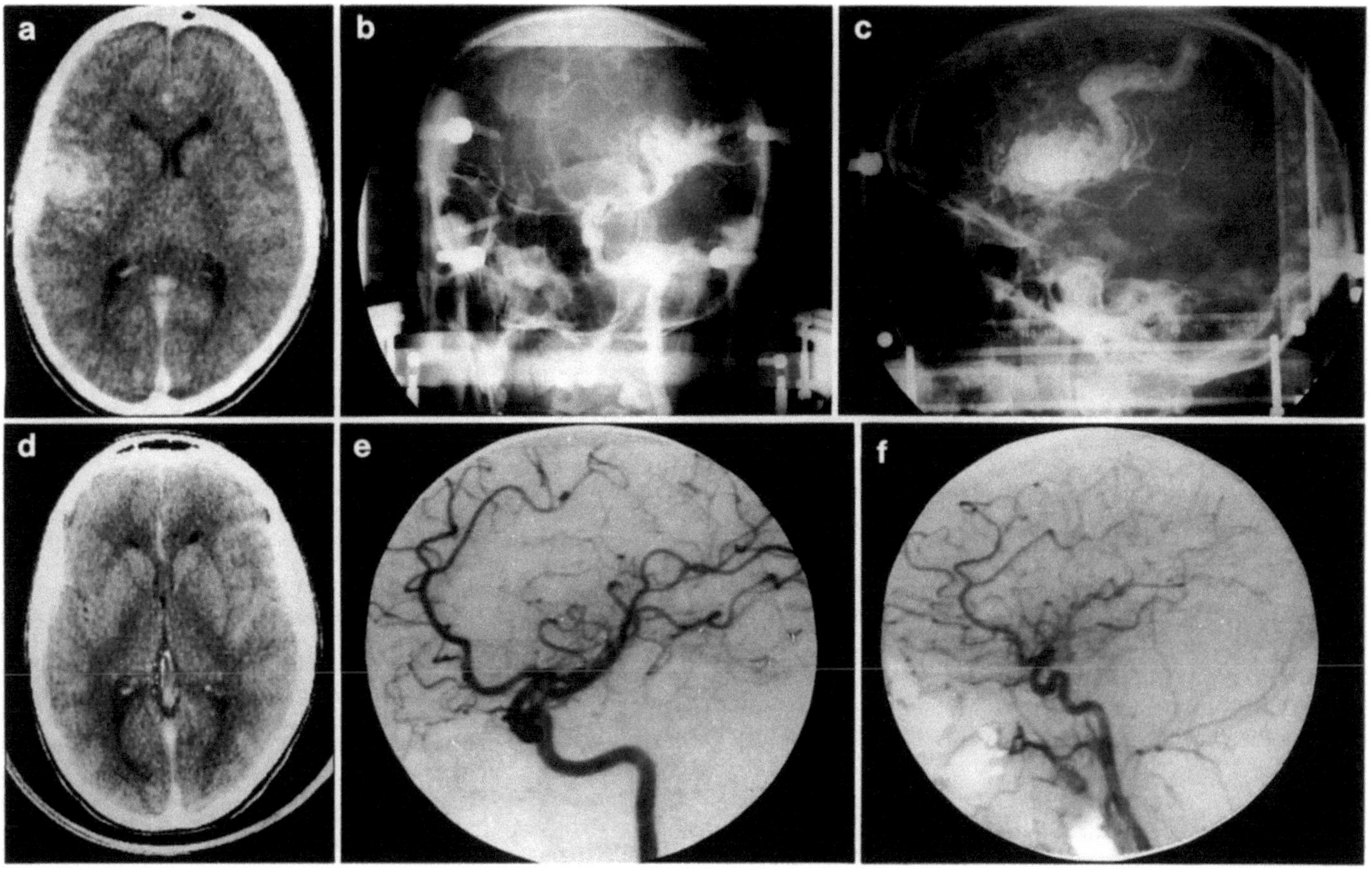

Fig. 1 a–f. Left frontal low convexity arteriovenous malformation (AVM): **a** contrast-enhanced CT; **b, c** stereotactic angiogram; **d** 2 year follow-up contrast-enhanced CT; **e, f** 2-year follow-up angiogram

out 5 years after the treatment and revealed total obliteration of the AVM (Fig. 2). Of the 194 patients, 5 (2.6%) suffered rebleeding before complete obliteration of the AVM; as a consequence 3 (1.5%) patients died (Table 2). Another 12 patients (6.2%) presented neurological deficits induced by the radiosurgical treatment. The symptoms were transient in 6 cases (3.1%) and permanent in 6 (3.1%) (Table 3).

Discussion

The term "radiosurgery" was first introduced in 1951 by Lars Leksell [1], describing single high external dose irradiation of small and medium-size intracranial structures by means of multiple beams of ionizing radiation in mechanically fixed positions [2]. The tool of this technique is the gamma knife, which consists of a heavily shielded unit with 201 ^{60}Co sources which direct beams to a target point. A two-section collimator system with an interchangeable external shield gives dose distributions of different shapes according to the shape and size of the lesion to be treated. The irradiation of small volumes of tissue with minimum damage in the adjacent areas indicates the measure of accuracy of the radiosurgical technique and its high safety rate. In any case, therapeutic doses with multiple targets for volumes larger than 35–40 mm diameter are not indicated because of the risk of radiation-induced damage [3]. The evidence of the changes induced by the ionizing radiation on the vascular endothelium and the subsequent vascular obliteration led Steiner et al. [4] to use the gamma unit for the treatment of AVMs. The mechanism of obliteration of the AVMs which have undergone radiosurgery is not still clearly elucidated. Nevertheless, there is enough evidence that suggests that the proliferation of the endothelial cells and the obliteration of vessels are due to a repair process in the endothelium and media triggered by the radiation. This happens progressively and in the latent period between the treatment and the obliteration of the AVM rebleeding may occur [5].

In our series, of 86 patients followed by angiography, 70 cases (81.4%) showed total and obliteration of the AVM 13 (15.2%) partial, and there was no change in 3 (3.4%). These results agree with other authors [3] (Table 1). The radiosurgical treatment can be repeated if only partial obliteration of the AVM takes place after the first treatment. In 11 cases the radiosurgery was repeated. Rebleeding rate in our series (Table 2) is comparable to that of the natural history of the illness [6]. The radiation-produced changes occurring between the 3rd and 12th month after irradiation produced new neurological deficits or deterioration of previous ones. In routine CT there is a low-density area which may show central contrast enhancement [3]. In our series 6 (3.9%) patients had radiation-induced neurological symptoms (Table 3).

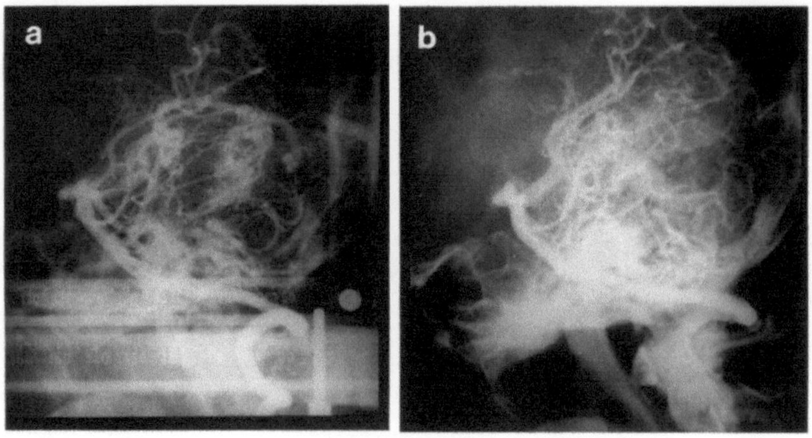

Fig. 2 a, b. Superior vermian AVM: **a** stereotactic angiogram in lateral view; **b** 5-year follow-up angiogram

In conclusion, the use of ionizing radiation from the gamma knife to an AVM achieves complete obliteration in a high percentage and with a low incidence of complications. Radiosurgery is suitable in an AVM which has bled and is not larger than 35–40 mm diameter, located in eloquent areas; in AVMs not larger than 35–40 mm, located in non-eloquent areas and presenting with seizures as a sole symptomatology; and as a complementary treatment after subtotal surgical resection or partial embolization of AVMs.

References

1. Leksell L (1951) The stereotaxic method and radiosurgery of the brain. Acta Chir Scand 103: 316–319
2. Leksell L (1983) Stereotaxic neurosurgery. J Neurol Neurosurg Psychiatry 46: 797–803
3. Steiner L (1988) Stereotactic radiosurgery with the cobalt 60 gamma unit. In: Schmidek H, Sweet W (eds) Operative neurosurgical techniques, vol 1. Grune and Stratton, New York, pp 515–529
4. Steiner L, Leksell L, Greitz T (1972) Stereotaxic radiosurgery for cerebral arteriovenous malformations. Report of a case. Acta Chir Scand 138: 459–464
5. Steiner L (1985) Radiosurgery in cerebral arteriovenous malformations. In: Fein J, Flamm E (eds) Cerebrovascular surgery, vol 4. Springer, New York Berlin Heidelberg, pp 1161–1215
6. Brown RD, Wiebens DO, Forbes G (1988) The natural history of unruptured intracranial arteriovenous malformations. J Neurosurg 68: 352–357

Dr. H. Bunge
Centro de Radiocirugía
Clínica del Sol
Arenales 1468
(1061) Buenos Aires
Argentina

SESSION 15
INTRACRANIAL INFECTIONS

Neuroradiology (1991) 33 [Suppl]: 210–212

Neuro radiology
© Springer-Verlag 1991

Indian experience of the controversies in CT morphology of infective brain lesions

S. Gupta

Department of Radiology, G. B. Pant Hospital, New Delhi, India

Summary. Two cases of solitary intracranial tuberculoma followed up by CT over the last 2 years are discussed because of their atypical appearances. One midline cerebellar lesion showed a speck of enhancement (followed up on MRI); after a shunt procedure the patient improved on antituberculous treatment. The second patient presented with a fit and had a normal CT initially. After a poor response to anticonvulsants, CT 18 weeks later showed homogeneous enhancement and oedema. On antituberculous treatment the response was encouraging at 4 months, but after 8 months of therapy a recurrence of the lesion was observed at the same site. A change in drug therapy produced the desired result.

Key words: Computed tomography morphology – Tuberculoma – Cerebellum – Homogeneous enhancement – Recurrence

CT appearances of intracranial tuberculomas have varied from a ring enhancement to a homogeneous disc enhancement [1, 2]. There is a variable degree of surrounding oedema – depending on the activity of the lesion and/or the response to antituberculous treatment. Van Dyk [3] suggested that a target sign was pathognomonic of an intracranial tuberculoma.

Chosen from more than 150 cases observed over a period of 2 years, the two cases illustrated here indicate the controversial and unusual CT appearances of tuberculoma.

Case reports

Case 1

A 35-year-old woman presented with a severe headache and marked cerebellar signs in July 1988. She was irregularly treated with broad-spectrum antibiotics for fever and sinusitis for 6 months. Fever upto 101°F and a raised erythrocyte sedimentation rate at 45 mm, were noted and examination of the cerebrospinal fluid (CSF) showed a mild increase in proteins (50 mg%). CT (Fig. 1) revealed dilatation of all four ventricles and a midline speck of enhancement in the cerebellum. No supratentorial lesion was observed. A diagnosis of posterior fossa tumour was made. A shunt was undertaken to relieve the intracranial pressure and MRI performed 2 weeks later (Fig. 2) showed the ventricles to be normal. The cerebellar signs had disappeared but there was an "isodense lesion in the posterior fossa close to the midline". Repeat CT at this stage (Fig. 3) revealed only a speck of enhancement in the posterior fossa, with normal ventricles. A planned craniotomy was postponed and the patient was started on antituberculous treatment. After 6 weeks, her temperature returned to normal and she went back to work. Treatment was continued until March 1990. CT in January 1987, MRI in June 1989 (Fig. 4) and further CT in February 1990 have continued to show the speck of enhancement faintly, but the patient has no symptoms.

Case 2

A 30-year-old woman presented with absence seizures in September 1988. CT at this stage was normal. She was put on anticonvulsants but did not respond well. In February 1989 CT revealed a solitary right parietal homogeneously enhancing lesion (Fig. 5) and a diagnosis of tuberculoma was considered. She was put on antituberculous drugs and reported after 18 weeks for follow-up. CT in June 1989 was normal (Fig. 6) and the treatment was continued. She then had another seizure in late October 1989 (while on treatment) and repeat CT showed recurrence of the lesion at the same site (Fig. 7). A change in therapy from ethambutol to streptomycin and thioacetazone produced marked improvement. She is symptom free and the most recent CT (March 1990) is normal. Serology for neurocysticercosis was negative.

Discussion

In the first of the two cases illustrated the presence of a solitary enhancing lesion in the midline of the posterior fossa presented a very unusual picture and a conservative approach with a carefully monitored response to treatment helped. It is noteworthy that there was no supratentorial lesion. In the second case recurrence of the lesion at the same site (on treatment) is most unusual. It has been reported that paradoxical expansion of intracranial tuberculomas can occur during chemotherapy [4], but a recurrence at the same site is a rare phenomenon. A change in drug therapy has helped the patient.

In a large series reported from India by Bhargava and Tandon [5], neither a solitary midline lesion in the posterior fossa nor a recurrence of the lesion at the same site (while the patient was on treatment) was observed. Furthermore, in neither of these cases was a target sign as described by Van Dyk [3] observed.

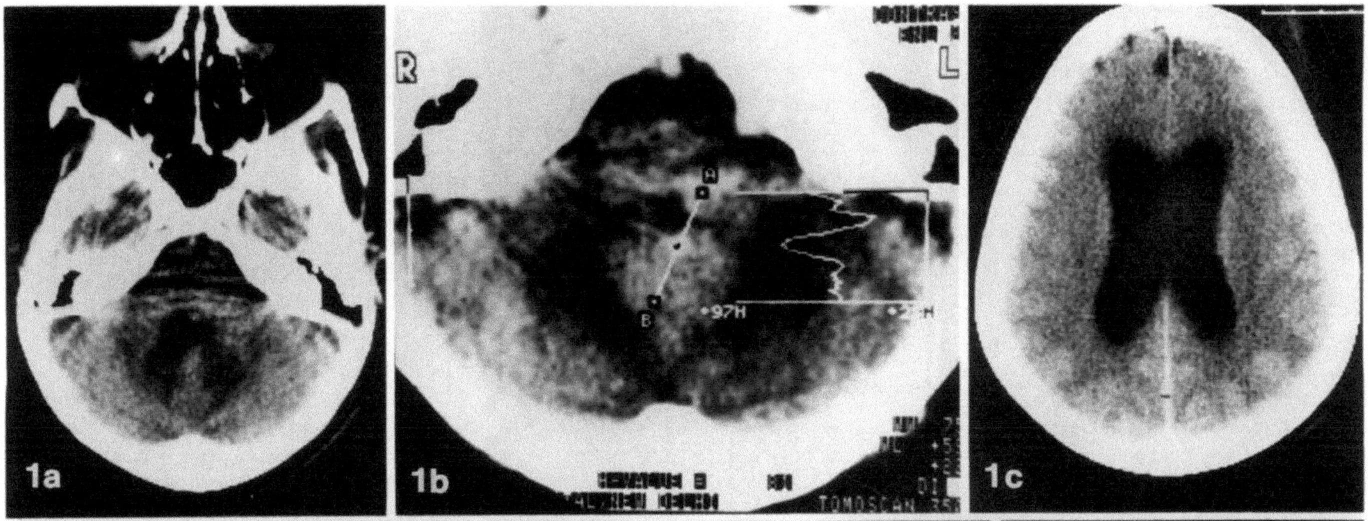

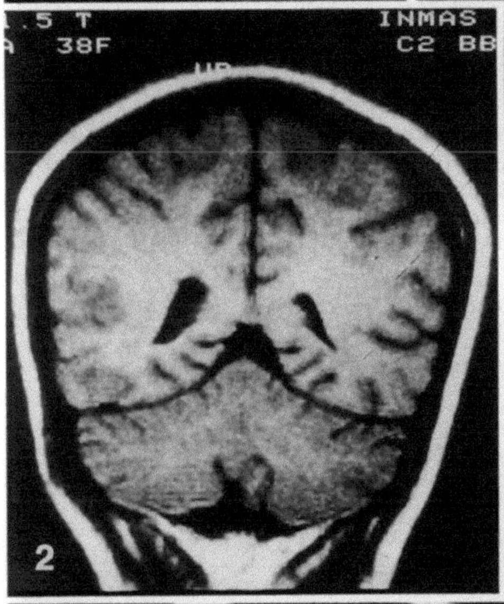

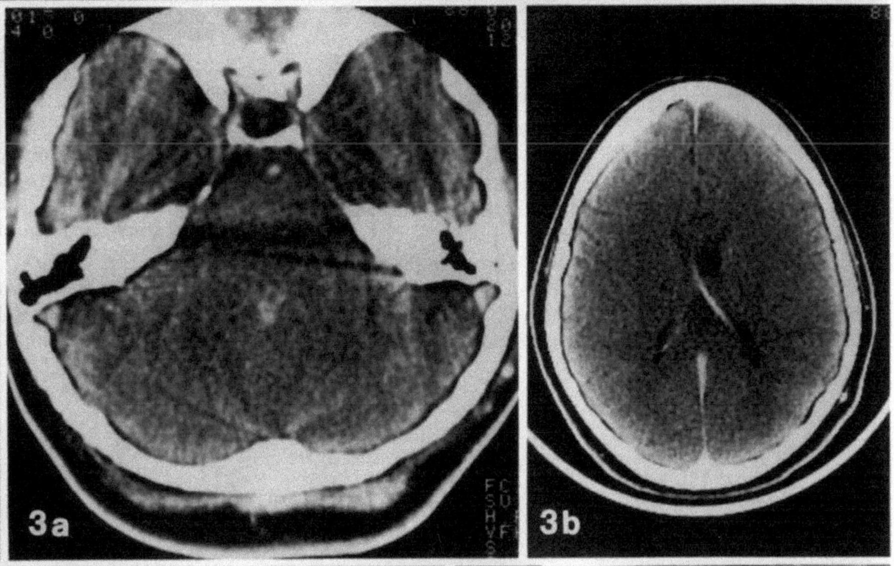

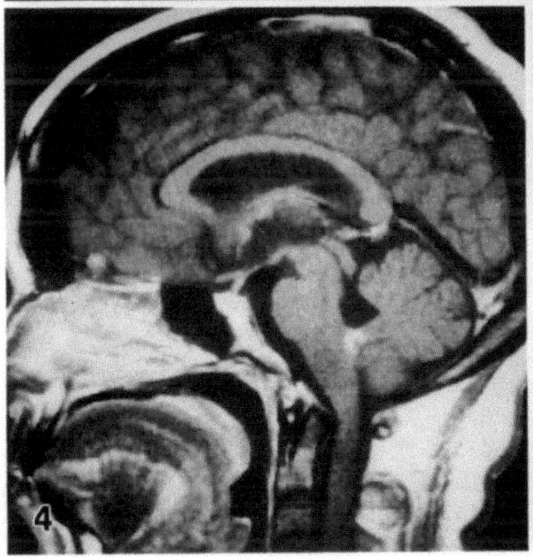

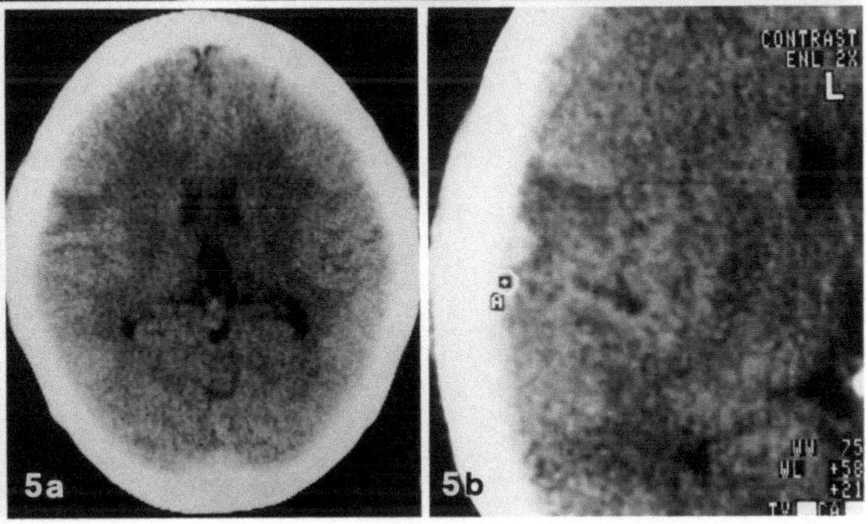

Fig. 1 a–c. CT of patient 1: **a** the posterior fossa shows a dilated fourth ventricle and marked surrounding oedema; **b** Following i. v. contrast medium, there is a midline speck of enhancement (81 HU); **c** symmetrical dilatation of the lateral ventricles

Fig. 2. MRI 2 weeks later, showing an isodence lesion close to the midline, below the fourth ventricle

Fig. 3. a CT (next day) showing only a speck of enhancement, without oedema; **b** the lateral ventricles are of normal size following shunting

Fig. 4. MRI with gadolinium after 11 months showing an enhancing lesion at the outlet of the fourth ventricle

Fig. 5. a CT scan showing a hypodense area in right frontal region; **b** After i. v. contrast medium, there is homogeneous enhancement of a superficial nodule

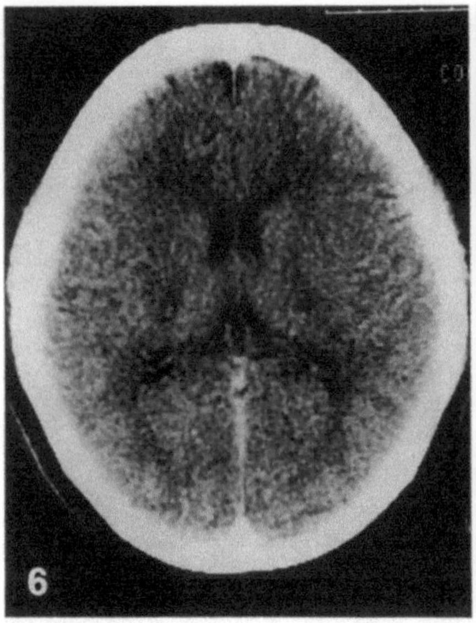

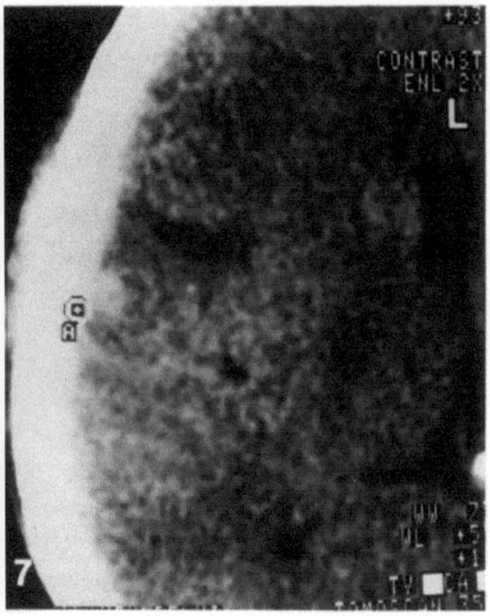

Fig. 6. Normal CT scan after 18 weeks of antituberculous therapy

Fig. 7. CT showing recurrence of the lesion at the same site

References

1. Claveria LF, du Boulay GH, Moseley IF (1976) Intracranial infections. Neuroradiology 12: 59–71
2. Welchman JR (1979) Comouterized tomography of intracranial tuberculomata. Clin Radiol 30: 567–573
3. Van Dyk A (1988) CT of intracranial tuberculomas with specific reference of the "target sign". Neuroradiology 30: 329–336
4. Chambers ST, Hendrickse WA, Record C, Rudge P, Smith H (1984) Paradoxical expansion of intracranial tuberculomas during chemotherapy. Lancet II: 181–184
5. Bhargava S, Tandon PN (1980) Intracranial tuberculomas: a CT-study. Br J Radiol 53: 935–945

Prof. Dr. Suvira Gupta
G. B. Pant Hospital
New Delhi, India

Neuroradiology (1991) 33 [Suppl]: 213–215

Neuro radiology
© Springer-Verlag 1991

Neuroimaging in neurocysticercosis before and after drug therapy

A. Khosla[1], R. K. Goulatia[1], M. K. Bihari[2], M. C. Maheshwari[2], A. Jena[3], and N. K. Mishra[1]

Departments of [1] Neuroradiology and [2] Neurology, Neurosciences Centre, All India Institute of Medical Sciences, New Delhi, India
[3] Institute of Nuclear Medicine and Allied Sciences, New Delhi, India

Summary. CT was carried out before and after intravenous contrast medium in a group of 50 randomly selected patients with neurocysticercosis, before and after drug therapy (praziquantel, albendazole). An attempt was made to correlate CT findings with the clinical presentation. The commonest CT abnormality was multiple high attenuating disciform lesions, with or without perifocal oedema. A high attenuation speck within a ring, suggestive of a scolex, was considered diagnostic. MRI was carried out in 5 cases. The morphology of the lesions was far better shown and more easily appreciated on MRI. Follow-up studies were carried out for 6–36 months after completion of drug therapy. Parenchymal lesions partially resolved in 68% of patients, remained unchanged in 28% and completely resolved in only 2 (4%).

Key words: Cysticercosis – Taeniasis

Cysticercosis is the most common parasitic cause of neurological disease in man [1] and neurocysticercosis (NCC) is caused by the larval form of *Taenia solium*. Clinical manifestations occur when the larvae are deposited in the parenchyma of the brain, spinal cord, meninges, eyes and skeletal muscle. NCC occurs worldwide; its incidence is highly variable and related mainly to sociocultural and economic factors. Its precise prevalence is not known even in endemic areas because the diagnosis can be confirmed only by CT and cerebrospinal fluid (CSF) studies and because of its protean clinical manifestations [2]. The disease has its own particular course in every patient depending upon the host's immune response, the number of parasites, viable or dead, and their location [3]. Improvements in neuroimaging techniques such as CT and MRI, immunological tests (enzyme immunoassay and radio-immunoassay) and the availability of cysticidal drugs (praziquantel and albendazole) have regenerated interest in this subject. We present our observations on pre- and post-treatment neuroimaging of 50 cases seen over the last 3 years.

Patients and methods

The study group includes 50 patients (age range 9 months to 58 years) and 36 of these were males. Most of the patients (88%) presented with a seizure disorder, followed by raised intracranial pressure in 16 patients (32%), intellectual deterioration in 6 (12%) and cortical venous thrombosis in 1 (2%). On clinical examination subcutaneous nodules were detected in 22 patients, focal neurological deficits in 8 and bilateral papilloedema in 20.

The patients included in this report had CT findings suggestive of NCC with biopsy-proven subcutaneous nodules and/or supportive cysticercosis serology (enzyme immunoassay). The CT patterns suggesting NCC were: (1) multiple hyperdense pinheads; (2) multiple focal, round, low density lesions (pockmarks); (3) multiple peripherally enhancing ring lesions with or without perifocal oedema. Signet rings, with an eccentrically placed hyperdense nodule suggestive of a scolex, were diagnostic; (4) diffuse brain swelling with slit ventricles and multiple, nodular or ring-like enhancing areas; (5) intraventricular filling defects on CT ventriculography.

CT (Somatom DRH scanner) was obtained in all cases and the patients were followed up for 6–36 months. For analytical purposes grading of the lesions on the initial CT study was as follows:

Grade I: 0–5 lesions; grade II: 6–10; grade III: 11–20; grade IV: 21–50; and grade V: in hundreds.

The response to treatment was evaluated: (1) no change in CT findings; (2) demonstrable reduction in number of disc lesions or ring lesions to at least one lower grade; (3) change from ring to disc lesions; (4) reduction or disappearance of low-density areas; (5) return to normal.

Twenty patients were treated with praziquantel 50 mg/kg per day for 15 days and 20 patients had albendazole 15 mg/kg per day for 10–30 days, while the remaining 10 patients had courses of both praziquantel and albendazole because of recurrence or non-remission of symptoms.

Three patients with intraventricular cysts had a dilated ventricular system with no parenchymal lesion and were diagnosed on ventriculography only. These patients did not respond to anticysticercal drug therapy.

Five patients underwent MRI. A 9-month-old girl with multiple ring lesions on CT was suspected to have multiple tuberculomas, but MRI demonstrated multiple cysts with scolices. Follow-up MRI after praziquantel therapy revealed a reduction in the number of lesions.

Results

We will discuss our observations according to the treatment.

Treatment with praziquantel (20 patients)

Nine patients were given oral steroids during the course of praziquantel therapy. Four patients had a severe reaction on starting treatment, in the form of raised intracranial pressure, recurrent seizures and marked deterioration of sensorium. Minor side-effects such as nausea, giddiness, anorexia, blurring of vision, paraesthesiae, etc., were observed in 14 patients. In 2 cases treatment was stopped within 72 h due to severe reactions. These side-effects

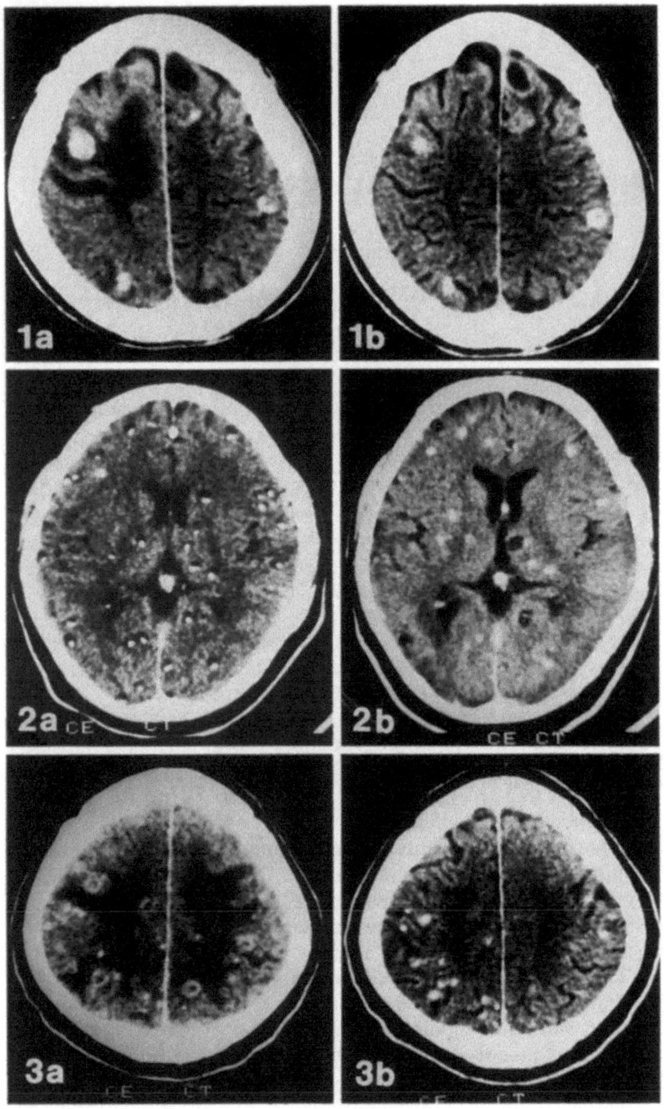

Fig. 1. **a** CT before treatment with praziquantel (October 1988); **b** CT after treatment (December 1988) demonstrates better defined ring lesions, reduction in size of disc lesions and disappearance of perifocal low density

Fig. 2. **a** CT before treatment with albendazole (April 1987); **b** CT following treatment (April 1989) reveals marked reduction in number of ring and disc lesions with conversion of ring lesions to discs

Fig. 3. **a** CT before treatment with praziquantel (September 1987). Following treatment (May 1988) CT was unchanged; **b** additional course of albendazole given (July 1989). CT shows marked reduction of white matter low density, conversion of ring lesions to discs and reduction in number of lesions

were managed conservatively, without significant morbidity in most cases.

There was no change in CT findings up to 1 year in 6 patients.

There was a demonstrable change in CT morphology after therapy in 14 patients: significant reduction in the number of disc or ring lesions in 6 (30%), conversion of signet ring/ring lesions to disc lesions (Fig. 1) in 5 (25%), and reduction in size or disappearance low-density areas in 7 (35%). None of our patient's CT studies returned to normal or near normal during 3–12 months follow-up.

Treatment with albendazole (20 patients)

In 5 patients oral steroids were added because of minor reactions on starting albendazole therapy, including headache, myalgia, vomiting and raised intracranial pressure. One patient developed drug-induced hepatitis. There was no change in CT appearances as compared with the pretreatment scan in 5 patients. There was a significant reduction in the number of disc and/or ring lesions in 10 patients, signet ring/ring lesions changed to discs in 5 and low-density areas disappeared or reduced significantly in 7 (Fig. 2). In 2 patients the CT returned to normal or near normal within a year.

Treatment with praziquantel and albendazole (10 patients)

Seven patients had a repeat course of albendazole at an interval varying from 6 months to 2 years. There had been no clinical or CT response to earlier praziquantel therapy in 3 patients and partial clinical and CT resolution of lesions with recurrence of symptoms had occurred in the 4 remaining patients.

On repeat therapy there was definite reduction in the number of lesions, disappearance or reduction in size of low-density areas and conversion of ring lesions to discs in all patients (Fig. 3), but in none of them did the CT return to normal.

Three patients treated with albendazole and steroids demonstrated partial resolution of lesions on CT and were given an additional course of praziquantel because of non-remission of symptoms.

Three patients who had cysts within the fourth ventricle, with hydrocephalus, did not respond to drug therapy and were subjected to surgery.

MRI delineated the scolex better and obviated a need to consider other diagnosis in 5 cases. Follow-up MRI in a 9-month-old girl showed definite reduction in the number of lesions after praziquantel therapy. Contrary to the popular belief that it takes a long time for the patient to become symptomatic after infestation, this 9-month-old child is possibly the youngest case of NCC to have been reported.

Discussion

Praziquantel is an isoquinoline of proven efficacy against a number of tape worm species including that of *T. solium* of pigs [4]. Several uncontrolled studies and reports have stressed the utility of praziquantel in NCC [2, 5–7]. It probably destroys the integument of cysticerci by blocking their ability to obtain nutrition from cyst fluid, thus killing the larvae [4].

Headache, nausea and seizures are common side-effects of praziquantel treatment, which can be managed conservatively. They are possibly due to a strong host-induced inflammatory reaction against the dying parasites and can be life threatening [3, 4]. Concomitant use of steroids in all patients undergoing praziquantel therapy is controversial [8] and there is no difference in cure rate when steroids are added to praziquantel [7]. Some

Table 1. Change in CT findings after drug therapy for neurocysticercosis

Change in CT findings	Drug therapy		
	Praziquantel treated (20)	Albendazole treated (20)	Both drugs (10)
No change	6 (30%)	5 (25%)	3 (30%)
Partial resolution	14 (70%)	13 (65%)	7 (70%)
(a) Reduction in number of discs and/or rings	6 (30%)	10 (50%)	4 (40%)
(b) Conversion from ring to disc lesions	5 (25%)	5 (25%)	7 (70%)
(c) Reduction in size or disappearance of low density areas	7 (35%)	7 (35%)	7 (70%)
Complete resolution	0	2 (10%)	0

workers believe that some lesions may be in a degenerate state, so that no change is evident after drug therapy. Similar observations were noted in 5 of our patients treated with albendazole and 6 of those treated with praziquantel. Albendazole, an imidazole derivative, has recently been demonstrated to be effective in treatment of parenchymal NCC [9, 10].

Comparing the effectiveness of albendazole and praziquantel in bringing about resolution of the various types of lesions seen in NCC we can make the following observations (Table 1).

Albendazole caused a demonstrable reduction in the number of disc and/or ring lesions seen on CT in 50% of patients as compared with 30% of patients treated with praziquantel. Similar observations were made in a previous study by Sotelo et al. [11]. However, there was no significant difference between the two drugs in conversion of ring into disc lesions or resolution of focal areas of low density.

Two of our patients (10%) treated with albendazole showed complete resolution of all lesions on CT; this did not occur in those treated with praziquantel. Robles et al. [7] reported 13% normal CT studies after praziquantel therapy. Multiple hyperdense pinhead lesions with or without calcification represent calcified cysts or granulomas, which are unaffected by these larvicidal drugs and may persist unchanged or resolve with time. Single or multiple cystic lesions, signet ring/rings usually represent viable cysts and respond favourably to larvicidal drugs by complete resolution or changing to discs [2].

This study and the previous study by Sotelo et al. [10] indicate that albendazole was slightly superior to praziquantel; it has the additional advantages of being less expensive and associated with fewer side-effects.

Our retrospective study includes no control group. We find it difficult to combine data from previous studies because of different methodology, different evaluation criteria and subjective interpretation. There is a need for further studies to establish guidelines for chemotherapy for NCC. It is well documented that some parenchymal NCC lesions resolve spontaneously [12], making accurate assessment of the efficacy of the various drugs difficult. It is also possible that new high density lesions may be seen in previously normal areas after therapy because some cysts may not have been visualized originally [7]. We found no significant difference in CT appearances in patients treated with albendazole for periods ranging from 10 to 30 days. To date, it has not been possible to stop antiepileptic medication in any of our patients.

To conclude, two-thirds of patients with parenchymal NCC show changes in CT findings after treatment with larvicidal drugs. There is no clear correlation between clinical status and persistence or disappearance of single or multiple cysts as seen on CT. We feel that parenchymal NCC should in the first instance be treated with albendazole, with follow-up CT after 3 months. If this shows only partial resolution, and symptoms persist, a trial of praziquantel may be attempted. Steroids and other drugs may be used for side-effects, if needed. Intraventricular forms of the disease will usually require surgical intervention. MRI is useful in parenchymal and intraventricular NCC and can be used for follow-up of treated patients.

References

1. Grisolia JS, Wiederholt WC (1982) CNS cysticercosis. Arch Neurol 39: 540–544
2. Del Brutto OH, Sotelo J (1988) Neurocysticercosis: an update. Rev Infect Dis 10: 1075–1087
3. Sotelo J, Guerrero V, Rubio F (1985) Neurocysticercosis: a new classification based on active and inactive forms: a study of 753 cases. Arch Intern Med 145: 442–445
4. Croll WE (1982) Chemotherapy of human cysticercosis with praziquantel. In: Flisser A, Williams K, Laclette JP, Larralde C, Ridaura C, Beltran F (eds) Cysticercosis: present state of knowledge and perspectives. Academic Press, New York, pp 207–218
5. Sotelo J, Escobedo F, Rodríguez-Carbajal J, Torres B, Rubio Donnadieu F (1984) Therapy of parenchymal brain cysticercosis with praziquantel. N Engl J Med 310: 1001–1007
6. Sotelo J, Torres B, Rubio-Donnadieu F, Escobedo F, Rodríguez-Carbajal J (1985) Praziquantel in the treatment of neurocysticercosis. Long term followup. Neurology 35: 752–754
7. Robles C, Sedano AM, Vargas Tentori N, Galindo-Virgens (1987) Long term results of praziquantel therapy in neurocysticercosis. J Neurosurg 66: 359–363
8. Nash TE, Neva FA (1984) Recent advances in the diagnosis and treatment of cerebral cysticercosis. N Engl J Med 311: 1492–1496
9. Escobedo F, Penagos P, Rodríguez J, Sotelo J (1987) Albendazole therapy for neurocysticercosis. Arch Intern Med 147: 738–741
10. Sotelo J, Penagos P, Escobedo F, Del Brutto OH (1988) Short course of albendazole therapy for neurocysticercosis. Arch Neurol 45: 1130–1133
11. Sotelo J, Escobedo F, Penagos P (1988) Albendazole vs praziquantel for therapy for neurocysticercosis; a controlled trial. Arch Neurol 45: 532–534
12. Miller B, Grinnell V, Goldberg MA, Heiner D (1983) Spontaneous radiographic disappearance of cerebral cysticercosis: three cases. Neurology 33: 1377–1379

Prof. Dr. R. K. Goulatia
Department of Neuroradiology
Neurosciences Centre
All India Institute of Medical Sciences
New Delhi – 110029 India

Neuroradiology (1991) 33 [Suppl]: 216–218

Neuro radiology

© Springer-Verlag 1991

MRI: more specific than CT in cranial tuberculomas

S. B. Desai[1], V. C. Shah[2], O. J. Tavri[2], and P. Rao[2]

[1] Jascor Hospital and Research Centre, Bombay, India
[2] Magnetic Resonance Imaging Department, Breach Candy Hospital and Research Centre, Bombay, India

Summary. A retrospective analysis of 16000 CT studies and 4000 MRIs was carried out. Ninety-seven patients with intracranial tuberculomas were studied by CT and MRI. Variously sized ring or solid enhancing lesions seen on CT showed characteristic uniform hypointense circular lesions or a hypointense lesion with central hyperintense nidus surrounded by high signal intensity oedema on T2-weighted MR images. MR appearances of tuberculomas were found to be specific and different from those of cysticercosis, gliomas, abscesses and metastases.

Key words: Brain infection – Computed tomography – Tuberculoma – Magnetic resonance imaging – T2-weighted images

Intracranial tuberculoma is secondary to haematogenous spread from a primary focus elsewhere in the body, which may be clinically evident or silent. The primary focus is usually pulmonary and is not always detected on chest radiographs [1]. CT continues to be the gold standard in diagnosing brain tuberculoma [2–6]. However, despite considerable experience obtained in the last 10 years, there appears to be no specific CT characteristic exclusive to tuberculoma [2]. We present a retrospective analysis of 97 cases of intracranial tuberculoma.

Materials and methods

Ninety-seven patients with various neurological presentations, usually focal epilepsy, and positive CT findings were studied with MRI (Table 1). Detailed clinical examination, routine investigations including chest radiographs and cerebrospinal fluid (CSF), were done in all cases. Eleven patients underwent surgical intervention (Table 2). The remainder received medical treatment (Table 2). CT was performed on a Siemens Somatom DR-3, a GE-9800, or a Hitachi Scanner.

MRI was obtained on a Siemens Magnetom superconducting magnet operating at 1.0 T. Multiple slice spin echo images were obtained with a short repetition time (TR) of 0.5–0.75 s and a long TR of 2.5–3.0 s. Echo-delay times (TE) of 17, 23 and 90 ms were used. Axial, coronal and sagittal images were obtained. Slice thickness was 5–8 mm with a 0.8–1.6 mm inter-slice gap. Images were acquired on a 256 × 256 or 128 × 256 matrix with a zoom factor of 1.0–1.4. MRI findings were compared with available CT studies.

Results

Prior to the advent of CT, diagnosis of intracranial tuberculoma was usually presumptive and confirmed only at surgery or at autopsy [7, 8].

CT appearances of intracranial tuberculomas have been extensively described in the literature [1–6]. Earlier publications described a solitary solid or ring-enhancing lesion on CT as characteristic of tuberculoma [1, 4–6, 9, 10]. However, many recent publications have discounted this theory [2, 11–14] and there appear to be no specific CT characteristics of tuberculoma.

In our series, we did not see any consistent CT density or enhancement pattern in intracranial tuberculomas. Some were interpreted as infiltrating gliomas (Fig. 1), ectopic pinealomas (Fig. 2) etc., as they presented an atypical CT appearance. Only excisional biopsy provided the answer in these cases. Whilst tuberculoma is a rare manifestation of tuberculosis in the developed countries, it is one of the common lesions seen in India [9]. Many disease processes may mimic the CT appearances of tuberculomas. Thus, even in post-CT days, CT diagnosis of tuberculoma remains essentially presumptive [2, 11, 14, 15]. It is usually based on findings such as a high degree of clinical suspicion supported by laboratory data, the age of the patient, and most important a positive therapeutic response to antituberculous treatment.

Histologically the mature tuberculomas are denser than the adjacent brain tissue. The rim formed by granulation tissue and compressed glial tissue is more dense than

Table 1. MR tuberculoma: signal intensity pattern (97 patients)

T1-weighted images	Hypo-to isointense	97
T2-weighted images	(a) Hypointense	72
	(b) Hypointense lesion with hyperintense nidus (target sign)	19
	(c) Irregular hyper-intensity	6
	(d) Perifocal oedema	97

Table 2. MR tuberculoma: 97 patients

Biopsy proven	– 11 (11.34%)
Therapeutic response	– 73 (75.26%)

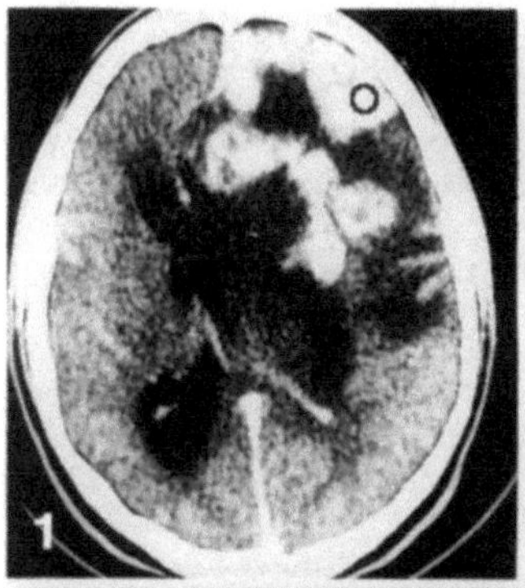

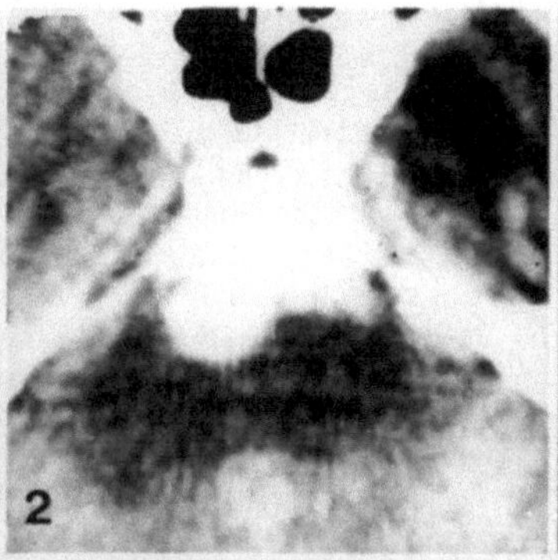

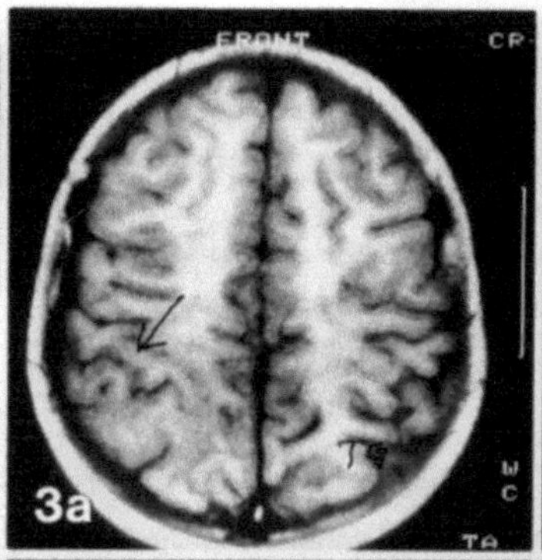

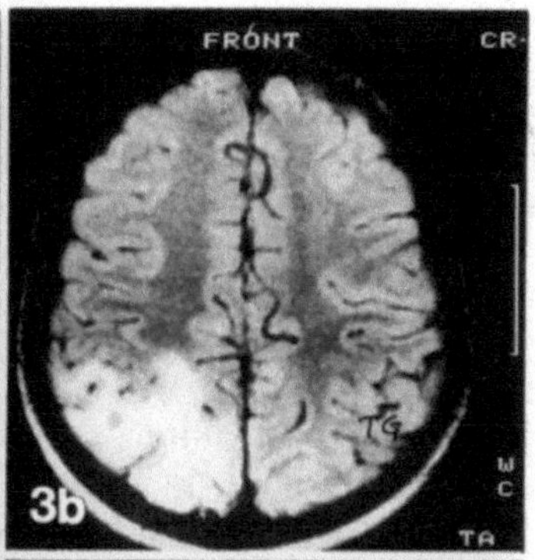

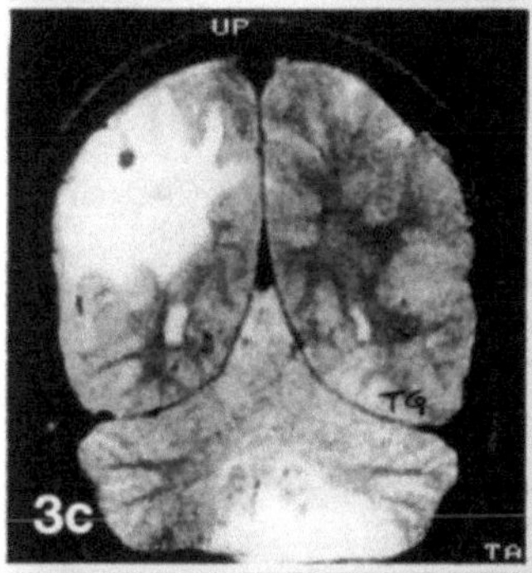

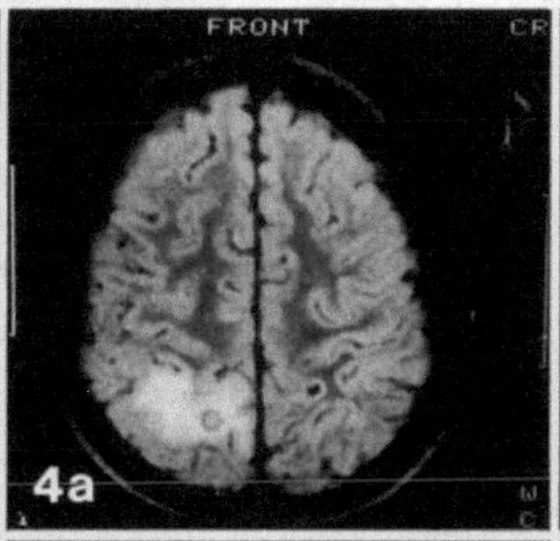

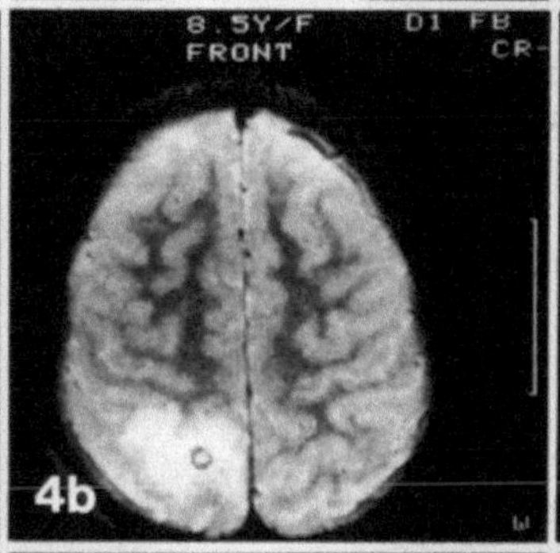

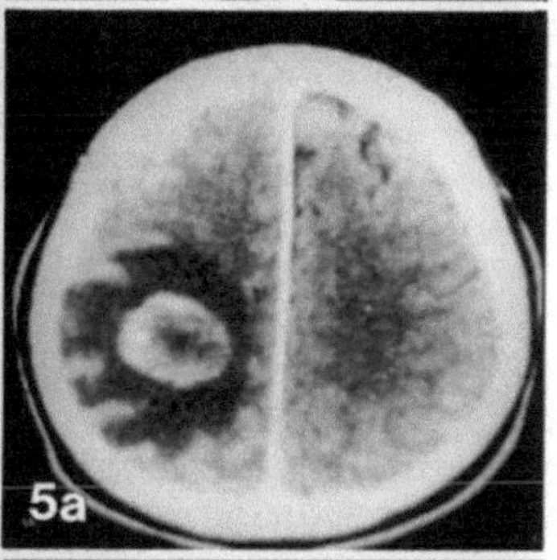

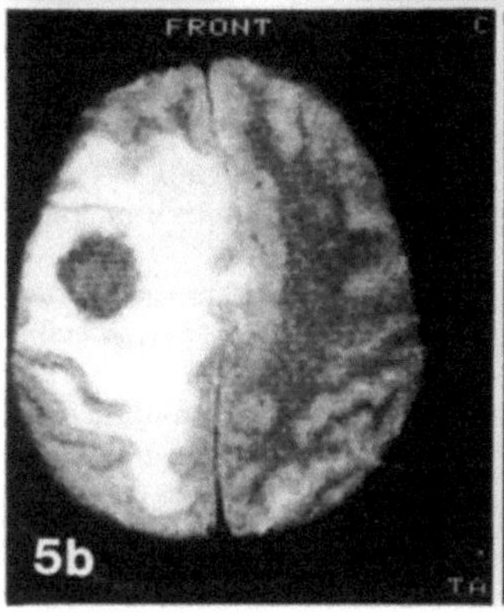

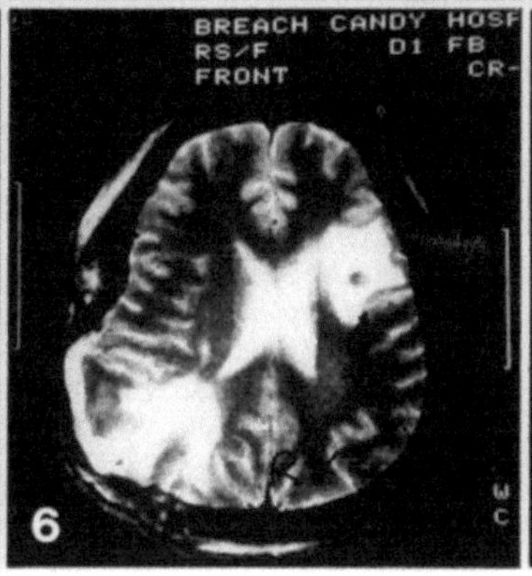

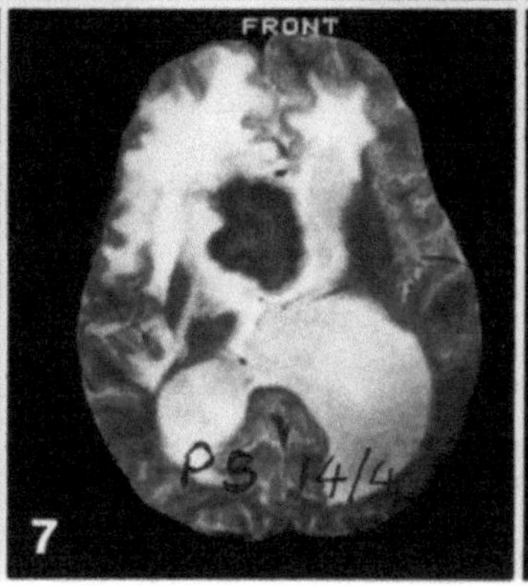

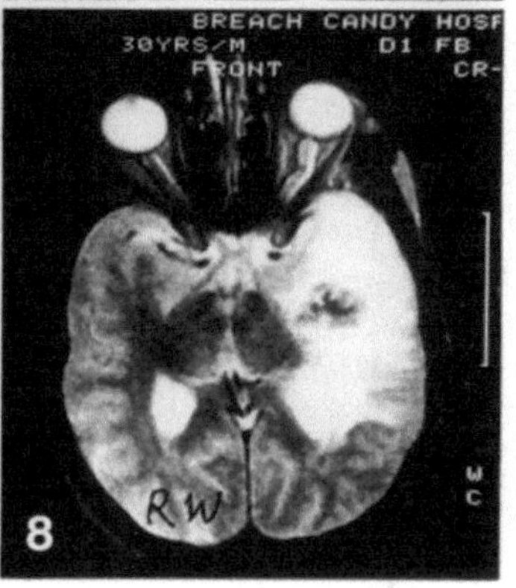

Fig. 1. Axial CT showing infiltrating and enhancing left frontal lobe tuberculoma

Fig. 2. Axial CT, irregular enhancing suprasellar tuberculoma

Fig. 3 a–c. Classical MR appearances in tuberculoma. **a** T1-weighted axial MRI: ill-defined hypointense lesion. **b** Proton density axial MRI: decreased signal intensity of lesion. **c** T2-weighted coronal image: marked hypointensity of lesion surrounded by perifocal hyperintense oedema

Fig. 4 a, b. First and second echo of axial MR of "target sign" – hyperintense nidus surrounded by hypointense lesion

Fig. 5. **a** Axial CT – ring enhancing mass. **b** Biopsy-proven T2-weighted axial MRI of tuberculoma

Fig. 6. T2-weighted axial MRI reveals classical hypointense tuberculoma

Fig. 7. T2 W1 axial MR – Tuberculoma

Fig. 8. T2W axial MR – left temporal hypointense tuberculoma

the centre. The tuberculoma has a gritty central core of caseation. The liquefaction usually starts in the centre.

Retrospective analysis of our 97 cases revealed specific appearances on MRI (Table 1). All of these patients showed the lesion(s) to be iso- to hypointense on T1-weighted images (Fig. 3 a) and it was difficult to appreciate the lesion separate from the surrounding hypointense oedema. On proton density images, all these lesions were better defined and appreciated separate from surrounding oedema (Fig. 3 b). On T2-weighted MR images, 72 of these 97 cases revealed a marked decrease in their signal intensity and appeared hypointense (Fig. 3 b) and the lesion stood out prominently against hyperintense oedema. These probably represented solid tuberculomas without central necrosis. In 19 patients a tuberculoma revealed a central hyperintense nidus within the hypointense lesion, surrounded by minimal hyperintense oedema. The central necrosis gave this bright signal. We called this a "target sign" (Fig. 4 a, b). This represents a mature tuberculoma.

Six patients revealed an irregular increase in the signal intensity of tuberculoma on T2-weighted images. There was an appreciable time gap between CT and baseline MRI studies. They had received anti-TB therapy, prior to MRI studies, which may explain the reversal of the classical pattern observed in these patients.

Biopsy confirmation of the lesion (interpreted as tuberculoma) based on the above MR criteria was obtained in 11 patients (Figs. 5, 6). The therapeutic response was an indicator in 73 patients; 13 patients have been lost to follow-up.

Discussion

The differential diagnosis of tuberculomas on CT includes other granulomas (cysticercosis being the commonest), abscess, glioma and metastases.

Cysticercosis has CSF-equivalent homogeneous intensity on both T1- and T2-weighted images, a demonstrable scolex and thin isointense rim distinguishing it from tuberculomas. Cerebral abscesses, on MRI, reveal a well-defined hypointense lesion, on T1-weighted images and homogeneous hyperintensity with an isointense rim and perifocal oedema on T2-weighted images. However, tuberculomas with large areas of central necrosis reveal a hypointense rim on T2-weighted images. Vascular malformations, glioma and metastasis have distinct MR appearances [17–19] and should not be confused with tuberculomas.

We feel that the MR appearance of iso- to hypointense lesion on T1-weighted images (intermediate T1) which becomes progressively hypointense from proton density to T2-weighted images (short T2) is pathognomonic of tuberculoma. The target sign visualised in some cases correlates with the maturity of tuberculomas.

In conclusion, the MRI appearances of cranial tuberculoma are more specific than CT. Intermediate T1 and short T2 are characteristics of tuberculoma and explain the pathological changes seen in tuberculomas.

References

1. Price HI, Danziger A (1978) Computed tomography in cranial tuberculosis. AJR 130: 769–771
2. Ganapathy K, Rajeshwari R, Kalyanaraman S (1989) Tuberculoma of the brain – recent concepts. Prog Clin Neurosci: 103–113
3. Bhargava S, Gupta AK, Tandon PN (1982) Tuberculous meningitis: a CT study. Br J Radiol 55: 189–196
4. Welchman JM (1979) Computerised tomography of intracranial tuberculomas. Clin Radiol 30: 567–573
5. Whelan MA, Stern J (1981) Intracranial tuberculoma. Radiology 138: 75–81
6. Draonat S, Abdenabi B, Ghenam M, Bourjat P (1987) Computed tomography of cerebral tuberculoma: J Comput Assist Tomogr 11: 594–597
7. Dastur HM, Desai AD (1965) A comparative study of brain tuberculomas and gliomas based upon 107 case records of each. Brain 88: 375–396
8. Dastur DK, Lalitha VS, Udani PM, Parekh U (1970) The brain and meninges in tuberculous meningitis – gross pathology in 100 cases and pathogenesis. Neurology (India) 18: 86–100
9. Wadia RS, Makhale CN, Kelkar AV, Grant KB (1987) Focal epilepsy in india with special reference to lesions showing ring or disc like enhancement on contrast computed tomography. J Neurol Neurosurg Psychiatry 50: 1298–1301
10. Bhargava S, Tandon PN (1980) CNS tuberculosis. Lessons learnt from CT studies. Neurology (India) 28: 212
11. Jain S, Mishra NK, Maheshwari MC (1989) Disappearing CT lesions in epileptic patients – Indian experience. Prog Clin Neurosci: 45–55
12. Bhatia S, Tandon PN (1988) Solitary microlesions in CT: a clinical study and follow-up. Neurology (India) 36: 139–150
13. Goulatia RK, Verma A, Mishra NK, Ahuja GK (1988) Disappearing CT lesions in epilepsy. Epilepsia 28: 523–527
14. Chandy MJ, Rajashekhar V, Prakash S, Ghosh S, Joseph T, Abraham T, Abraham J, Chandy SM (1989) Cysticercosis causing single small CT lesions in Indian patients with seizures. Lancet I: 390–391
15. Gupta RK, Jena A, Sharma A, Guha DK, Khushru S, Gupta AK (1988) MR imaging of intracranial tuberculomas. J Comput Assist Tomogr 12: 280–285
16. Davidson HD, Steiner RE (1985) Magnetic resonance imaging in infections of the central nervous system. AJNR 6: 499–504
17. Kortman KE, Bradley WG (1988) Supratentorial neoplasms. In: Stark DD, Bradley WG (eds) Magnetic resonance imaging. Mosby, St. Louis, pp 375–424
18. Hasso AN, Fahmy JL, Hinshaw DB (1988) Tumors of posterior fossa. In: Stark DD, Bradley WG (eds) Magnetic resonance imaging. Mosby, St. Louis, pp 425–450
19. Rao KCVG, Lee SH (1988) Cerebrovascular anomalies. In: Stark DD, Bradley WG (eds) Magnetic resonance imaging. Mosby, St. Louis, pp 473–505

Viral Shah
MRI Center
Breach Candy Hospital
60 B Bhulabhai Desai Rd
Bombay 400-026, India

Neuroradiology (1991) 33 [Suppl]: 219–221

Neuro radiology

© Springer-Verlag 1991

Cerebral sparganosis: CT characteristics and pathological correlation

K. H. Chang[1], J. G. Chi[2], S. Y. Cho[5], M. H. Han[1], J. H. Suh[4], D. H. Han[3], K. S. Choi[3], and M. C. Han[1]

Departments of [1] Radiology, [2] Pathology and [3] Neurosurgery, Seoul National University College of Medicine, Seoul, Korea
[4] Department of Radiology, Yonsei University College of Medicine, Seoul, Korea
[5] Department of Parasitology, Chung-ang University College of Medicine, Seoul, Korea

Summary. Fifty CT studies of 34 patients with cerebral sparganosis were retrospectively analysed and correlated with pathological findings. On initial CT, the following characteristics were noted: (1) low density in white matter and cerebral hemisphere associated with ipsilateral ventricular dilatation (30/34, 88%); (2) irregular focal contrast enhancement in cortical or subcortical areas (30/34, 88%); (3) a few small, punctate calcifications (26/34, 76%). On follow-up studies the focal enhancing nodule appeared to change in location (5/16, 31%). The CT findings correlated well with pathological findings showing a chronic inflammatory process with active granulomatous lesions and co-existing encephalomalacia, probably caused by migration of the long-surviving sparganum.

Key words: Brain computed tomography – Brain infection – Brain parasites – Sparganosis

Human sparganosis is a rare parasitic infection caused by a migrating tapeworm larva (sparganum) of the genus *Spirometra*, which has been reported worldwide, but more commonly in East Asia [1–3]. It usually involves the subcutaneous tissue or muscle of the chest, abdominal wall or limbs. Intracranial involvement is extremely rare [2, 4, 5–8]. We present the CT characteristics of cerebral sparganosis with pathological correlation.

Materials and methods

CT studies of 34 patients with cerebral sparganosis, collected in Korea over the 7-year period 1984–1990, were retrospectively analysed and correlated with the histopathological findings. The study included 26 men and 8 women with a mean age of 36 years (range, 7–59 years). A total of 50 CT studies was available; 11 patients underwent more than one CT examination. The diagnosis was made by a positive enzyme-linked immunosorbent assay (ELISA) for sparganum-specific immunoglobulin G antibody in cerebrospinal fluid (CSF) and serum, and was surgically confirmed in 15 patients. The present study includes 12 patients reported previously [9].

All CT studies were performed in the axial plane, using 10-mm-thick contiguous sections, on GE 8800, 9800, or equivalent third-generation scanners, and included pre- and post-contrast scans.

Results

CT features

The most common and characteristic CT findings were a low density area of variable extent in the cerebral white matter (seen in all patients), ipsilateral ventricular dilatation (30/34, 88%) and focal contrast enhancement in the cortical or subcortical areas (30/34, 88%) (Figs. 1, 2). The abnormalities were unilateral in 25 patients (74%), involving the right hemisphere in 9 patients (26%) and the left in 16 (48%). The low-density area was extensive, involving the cerebral white matter including the centrum semiovale, periventricular white matter, the external and/or internal capsule in 17 patients (50%), and was more localised in 6 (18%). In the remaining 11 patients (32%) the lesions were apparently multiple (Fig. 2). The lesions were most frequently observed in the cerebral hemispheres, particularly the frontal lobes and/or parietal lobes. Extension into the external capsule and basal ganglia was not uncommon. The midbrain and cerebellum were rarely affected. The focal area of contrast enhancement seen in 30 patients was approximately 1–3 cm in diameter, and usually present in the cortex or subcortex of the cerebral hemispheres. Another characteristic CT finding was multiple small, punctate areas of calcification, seen in 26 patients (76%) (Figs. 1, 2). In 16 follow-up CT studies on 11 patients, 5 revealed change in location of an enhancing nodule.

CT-pathological correlation

White matter low density with ipsilateral ventricular dilatation. White matter around the worm itself or worm tract showed organising oedema and fibrillary gliosis associated with a considerable loss of myelin.

Enhancing areas of the lesion. The worm was surrounded by a dense collagenous wall which varied in thickness and maturity from case to case and in areas in the same case. Next to the collagenous wall was a zone of granulation tissue with many newly formed capillaries, macrophages and lymphocyte/plasma cell infiltration. Highly vascular granulation tissue zone and surrounding gliotic white matter could account for the enhancement.

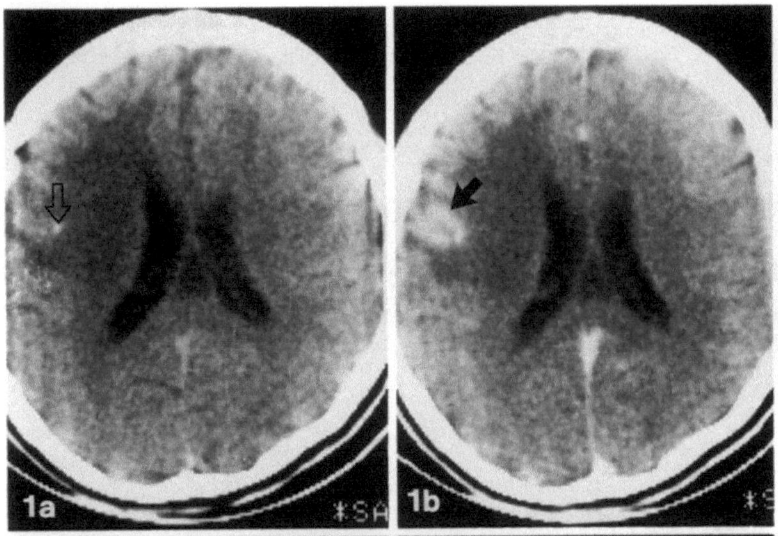

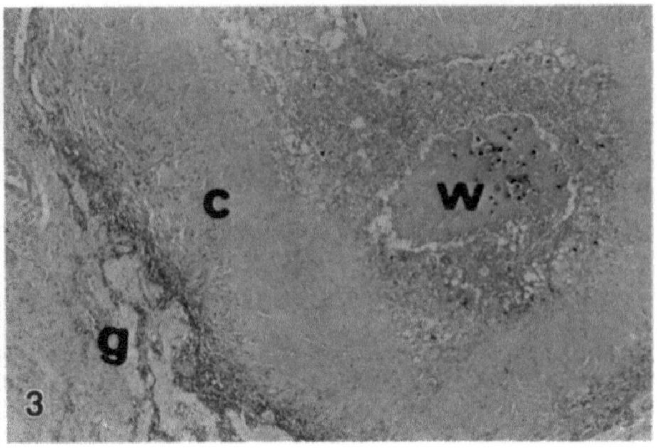

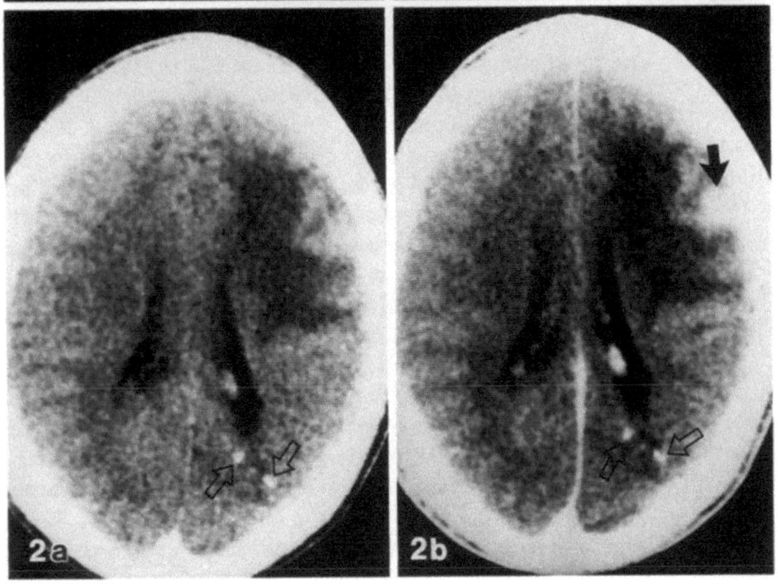

Fig. 1. CT before (**a**) and after (**b**) i. v. contrast medium reveals punctate calcification *(open arrow)*, an extensive low-density area in the white matter and nodular cortical enhancement *(arrow)* in the right frontal and parietal lobes. The enhancing area proved to be a granulomatous lesion surrounding a dead worm

Fig. 2. CT before (**a**) and after (**b**) i. v. contrast medium shows a large area of low density in the white matter associated with irregular nodular cortical enhancement *(arrow)* in the left frontal lobe. There are two small areas of calcification *(open arrows)* with a focal low-density area in the left parieto-occipital region. The ipsilateral lateral ventricle is slightly dilated. Sparganosis was confirmed at surgery

Fig. 3. Histological specimen of the brain shows a worm granuloma consisting of a dead worm *(w)*, surrounding dense collagen tissue *(c)* and glial inflammatory reaction *(g)* (haematoxylin and eosin, × 40)

Punctate calcification. The degenerated worm contained a large number of calcospherules in its parenchyma and abundant smooth muscle bundles which can calcify after degeneration. Minimal haemosiderin deposits could also be seen near the worms and the tunnels they had made.

Discussion

Man can be infected in three ways: (1) by drinking untreated water with infected copepods (1st intermediate host); (2) by ingesting raw or inadequately cooked flesh of snakes or frogs (2nd intermediate host) infected with the sparganum; and (3) by applying the flesh of an infected intermediate host as a poultice to the wound. In the present study, 75% of the patients gave a history of eating frogs and/or snakes, suggesting that the most common source of human infection in Korea is ingestion of these reptiles.

The clinical symptoms and signs varied depending upon the location and extent of the lesions. Seizure is the most common clinical manifestation, and is usually followed after some years by progressive hemiparesis. No patient in the present series had the acute form of the disease.

Preoperative diagnosis is known to be extremely difficult, because of the rarity of the disease, even in the endemic areas. Since characteristic CT findings were reported [9], and ELISA for sparganosis was found highly sensitive and specific [10], cerebral sparganosis has increasingly been diagnosed and confirmed at surgery in Korea. We believe that the CT triad of extensive low density of white matter with adjacent ventricle dilatation, irregular nodular enhancing lesion(s) and punctate calcification, is virtually pathognomonic of cerebral sparganosis, especially in endemic areas. In fact, 9 of 15 cases confirmed at surgery were correctly diagnosed on CT findings without clinical or serological information preoperatively. The CT triad represents widespread degeneration of the white matter associated with an active inflammatory process around the worm, alive or dead, as shown by the pathological specimens. These particular CT findings are considered to be related to a combined effect of long survival and active movement of the worm in the brain tissue and probably also to histotoxic effects of proteases secreted by the worm [11].

References

1. Cho SY (1983) Diphyllobothriasis and sparganosis. In: Weatherall DJ, Ledingham JGG, Warrell DA (eds) Oxford textbook of medicine. Oxford University Press, Oxford, pp 5448–5449
2. Cho SY, Bae JH, Seo BS, Lee SH (1975) Some aspects of human sparganosis in Korea. Korean J Parasitol 13: 60–77
3. Muller JF, Hart EP, Walsh WP (1963) Human sparganosis in the United States. J Parasitol 49: 294–296
4. Chi JG, Chi HS, Lee SH (1980) Histopathologic study on human sparganosis. Korean J Parasitol 18: 15–23
5. Anders K, Foley K, Stern E, Brown WJ (1984) Intracranial sparganosis: an uncommon infection – case report. J Neurosurg 60: 1282–1286
6. Fan KJ, Pezeshkpour GH (1986) Cerebral sparganosis. Neurology 36: 1249–1251
7. Anegawa S, Hayashi T, Ozuru K (1989) Sparganosis of the brain. Case report. J Neurosurg 71: 287–289
8. Yamashita K, Akimura T, Kawano K, Wakuta Y, Aoki H, Gondou T (1990) Cerebral sparganosis mansoni. Report of two cases. Surg Neurol 33: 28–34
9. Chang KH, Cho SY, Chi JG (1987) Cerebral sparganosis: CT characteristics. Radiology 165: 505–510
10. Kim H, Kim SI, Cho SY (1984) Serological diagnosis of human sparganosis by means of micro-ELISA. Korean J Parasitol 22: 222–228
11. Fukase T, Matsuda Y, Akihama S, Itagaki H (1985) Purification and some properties of cysteine protease of Spirometra erinacei plerocercoid (Cestoda; Diphyllobothriidae). Jpn J Parasitol 34: 351–360

Dr. K. H. Chang
Department of Diagnostic Radiology
Seoul National University Hospital
28 Yongon-dong Chongno-gu
Seoul 110-744, Korea

Neuroradiology (1991) 33 [Suppl]: 222–224

Neuro radiology
© Springer-Verlag 1991

Impairment of central nervous system in leprosy: CT and MRI

J. L. Dumas[1, 2], J. Hugon[1], P. Brugieres[2], O. Barbancon[3], Y. Al Qubati[4], A. Gaston[2], and J. Laffont[5]

[1] Institute of Tropical Neurology, Limoges, France
[2] Department of Neuroradiology, Hôpital Henri Mondor, Créteil, France
[3] French Medical Mission, Taez, Yemen Arab Republic
[4] City of Light Hospital, Taez, Yemen Arab Republic
[5] Department of Neuroradiology, Hôpital Bretonneau, Tours, France

Summary. Leprosy is an infectious disease which induces hypertrophic neuropathy. Impairment of the central nervous system (CNS) is exceptional and not documented in the radiological literature. Results of brain CT in six Yemeni leprosy patients with clinical signs of corticospinal tract involvement and prolonged central conduction times in motor evoked potentials are reported. Two patients aged 45 and 48 years had a lacunar lesion in the external part of the lentiform nucleus; neither had evidence of cardiovascular disease or metabolic disorder. Another 51-year-old leprosy patient without evidence of CNS impairment showed on MRI a lacunar lesion below the lentiform nucleus with a normal cardiovascular status. In the early literature, the presence of Hansen bacillus in brain perivascular spaces associated with endothelial lesions was described. Lacunar type infarction (type I lacunae of Poirier neuropathological classification) or dilatation of Virchow-Robin spaces (type IIIc lacunae) could account for these lacunar lesions observed in our leprosy patients.

Key words: Leprosy – Central nervous system – Computed tomography – Magnetic resonance imaging – Lacunar lesions

Leprosy is still of world-wide importance; it is a chronic disease due to Hansen bacillus infection, characterized by peripheral nerve involvement. Impairment of the central nervous system (CNS) is usually considered unusual [1]. It has not been documented in the radiological literature.

This study was designed to investigate CNS lesions in leprosy. We report the results of brain CT carried out in a selected leprosy population with suspected lesions of CNS on a clinical and neurophysiological grounds. A case of brain magnetic resonance imaging (MRI) is also included.

Patients and methods

In a population of 30 Yemeni and Senegalese patients suffering from lepromatous and tuberculoid forms of leprosy we first carried out a clinical and neurophysiological study. All patients had a neurological examination.

Central motor pathway assessment using motor evoked potentials was used [2]. Eighteen of the patients (60%) had prolonged central motor conduction times. Results were compared to those in 16 control subjects from Yemen and Senegal living close to the leper colonies [3]. The location and aetiology of the detected abnormality is unknown but these results indicate that subclinical lesions of the CNS may be present in these patients with leprosy.

In this selected group of 18 patients with prolonged central motor conduction times, CT was carried out in 11, 6 of whom had clinical corticospinal tract involvement. We used a CGR CE 10000 CT scanner, axial adjacent sections of 5 mm, 512 matrix reconstruction, before and after intravenous contrast medium.

In addition, a 51-year-old white leprosy patient with multiple peripheral nerve involvement underwent brain MRI (Thomson CGR Magniscan, 1.5 T) with a sagittal T1-weighted sequence and axial and coronal T2-weighted sequences.

Results

CT was normal in 7 patients. In 2 patients aged 48 and 25 years cerebral atrophy was observed. Two patients had unilateral hypodense zones of lacunar type in the external part of the lentiform nucleus, not enhanced by contrast medim. They were 48 and 45 years old and both demonstrated corticospinal tract involvement (Fig. 1, 2). The white patient, without clinical evidence of CNS impairment, showed on brain MRI a lacunar lesion in the inferior third of the corpus striatum. Its signal was identical to that of cerebrospinal fluid in every echo of each sequences (Fig. 3). CT failed to detect this lacunar lesion.

Discussion

There was no significant difference between the type and the evolution of the disease in the groups of patients with normal and abnormal brain CT. Analysis of the correlation between neurological signs and CT results shows that 3 patients with obvious clinical signs of CNS impairment had normal CT. However, there is a good correlation for the 2 patients with lacunae.

CT demonstrated low-attenuation areas of uncertain significance and MRI displayed location and signal characteristics suggesting an enlarged perivascular space. In the radiological literature MRI and histopathological findings of normal perivascular spaces mimicking lacunar infarction are described [4]. Nevertheless on our CT results the diagnosis of lacunar type infarcts cannot be excluded. Lacunar type infarction (type I lacunes from Poi-

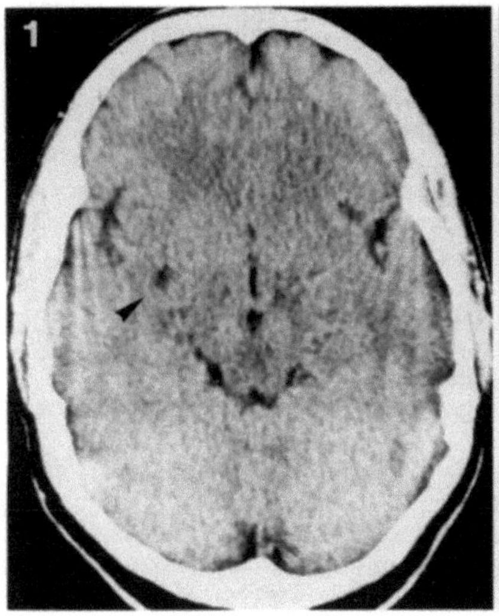

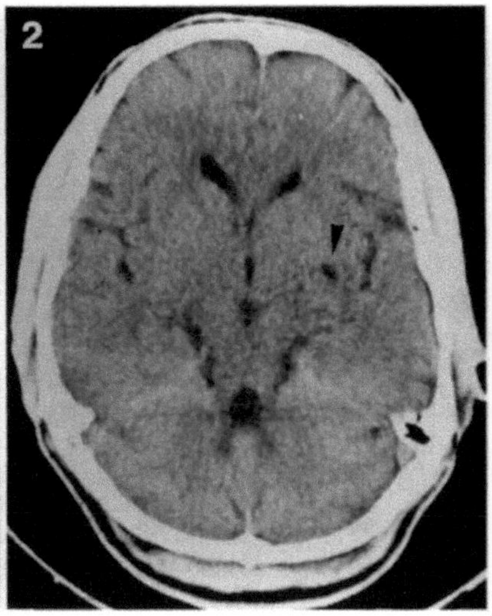

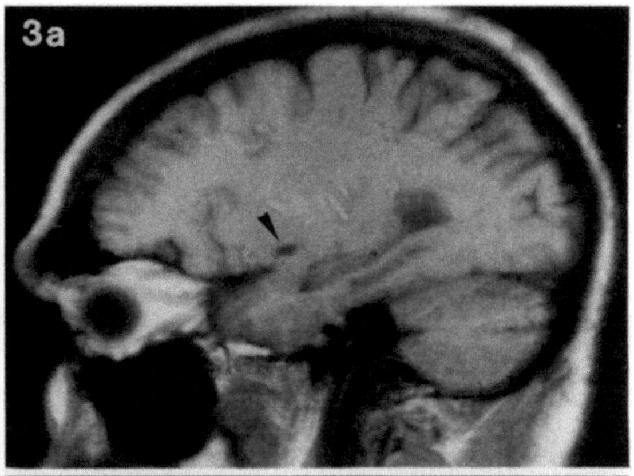

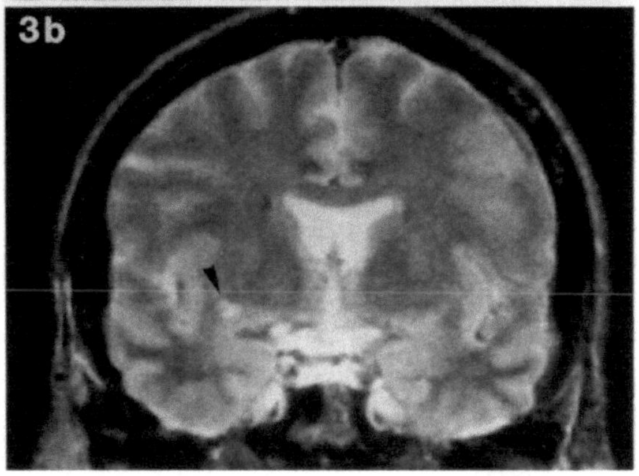

Fig. 1. CT in a 48-year-old Yemeni patient with a borderline tuberculoid form of leprosy and 26-year course. Signs of corticospinal tract involvement were brisk tendon reflexes. CT demonstrates a lacune along the lateral margin of the right putamen *(arrowhead)*

Fig. 2. CT in a 45-year-old Yemeni patient with a lepromatous form of leprosy and 30-year course. Clinical signs of corticospinal tract involvement were diffuse tendon reflexes on the right side with epileptiform jerks of the foot. CT demonstrates a lacune along the lateral margin of the left putamen

Fig. 3 a, b. MR images in a 51-year-old white leprosy patient without clinical evidence of central nervous system impairment. **a** T1-weighted sagittal image shows an oval focus of low-intensity signal. **b** T2-weighted coronal image of same area demonstrates a high-intensity signal in the inferior third of the right putamen. Signal in lacune is identical to cerebrospinal fluid signal in ventricles. MRI displays location and signal characteristics typical of an enlarged perivascular space

rier [5] neuropathological classification) or dilatation of Virchow-Robin spaces (type IIIc lacunes) could account for these possible vascular lesions in lateral striate artery distribution observed in our leprosy patients. In previous studies of relative prevalence both types of lacunar lesions were seen in specimens from predominantly elderly, hypertensive subjects [6]. Lacunar type infarcts are due to the occlusion of a single small penetrating artery by atheroma, lipohyalinosis, fibrinoid necrosis or embolization and involve mainly the basal ganglia. Virchow-Robin space dilatation corresponds to a single large perivascular dilatation at the entrance of a perforating artery into the lentiform nuclei. It occurs more frequently in association with hypertension, cortical and subcortical atrophy, and Binswanger's encephalopathy. The mechanisms involved in the formation of these type III lacunes are not clearly understood. An abnormality of arterial wall permeability was suggested by Poirier et al. [7] in a particular case of extensive lacunes with lesions of segmental necrotizing angiitis of the artery supplying the involved territory.

The leprosy patients with lacunar lesions were not elderly, and cardiovascular examination was normal; serological tests for syphilis and retrovirus were negative; and none had evidence of a metabolic disorder.

The relationship between these lacunes and the leprosy is uncertain but involvement of the CNS is supported by the following observations.

Concerning the pathogenesis of leprosy Ridley [8] emphasized that "leprosy cannot be understood without recognition that it is a systemic disease". There is a predilection for cool sites which provide suitable conditions for microbial growth but other tissues often become involved. Bacteraemia occurs in both lepromatous and tuberculoid forms of leprosy and is the main cause of the dissemination of the disease; it results in the bacterial colonization of small blood vessel endothelium. Bacilli are more often present in arterioles and venules than in the capillary endothelium, producing changes of chronic inflammation with endarteritis, thrombosis and recanalization. Hyalinization and fibrosis of arteriole wall can also appear. Vascular lesions are documented in the radiological literature as terminal arteritis [9].

In the early literature some publications reported clinical corticospinal tract impairment in patients with leprosy (Hudelo et al. 1926 [10], Hesse 1934 [11]) and a syndrome of spastic paraplegia among Melanesian leprosy patients in New Caledonia was described by Desmoulins and Zeldine in 1967 [12]. Hansen meningitis was described by Beurman in 1909, then by Touraine in 1918. There are a few reports of anatomical or bacteriological involvement of central nervous structures in leprosy: degeneration of posterior ascending tracts (Jeanselme and Pieere-Marie in 1898), presence of Hansen bacillus in spinal cord [13] (Chassiotis in 1887, Garcin in 1961) in brain cortex (Babes in 1889, Collela in 1890) and thalamus wall (Lie in 1930). The most famous observation is the one of

Grieben in 1960 [14], who described a case of intracerebral lepromatous abscess, Moreover, brain perivascular lesions have been reported. Zenoni in 1904 described the presence of Hansen bacillus in the brain perivascular spaces and observed a perivascular hyperplasia of the glia. Stahlberg in 1906 described thickened cerebral vessels; their endothelium had proliferated and contained pigmentary bodies. Harada and Takashima in 1956 reported a case of meningo-encephalitis in a patient with lepromatous leprosy and observed bacilli in the perivascular macrophages of the frontal cortex.

Recently, Job et al. [15] showed neuronal cells and glial cells containing intracellular bacilli in brains from nine-banded armadillos with lepromatous leprosy.

Conclusion

This study indicates that vascular lesions of central nervous structures may be present in patients with leprosy. It emphasizes the need to carry on neuroradiological and histopathological studies of the CNS in Hansens disease to confirm this suspected involvement.

References

1. Sebille A (1983) Multinévrites lépreuses. Encyclopédie Médico-chirurgicale, Neurologie, Paris, pp 1–4
2. Hugon J, Lubeau M, Tabaraud F, Chazot F, Vallat JM, Dumas M (1988) Potentiels évoqués moteurs. Technique, résultats chez le sujet normal. Rev Neurol (Paris) 144: 91–95
3. Dumas JL, Hugon J, Al-Qubati Y, Barbancon O, Petit G, Vialard Y (1989) Prolonged central motor conduction time in leprosy patients. XIVth World Congress of Neurology, New Delhi, 22–27 October 1989. Neurology (India) 37 [Suppl]: 276
4. Jungreis CA, Kanal E, Hirsch WL, Martinez AJ, Moossy J (1988) Normal perivascular spaces mimicking lacunar infarction: MR imaging. Radiology 169: 101–104
5. Poirier J, Derouesne C (1984) Cerebral lacunae. A proposed new classification. Clin Neuropathol 3: 266
6. Braffman BH, Zimmerman RA, Trojanowski JQ, Gonatas NK, Hickey WF, Schlaepfer WW (1988) Brain MR: pathologic correlation with gross and histopathology. 1. Lacunar infarction and Virchow-Robin spaces. AJR 151: 551–558
7. Poirier J, Barbizet J, Gaston A, Meyrignac C (1983) Démence thalamique. Lacunes expansives du territoire thalamo-mésencéphalique paramédian. Hydrocéphalie par sténose de l'aqueduc de Sylvius. Rev Neurol (Paris) 139: 349–358
8. Ridley DS (1988) Pathogenesis of leprosy and related diseases. Wright, London
9. Pietra R, Mauduit A (1962) Les lésions artérielles dans la lèpre. Ann Radiol 5: 705–710
10. Hudelo MM, Mouzon, Duhamel (1926) Sur un cas de lèpre nerveuse avec tremblement et symptomes de la série spasmodique (lèpre à forme mixte d'emblée). Bull Mém Soc Méd Hôp Paris 50: 971–976
11. Hesse J (1934) Contribution à l'étude des troubles nerveux de la lèpre. La lèpre du système nerveux central. Thesis, Paris
12. Desmoulins G, Zeldine G (1967) Syndromes paraplégiques en milieu lépreux. A propos de 12 cas observés en Nouvelle-Calédonie. Bull Soc Pathol Exot 60: 482–497
13. Garcin R, Layani F, Lapresle J, Margairaz A, Chaouat Y (1961) Lèpre nerveuse à type de polynévrite sensitivo-motrice des quatre membres. Presse Méd 69: 2597–2600
14. Grieben L (1960) Lepromatous cerebral abscess; bibliography revew and repport of a case. J Int Coll Surg 33: 700–712
15. Job CK, Sanchez RM, Hastings RC (1988) Lepromatous meningoencephalitis in the nine-banded armadillo (Dasypus novemcinctus). Int J Lepr 56: 291–295

Dr. J. L. Dumas
Institute of Tropical Neurology
Faculty of Medicine
2 rue du Docteur Marcland
F-87025 Limoges cedex, France

Neuroradiology (1991) 33 [Suppl]: 225–228

Neuro radiology
© Springer-Verlag 1991

Clinical and radiological aspects of extracerebral empyemas: 39 cases

S. Chanalet[1, 2], D. Gense de Beaufort[1], J. F. Gréselle[1], C. Louail[1], B. Padovani[2], and J. M. Caillé[1]

[1] Service de Neuroradiologie, C. H. R. Pellegrin-Tripode, Bordeaux Cédex, France
[2] Service de Radiologie, C. H. R. Pasteur, Nice Cédex, France

Summary. The authors reviewed 39 cases of extracerebral empyemas with emphasis on clinical and radiological findings. Extracerebral empyemas represent a small percentage of intracranial infections. The erstwhile poor prognosis has been inproved by: (1) early radiological diagnosis with CT and/or MRI; (2) radiological follow-up and early detection of complications such as thrombophlebitis; (3) modifications of surgical treatment and progress of antimicrobial-therapy.

Key words: Empyema – Cerebral thrombophlebitis – Infectious brain diseases

Extracerebral empyemas (ECEs) are extraaxial intracranial purulent collections. They are rare (13%–20% of intracranial suppurations [1, 2]) and serious (8%–12% mortality [3]). Early diagnosis is required to determine appropriate treatment. Modern imaging, together with progress in antibiotic therapy, has considerably improved the prognosis by permitting early diagnosis. However, certain lesions are not detected by the initial CT examination. In these cases, MRI appears a promising technique. ECEs can be classified into four aetiological groups with different clinical characteristics, diagnostic problems and evolution: (1) ENT origin; (2) postcraniotomy and post-traumatic; (3) postmeningitis; (4) unknown.

Patients and methods

The clinical and radiological data of 39 patients with CT diagnosed ECE were analysed in this 10-year retrospective study. CT was performed before and after i. v. contrast medium.

Eight patients underwent angiography, 4 MRI with a Magniscan CGR 0.5 Tesla. No patient received gadolinium (Gd).

Twenty-nine patients were operated upon. In 26, the diagnosis of ECE was confirmed by surgery; in 2, empyema was a surgical finding; the last case was a false positive, clinically and radiologically.

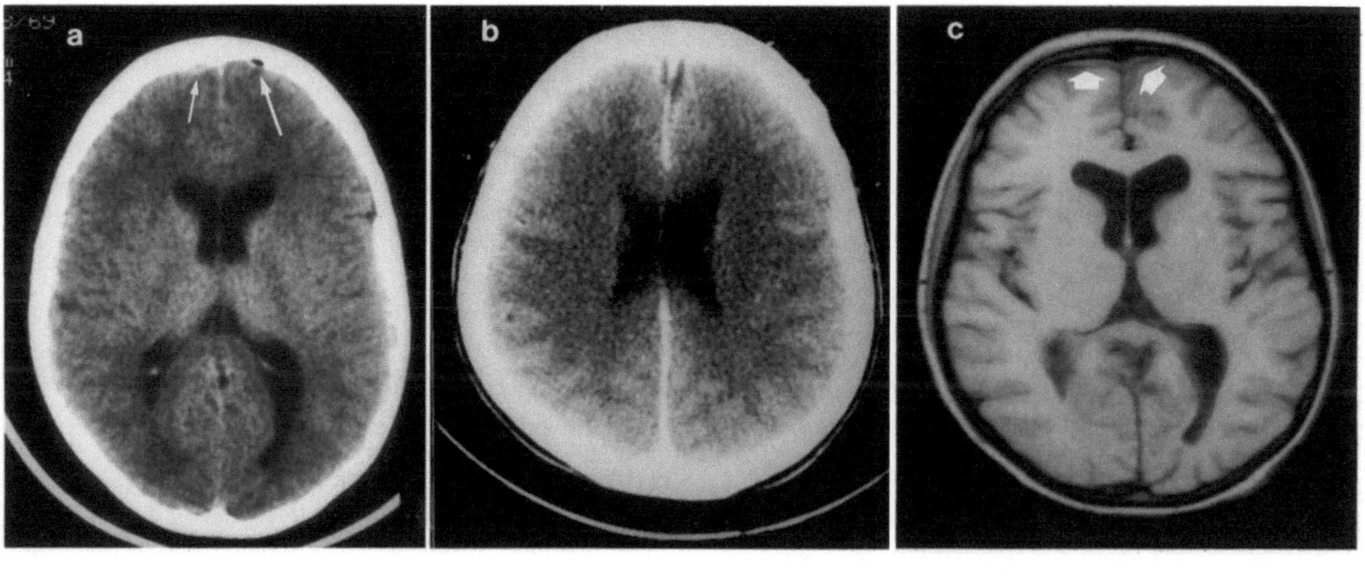

Fig. 1 a–c. Case 9: **a** CT 2 days before hospitalization. Note the left subdural frontal air and the right frontal contrast enhancement. **b** After contrast medium, extracerebral empyemas (ECEs) on both sides of the falx. **c** MRI (TR 500 ms, TE 28 ms). The lateral extension (under the skull vault) is better seen than on CT

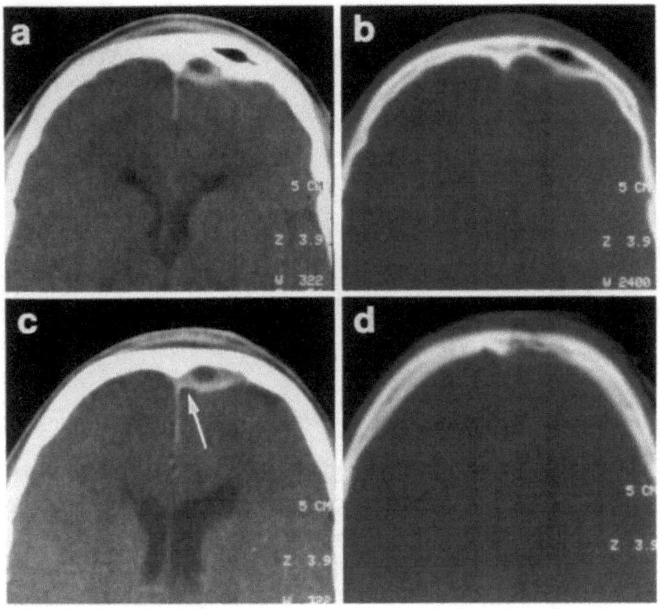

Fig. 2 a–d. CT after contrast medium. ECE after frontal sinusitis. The contrast enhancement of the wall of the ECE (**a**) and the elevation of the superior sagittal sinus on its left side confirm the extradural location of the empyema (**c**). Note the frontal bone osteitis on wide window (**d**)

Results

The 39 patients, 28 men and 11 women, fell into four groups according to the site of origin of the infection.

ECEs of ENT origin (Figs. 1, 2)

There were 17 patients, 13 men and 4 women, 8–72 years old (15 less than 30 years old). All had an acute ENT infection for at least 8 days, most commonly sinusitis or chronic mastoiditis with acute manifestations. Fifteen patients had a fever higher than 38 °C. Fourteen were receiving antibiotics (β-lactamine or macrolide) in the correct dosage with persistence or aggravation of signs of infection.

CT was performed for meningeal inflammatory symptoms (fever higher than 40 °C) accompanied by focal neurological signs in 12 cases, without focal signs in 3 cases and subgaleal empyema in 2 cases. The organisms responsible were found in 10 cases: in 7 from the empyema, in 4 from the cerebrospinal fluid and in 4 from the ENT focus. Leucocytosis and erythrocyte sedimentation rate greater than 40 were common.

CT was performed between the 1st and 8th days after the onset of clinical signs. An extradural empyema was found in 4 cases, a subdural empyema in 11 patients and 2 false negatives were found at surgery. The first was a patient whose CT was severely degraded by motion artefacts that suggested a frontal cortical abscess. The second had an extradural empyema on the lateral sinus and CT suggested a thrombophlebitis. Three patients with mastoiditis had an empyema in the posterior fossa (Fig. 3), and in 1 patient an associated subdural empyema beneath the tentorium. There was associated thrombophlebitis in 4 patients confirmed by angiography in 2 and by MRI in 1. One of these patients died. Three cases had an associated encephalitis, 3 a parenchymal abscess. In only 2 cases did we find isolated hemisphere oedema, without an associated parenchymal lesion.

Postcraniotomy empyemas

There were 12 patients, 6 men and 6 women, with ages ranging from 9 to 71 years. Three had chronic suppuration 2 months to 3 years old, manifest by local signs only. These patients had a bone flap osteitis associated with an extradural empyema, and CT showed an extremely thick dura mater underlying the collection which enhanced considerably with contrast medium.

The other 9 patients had evidence of infection confirmed by bacteriology 8–13 days after surgery and manifest in 6 as neurological deterioration and high fever. CT revealed 7 subdural empyemas and 1 abscess at the surgery site. The organism was identified in all patients: 6 had *Staphylococcus aureus* and 6 *Enterobacter, Acinetobacter* or *Pseudomonas*.

Postmeningitis empyemas

There were 5 boys and 1 girl, 10 days to 1 year old. Five patients had meningitis with 4–12 days duration; the 6th had a month history. CT was performed to find a lesion that could explain persistent fever, sleepiness and seizures, despite appropriate antibiotic therapy. Four children were operated upon. In 1, despite typical clinical and radiological features the bacteriology of the subdural collection was negative. This was the only false positive of our series.

ECEs of unknown origin

Four men, 39–69 years old had neurological symptoms and evidence of infection evolving over 8–15 days, and no known site of entry. CT revealed 4 subdural empyemas. All 4 were operated upon; 1 patient had a secondarily infected chronic subdural hematoma. A right frontoparietal subdural empyema was associated with a right frontal lobe abscess. An extradural empyema at the site of osteitis of the left frontal inner table was associated with thrombophlebitis of the anterior two-thirds of the superior sagittal sinus.

Discussion

ECE remains a serious disease. In our series, there were 3 deaths (8%). Two were old, in poor general state and the other an 11-year-old girl with an empyema associated with extensive thrombophlebitis of the superior sagittal sinus. This mortality rate is low in comparison to older series

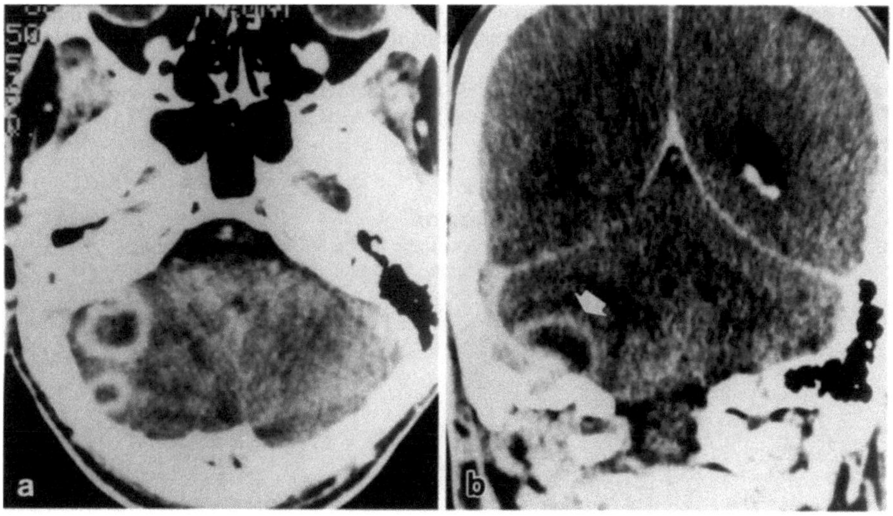

Fig. 3 a, b. CT after contrast medium. **a** This axial slice shows two abscess cavities with enhancing walls in the right cerebellar hemisphere. **b** The subdural empyema is evident on this coronal slice. Note displacement of the cerebellar cortex, and right mastoid opacification

(26% reported by Mauser et al. [4], 12% in a more recent series of 49 patients [3]).

This condition affects young men: the mean age was 23.5 years [1]. The male predominance is more apparent in the empyemas of ENT origin, with 70% of cases in the study by Mauser et al. [4]. In our series, 28 patients (72%) were men, and 13 of 17 empyemas of ENT origin (76%) were in men.

In the empyemas of ENT origin, frontal sinusitis is more commonly encountered. Four to 10% of sinusitis result in intracranial complications and 40%–90% of ECEs are secondary to sinusitis [5]. There are two main mechanisms: retrograde venous spread following thrombophlebitis and spread through bone following an osteitis, which carries a risk of thrombophlebitis if in contact with a venous sinus. The responsible organisms were anaerobic in 78% of cases, 12% were *Staphylococcus* [6].

The frequent presence of multiple organisms should be emphasized. The two main reasons are blind antibiotic therapy and the lack of routine search for anaerobic bacteria [7]. In chronic ENT infections one can find anaerobic bacteria that produce β-lactamase and inhibit phagocytosis. Moreover, antibiotics have poor penetration to regions affected by osteitis. This explains persistent infection and development of an empyema despite antibiotic treatment.

Postcraniotomy ECEs appear in specific compartments, so extension is limited and the risk of thrombophlebitis is low. However, extension to the operative site is possible. The most frequently encountered microbes are *Staphylococcus* (50%) and nosocomial micro-organisms causing problems of antibiotic resistance.

Postmeningitis empyemas complicate subdural effusions. Twenty to 50% of cases of meningitis in children less than 1 year old are complicated by sterile subdural effusions; 2% of these are secondarily infected and become subdural empyemas. The organisms responsible are those that produce meningitis: *Haemophilus influenzae* is most commonly found. The risk of thrombophlebitis is minimal.

The contribution of radiology to the management of ECE is very important. CT makes possible early diagnosis in the majority of cases; the site of entry and the extent of the lesion can be shown. It also allows identification of associated lesions (abscess, thrombophlebitis). MRI has proved to be superior to the CT in the diagnosis of empyemas as for all extra-axial lesions [8, 9]. It shows associated lesions in a more precise manner than CT revealing thrombophlebitis, abcesses and parenchymal oedema. In contrast to Zimmerman et al. [3] and in agreement with Weisberg [10], we think that cerebral oedema is not common in empyemas, due to parenchymal contamination or cortical thrombophlebitis. The injection of Gd should further improve the visualization of empyemas. Angiography is no longer used for the diagnosis of ECE, but allows analysis of the venous drainage when there is cerebral thrombophlebitis.

There are two different types of empyema. In the first, empyemas are secondary to a pre-existing subdural effusion and present the same diagnostic, prognostic and therapeutic problems as cerebral abscesses. In the second, empyemas appear de novo and are frequently of venous origin, giving a high risk of cerebral thrombophlebitis.

Imaging represents the most important step for the diagnosis and management of patients with suspected ECE. Improvement of prognosis of this disease in the past 10 years reflects the spectacular progress of antibiotic therapy and imaging.

References

1. Danziger A, Price H, Schechter MM (1980) An analysis of 113 intracranial infections. Neuroradiology 19: 31–34
2. Morgan DW, Williams B (1985) Posterior fossa subdural empyema. Brain 108: 983–992
3. Zimmerman RD, Leeds NE, Danziger A (1984) Subdural empyema: CT findings. Radiology 150: 417–422
4. Mauser HW, Van Houwelingen HC, Tulleken CAF (1987) Factors affecting the outcome in subdural empyema. J Neurol Neurosurg Psychiatry 50: 1136–1141

5. Carter BL, Bankoff MS, Fisk JD (1983) Computed tomographic detection of sinusitis responsible for intracranial and extracranial infections. Radiology 147: 739–742
6. Kaufman DM, Litman N, Miller MH (1983) Sinusitis: induced subdural empyema. Neurology 33: 123–132
7. Miller ES, Dias PS, Uttley D (1987) Management of subdural empyema: a series of 24 cases. J Neurol Neurosurg Psychiatry 50: 1415–1418
8. Weingarten K, Zimmerman RD, Becker RD, Heier LA, Deck MDF (1989) Subdural and epidural empyemas: MR imaging. AJNR 10: 81–87
9. Sze G, Zimmerman RD (1988) The magnetic resonance imaging of infections and inflammatory diseases. Radiol Clin North Am 26: 839–859
10. Weisberg LA (1986) Subdural empyema: clinical and computed tomographic correlations. Arch Neurol 43: 497–500

Dr. D. Gense de Beaufort
Service de Neuroradiologie. C. H. R. Pellegrin-Tripode
F-3076 Bordeaux Cédex, France

Neuroradiology (1991) 33 [Suppl]: 229–231

Neuro radiology

© Springer-Verlag 1991

Radiological features of adhesive optochiasmatic arachnoiditis

An analysis of 25 cases

K. F. Lee[1,3], Y. E. Lee[4], R. Tang[4], W. S. Fields[5], N. J. Schatz[2], M. J. D. Post[1], and R. Quencer[1]

Departments of [1] Radiology, and [2] Ophthalmology, University of Miami School of Medicine, Miami, Florida, USA
Departments of [3] Radiology, [4] Ophthalmology, and
[5] Neurology, The University of Texas Health Science Center At Houston, Houston, Texas, USA

Summary. Adhesive optochiasmatic arachnoiditis (AOCA) was found to be the most common cause of an ischemic chiasmal syndrome. The etiology of AOCA is diverse: closed head injury, meningitis, radiation therapy, craniotomy for aneurysm, arteriovenous malformation or tumor, sarcoidosis, rheumatoid arthritis, or allergy to myelographic contrast medium appeared to be the cause of fibrosis and scar formation in 23 of 25 cases, while the etiology of the remaining 2 cases is unknown. The radiological features of AOCA are as follows: partial or total obliteration of suprasellar cisterns and the recesses of the third ventricle, atrophy and irregular configuration of the optic chiasm and nerves, fibrous retraction with intrasellar herniation of the optic chiasm, which often shows a "V" shape, occasional arachnoid cyst formation with elevation of the chiasm and indentation of the rostral third ventricle, segmental attenuation of the supraclinoid portion of the carotid, and/or main trunk of the anterior cerebral arteries, and a high incidence of empty sella (89%).

Key words: Optochiasmatic arachnoiditis – Computed tomography – Magnetic resonance imaging – Angiography

Since 1968, we have seen 25 patients diagnosed as having adhesive optochiasmatic arachnoiditis (AOCA). The diagnosis was established by clinicoradiological correlation and long-term follow-up, with surgical or post mortem confirmation in more than three-quarters of cases. The purpose of this communication is to present the radiological features of AOCA on the various imaging procedures performed on our patients.

Materials and methods

Prior to 1974, the mainstay of radiological studies of AOCA was Polytome encephalography with continuous insufflation of nitrous oxide, and 12 patients were investigated by this method and by magnification angiography (Fig. 1). High resolution CT with multiplanar reformation was performed with or without subarachnoid contrast medium (Fig. 2). Since the early 1980s, MRI has been used extensively for multiplanar imaging (Fig. 3). Eight patients had autopsy, and 11 underwent surgery (8 craniotomies and 3 transphenoidal explorations). This series consists of 14 males and 11 females ranging from 8 to 69 years of age, the mean age being 43.2 years.

Results

The etiology of AOCA varies; closed head injury (5 cases), meningitis (4), postoperative radiation therapy (4), craniotomy for tumor (3), subarachnoid hemorrhage from aneurysm or arteriovenous malformation (3), sarcoidosis (2), rheumatoid arthritis (1), exposure to iodinated myelographic, contrast medium (1), and unknown (2).

Clinical findings included headache, progressive visual impairment, visual field constriction, and optic atrophy.

The radiological findings are shown in Table 1.

Discussion

AOCA may produce signs of chiasmal compression, simulating a suprasellar tumor [1, 2]. At the X and XII Symposia Neuroradiologica, we proposed an ischemic chiasmal syndrome (ICS) consisting of five categories [3, 4]. We designated AOCA as type III ICS, the most common cause of a non-tumoral chiasmal syndrome. Polytome encephalography with continuous insufflation of nitrous oxide was employed in the first 12 patients [4], prior to the CT era. This technique provided most useful information as to the pathways of the cerebrospinal fluid (CSF), so that any block of gas or CSF due to AOCA could be readily identified (Fig. 1 A). Magnification angiography was used to demonstrate constriction of the

Table 1. Radiological features of adhesive optochiasmatic arachnoiditis

Distortion/obliteration of basal cisterns	25/25
Deformed and indistinct optic structures	25/25
Empty sella with marked flattening of the pituitary	21/25
Intrasellar retraction of the chiasm	19/25
Obliteration of the third ventricular recesses	18/25
Atrophy of the optic nerves/chiasm	17/25
Segmental constriction of arteries	6/12
Arachnoid fluid collection ("cyst")	3/25

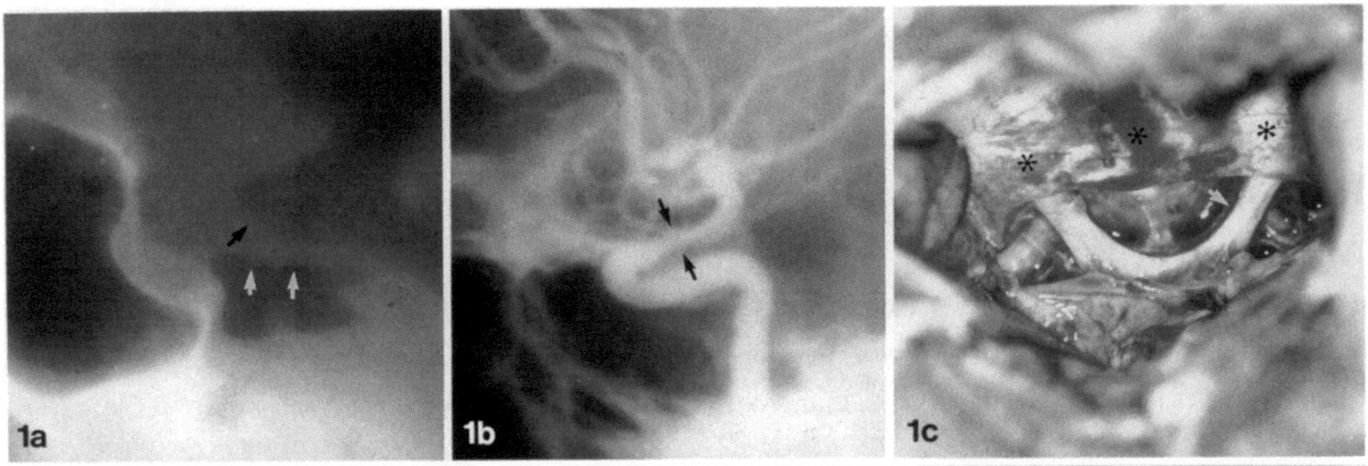

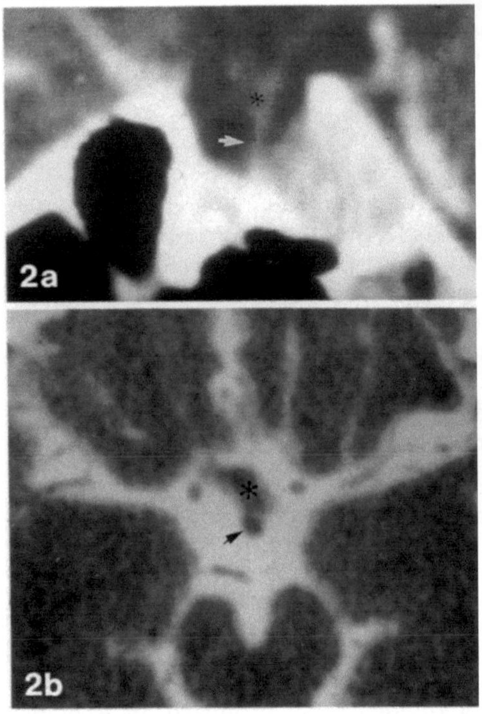

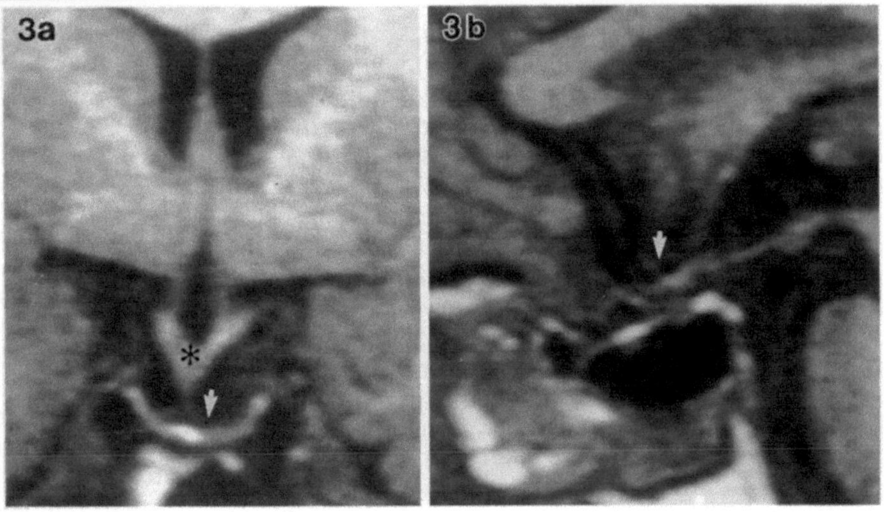

Fig. 3 a, b. A 43-year-old woman with closed head injury. **a** Coronal T1-weighted image shows intrasellar herniation of the chiasm *(asterisk)* with a "V" configuration. Marked flattening of the pituitary gland *(arrow)* is noted, indicating an empty sella. **b** Sagittal T1-weighted image shows low-lying chiasm and anterior cerebral anteries secondary to fibrous retraction. Diffuse fibrosis with thickened arachnoid mater encasing the optic and vascular structures was found at surgery

Fig. 1 a–c. A 31-year-old man with syphilitic meningitis. **a** Polytome encephalography with nitrous oxide insufflation shows obliteration of the recesses of the third ventricle *(black arrow)*, associated with non-filling of the chiasmatic cistern and cisterna lamina terminalis. Gas is trapped in the interpeduncular fossa *(white arrows)*. **b** Carotid arteriogram shows segmental narrowing of the supraclinoid portion of the internal carotid artery *(arrows)* due to fibrous constriction. **c** A surgery, marked thickening of the arachnoid mater *(asterisks)* was noted, associated with atrophy of the left optic nerve *(arrow)*

Fig. 2 a, b. A 34-year-old women with sarcoidosis. **a** CT, sagittal reformatted image, shows intrasellar herniation of the optic chiasm *(asterisk)* associated with elongation of the pituitary stalk *(arrow)* and flattening of the pituitary gland, indicating an empty sella. **b** Metrizamide CT cisternogram shows distortion of the chiasm *(asterisk)*. The *arrow* indicates the pituitary stalk

supraclinoid segment of the internal carotid and/or main trunk of the anterior cerebral arteries (Fig. 1 B).

CT usually shows partial or total obliteration of the pentagonal CSF space in the suprasellar region with an indistinct distorted chiasm, often herniated into the pituitary fossa (Fig. 2 A) in 19 cases; the chiasm was elevated in 3 cases, due to an arachnoid cyst. Accumulation of fluid within the arachnoid, frequently described as a "cyst", may rupture unnoticed at the time of craniotomy since the fluid within the arachnoid does not have a cyst wall but lies enmeshed between the two layers, namely dura mater and pia mater [5, 6].

MRI has a multiplanar imaging capability with excellent delineation of the nervous and vascular structures [7, 8], and it provided most useful information as to the status of the optic nerves and chiasm (Fig. 3); CT with intrathecal nonionic contrast medium (Fig. 2 B) was performed prior to the MRI era. The optic nerves and chiasm usually show more or less profound atrophy; the nerves in particular may be reduced in caliber, and may be flattened. A high incidence of empty sella (21/25) was associated with AOCA. Visual field defect may or may not be present in the presence of empty sella, with intrasellar herniation or fibrous retraction of the chiasm, which often shows a "V" deformity [8, 9]. The visual impairment in AOCA, however, like other types of ischemic chiasmal syndrome, is most likely to be related to the degree of optic nerve or chiasmal ischemia [3, 4, 10]. Surgical treatment of AOCA appears to have a limited success rate, as recurrence of symptoms is not uncommon [9, 11].

References

1. Walsh FB, Hoyt WF (1969) Clinical neuro-ophthalmology, 3rd edn. Williams and Wilkins, Baltimore, pp 2100–2105
2. Vail D (1938) Optochiasmatic arachnoiditis. Arch Ophthalmol 20: 384–394
3. Lee KF, Schatz NJ (1975) Ischemic chiasmal syndrome. Acta Radiol Suppl (Stockh) 347: 131–148
4. Lee KF (1983) Ischemic chiasma syndrome. AJNR 4: 777–780
5. Iraci G, Pellone M, Scuccimarra A (1976) Post-traumatic opto-chiasmatic arachnoiditis. Ann Ophthalmol 8: 1313–1328
6. Walker EA (1962) The neurosurgical evaluation of the chiasmal syndrome. Am J Ophthalmol 54: 563–581
7. Daniels DL, Herfkins R, Gager WE (1984) Magnetic resonance imaging of the optic nerves and chiasm. Radiology 152: 79–83
8. Kaufman B, Tomsak RL, Kaufman BA (1989) Herniation of the suprasellar visual system and third ventricle into empty sellae: morphologic and clinical considerations. AJNR 10: 65–76
9. Lee KF, Richter HA, Tsai FY (1975) Secondary empty sella syndrome. Acta Radiol [Suppl] (Stockh) 347: 313–326
10. Matsumoto M, Miura N, Takinawa T, Yamazaki T (1976) Vascular factor in the adhesive arachnoiditis of the optic-chiasmatic region. Brain Nerve 28: 549–555
11. Welch HL, Stears (1971) Chiasmapexy for the correction of traction on the optic nerves and chiasm associated with their descent into an empty sella turcica. Case report. J Neurosurg 35: 760–764

Dr. K. F. Lee
Department of Radiology
University of Miami School of Medicine
Miami, Florida, USA

SESSION 16
BRAIN DISEASES

Neuroradiology (1991) 33 [Suppl]: 234–237

Neuro radiology
© Springer-Verlag 1991

Acute facial nerve paralysis: gadolinium-DTPA-enhanced MRI

A. M. Wang[1], R. M. Ernstoff[2], D. I. Bojrab[3], D. P. Wesolowski[1], and J. Farah[1]

Departments of [1]Diagnostic Radiology, [2]Neurology, and [3]Otology, William Beaumont Hospital, Royal Oak, Michigan, USA

Summary. T1-weighted (TR 500 ms/TE 15 ms) magnetic resonance (MR) images of the facial nerve before and after intravenous gadolinium were studied in 22 patients with acute facial nerve paralysis (1 patient with acute trauma, 21 patients with Bell's palsy). A total of 33 studies was performed (one-half of the patients had a single study; the others had two studies). Proton density and T2-weighted axial brain MRI was also performed in all the patients. Eighteen patients with Bell's palsy (85.7%) had enhancement of the distal meatal portion of the facial nerve on the symptomatic side (6 patients had enhancement of the meatal portion only, 12 patients had enhancement of the entire intratemporal facial nerve, i.e. meatal, labyrinthine, geniculate ganglion, tympanic and mastoid portions of facial nerve). No enhancement was seen in the normal facial nerve. The brain, pons and cerebellopontine angle were all normal. The facial nerve enhancement demonstrated by MR images is nonspecific; the enhancement patterns of the facial nerve seen in the patients with Bell's palsy with complete or near complete recovery could not be separated from that of the patients with permanent damage.

Key words: Acute nerve paralysis – Bell's palsy – Acute trauma – Magnetic resonance imaging – Gadolinium

---

MRI has been reported to be useful for demonstration of the anatomy of the facial nerve, particularly in its intratemporal portion [1, 2]; in addition, gadolinium(Gd)-enhanced T1-weighted (short TR, short TE) MR images have been shown to be useful for evaluation of facial nerve pathology, by showing enhancement of facial nerve neuromas, of the nerve in Bell's palsy and after temporal bone surgery [3–5]. The object of this study is to utilize Gd-DTPA-enhanced T1-weighted MRI to evaluate the presence and extent of facial nerve enhancement as well as to monitor progression or regression of the disease process in patients with acute facial nerve paralysis.

Patients and methods

The study concerned 22 patients (10 males, 12 females) with ages ranging from 12 to 80 years; 21 patients had Bell's palsy and 1 had acute trauma. All the patients presented with acute unilateral facial nerve paralysis (14 right-sided, 8 left-sided). The patients were divided into two groups; group 1 (11 patients) with only one MRI study and group 2 (11 patients) with two MRI studies. The interval between the acute facial nerve paralysis and the first MRI study ranged from 3 days to 1 month.

The MRI study was performed using a Siemens Magnetom unit operated at 1.0 T with 6 mT/m gradient capability. A circularly polarized head coil was used. In addition to routine axial double spin-echo brain MRI studies (TR 3000 ms/TE 30,90 ms), thin slices (3 mm thickness per slice without gap) of axial and coronal T1-weighted (TR 500 ms/TE 15 ms) MR images with acquisition matrix of 256 × 512 and four acquisitions of each study were obtained through the intratemporal portion of the facial nerve and brain stem before and after intravenous gadolinium.

Results

No abnormality was found in the brain, pons, cerebellopontine angle cistern or proximal internal auditory meatal portion of the facial nerves, or the fallopian canal portion of the facial nerve of the asymptomatic side. In group 1, 3 patients had a normal study and 8 patients had abnormal studies: in 3 patients there was enhancement of the distal meatal portion only and in 5 enhancement of the distal meatal and fallopian canal portions of the symptomatic facial nerve. One patient who showed enhancement of the entire meatal and fallopian canal portions of the right facial nerve underwent surgical decompression, without improvement in the facial paralysis (Fig. 1). The rest of the patients in group 1 made a complete or nearly complete recovery.

In group 2, one patient (acute trauma) with two normal studies had complete recovery of his right-sided facial nerve paralysis. One patient had a normal first study and an abnormal second (enhancement of the meatal and fallopian canal portions of the facial nerve) during a recurrence of the facial paralysis. Nine patients had abnormal first studies; 4 showed enhancement of only the meatal portion of the facial nerve, with a normal second study and complete recovery, and 5 showed enhancement of the meatal and fallopian canal portions of the facial nerve. This resolved at the time of the second study in 4 (including 1 who underwent surgical decompression) who showed complete or moderate recovery, while 1 patient whose second study was still abnormal, but improving, (Fig. 2) showed almost complete recovery.

Discussion

The facial nerve is the longest nerve lying within bone and is the most frequently paralyzed nerve [1]. Its nucleus is located in the pons. It enters the internal auditory meatus accompanied by the cochlear and vestibular divisions of

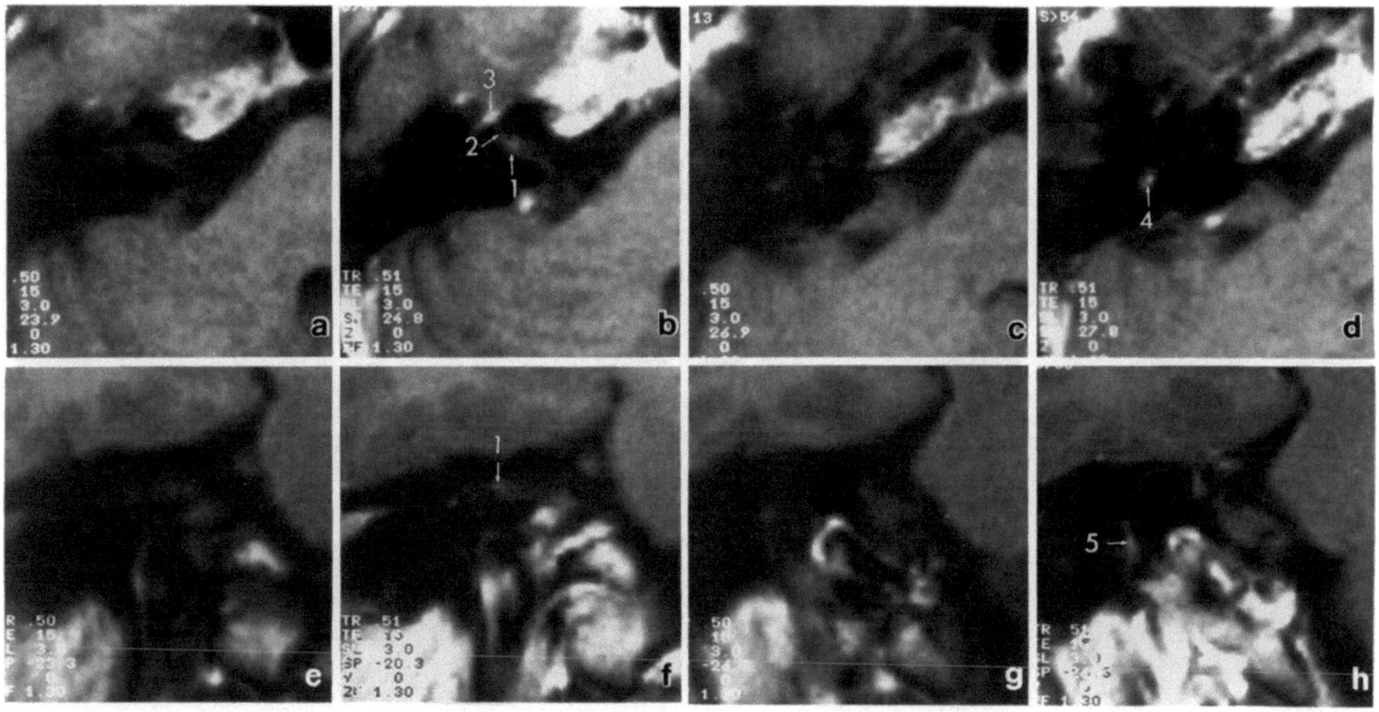

Fig. 1a–h. A 48–year–old female presented with complete right facial nerve paralysis for 1 week. High dose steroids were given without clinical improvement. Electroneuronography of the right facial nerve demonstrated almost 100% degeneration. The patient underwent a surgical decompression without any improvement. T1–weighted MR images of the right facial nerve prior to surgical decompression before (**a, c** for axial; **e, g** for coronal) and after (**b, d** for axial; **f, h** for coronal) gadolinium enhancement show abnormal enhancement of the meatal and fallopian portions of the right facial nerve. Facial nerve: 1, meatal portion; 2, labyrinthine portion; 3, geniculate ganglion; 4, tympanic (horizontal) portion; 5, mastoid (vertical) portion

the vestibulocochlear nerve. The facial nerve is located in the anterior and superior quadrant of the internal auditory canal, in which its entire course can be visualized on images in coronal and axial planes. It then enters the fallopian canal at the meatal foramen, which is surrounded by a fibrous ligament and is the narrowest point of the fallopian canal. This anatomic relationship may explain why the most common site of enhancement in Bell's palsy observed in this study is the distal meatal portion of the facial nerve. The fallopian (or facial nerve) canal is approximately 30 mm in length and is divided into labyrinthine, tympanic and mastoid sections. The labyrinthine portion of the facial nerve passes anteriorly around the basal turn of the cochlea and expands to form the geniculate ganglion at which level the greater superficial petrosal nerve branches from the main trunk of the facial nerve, coursing to the pterygopalatine fossa. The facial nerve then descends through the mastoid (vertical) portions of the fallopian canal toward the stylomastoid foramen. The labyrinthine, geniculate ganglion and tympanic portions of the facial nerve are best visualized in the axial plane. The vertical portion of the facial nerve can be visualized in its entire course on coronal or sagittal images.

Because of the lack of bone artifact, MRI of the facial nerve appears to be the procedure of choice for evaluation of facial nerve palsy [1–5]; Gd–enhanced T1–weighted sequences are particularly helpful for identifying abnormal enhancement of the facial nerve [3–5]. The mechanism of facial nerve enhancement is uncertain; a possible explanation is that with inflammation or injury, the facial nerve becomes edematous, with increased permeability of adjacent vascular structures and an increase of extracellular fluid [5]. The facial nerve enhancement observed in this study appears to be uniform, without the nodularity reported in facial nerve neuroma [3, 5]. Acute facial nerve paralysis is usually unilateral and can be seen in patients with acute trauma and Bell's palsy. Bilateral facial nerve paralysis (facial diplegia) can be seen in patients with acute inflammatory polyradiculoneuritis, Lyme disease, sarcoidosis and rarely with Bell's palsy. In acute trauma, facial nerve paralysis is most commonly associated with a temporal bone fracture, and its severity is related to the location of the fracture. Our patient had only a linear fracture through the mastoid, without transection of the facial nerve; the MRI study showed no abnormal enhancement of the facial nerve, although its mastoid portion could not be evaluated due to hemorrhage. This patient's facial nerve paralysis recovered completely. The most common form of acute facial nerve paralysis is Bell's palsy (idiopathic facial paralysis). The incidence of Bell's palsy is 23/100,000 annually or 1 in 60 or 70 persons in a lifetime [6]. The pathogenesis is unknown, although inflammatory changes are commonly presumed. The maximum facial weakness occurs within 4–8 h. Eighty–five per cent of patients with Bell's palsy recover comletely without treatment; however, the recommended medical treatment for Bell's palsy is high doses of steroids (prednisone 1 mg/kg daily for 7 days, followed by a tapering dose). Surgical decompression is controversial and is based on the assumption that compression

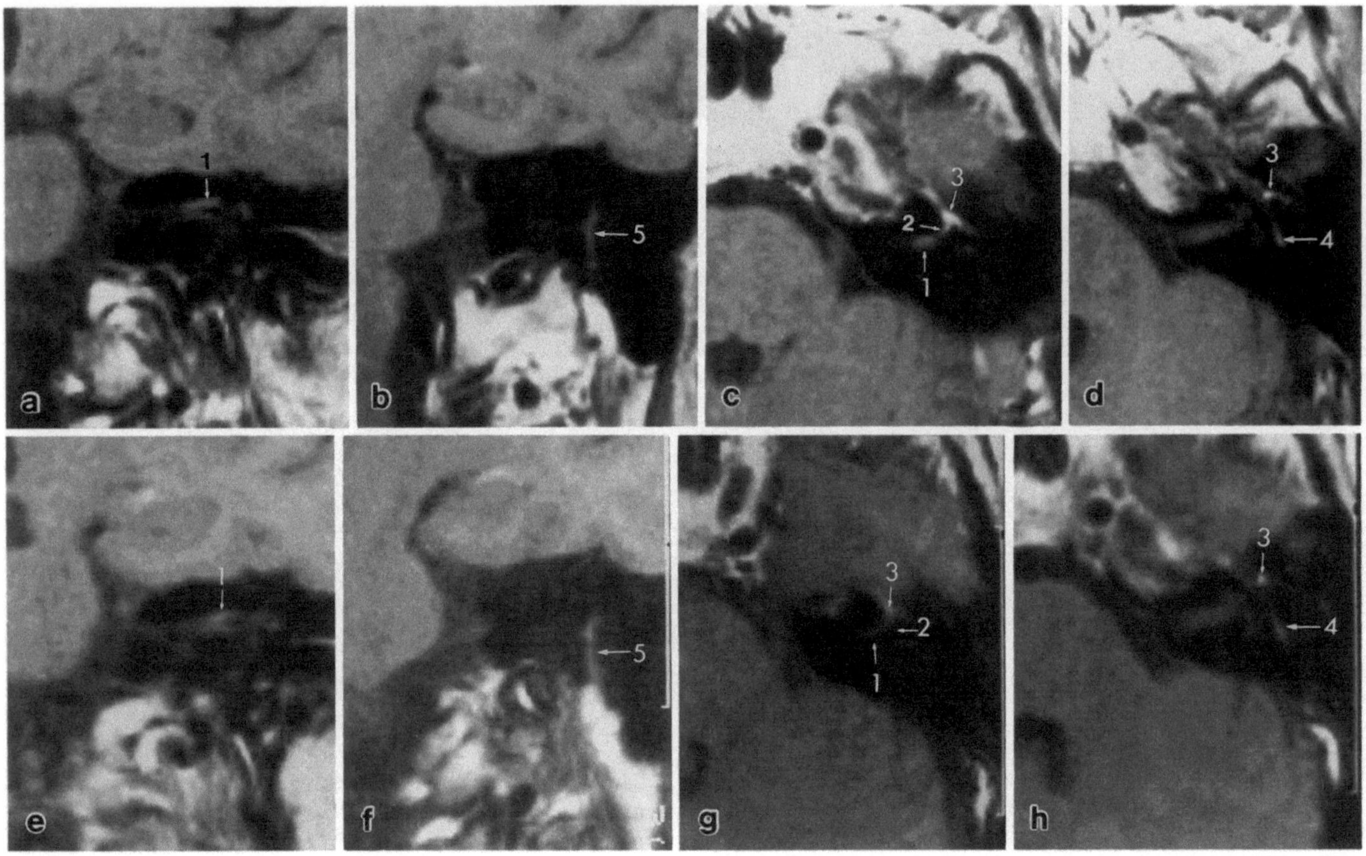

Fig. 2a–h. A 46-year-old female was exposed to chicken pox 3 weeks prior to her acute onset of complete left facial nerve paralysis. She had a suboptimal response to steroid treatment. T1-weighted MR images with gadolinium-enhancement (**a, b** coronal), (**c, d** axial) obtained 3 weeks after the onset of symptoms show marked enhancement of the meatal and fallopian portion of the left facial nerve. High dose steroids and Zovivax were then given for 2 weeks, with 95% recovery. Two months later, follow-up gadolinium-enhanced T1-weighted MR images (**e, f** coronal; **g, h** axial) show persistent but diminished left facial nerve enhancement

of the swollen facial nerve within the fallopian canal may result in permanent injury, so that surgical release of the compression of the entire facial nerve by the middle cranial fossa and transmastoid route improves the recovery of facial movements. Intraoperative evoked electromyography has shown that the lesion producing Bell's palsy lies within the fallopian canal and is situated at the meatal foramen in 94% of the cases [7]. Electroneuronographic studies of the spontaneous course of Bell's palsy [8] indicate that the destiny of the facial nerve in patients with Bell's palsy is decided within 2–3 weeks after the onset of symptoms. All patients who had less than 90% maximal degeneration of facial nerve fibers within 3 weeks of onset of Bell's palsy experienced a satisfactory recovery without any form of treatment. Fifty per cent of patients with 95%–100% degeneration within 2 weeks of onset of Bell's palsy had a permanent unsatisfactory recovery of facial nerve function. Therefore, it seems that as long as 10% of the facial nerve fibers remain conductive for electrically evoked nerve impulses, a sufficient number of endoneural tubes remain intact and ensure proper regeneration of the degenerated nerve fibers. As a result of this study, Fisch [9] recommended immediate surgical decompression as soon as 90% of the facial nerve fibers are shown to have undergone degeneration within 2 weeks of the onset of Bell's palsy. In our study, only a few cases of MRI were correlated with electroneuronography; the data are not sufficient to draw a conclusion as to whether facial nerve enhancement is related to the severity of facial nerve degeneration. However, localizing the site of facial nerve enhancement could assist the surgeon in surgical planning.

In summary, the facial nerve in the internal auditory and fallopian canals can be evaluated well by Gd-enhanced T1-weighted MRI in the axial and coronal planes. Gd-enhanced MRI is very sensitive but not specific, demonstrating facial nerve enhancement in patients with acute facial nerve paralysis. The meatal portion of the facial nerve is the most common site of enhancement in Bell's palsy (85.7% of all Bell's palsy patients, 100% of all positive studies). There is never enhancement of normal facial nerves. The enhancement of the facial nerve on a single MRI study does not indicate prognosis in Bell's palsy; however, a follow-up MRI study showing resolution or improvement of the facial nerve enhancement seens to indicate a better prognosis. Since 85% of patients with Bell's palsy will spontaneously recover completely, MRI is not recommended for routine work-up in this condition However, Gd-enhanced MRI still plays a role in the differential diagnosis of facial paralysis, to rule out facial nerve neuroma or other central nervous system cause of facial paralysis.

References

1. Teresi L, Lufkin R, Wortham D, Flannigan B, Reicher M, Halbach V, Bentson J, Wilson G, Ward P, Hanafee W (1987) MR imaging of the intratemporal facial nerve using surface coils. AJNR 8: 49–54
2. Wortham DG, Teresi LM, Lufkin RB, Hanafee WN, Ward PH (1989) Magnetic resonance imaging of the facial nerve. Otolaryngol Head Neck Surg 101: 295–301
3. Daniels DL, Czervionke LF, Pojunas KW, Meyer GH, Millen SJ, Williams AL, Haughton VM (1987) Facial nerve enhancement in MR imaging. AJNR 8: 605–607
4. Kilgore DP, Breger RK, Daniels DL, Pojunas KW, Williams AL, Haughton VM (1986) Cranial tissues: normal MR appearance after intravenous injection of Gd–DTPH. Radiology 160: 757–761
5. Daniels DL, Czervionke LF, Millen SJ, Haberkamp TJ, Meyers GA, Hendrix LE, Mark LP, Williams AL, Haughton VM (1989) MR imaging of facial nerve enhancement in Bell palsy or after temporal bone surgery. Radiology 171: 807–809
6. Victor M, Martin JB (1987) Bell's palsy. In; Braunwald E, Isselbacher KJ, Petersdorf RG, Wilson JD, Martin JB, Fauci AS (eds) Harrison's principles of internal medicine, 11th edn. McGraw–Hill, New York, p 2038
7. Fisch U, Esslen E (1972) Total intratemporal exposure of the facial nerve. Arch otolaryngol 95: 335–341
8. Fisch U (1977) Total facial nerve decompression and electroneuronography. In: Silverstein H, Norrell H (eds) Neurological surgery of the ear. Aesculapius, Birmingham, Ala., pp 21–23
9. Fisch U (1981) Surgery for Bell's palsy. Arch Otolaryngol 107: 1–11

Dr. Ay–Ming Wang
Department of Diagnostic Radiology
William Beaumont Hospital
3601 West 13 Mile Road
Royal Oak, MI 48073, USA

Neuroradiology (1991) 33 [Suppl]: 238–240

Neuro radiology
© Springer-Verlag 1991

Early caudate nucleus atrophy in Huntington's disease: does it correlate with presenting symptoms?

J. M. Wardlaw and R. J. Sellar

Department of Neuroradiology, Western General Hospital, Edinburgh, UK

Summary. Atrophy of the caudate nucleus in Huntington's disease, measured as a decrease in cross-sectional area on axial CT brain scan, correlates with severity of symptoms, but not their duration, nor whether clinical presentation was predominantly with cognitive impairment or movement disorder. The implications are discussed.

Key words: Huntington's disease – Chorea – Caudate nucleus.

Huntington's disease (HD) is a progressive fatal neurological disorder with dominant inheritance and complete penetrance. It manifests clinically as dementia, psychiatric disturbance and choreiform movement disorder, beginning insidiously in early adult life, and progressing over 10–15 years to a severely debilitated state, although symptoms and rate of progression vary [1]. It is surprisingly common, the incidence being 1 in 10000 in Britain. Pathologically there is global cerebral atrophy, the caudate nucleus (CN) and putamen being particularly affected, losing up to 60% of their volume by neuronal loss [2].

Attempts to identify the HD gene show promise, but a routine genetic test is not yet available, nor are there any other reliable means of identifying affected individuals before development of symptoms [3].

Radiological methods of measuring CN atrophy have been described, notably the bicaudate ratio [4], and the ratio of the distance between the frontal horns (FH) to the distance between the CN heads (CC) at the foramen of Monro [5], but these are indirect (Fig. 1). We therefore measured CN on axial CT brain scans in 30 subjects with or at risk of HD, and 100 age-matched controls (the lower limit of normal CN area for the age group 20–40 years was 1.0 cm^2). We found this to be more sensitive and specific (91% and 100% respectively on analysis of the 24 of 30 cases with known outcome) for HD than the FH: CC ratio in either our own series or by comparison with figures quoted inthe literature (Wardlaw and Sellar, in preparation). We correctly identified 3 presymptomatic cases, and 3 DNA–negative cases. This method was also previously described by Lang in 5 patients [6].
Work in primates has suggested that the main connections of the CN are to areas of cerebral cortex involved in cognitive functions and eye movements, but not to other motor areas [7]. Starkstein et al. [8] showed a correlation between caudate atrophy, eye movement disorders and intellectual dysfunction in 34 patients with established HD. Our impression was that patients who presented with cognitive impairment had smaller CN area than those presenting with movement disorder. If this observation were true, then CN size at presentation might have useful predictive value for progression and pattern of HD in that patient. We have therefore examined this in more detail.

Subjects and methods

The subjects had definite symptoms of HD, although some underwent CT brain scanning shortly before these developed. All had detailed examination by an experienced clinical geneticist, and in addition those with early symptoms were examined by a clinical neuropsychologist according to the "Baltimore Huntington's disease protocol" [1]. They also had genetic counselling, and where appropriate family structure existed, genetic testing for the HD gene.

All had CT of the brain (axial, 10 mm slice interval and thickness) from base of skull to vertex, with additional slices at 3 mm intervals through the CN. The area of both CN and the FH: CC ratio were measured on all slices on which the CN were visible using the programmes available on the CT consul. The mean of the largest right and left CN areas was used in the calculations. The measurements were made "blind" by one of the two authors. We have previously calculated intra– and inter–observer error for this method to be less than 10% (Wardlaw and Sellar, in preparation).

In the present study, we compared CN area with the duration of symptoms, presenting symptom (i.e. predominantly dementia or

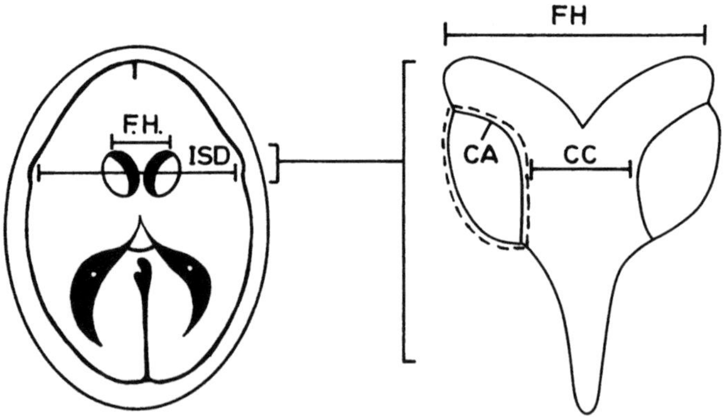

Fig. 1. Method of obtaining FH: CC ratio, bicaudate ratio, and caudate area measurements. *FH,* Maximum distance between the tips of the frontal horns of the lateral ventricles; *CC,* minimum distance between the heads of the caudate nuclei at the level of the foramen of Monro. Bicaudate ratio = CC/ISD × 100; *ISD,* inner skull diameter at level of CC

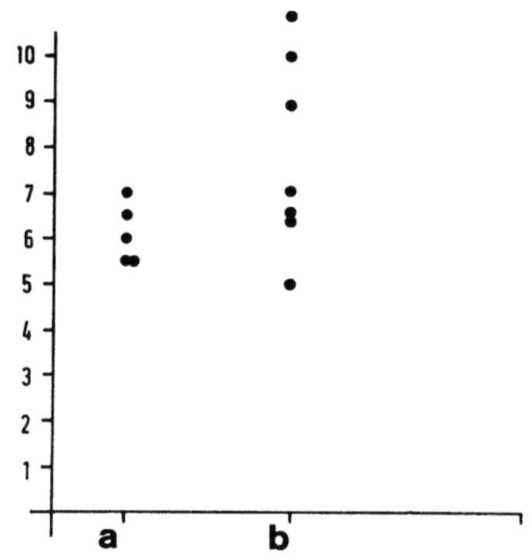

Fig. 2a, b. Graph demonstrating the relationship between caudate nucleus area in square millimetres (y axis) and presentation with intellectual impairment (**a**) or movement disorder (**b**)(x axis) in patients scanned within 2 years of presentation

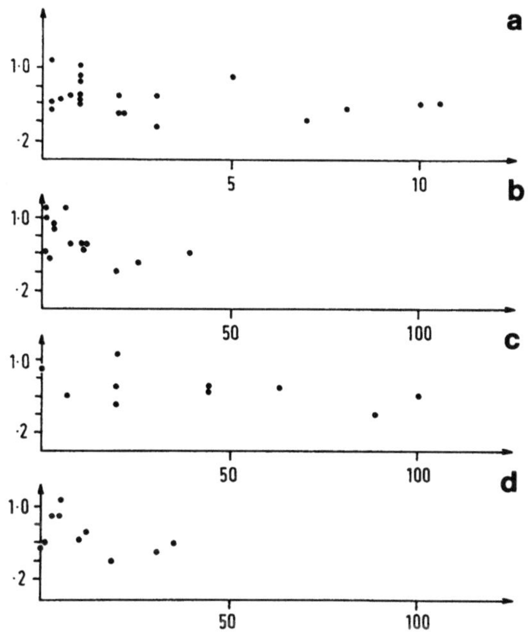

Fig. 3a–d. Graphs demonstrating the relationship between caudate nucleus area (cm^2; y axis) and on the x axis (**a**) duration of symptoms in years ($k = -0.32$, $p > 0.05$), **b** total symptom score ($k = -0.44$, $p < 0.05$), **c** intellectual dysfunction score ($k = -0.39$, $p > 0.05$) and **d** motor impairment score ($k = -0.59$, $p > 0.05$), the latter three expressed as a percentage of the possible score on the Baltimore Huntington's disease test

movement disorder), and severity of symptoms as expressed by the Baltimore HD test score. For this purpose, we amalgamated all movement scores (voluntary and involuntary), except for eye movement. Statistical analysis was by Student's t–test and Kendall coefficient of rank correlation.

Results

There were 25 subjects, 13 female and 12 male. Ages ranged from 22 to 61 years (mean 42.6 ± 12). Clinical details were available from presentation, and 14 had also had the Baltimore HD test for which a score was available. Twelve had a CT of the brain within 2 years of developing symptoms; 3 were asymptomatic (2 tested positive for the HD gene) and have since developed symptoms. The other 13 had had symptoms for more than 2 years, mean 6 ± 4 years, maximum duration 16 years.

Of the 12 scanned within 2 years of clinical presentation, 5 had cognitive impairment and 7 movement disorder as the predominant symptom. There was no significant difference in the CN area between the two groups (Fig. 2).

In the 14 subjects with Baltimore HD test scores there was no significant association between small CN area and score for intellictual impairment, intellectual and eye movement abnormalities, voluntary motor/movement disorder, or duration of symptoms. This was true for score expressed as absolute value or as percentage of possible score for that category. There was, however, a significant association between small CN area and high total Baltimore HD test score ($p < 0.05$) (Fig. 3). However there was no significant association between a high Baltimore HD test score and duration of symptoms as some subjects had a high score with relatively short history, and others with a longer history had lower scores. This suggests that small CN area is associated with a worse prognosis. Analysis of duration of symptoms and presenting symptom for all 25 subjects showed no association between CN size and either of these parameters.

Discussion

We have previously assessed our method of measuring CN atrophy and found good reproducibility and ease of use without image edge enhancement. We believe that it is a more direct measure of CN size than the FH: CC or the bicaudate ration.

Our results indicate that CN atrophy in HC, as measured by a decrease in cross–sectional caudate area on axial CT, is not associated with any predominant presenting symptom. Nor does there appear to be any correlation with the main symptom in established HD, be it cognitive impairment or movement disorder, or with duration of symptoms. However, we have found a significant correlation between total symptom score (i. e. more severe symptoms) and small CN area, suggesting that patients presenting with small caudates may have a more rapid disease course. This differs with the findings of Starkstein et al. [9], who showed a positive correlation between bicaudate ratio and eye movement and cognitive abnormalities, and duration of symptoms in established HD. However, they did not correlate caudate atrophy with presenting symptom.

Our results are in agreement with those of Shoulson et al. [9], who found that caudate atrophy (measured by FH: CC ratio) correlated with total functional impairment and severity of HD symptoms, also with the results of post–mortem studies of patients who had established HD in life, which showed that the more severe grades of CN atrophy were associated with more severe symptoms (of all kinds) [2, 10]. This may have useful predictive value for the clinical course of HD. Follow–up of the subjects who are now just developing symptoms of HD is required before this can be confirmed.

In conclusion, our study of this small series of HD patients shows that a decrease in the area of the CN on axial CT brain scan is associated with more severe symptoms of HD, but not with the duration of symptoms or the presenting symptom. This may have useful predictive value for disease course.

References

1. Folstein SE, Jensen B, Leigh RJ, Folstein MF (1983) The measurement of abnormal movement: methods developed for Huntington's disease. Neurobehav Toxicol Teratol 5: 605–609
2. Monte SM de la, Vonsattel J–P, Richardson EP (1988) Morphometric demonstration of atrophic changes in the cerebral cortex, white matter and neostriatum in Huntington's disease. J Neurol Exp Psychol 47: 516–525
3. Harper PS, Morris MJ (1989) Predictive testing for Huntington's disease. Br Med J 298: 404–405
4. Starkstein SE, Folstein SE, Brandt J, Pearlson GD, McDonnell A, Folstein M (1989) Brain atrophy in Huntington's disease. Neuroradiology 31: 156–159
5. Neophytides AN, DiChiro G, Barron SA, Chase TN (1979) Computed axial tomography in Huntington's disease and persons at risk of Huntington's disease. Adv Neurol 28: 185–191
6. Lang C (1985) Is direct CT caudatometry superior to indirect parameters in confirming Huntington's disease? Neuroradiology 27: 161–163
7. Selemon LD, Goldman–Rakic PS (1985) Longitudinal topography and interdigitation of corticostriatal projections in the rhesus monkey. J Neurosci 5: 776–794.
8. Starkstein SE, Brandt J, Folstein S, Strauss M, Berthier ML, Pearlson GD, Wong D, McDonnell A, Folstein M (1988) Neuropsychological and neuroradiological correlates in Huntington's disease. J Neurol Neurosurg Psychiatry 51: 1259–1263
9. Shoulson I, Plassche W, Odoroff C (1982) Huntington disease: caudate atrophy parallels functional impairment. Neurology 32: 143
10. Vonsattel J–P, Myers RH, Stevens TJ, Ferrante RJ, Bird ED, Richardson EP (1985) Neuropathological classification of Huntington's disease. J Neurol Exp Psychol 44: 559–577

J. M. Wardlaw
Department of Radiology
Royal Infirmary of Edinburgh
1 Lauriston Place
Edinburgh EH3 9YW, UK

Neuroradiology (1991) 33 [Suppl]: 241–243

Neuro radiology
© Springer-Verlag 1991

Deep cerebral vein thrombosis

A. S. Sandhu[1], D. Johns[2], and L. E. Albertyn[2]

[1] Department of Radiology, Royal Adelaide Hospital, Adelaide, South Australia
[2] Department of Radiology, Queen Elizabeth Hospital, Woodville, South Australia

Summary. Four cases of deep cerebral venous thrombosis are presented. Direct evidence on CT consists of hyperdense thrombus in the deep veins and/or straight sinus, with indirect changes of ganglionic low density and/or parenchymal haemorrhage. MRI offers direct visualisation of blood flow and its cessation, with more sensitive demonstration of the deep grey matter changes, and may thereby obviate angiography.

Key words: Cerebral blood vessels, thrombosis – Venous infarction – Head, computed tomography – Venous thrombosis – Magnetic resonance imaging – Infarction

Thrombosis of the deep cerebral veins is an infrequent form of stroke in adults [1]. It is well recognised in children, usually associated with sepsis [2] but the incidence in adults is uncertain and it probably occurs more often than it is diagnosed. Antemortem diagnosis is difficult and frequently delayed.

CT is still the main imaging modality, but MRI offers distinct advantages, allowing direct visualisation of blood flow and its cessation, and is more sensitive in demonstrating the deep basal ganglia changes. The clinical and radiological features of four adults with deep cerebral vein thrombosis (DCVT) are presented.

Materials and methods

CT was performed before and after intravenous contrast medium on modern generation scanners. Selective arterial angiography was carried out in three patients. MRI was performed on Siemens 1.0T (case 1) and Picker 0.5T (case 3) imagers using T1- and T2-weighted spin echo pulse sequences.

Results

Tables 1 and 2 detail the clinical and radiological features at presentation. Case 1 had a further two CT and MRI scans. Early CT showed progression of thrombus into the thalamostriate (TSV) and internal cerebral veins (ICV) (Fig. 1 b). Delayed CT showed absence of hyperdense thrombus and resolution of ganglionic low densities. MRI on day 6 demonstrated iso- and hyperintense thrombus in the ICV, vein of Galen (VG), straight sinus (SS) and right transverse sinus on T1-weighted coronal and sagittal images (Fig. 2 c), and in the SS on T2-weighted images.

Early repeat CT in case 2 showed more extensive bilateral deep hemispheric low density, mass effect and pronounced hyperdensity of the TSVs. There was also tentorial enhancement. Autopsy revealed bilateral haemorrhagic infarction of the central grey matter and thrombus in the TSVs, ICVs and VG.

Follow-up CT showed resolution of the basal ganglia changes in case 3 and the usual evolution of parenchymal haemorrhages in case 4.

The cerebrospinal fluid (CSF) was examined in three patients and showed increased numbers of red cells and elevation of protein.

Discussion

The common conditions predisposing to central sinovenous thrombosis are aseptic primary thrombosis of unknown aetiology, pregnancy and the puerperium, exogenous steroids, dehydration (especially in children), hypercoagulable states, local neoplasm, trauma, surgery and sepsis.

The predisposing condition in three of our four patients was oestrogen ingestion. No cause was identified in the one male patient.

The non-specific clinical features include raised intracranial pressure, headache, nausea, vomiting, drowsiness and fever [1–3]. Of interest is the variable paresis present

Table 1. Four patients and their presenting symptoms

Case/age (years)/sex	Signs/symptoms	Probable aetiology	Outcome
1/25/F	Headache, aphasia, catatonia, vomiting, right hemiparesis	Low-dose contraceptive pill – 4 years	Short-term memory loss; full physical recovery
2/41/M	Headache, confusion, left hemiparesis	Idiopathic	Autopsy diagnosis
3/26/F	Headache, vomiting, confusion, hysteria, bilateral paresis R > L	Low-dose contraceptive pill – 3 months	Short-term memory loss; some extrapyramidal signs
4/52/F	Headache, unsteady gait, drowsy, left haemianopia and paresis	Oestrogen/progesterone replacement – 5 weeks	Full recovery

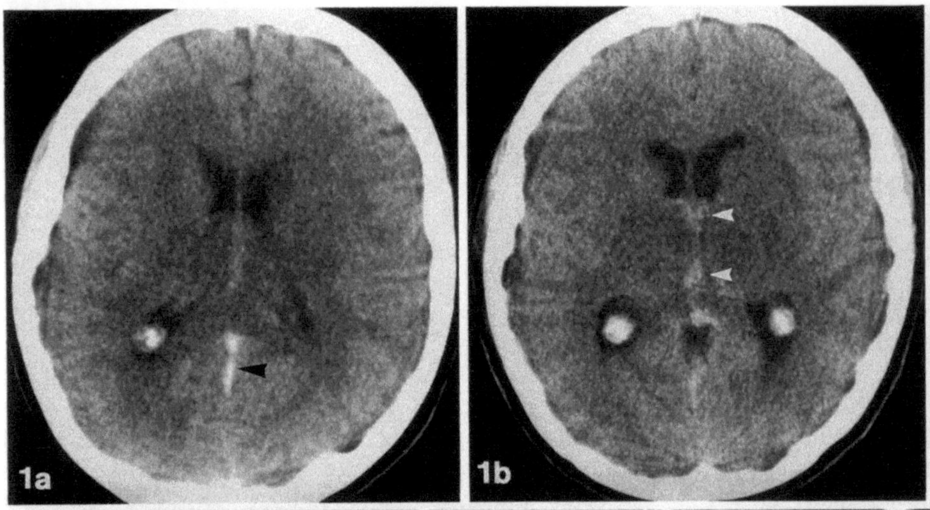

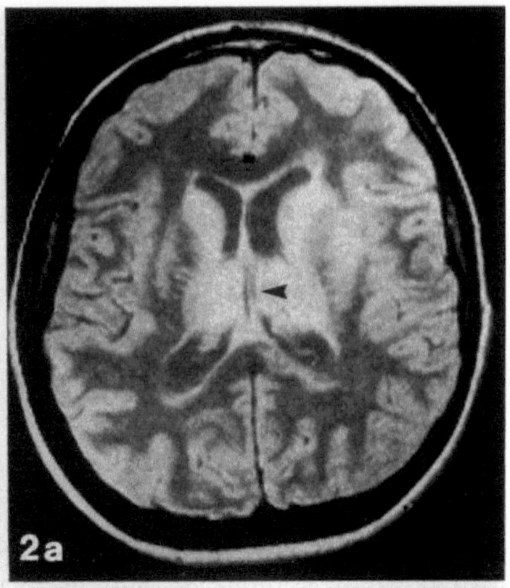

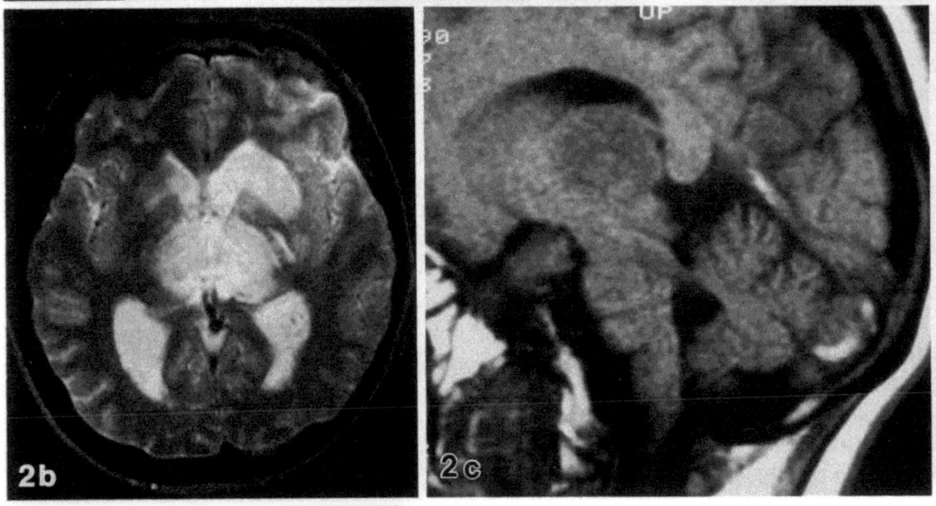

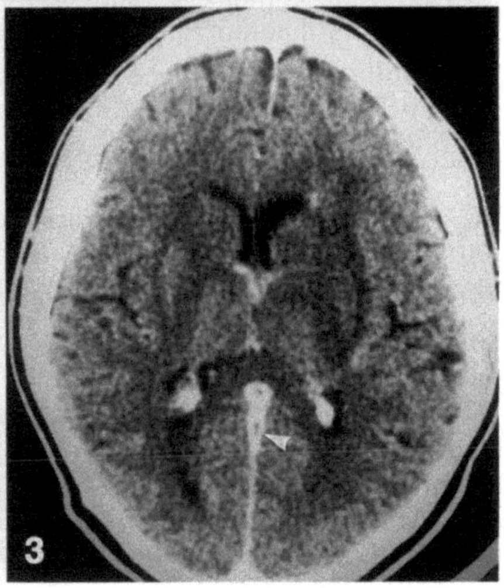

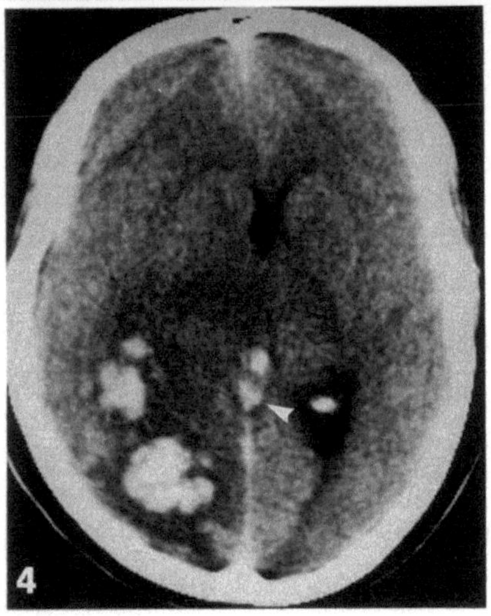

Fig. 1a, b. Case 1, precontrast CT. **a** Day 1, hyperdense anterior straight sinus (SS) *(arrow)*. **b** Day 2, anterior progression of hyperdense thrombus into thalamostriate vein, internal cerebral vein (ICV) *(arrow)* and vein of Galen (VG). Bilateral ganglionic low density, L > R

Fig. 2a–c. Case 1, MRI (spin echo). **a** Proton density, isointense signal ICV *(arrow)*. **b** T2-weighted image signal void in the ICV and VG, bilateral ganglionic infarcts. **c** T1-weighted image day 6, iso- and hyperintense thrombus in SS and right transverse sinus

Fig. 3. Case 3, postcontrast CT. Non-opaque thrombus in the anterior SS *(arrow)*, bilateral basal ganglia low density

Fig. 4. Case 4, precontrast CT. Hyperdense thrombus in the VG *(arrow)*. Right occipital, temporal and ganglionic low density and parenchymal haemorrhage; midline shift

in all four cases, as described by Kim and Walczak [1] but not by others [2–5].

Direct evidence of thrombosis on CT is the presence of high density within the deep veins and sinuses on unenhanced images in the acute stage, and subsequent contrast enhancement around lucent clot within the sinuses. Indirect evidence includes infarction without apparent arterial distribution, areas of parenchymal haemorrhage, gyral enhancement, cerebral oedema, small ventricles, dilated transcerebral medullary veins and tentorial enhancement.

In all four cases thrombus within the deep veins was visualised on non-contrast scans. A 'V'-shaped high density in the TSVs was present in two patients (cases 2, 3) on the first study and subsequently in case 1 on the second (Fig. 1b), probably indicating anterior propagation. Invol-

Table 2. Radiological findings at presentation

Case	Interval from symptoms to CT	CT		Angiography/MRI
1	48 h	C –[a]	Hyperdense thrombus in VG and anterior SS (Fig. 1 a); bilateral low density in thalamic and basal ganglia L > R	MRI (60 h) Absence of flow void IVC (proton density) (Fig. 2 a) isointense SS on T1 WI but flow void in IC and VG on T2WI. Bilateral ganglionic high signal on T2WI L > R (Fig. 2 b)
		C +[b]	Collateral medullary veins and marked choroid plexus blush	Angiography (64 h) Bilateral non-filling of deep veins and SS + collaterals
2	72 h	C –	Hyperdense thrombus in TSV, ICV, VG and anterior SS; left ganglionic low density	Not performed
3	1 week	C –	Hyperdense thrombus in TSVs. Bilateral basal ganglia low density L > R	MRI Bilateral ganglionic high signal on T2WI
		C +	Non-opaque filling defect in SS (Fig. 3)	Angiography Bilateral non-filling of deep veins and SS + thrombus right transverse sinus
4	5 days	C –	Multiple intracerebral temporal and occipital haemorrhages. Right ganglionic and occipital low density. Hyperdense thrombus right basal and VG (Fig. 4)	Angiography (at 7 days) Non-filling of deep veins, SS + superficial collaterals to right sylvian fissure

[a] Without contrast medium
[b] With contrast medium
VG, Vein of Galen; SS, straight sinus
TSV, thalamostriate vein; ICV, internal cerebral vein; T1 WI, T1-weighted image; T2WI, T2-weighted image

vement of the VG and the SS was present in cases 1–3, the last showing a non-opaque filling defect on the contrast-enhanced scan (Fig. 3). Indirect evidence of thalamic and basal ganglion low density was present in all cases, with unilateral preponderance on the side opposite to the paresis. Cases 1 and 3 had delayed CT showing resolution of the hyperdense thrombus and almost complete resolution of the ganglionic low density, commensurate with clinical improvement. Multiple separate regions of haemorrhage, presumably due to venous infarction, were seen in case 4 (Fig. 4).

Macchi et al. [4] claimed that MRI demonstrates a stepwise evolution of signal intensity in venous thrombosis, as has been described in intracranial haemorrhage [5]. Case 1 demonstrated the loss of flow void in the SS on the T1-weighted sagittal image and hypointense internal cerebral veins on the proton density MRI (TR 2,500/TE 25 ms) (Fig. 2 a) but flow void was clearly present in the posterior IC and VG on the second echo T2-weighted image (2,500/90 ms) (Fig. 2 b). The second MRI demonstrated the conversion to hyperintensity intermediate stage on the T1-weighted coronal and sagittal (Fig. 2 c) sequences. The anterior SS (corresponding to the hyperdensity on the CT) was hypointense on the T2-weighted image on day 1 and was hyperintense on day 6. However, flow signal void was again present in the posterior ICVs and VG on delayed T2-weighted images. The signal void on the first MRI study had cast doubt on the diagnosis and prompted angiography 4 h later. This confirmed bilateral non-filling of the entire deep venous system and SS, with normal cortical and sagittal sinus filling, and dilated collateral medullary veins.

Carotid angiography is still considered definitive, showing no filling of the deep cerebral veins and/or dural sinuses but may become unnecessary with increasing availability of MRI and its ability to demonstrate intravascular thrombus.

All our patients had direct and indirect CT evidence at the time of presentation. In the clinical setting, the diagnosis of DCVT should be considered, as it alters the management and prognosis. MRI would confirm the early ganglionic changes and allow direct visualisation of the vessels on the T1-weighted image. In our experience hypointensity on the T2-weighted image was not universal and caution should be exercised in its interpretation. With increasing use of gradient echo, flow-sensitive sequences, patency of the vessels would be confidently demonstrated, thereby obviating angiography.

References

1. Kim KS, Walczak TS (1986) CT of deep cerebral venous thrombosis. J Comput Assist Tomogr 10: 386–390
2. Eick JJ, Miller KD, Bell KA, Tutton RH (1981) CT of deep cerebral venous thrombosis in children. Radiology 140: 399–402
3. Gabrielsen TO, Seeger JF, Knake JE, Stilwell EW (1981) Radiology of cerebral vein occlusion without dural sinus occlusion. Radiology 140: 403–408
4. Macchi PJ, Grossman RI, Gomori JM, Goldberg HI, Zimmerman RA, Bilaniuk LT (1986) High field MR imaging of cerebral venous thrombosis. J Comput Assist Tomogr 10: 10–15
5. Gomori JM, Grossman RI, Goldberg HI, Zimmerman RA, Bilaniuk LT (1985) Intracranial haematomas: imaging by high field MR. Radiology 157: 87–93

Dr. A. S. Sandhu
Department of Radiology
Royal Adelaide Hospital
North Terrace
Adelaide S. A. 5000, Australia

Neuroradiology (1991) 33 [Suppl]: 244–246

Neuro radiology
© Springer-Verlag 1991

Cerebral MRI findings in patients with eclampsia

J. R. Bentson[1], T. M. Koci[2], C. M. Mehringer[2], F. T. Chang[2], B. D. Pressman[3], and F. Kioumehr[4]

Departments of Radiology, [1] UCLA Medical Center, [2] UCLA-Harbor Medical Center, [3] Cedars-Sinai Medical Center, and [4] Olive View Medical Center, Los Angeles, California, USA

Summary. MRI was abnormal in six patients with pre-eclampsia/eclampsia. The abnormal areas were hyperintense on T2-weighted images, and their locations correlated well with neurologic dysfunction. Several characteristic features of these lesions were apparent: they occur most often in the occipital lobes and watershed zones; the subcortical white matter is primarily involved, with some cortical involvement in addition; symmetry is the rule. Rapid disappearance of the lesions is consistent with a vasospastic causation.

Key words: Eclampsia – Convulsions – Epilepsy

Toxemia of pregnancy includes pre-eclampsia and eclampsia. Pre-eclampsia is a syndrome of hypertension, proteinuria and peripheral edema occurring after the 20th week of gestation. When convulsions occur in a patient with pre-eclampsia, the condition is termed eclampsia. Other neurological manifestations of pre-eclampsia/eclampsia include headache, confusion, obtundation, hemiparesis, and loss of vision. Temporary blindness occurs in 1%–3% of patients with pre-eclampsia/eclampsia and may be related to retinal or occipital cortical abnormalities [1]. The understanding of this and other neurologic deficits in pre-eclampsia/eclampsia has been aided in recent years by cross-sectional imaging of the brain. The importance of CT in demonstrating hypodense areas in the brain and ruling out large hematomas in pre-eclampsia/eclampsia has been emphasized by some authors [2, 3], while others have found it insensitive and have questioned its utility [4]. More recently, case reports of positive MRI in toxemic patients have appeared, with claims of increased sensitivity in demonstrating the pathologic findings. We describe six patients with pre-eclampsia/eclampsia who had abnormal MRI, with further analysis of the pattern of involvement in this condition.

Case reports

The ages of these six women ranged from 18 to 39 years, with a mean of 22 years. Three were Hispanic, two white, and one black. Only two were primigravidae. Gestational age at onset of toxemic symptoms ranged from 31 to 39 weeks. All these women developed hypertension, with blood pressures of 140–190/80–110 mmHg, and all had proteinuria, but the degree of hypertension and proteinuria did not correlate with the severity of neurologic symptoms. Five of the six had one or more seizures, placing them in the eclampsia category. To aid correlation of the neurologic dysfunction and MRI findings, a brief description of each patient will be given.

Case 1 developed pre-eclampsia at term and had a caesarean section. She had marked loss of vision (finger counting only) 48 h after the operation, and a single seizure the next day. MRI revealed bilateral hyperintensity of the occipital lobes on T2-weighted images (Fig. 1). Venous sinus thrombosis suspected clinically was excluded by the same study. Follow up MRI 7 days later was nearly normal and her vision was normal at discharge, 11 days postpartum.

Case 2 developed pre-eclampsia at the time of delivery, progressing to loss of vision, obtundation, and seizures 2 days postpartum. MRI and CT showed extensive bilateral abnormalities in the frontal and parietal lobes, in a watershed zone distribution, as well as bilateral occipital lesions (Fig. 2). Recovery was complete within 2 weeks, with return of the MRI to normal.

Case 3 experienced onset of focal seizures 5 days postpartum, with no visual changes. On MRI, the occipital lobes were normal but there were bilateral frontal lobe lesions (Fig. 3).

Case 4 was near term when she awoke blind, had a single seizure, and required a caesarian section. In addition to bilateral occipital lobe lesions, MRI demonstrated subtle regions of high intensity in the basal ganglia.

Case 5 presented with headaches and seizures, but no visual loss. Small areas of hyperintensity were seen in the upper portions of the occipital lobes, not involving the visual cortex.

Case 6 had neither visual loss nor seizures, but developed a right hemiparesis and slurred speech 2 h following a caesarean section which had been prompted by pre-eclamptic symptoms. MRI demonstrated two areas of hyperintensity, one in the left frontal lobe, the other in the lateral portion of the left occipital lobe.

Discussion

Pathologic studies of the brains of patients dying as the result of toxemia of pregnancy have shown cerebral and brain stem hematomas, patches of petechial hemorrhage, zones of infarction and venous thromboses [5]. However, CT has demonstrated that the majority of patients with pre-eclampsia/eclampsia have neither hemorrhage nor infarction, but rather areas of abnormally low intensity implying increased tissue fluid. These lesions clear with surprising rapidity on treatment, usually leaving no trace of abnormality. There have been several reports of cerebral

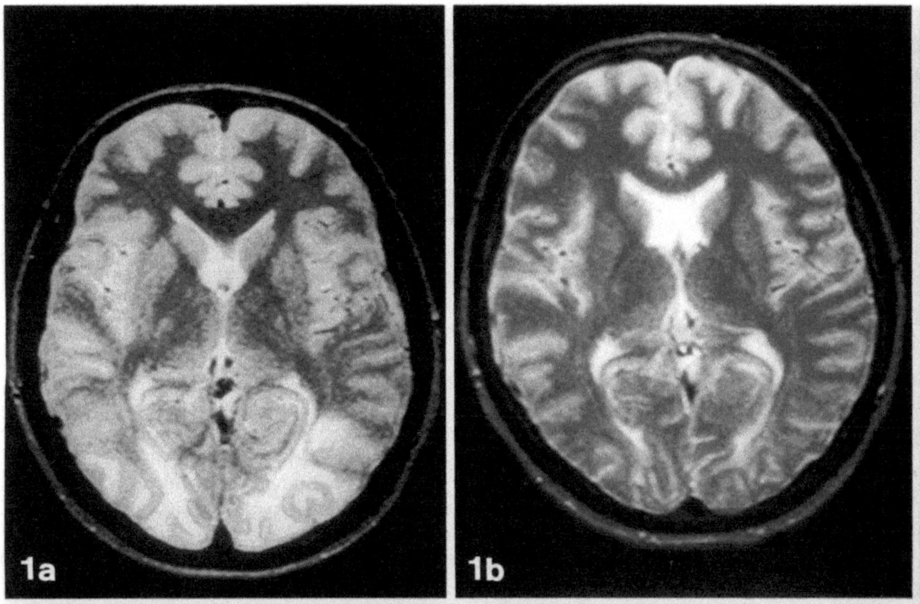

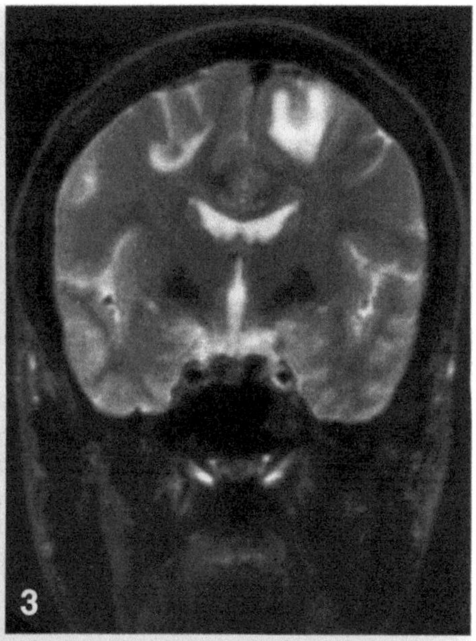

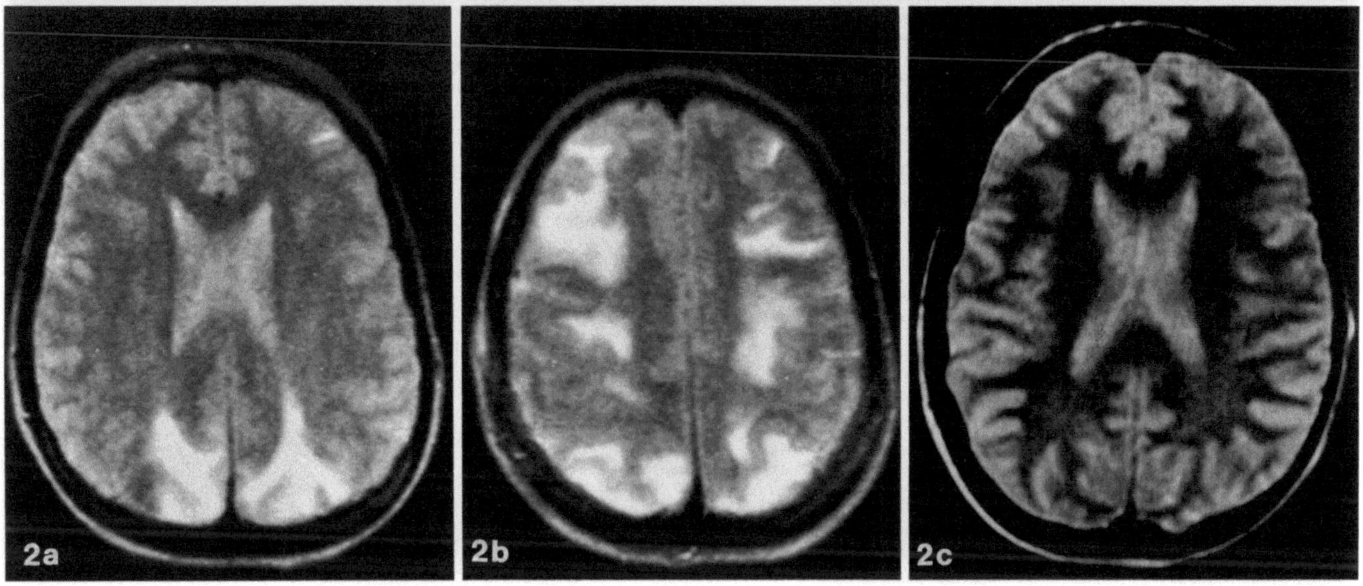

Fig. 1. **a** Axial T2-weighted (2600/100) MRI demonstrates bilateral symmetric hyperintensity in the occipital lobes, affecting mainly white matter. **b** MRI 1 week later shows only minimal residua of the occipital lesions

Fig. 2. **a** Axial T2-weighted image shows bilateral occipital lesions. **b** There are also bilateral symmetrical frontal and parietal lesions in a watershed zone distribution. **c** T2-weighted MRI 3 weeks after the initial examination is normal

Fig. 3. Coronal T2-weighted image shows bilateral frontal lobe lesions; this patient's MRI was otherwise normal. Note the subcortical white matter location of these lesions and the low signal (flow-void) in the superior sagittal sinus, indicating its patency

angiography in eclamptic patients, demonstrating widespread vasoconstriction, involving mainly the peripheral vascular territories [6, 7]. The vessel wall damage associated with this vasospasm apparently produces a defect in the blood-brain barrier and results in vasogenic edema. Whether certain portions of the brain should be more likely to be involved is not clear, but it is of interest that the higher and more posterior portions of the cerebral hemispheres are also the areas most commonly involved in hypertensive encephalopathy unassociated with pre-eclampsia/eclampsia [8].

When MRI and CT are compared in the same cases of pre-eclampsia/eclampsia, it is obvious that MRI is superior, that it demonstrates more areas of abnormality with greater clarity, and that it also has other valuable features such as its ability to rule out venous sinus thrombosis; the latter possibility continues to arouse considerable clinical concern in these cases. MRI is also very sensitive to the signs of subacute hemorrhage.

The cases described here demonstrate the major MRI findings in pre-eclampsia/eclampsia; hemorrhage is uncommon. The lesions have a strong tendency to be bilateral and symmetrical, although not always so. The occipital lobes are most often involved, explaining the high frequency of cortical blindness. Bilateral occipital involvement may spare the occipital cortex, in which case vision may not be affected. The temporal lobes are seldom involved. Frontal and parietal lobe involvement is relatively common, often in a watershed zone distribution.

There has been disagreement in the literature as to whether the abnormalities seen on imaging pre-eclampsia/eclampsia involve primarily the white matter [2, 9] or the cerebral cortex [10]. The patients in this series had lesions primarily involving the subcortical white matter, although there was also some gray matter involvement, seen more often in the larger lesions. While most lesions are located peripherally in the cerebrum, they may also occur in the brain stem or basal ganglia. The basal ganglia were affected in only one of these six cases.

The rapid disappearance of the subcortical white matter lesions following treatment supports the hypothesis that arterial spasm is the causative factor. Other pathologic processes that result in white matter edema, such as infarction, would not be expected to clear so rapidly, without leaving any residuum. The cause of the spasm, which can be observed in arterial systems beside that of the brain in pre-eclampsia/eclampsia, has not been clearly identified, but it is postulated that vasoconstrictive factors are released in the later stages of pregnancy [2]. It has been suggested that transitory platelet-rich intravascular occlusions may combine with vasospasm to produce the edematous lesions of the brain seen on CT and MRI [11]. It does not appear at this time that this can be confirmed or ruled out by MRI findings alone.

References

1. Beeson JH, Duda EE (1982) Computed axial tomography scan demonstration of cerebral edema in eclampsia preceded by blindness. Obstet Gynecol 60: 529–532
2. Colosimo C, Fileni A, Moschini M, Guerrini P (1985) CT findings in eclampsia. Neuroradiology 27: 313–317
3. Naheedy MH, Biller J, Schiffer M, Azan-Kia B, Gianopoulous J, Zarandy S (1985) Toxemia of pregnancy: cerebral CT findings. J Comput Assist Tomogr 9: 497–501
4. Sibai BM, Spirnato JA, Watson DL, Lewis JA, Anderson GD (1985) Eclampsia. IV. Neurological findings and future outcome. Am J Obstet Gynecol 152: 184–192
5. Sheehan HL, Lynch JB (1973) Pathology of toxaemia of pregnancy. Williams and Wilkins, Baltimore
6. Trommer BL, Homer D, Mikhael MA (1988) Cerebral vasospasm and eclampsia. Stroke 19: 326–329
7. Lewis LK, Hinshaw DB, Hasso AN, Thompson JR (1988) CT and angiographic correlation of severe neurological disease in toxemia of pregnancy. Neuroradiology 30: 59–64
8. Rail DL, Perkin GD (1980) Computerized tomographic appearance of hypertensive encephalopathy. Arch Neurol 37: 310–311
9. Coughlin WF, McMurdo SK, Reeves T (1989) MR imaging of postpartum cortical blindness. J Comput Assist Tomogr 13: 572–576
10. Schwaighofer BW, Hesselink JR, Healy ME (1989) MR demonstration of reversible brain abnormalities in eclampsia. J Comput Assist Tomogr 13: 310–312
11. Fredriksson K, Linvall O, Ingemarsson I, Astedt B, Cronquist S, Goltas S (1989) Repeated cranial computed tomographic and magnetic resonance imaging scans in two cases of eclampsia. Stroke 20: 547–553

Dr. John R. Bentson
Department of Radiological Sciences
UCLA Medical Center
Los Angeles, CA 90024, USA

SESSION 17
PAEDIATRICS

Neuroradiology (1991) 33 [Suppl]: 248–250

Neuro-radiology
© Springer-Verlag 1991

Periventricular leukomalacia: a common CT finding in full-term children with congenital hemiplegia

L.-M. Wiklund[1], O. Flodmark[3], and P. Uvebrant[2]

Departments of [1] Diagnostic Radiology and [2] Pediatrics, Children's Hospital, Östra Sjukhuset, Gothenburg, Sweden
[3] Department of Neuroradiology, Karolinska Hospital, Stockholm, Sweden

Summary. CT studies of 83 children born at term with congenital hemiplegic cerebral palsy (CP) were reviewed. The children belonged to a Swedish population-based series of a total of 115 children with congenital hemiplegic CP born at term, aged 5–15 years. The CT images were analysed for morphological evidence of periventricular leukomalacia (PVL) and the medical records scrutinised for risk factors and causes of hemiplegia. Although PVL is considered to be typical of the preterm infant it was the most prevalent CT finding in these term born hemiplegic children, being seen in 33 cases (40%). The presence of PVL suggests that the injury, caused by an hypoxic-ischaemic event, occurs in utero. This was supported by clinical data in 25 children.

Key words: Cerebral palsy – Hemiplegia – Periventricular leukomalacia

Congenital hemiplegic cerebral palsy (CP) is the most common CP syndrome among children born at term [1]. It has been thought to be of perinatal origin, but recent studies have suggested that prenatal events may be more common causes [2, 3].

Periventricular leukomalacia (PVL) is a vascular injury to the immature brain, occurring in the periventricular white matter, predominantly adjacent to the upper lateral angles of the lateral ventricles [4, 5]. In most cases, PVL has been reported to be bilateral, and usually associated with spastic diplegia. It is considered to be the most common cause of CP in children born preterm. Although PVL has been a well-known neuropathological entity for many years it is not until recently that it has been possible to make the diagnosis by computed tomography (CT) [6]. The criteria used to make the diagnosis on CT are reduction of periventricular white matter and ventriculomegaly with irregular ventricular outline. However, PVL can take many forms. The periventricular lesions may be regional and located anteriorly at the upper lateral angles of the frontal horns, intermediately at the cella media, posteriorly at the trigone, or they can be extensive, with a reduction of the entire lateral periventricular white matter. Some examples of PVL are illustrated in Figs. 1–3.

Materials and methods

The material for this study was a population based series from the south-western region of Sweden, comprising 25% of the total Swedish population. All children born during a decade (1969–1978) were included, giving a total of 115 full-term children with hemiplegic CP. Eighty-three (72%) of the 115 children were studied with at least one CT examination. The missing children did not differ from the total group in any of the clinical parameters.

All the CT studies were reviewed and morphological signs of PVL were specially looked for. The medical records were scrutinised for the presence of obvious causes of or risk factors for hemiplegia. Any history of a postnatal cause of hemiplegia disqualified the child from the study. The size and location of the PVL were correlated with clinical parameters, such as the distribution of hemiplegia, motor impairment, sensory impairment, additional impairments and total handicap.

Results

The CT examinations showed that PVL was the most prevalent morphological finding, being seen in 33 children (40%). In 14 children (17%) CT showed congenital malformations and in 11 (13%) cortical/subcortical injuries. Three children (3%) had miscellaneous abnormal findings, and in 22 (27%) CT showed no abnormality.

The distribution of CT findings did not differ from those found in a comparable group of hemiplegic children born preterm. In 19 children we found a prenatal risk factor or cause for hemiplegia, in 8 a perinatal risk factor or cause, and in 6 no adverse factor could be found.

Anteriorly located PVL correlated to arm-dominated hemiplegia. Besides distribution of hemiplegia, the clinical manifestations were very variable, and not predictable from the finding of PVL. Hand function, overall motor impairment, epilepsy, intellectual impairment and total handicap were all features that varied from mild to severe. Although extensive lesions often corresponded to severe impairments, no statistical correlation could be confirmed.

Discussion

What conclusions may be drawn from the finding of PVL in 40% of hemiplegic children born at term? When reviewing the pathophysiology of PVL, its origin is still

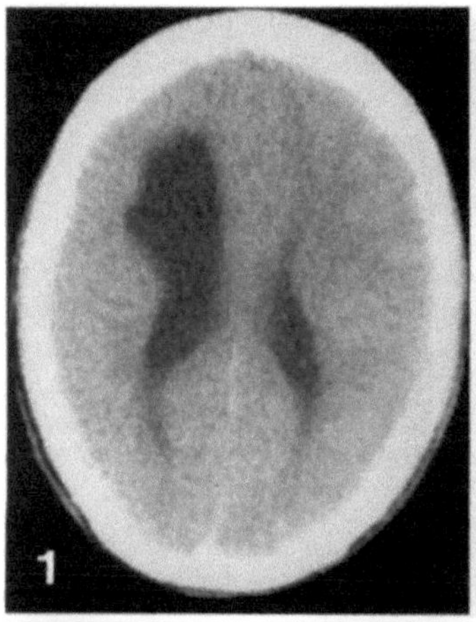

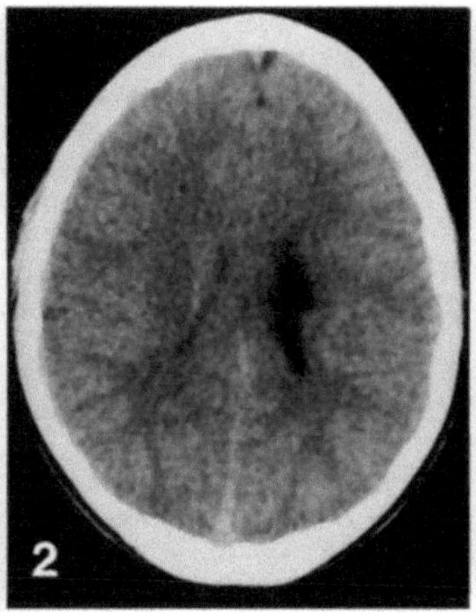

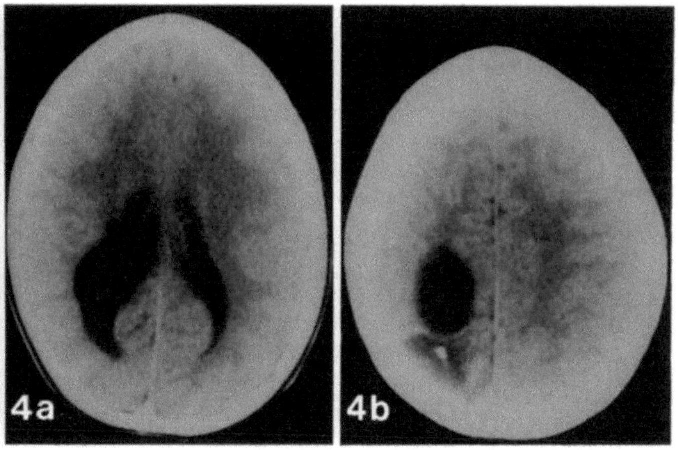

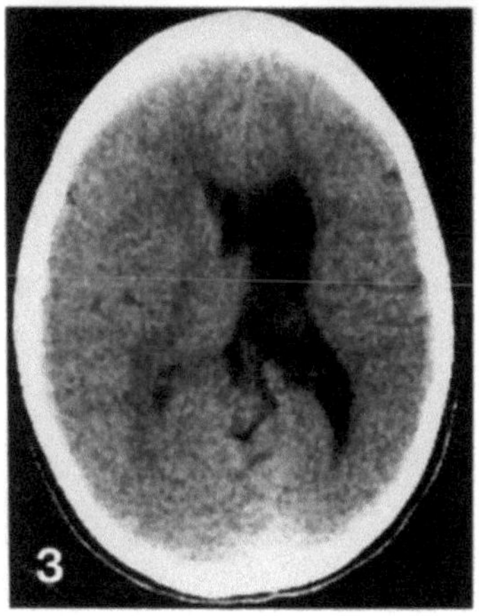

Fig. 1. Axial CT shows periventricular leukomalacia (PVL) located anteriorly, at the upper lateral angle of the right frontal horn. This boy with left-sided hemiplegia, was born at gestational age (GA) 42 weeks. The cause of the hemiplegia was clinically untraceable

Fig. 2. Axial CT shows PVL located at the left cella media. This boy with right-sided hemiplegia was born at GA 40 weeks. The mother had hypothyroidism, for which she was treated during the entire pregnancy. The obstetric and perinatal history was uneventful.

Fig. 3. Axial CT shows extensive left-sided PVL, with loss of the entire periventricular white matter and atrophy of the thalamus and basal ganglia. This girl with right-sided hemiplegia was born at GA 37 weeks after a period of 10 weeks of threatened abortion. The perinatal history was uneventful

Fig. 4a, b. Axial CT shows right-sided PVL located at the trigone, separate from a small parietal infarct. This boy with left-sided hemiplegia was born at GA 39 weeks. The perinatal history was that of a cerebral irritation, apnoea and lumbar puncture showed blood; an intracranial haemorrhage was considered clinically

somewhat obscure. Hypoperfusion is considered to be of importance, causing ischaemia of the watershed area between the ventriculofugal and ventriculopetal arteries [7, 8]. This watershed area corresponds in the immature brain to the periventricular white matter. With the maturation of the vascular supply, the development of the ventriculofugal cerebral vessels causes the watershed area to migrate from the periventricular zone to the subcortical. This explains why PVL is seen predominantly in preterm infants. It also implies that PVL should be considered as occurring prenatally when seen in children born at term, as in this series.

Did the medical records provide any clinical support for a prenatal origin in our 33 children with a CT finding of PVL? Evidence of a prenatal origin, based on risk factors, was found in 19 cases. The untraceable origin in 6 children also supports a prenatal cause. It is very unlikely that a full-term infant would suffer from a perinatal insult, sufficient to cause a manifest brain lesion, without showing any clinical deterioriation [9]. This is in contrast to the preterm infant, which may develop PVL without any clinical sign [10]. Thus, evidence for a prenatal origin was encountered in 76% (25/33).

In 2 cases CT showed small infarcts, in addition to and separate from the lesions representing PVL, as illustrated in Fig. 4. This child was known to have had a perinatal, intracranial haemorrhage, an event clinically considered to be of crucial importance [11]. The diagnosis was indicated by a lumbar puncture showing blood. However, the CT findings tell us that the brains have been exposed to insults on two different occasions, one to the immature brain and a second one to the more mature. The first insult may predispose to the second. This example further illustrates that perinatal clinical symptoms indicate a peri- or prenatal process. On the other hand, the CT finding of PVL strongly suggests a prenatal injury to the immature brain [12].

Although PVL has been claimed to correlate to the type and severity of impairment [13, 14] we could not establish any statistical correlation. The correlation shown by us between PVL located at the frontal horns and arm-dominated hemiplegia can be explained by the topographic representation within the corticospinal tracts.

Conclusion

Our results suggest that a cerebral injury, manifest as PVL on CT, is a common cause of congenital hemiplegic CP. In hemiplegic children born at term, the presence of PVL suggests that the brain injury was sustained in utero.

References

1. Hagberg B, Hagberg G, Olow I, Wendt L (1989) The changing panorama of cerebral palsy in Sweden. V. The birth year period 1979–82. Acta Paediatr Scand 78: 283–290
2. Hagberg B, Hagberg G (1984) Prenatal and perinatal risk factors in a survey of 681 Swedish cases. In: Stanley F, Alberman E (eds) Epidemiology of the cerebral palsies. Clinics in developmental medicine 87. Heinemann, London, pp 116–134

3. Uvebrant P (1988) Hemiplegic cerebral palsy – aetiology and outcome. Acta Paediatr Scand [Suppl]: 345
4. Banker BQ, Larroche J-C (1962) Periventricular leukomalacia of infancy. Arch Neurol 7: 386–410
5. Shuman RM, Selednik LJ (1980) Periventricular leukomalacia: a one-year autopsy study. Arch Neurol 37: 231–235
6. Flodmark O, Roland EH, Hill A, Whitfield MF (1987) Periventricular leukomalacia: radiologic diagnosis. Radiology 162: 119–124
7. Pape KE, Wigglesworth JS (1979) Haemorrhage, ischaemia and the perinatal brain. Clinics in developmental medicine 69/70. Spastics International Medical Publications. Heinemann, London
8. De Reuck J, Chattha AS, Richardson EP (1972) Pathogenesis and evolution of periventricular leukomalacia in infancy. Arch Neurol 27: 229–236
9. Towbin A (1986) Obstetric malpractice litigation: a pathologist's view. Am J Obstet Gynecol 155: 927–935
10. Vries LS de, Regev R, Dubowitz LMS (1986) Late onset cystic leucomalacia. Arch Dis Child 61: 298–299
11. Volpe JJ (1987) Intracranial hemorrhage: subdural, primary subarachnoid, intracerebellar, intraventricular (term infant), and miscellaneous. In: Neurology of the newborn, 2nd edn. Saunders, Philadelphia, pp 282–310
12. Volpe JJ (1987) Hypoxic-ischemic encephalopathy: clinical aspects. In: Neurology of the newborn, 2nd edn. Saunders, Philadelphia, pp 236–279
13. Picard A, Brentanos E, Schouman-Claeys E, Lacert P (1987) Delayed motor and intellectual sequelae in thirty-four children with cerebral palsy and CT scan evidence of periventricular leukomalacia (in French). Ann Pédiatr (Paris) 34: 615–621
14. Yokochi K, Horie M, Inukai K, Kito H, Shimabukuro S, Kodama K (1989) Computed tomographic findings in children with spastic diplegia: correlation with the severity of their motor abnormality. Brain Dev 11: 236–240

Dr. L.-M. Wiklund
Department of Diagnostic Radiology
Children's Hospital, Östra Sjukhuset
S-416 85 Gothenburg, Sweden

Neuroradiology (1991) 33 [Suppl]: 251–253

Neuro-radiology
© Springer-Verlag 1991

Thalamic atrophy in periventricular leukomalacia

K. J. Poskitt, C. O. Flodmark, E. H. Roland, and A. Hill

Departments of Radiology and Pediatrics, University of British Columbia, British Columbia's Children's Hospital, Vancouver, B. C., Canada

Summary. Sixty-five cases of periventricular leukomalacia (PVL) documented by CT were assessed in terms of the location and severity in reduction of periventricular white matter. CT studies of these and 75 age-matched controls were assessed for thalamic volume. The thalamic volume estimates were correlated with the location and severity of PVL on CT, and with clinical features. Asymmetric loss of thalamic volume was a frequent observation in PVL (38%) and correlated well with both clinical findings and asymmetry of periventricular white matter loss. Symmetric absolute loss of thalamic volume was common and was directly proportional to the severity of PVL. These observations support the hypothesis that neuronal injury and Wallerian degeneration following the hypoxic-ischemic insult cause secondary thalamic atrophy proportional to the severity of periventricular atrophy.

Key words: Thalamic atrophy – Periventricular leukomalacia – Wallerian degeneration

Hypoxic-ischemic cerebral insults in premature infants often result in periventricular leukomalacia (PVL), a specific pattern of periventricular infarction [1–3]. At the XIII Symposium Neuroradiologicum we reported characterstic CT findings in PVL that included: (1) ventriculomegaly with irregular lateral walls, (2) reduced periventricular white matter at the trigones, and (3) deep sulci with subcortical grey matter abutting the ventricles directly without intervening white matter [4, 5]. The classic sequelae of PVL include cerebral palsy with bilateral, although frequently asymmetric, spastic diplegia or quadriplegia [6]. In addition, we reported good correlation between the clinical findings and location of CT abnormalities in all cases [4]. Subsequent observation of cases with asymmetric PVL suggested that thalamic volume loss was ipsilateral to the most severely affected side. We hypothesized that thalamic volume loss was secondary to injury of the periventricular white matter and that therefore the volume loss should be proportional to the degree and severity of PVL, whether asymmetric or symmetric.

Patients and methods

All patients with PVL confirmed by CT for whom contiguous 5 mm images through the midbrain to the level of the centrum semiovale had been performed in the last 5 years were accepted for study. Sixty-five patients were assessed for the distribution and severity of PVL. Each hemisphere was assessed and graded as normal, mild, moderate or severe (Fig. 1). Estimates of thalamic volume were carried out using double magnification and identical narrow window and level settings (W 40 L 37) to delineate regions of interest (ROIs). Thalamic volume was calculated by summation of contiguous ROIs and dividing by 2, while relative size was determined by a ratio of smaller/larger thalamic volume. Seventy-five age-matched controls with normal CT underwent an identical prospective assessment in order to develop normative data. Because the estimates of thalamic volume were performed separately from the diagnostic study on the population with both normals and abnormal studies, the severity of PVL was usually unknown to the observer. Finally, 20 cases were double entered in a random fashion in order to determine the reproducibility of thalamic volume estimations. On completion, thalamic volumes, patient's birth weight, gestational age and corrected chronologic age were entered alongside the previously recorded CT assessment of extent and severity of PVL and clinical examination of the patient.

Results

The 65 patients with PVL included 35 males and 30 females with an average birth weight of 1197 g (range 580–2275), and gestational age of 28.5 weeks (range 24–40). Seventy-five diagnostic CT studies were performed at an average corrected age of 16 months, with 10 patients having two studies.

The validity and reproducibility of the method were tested in two ways. First, estimates of relative thalamic symmetry in normal children ($n = 75$) varied less than 10% which was then accepted as the upper limit of normal variation. Second, unknown to the observer, 20 patients had repeat volume calculations with a variance of 2%–14% (mean 5%) for absolute volume estimates and less than 7% for relative thalamic symmetry. Four double calculations occurred in patients with asymmetric PVL and in all, the thalamic asymmetry remained constant.

Twenty-five of 65 cases of PVL (38%) showed relative thalamic asymmetry greater than 10%, with an average asymmetry of 33% (Fig. 2). Of these, 23 correlated strongly with the clinical findings consistent with asymmetric PVL. However in 2 cases of asymmetry (12%, 16%) there was poor agreement. In 1 (12%), the smaller thalamus was contralateral to the most affected clinical side, while in the second (16%), asymmetric clinical findings were not elicited. With one exception, the small thalamus was ipsilateral to the most severe periventricular atrophy. However, detectable thalamic asymmetry was identifiable only if there were at least two grades of severity difference in hemispheric periventricular tissue loss. Thus measurable thalamic asymmetry was identified only in cases with mild hemispheric PVL and contralateral severe changes or

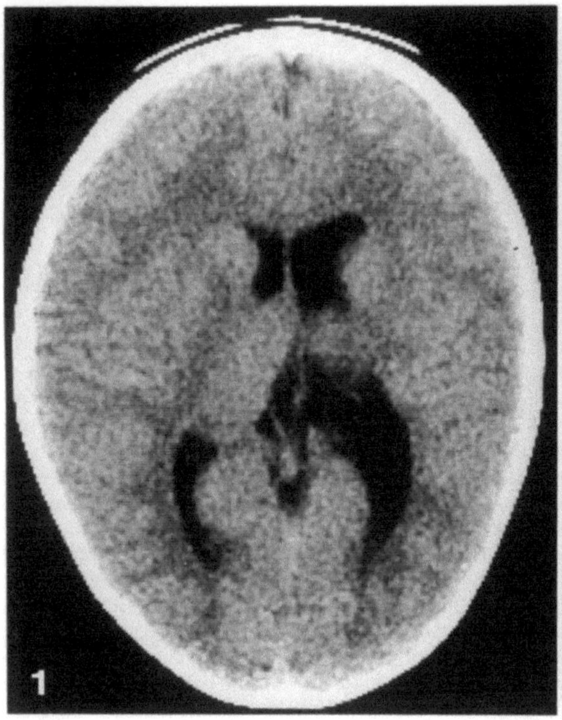

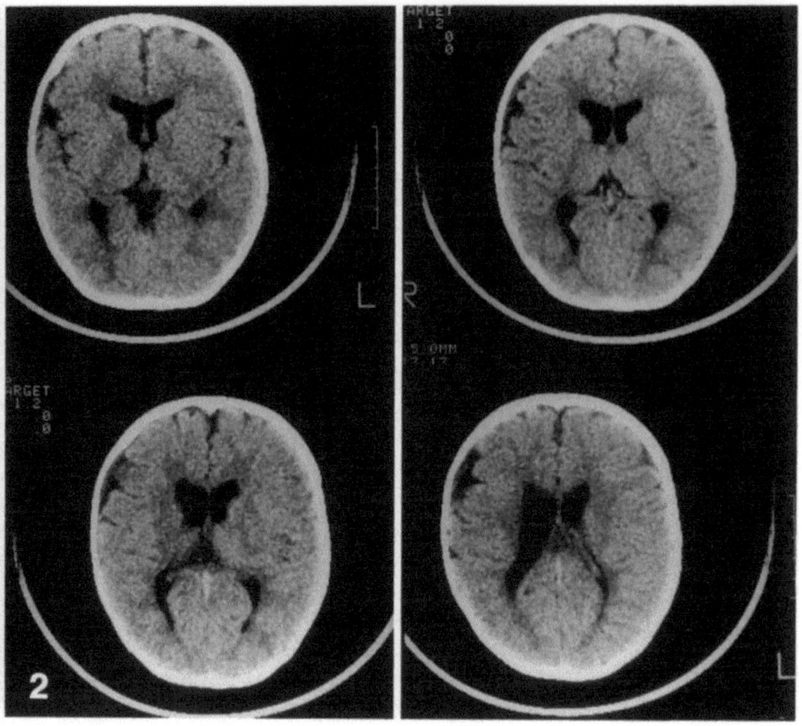

Fig. 1. Volume loss in the left thalamus and moderate, ipsilateral changes characteristic of periventricular leukomalacia (PVL)

Fig. 2. Minimal left-sided periventricular changes and moderate/severe right sided PVL associated with asymmetric volume loss of the right thalamus

moderate/severe disease associated with a contralateral normal hemisphere.

Calculations of absolute thalamic volume in patients with PVL were compared with those in age-matched children who, although being studied for possible neurologic disease, were considered to have normal CT studies. Each cerebral hemisphere was graded for severity of PVL with the following results; normal 5, mild 38, moderate 49, and severe 38. These groups were then compared with their age-matched controls. Thalamic volumes ipsilateral to mild PVL were 92% of normal compared to 70% for thalamic volumes ipsilateral to moderate PVL. Severe PVL was associated with thalamic volumes 54% of normal. Serial studies in 10 cases of PVL demonstrated absolute thalamic volume loss in 5 patients. The loss of thalamic volume was greater than 10%, with an average of 22%.

Discussion

PVL is a result of hypoxic-ischemic injury to watershed zones of arterial supply located in a periventricular distribution in the immature brain. These zones are most prominent adjacent to the trigone of the lateral ventricle and in the white matter at the level of the foramina of Monro [1–3, 7]. It is precisely the anatomic location of the insult that determines the neurologic sequelae. If the lesions affect the geniculocalcarine tract or corticospinal tracts the child will exhibit the classical features of PVL, e.g., cortical blindness and spastic diplegia or quadriplegia with relative preservation of cognitive functions. In instances where the cerebral injury is severe and diffuse, multiple handicaps occur [1, 2].

Thalamic injury associated with PVL has been recognized in the pathology literature. Thus, Rorke [8] states ... "the most common lesions in low birthweight infants are intraventricular hemorrhages, necrosis of the white matter and neuronal destruction in deep grey nuclei and thalamus". She also points out that ... "it is infrequently emphasized that other structures such as thalamus or cortex are also damaged . . . Hence a distorted concept of the nature and distribution of hypoxic-ischemic injury in both animals and humans prevails". Prior radiological works outlining the characteristic features of PVL have not described thalamic changes.

The preliminary observation of occasional asymmetric thalami in association with PVL led us to postulate that thalamic atrophy was likely to be secondary to the hypoxic-ischemic insult involving the periventricular white matter. We postulated that decreased thalamic volume would correlate with the location and severity of periventricular atrophy. First we documented relative thalamic volume loss in cases of asymmetric PVL, which constituted 38% of our patient population. In addition, absolute loss of thalamic volume proportional to the severity of symmetric periventricular atrophy was observed in cases with symmetric PVL. Finally, we were able to demonstrate absolute and progressive thalamic volume loss in 5 of 10 patients with PVL. Although these findings do not clearly separate primary from secondary thalamic injury, the constant relationship to severity and clinical findings argues in favour of a secondary mechanism.

Atrophy has been described as a secondary process in other vascular insults e.g., thalamic volume reduction following spontaneous intracerebral hemorrhage [9] as well as crossed cerebellar atrophy in infantile hemiplegia [10]. Similarly, numerous articles [11–16] have reported secondary atrophic change caused by Wallerian degeneration of corticospinal and descending tracts. It is tempting to speculate that Wallerian degeneration may be the underlying mechanism of the thalamic atrophy observed in association with PVL. Our data are consistent with this notion but do not distinguish between a primary or secondary insult to the thalami. Nonetheless, it is important to stress that loss of thalamic volume is common in patients with PVL and has not been described previously in the radiologic literature. Finally, we endorse the statement of Rorke [8] that structures other than the periventricular white matter are affected by hypoxic-ischemic cerebral insults causing PVL. They include grey matter such as thalamus and cortex and we must be careful not to misrepresent the nature and distribution of neuronal injury in hypoxic-ischemic injury in preterm infants. Thalamic injury may be primary and occur at the same time as the injury to the periventricular white matter; it may be secondary to Wallerian degeneration or may be a combination of both. Based on our finding that loss of thalamic volume is invariably proportional to the severity of periventricular atrophy it would appear that secondary atrophy is the dominant effect.

References

1. DeReuck J, Chatta AS, Richardson EP Jr (1972) Pathogenesis and evolution of periventricular leukomalacia in infancy. Arch Neurol 27: 229–236
2. Banker BQ, Larroche JC (1962) Periventricular leukomalacia of infancy. Arch Neurol 7: 386–410
3. Shuman RM, Selednik LJ (1980) Periventricular leukomalacia; a one-year autopsy study. Arch Neurol 37: 231–235
4. Flodmark O, Roland EH, Hill A, Whitfield M (1986) Radiologic diagnosis of periventricular leukomalacia. Acta Radiol (Stockh) [Suppl] 369: 664–666
5. Flodmark O, Roland EH, Hill A, Whitfield M (1986) Periventricular leukomalacia: radiologic diagnosis. Radiology 160: 507–511
6. Weindling AM, Rochefort MJ, Calvert SA, Fok TF, Wilkinson A (1985) Development of cerebral palsy after ultrasonographic detection of cysts in the newborn. Dev Med Child Neurol 27: 800
7. Armstrong D, Norman MG (1974) Periventricular leukomalacia in neonates: complications and sequelae. Arch Dis Child 49: 367–375
8. Rorke L (1982) Pathology of perinatal brain injury. Raven Press, p 4
9. Skriver EB, Olsen TS (1986) Tissue damage at computed tomography following resolution of intracerebral hematomas. Acta Radiol 27: 495–500
10. Hyung DC (1985) Retrograde crossed cerebellar atrophy. Brain 108: 881–895
11. Rafto SE, Wallace SF, Grossman RI, Rosenquist AC, Kundel HL (1988) Magnetic resonance imaging: an animal model of wallerian degeneration. AJNR 9: 1025
12. Schrodt JF (1988) MRI of brainstem corticospinal tract wallerian degeneration. AJNR 9: 1025
13. Kuhn MJ, New PFJ, Davis KR (1988) Neuroanatomic mapping of corticofugal tracts in the internal capsule and brain stem on MRI by wallerian degeneration. AJNR 9: 1026
14. Bouchareb M, Moulin T, Cattin F, Dietemann JL, Racle A, Verdot H, Bonneville JF (1988) Wallerian degeneration of the descending tracts. J Neuroradiol 15: 238–252
15. Kuhn MJ, Johnson KA, Davis KR (1988) Wallerian degeneration: evaluation with MR imaging. Radiology 168: 199–202
16. Stovring J, Fernando LT (1983) Wallerian degeneration of the corticospinal tract region of the brainstem: demonstration by computed tomography. Radiology 149: 717–720

Dr. K. J. Poskitt
British Columbia's Childrens Hospital
4480 Oak Street
Vancouver, B. C. V6H 3V4, Canada

Neuroradiology (1991) 33 [Suppl]: 254–256

Neuroradiology
© Springer-Verlag 1991

Myelination, structural abnormalities and diseases of white matter – an assessment using high field MRI

J. P. Finn, B. E. Kendall, D. M. K. Kingsley, M. A. Hall-Craggs, and A. Connelly

The Hospital for Sick Children, London, UK

Summary. Comparison between a double-echo short tau inversion recovery (DESTIR) [1, 2] sequence and a combination of T1- and T2-weighted spin echo sequences was performed in a series of 120 children aged 6 weeks to 4 years. The effects of myelination could be seen with greater clarity on the DESTIR sequence and using it structural lesions were consistently demonstrated to better advantage. The DESTIR sequence is suitable for routine cranial MRI in paediatrics.

Key words: Myelination – Magnetic resonance imaging – Short tau inversion recovery sequences

In infants and young children structural abnormalities and diseases of the brain, particularly those involving the white matter, must be diagnosed against a changing pat-

Fig. 1a–c. "Normal" 2 month-old-child; 5-mm thick sections through internal capsules. **a** Spin echo (SE) 3000/90/1; **b** short tau inversion recovery (STIR) 3000/145/23/1; **c** STIR 3000/145/85/1. Note increased conspicuity of posterior limb and visibility of anterior limb of internal capsule on DESTIR sequences

Fig. 2a, b. A 3-year-old child with methionine adenosyl-transferase deficiency, myelination mature; 5-mm thick sections through centra semiovale. **a** SE 3000/90/1; **b** STIR 300/145/85/1. Note myelin is visualised further out into some of the gyral cores and contrast between myelinated white matter and the peritrigonal and multifocal white matter lesions is greater in Fig. 2b

Fig. 3a–c. A 7-year-old female with neurofibromatosis; 5-mm thick sections through internal capsules. **a** SE 3000/90/1; **b** STIR 3000/145/15/1; **c** STIR 3000/145/85/1. Note increased contrast between myelinated white matter and both grey matter and typical lesions in **c**. Myelination well shown in **b**, but contrast between grey matter, lesions and cerebrospinal fluid is poor

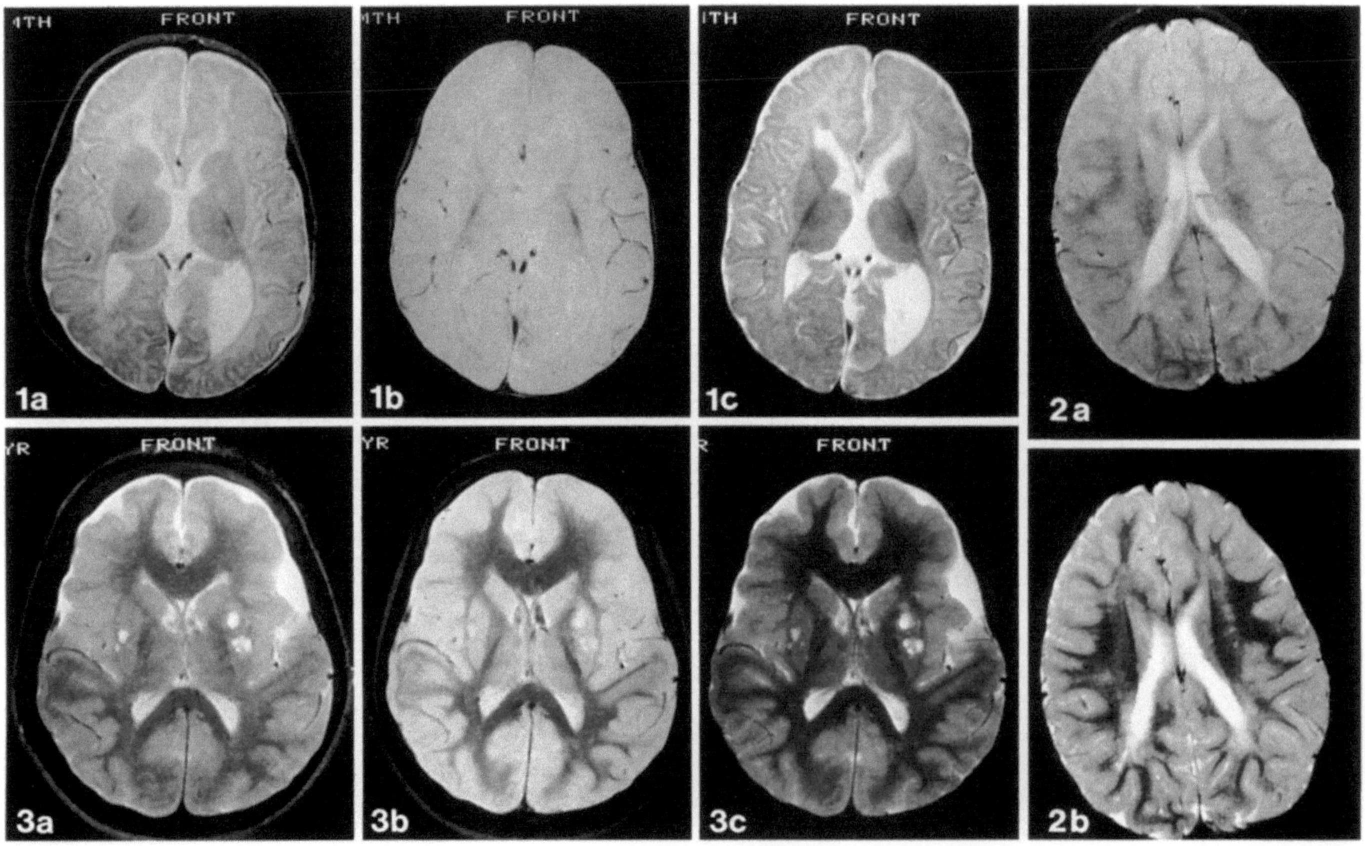

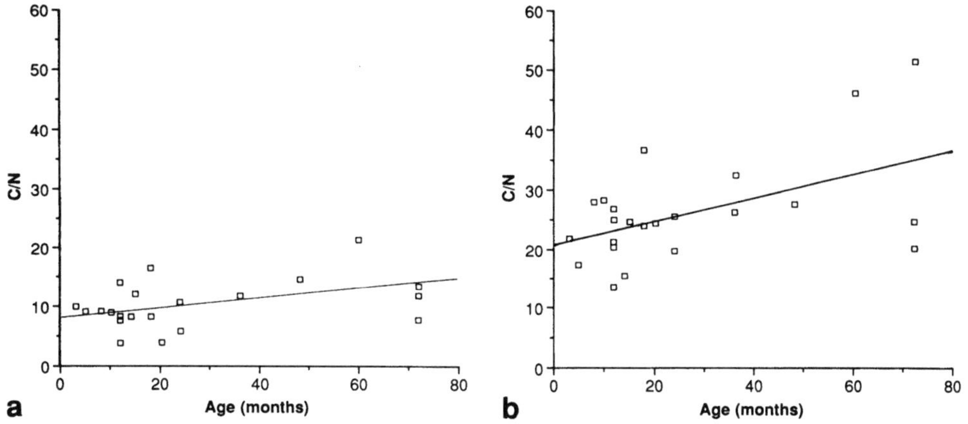

Fig. 4 a, b. Graphs of contrast/noise (*C/N*) against age in months. **a** SE 3000/90/1; **b** STIR 3000/145/23/1. Note C/N in **b** is over twice that in **a** and increases further with age

tern caused by the normal processes of myelination. The normal progression of myelination at high field is characterised by an orderly sequence of changes [3]: initial shortening of T1 is followed by shortening of T2 and fall in proton density. The process begins in the dorsal brain stem, advances through the posterior limbs of the internal capsules into the sensory radiations and progresses anterosuperiorly. Based on the recommendations of Barkovich et al. [3] it is conventional to use spin echo (SE) short TR short TE sequences (T1-weighted) for assessing myelination up to 6 months of age and long TR long TE sequences (T2-weighted) after 6 months of age.

This approach has certain disadvantages. Signal intensity on T1-weighted sequences increases as T1 decreases with myelination but as shortening of T2 and decrease in proton density supervene signal intensity diminishes and this adversely affects grey, white matter contrast. Converse effects occur on the T2-weighted sequence. Also the two sequences are necessary for full evaluation of developmental status and this results in prolongation of imaging, thus increasing the risk of movement and therefore of an unsatisfactory study.

Signal on both echoes of a double echo short tau inversion recovery (DESTIR) sequence decreases with reduction in T1 or T2 or proton density so that decreasing white matter signal should be a monotonic function of increasing brain maturation, making it a more suitable sequence for routine use in a paediatric population. We have verified this in practice.

Materials and methods

A multi-slice optimised band width double-echo STIR sequence (TR/TI/TE = 3,000/148/23/85) was compared with a combination of SE (TR/TE/NEX) 600/15/2 and SE (TR/TE/TE/NEX) 3000/15/90/1 sequence in the axial plane using a 1.5 T Siemens Magnetom. Second order gradient motion rephasing was used on the longer echoes and all sequences utilised the same slice thickness (5 mm) and slice gap (2 mm).

The use of an asymmetrical field of view made it possible to acquire 12 slices in 7 min on a 256 × 180 matrix and 16 slices in a little under 9 min. Post-processing by adding the first and second echoes of the STIR to produce higher signal to noise and improve definition of the interface between brain and cerebrospinal fluid was performed off-line in appropriate cases.

All the sequences were performed on 120 children aged between 1 week and 10 years of age and the images obtained in this consecutive series were assessed by two observers independently for conspicuity of myelination in 14 anatomical regions as described by Barkovich et al. [3], as well as for visibility of structural lesions and abnormalities of the white matter. In 30 of these patients grey-white matter contrast to noise measurements were made on corresponding slices for each echo of the T2W sequence and for each echo of the DESTIR.

Results

Myelination was in all cases more conspicuous on DESTIR than on T2W SE sequences (Fig. 1) and grading of myelination was easier on STIR than on the T1-weighted SE sequence. Under 2 years of age arborisation of myelin was more clearly shown on STIR than on the T2-weighted sequence in most patients (Fig. 2) and in 10 patients arborisation could be seen more peripherally on the STIR sequence.

The average contrast-to-noise ratio for the first echo of the DESTIR sequence was twice that for the T2-weighted SE sequence and high contrast levels were present at an earlier age on the STIR sequence (Fig. 4, $P < 0.001$). Abnormalities were present in 91 patients and these were shown at least as well in all cases (Fig. 3) and in 10 cases better on the STIR than on other sequences. The relationship of lesions to vascular structures and anatomical landmarks could be seen on all sequences but in no case was it less well shown on the long-echo STIR sequence than on any other sequence.

Discussion

The results confirm the theoretical advantage of the modified STIR sequence in routine paediatric clinical practice. Structural and white matter lesions were consistently demonstrated and often to better advantage on the DESTIR sequence and fine details were more definitively shown with this sequence on several occasions. In this series no pathological process was obscured, although signal changes in certain pathologies are modified and this could be confusing. This will particularly apply to fat-containing lesions such as dermoids and lipomas, in which the suppressed signal from fat could theoretically be mistaken for signal void, as may occur in aneurysm or angioma.

The DESTIR sequence is recommended for routine practice, particularly in paediatrics, to be supplemented as indicated by other sequences to clarify abnormalities revealed by the study, or in relation to clinical diagnosis.

References

1. Bydder GM, Young IR (1985) MR imaging: clinical use of the inversion recovery sequence. J Comput Assist Tomogr 9: 659–675
2. Finn JP, Hall-Craggs MA, Connelly A (1989) A modified inversion recovery sequence for high contrast brain imaging. 8th Meeting of SMRM, 722
3. Barkovich AJ, Kjos BO, Jackson DE, Norman D (1988) Normal maturation of the neonatal and infant brain: MR imaging at 1.5 T. Radiology 166: 173–180

Dr. B. E. Kendall
Radiology Department
National Hospital for Nervous Diseases
Queen Square
London WC1N 3BG, UK

SESSION 18
CEREBROVASCULAR DISEASE, FUNCTIONAL

Neuroradiology (1991) 33 [Suppl]: 258–259

Neuro radiology
© Springer-Verlag 1991

Non-invasive methods for identifying major vessel occlusion in acute cerebral infarction: correlation between CT findings and Doppler patterns of underlying vascular pathology

A. R. Naylor[1], R. J. Sellar[2], P. A. G. Sandercock[1], M. V. Merrick[3], and C. P. Warlow[1]

Departments of [1] Clinical Neurosciences, [2] Neuroradiology and [3] Nuclear Medicine, The Western General Hospital, Edinburgh, Scotland

Summary. We have correlated Doppler patterns of underlying vascular pathology [using duplex and transcranial Doppler sonography (TCD)] with CT findings in 28 patients with acute, first-ever cerebral infarction affecting the carotid territory. Patients with extensive middle cerebral artery (MCA) territory infarction or oedema had the worst prognosis and almost invariably had an underlying major vessel occlusion (internal carotid artery and/or MCA). Patients with partial MCA territory infarction generally had patent major vessels. One patient with capsulostriate infarction had MCA hyperaemia on TCD suggesting an initial MCA occlusion, spontaneous lysis and secondary hyperaemia. The majority of patients with normal CT had normal TCD examinations.

Key words: Acute cerebral infarction – Duplex scan – Transcranial Doppler sonography – Computed tomography

Twenty-eight patients with first-ever acute cerebral infarction (ACI) were assessed by duplex scan [extracranial internal carotid artery (ICA)], transcranial Doppler (TCD) examination of the basal cerebral arteries and CT. The median time from onset of symptoms to CT was 34 h (95% CI 24–50). Specific attention was directed towards identifying major vessel occlusion (Doppler) and CT was classified as extensive middle cerebral artery (MCA) territory infarction or oedema, partial MCA territory infarction, lacunar infarction, capsulostriate infarction or normal. There was no significant difference in the time interval between onset of symptoms and CT in any of the subgroups.

Results

Eleven patients (39%) had extensive MCA territory infarction or oedema, of whom 4 died and 5 remained dependent in hospital at 30 days. Table 1 details the Doppler patterns of vascular pathology in this subgroup; all had major vessel occlusion or some other significant pathology in the main stem of the MCA. Of the 6 patients (21%) with partial MCA territory infarction, none died and all were discharged home within 30 days. Table 2 details the Doppler findings in this subgroup; the majority had patent major vessels although 3 had MCA abnormalities. One patient had ICA occlusion and showed the largest area of infarction in this subgroup. One patient had a lacunar infarct on CT and had no evidence of major vessel occlusion, while another had an area of capsulostriate infarction with preservation of the overlying cortex in association with MCA hyperaemia. The features in the latter patient are consistent with an initial MCA occlusion, spontaneous lysis and secondary hyperaemia. Nine patients (32%) had normal CT at a median interval of 46 h after onset of symptoms. In 7 the ICA was patent and there was no TCD abnormality; all were discharged home within 30 days. However, 2 patients had MCA occlusion; CT remained normal at 7 days in 1, while in the other CT was performed within 6 h of onset, and he died at 36 h.

Discussion

CT performed within 6 h of ACI permits exclusion of haemorrhage but cannot subclassify ACI with respect to patterns of vascular pathology [1]. However, in order to identify appropriate patients for future trials of thrombolysis, it is important to know the relationship between vas-

Table 1. Doppler patterns of vascular pathology in patients with extensive infarction or oedema throughout the middle cerebral artery (MCA) territory on CT

Cervical ICA	Main MCA	No.
Occluded	Reduced velocity	3
Occluded	Occluded	3
Patent	Occluded	3
Patent	Reduced velocity	1
Patent	Stenosis	1

ICA, Internal carotid artery

Table 2. Doppler patterns of vascular pathology in patients with partial MCA territory infarction on CT

Cervical ICA	Main MCA	No.
Occluded	Reduced velocity	1
Patent	Reduced velocity	1
Patent	Stenosis	2
Patent	Normal	2

cular pathology and established infarction on MCA territory, as the latter has been shown to correlate with clinical outcome [2]. Doppler techniques are non-invasive and not associated with the risk of precipitating further neurological deterioration [1]. Moreover, TCD is reproducible [3] and shows good interobserver reliability [4]. This study has shown that patients with the most extensive area of infarction have the worst prognosis and, almost invariably, an underlying major vessel occlusion that might be suitable for thrombolysis. Patients with partial MCA territory infarction tend to have patent major vessels (suggesting distal MCA disease as the aetiology) and TCD could be used to identify appropriate patients for thrombolysis. The CT and TCD features in the 2 patients with lacunar or capsulostriate infarction indicate that thrombolytic therapy would not be indicated. The combination of CT and normal TCD indicates a good prognosis and thrombolytic therapy is therefore probably not indicated. Two patients, however, had normal CT and an occluded MCA. In 1, CT was clearly performed too early, while a normal repeat scan in the second suggests that collateral circulation was excellent. In both, however, decisions with regard to the use of thrombolytic therapy could be made on the basis of the TCD findings.

Acknowledgements. Mr. Naylor is a research fellow sponsored by the UK Chest, Heart and Stroke Association.

References

1. Fieschi C, Argentino C, Lenzi GL, Aacchetti ML, Toni D, Bozzao L (1989) Clinical and instrumental evaluation of patients with ischaemic stroke within the first 6 hours. J Neurol Sci 91: 311–322
2. Brott T, Marter JR, Olinger CP, Adams HP, Tomsich T, Barsan WG, Biller J, Hertzberg V, Walker M (1989) Measurement of acute cerebral infarction: lesion size by computed tomography. Stroke 20: 871–875
3. Merrick MV, Naylor AR, Miller JD, Notghi A, Slattery J (1989) Validation of a new method for demonstrating regional differences in cerebral perfusion reserve. J Cereb Blood Flow Metab 9 [Suppl 1]: S431
4. Minciotti P, Ceravalo G, Orlandini M, Provinciali L (1990) Interobserver reliability of transcranial Doppler examination. J Neurol 237: 137

Dr. R. J. Sellar
The Western General Hospital
Crewe Road, Edinburgh, Scotland

Neuroradiology (1991) 33 [Suppl]: 260–262

Neuro radiology
© Springer-Verlag 1991

Changes of haemorheological factors induced by Magnevist and the influence of blood flow stimulation in magnetic field 2.5 T

R. Schickerova, Y. Shinohara, M. Yamamoto, and H. Ohsuga

Department of Neurology, School of Medicine, Tokai University, Japan

Summary. Magnevist (gadolinium-DTPA) has been used as an MRI contrast agent in patients with limited brain perfusion, where rheological properties of blood play an important role. The dose-dependent effects of Magnevist on red blood cell aggregability (RBCA), deformability and blood viscosity were measured. To check the influence of the magnetic field (MF) we simulated blood flow using a cannula placed in MF 2.5 T. Magnevist has a dose-dependent effect of prolonging of aggregation time and this is further significantly prolonged after simulation of flow in MF. In concentrations used in patients the prolongation is more than 20%. There is no significant influence on deformability. Slight decrease in viscosity was observed with low doses. The possible mechanisms of influence of Magnevist on RBCA and its potentiation after blood flow simulation in MF are discussed.

Key words: Gadolinium-DTPA – Haemorheology – Magnetic field, influence of – Magnetic resonance imaging – Contrast media

Magnevist gadolinium(Gd)-DTPA is useful for increasing the diagnostic yield of MRI and therefore is being increasingly used in patients with limited brain perfusion, in whom the rheological properties of blood play an important role. Red blood cell aggregability (RBCA), deformability and blood viscosity are the main haemorheological parameters, which can be influenced both positively and negatively by different drugs. Firstly, from this point of view, the dose-dependent effect of Gd-DTPA on these factors was studied.

The magnetic field (MF) encountered during the MRI examination is considered to have no effect on biological systems and when studying global changes in blood cell count, enzyme and glucose levels, no significant changes were found [1]. Other reports now suggest that steady MF in the range used clinically can directly affect the functional activity of biologically important molecules [2]. Deoxygenated sickle erythrocytes have also been shown by in vitro studies to align perpendicular to relatively low MF (0.35 T), due to the paramagnetic properties of ferrohaemoglobin, while normal human erythrocytes containing oxygenated or deoxygenated haemoglobin do not show any apparent orientation in MF [3].

Gd-DTPA is a paramagnetic agent, which, when placed in MF, develops a relatively large magnetic moment, resulting in a relatively large local MF, with enhancement of water proton relaxation rates.

The effect of Magnevist on RBCA after flow simulation in 2.5 T MF was studied.

Patients and methods

Fresh blood samples were placed in heparinised tubes and all measurements were made within 2 h. RBCA was measured using a photometric aggregometer [4]. We used the RBC aggregation time ($t_{1/2}$), defined as the time required for the intensity of light transmission through blood in a transparent tube to increase by half the total increment after stopping the flow, as an index of RBCA. Blood obtained from each of ten patients was divided into six 3-ml samples. One was used as a control, and the others were incubated for 20 min with 5, 10, 20, 30 and 40 µl of Magnevist and examined at room temperature, three times for each sample to confirm reproducibility.

RBC deformability was estimated using a conventional microporous filtration method, expressed as filtrability (the time necessary for filtration). The haematocrit from each patient was adjusted to 30% and the 3-ml samples were incubated with 5, 10 and 20 µl of Magnevist. Measurement of control and incubated samples was carried out twice at room temperature. Whole blood viscosity was measured using a cone plate viscometer with a shear rate of 150/s. The temperature was maintained at 37 °C. Blood samples were prepared in the same way as for measurement of deformability.

To study the effect of Magnevist on RBCA after blood flow simulation in MF the blood of each patient was divided into six 3-ml samples. The first sample was measured as a control, the second after 10 min flow simulation in room conditions. Two remaining samples were incubated with 10 µl and other two with 30 µl of Magnevist. In both concentrations one sample was examined 10 min after incubation and the second after 10 min of flow simulation in MF. To compare the effect of flow simulation in room conditions and in MF the obtained blood was divided into five 3-ml samples, one measured as a control, two incubated with 10 µl and two with 30 µl of Magnevist. In both concentrations RBCA was measured after 10 min of flow simulation in room conditions and after 10 min of flow simulation in magnetic field.

A coiled cannula 50 cm long and 3.3 mm in diameter was placed in an MF of 2.5 T or in room conditions. The blood was moved backwards and forwards at a mean flow speed of approximately 20 cm/s.

Haematocrit, pH and PO_2 were measured to check the effect of oxygenation and haemolysis after blood flow simulation.

Results

In vitro Magnevist has a dose-dependent effect, prolonging RBC aggregation time ($t_{1/2}$). Significant prolongation was found with the lowest concentrations used. In a con-

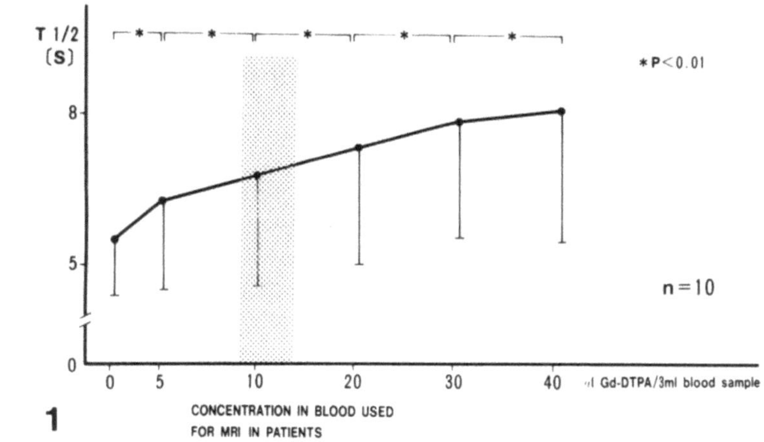

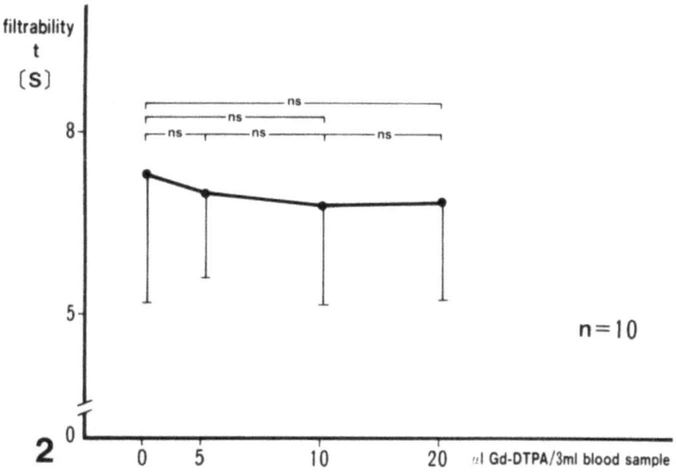

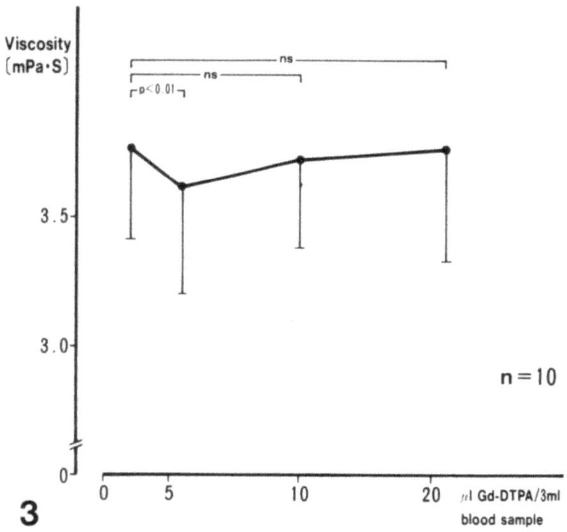

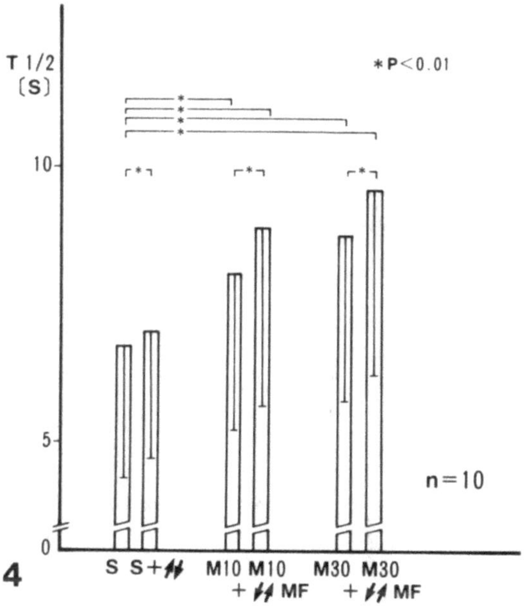

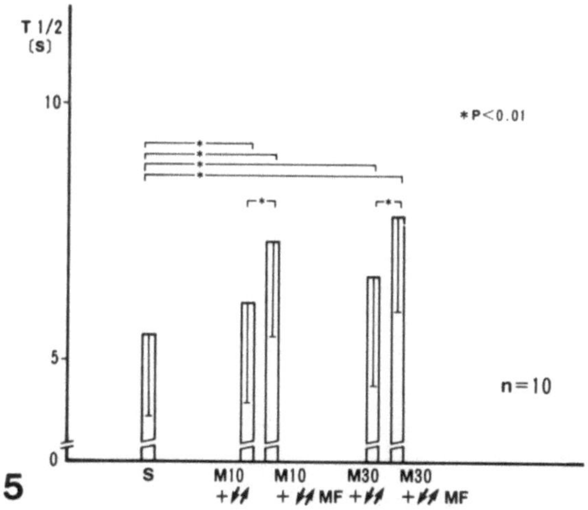

Fig. 1. Dose-dependent effect of Gd-DTPA on red blood cell aggregability (RBCA $t_{1/2}$): in vitro study

Fig. 2. Effect of Gd-DTPA on blood cell deformability (expressed as a time necessary for filtration): in vitro study

Fig. 3. Effect of Gd-DTPA on blood viscosity (in vitro study)

Fig. 4. Changes in RBCA $t_{1/2}$ after administration of Gd-DTPA and influence of flow simulation in magnetic field 2.5 T: in vitro study

Fig. 5. Changes in RBCA $t_{1/2}$ after administration of Gd-DTPA and influence of flow simulation in room conditions and magnetic field 2.5 T: in vitro study

centration of 10 µl (3 ml blood sample), corresponding approximately to the levels after administration of 0.2 mg/kg i. v., routinely used in patients, the prolongation is more than 20%, as shown in Fig. 1.

The filtration time was slightly but not significantly shortened by all concentrations used (Fig. 2). Whole blood viscosity was significantly lowered by low doses (5 µl/3 ml blood sample) but no significant changes were found with higher concentrations (Fig. 3). There was a small but significant prolongation of RBCA $t_{1/2}$ in control samples after flow simulation in room conditions. The prolongation of RBCA $t_{1/2}$ was significantly higher with both concentrations after 10 min flow simulation in MF (Fig. 4).

Significant changes in pH and PO_2 before and after flow simulation were revealed in all samples, but no significant differences were observed between control samples and samples incubated with Magnevist. The prolongation of RBCA $t_{1/2}$ was significantly higher when flow simulation was in MF than in room conditions, although the changes of pH and PO_2 were similar (Fig. 5).

Discussion

Erythrocyte aggregation is a major determinant of the rheological properties of blood. The mechanisms involved in RBCA are highly complex. It has been proposed that aggregation is due to adsorption and reversible "cross-bridging" of the membrane components of adjacent cells by macromolecules. This theory may explain the effect of different plasma proteins on changes of RBCA [5], but other authors stress the role of cellular factors [6]. The effects of albumin, glycerol and high doses of urokinase on improving RBCA are well known [7]. On the other hand, high fibrinogen levels, citrate and high molecular dextran contribute to hyperaggregability [8].

Our results do not explain the mechanism of prolongation of RBCA $t_{1/2}$ but an effect on the plasma or on the RBC membrane is possible.

The lack of effect on deformability even with high doses suggests that there is no effect on the rigidity of the RBC membrane, as is usually found after glycerol treatment in levels effective in improving RBCA. The viscosity was significantly decreased only by low doses of Magnevist and there was no correlation between blood viscosity and RBCA with high doses when measured only using a high shear rate. This is partially in agreement with the findings of Shinohara et al. [9], who found no correlation between blood viscosity and RBCA in patients with cerebrovascular disease at wall shear rates from 30 to 130/s, although the blood viscosity may correlate with wall shear rates lower than 30/s.

Our data indicate that there is a significant prolongation of RBCA $t_{1/2}$ in blood samples containing Magnevist after flow simulation in MF when compared with samples with the same concentration of Magnevist but without flow simulation or with simulation in room conditions. Budinger [10] proposed four mechanisms whereby MFs might influence biological processes, one of which was changes of macromolecular orientation leading to changes in chemical kinetics and membrane permeability. Effects on molecules and some organized cellular structures are dependent on sufficiently great anisotropy in magnetic susceptibility and sufficient numbers of these structures. As mentioned above, relatively low fields (0.35 T) were effective.

Two aspects must be considered in our study; firstly the effect of Magnevist as a chemical agent and secondly the influence of the paramagnetic effect of Gd, which probably increases electromagnetic field potentials induced by the rapid perpendicular flow of the blood in MF. Increased electrical charge of the RBC membrane, increasing the electrostatical forces between cells seems possible.

We can conclude that from the haemorheological point of view Magnevist seems to be safe, tending to have a favourable effect on some parameters, but further investigation is necessary.

References

1. Battocletti JH, Salles-Cunha S, Halbach RE, Nelson J, Sances A, Antonich FJ (1981) Exposure of rhesus monkeys to 20000 G steady magnetic field: effect on blood parameters. Med Phys 8: 115–118
2. Chiles C, Hawrot E, Gore J, Byck R (1988) Magnetic field modulation of receptor binding. Magn Reson Med 10: 241–245
3. Murayama M (1965) Orientation of sickled erythrocytes in a magnetic field. Nature 206: 420–422
4. Yamamoto M (1986) Effects of fibrinogen, globulin, albumin and hematocrit on the kinetics of erythrocyte aggregation in man. Angiology 37: 663–671
5. Donner M, Mills P, Stoltz JF (1989) Influence of plasma proteins on erythrocyte aggregation. Clin Hemorheol 9: 715–721
6. Sowemimo-Coker SO, Whittingstall P, Pietsch L (1989) Effects of cellular factors on the aggregation behavior of human, rat and bovine erythrocytes. Clin Hemorheol 9: 723–737
7. Shinohara Y (1986) Some rheological considerations of the treatment of acute and chronic stages of cerebrovascular disease. In: Gotoh F, Lechner H (eds) Clinical haemorheology, pp 89–95
8. Janzen J, Brooks DE (1989) Do plasma proteins adsorb to red cells? Clin Hemorheol 9: 695–714
9. Shinohara Y, Yamamoto M, Saitoh H, Yoshitoshi M (1987) Some rheological considerations in ischemic cerebrovascular disease. In: Hartmann A, Kuschinsky W (eds) Cerebral ischemia and hemorheology, pp 514–519
10. Budinger FT (1981) Nuclear magnetic resonance (NMR) in vivo studies: known thresholds for health effects. J Comput Assist Tomogr 5: 800–811

R. Schickerova
Department of Neurology
Postgraduate Medical School
Videnska 800
Prague 4, Czechoslovakia

Neuroradiology (1991) 33 [Suppl]: 263–266

Neuro-radiology
© Springer-Verlag 1991

Changes in right-left asymmetry and sex differences of regional cerebral blood flow with ageing evaluated by the ^{133}Xe inhalation method*

Y. Tsuda[1, 2], A. Hartmann[1], and H. Matsuo[2]

[1] Neurology Clinic, University of Bonn, Bonn, Federal Republic of Germany
[2] Second Department of Internal Medicine, Kagawa Medical School, Kagawa, Japan

Summary. Regional cerebral blood flow distributions were evaluated in 45 right-handed normal subjects, 23 women, 22 men (mean: 42 years), including 15 young normals below the age of 30 years, 11 women, 4 men (mean: 24 years), 15 middle-aged normals 30–50 years, 5 women, 10 men (mean: 40 years), and 15 elderly normals above the age of 50 years, 7 women, 8 men (mean: 62 years), by the ^{133}Xe inhalation technique. Measurements were made in the four vascular territories of anterior, anterior middle, posterior middle, and posterior cerebral arteries, in addition to the anterior precentral and postcentral temporooccipital regions. Significantly higher values of cerebral blood flow in the right frontal region than in the left were observed only in the middle-aged normal men. Lower values of cerebral blood flow were observed in men, particularly in the elderly, as compared with the values in women in every region and territory. The results show that the right-left asymmetry and sex differences of regional cerebral blood flow change with ageing.

Key words: Ageing – Cerebral blood flow – Right-left asymmetry – Sex differences – Xenon-133 inhalation

---

High frontal regional cerebral blood flow (rCBF) in normal subjects has often been reported [1–3]. It is also reported that the right frontal lobe shows higher rCBF than the left [4–8]. Sex differences of rCBF values are also reported, i. e. significantly higher values of rCBF in women than men [9–11]. Right-left asymmetry and sex differences of rCBF might be influenced by ageing. We examined the effects of ageing on the right-left asymmetry and sex differences of rCBF.

Subjects and methods

The topographical distribution of rCBF was studied in 45 right-handed normal subjects, 23 women, 22 men (mean age: 42 years) by the ^{133}Xe inhalation technique and expressed as the initial slope index. The details of the rCBF study have been reported previously [3]. The normal subjects were divided by age into 15 young subjects less than 30 years old, 11 women, 4 men, (mean: 24 years), 15 middle-aged subjects (30–50 years old), 5 women, 10 men, (mean: 40 years), and 15 elderly subjects, 7 women, 8 men (mean: 62 years) more than 50 years old, as shown in Table 1. No significant differences of the end expiratory CO_2 tension (p_ECO_2) were observed between the groups of subjects. Mean rCBF was measured in the anterior precentral region using seven detector pairs and in the postcentral temporo-occipital region, with eight detector pairs. Each cerebral hemisphere was also divided into four vascular territories of anterior, anterior middle, posterior middle, and posterior cerebral artery, consisting of 4, 3, 4, and 3 detector pairs in each hemisphere (Fig. 1). Left-sided and corresponding right-sided values were compared using two-tailed, paired t-tests, and the differences between women and men were compared using two-tailed, independent t-tests.

Results

There were no significant right-left differences of rCBF in the whole group of 45 normal subjects (Fig. 2 a), including 15 young and 15 elderly subjects (Fig. 3 a, 5 a), but in the 15 middle-aged subjects (Fig. 4 a) there were significant right-left differences of mean rCBF in the anterior precentral region (right 55.5, left 54.3) and in the anterior cerebral artery territory (right 55.6, left 54.0) ($p < 0.001$, respectively), i. e. the right frontal region showed higher

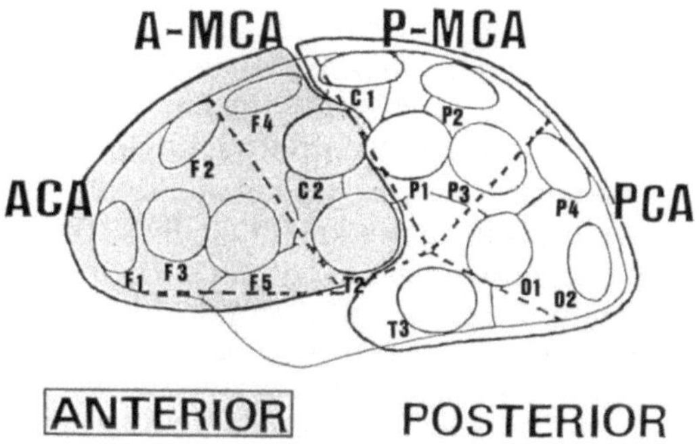

Fig. 1. Diagram showing locations of detectors over cerebral hemisphere. *Shaded areas* show anterior precentral region; *unshaded areas* show postcentral temporo-occipital region. ACA, A-MCA, P-MCA, PCA: territories of anterior, anterior middle, posterior middle, posterior cerebral arteries, respectively. *F*, Frontal; *P*, parietal; *C*, central; *T*, temporal; *O*, occipital

* This study was supported in part by a Research Fellowship from the Alexander von Humboldt-Foundation, FRG (to Y. T.).

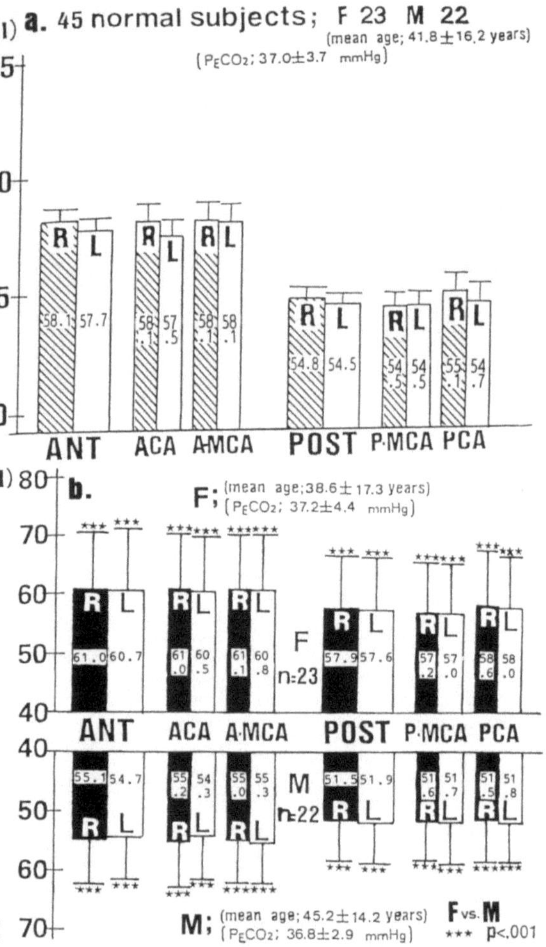

2

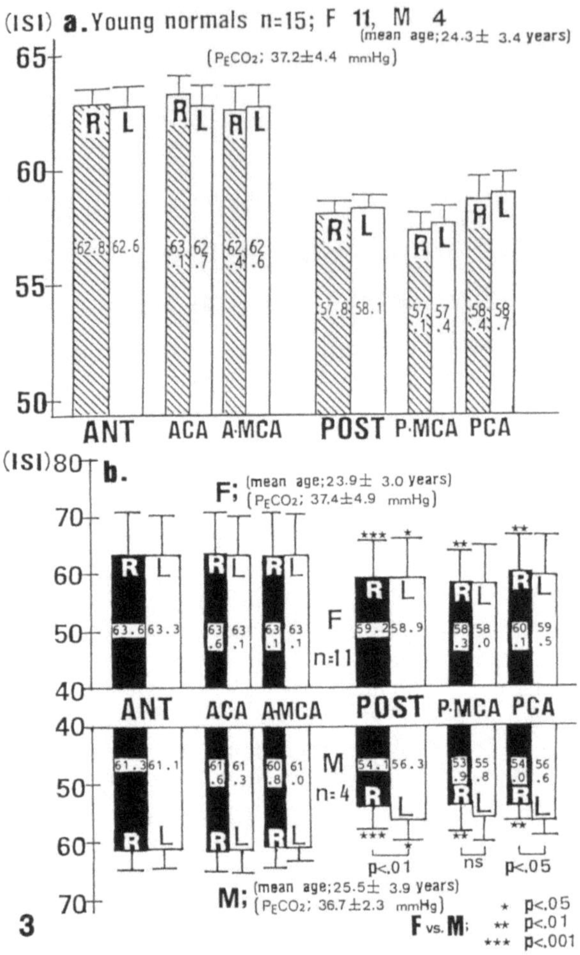

3

Fig. 2 a, b. Distribution of the mean regional cerebral blood flow (rCBF) **a** in 45 normal subjects and **b** in the 23 women and 22 men. *F*, women; *M*, men

Fig. 3 a, b. Distribution of the mean rCBF **a** in the 15 young subjects (below 30 years of age) and **b** in the 11 women and 4 men of this group. *F*, Women; *M*, men

rCBF than the left. These differences of rCBF were observed only in men (Fig. 4b). Moreover, we observed lower values of rCBF in the normal men overall, particularly, in the elderly, as compared with the women, in every region and vascular territory ($p < 0.05$–0.001) (Figs. 2b, 5b). On the other hand, significantly higher values of rCBF were observed in the postcentral region in young women as compared with men, and the left-sided values of the young men were significantly higher than those on the right in the postcentral region (left 56.3, right 54.1; $p < 0.001$), including the posterior cerebral artery territory (left 56.6, right 54.0; $p < 0.05$), although the number of the young normal men was small (Fig. 3b).

Discussion

It is reported that the right frontal lobe shows higher rCBF than the left [4–7], particularly in the superior frontal regions [5, 6]. It is also reported that this predominance persists in older normal subjects [7]. Moreover, the right sensorimotor regions are reported to show higher values of regional cerebral metabolic rate for oxygen, in addition to higher rCBF values [8]. The explanation of this side to side difference may be that the left sensorimotor region is larger than the right. However, right-sided rCBF is slightly higher than the left in all regions except for the frontal and

Table 1. Normal subjects in resting regional cerebral blood flow study

			Age (years)	p_ECO_2 (mm Hg)
		n	Mean ± SD	Mean ± SD
Total subjects		45	41.8 ± 16.2	37.0 ± 3.7
	Women	23	38.6 ± 17.3	37.2 ± 4.4
	Men	22	45.2 ± 14.2	36.8 ± 2.9
Young subjects		15	24.3 ± 3.4	37.2 ± 4.4
< 30 years	Women	11	23.9 ± 3.0	37.4 ± 4.9
	Men	4	25.5 ± 3.9	36.7 ± 2.3
Middle-aged subjects		15	39.8 ± 5.2	36.2 ± 2.8
30–50 years	Women	5	38.6 ± 5.5	36.0 ± 2.7
	Men	10	40.4 ± 4.9	36.3 ± 2.9
Elderly subjects		15	61.5 ± 7.6	37.6 ± 3.4
> 50 years	Women	7	61.8 ± 8.5	37.8 ± 3.8
	Men	8	61.2 ± 6.6	37.5 ± 3.0

p_ECO_2, End expiratory CO_2 tension

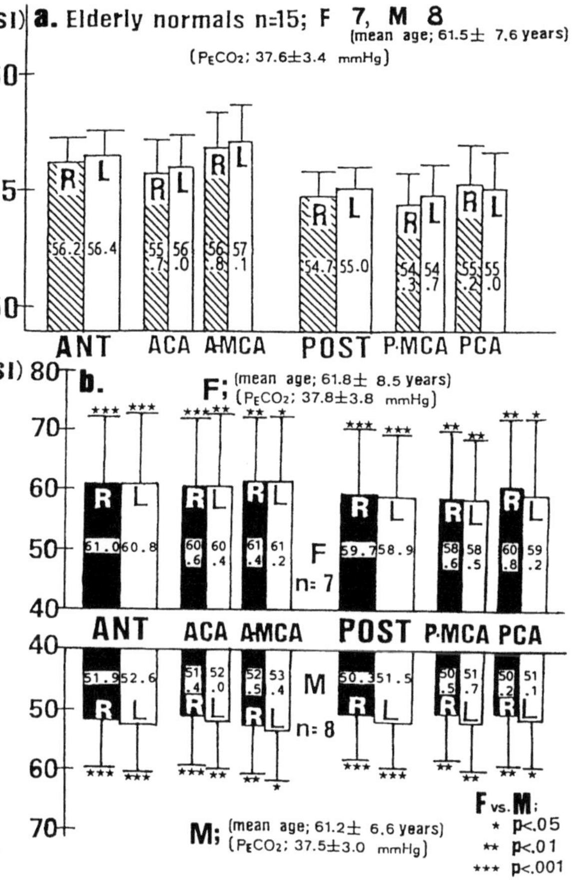

4

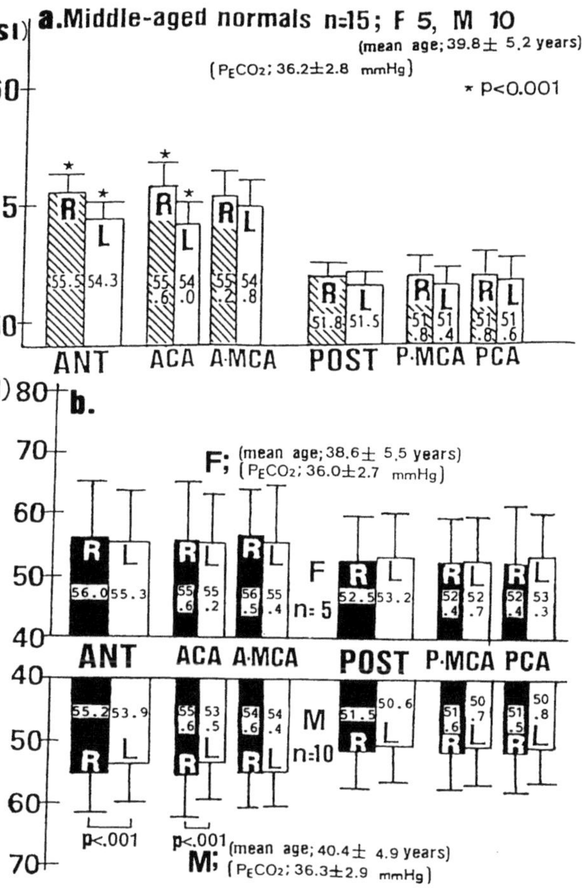

5

Fig. 4 a, b. Distribution of the mean rCBF **a** in the 15 middle-aged subjects (30–50 years old) and **b** in the 5 women and 10 men of this group. *F*, Women; *M*, men

Fig. 5 a, b. Distribution of the mean rCBF **a** in the 15 elderly subjects (above 50 years of age) and **b** in the 7 women and 8 men of this group. *F*, Women; *M*, men

parietal lobes [9]. In our study, significantly higher values of rCBF in the right frontal region, including the right anterior cerebral artery territory, as compared with the left were observed only in the middle-aged men. This might be in accordance with a previous report [10], in which the right frontal region showed higher mean rCBF than the left in men ($n = 38$, mean age 38 years) but not in women ($n = 38$, mean age 38.4 years). In most reports which show significant right-left differences of mean rCBF in the frontal region, the mean age of the subjects is 30–40 years, which might be in accordance with the results of our study.

With respect to sex differences of rCBF, lower values of rCBF were observed in normal men than in women in every region and vascular territory, which is in agreement with previous studies showing that flow is higher in women than in men at all ages [9–11], and that it falls with age in both sexes [9]. In elderly men we observed significantly higher values of mean rCBF in every region and vascular territory than those in elderly women, which has never been reported previously. On the other hand, in the young women we observed significantly higher values of mean rCBF in the postcentral region, particularly on the right, in the postcentral region as compared with the young men. Left-sided mean rCBF values in the young normal men were significantly higher than those in the right ($p < 0.01$), although the number of the young normal men is small. The reason for the sex differences of cerebral blood flow may be explained in part by anatomical differences of the brain: in general, the brains of women weigh 10% less than those of men, in particular in the elderly, which may result in a higher rate of cerebral blood flow per unit weight of the brain in women [10]. The fact that the cardiac index is larger in women than in men [10] could also affect sex differences of cerebral blood flow.

References

1. Ingvar DH (1979) "Hyperfrontal" distribution of the cerebral grey matter flow in resting wakefulness; on the functional anatomy of the conscious state. Acta Neurol Scand 60: 12–25
2. Mamo H, Meric P, Luft A, Seylaz J (1983) Hyperfrontal pattern of human cerebral circulation. Variations with age and atherosclerotic state. Arch Neurol 40: 626–632
3. Tsuda Y, Hartmann A (1989) Changes in hyperfrontality of cerebral blood flow and carbon dioxide reactivity with age. Stroke 20: 1667–1673
4. Blauenstein UW, Halsey JH, Wilson EM, Willis EL, Risberg J (1977) Xe-133 inhalation method: analysis of reproducibility: some of its physiological implications. Stroke 8: 92–102

5. Prohovnik I, Hakansson K, Risberg J (1980) Observations of the functional significance of regional cerebral blood flow in 'resting' normal subjects. Neuropsychologia 18: 203–217
6. Matsuda H, Maeda T, Yamada M, Gui LX, Tonami N, Hisada K (1984) Age-matched normal values and topographic maps for regional cerebral blood flow measurements by Xe-133 inhalation. Stroke 15: 336–342
7. Bes A, Guell A, Arne-Bes MC, Dupui P, Geraud G (1985) Hyperfrontal distribution of cerebral blood flow: correlation with computerized EEG and relationship with handedness. J Cereb Blood Flow Metab 5 [Suppl 1]: S209–210
8. Perlmutter JS, Powers WJ, Herscovitch P, Fox PT, Raichle ME (1987) Regional asymmetries of cerebral blood flow, blood volume, and oxygen utilization and extraction in normal subjects. J Cereb Blood Flow Metab 7: 64–67
9. Devous MD, Stokely EM, Chehabi HH, Bonte FJ (1986) Normal distribution of regional cerebral blood flow measured by dynamic single-photon emission tomography. J Cereb Blood Flow Metab 6: 95–104
10. Rodriguez G, Warkentin S, Risberg J, Rosadini G (1988) Sex differences in regional cerebral blood flow. J Cereb Blood Flow Metab 8: 783–789
11. Gur RC, Gur RL, Obrist WD, Hungerbuhler JP, Youkin D, Rosen AD, Skolnick BE, Reivich M (1982) Sex and handedness differences in cerebral blood flow during rest and cognitive activity. Science 217: 659–661

Assistant Professor Dr. Yoshiyasu Tsuda
Second Department of Internal Medicine
Kagawa Medical School
1750-1 Ikenobe, Miki-cho
Kagawa 761-07, Japan

Neuroradiology (1991) 33 [Suppl]: 267–268

Neuro radiology
© Springer-Verlag 1991

Echo planar imaging with a contrast medium in studying brain perfusion

N. J. Patronas[1,4], R. Turner[2], D. Le Bihan[1], M. Fulham[3], D. Schellinger[4], and G. Di Chiro[3]

[1] Department of Diagnostic Radiology, [2] Biomedical Engineering and Instrumentation Program,
[3] National Institute of Neurological Disorders and Stroke, National Institutes of Health, Bethesda, Maryland, USA
[4] Department of Radiology, Georgetown University Medical Center, Washington, D. C., USA

Summary. Echo planar imaging is a new MRI technique capable of producing images in short periods of time. This type of examination has the time resolution required to study the first passage of contrast medium through an organ. We report observations using this technique in 12 patients with regional variations in perfusion due to cerebral gliomas.

Key words: Cerebral gliomas – Perfusion – Echo planar imaging

MRI of capillary perfusion is a new area of investigation which appears to be promising in the study of cerebral circulatory disorders. A major breakthrough in this field was made with the invention of the echo planar technique which allows imaging in extremely short periods of time [1]. Using the echo planar technique, MR images can be obtained in 50 ms, separated from each other by a period of 1–4 s. If during this type of imaging we administer intravenously a paramagnetic compound such as gadolinium (Gd)-DTPA (Magnevist), the magnetic susceptibility effect in the tissues produces a fall in signal which is proportional to the amount of Gd-DTPA passing through the capillaries, provided that the capillaries occupy a small fraction of the tissue volume. This in turn is proportional to the density of the functional capillaries in the tissue under question [2, 3].

It is known from pathological studies that the capillary density and the flowing blood volume vary in gliomas of different histological grade.

We report assessment of capillary perfusion in 12 patients with gliomas of the brain studied with echo planar MRI and intravenous Gd-DTPA injection.

Materials and methods

Twelve patients, 9 males and 3 females, ranging in age from 34 to 65 years (mean 46 years), were included. Seven patients had high-grade gliomas (III or IV) and 5 had low-grade gliomas (II); in every case the grade of the tumor was verified histologically. All 12 patients had conventional precontrast T1- and T2-weighted MRI. Echo planar imaging was also performed during an intravenous bolus injection of Gd-DTPA (0.1 mM/kg). We used a variant of the echo planar sequence on an imager fitted with a special high-efficiency head gradient coil. Images of a selected plane were obtained every second, each taking 100 ms to acquire. Sixty images were generated over a period of 1 min.

Image analysis was performed by averaging the signal inside a region of interest (ROI) in such areas as normal gray and white matter, tumor parenchyma, necrotic tissues and ventricular cavities. From these measurements, curves were reconstructed that showed signal changes during the first passage of Gd through the capillaries. Post-Gd T1-weighted spin-echo scans were then obtained.

Results

The arrival of contrast medium in the cerebral circulation occurred within about 10 s of injection and resulted in a diffuse fall in signal throughout the examined area, and marked loss of signal in larger blood vessels. The signal loss lasted 10–15 s and had a magnitude of 15%–25% in the gray matter and of 5%–10% in the white matter. No signal change occurred within the ventricles. ROI measurement in the parenchyma of high-grade gliomas showed loss of signal ranging from 25% to 50% (Fig. 1). The fall of signal in low-grade gliomas ranged from 5% to 15%.

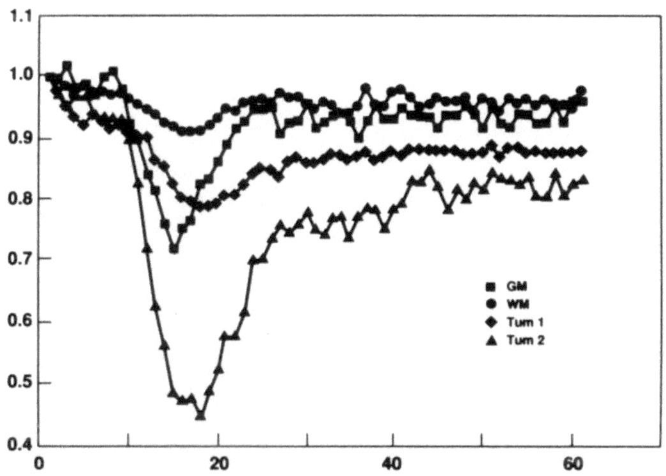

Fig. 1. Dynamic perfusion of MRI glioma, grade IV. Gadolinium-DTPA echo planar study in a patient with a high-grade glioma. Note the variable loss of signal in two areas of the tumor, reflecting differences in vascularity within the same lesion. Note also, the difference in vascularity between white and gray matter

Discussion

Echo planar imaging during intravenous bolus injection of Gd-DTPA enables assessment of cerebral microcirculation. We selected patients with lesions that are known to have different vascular patterns in terms of both capillary density and flowing blood volume. Thus, low-grade gliomas with poor blood supply showed only a small decrease in signal during the first pass of Gd through the capillaries. On the other hand, all tumors of high grade (III or IV) showed a decrease of signal intensity within the highly vascular regions which ranged from 25% to 50% as compared with baseline values prior to arrival of the contrast medium in the tissue in question. The superior temporal resolution of the echo planar technique allows, at the present time, qualitative assessment of hypervascular or hypovascular lesions. Therefore, this technique can be used to diagnose focal lesions with different perfusion patterns. Problems are encountered in quantitation of the findings since the concentration of Gd in tissue and flowing blood must be known before one can attempt to measure flowing blood volume and blood flow.

References

1. Mansfield P (1988) Imaging by nuclear magnetic resonance. J Phys E Sci Instrum 21: 18–30
2. Rosen BR, Belliveau JW, Chien D (1989) Perfusion imaging by nuclear magnetic resonance. Magn Res Q 5: 263–281
3. Turner R, Patronas N, Le Bihan D (1990) Dynamic MRI of brain perfusion using Gd-DTPA enhanced EPI. Magn Reson Imaging 8: 29

Dr. Nicholas J. Patronas
Diagnostic Radiology Department
National Institutes of Health
Bldg. 10, Rm. 1C-660
Bethesda, MD 20892, USA

SESSION 19
PAEDIATRICS

Neuroradiology (1991) 33 [Suppl]: 270–272

Neuro radiology
© Springer-Verlag 1991

CT analysis of the pituitary gland and stalk in pituitary dwarfism and in children without pituitary disorders

M. Lovrencic[1], M. Kalousek[1], and M. Kadrnka-Lovrencic[2]

Departments of [1] Radiology and [2] Pediatrics, "Dr. M. Stojanovic", University Hospital, Zagreb, Yugoslavia

Summary. A CT study of the pituitary gland and stalk has been performed in 23 children with pituitary dwarfism and the findings compared with those in 7 patients without pituitary disorders. The pituitary dwarfism group consisted of 5 children with multiple hypothalamic, 13 with multiple pituitary and 5 with isolated growth hormone deficiencies. In pituitary dwarfism the height of the pituitary gland (1.46 mm ± 1.4) was found to be significantly lower than in the control group (3.6 mm ± 1.4). The diameter of the pituitary stalk was also smaller in pituitary dwarfism (0.85 mm ± 0.84) than in the control group (1.18 mm ± 0.63).

Key words: Pituitary dwarfism – Computed tomography – Pituitary gland

High-resolution CT has been established as a method for evaluation of sellar and perisellar morphology [1–3]. It has yielded valuable results in the investigation of patients with pituitary secreting adenomas [4–6]. The cause of congenital pituitary dwarfism is impaired function of the hypothalamus, which is responsible for deficiency of growth hormone [7]. Current imaging techniques (CT and MRI) failed to demonstrate any abnormality of the hypothalamus in patients with idiopathic pituitary dwarfism [8]. Recently a CT study of pituitary dwarfism showed evidence of pituitary gland and stalk hypoplasia [9], while MRI studies revealed a hypoplastic or aplastic pituitary stalk with ectopic posterior lobe of the pituitary gland probably as a result of transection [10, 11].

A high-resolution CT study of the pituitary gland and its stalk has been performed in 30 children. Measurements in 23 patients with pituitary dwarfism were compared to those in 7 children without pituitary disorders.

Patients and methods

Twenty-three patients with growth retardation were included in this study: 19 males and 4 females ranging in age from 2 to 15 years. The diagnosis of pituitary dwarfism was made on the basis of bodily characteristics such as growth retardation, with short stature, immature body proportions and truncal obesity. None of the patients had a family history of dwarfism.

In each case laboratory tests revealed low or absent plasma growth hormone (GH) which failed to respond to challenges with insulin, arginine and L-dopa. Serum T_3 and T_4 were estimated. A TRH test was performed in order to evaluate the thyroid axis. The adrenal axis was evaluated by cortisol and ACTH rhythm. Three groups of patients were defined according to their endocrine status. Isolated GH deficiency was found in 5 patients, multiple pituitary deficiency in 13 and multiple hypothalamic deficiency in 5. Hand and wrist radiography demonstrated a delay of bone age from 1.6 to 8.5 SD.

Replacement therapy of deficient hormones had not begun or had just started at the time of the CT study.

Seven control patients, 4 males and 3 females aged 6–15 years, without clinical or laboratory features suggestive of pituitary or hypothalamic disorder, were used for analysis of the normal pituitary gland.

High-resolution CT was performed on a Somatom DRH (Siemens) using 2-mm-thick sections. Immediately after the intravenous injection of 40 ml iohexol, 28 CT sections were obtained in the coronal plane. In 6 young children axial scans with sagittal and coronal reformation were obtained after contrast medium administration. A magnification factor of 3 was employed.

Thirty-four studies were performed in 30 patients. The CT images were analysed with regard to the size of the pituitary gland and stalk. The height and diameter of the pituitary gland were measured.

Results

In the control group the pituitary gland was visualised in 7 and the pituitary stalk in 6 enhanced CT studies (Fig. 1). The height and diameter of the pituitary stalk are listed in the Table 1.

Table 1. Visualisation and size of the pituitary gland and stalk on 30 CT studies

	Pituitary gland	Height		Pituitary stalk	Diameter	
	Visualisation	Range	Mean ± SD	Visualisation	Range	Mean ± SD
Control group (n = 7)	7	2–6.1 mm	3.6 mm ± 1.4	6	0–1.8 mm	1.18 mm ± 0.63
Pituitary dwarfism (n = 23)	13	0–4.2 mm	1.46 mm ± 1.4	13	0–2.3 mm	0.85 mm ± 0.84
			$P < 0.005$			

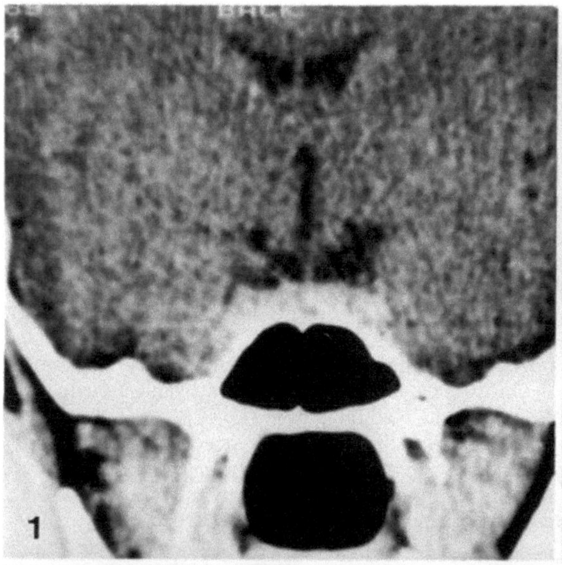

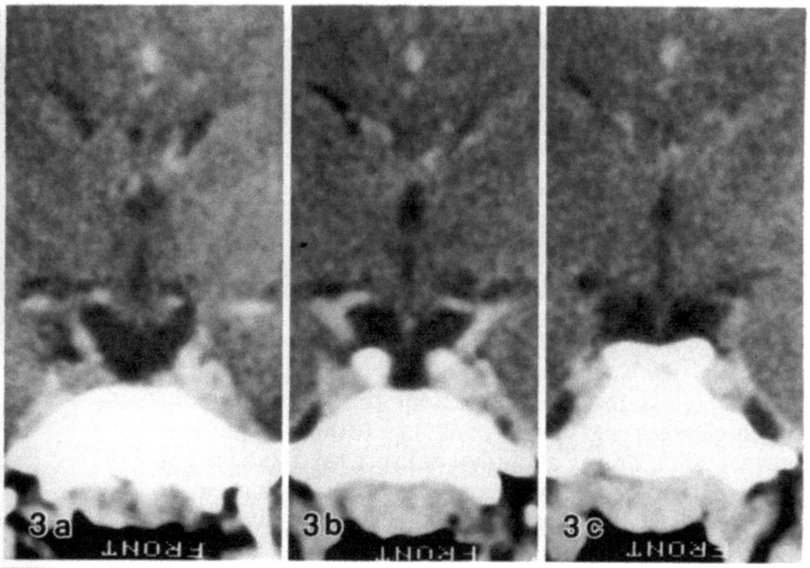

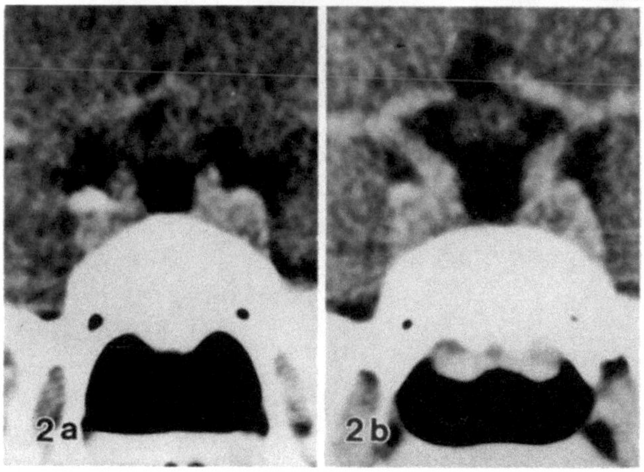

Fig. 1. CT of a 14-year-old boy. Normal pituitary gland seen in coronal section. Height of the gland is 4 mm and diameter of the stalk 1.5 mm

Fig. 2 a, b. CT of a 10-year-old boy with pituitary dwarfism. No visualisation of pituitary gland and stalk on 2-mm coronal sections

Fig. 3 a–c. CT of a 12-year-old boy with pituitary dwarfism. **a** Small pituitary gland seen on sellar floor in coronal section. **b, c** Evidence of the pituitary stalk on a 2-mm section posteriorly

In 8 of the 23 patients with pituitary dwarfism, neither the pituitary stalk nor gland were visualised on enhanced CT, while either pituitary gland or pituitary stalk were not demonstrated in another 2 patients (Fig. 2). In the remaining 13 patients pituitary gland and stalk were visualised (Fig. 3). The mean values of the height of the pituitary gland and diameter of stalk in the group of the patients with pituitary dwarfism are listed in Table 1. The mean height of the pituitary gland in pituitary dwarfism vs the control group was significantly smaller ($p < 0.005$).

Discussion

The size of the normal pituitary gland has been the subject of several studies in which the mean height of the pituitary gland was found to be 3.5 mm ± 1.5 in boys and 4.3 mm ± 1.5 in girls [6]. Very similar results were described in another study of 30 healthy patients [12]. In our control group of 7 patients (4 males, 3 females) aged 6–15 years, the pituitary gland was seen in all enhanced CT studies. Its mean height was 3.6 mm ± 1.4, in agreement with the previous studies. The pituitary stalk was seen in 6 of 7 enhanced CT studies with an average diameter of 1.18 mm ± 0.63. Another study of 127 enhanced CT studies in the axial plane using 5-mm section thickness revealed a 2.1 mm ± 0.7 diameter of the pituitary stalk at the dorsum sellae [13]. The results of this study differ from ours, probably due to the age of our group, and the fact that measurement of the pituitary stalk was made on coronal sections, with 2-mm section thickness and magnification. In 23 patients with pituitary dwarfism, the pituitary gland was not seen in 10 patients and 8 of them did not have a visible pituitary stalk either (Fig. 2). The average height of the pituitary gland was 1.46 mm ± 1.4, significantly smaller than in the control group. This is in accordance with another study in which the height of the pituitary gland, when seen, was less than 2 mm [9]. The average diameter of the pituitary stalk in pituitary dwarfism was 0.85 mm ± 0.84, smaller than in the control group, but the difference is not statistically significant. MRI studies in pituitary dwarfism revealed a very thin, hypoplastic, or even absent pituitary stalk [8, 10, 11]. In order to avoid intrasellar artefacts in the axial plane and to assess the size of the pituitary gland and stalk we preferred coronal CT scanning in our study. Measurements of the height of the pituitary gland and diameter of the stalk seem to be reliable, since they are similar to those obtained in other studies.

The pituitary gland and stalk were not visualized in 43% of patients with pituitary dwarfism. However, this does not prove the absence of the gland. The hormonal responses of the anterior lobe following stimulation indicate functional and probably anatomical existence of a very small, paper thin gland that is below the spatial resolution capability of the CT scanner. Even MRI, the technique with best spatial resolution, can not ensure visualisation of the gland in some patients with pituitary dwarfism, while the bright spot representing the posterior lobe can be seen in an aberrant position.

An attempt to elucidate functional disturbance and structural defects such as a hypoplastic or aplastic pituitary stalk suggests that they represent the residua of embryological derangement of or damage to the hypophyseal-portal system during abnormal delivery [8]. Increased incidence of breech delivery and birth asphyxia have been reported in newborns who have later developed pituitary dwarfism [9, 10]. Pathological proof of damage to the hypothalamus is missing in pituitary dwarfism.

References

1. Bonneville JF, Cattin F, Dietemann JL (1986) Computed tomography of the pituitary gland. Springer, New York Berlin Heidelberg
2. Chambers EF, Turski PA, Le Masters D, Newton TH (1982) Regions of low density in contrast enhanced pituitary gland: normal and pathologic processes. Radiology 144: 109-113
3. Lovrencic M, Kalousek M, Klaric R, Sekso M (1984) Computertomographie des Inhaltes der sella turcika in transversaler und frontaler Ebene. Fortschr Röntgenstr 141: 417–422
4. Hemminghytt HS, Kalkhoff RK, Daniels DL, Williams AL, Grogan JP, Haughton VM (1983) Computed tomographic study of hormone-secreting microadenomas. Radiology 146: 65–69
5. Lovrencic M, Kalousek M, Sekso M, Vizner B, Gnjidic Z (1987) CT in pituitary tumors with emphasis on prolactinomas and growth-hormone secreting adenomas. In: Calabro AM, Leonardi M (eds) Computer aided neuroradiology. CIC, Rome, pp 431–434
6. Syvertsen A, Haughton VM, Williams AL, Cusik JF (1979) The computed tomographic appearance of the normal gland and pituitary microadenomas. Radiology 133: 385–391
7. Di George AM (1987) The endocrine system. In: Behrman RE, Vaughan VC (eds) Nelson's textbook of pediatrics. Saunders, Philadelphia, pp 1176–1192
8. Kelly WM, Kucharczyk J, Kjos B, Peck WW, Norman D, Newton TH (1988) Posterior pituitary ectopia: an MR feature of pituitary dwarfism. AJNR 9: 453–460
9. Inoue Y, Nemoto Y, Fujita K, Aoki H, Takemoto K, Tsukamoto Y, Oda J, Onoyama Y (1986) Pituitary dwarfism: CT evaluation of the pituitary gland. Radiology 159: 171–173
10. Triulzi F, Scotti G, Pieralli C, Righi C, Visciani A, Livian S (1989) MR imaging detection of pituitary and brain anomalies in pituitary dwarfs. In: Nadjmi M (ed) Imaging of the brain metabolism, spine and cord. Springer, Berlin Heidelberg New York, pp 469–472
11. Fujisawa I, Kikuchi IK, Nishimura K, Togashi K, Itoh K, Noma S, Minami S, Sagoh T, Hiraoka T, Mamoi T, Mikawa H, Nakano Y, Itoh H, Konishi J (1987) Transection of the pituitary stalk: development of the ectopic posterior lobe assessed with MR imaging. Radiology 165: 487–489
12. Roppolo HM, Latchaw RE, Meyer JD, Curtin HD (1983) Normal pituitary gland. 1. Macroscopic anatomy – CT correlation. AJNR 4: 927–935
13. Peyster RG, Hoover ED, Adler LP (1984) CT of the normal pituitary stalk. AJNR 5: 45–47

Dr. M. Lovrencic
Department of Radiology
"Dr. M. Stojanovic" University Hospital
4100 Zagreb, Vinogradska 29
Yugoslavia

Neuroradiology (1991) 33 [Suppl]: 273–275

Neuro-radiology
© Springer-Verlag 1991

Anterior pituitary hyperintensity on T1-weighted MRI in the newborn

F. Triulzi, G. Scotti, L. Beccaria, E. Bianchini, E. Corbella, and C. Bianchi

Departments of Neuroradiology and Paediatrics, Scientific Institute, H. S. Raffaele, University of Milan, Milan, Italy

Summary. In order to assess the prevalence and significance of a previously reported anterior pituitary (AP) hyperintensity on T1-weighted MRI a semiquantitative MRI analysis was performed in 27 infants aged from 2 to 45 days. The differences between the signal intensity of the AP and pons and the suprasellar cerebrospinal fluid (CSF) were calculated and correlated with age. Signal intensity of the AP was found always to be higher than the chosen references: values ranged from 7% to 61% with respect to the pons and from +86% to 216% with respect to the CSF. However hyperintensity of the AP with respect to the pons could be perceived visually only when it was greater than +25%–30%. Both AP/pons and AP/CSF values correlated strictly with age (correlation coefficient $r = 0.81$ and 0.86, respectively). We concluded that hyperintensity of the AP is a striking MRI feature in the 1st week of life, which disappears within 2 months.

Key words: Pituitary gland – Anterior pituitary – Newborns – Magnetic resonance imaging – Delivery

It is well kown that in a T1-weighted midsagittal MRI section the pituitary gland can be subdivided in two different parts: the anterior pituitary (AP) is isointense with brain parenchyma and the posterior pituitary is hyperintense [1, 2]. It is also known that hyperintensity of the posterior pituitary is related to the function of the neurohypophysis and vasopressin secretion: in patients with diabetes insipidus and failure of vasopressin secretion the posterior pituitary gives the same intensity signal as the AP ([3]; Triulzi et al., unpublished data). Recently Wolpert et al. [4] reported some cases of totally bright pituitary in MRI of neonates. In these cases not only the posterior pituitary but also the anterior is hyperintense with respect to brain parenchyma. In order to assess the prevalence and significance of this finding we studied 27 infants aged 2–45 days by 1.5 T MRI, using a semiquantitative procedure.

Patients and methods

Twenty-seven infants (13 males, 14 females) aged from 2 to 45 days, clinically and biochemically normal, were admitted to the study.

MRI (at 1.5 T), with sagittal and coronal, 4-mm contiguous T1-weighted sections, 186 mm field of view, was performed on all subjects. Informed consent was obtained from the parents and in no case was anaesthesia or sedation employed.

Semiquantitative analysis was carried out on the midsagittal section, where circular or elliptical regions of interest (ROIs), containing at least 61 pixels, were selected in the AP, the pons, and in the suprasellar cerebrospinal fluid (CSF) for each patient. For each ROI the mean of signal intensity (SI) values was calculated.

The AP hyperintensity was referred to the SI of brain parenchyma; thus the SI of the pons, almost fully myelinated in newborns, was taken as a reference. However, in order to avoid any change in SI in the pons with age, the suprasellar CSF was also taken as a reference for AP ROI values.

For each subject the difference between the mean value of the ROI of the AP and that of the pons and CSF were expressed as a percentage according to formula:

$$\frac{\text{Mean value of ROI of AP} - \text{mean value for pons (or CSF)}}{\text{Mean value for pons (or CSF)}} \times 100$$

In order to assess any SI change with age of the pons the same procedures were used to compare the mean values of pons and CSF. The correlation coefficient (r) between the values obtained and chronological age was than calculated.

Results

The AP was always more intense than the chosen references (Fig. 1), values ranging from +7% to +61% with respect to the pons and from +86% to 216% with respect to the suprasellar CSF. However the hyperintensity of the AP with respect to the pons could be appreciated visually only when it was more than 25%–30%.

The correlation coefficients were: AP/pons versus age = −0.81 (Fig. 2); AP/CSF versus age = −0.86 (Fig. 3); pons/CSF versus age = −0.56 (Fig. 4). Hyperintensity of the AP correlated strictly with age, but also a value of −0.56 suggests some correlation between pons SI and age. However, excluding the pons SI values of the children less than 1 week old and correlating pons/CSF values with age, we found no correlation ($r = -0.04$, Fig. 5).

Discussion

Our results confirm that on T1-weighted MRI, the AP is hyperintense in the newborn, and that the hyperintensity correlates strictly with age. SI of the AP is maximal in the days after birth and decreases rapidly (Fig. 5). At about 1.5 months of age the AP appears isointense with brain parenchyma, even though semiquantitative measurement shows up to 25%–30% of SI difference.

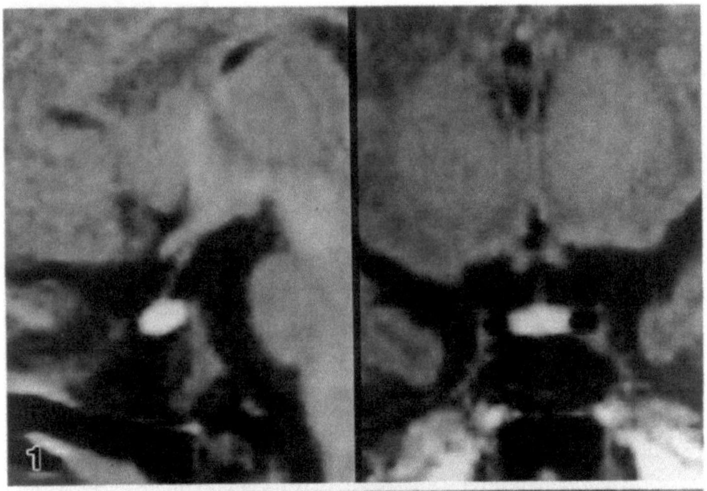

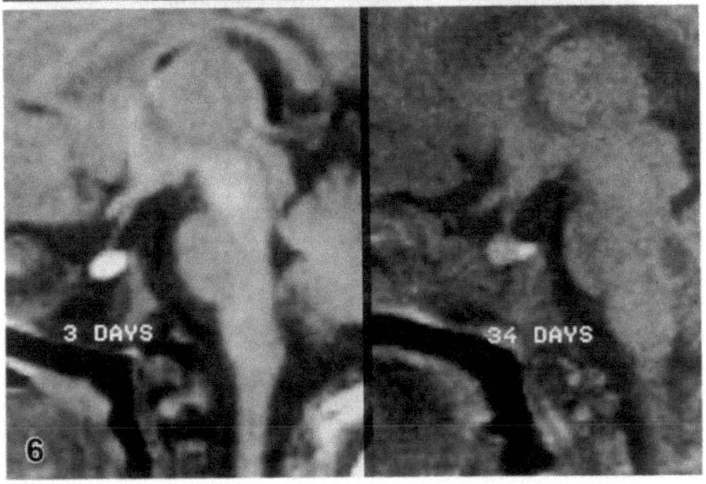

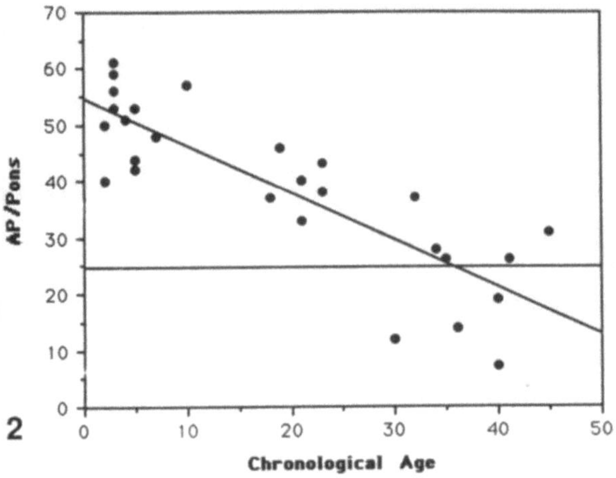

2

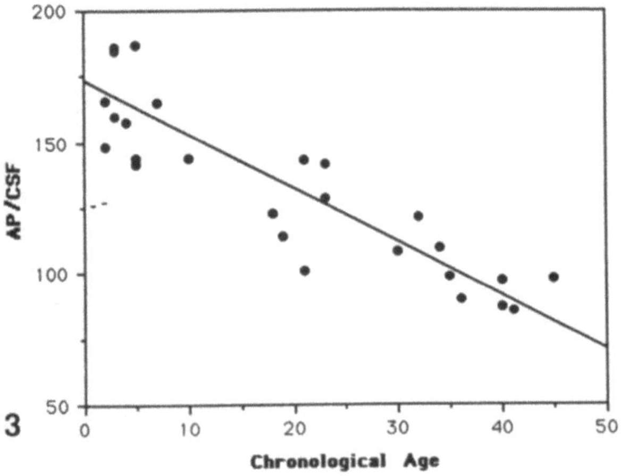

3

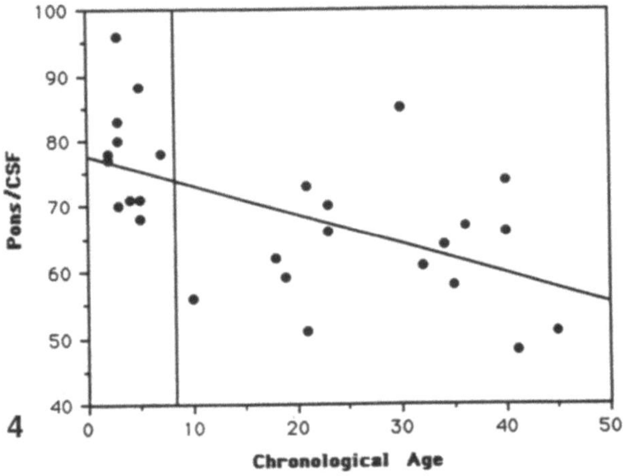

4

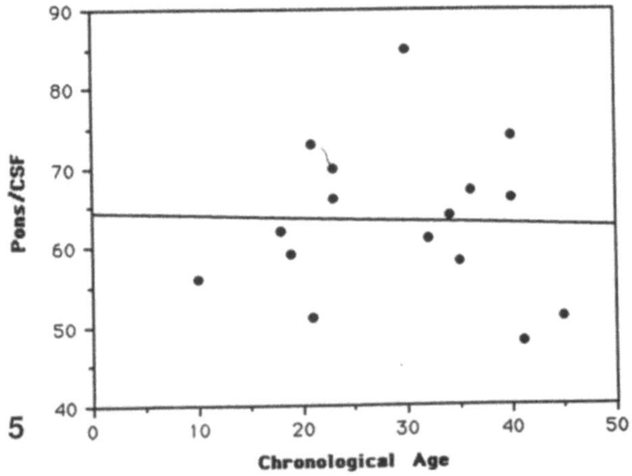

5

Fig. 1. A 3-day-old child: MRI midsagittal (left) and coronal (right) T1-weighted images clearly show diffuse hyperintense signal in the pituitary gland

Fig. 2. Linear regression graph of anterior pituitary *(AP)*/pons percentage values and chronological age. The correlation coefficient is −0.81. The line parallel to the abscissa indicates the threshold of visually perceptable *AP* hyperintensity

Fig. 3. Linear regression graph of *AP*/cerebrospinal fluid *(CSF)* percentage values and chronological age. The correlation coefficient is −0.86

Fig. 4. Linear regression graph of pons/*CSF* percentage values and age. The correlation coefficient is −0.56. The line parallel to the ordinate divides children less than 1 week old from the older children. A difference between the values of these two group is evident

Fig. 5. Linear regression graph of pons/*CSF* percentage values of children aged more than 1 week and age. The correlation coefficient is −0.04

Fig. 6. A 3-days-old child (left) and 34-days-old child (right)

Fat, slowly flowing blood and natural paramagnetic substances like methaemoglobin are the main sources of short T1 values. As pointed out by Wolpert et al. [4] none of these potential causes of T1 relaxation shortening can reasonably be assumed to be responsible for AP hyperintensity. They argue that the remarkable increase in protein synthetic activity of the newborn's pituitary could account for the short T1 values of both anterior and posterior pituitary. Although this hypothesis could be accepted, it recognised that the source of posterior pituitary hyperintensity is still extremely controversial [5, 6] and no definite cause has been documented or proved. We suggest that in the absence of experimental models we must include AP hyperintensity in the group of unsolved function-related T1 hyperintensities, together with hyperintensity in the normal posterior pituitary and in the basal ganglia of patients with chronic liver failure [7].

Semiquantitative analysis reveals also a weak correlation between pons SI and age; however, as shown in Fig. 5, this change is appreciable only in the 1st week of life. In an attempt to perform a semiquantitative assessment of the AP hyperintensity, a brain parenchyma SI reference which does not change with age must be chosen in the midsagittal section. The anterior pons was selected as a reference because it contains gray and white matter that is almost fully myelinated in newborn [8, 9].

A residual myelination process could probably account for the slight SI change of the pons in the 1st week of life. However, use of the suprasellar CSF reference guaranteed control not related to age.

References

1. Fujisawa I, Asato R, Nishimura K (1987) Anterior and posterior lobes of the pituitary gland: assessment by 1.5 T MR imaging. J Comput Assist Tomogr 11: 214–220
2. Nishimura K, Fujisawa I, Togashi K (1986) Posterior lobe of the pituitary: identification by lack of chemical shift artifact in MR imaging. J Comput Assist Tomogr 10: 899–902
3. Fujisawa I, Nishimura K, Asato R (1987) Posterior lobe of the pituitary in diabetes insipidus: MR findings. J Comput Assist Tomogr 11: 221–225
4. Wolpert SM, Osborne M, Anderson M, Runge VM (1988) The bright pituitary gland – a normal MR appearance in infancy. AJNR 9: 1–3
5. Kucharczyk J, Kucharczyk W, Berry I (1988) Histochemical characterization and functional significance of the hyperintense signal on MR images of the posterior pituitary. AJNR 8: 1079–1083
6. Fujisawa I, Asato R, Kawata M (1989) Hyperintense signal of the posterior pituitary on T1-weighted MR images: an experimental study. J Comput Assist Tomogr 13: 371–377
7. Levy LM, Yang A, Kumar AJ (1989) The brain and hepatic failure: MR abnormalities. AJNR 10: 904
8. Barkovich AJ, Kjos BO, Jackson DE, Norman D (1988) Normal maturation of the neonatal and infant brain: MR imaging at 1.5 T. Radiology 166: 173–180
9. Martin E, Kikinis R, Zuerrer M (1988) Developmental stages of human brain: an MR study. J Comput Assist Tomogr 12: 917–922

Dr. F. Triulzi
Department of Neuroradiology
H. S. Raffaele
via Olgettina 60
20132 Milano, Italy

SESSION 20
MAGNETIC RESONANCE: TECHNICAL ASPECTS

Neuroradiology (1991) 33 [Suppl]: 278

Neuroradiology
© Springer-Verlag 1991

The value of real time adjustment of T1 weighting in ultra high speed IR-EPI of the brain

B. S. Worthington[1], J. L. Firth[2], R. Ordidge[3], M. K. Stehling[3], R. Coxon[3], P. Gibbs[3], A. Blamire[3], and P. Mansfield[3]

Departments of [1] Radiology, [2] Neurosurgery, and [3] Physics, University of Nottingham, Nottingham, UK

Summary. Inversion recovery can be readily combined with the basic echo planar imaging experiment. The facility of real time adjustment of the inversion time has been found to be valuable in a wide variety of clinical studies.

Key words: Magnetic resonance imaging – Echo-planar imaging – Sequence – Inversion recovery

The echo planar imaging (EPI) technique and the several variants which have been developed allow the collection of data for a complete two-dimensional image in a single shot experiment typically lasting between 64 and 128 ms. A full description of the technique is given in the appended references [1–4].

Methods and results

By first preparing the spin system with a 180° spin inversion pulse, inversion recovery (IR) can be added to the basic EPI experiment so that their respective advantages of high speed and wide range of T1 contrast are combined. Imaging is carried out at 0.52T employing a low inductance actively screened coil system and high-quality images of 5–10 mm thickness, with a resolution better than 2 mm, are obtained without the need for signal averaging in a time of 128 ms plus the inversion time. Optimisation of contrast within the resulting images to give maximal conspicuity of particular features is achieved simply and interactively by real time adjustment of the inversion time, whereas choice of a single inversion time in conventional imaging invariably means that the resulting images are a compromise in providing optimal contrast between pathology and adjacent brain tissue, or information on any internal structure, surrounding reaction or mass effect on the cerebrospinal fluid pathways. In dynamic studies assessing tissue perfusion and distribution of intravenous gadolinium-DTPA in intracranial tumours, prior signal nulling of the tissue of interest maximises sensitivity to the T1 shortening produced.

Conclusion

Examination of over 30 patients with a wide range of pathology illustrates the benefits of reduced examination time and the clinical value of this facility, and a full description of this work will be presented elsewhere.

References

1. Mansfield P, Morris PG (1982) NMR imaging in biomedicine. Academic Press, London
2. Mansfield P (1988) Imaging by nuclear magnetic resonance. J Phys E Sci Instrum 21: 18–30
3. Ordidge RJ, Coxon R, Howseman A, Chapman B, Turner R, Stehling M, Mansfield P (1988) Snapshot head imaging at 0.5T using the echo-planar technique. J Magn Reson Med 8: 110–115
4. Howseman AM, Stehling MK, Chapman B, Coxon R, Turner R, Ordidge RJ, Cawley MG, Glover P, Mansfield P, Coupland RE (1988) Improvements in snap-shot nuclear magnetic resonance imaging. Br J Radiol 61: 822–828

Dr. B. S. Worthington
Department of Radiology
University Hospital
Nottingham, UK

Neuroradiology (1991) 33 [Suppl]: 279–281

Neuro radiology
© Springer-Verlag 1991

Non-invasive assessment of brain lesions by fast scan MRI and localized proton spectroscopy

H. Bruhn, M. L. Gyngell, K. D. Merboldt, W. Hänicke, and J. Frahm

Max-Planck-Institut für biophysikalische Chemie, Göttingen, Federal Republic of Germany

Summary. Fast scan MRI and image-guided localized proton spectroscopy were employed to assess both the morphology and the metabolic characteristics of brain lesions in a single investigation. Recent progress in the development of STEAM localization techniques allows the acquisition of proton MR spectra from volumes of interest as small as 1–8 ml within measuring times of 5–10 min. This enables the study of tumour heterogeneity to be done by proton spectroscopy, e.g. by monitoring variations in N-acetyl aspartate (NAA) and lactate levels between central necrosis and the surrounding portion of an astrocytoma. Metabolic alterations in small plaques of multiple sclerosis can also be studied without the results being compromised by partial volume effects. Typical findings include decreased levels of NAA and total creatine indicative of degeneration of the neuronal parenchyma, and increased choline consistent with membrano-proliferative gliosis.

Key words: Magnetic resonance spectroscopy – Magnetic resonance, tissue characterization – Brain neoplasms – Multiple sclerosis

The neuroradiological assessment of brain lesions may benefit from non-invasive determination of focal metabolite levels by localized proton MR spectroscopy (MRS). Clinical requirements are reasonable examination times, certainty about the origin of the spectral data, and access to small volumes of interest (VOIs) matching the pathology. These aspects have been addressed by a specially designed fast scan MRI protocol (Brühn et al., to be published), followed by single voxel localized proton MRS using STEAM sequences [1–3].

Methods

All studies have been carried out at 2.0 T (Siemens Magnetom) using the standard circularly polarized head coil for both MRI and MRS. Prior to spectroscopy the lesions were identified by T1- and T2-weighted fast scan images using FLASH [4] and CE-FAST [5] sequences, respectively. These allow a complete brain MRI study to be completed within 5–10 min. Localized STEAM spectra were obtained [1, 3] using repetition times of 1500–3000 ms, echo times of 20–270 ms, and 128–256 acquisitions. In general, total examination times were 60–90 min. Informed consent was obtained prior to the investigations.

Results and discussion

Figure 1 shows a transverse T2-weighted CE-FAST image of a heterogenous lesion in the right hemisphere of a 79-year-old patient. The mass has a hyperintense core indicative of cyst fluid. It is medially demarcated by a thin hypointense margin (probably consisting of a haemosiderin-laden macrophages), and by a moderately hyperintense region typical of surrounding parenchymal oedema. For spectroscopy, multiple VOIs (5.8 ml or $18 \times 18 \times 18$ mm^3) including a contralateral control (16 ml or $25 \times 25 \times 25$ mm^3), were selected as indicated. The corresponding proton spectra are shown in Fig. 2. In comparison with the normal control (Fig. 2c) the spectrum from the border zone (Fig. 2b) shows a marked decrease in the *N*-acetyl aspartate (NAA) concentration and the emergence of a lactate (Lac) signal. In the spectrum of the tumour core (Fig. 2a) the NAA concentration is below the level of detectability. The creatine pool is drastically reduced, whereas the resonance due to cholines remains almost normal. The doublet resonance of the lactate CH_3 group is even further increased when compared with the spectrum from the border zone (Fig. 2b). Obviously, localized proton spectroscopy using small VOIs enables the resolution of metabolite variations within heterogeneous regions of a brain tumour to be made. The long echo time of 270 ms used in these experiments emphasizes metabolite resonances with long T2 relaxation times. The results are characteristic of a high-grade astrocytoma with central necrotic cyst formation and extensive use of anaerobic glycolysis to fulfill its energy requirements [6].

Another example of the progress in spectroscopic analysis of focal brain lesions is the investigation of multiple sclerosis (MS) plaques. Figure 3 shows proton spectra of a periventricular MS plaque (VOI = 4 ml) in a 14-year-old patient and of a healthy control. The use of a short echo time of 20 ms results in a significant increase in the number of accessible metabolites. As shown in Fig. 3b the resonances of NAA, creatine, and choline are complemented by inositols, taurine, and glutamate. When comparing the proton spectrum of the MS plaque (Fig. 3a) with that of normal brain it is noted that NAA is decreased by more than 50%. The creatine pool is also markedly diminished, whereas cholines and inositols are moderately increased. These findings are consistent for all patients investigated so far ($n = 6$). Data established in the investigation of cerebral infarcts suggest [7] diminished NAA

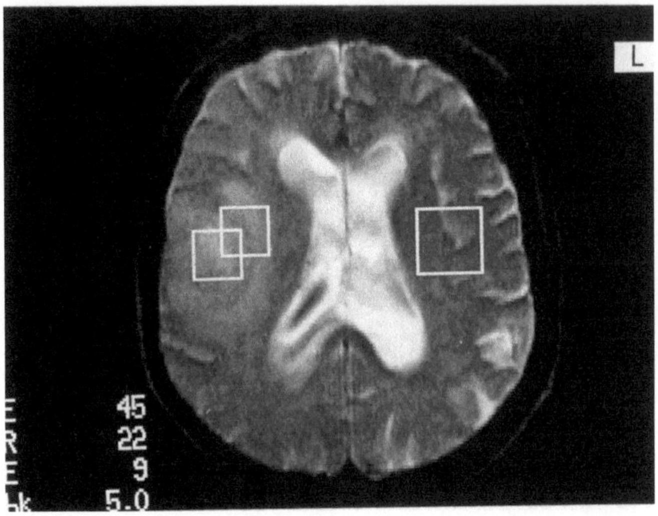

Fig. 1. Transverse T2-weighted CE-FAST image (2.0-T) of a patient with a high-grade astrocytoma showing tumour heterogeneity. The volumes of interest (VOI) selected for localised proton MR spectroscopy are indicated by squares. Parameters are: TR = 22 ms, TE = −9 ms, 45 °, slice thickness 4 mm, total imaging time 12 s

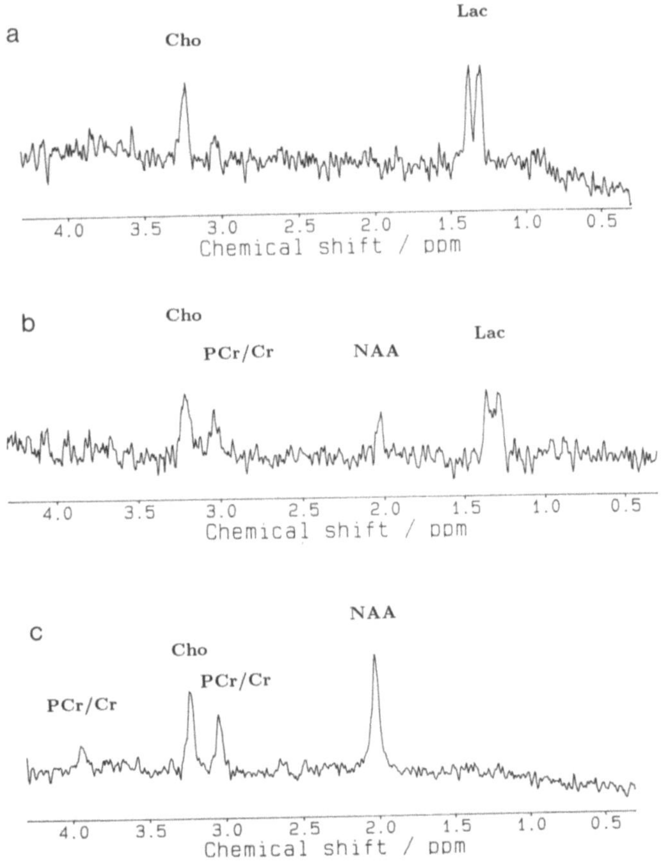

Fig. 2 a–c. Localised proton MR spectra (2.0-T) of the patient shown in Fig. 1: **a** spectrum from the cystic tumour core (VOI = 5.8 ml); **b** spectrum from the tumour border zone (VOI = 5.8 ml); **c** spectrum from a contralateral control (VOI = 16 ml). Spectral parameters are TE = 270 ms, TR = 1500 ms, TM = 30 ms, and 256 scans. *Lac,* Lactic acid; *NAA,* N-acetyl aspartate; *PCr,* phosphocreatine; *Cr,* creatine; *Cho,* choline-containing compounds. Chemical shifts are given in parts per million (ppm) and referenced to 2.01 ppm for the CH_3 group of NAA. The spectra are scaled for direct comparison

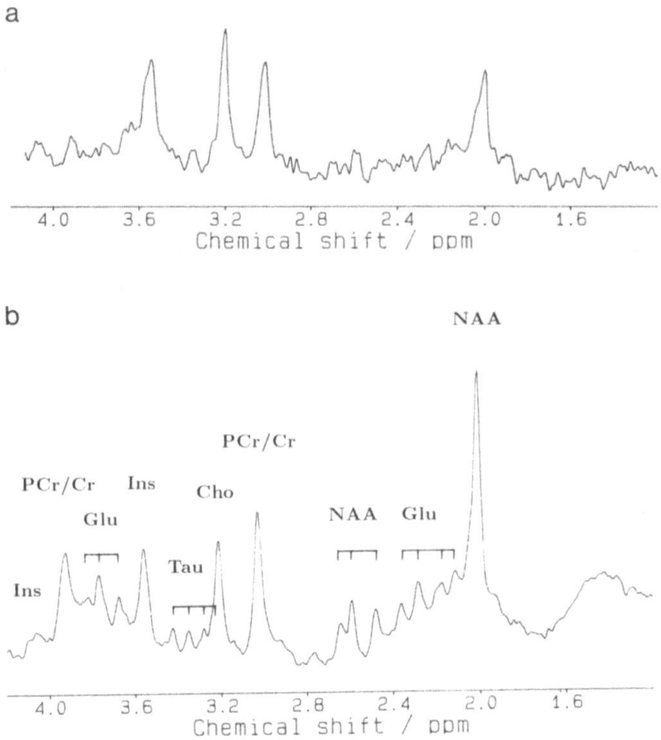

Fig. 3 a, b. Localized proton MR spectra (2.0-T) of **a** a periventricular plaque of a patient presenting with multiple sclerosis and **b** normal white matter of a control subject. Spectral parameters are TE = 20 ms, TR = 1500 ms, TM = 30 ms, 256 scans, VOI = 4 ml (8 ml for the control). Further resonances visible at the short echo time of 20 ms are due to glutamate *(Glu),* taurine *(Tau),* and inositols *(Ins).* Chemical shifts are given in ppm and referenced to 2.01 ppm for the CH_3 group of NAA. The spectra are scaled for direct comparison

and probably indicate neuronal cell death. The observed metabolic alterations, therefore, are in agreement with neuropathological findings of secondary loss or shrinkage of neurons in the MS plaque and fibrous gliosis [8]. Since choline-containing compounds are representative of membrane constituents, their increase could be expected in a membrano-proliferative mechanism such as gliosis. An increase in lactate was not observed in moderate cases but was instead seen in confluent lesions of the white matter in a 31-year-old woman who suffered from severe MS with large regions of demyelination.

In conclusion the spectral, temporal, and spatial resolution of STEAM proton MRS have matured to a degree that a role in neuroradiological diagnostics is foreseeable.

Acknowledgement. Financial support by the Bundesminister für Forschung und Technologie (BMFT) of the Federal Republic of Germany (grant 01 VF 8606/6) is gratefully acknowledged.

References

1. Frahm J, Bruhn H, Gyngell ML, Merboldt KD, Hänicke W, Sauter R (1989) Localized high-resolution proton NMR spectroscopy using stimulated echoes. Initial applications to human brain in vivo. Magn Reson Med 9: 79–93

2. Frahm J, Michaelis T, Merboldt KD, Hänicke W, Gyngell ML, Chien D, Bruhn H (1989) Localized NMR spectroscopy in vivo. Progress and problems. Nucl Magn Reson Biomed 2: 188–195
3. Frahm J, Michaelis T, Merboldt KD, Bruhn H, Gyngell ML, Hänicke W (1990) Improvements in localized proton NMR spectroscopy of human brain. Water suppression, short echo times, and 1 ml resolution. J Magn Reson (in press)
4. Frahm J (1987) Rapid FLASH NMR imaging. Naturwissenschaften 74: 415–422
5. Gyngell ML (1988) The application of steady-state free precession in rapid 2DFT NMR imaging: FAST and CE-FAST sequences. Magn Reson Imaging 6: 415–419
6. Bruhn H, Frahm J, Gyngell ML, Merboldt KD, Hänicke W, Sauter R, Hamburger C (1989) Noninvasive differentiation of tumors with use of localized H-1 MR spectroscopy in vivo: initial experience in patients with cerebral tumors. Radiology 172: 541–548
7. Bruhn H, Frahm J, Gyngell ML, Merboldt KD, Hänicke W, Sauter R (1989) Cerebral metabolism in man after acute stroke. New observations using localized proton NMR spectroscopy. Magn Reson Med 9: 126–131
8. Prineas J (1975) Pathology of the early lesion in multiple sclerosis. Hum Pathol 6: 531–554

Dr. Harald Bruhn
Max-Planck-Institut für biophysikalische Chemie
Postfach 2841
W-3400 Göttingen, Federal Republic of Germany

Neuroradiology (1991) 33 [Suppl]: 282–285

Neuro-radiology
© Springer-Verlag 1991

Improved contrast and temporal resolution with MR snapshot FLASH imaging of the brain

W. Grodd, U. Klose, D. Petersen, and T. Nägele

Department of Neuroradiology, University of Tübingen, Tübingen, Federal Republic of Germany

Summary. The lack of tissue contrast in gradient echo sequences with very short repetition times can be resolved by using a single inversion pulse prior to the whole image sequence. The contrast can be changed by varying the time delay between the inversion and first excitation pulses. This technique was implemented on a conventional whole body imager and evaluated for clinical utility in volunteers and patients with different diseases of the brain. The large variation of T1 tissue contrast permits excellent delineation of normal and pathological structures and the high temporal resolution allows dynamic studies of contrast enhancment in a variety of diseases.

Key words: Magnetic resonance imaging – Magnetic resonance technique – Snapshot FLASH – Brain tumours – Gadolinium

Gradient echo sequences in MRI with very short repetition times (TR) and low flip angles allow a reduction of measurement time but lack contrast due to equilibrated tissue magnetisation. Improved contrast can be achieved by using a single shot FLASH image acquisition with a preceding inversion pulse prior to the imaging sequence, as first proposed by Haase et al. [1, 2]. With this so-called "snapshot-FLASH", technique good tissue contrast and short measurement times, of approximately 1 s, can be combined with satisfactory spatial resolution and implemented on a conventional whole body system [3, 4].

Materials and methods

To ensure that the image contrast is affected by the preceding inversion signal, the measurement time has to be shortened to the range of proton relaxation times. The snapshot-FLASH technique (Fig. 1) was therefore tested for a desired spatial resolution of 0.8 mm^2 with a flip angle of 7°, a TR of 9 ms, a field of view of 200×200 mm^2, a 256×256 matrix and a slice thickness of 4 mm, as in standard sequences. In conjunction with a half-Fourier space reconstruction technique (symmetrical acquisition of the central k-space lines) the measurement time was 1.2 s. For repeated measurements the minimal repetition time between two consecutive scans was approximately 3 s, because of the soft- and hardware equipment used. Magnitude reconstruction of images was used in order avoid phase errors. The smallest inversion time (TI) was 9 ms and the echo time (TE) of the gradient echo 4.7 ms.

For signal intensity and contrast calculations one has to distinguish between the inversion time TI (the time between inversion and the first excitation pulse) and the effective inversion interval TI_{eff} (the time interval between the inversion pulse and the central lines of the k-space), because the central k-lines carry most of the signal intensity. This intrinsic delay time was minimised by an asymmetrically scanned k-space to 400 ms in our case, which has to be added to the choosen inversion time (Fig. 2). The sequence was implemented on a whole body imager (Siemens, Magnetom) at 1.5 T and tested for clinical utility in volunteers and more than 60 patients with various diseases of the brain.

Results

Image contrast

The image contrast of the snapshot technique depends on the difference in T1 relaxation of the tissues and is similar to an inversion recovery sequence. Therefore it can be calculated qualitatively in the same manner if the relaxation times T1 and T2 and the proton density ρ are known. In Fig. 2 the signal intensity of cerebrospinal fluid (CSF) and grey and white matter are calculated with fixed T1, T2 and ρ values (T1/T2/ρ: CSF 3000/1500/1, grey matter 900/115/0.85, white matter 600/85/0.72) for increasing in-

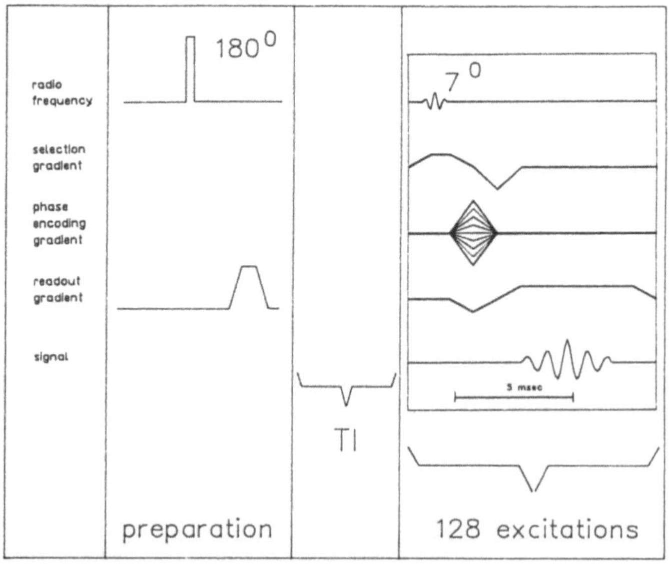

Fig. 1. Diagram of the snapshot FLASH sequence with a TE of 5 ms. After the inversion pulse a gradient pulse is applied to dephase residual transverse magnetisation. The inversion time is variable, with a minimum of 9 ms

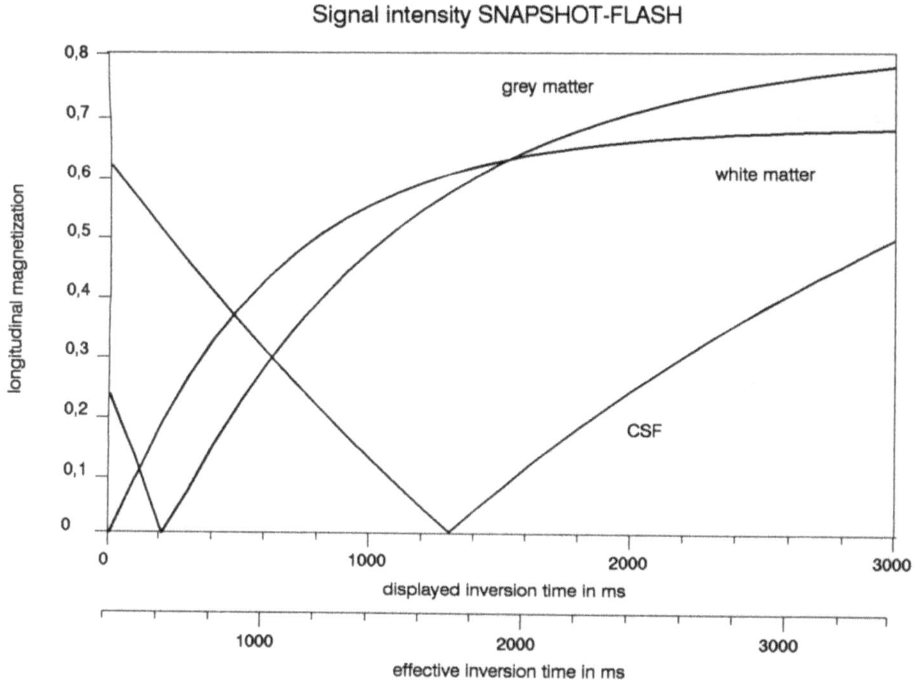

Fig. 2. Calculated signal intensity graph of cerebrospinal fluid (CSF), grey and white matter for different inversion times and an effective minimum inversion time of minimal 400 ms

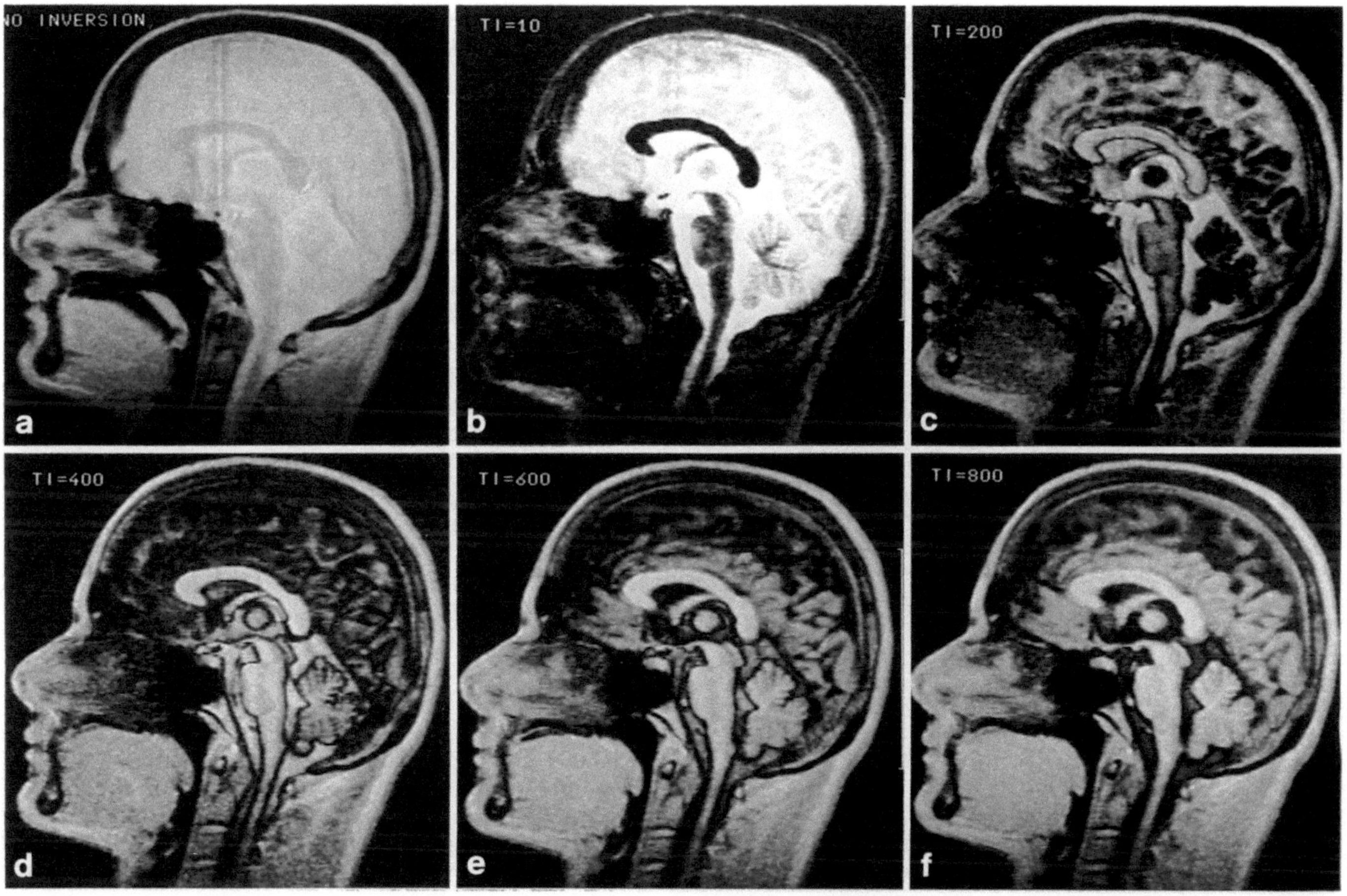

Fig. 3a–f. Sagittal snapshot images of a volunteer, using different inversion times: **a** no inversion pulse; **b** TI 10 ms; **c** TI 200 ms; **d** TI 400 ms; **e** TI 600 ms; **f** TI 800 ms. Note the lack of contrast with no inversion pulse, the decay of signal intensity of the CSF and the decreasing contrast between grey and white matter with increasing inversion times

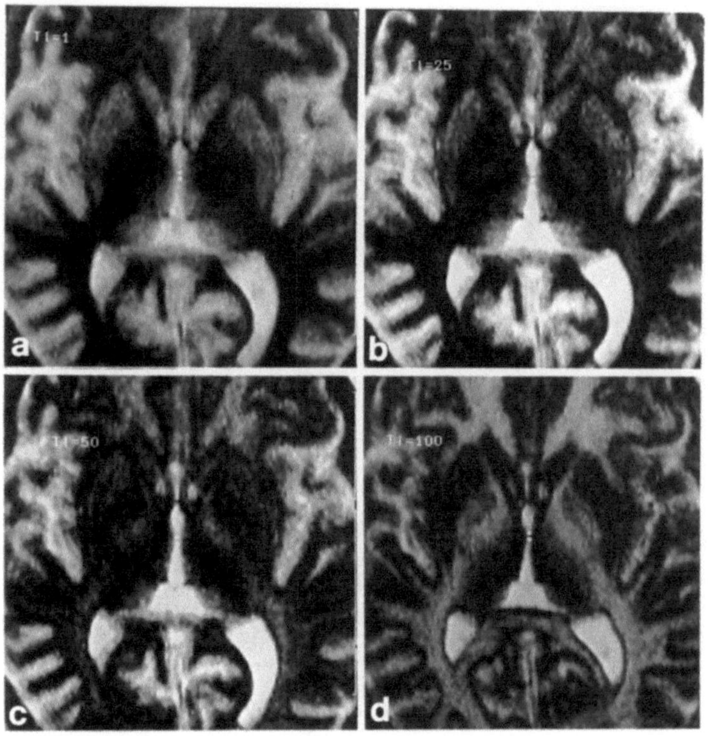

Fig. 4a–d. Magnified axial snapshot images at the level of the basal ganglia in a volunteer, using different inversion times: **a** TI 10 ms; **b** TI 25 ms; **c** TI 50 ms; **d** TI 100 ms. Note the differences in signal intensity of the putamen, the globus pallidus and the internal capsula, best separated at TI = 100 ms

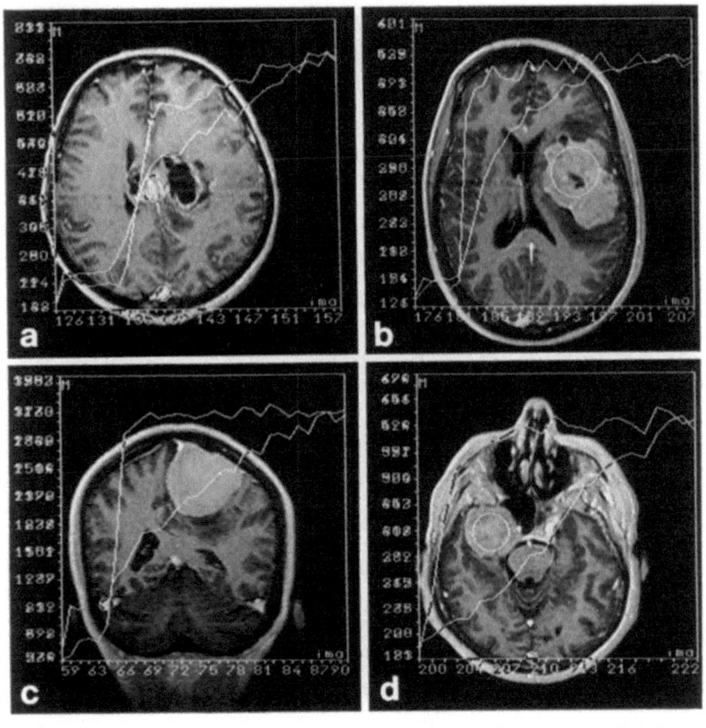

Fig. 5a–d. Dynamic contrast medium studies with 3 s interval snapshot images in four different brain tumours with signal intensity slopes for the tumour and a venous sinus: **a** glioblastoma 32 scans; **b** haemangiopericytoma 32 scans; **c** meningioma 32 scans **d** neuroma 22 scans. Note the rapid enhancement of the glioblastoma and haemangiopericytoma and the difference in slope between the meningioma and the neuroma

version times. As magnitude images are acquired, a negative longitudinal magnetisation after the inversion pulse leads to a positive signal. No signal is detected for certain inversion times with vanishing longitudinal magnetisation (white matter at 10 ms, grey matter at 200 ms), as when using the STIR technique [5]. For inversion times up to 600 ms with a bright CSF signal a boundary effect between the brain parenchyma and the adjacent CSF is produced (Fig. 3). To optimize the T1 contrast within certain brain structures, the inversion time has to be in the lower range of 20–100 ms. As shown in Fig. 4 a reversal in contrast between putamen, globus pallidus and internal capsule occurs with 100 ms TI and this allows excellent delineation, comparable with that given by T2-weighted spin echo images.

Dynamic studies

The short acquisition time of 1 s and the achievable repetition rate of 3 s are favourable for dynamic studies. The sequence was tested with up to 32 repeated scans in vascular malformations and brain tumours after intravenous administration of 0.1 mmol gadolinium-DTPA (Magnevist)/kg body weight within 10 s. For quantitation and comparison between different patients the signal enhancement of the venous sinuses (sagittal, transversal or cavernous sinus) was used as reference. Typical results in four different brain tumours (glioblastoma, haemangiopericytoma, meningioma and neuroma) with the region of the tumour examined and the venous sinuses are shown in Fig. 5.

The measurements of signal intensity of these tumours normalised against the venous sinus are shown in Fig. 6. The steepest initial slope and the earliest onset of enhancement are found in the glioblastoma. This is compatible with the findings of pathological arteries and arteriovenous shunts on angiography [6]. The haemangiopericytoma and the meningioma show an identical onset within the first 10 s but differ in the extent of the later enhancement, probably due to initial lower tumour signal intensity of the haemangiopericytoma. The neuroma has the lowest slope but a continuous increase of enhancement, as is known from other MRI dynamic contrast medium studies [7].

Discussion

The MR snapshot technique allows imaging within seconds with preservation of spatial resolution on conventional imaging systems and offers excellent T1 contrast, which can be optimised for different structures and is comparable with the T2 contrast in spin echo sequences. This is of special interest as until now T1 contrast of brain pathology has not been fully studied due to the limitations of conventional inversion recovery sequences, i.e. long acquisition time, low signal/noise ratio and limited multislice capability on some imagers. The snapshot technique is helpful for rapid localisation of circumscribed lesions in additional planes to display their exact anatomical rela-

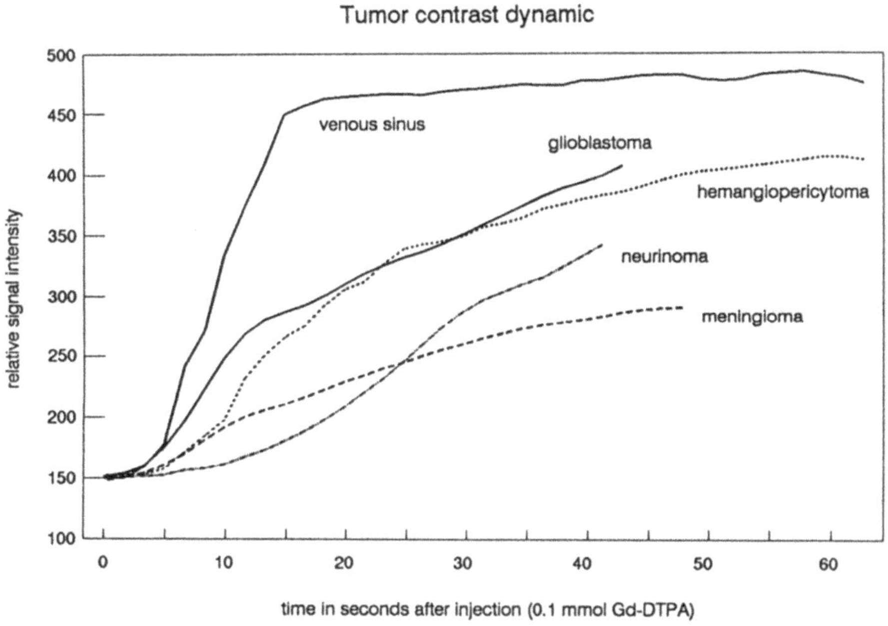

Fig. 6. Signal intensity versus time after bolus injection of 0.1 mmol gadolinium-DTPA for four different brain tumours standardised against signal intensity of the sagittal or transverse sinuses

tionships. The technique is particularly suited for dynamic contrast medium studies of brain tumours and may allow greater characterisation by differences in contrast kinetics. A more detailed study of temporal contrast behaviour in intra- and extra-axial tumours is under way.

However, with the given hard- and software equipment there are some restrictions, which should be solved by manufacturers to allow widespread use of this technique. For example, handling of raw data in our system permits no multislice acquisition and no direct averaging, and operation of the hardware is extremely noisy. Nevertheless we are confident, that with further progress in the MRI technology these problems will be solved and snapshot imaging will become part of clinical routine for dynamic studies not only in the brain: its simple concept, on the basis of two-dimensional Fourier imaging, is easy to implement and to use in conventional whole-body systems.

References

1. Haase A (1990) Snapshot FLASH MRI. Applications to T1, T2 and chemical shift imaging. Magn Reson Med 13: 77–89
2. Haase A, Matthaei D, Bartkowski R, Dühmke E, Leibfritz D (1989) Inversion recovery snapshot FLASH MR imaging. J Comput Assist Tomogr 13: 1036–1040
3. Frahm J, Merboldt KD, Bruhn H, Gyngell ML, Hänicke W, Chien D (1990) 0.3 second FLASH MRI of the human heart. Magn Reson Med 13: 150–157
4. Klose U, Nägele T, Grodd W, Petersen D (1990) Contrast variation of brain tissues with an MR snapshot technique. Radiology (in press)
5. Young IR (1988) Special pulse sequences and techniques. In: Stark DD, Bradley WG (eds) Magnetic resonance imaging. Mosby, St. Louis
6. Krayenbühl H, Yasargil MG, Huber P (1979) Zerebrale Angiographie für Klinik und Praxis. Thieme, Stuttgart
7. Laniado M, Claussen C, Weinmann H, Schörner W (1990) Paramagnetic contrast media in magnetic resonance imaging of the brain. In: Taveras JM, Ferucci JT (eds) Radiology: diagnosis/imaging/intervention, vol 3. Lippincott, Philadelphia

Dr. Wolfgang Grodd
Department of Neuroradiology
Radiological Clinic
Hoppe-Seyler-Str. 3
W-7400 Tübingen, Federal Republic of Germany

Neuroradiology (1991) 33 [Suppl]: 286–288

Neuro radiology

© Springer-Verlag 1991

T1 and T2 shortening associated with iodinated contrast media in MRI of the central nervous system

J. R. Jinkins, L. Sisk, J. W. Robinson, G. D. Fullerton, and R. F. Williams

Department of Radiology, University of Texas Health Science Center, San Antonio, USA

Summary. MRI was utilized to investigate the effects of iodinated radiographic contrast media in the central nervous system. Patients were studied both after intrathecal administration of an iodinated non-ionic contrast medium (Isovue) and following i. v. administration of an iodinated ionic contrast medium (Renografin). Two patients with subarachnoid iodinated contrast medium showed T1 and/or T2 shortening on spin echo acquisitions, while four of the five subjects with intracranial tumors and i. v. enhancement demonstrated a similar effect on MRI. In vitro experiments revealed that all iodinated contrast media manifested greater T1 and T2 shortening as the concentration of the agent was increased. It is proposed that the largest contributing mechanism is that of dipolar relaxation on the protons in the surrounding water. These effects suggest that the administration of iodinated contrast media during the period immediately prior to MR scanning may be contraindicated because of the demonstrated alteration of MR signal intensity, which may lead to inaccurate diagnostic conclusions.

Key words: Magnetic resonance imaging – Radiologic iodinated contrast media

When one radiologic examination quickly follows another, the possible adverse effect of one procedure upon interpretation of the other sometimes comes into question. Such a consideration is particularly relevant because of the necessity for timely patient diagnosis and treatment during a period of rapidly escalating cost of medical care. A study was therefore initiated to assess the possible effect of commonly used iodinated radiologic contrast media both in vitro and in clinical MRI of the central nervous system.

Materials and methods

All MRI studies were performed with a 1.5T GE Signa clinical unit utilizing spin-echo acquisitions with T1- (500/15/2: TR/TE/NEX) and/or T2- (2500/30–80/1) weighting. Two patients were studied

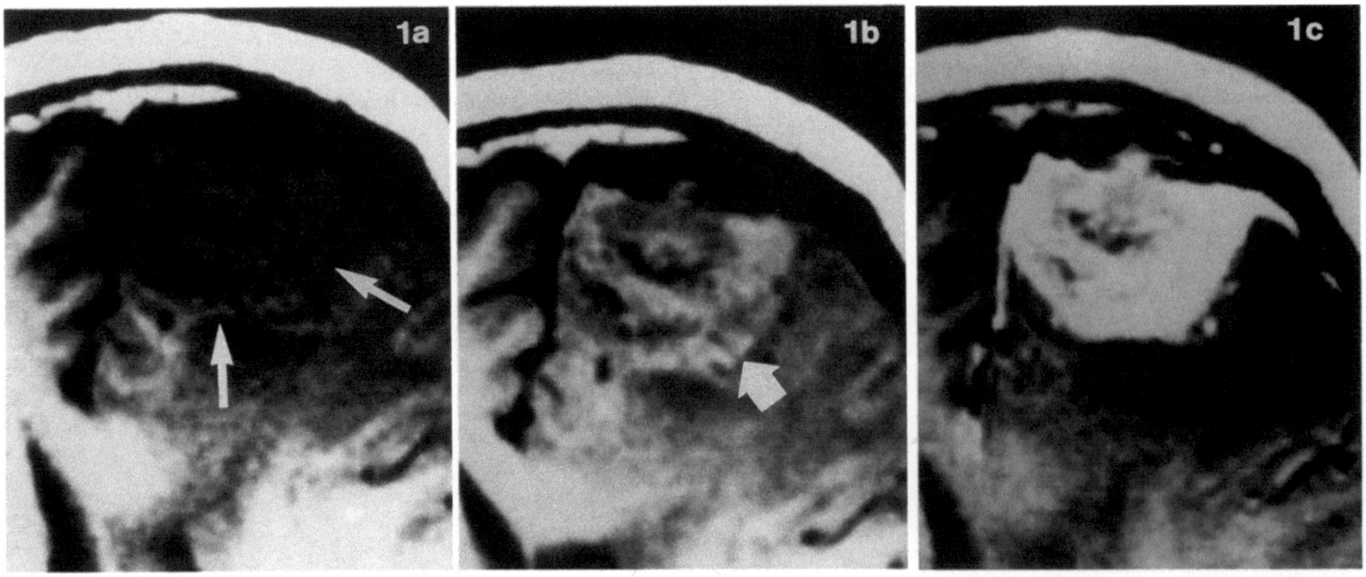

Fig. 1a–c. Calcified frontal meningioma: **a** detail from axial T1-weighted precontrast section showing low intensity in the region of the poorly defined tumor *(arrows)* (calcification proven by prior CT); **b** post-intravenous iodinated contrast-enhanced (100 cc Renografin-76). T1-weighted image demonstrates T1 shortening induced within the tumor by showing an increase in intensity (over that observed in a) to become nearly isointense with surrounding gray matter *(arrow)*; **c** subsequent gadopentetate dimeglumine (0.1 mmol/kg Magnevist) enhanced T1-weighted image illustrating intense enhancement of the tumor

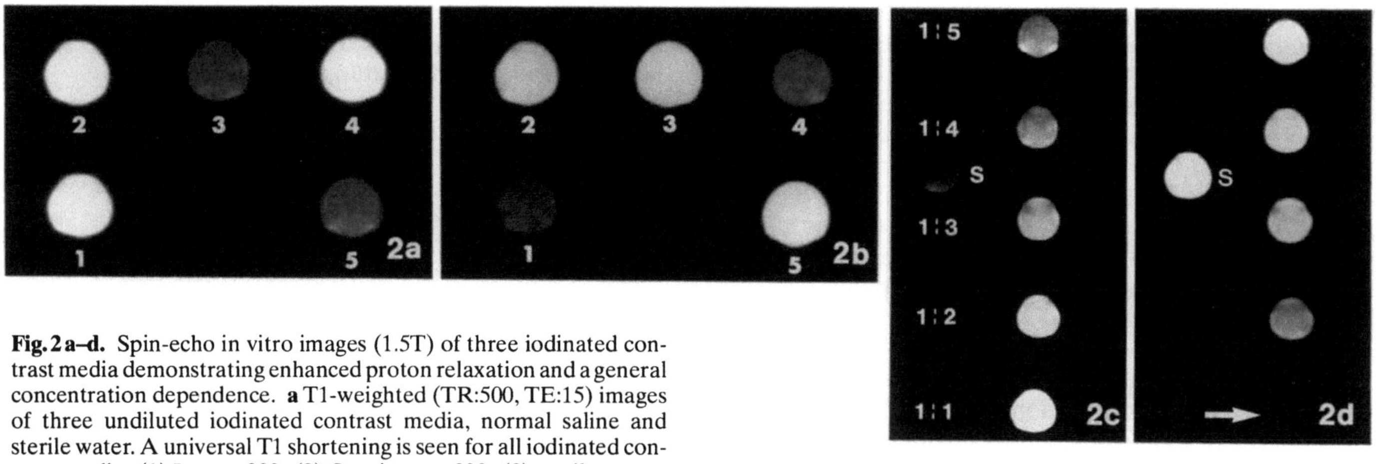

Fig. 2 a–d. Spin-echo in vitro images (1.5T) of three iodinated contrast media demonstrating enhanced proton relaxation and a general concentration dependence. **a** T1-weighted (TR:500, TE:15) images of three undiluted iodinated contrast media, normal saline and sterile water. A universal T1 shortening is seen for all iodinated contrast media. (1) Isovue-300; (2) Omnipaque-300; (3) sterile water; (4) Renografin-76; (5) normal saline. **b** T2-weighted (TR:2500, TE:80) images of the same samples as in a. A universal T2 shortening is seen for all iodinated contrast media. **c** T1-weighted (TR:500, TE:15) images of serial dilutions of Iopamidol-300 showing the marked effect of concentration upon T1 shortening, compared to that of normal saline *(S)*. **d** T2-weighted (TR:2500, TE:80) images samples seen in **c.** A similar concentration dependence upon T2 shortening for iodinated contrast media is shown in comparison to normal saline *(S)*. Note the almost complete signal void due to marked T2 shortening at the highest concentration *(arrow)*

after the instillation of non-ionic radiographic contrast medium (Isovue-300: 3–10 cc) into the subarachnoid space. Five additional subjects with cranial neoplasms were studied following i. v. injection of an ionic contrast medium (Renografin-76: 100 cc). Each MRI examination was performed within 2 h of administration of the iodinated contrast medium.

T1-weighted MR acquisitions were also performed after i. v. injection of gadopentetate dimeglumine (Magnevist: 0.1 mmol/kg) in the individuals with cranial tumors. Follow-up T1- and T2-weighted MRI studies were acquired for comparison after excretion of the iodinated contrast medium in all cases.

The in vitro relationship of T1 and T2 relaxation on imaging was studied in a 1.5T clinical magnet (GE Signa) with regard to several commonly used iodinated contrast media at full strength (Isovue, Omnipaque, and Renografin) and compared with normal saline and sterile water as a reference. In addition, imaging of serial saline dilutions of Isovue-300 over a range of concentrations (1:1–1:5) was performed in order to estimate the effect of dilution on possible visible T1 and T2 effects of iodinated contrast media.

Results

Both patients with subarachnoid non-ionic iodinated contrast medium, and four of five subjects with cranial neoplasms and i. v. administered ionic iodinated contrast medium demonstrated visible T1 and/or T2 shortening on the MR images when compared with precontrast images obtained under identical conditions. The T1 shortening was noted to produce hyperintensity on a T1-weighted acquisition, and the T2 shortening produced variable hypointensity on T2-weighted images (Fig. 1). In one case of dural metastasis, the T1 shortening induced by the iodinated agent raised the intensity of the tumor to isointensity with surrounding brain and thus masked its presence.

Imaging of three commonly used iodinated contrast media at full strength in the clinical GE 1.5T Signa MR unit showed marked T1 and T2 shortening on the images with reference to sterile water and normal saline (Fig. 2a, b). In addition, the serial dilutions of iodinated contrast medium (Isovue) studied showed a concentration-dependent effect on both T1 and T2 relaxation rates (Fig. 2c, d).

Discussion

When consecutive diagnostic studies are being performed on the same individual, there should always be a concern that one examination might have a more or less profound effect upon the interpretation of another. The assumption that conventional iodinated radiologic contrast media are without effect on T1 and T2 relaxation times in clinical MRI is incorrect.

The proposed mechanism for this proton relaxation phenomenon is based upon the molecular structures of the iodinated contrast media. Examination of the various contrast medium molecules reveals that each possesses an iodinated aromatic ring as well as polar hydrophilic chains that extend away from the hydrophobic aromatic region. These hydrophilic hydroxyl(OH)-containing portions of the molecule can form hydrogen bonds to water. The larger the number of OH moieties in the iodinated contrast agent, the larger will be the aqueous solvation shell that forms around the molecule.

The simplest explanation for the observed effects of the iodinated contrast media on both T1 and T2 relaxation rates concerns the electrostatic dipolar field generated by the iodinated aromatic ring of the molecules. In the case of Renografin-76 an ionic salt bridge further increases the effective dipole. In other words, a dipole/dipole relaxation mechanism best describes the observed relaxation effects upon the surrounding hydrogen-bonded water [1, 2]. The iodinated contrast medium that best supports extensive hydrogen bonding (e.g., Renografin-76) also shows greater shortening of T1 and T2 compared to the non-ionic agents (Iopamidol and Isovue), which have lesser hydrogen-bonding capability [3, 4].

The change in the MRI signal induced by the iodinated contrast medium becomes important when the characteristic appearance of a tissue or lesion deviates from its precontrast state. For example, some of the alterations in MRI signal in this series revealed characteristics which, in any other setting, would have been interpreted as complicating factors such as hemorrhage, calcification, or perhaps abnormal flow phenomena. A consideration of greater concern is that of unsuspected enhancement of a lesion to isointensity with surrounding cerebral tissue. Such an observation leads to the conclusion that there is a real possibility of lesion masking by iodinated contrast media in MR imaging of the CNS.

Based upon these investigations, it is recommended that all patients having MRI examinations of any part of the body be questioned as to the possibility of recent administration of iodinated contrast media by any route. If such agents have been administered, the presence of possible superimposed alterations in MRI signal induced by the iodinated contrast medium should be taken into account when interpreting the images. Perhaps in some instances a delay in the MRI study might be requested in order to allow the iodinated contrast medium to clear the body. The final goal should be a more precise representation and understanding of the unadulterated MRI signal of the normal and pathologic tissue. In this way a more accurate radiologic diagnosis will result.

References

1. Gunther H (1980) NMR spectroscopy: an introduction. Wiley, New York, pp 377
2. Shaw D (1984) Fourier transform N.M.R. spectroscopy. Elsevier, New York, pp 256–260
3. Ling GN (1984) In search of the physical basis of life. Plenum Press, New York, pp 1–53, 437–462
4. Daskiewicz OK, Hennel JW, Lubas B, Szczepkowski TW (1963) Proton magnetic relaxation and protein hydration. Nature 200: 1006–1007

Dr. J. Randy Jinkins
Department of Radiology
The University of Texas Health Science Center
at San Antonio
7703 F. Curl Drive
San Antonio, TX 78284-7800, USA

POSTER SESSION 1

Neuroradiology (1991) 33 [Suppl]: 290–292

Neuro radiology
© Springer-Verlag 1991

MRI of the displaced and distorted optic chiasm and adjacent visual pathways

T. El Gammal[1], B. Brooks[1], R. Harbour[2], P. Jacob[1], E. R. Duvall[1], and L. Kline[3]

[1] University of Alabama at Birmingham, Street, Birmingham, Alabama, USA
[2] Northwest Florida Eye Associates, Pensacola, Florida, USA
[3] Children's Hospital of Alabama, Department of Ophthalmology, Birmingham, Alabama, USA

Summary. The MRI features of chiasmal and adjacent visual pathway displacement and distortion have not been emphasized to date. We have retrospectively studied 58 patients to compare and contrast the frequency and appearance of the morphologic changes and the presence or absence of consequent visual disturbances. This material included 9 mass lesions (6 neoplasms and 3 aneurysms) and other non-neoplastic lesions: 15 cases of severe hydrocephalus, 14 of advanced primary empty sella turcica and 20 of secondary empty sella and leptomeningeal inflammation. There was a general correspondence of anatomic change and abnormal ophthalmologic examination in patients with mass lesions. There was no correlation of visual disturbances with anatomic abnormalities found in the non-neoplastic group.

Key words: Optic chiasm – Optic nerve – Empty sella – Hydrocephalus – Magnetic resonance imaging

MRI affords precise delineation of chiasmal compression and/or displacement by tumors, and of distortion and intrasellar translocation in patients with hydrocephalus, primary and secondary empty sella turcica, and leptomeningeal inflammatory disease.

Patients and methods

Patients noted to have an advanced degree of anatomic abnormality of the chiasm and/or optic nerves and tracts in these conditions were selected for study by MRI reviewed over a 3-year-period. The morphologic changes and imaging features were analyzed and, when available, the clinical information, including the ophthalmologic examination, was reviewed.

The patients were divided into categories of tumoral and non-tumoral causes of distortion and displacement of the chiasm and adjacent visual pathways (Table 1). Included in the tumoral group were 6 patients with neoplasms and 3 with aneurysms. Non-tumoral etiologies included marked hydrocephalus, advanced changes of primary empty sella, secondary empty sella, and leptomeningeal inflammatory disease.

Results and discussion

The normal appearance of the chiasm on sagittal images is of an oblique line from inferiorly to superiorly within the chiasmatic cistern [1]. Morphologic changes in the chiasm tended to show characteristic features depending on the

Table 1. MRI of displacement and distortion of the optic chiasm and adjacent visual pathways ($n = 58$)

Nontumoral ($n = 49$)	Tumoral ($n = 9$)
Advanced hydrocephalus ($n = 15$)	Neoplasm ($n = 6$)
	Pituitary adenoma[b] 2
Advanced primary empty sella ($n = 14$)	Temporal lobe tumors[b] 2
	Ethmoid chondrosarcoma[a] 1
	Esthesioneuroblastoma[a] 1
Secondary empty sella ($n = 18$)	
Postoperative 17	Aneurysm ($n = 3$)
After hemorrhage with pituitary apoplexy 1	Posterior communicating[c] 1
	Terminal internal carotid[b] 1
	Terminal internal carotid[a] 1
Leptomeningeal inflammation ($n = 2$)	
Meningitis with intrasellar infection 1	
CNS sarcoidosis with pituitary sarcoid granuloma 1	

Compression and/or displacement of: [a] Optic nerve [b] Optic chiasm [c] Optic tract

Table 2. MRI morphology of abnormal chiasm in hydrocephalus, primary and secondary empty sella and leptomeningeal inflammation

Patients with advanced changes of hydrocephalus – 15	
Chiasm normal	3
Chiasm horizontally oriented, low in position	6
Chiasm compressed against bone by dilated anterior third ventricle	6
Patients with advanced changes of primary empty sella – 14	
Chiasm normal	7
Normal chiasm, low in position	5
Mild inferior bowing of chiasm	1
Chiasm low in position with "V"-shaped deformity	1
Patients with secondary empty sella – 18	
Chiasm normal	3
Normal chiasm, low in position	2
Inferior bowing of chiasm	3
"V"-shaped deformity of chiasm	4
Marked chiasmal deformity with intrasellar herniation	6
Patients with leptomeningeal inflammation – 2	
Non-visualization of chiasm	1
Marked chiasmal deformity with intrasellar herniation	1

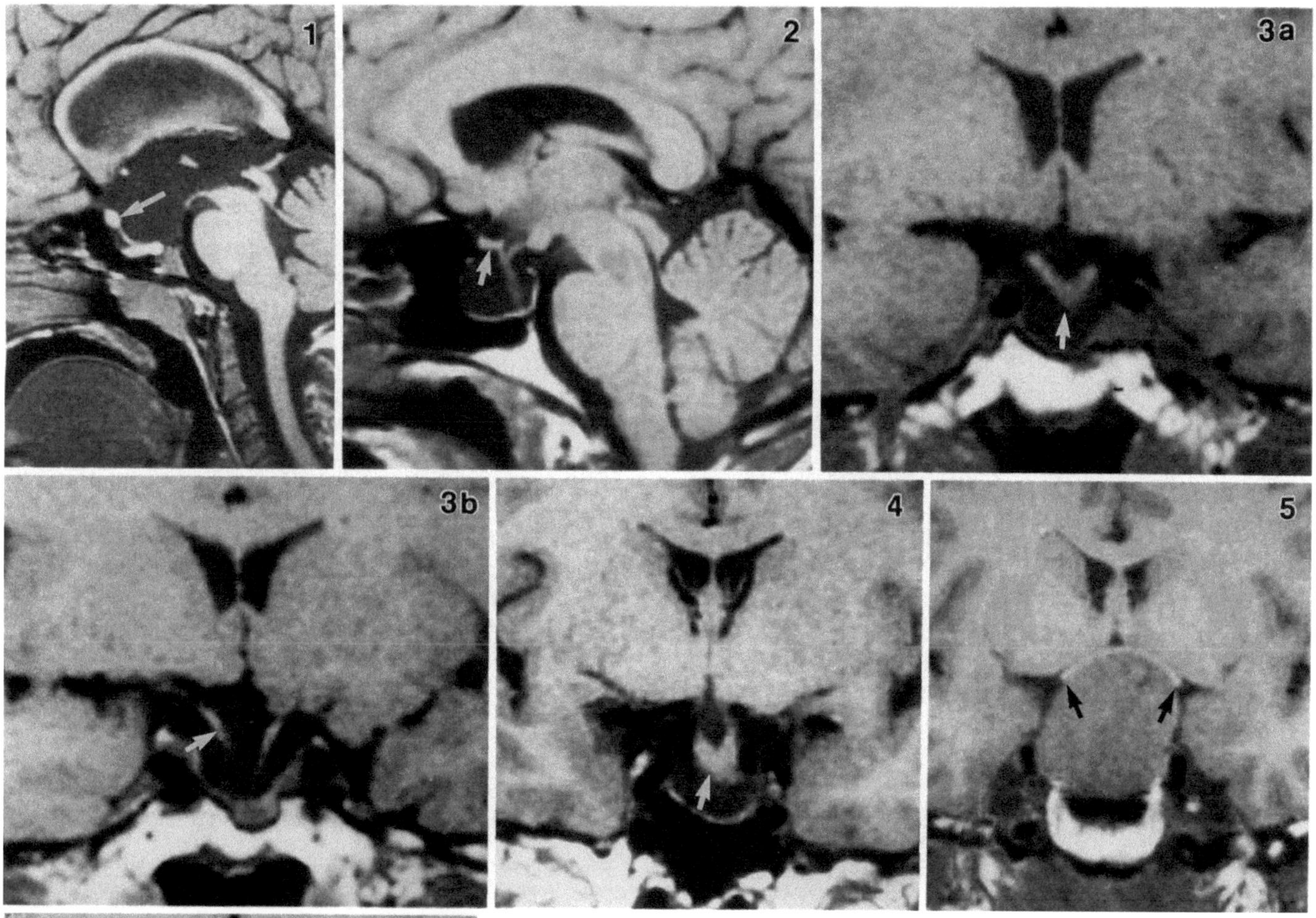

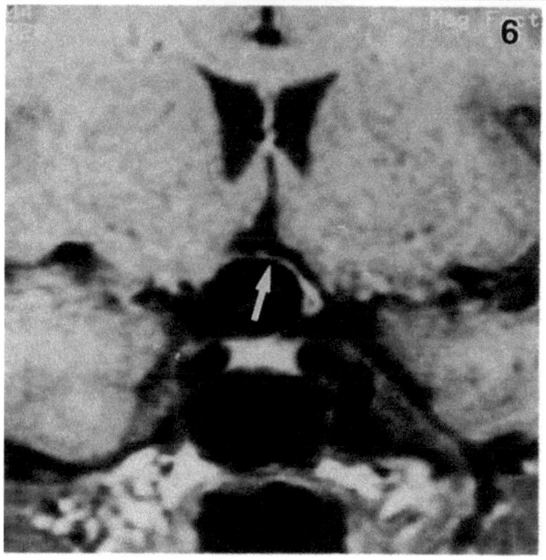

Fig. 1. Hydrocephalus with ballooned anterior third ventricle compressing the chiasm against the tuberculum sellae *(arrow)*. Sagittal T1-weighted images. Patient had a normal ophthalmologic examination

Fig. 2. Advanced primary empty sella with low, horizontal chiasm *(arrow)*. Sagittal T1-weighted images

Fig. 3. a Advanced primary empty sella. There is a low "V"-shaped chiasm *(arrow)*. **b** The distorted optic nerves are herniated into the upper part of the sella turcica *(arrow)*. Patient had normal ophthalmologic examination. Coronal T1-weighted images

Fig. 4. Postoperative secondary empty sella with a low, distorted chiasm *(arrow)*. Coronal T1-weighted images

Fig. 5. Large suprasellar extension of chromophobe adenoma. Note upward bowing of a severely compressed and elongated chiasm *(arrows)*. Coronal T1-weighted images

Fig. 6. Terminal right internal carotid aneurysm produces displacement and severe narrowing of the right side of the optic chiasm *(arrow)*. Coronal T1-weighted images

presence of hydrocephalus or of a primary or a secondary empty sella (Table 2). In patients with third ventricular dilatation, the chiasm may be flattened and displaced forwards against the bone of the tuberculum sellae or the dorsum sellae or, less frequently, displaced posteroinferiorly against the dorsum sellae. The chiasm most often remained normal or nearly normal, except for assuming a more horizontal and somewhat low position (Fig. 2) in cases of primary empty sella. In 14 cases of primary empty sella, only 1 patient was found to have a marked degree of distortion of the chiasm with a "V"-shaped configuration and translocation into the uppermost part of the sella turcica (Fig. 3).

In contrast, a normal or only somewhat low position of the chiasm was seen in the minority of patients with a secondary empty sella (Table 2). Varying degrees of deformity occurred in 13 of 18 cases, with marked intrasellar herniation in many (Fig. 4). A traction mechanism occurring consequent to postsurgical inflammatory changes probably accounts for these different appearances. In the

Table 3. Ophthalmologic examination in 37 patients with displaced and/or distorted optic nerves, chiasm, or tract

Neoplastic or aneurysmal compression ($n = 9$)	
Normal	3
Correlative abnormality	3
Partially correlative abnormality	3
Advanced hydrocephalus ($n = 4$)	
Normal	3
Non-correlative abnormality in one eye due to retinal scar	1
Primary empty sella ($n = 11$)	
Normal	9
Non-correlative abnormality due to cataract (1) and arteriosclerosis (1)	2
Secondary empty sella[a] ($n = 12$)	
Normal	8
Pre- and postoperative visual field defects	3
Questionable decreased visual acuity bilaterally	1
Leptomeningeal inflammation ($n = 1$)	
Left homonymous hemianopsia	1

[a] Two other patients had no formal ophthalmologic examination, but had no visual complaints

2 patients with leptomeningeal inflammatory disease, the chiasm could not be seen distinct from adjacent isointense inflammatory tissue in a patient with meningitis, and showed a markedly distorted configuration and intrasellar herniation in a patient with sarcoidosis.

Abnormalities on ophthalmologic examination correlated reasonably well in 6 of 9 patients with tumoral causes of chiasmal distortion (Fig. 5, 6). Of more interest are the results in the patients reviewed with hydrocephalus and primary and secondary empty sella turcica (Table 3). In patients with hydrocephalus and with primary empty sella, the ophthalmologic examinations were normal in 12 of 15 cases, and demonstrated abnormalities consequent upon ocular pathology unrelated to the intracranial abnormalities in the other 3. In many patients in the secondary empty sella group, a striking degree of deformity of the optic nerves and/or chiasm was present in the face of a completely normal ophthalmologic examination. The single patient with primary empty sella and significant chiasmal deformity with intrasellar herniation similarly had a normal ophthalmologic examination (Fig. 3). In a small number of patients (3/12) with postoperative secondary empty sella, visual field defects remained but were less extensive than prior to surgery. A number of the secondary empty sella patients also had atrophy of the optic nerve and/or chiasm or tract as an associated finding and still had normal ophthalmologic examinations. These results are similar to those of Kaufman et al. [2] who found a lack of correlation between visual disturbances and intrasellar herniation in their review of primary and secondary empty sella turcicas.

In conclusion, in this study the extensive anatomic abnormalities of the chiasm and adjacent visual pathways seen with MRI in cases of hydrocephalus and in primary and secondary empty sella turcica are not usually associated with ophthalmologic findings. This information may be reassuring when assessing MRI studies demonstrating such changes in these patients.

References

1. Langer BG, Mafee MF, Pollack S, Spigos DG, Gyi B (1987) MRI of the normal orbit and optic pathway. Radiol Clin North Am 25: 429–446
2. Kaufman B, Tomsak RL, Kaufman BA, Arafah BU, Bellou EM, Selman WR, Modic MT (1989) Herniation of the suprasellar visual system and third ventricle into empty sellae: morphologic and clinical considerations. AJR 152: 597–608

T. El Gammal
University of Alabama at Birmingham
619 South 19th Street
Birmingham, Alabama 35233, USA

Neuroradiology (1991) 33 [Suppl]: 293–295

Neuroradiology
© Springer-Verlag 1991

Gadolinium-enhanced MRI of the intracranial visual pathways

T. El Gammal[1], B. S. Brooks[1], P. Jacob[1], E. R. Duvall[1], L. Kline[2], and R. C. Harbour[3]

[1] Department of Radiology, The University of Alabama at Birmingham, Birmingham, Alabama, USA
[2] Department of Ophthalmology, The Children's Hospital of Alabama, Birmingham, Alabama, USA
[3] The Northwest Florida Eye Associates, Pensacola, Florida, USA

Summary. MRI with gadolinium (Gd) showed abnormal enhancement in the optic nerves and/or chiasm and tract in three patients with multiple sclerosis and three with neurosarcoidosis. Postoperative enhancement in the chiasm was seen in two patients, possibly due to postsurgical inflammatory reaction. Gd increases the sensitivity of MRI in demonstrating involvement of the optic nerves and intracranial optic pathways in inflammatory diseases and systemic disease with suspected visual pathway involvement.

Key words: Gadolinium – Multiple sclerosis – Central nervous system sarcoidosis – Optic nerve – Optic chiasm – Optic tract

Previous reports have documented the utility of MRI for demonstrating involvement of the intraorbital optic nerve in patients with multiple sclerosis (MS), neurosarcoidosis, and other inflammatory diseases. However, the value of MRI with gadolinium (Gd) contrast enhancement in the evaluation of not only the optic nerves but also the intracranial visual pathways has not been emphasized to date. We present our experience in eight patients with comparison of clinical and MRI features in each case.

Patients and methods

The eight patients, ranging in age from 26 to 54 years, included seven females and one male. A diagnosis of clinically definite MS in one patient was based upon the characteristic course of the disease and laboratory data, while the diagnosis of clinically probable MS in another was made on the basis of presenting symptoms and signs and MRI findings typical of the disease. A third patient, who presented with brain stem and cerebellar symptoms is considered as having clinically possible MS at the present time. Neurosarcoidosis was proven by trans-sphenoidal biopsy in one patient and was a presumptive diagnosis in two, based upon clinical presentation and response to corticosteroid therapy, and the MRI appearance and location of the intracranial lesions and their subsequent resolution on follow-up examination after treatment. Two other patients were included as examples of postsurgical (inflammatory) changes after operation for a suprasellar meningioma and a pituitary adenoma respectively. A representative case history for each of the MS and neurosarcoidosis groups of patients follows.

Case reports

A 40-year-old female was examined in May 1989 for complaints of visual blurring and diminished vision of the right eye. Ophthalmologic examination confirmed an incongruous left homonymous hemianopia and MRI (Fig. 1) showed focal enlargement of the right side of the optic chiasm and abnormal enhancement of the right optic nerve, chiasm, and tract. There were no cerebral parenchymal lesions. The cerebrospinal fluid (CSF) showed oligoclonal bands and an increased immunoglobulin synthesis rate. Repeat MRI 1 month later did not demonstrate any abnormality. Two months later the patient's visual complaints had almost completely resolved, but she began to complain of paresthesiae and diminished balance and coordination in her legs. These complaints slowly resolved over 3 months, but in December the patient noted paresthesiae in the hands with diminished dexterity on the right. To date, there has been a gradual improvement in these symptoms, but the patient still retains trace sensory disturbances in both hands and complains of occasional burning sensations in the fingertips and soles of the feet. In early 1990, an episode of left hemianesthesia and a left facial burning sensation occurred, which resolved after 2 weeks. The family history includes MS in two paternal first cousins.

A 33-year-old female presented with a 2-month history of severe headaches, described as stabbing in character, behind the left eye, scintillating scotomata, photophobia, and intermittent fever. The patient had normal visual acuity and normal visual fields on ophthalmologic examination, and CSF findings of a lymphocytic pleocytosis. Endocrinologic evaluation disclosed mild panhypopituitarism. Cranial MRI demonstrated a hypothalamic mass extending into the optic chiasm with central enhancement and a second enhancing mass with central low signal within the pituitary gland. Non-enhancing swelling of the left optic tract was also noted. Trans-sphenoidal biopsy of the pituitary mass revealed a florid granulomatous inflammation negative on acid fast and fungal stains and cultures. The patient received corticosteroid therapy. Follow-up ophthalmologic examinations remained normal and postoperative MRI after 3 and 6 months showed progressive resolution of the hypothalamic and intrasellar masses. At the time of the last (6 month) MRI, abnormal intracranial enhancement was no longer evident.

Discussion

Until recently, imaging investigation of suspected inflammatory lesions involving the optic nerves and intracranial visual pathways has been limited to contrast-enhanced CT and MRI without contrast media [1]. The use of STIR sequences for the demonstration of demyelinated plaques in optic neuritis patients was described by Miller et al. [2] and, subsequently, Grossman et al. [3] reported their ex-

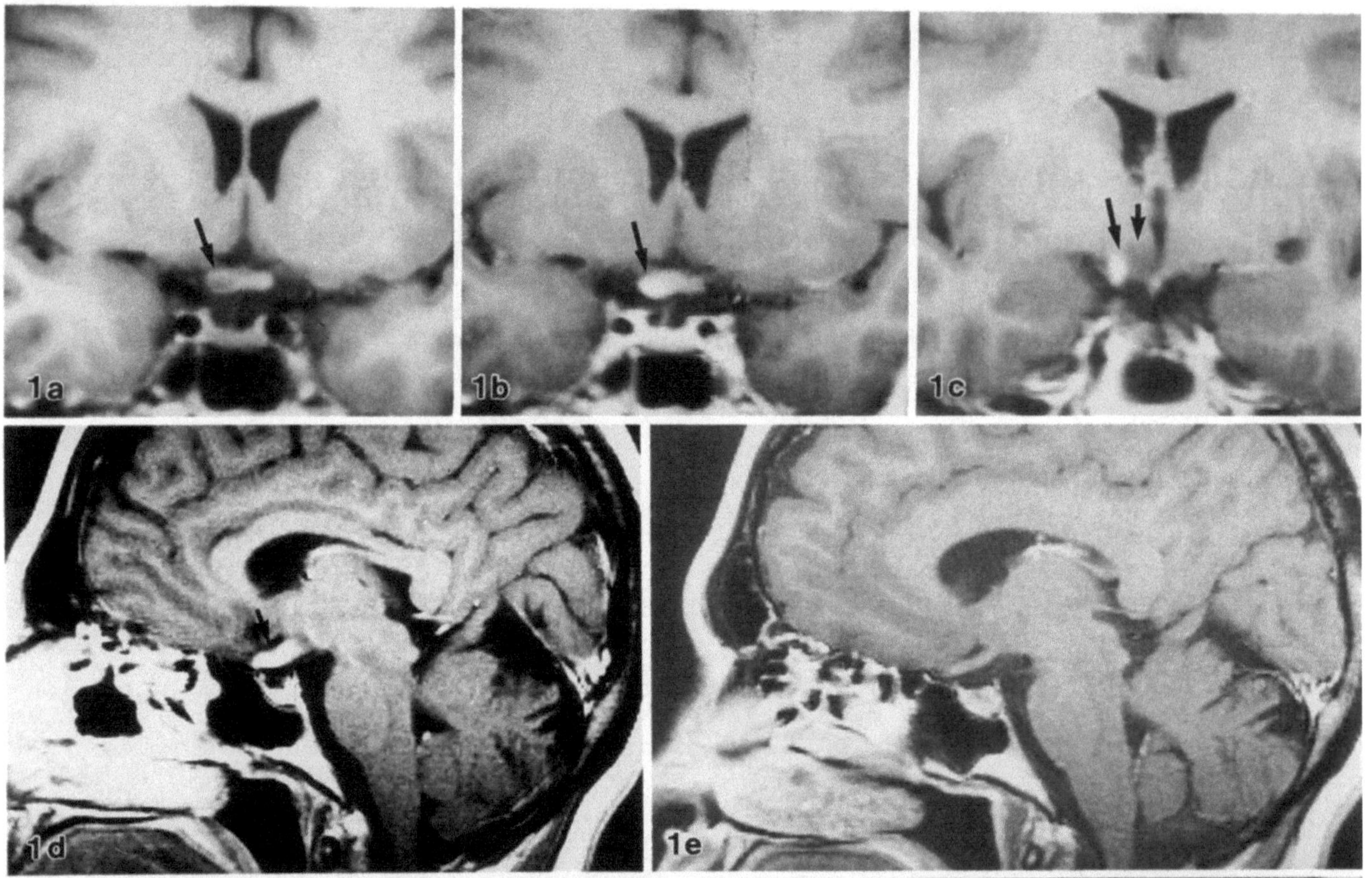

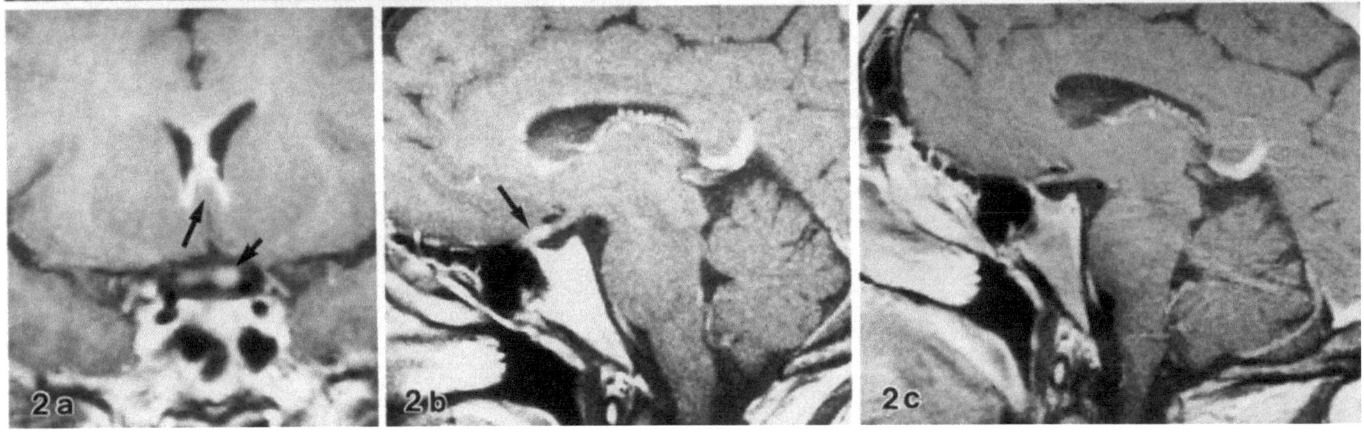

Fig. 1 a–e. A 40-year-old female with clinically definite multiple sclerosis presenting with acute optic neuritis (case 3, Table 1). **a** Unenhanced coronal T1-weighted image shows enlargement of the optic chiasm on the right with a low signal area within it *(arrow)*. **b** Coronal section after gadolinium (Gd) shows abnormal enhancement in the same location *(arrow)*. **c** More posterior coronal section demonstrates enhancement in the right optic tract *(arrow)* with adjacent low signal in the hypothalamus and compression of the lower third ventricle *(small arrow)*. **d** Parasagittal image after Gd demonstrates enlargement and enhancement of right optic nerve, chiasm, and tract. **e** One month follow-up parasagittal image after Gd. Note absence of abnormal enhancement of right optic nerve, chiasm, and tract

Fig. 2 a–c. A 54-year-old female with probable CNS sarcoidosis. **a** Contrast-enhanced coronal MRI section reveals subependymal enhancement around the frontal horns of the lateral ventricles *(upper arrow)* with enlargement of and enhancement in the left optic nerve and chiasm *(lower arrow)*. **b** Enhanced parasagittal section shows left optic nerve enhancement. **c** Five-month follow-up enhanced parasagittal image shows no abnormal enhancement and possible left optic nerve atrophy

perience with Gd-enhanced MRI in MS patients and illustrated abnormal enhancement in the optic tract in one patient. In two patients with MS and visual field defects MRI without Gd also showed lesions in or near the optic tract [4]. Therefore, although autopsy studies of patients with MS have revealed frequent involvement of the optic chiasm, tract and radiations [5], MRI demonstration of lesions in these locations has up to now been described in only a very few cases. However, previous studies have shown that abnormal enhancing lesions elsewhere in the brain do correlate with activity of the disease at least at high field strengths [3]. As the use of Gd-enhanced MRI for MS patients increases, it can be expected that visual pathway pathology will be seen with greater frequency. In patients with neurosarcoidosis, two hypothalamic sarcoid granulomas were illustrated by Karnaze et al. [6] using MRI without Gd, and a pituitary mass with infiltration of the chiasm due to sarcoidosis was shown on non-enhanced MRI by Naheedy et al. [7]. Although sarcoidosis has a well-known predilection for involvement of the basal leptomeninges and cranial nerves, with frequent occurrence of chiasmal and hypothalamic lesions, demonstration of abnormal contrast enhancement of the optic nerves and intracranial visual system with enhanced MRI studies has not, to our knowledge, been previously reported in CNS sarcoidosis.

Abnormal enhancement of the optic nerve and/or chiasm and tract was found in three of our patients (cases 1, 4, 5) who did not have visual complaints at the time of their imaging studies. The MRI findings in these three patients may have represented subclinical involvement with their disease at the time of the imaging studies. In two other patients, (cases 3, 7) correlation of the MRI findings with the ophthalmological examination was precise. In case 6 of this series, the initial presentation of relatively sudden onset of severely diminished visual acuity of the left eye corresponded with MRI demonstration of abnormal enhancement of the left optic nerve, chiasm and tract (Fig. 2). MRI in this patient also revealed enhancing subependymal lesions and all the MRI abnormalities were steroid responsive with complete resolution on a 5-month follow-up study. However, in this patient, the clinical course was that of progressive visual loss affecting both eyes, possibly due to optic atrophy (Fig. 2c). Cases 7 and 8 demonstrate the importance of awareness that abnormal Gd enhancement can be seen in the postoperative state as a sequela of surgery alone when utilizing contrast-enhanced MRI to assess for residual or recurrent tumor.

Our findings not only reveal the expanded sensitivity of Gd-enhanced MRI in patients with MS and neurosarcoidosis, but also predict that MRI with Gd will prove extremely helpful for assessing the extent of disease and response to therapy in other inflammatory conditions and systemic diseases with suspected visual pathway involvement.

References

1. Rubenfeld M, Wirtschafter JD (1987) The role of medical imaging in the practice of neuro-ophthalmology. Radiol Clin North Am 25: 863–876
2. Miller DH, Johnson G, McDonald WI (1986) Detection of optic nerve lesions in optic neuritis with magnetic resonance imaging (letter). Lancet I: 1490–1491
3. Grossman RI, Gonzalez-Scarano F, Atlas SW (1986) Multiple sclerosis: gadolinium enhancement in MR imaging. Radiology 161: 721–725
4. Rosenblatt MA, Behrens MM, Zweifach PH (1987) Magnetic resonance imaging of optic tract involvement in multiple sclerosis. Am J Ophthalmol 104: 74–79
5. Hawkins K, Behrens MM (1975) Homonymous hemianopsia in multiple sclerosis with report of bilateral case. Br J Ophthalmol 59: 334–337
6. Karnaze MG, Sartor K, Winthrop JD (1986) Suprasellar lesions: evaluation with MR imaging. Neuroradiology 161: 77–82
7. Naheedy MH, Haag JR, Azar-Kia B (1987) MRI and CT of sellar and parasellar disorders. Radiol Clin North Am 25: 819–847

T. El Gammal
The University of Alabama at Birmingham
Department of Radiology
619 South 19th Street
Birmingham, Alabama 35233, USA

Neuroradiology (1991) 33 [Suppl]: 296–297

Neuro radiology
© Springer-Verlag 1991

MRI of pituitary adenomas using gadolinium-DTPA

A. L. Agnoli[1], T. Bauer[1], and G. Hildebrandt[2]

Departments of [1] Neuroradiology and [2] Neurosurgery, Justus-Liebig-University of Giessen, Giessen, Federal Republic of Germany

Summary. In 90 patients with pituitary adenomas gadolinium (Gd)-DTPA-enhanced MRI was more sensitive for delineating microadenomas (82%) than plain MRI. In macroadenomas delineation of cavernous sinus from adjacent brain tissue and tumour regression or necrosis was improved. In patients with prolactinomas after surgery and for medical therapy, Gd-DTPA-enhanced MRI provided additional information on shrinkage. The MRI patterns were not related to endocrine findings.

Key words: Pituitary adenoma – Magnetic resonance imaging – Gadolinium-DTPA

In investigating pituitary adenomas high-resolution MRI is widely regarded as the method of choice [1–3]. Better visualization is described using gadolinium (Gd)-DTPA [4, 5]. We report on our results of MRI diagnosis and follow-up in a group of 90 patients with pituitary adenomas, using Gd-DTPA.

Patients and methods

Ninety patients (aged 17–85 years, mean 48 years) had 136 MRI examinations performed, 90 before therapy, 46 during dopamine agonist therapy for prolactinoma. The MRI parameters on 0.5 T and 1.5 T superconducting systems were T_1-weighted spin-echo sequences (TR/TE 420–600 ms/15–40 ms) in coronal and sagittal sections (3–5 mm thick without spacing, matrix 256 × 256) before and after i. v. injection of Gd-DTPA (Schering).

Results

Of the 90 adenomas, 45 (50%) were non-functioning, 31 (34%) prolactinomas and 14 (16%) growth-hormone secreting adenomas. There were 17 (19%) microadenomas and 73 (81%) macroadenomas. Table 1 shows the most frequent intra- and extrasellar changes induced by the tumours. As indirect signs of tumour *microadenomas* showed an asymmetrical superior convexity in 13 (76%), displacement of pituitary stalk in 11 (65%) and asymmetrical sellar floor changes in 6 cases (35%). Fourteen microadenomas were hypointense or isointense with absent or only slight contrast enhancement compared with adjacent tissue; only 3 adenomas had higher signal intensity. In Gd-DTPA-enhanced studies 14 (82%) microadenomas could be delineated from the visibly enhancing normal pituitary gland or stalk and the cavernous sinus (Fig. 1). One case showed unilateral cavernous sinus invasion. *Macroadenomas* were all demonstrated on pre-contrast MRI studies. Forty-two cases (58%) showed hypo- or isointense tumour signal; 24 (33%) were inhomogeneous and 7 (9%) hyperintense relative to white matter. On post-Gd images 15 cases (21%) had little or no, 58 (79%) moderate or intense enhancement. In 27 cases (37%) demarcation of cystic or necrotic areas was visible due to inhomogeneous enhancement.

Post-Gd studies improved demarcation of the cavernous sinus in 48 (66%) and adjacent brain tissue in 8 cases (11%), while pre-Gd images were not conclusive in these patients (Fig. 2). As in patients with microadenomas, correlation between endocrine activity, signal intensity or Gd enhancement was not found. In prolactinomas shrinkage was documented in 84% of cases within 4 weeks after treatment with a dopamine agonist. Adenomas with a homogeneous tumour matrix demonstrated a greater degree of tumour shrinkage than those with large cystic or necrotic areas (Fig. 3). Post-Gd studies outlined regression of unenhancing tumour in 32% of cases, not as clearly seen in the pre-Gd images (Fig. 4). Tumour shrinkage did not always correlate with decreasing serum prolactin levels.

Discussion

MRI is widely regarded as the method of choice in the diagnosis of pituitary adenomas. In our study additional use of Gd-DTPA improved visualization of most microadenomas (82%) and more than two-thirds of macroadenomas. The differentiation between cavernous sinus and tumour

Table 1. Frequency of intra- and extrasellar changes caused by pituitary adenomas seen using gadolinium-DTPA-enhanced MRI

Microadenomas (n = 17)	n	%
Asymmetrical superior convexity	13	76
Displacement of pituitary stalk	11	65
Sellar floor changes	6	35
Invasion of cavernous sinus[a]	1	6
Macroadenomas (n = 73)		
Compression/displacement of pituitary stalk	68	93
Compression of chiasm	46	63
Invasion of cavernous sinus[a]	40	55
a) unilateral	25	34
b) bilateral	15	21
Sellar floor changes	32	44
Displacement of carotid arteries	27	37
Compression of third ventricle	26	36

[a] Signs of cavernous sinus invasion: encasement of cavernous carotid artery; displacement of lateral sinus margin; diminished enhancment after Gd-DTPA

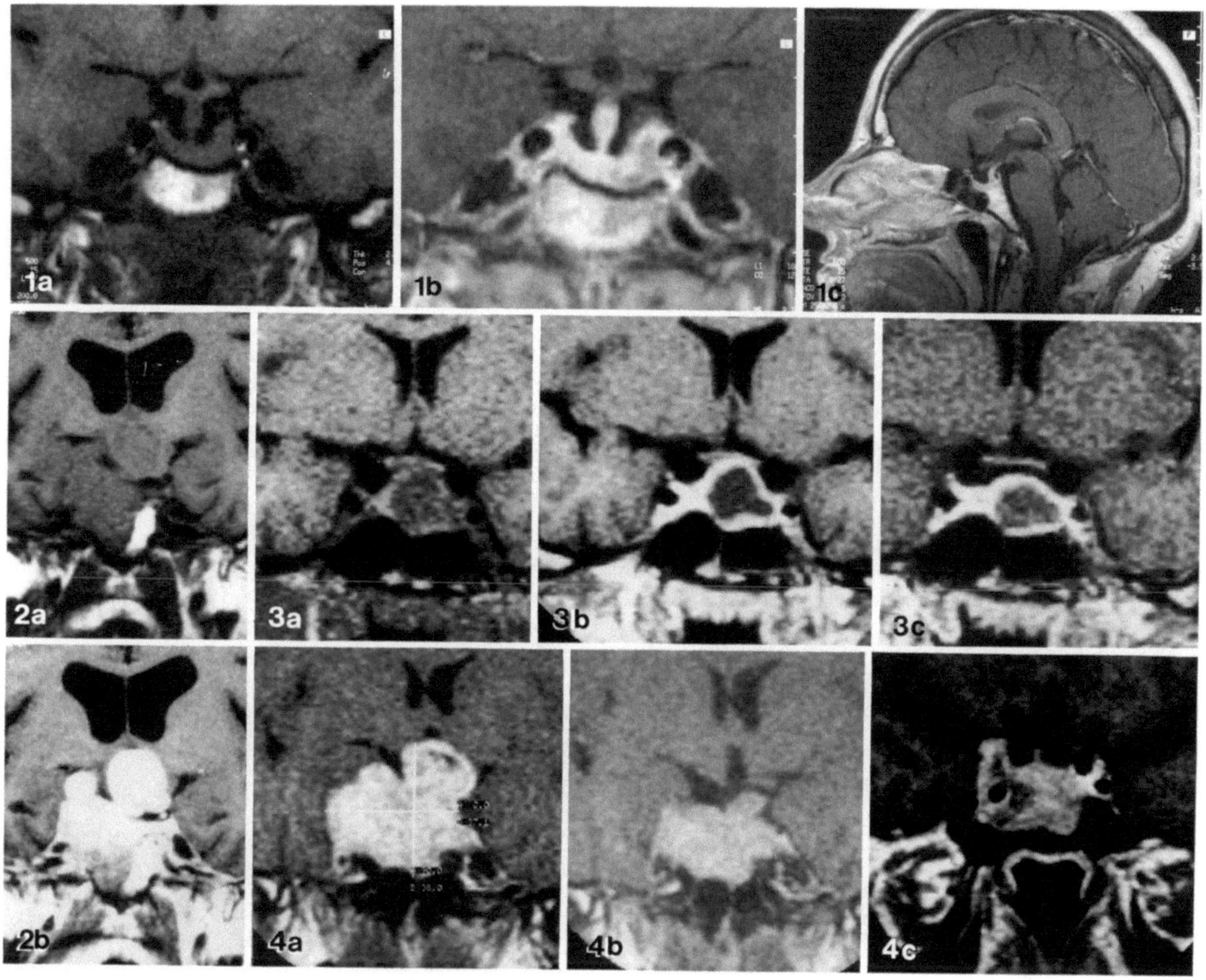

Fig. 1a–c. Growth-hormone-secreting microadenoma showing displaced pituitary stalk. Post-gadolinium (Gd)-DTPA images differentiate between adenoma, pituitary gland, and medial wall of cavernous sinus (surgically and histologically proved)

Fig. 2a, b. Non-functioning macroadenoma before and after Gd-DTPA injection: post-Gd image improves delineation of adenoma from adjacent brain tissue due to increase of tumour signal intensity

Fig. 3. a, b The pretreatment MRI of this female patient (galactorrhoea/amenorrhoea syndrome) shows a cystic-appearing prolactin secreting macroadenoma in contact with the optic chiasm. **c** After i. m. 50 mg bromocriptine-retard tumour volume was only slightly reduced

Fig. 4 a, b Macroprolactinoma before and 4 weeks after medical therapy (i. m. bromocriptine 50 mg retard). Shrinkage of the age of the adenoma is seen. **c** Four months later the post-Gd image shows involution of adenoma with regressive intratumoural areas

mass was better. In the follow-up of medically treated prolactinoma patients tumour shrinkage was documented in over 80%. Post-Gd images demonstrated tumour regression more often than MRI studies without contrast medium [6].

Despite the additional time, we regard Gd-enhanced MRI studies as superior in the diagnostic work-up and follow-up of pituitary adenomas.

References

1. Davis PC, Hofmann JC Jr, Spencer T, Tindall GT, Braun IF (1987) MR imaging of pituitary adenoma: CT, clinical and surgical correlation. AJR 148: 797–802
2. Kucharczyk W, Davis DO, Kelly WM, Sze G, Norman D, Newton DH (1986) Pituitary adenomas: high-resolution MR imaging at 1.5 T. Radiology 161: 761–765
3. Mikhael MA, Ciric MS (1988) MR imaging of pituitary tumors before and after surgical and/or medical treatment. Comput Assist Tomogr 12: 441–445
4. Nakamura T, Schörner W, Bittner RC, Felix R (1988) The value of paramagnetic contrast agent gadolinium-DTPA in the diagnosis of pituitary adenomas. Neuroradiology 30: 481–486
5. Macpherson P, Hadley DM, Teasdale E, Teasdale G (1989) Pituitary microadenomas. Does gadolinium enhance their demonstration? Neuroradiology 31: 293–298
6. Bauer T, Agnoli AL, Hildebrandt G (1990) MRT und CT bei Patienten mit Hypophysenprolaktinomen unter pharmakologischer und operativer Therapie. Zentralbl Radiol 141: 174

Prof. A. L. Agnoli
Neuroradiologische Abteilung des Zentrums für Radiologie
der Justus-Liebig-Universität
Am Steg 22
W-6300 Giessen
Federal Republic of Germany

Neuroradiology (1991) 33 [Suppl]: 298–299

Neuroradiology
© Springer-Verlag 1991

Assessment of osteolytic space-occupying lesions involving the parasellar region and/or the middle cranial fossa

R. Stiglbauer[1], E. Schindler[2], and P. Barton[1]

[1] Department of Radiology and
[2] Division of Neuroradiology, Department of Neurosurgery, University of Vienna Medical School, Vienna, Austria

Summary. The MRI and CT findings in 18 patients with osteolytic lesions involving the parasellar region and/or the floor of the middle cranial fossa were compared with neurosurgical findings to determine the diagnostic efficacy of these imaging methods. MRI was found to be superior for precise demonstration of intra- and extracranial tumour extent, and for showing the lesion's relationship to essential parasellar structures (cavernous sinus, internal carotid artery, Gasserian ganglion). CT, particularly in the high resolution mode, however, proved to be superior for precisely visualising skull-base involvement and tumour calcification.

Key words: Parasellar lesions – Computed tomography – Magnetic resonance imaging – Skull base – Osteolytic lesions

In assessing parasellar lesions the following questions should be answered: (1) Is there an intra- and/or extracranial extension of the lesion? (2) Is there involvement of adjacent vessels or of cranial nerves? (3) What is the size of the bone defect? (4) Is osteolysis caused by expanding tumour growth or is the skull base infiltrated by the tumour? (5) Can the histology of the tumour be predicted?

In order to answer these questions we have retrospectively reviewed the MRI and CT findings in 18 patients with parasellar lesions, surgically verified in all cases (Table 1).

Table 1. Surgically verified diagnoses in 18 patients

Chordoma	4
Chondrosarcoma	3
Osteolytic meningioma	3
Nasopharyngeal carcinoma	2
Giant aneurysm of the internal carotid artery	2
Pituitary adenoma	1
Adenoid cystic carcinoma	1
Mucocoele	1
Meningoencephalocoele	1

Patients and methods

Eighteen patients (8 male, 10 female, age 20–66 years) were examined by MRI [1.5 T superconductive unit, head coil, two imaging planes, T1- and T2-weighted spin echo sequences (TR/TE: 700/15, 2500/15,90), slice thickness 3–5 mm, i. v. administration of 0.1 mmol gadolinium-DTPA/kg body weight in selected cases] as well as by CT (third-generation scanner, two imaging planes, slice thickness 2–4 mm, i. v.-administration of 90 ml non-ionic contrast medium in all patients). The MRI and CT findings were compared with the neurosurgical reports.

Results and discussion

Because of the complex anatomy of the parasellar region the diagnostic work-up of lesions involving this area is a challenge for the neuroradiologist, who has to provide

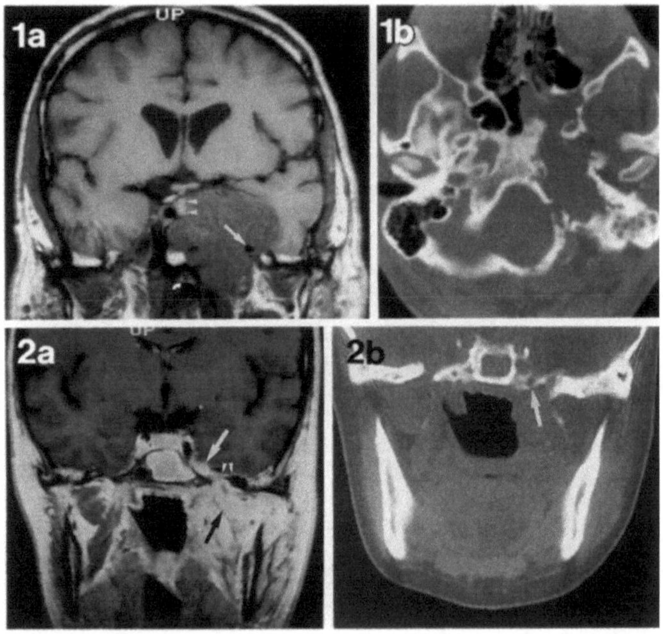

Fig. 1a, b. A 47-year-old man with a chordoma of the skull base. **a** T1-weighted coronal image: intra- and extracranial tumour extent, encasement and displacement of the left internal carotid artery *(arrow)*, intrasellar extension *(arrowheads)* are shown. **b** Axial CT, high-resolution mode: large, irregularly outlined skull base defect

Fig. 2a, b. A 48-year-old woman with a partially resected adenoid cystic carcinoma of the left maxillary sinus. **a** T1-weighted coronal image following i. v. administration of 0.1 mmol gadolinium (Gd)-DTPA/kg body weight: markedly enhancing parasellar lesion on the left side *(arrow)*, linear enhancement along the floor of the middle cranial fossa, consistent with meningeal tumour spread *(arrowheads)*. Residual tumour mass located in the infratemporal fossa *(black arrow)*. **b** Coronal CT, high-resolution mode: localised infiltration/destruction of the parasellar portion of the skull base on the left *(arrow)*

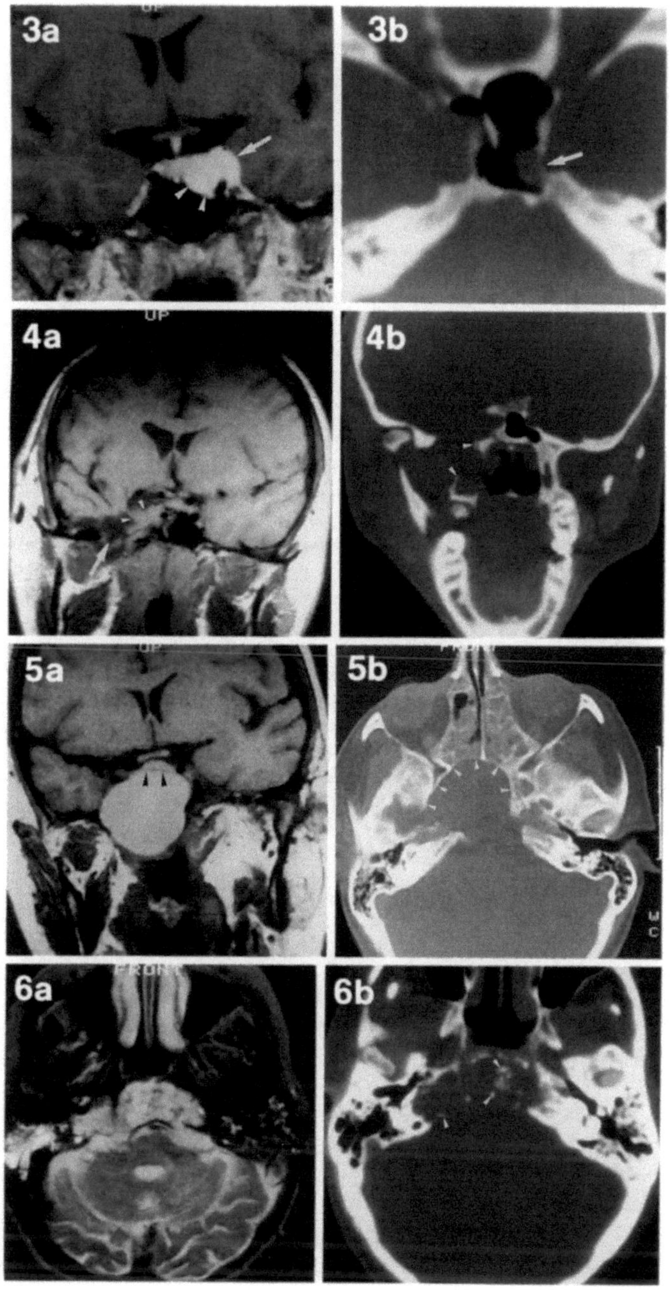

Fig. 3a, b. A 39-year-old woman with an osteolytic meningioma. **a** T1-weighted coronal image following i.v. administration of 0.1 mmol Gd-DTPA/kg body weight: hyperintense lesion *(arrow)* in the para/ suprasellar region on the left side, in close proximity to the cavernous sinus. There is apparent extension of tumour into the left sphenoid sinus *(arrowheads)*. **b** Axial CT, high-resolution mode: small bone defect in the roof of the left sphenoid sinus *(arrow)*; the adjacent bone appears normal

Fig. 4a, b. A 20-year-old man with a meningoencephalocoele. **a** T1-weighted coronal image: lesion predominantly isointense with cerebrospinal fluid involving the floor of the middle cranial fossa on the right *(arrow)*. Dysplastic changes are present within the medial portion of the right temporal lobe *(arrowheads)*. **b** Coronal CT, high-resolution mode: large bone defect, also involving the lateral aspect of the pterygoid process *(arrowheads)*

Fig. 5a, b. A 42-year-old woman with a mucocoele of the sphenoid sinus. **a** T1-weighted coronal image: well-defined, hyperintense lesion involving the sphenoid sinus, displacing the pituitary gland *(arrowheads)* upwards and compressing the air in the pharynx. **b** Axial CT, high-resolution mode: sharply outlined skull base lesion with a sclerotic rim *(arrowheads)* indicating pressure erosion

Fig. 6a, b. A 75-year-old woman with a chondrosarcoma of the skull base. **a** T2-weighted axial image: inhomogeneously hyperintense tumour affecting predominantly the clivus. **b** Axial CT: extensive skull base destruction and characteristic calcification of the tumour *(arrowheads)*

precise information for neurosurgical planning. MRI and CT are the most useful imaging methods to assess parasellar lesions [1–6]. In all our cases the intra- and/or extracranial extent of the lesion was exactly demonstrated by means of MRI (Figs. 1–6), particularly in coronal images. MRI also showed the relationship of soft tissue masses to adjacent structures such as the carotid arteries, pituitary gland and cavernous sinus (Fig. 1) [6], and these findings were confirmed at surgery. Furthermore, tumour involvement of the meninges could be detected by contrast-enhanced MRI (Fig. 2). On the other hand, definitive assessment of bone defects was possible only with CT (Figs. 3, 4). On the basis of CT findings, expanding lesions (Fig. 5) could be differentiated from tumours infiltrating bone (Fig. 2). Tumour calcification was visualised by means of CT, and this contributed to specific tumour diagnosis (Fig. 6). The CT findings of bone involvement were verified at operation. Tumour histology, however, could not be predicted exactly with MRI nor with CT, except in a few cases.

MRI seems to be the most useful diagnostic tool for assessing parasellar space-occupying lesions. This modality provides essential information concerning tumour extent and involvement of adjacent structures. CT, however, is required as well in these cases for visualising bone involvement. The knowledge of skull base involvement is indispensable for planning the adequate neurosurgical procedure precisely.

References

1. Goldstein SJ, Lee C, Carr WA, Rosenbaum HD, Tibbs PA, Walsh JW (1986) Magnetic resonance imaging of the sella turcica and parasellar region. A clinical-radiographic evaluation with computed tomography. Surg Neurol 26: 330–337
2. Karnaze MG, Sartor K, Winthrop JD, Gado MH, Hodges FJ (1986) Suprasellar lesions: evaluation with MR imaging. Radiology 161: 77–82
3. Lee BC, Deck MD (1985) Sellar and juxtasellar lesion detection with MR. Radiology 157: 143–147
4. Sartor K, Karnaze MG, Winthrop JD, Gado MH, Hodges FJ (1987) MR imaging in infra-, para- and retrosellar mass lesions. Neuroradiology 29: 19–29
5. Wolfman NT, Boehnke M (1978) The use of coronal sections in evaluating lesions of the sellar and parasellar regions. J Comput Assist Tomogr 2: 308–313
6. Young SC, Grossman RI, Goldberg HI, Spagnoli MV, Hackney DB, Zimmerman RA, Bilaniuk LT (1988) MR of vascular encasement in parasellar masses: comparison with angiography and CT. AJNR 9: 35–38

Dr. R. Stiglbauer
Univ. Klinik für Radiodiagnostik der
Universität Wien, Allgemeines Krankenhaus
Alserstraße 4
A-1097 Vienna, Austria

Neuroradiology (1991) 33 [Suppl]: 300–301

Neuro radiology
© Springer-Verlag 1991

Orbital trauma: CT or MRI for medial wall assessment?

D. M. Hadley[1], V. Ilankovan[2], K. F. Moos[2], and P. Macpherson[1]

[1] Department of Neuroradiology, Institute of Neurological Sciences, Glasgow, UK
[2] West of Scotland Regional Plastic and Oral Surgery Unit, Glasgow, UK

Summary. Fifteen consecutive patients with clinically suspected medial orbit blow-out fractures and soft tissue entrapment were examined with CT and surface coil MRI. Prospective analysis of the cross-sectional images was carried out blind to clinical data. MRI was found to be superior to CT in the assessment of fracture site, and identification of prolapsed orbital fat and muscle entrapment. It should therefore be the initial investigation, as positioning is easier and more comfortable for the traumatised patient.

Key words: Orbital fractures – Facial trauma – Naso-ethmoidal trauma – Computed tomography – Magnetic resonance imaging

Clinical examination and conventional radiography of the orbit following trauma often underestimate the damage present. Blow-out fractures of the medial wall of the orbit are rare, but they can occur alone or in conjunction with fractures of the zygomatic complex, Le Fort II, III fractures or nasoethmoidal fractures. Damage to the medial orbital wall can result in prolapse of fat or muscle and sometimes tagging of orbital contents into the maxillary and ethmoidal air sinuses. Early detection and surgical treatment have been recommended to avoid late residual enophthalmos, diplopia and restricted eye movements [1]. CT has markedly improved the accuracy of diagnosis of fractures but less readily identifies prolapsed soft tissue. The improved soft tissue characterisation possible with MRI may allow better overall assessment of medial orbital wall injury [2].

We present a comparison of the usefulness of CT and MRI examinations for preoperative assessment of fractures, suspected soft tissue herniation and entrapment in the medial orbital wall after facial trauma.

Patients and methods

Fifteen consecutive patients (13 male, 2 female) aged 17–32 years (mean 29.7 years) who presented with clinically suspected medial orbit blow-out fractures and soft tissue entrapment underwent CT and MRI examinations. These were completed within 24 h of each other and the interval after trauma varied between 18 h and 30 days.

CT was performed on a Philips Tomoscan 350 with 3-mm-thick direct coronal sections (pixel size 0.38 mm^2) or, in 3 patients whose head and chest injuries precluded this, supine axial sections with coronal reformatting.

MRI was performed with a Picker 0.15 T resistive magnet. A "balanced" spin echo pulse sequence with a TR of 700 ms and TE of 32 ms was used. Contiguous 5-mm thick coronal sections were obtained with a purpose-built facial surface coil (pixel size 1.37 mm^2) from the inferior orbital margin to the optic apex. The patients were asked to keep their eyes closed during the examination and to refrain from moving them. The study was approved by the Institute's Research Ethics Committee and informed consent was obtained from the patients or, if they were unconscious or confused, from their next of kin.

Prospective analysis of the cross-sectional images was carried out by two neuroradiologists blind to the clinical data and with the CT and MRI examinations randomised. The results were recorded on proformas and compared with the findings recorded at surgical exploration and repair with respect to the presence or absence of fractures, soft tissue (fat and muscle) herniation, muscle tagging, sinus fluid and haemorrhage.

Results

Technically adequate images were obtained in all patients (Fig. 1) although in 3, head and neck injuries precluded prone direct coronal CT. The comparison of imaging results with surgical findings is shown in Table 1 (fractures) and Table 2 (medial soft tissue herniation, tagging and/or entrapment). For demonstrating or excluding fractures, MRI (13/15 correct) was superior to CT (11/15 correct) (Fig. 2) but MRI underestimated the degree of comminution in many of these fractures. In 1 patient both modalities overestimated the extent of soft tissue herniation.

Table 1. Medial wall fracture: CT and MRI compared with surgical findings

(n = 15 patients)	CT	MRI
True +ve	8	10
True −ve	3	3
False +ve	0	0
False −ve	4	2

Table 2. Medial soft tissue herniation (with tagging or entrapment): CT and MRI compared with surgical findings

(n = 14 patients[a])	CT	MRI
True +ve	5 (1)	8 (2)
True −ve	6 (9)	5 (8)
False +ve	0 (0)	1 (1)
False −ve	3 (4)	0 (3)

[a] Unrecorded in 1 patient

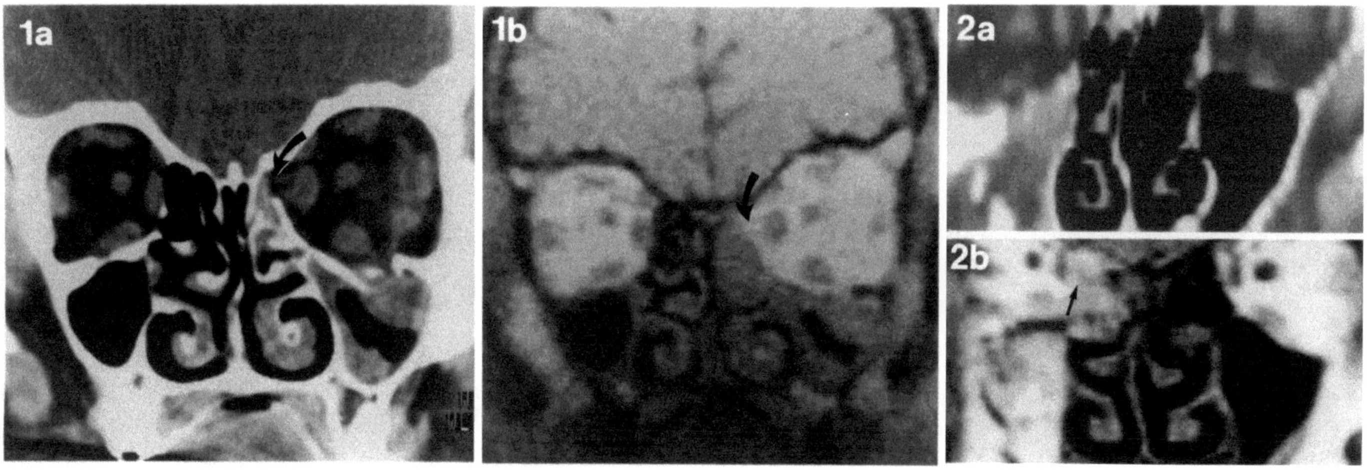

Fig. 1 a, b. Medial orbital wall fracture with prolapse of fat and tagging of fibres of the medial rectus muscle *(arrows)* correctly identified on **a** CT and **b** MRI (SE 700/32)

Fig. 2. **a** Reformatted axial CT reported as normal; **b** MRI (SE 700/32) demonstrated medial wall fracture with subtle herniation of fat *(arrow)*, confirmed at operation

MRI suggested fat herniation when it was not present at operation in a further patient, while CT failed to show fat herniation in 3 patients. The degree of herniation was unrecorded at operation in 1 patient. Tagging or entrapment of herniated soft tissue was seen slightly better on MRI than an CT but both modalities yielded false-negative findings. Orbital gas was noted only on CT in 1 patient but both modalities agreed on the presence or absence of haemorrhage into the paranasal sinuses.

Discussion

Surgical exploration is not desirable in every case of blow-out fracture and orbital exploration alone carries with it an increase in morbidity. An accurate method of diagnosis is therefore required in many cases before the resolution of facial oedema and other injuries [1]. Until recently CT has proved to be the most accurate diagnostic method with the use of direct coronal scans and computer reformatted images, but these may fail to demonstrate lesions because of dental filling artefacts and the obvious loss of spatial resolution when computer reformatting is required [1, 3].

MRI of the orbit allows direct multiplaner imaging and gives a high soft tissue contrast resolution, with the added advantage of reducing ionising radiation to the lens.

In this study MRI provided an overall improvement over CT in the evaluation of medial wall fractures. Although MRI does not show the displaced cortical bony fragments, a fracture can be diagnosed by the indentation of prolapsed orbital fat and bulge of nasal mucosa. Orbital fat contains numerous fibrous bands that connect the muscle sheath to the periosteum which, when caught in the fracture, may cause diplopia and restricted eye movement. Although MRI gave useful information on the appearance of the extraocular muscles and the degree of orbital fat prolapse, both modalites underestimated the degree of tagging or entrapment.

In the appropriate clinical setting, surface coil MRI may be performed in the coronal plane using a multisection technique soon after trauma. MRI proved to be better than CT for demonstration of medial orbital wall fractures and soft tissue herniation. However, both modalites underestimated the degree of tagging or entrapment subsequently found at operation. MRI should therefore be used as the initial imaging modality and CT held in reserve for confirmation, as positioning in the MRI unit is easier and more comfortable for the recently traumatised patient, who may well have multiple other injuries.

References

1. Moos KF, Le May M, Ord RA (1981) Investigation and management of orbital trauma. Int J Oral Surg 1: 229–234
2. Tonami H, Nakagawa T, Ohguchi M, Takarada A, Yamamoto I, Karino K, Sasaki K (1987) Surface coil MR imaging of orbital blow-out fractures: a comparison with reformatted CT. Am J Neuroradiol 8: 445–449
3. Daly BD, Russell JL, Davidson MJ, Lamb JT (1990) Thin section computed tomography in the evaluation of naso-ethmoidal trauma. Clin Radiol 41: 272–275

Dr. D. M. Hadley
Department of Neuroradiology
Institute of Neurological Sciences
1345 Govan Road
Glasgow G51 4TF, UK

Neuroradiology (1991) 33 [Suppl]: 302

Neuro radiology
© Springer-Verlag 1991

MRI of small pituitary adenomas

H. Shiga, S. Momoshima, H. Kayama, and T. Ushioda

Department of Diagnostic Radiology, Keio University, Tokyo, Japan

Summary. Thirty cases of functioning pituitary adenoma less than 15 mm in diameter were studied on a 1.5 T MR imager. Sensitivity for adenomas in pre- and post-contrast images was 30% and 67% respectively, which was further increased to 87% by additional dynamic-enhanced and SPGR imaging. Our standard protocol for small adenomas takes 30 min and is of high sensitivity.

Key words: Pituitary adenoma – Magnetic resonance imaging

Subjects and methods

Thirty cases of small pituitary adenoma were studied by MRI. Only tumours less than 15 mm in diameter were included, so as to permit comparison of signal intensity with that of the normal anterior pituitary gland. All the adenomas were endocrinologically active (prolactin-producing 13, growth hormone (GH)-producing 9, adrenocorticotrophin (ACTH)-producing 7, thyroid stimulating hormone (TSH)-producing 1). MRI studies were performed on a 1.5 T MR imager (Signa, GE) according to the standard protocol shown in Table 1. Gadolinium (Gd)-DTPA was used in all cases (0.1 mmol/kg). Dynamic studies were performed as follows: Gd-DTPA was rapidly injected intravenously. The first acquisition was started simultaneously with the contrast medium injection, and followed by another seven acquisitions at 10-s intervals; thus eight sequential images were obtained.

Table 1. Imaging protocol for small pituitary adenomas

Sequence		Section	FOV (cm)	THK (mm)	Time
1 – GRASS	140/5/90	Sagittal	24	5	0′29″
2 – SE	400/11	Coronal	14	3	3′27″
3 – 2D SPGR[a]	60/5/30	Coronal	14	4	0′16″ × 8
4 – SE	400/11	Coronal	14	3	3′27″
5 – 3D SPGR	45/5/30	Coronal	18	2	4′37″
6 – 3D SPGR	45/5/30	Sagittal	18	2	4′37″

FOV, Field of vision; THK, Slice thickness
[a] Dynamic study

Table 2. Signal intensity of adenomas

	Pre-contrast	Post-contrast		
	T1W-SE ($n = 30$)	Dynamic ($n = 11$)	T1W-SE ($n = 30$)	SPGR ($n = 11$)
Hyperintense	1	0	0	0
Isointense	21	3	10	6
Hypointense	8	8	10	5

T1W, T1-weighted

Table 3. Detection of small pituitary adenomas by the standard protocol

	Pre	Post-contrast		
	T1W – SE	Dynamic	T1W – SE	SPGR
30 Adenomas	9[a]	11[a]	3[a]	3[a]
	21[b]	10[b]	7[b]	4[b]

[a] Adenoma visualized [b] Adenoma not visualized

Results and discussion

Our results are summarised in Tables 2 and 3. Although Macpherson et al. [1] reported that CT and unenhanced MRI were comparable for detection of microadenomas, only 30% (9/30) of the lesions were visualised on unenhanced MRI in our series. Sensitivity of post-contrast T1-weighted images was 67% (20/30) and overall sensitivity, including a dynamic study and three-dimensional Fourier transfer spoiled grass (3DFT SPGR) imaging was 87% (26/30). This result is consistent with that reported by Newton et al. [2].

Our protocol for small pituitary adenomas is based on T1-weighted coronal and sagittal images. It can be completed in 30 min and yields sensitivity as high as 87%. Administration of Gd-DTPA is mandatory and sequential dynamic study significantly increases the yield. With 3DFT SPGR, thin-slice T1-weighted images of high quality can be obtained and these further facilitate the diagnosis of adenomas. The additional contribution of T1-weighted axial images and T2-weighted images to diagnostic sensitivity was insignificant.

In our series the sensitivity of MRI for prolactinomas was 77% while that for GH, ACTH and TSH-producing adenomas was 94%. The exact cause of this relative low sensitivity for prolactinomas is unclear, but some patients had been on bromocriptine for various periods and the effect of this on imaging remains to be clarified.

References

1. Macpherson P, Hadley DM, Teasdale E (1989) Pituitary microadenomas. Does gadolinium enhance their demonstration? Neuroradiology 31: 293–298
2. Newton DR, Dillon WP, Norman D (1989) Gd – DTPA – enhanced MR imaging of pituitary adenoma. AJNR 10: 949–954

Dr. H. Shiga
Keio University
Department of Diagnostic Radiology
35 Shimamomachi, Shinjuku-ku
Tokyo 160, Japan

Neuroradiology (1991) 33 [Suppl]: 303–304

Neuro-
radiology
© Springer-Verlag 1991

MRI of symptomatic Rathke's cleft cysts

M. Hermes and U. Piepgras

Institute for Neuroradiology, Saarland University Hospital, Homburg-Saar, Federal Republic of Germany

Summary. The cystic remnants of Rathke's pouch can cause visual disturbances or hypopituitarism by compressing surrounding intracranial structures. With MRI it is possible in many cases to distinguish between Rathke's cleft cysts and other sellar cysts or cystic tumours. Rathke cysts have intra- and suprasellar components. They are almost spherical with well-defined contrast-enhanced margins, and the pituitary stalk and gland are displaced posteriorly. The signal from the cysts is slightly more intense than cerebrospinal fluid on both T1- and T2-weighted images. The cyst contents are very homogeneous and show no contrast enhancement. Morphological features and signal intensity are generally characteristic of Rathke's cleft cysts.

Key words: Rathke's cleft cysts – Pituitary cysts – Suprasellar cysts – Sella turcica – Magnetic resonance imaging

The cystic lesions of the sellar region include the remnants of Rathke's pouch. These cysts have intra- and suprasellar components [1] and are lined by an ectodermal epithelial layer [2]. Small cysts are usually asymptomatic, but larger cysts can swell because of fluid retention and compress the surrounding structures [3]. They can thus cause headaches, visual impairment or hypopituitarism [4–6].

We used a 1.0 T MRI system with proton density, T1- and T2-weighted spin echo and gradient echo sequences and gadolinium (Gd) enhancement.

Four of our patients had headaches and visual disturbances in the form of a bitemporal visual field defect, and one had headaches and hypopituitarism.

The cysts can be readily demonstrated by CT; with density values of about 28 Hounsfield units, they are slightly denser than cerebrospinal fluid (CSF). There is marginal contrast enhancement, but not in the cyst itself. Intrathecal administration of contrast medium shows that there is no connection between the cyst and the subarachnoid space.

MRI affords much better demonstration of Rathke cysts because of the ability to obtain coronal and sagittal sections. The elevation of the optic chiasm, which lies like an arch on the spherical cyst, and which is responsible for the clinical deficits, is shown much more clearly by MRI than by CT. The relationship to the pituitary gland is shown best in the sagittal MR images. The pituitary tissue is slightly compressed against the floor and lateral walls of the sella turcica. The pituitary stalk is displaced posteriorly against the dorsum sellae and is also slightly elevated.

Administration of Gd-DTPA causes an increase in signal intensity in only parts of the capsule-like margin of the cyst, especially the lower and posterior portions, which represent the normal pituitary tissue, including the stalk. As stated previously, they form part of the capsule and have a normal Gd uptake. The upper and anterior parts of the cyst include no pituitary tissue and consist only of a thin membrane, which does not show Gd enhancement. Thus we can clearly distinguish the cyst from normal pituitary tissue.

The cyst is slightly more intense than CSF on proton density and T1-weighted images. On T2-weighted images the signal is much more intense than that of CSF because of its high content of mucopolysaccharide [4]. The secretion of mucopolysaccharide from the ciliated ectodermal epithelial cells is characteristic of Rathke's cleft cysts [6]. The contents of the cyst are very homogeneous on all imaging sequences.

Discussion

MRI appears to be much better than CT for the identification of a Rathke's cleft cyst. The differential diagnosis is based on the signal intensity of the cyst. T1-weighted and proton density images show an intermediate signal intensity, only slightly higher than that of CSF. In T2-weighted images the signal intensity is considerably higher than that of CSF. These signal properties indicate a cyst with mucous contents, and this is the case in Rathke's cleft cysts [2, 4, 6]. We found few cases with similar signal characteristics that proved to be other types of cystic tumour.

The other important point for the identification of a Rathke cyst is the excellent demonstration of the cyst itself and of its surroundings by MRI. A very symmetrical, usually spherical cyst, exactly in the midline, with a very even capsule is characteristic of a Rathke cyst, especially when the cyst lies both within and above the sella turcica and shows no tissue proliferation in its neighbourhood.

Even if all these criteria are met, a cyst may not necessarily be a Rathke cyst. MRI orientates the diagnosis much better than CT, but definitive diagnosis requires histological examination. Our patients underwent surgery, and histological examination revealed among them one craniopharyngioma and one pituitary adenoma.

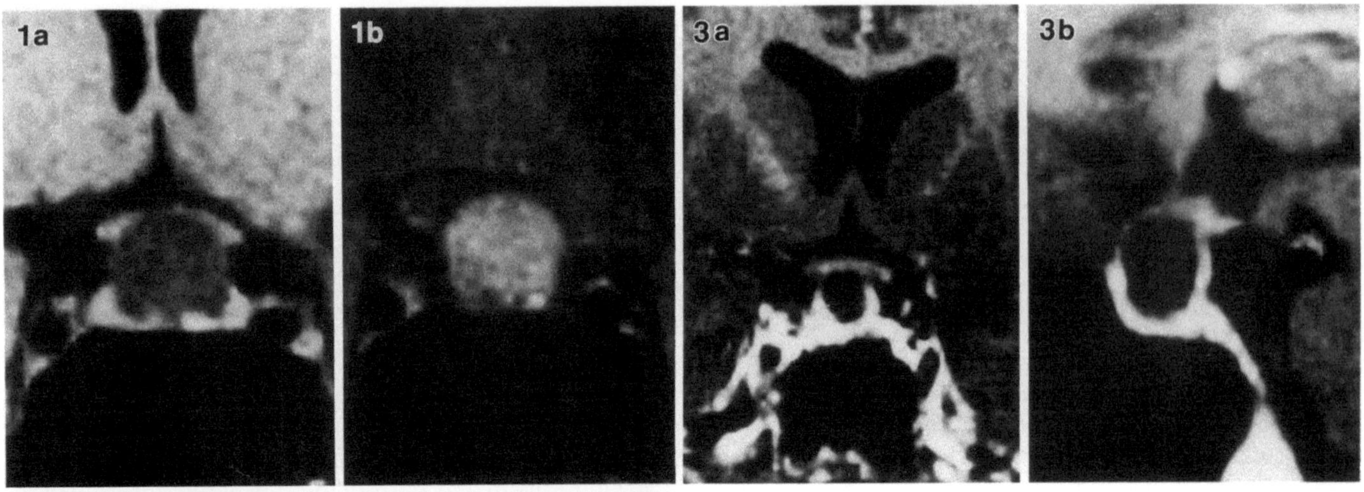

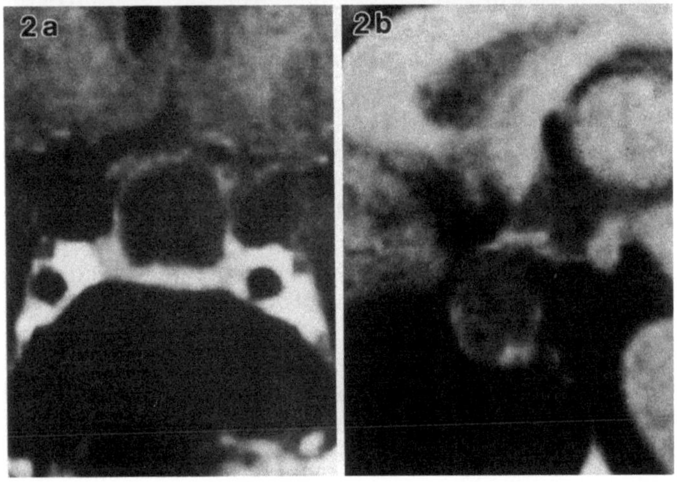

Fig. 1. **a** Proton density and **b** T2-weighted image, coronal view. The signal intensity of the cyst is higher than that of cerebrospinal fluid because of mucopolysaccharides

Fig. 2. **a** Coronal and **b** sagittal T1-weighted images. The optic chiasm is symmetrically elevated. The pituitary gland is compressed against the floor of the sella, and the pituitary stalk is displaced posteriorly

Fig. 3. **a** Coronal and **b** sagittal Gd-enhanced T1-weighted images. Gd enhances the normal pituitary tissue, but not the cyst itself. The anterosuperior part of the capsule contains no pituitary tissue, and does not enhance

References

1. Yoshida J, Kobayshi T, Kageyama N, Kanzaki M (1977) Symptomatic Rathke's cleft cyst: morphological study with light and electron microscopy and tissue culture. J Neurosurg 47: 451–458
2. Okamoto S, Handa H, Yamashita J, Ishikawa M, Nagasawa S (1985) Computed tomography in intra- and suprasellar epithelial cysts (symptomatic Rathke cleft cysts). AJNR 6: 515–519
3. Weber EL, Vogel FS, Odom GL (1970) Cysts of the sella turcica. J Neurosurg 33: 48–53
4. Steinberg GK, Koenig GH, Golden JB (1982) Symptomatic Rathke's cleft cysts. Report of two cases. J Neurosurg 56: 290–295
5. Nemoto Y, Inone Y, Fukuda T, Shakudo M, Katsuyama J, Hakuba A, Nishimura S, Onoyama Y (1988) MR appearance of Rathke's cleft cysts. Neuroradiology 30: 155–159
6. Kucharczyk W, Peck WW, Kelly WM, Norman D, Newton TH (1987) Rathke cleft cysts: CT, MR imaging and pathologic features. Radiology 165: 491–495

Dr. M. Hermes
Institut für Neuroradiologie
Universitätskliniken
W-6650 Homburg-Saar
Federal Republic of Germany

Neuroradiology (1991) 33 [Suppl]: 305–306

Neuro radiology

© Springer-Verlag 1991

Biochemical analysis and MRI characterisation of craniopharyngiomas

F. Di Salle, R. Morrone, F. Golia, S. Cirillo, R. Elefante, and F. Smaltino

Department of Radiology and Neuroradiology, Faculty of Medicine, University of Naples II, Naples, Italy

Summary. The authors propose a two-step biochemical procedure able to provide information concerning T1 relaxation of biological systems. This method has been applied to the study of cystic craniopharyngiomas. The cyst fluid has been fractionated on a sucrose-gradient; the fractions have been examined by MRI and their composition has been determined. While fractions deriving from a control sucrose gradient showed a regular decrease of T1-weighted signal intensity, the tumour fractions have shown particular intensity patterns. The hyperintense fractions were believed to contain molecular components able to shorten T1 relaxation time. A significant correlation between signal intensity and molecular composition has been constant for haemoglobin, methaemoglobin and iron.

Key words: Magnetic resonance imaging – Craniopharyngioma, Molecular composition

Because of the molecular complexity of biological systems, it is difficult to find correlations between biochemical composition and signal intensity [1, 2]. It could be useful to reproduce in vitro lower complexity systems in order to investigate the molecular basis of T1 relaxation [1].

Materials and methods

The cyst fluid from five craniopharyngiomas appeared hyperintense in both T1-weighted and T2-weighted images in three cases (Figs. 1, 2, samples 2, 5, 6) and hypointense in the other two (Fig. 2, samples 3, 4). The fluid has undergone a preparative sucrose-gradient ultracentrifugation able to separate the molecular components [1]. From each gradient 12 fractions (1 ml) have been collected and examined by T1- and T2-weighted SE sequences (Figs. 3, 4). Each fraction's content of total protein, haemoglobin, methaemoglobin and iron has been measured by microanalytical procedures and has been com-

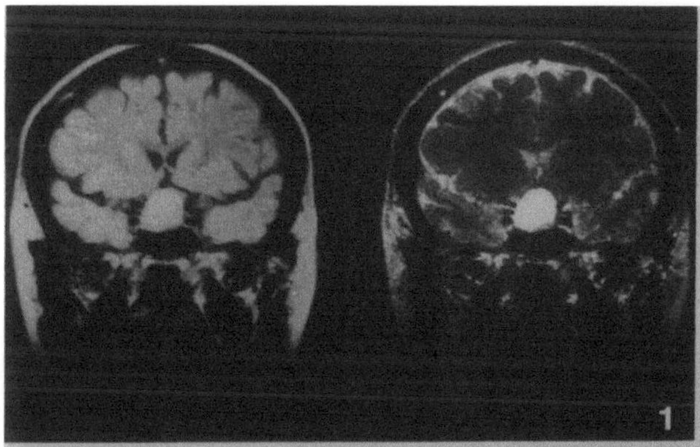

Fig. 1. Coronal T1-weighted (TR 450; TE 20) and T2-weighted (TR 2000; TE 100) MRI of hyperintense craniopharyngioma

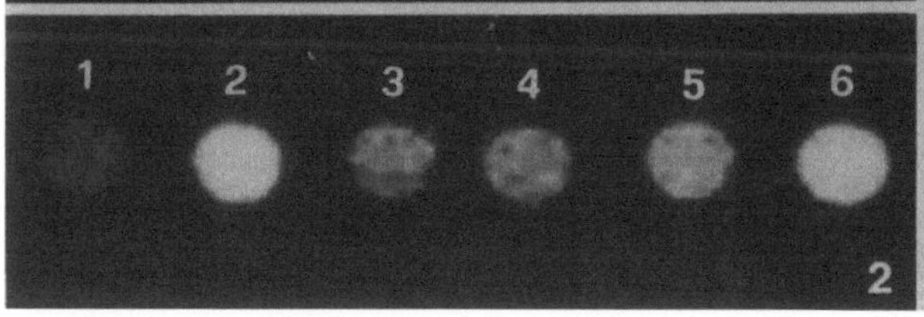

Fig. 2. T1-weighted (TR 450; TE 20) image of tubes containing: (1) normal saline solution; (2), (5), (6) cyst fluid of hyperintense craniopharyngiomas; (3), (4) cyst fluid of hypointense craniopharyngiomas

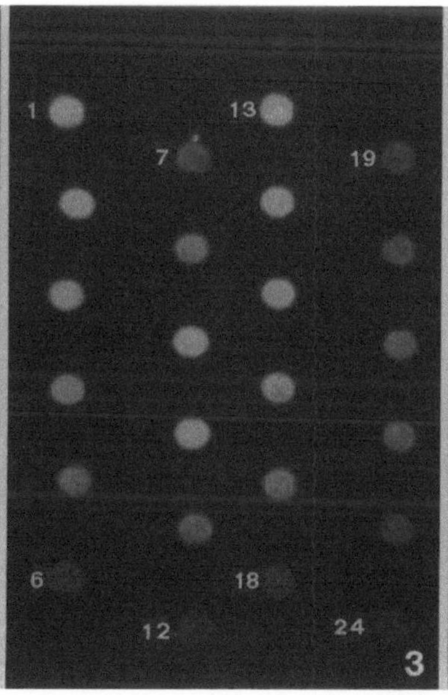

Fig. 3. T1-weighted image of sucrose gradient fractions carrying (1–12) and not carrying (13–24) cyst fluid from the first hyperintense craniopharyngioma. Signal of fractions 9 and 10 is clearly hyperintense in comparison with controls in 21 and 22

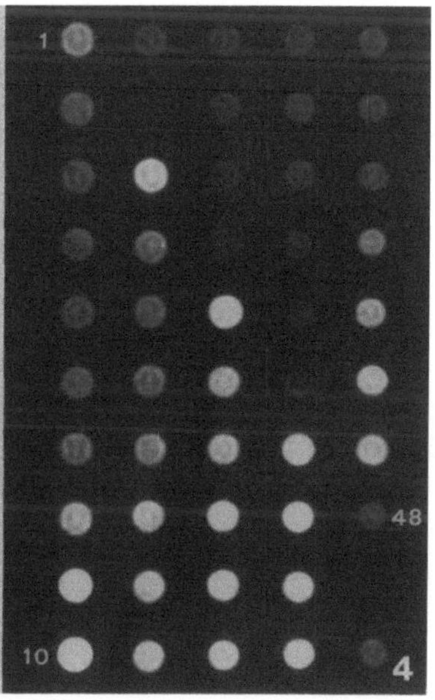

Fig. 4. T1-weighted image of sucrose gradient fractions carrying cyst fluid from the second (1–12) and the third (37–48) hyperintense craniopharyngiomas and from the two hypointense tumours (13–24 and 25–37). Fractions 1–12 and 37–48 show nearly the same intensity pattern as the first tumour

pared as to T1-weighted signal intensity and spectroscopy-determined T1 relaxation time [1].

Results and discussion

The problem of the high molecular heterogeneity of biological systems can be resolved by various preparative biochemical procedures; for this purpose the fluid from cystic craniopharyngiomas has been collected in virtual absence of external contamination and stored at −20 °C in test tubes. Fractions from sucrose-gradient ultracentrifugation have undergone an MRI spin-echo T1- and T2-weighted examination. Hyperintense tumours have shown a higher signal intensity in two fractions from the sample gradient (Fig. 3) that were hypointense both in sucrose controls and in hypointense tumour gradients. A MRI spectroscopy check has shown a statistically significant T1 shortening in the high signal fractions. In our opinion the short T1 relaxation time of hyperintense tumours could be explained by molecular composition differences in the high signal-low sucrose concentration fractions. Total protein [3], iron, haemoglobin, methaemoglobin, lipids, cholesterol, and ferritin concentrations have been determined in all gradient fractions. Iron, haemoglobin, methaemoglobin and protein concentrations have shown peak values corresponding to high signal fractions. Lipids and cholesterol did not correlate with T1-weighted signal intensity. The correlation with proteins seems to be of less significance because a peak in the same gradient position is also present in hypointense tumour gradient fractions.

While the analysis of hyperintense craniopharyngiomas suggests that protein, haemoglobin, methaemoglobin and iron correlate with signal intensity, the study of hypointense tumours allowed the exclusion of proteins as significant in T1 shortening. The close molecular relationship that links haemoglobin, methaemoglobin and iron, and the strong paramagnetic properties exhibited by methaemoglobin, could support this molecule as being the main factor of T1 hyperintensity. Other substances might contribute to the T1 shortening and further studies will be able to provide more detailed information about the role of each biomolecule in T1 relaxation.

References

1. Di Salle F, Simonetti L, Caranci F, Cirillo S, Elefante R, Smaltino F (1990) A biochemical approach to the interpretation of MRI images: in vitro study on a craniopharyngioma. In: Higer HP, Bielke G (eds) Tissue characterization in MR imaging. Springer, Berlin Heidelberg New York, pp 59–62
2. Bradley WG (1987) Pathophysiologic correlation of signal alteration. In: Brant-Zawadzki M, Norman D (eds) Magnetic resonance imaging of the central nervous system. Raven Press, New York, pp 23–42
3. Hackney DB, Grossman RI, Zimmermann RA, Joseph PM, Goldberg HI, Bilaniuk LT, Spagnoli MV (1987) Low sensitivity of clinical MR imaging to small changes in the concentration of non-paramagnetic protein. AJNR 8: 1003–1008

Dr. F. Di Salle
Department of Radiology and Neuroradiology
II. Faculty of Medicine
University of Naples
Naples, Italy

Neuroradiology (1991) 33 [Suppl]: 307–308

Neuro-radiology
© Springer-Verlag 1991

MRI of acoustic neuromas

K. Ishii[1], S. Takahashi[1], K. Matsumoto[1], T. Ishibashi[1], S. Tazawa[1], K. Sakamoto[1], S. Hashimoto[2], R. Katakura[3], and T. Yuasa[4]

Departments of [1] Radiology, [2] Otolaryngology and [3] Neurosurgery, Tohoku University, Sendai, Japan
[4] Department of Otolaryngology, Tohoku Rosai Hospital, Sendai, Japan

Summary. MRI of 51 acoustic neuromas verified surgically or neuro-otologically was reviewed. Tumours were classified according to their size into small (< 10 mm), medium (< 25 mm) and large (> 25 mm). Twenty-two small neuromas were best demonstrated on T1-weighted images (T1WI) with gadolinium-DTPA. Nineteen medium-sized tumours appeared hypo- to isointense on T1WI and iso- to hyperintense on T2-weighted images (T2WI), and half of them appeared heterogeneous on both T1WI and T2WI. Ten large tumours appeared heterogeneous on both sequences. In 4 of these a hypointense area was seen on T2WI, representing haemosiderin deposition, verified histologically. Signal void was noted at the periphery of 8 tumours, representing the "abnormal veins" described in earlier angiographic studies of acoustic neuroma.

Key words: Acoustic neuroma – Magnetic resonance imaging – Haemorrhage

MRI with thin, contiguous sections has replaced CT for diagnosis of acoustic neuromas. However, there have been few papers on MRI evaluation of a large number of these tumours [1–4]. We reviewed MRI at 1.5 T of 51 acoustic neuromas and discuss the characteristic MRI features of this tumour.

Materials and methods

MRI findings of 51 acoustic neuromas verified at surgery or neuro-otologically were reviewed. MRI was performed at 1.5 T with spin-echo sequences, 500/15 for T1-weighted images (T1WI), 2500/90 for T2-weighted images (T2WI) and 2500/15 for proton-density weighted images (PDWI), with contiguous 3-mm slice thickness. T1WI of 36 tumours were obtained after injection of 0.1 mmol/kg of gadolinium (Gd)-DTPA. Tumours were classified into small (< 10 mm), medium (< 25 mm) and large (> 25 mm). The MR images were reviewed as regards signal intensity of the tumours before and after injection of Gd-DTPA and abnormalities of the adjacent structures.

Results

The MRI findings in 51 acoustic neuromas are shown in Table 1. Twenty-two small neuromas appeared hypointense on T1WI, iso- to hyperintense on T2WI and PDWI, and enhanced homogeneously with Gd-DTPA. Tumours located within the internal auditory canal were best demonstrated on T1WI with Gd-DTPA (Fig. 1). Nineteen medium-sized tumours were hypo- to isointense on T1WI and iso- to hyperintense on T2WI; half were heterogeneous on all sequences. Ten large tumours were heterogeneous on all sequences. Hypointense areas were seen in 4 large tumours on T2WI, representing haemosiderin deposits, verified histologically (Fig. 2). Signal void was seen at the periphery of 8 tumours, representing displaced veins, which were demonstrated on vertebral angiography (Fig. 3). The tumour could be seen to extend into the internal auditory canal in all but 1 case, a large tumour.

Discussion

Many publications describe MRI findings in acoustic neuroma, but how few papers have dealt with large numbers [1–4]. In our series the signal intensities of the tumours were more or less the same as those in previous reports. As tumours grow larger, they appear heterogeneous on all sequences. It is well known that de-

Table 1. MRI findings of 51 acoustic neuromas

Sequence	Signal intensity	Size[a] Small (n = 22)	Medium (n = 19)	Large (n = 10)
T1WI	Low	18/22	11/19	
	Low-iso	4/22	8/19	10/10
Gd-T1	Enhancing	16/16	13/13	7/7
T2WI	Iso	4/8	6/13	
	Iso-high	4/8	7/13	3/7
	Low-high			4/7[b]
PDWI	Iso	8/8	11/13	1/7
	Low-iso		2/13	5/7
	High			1/7
Abnormal vein[c]			3/19	5/10
Tumour in IAC		22/22	19/19	9/10

T1WI, T1-weighted image; Gd-T1, T1-weighted image after gadolinium DTPA; T2WI, T2-weighted image; PDWI, proton density weighted image; IAC, internal auditory canal
[a] Small, < 10 mm; medium, < 25 mm; large > 25 mm
[b] Low intensity areas on T2WI in large tumours represented haemosiderin, verified histologically
[c] Signal void seen at the periphery of the tumours corresponded with abnormal veins on vertebral angiography

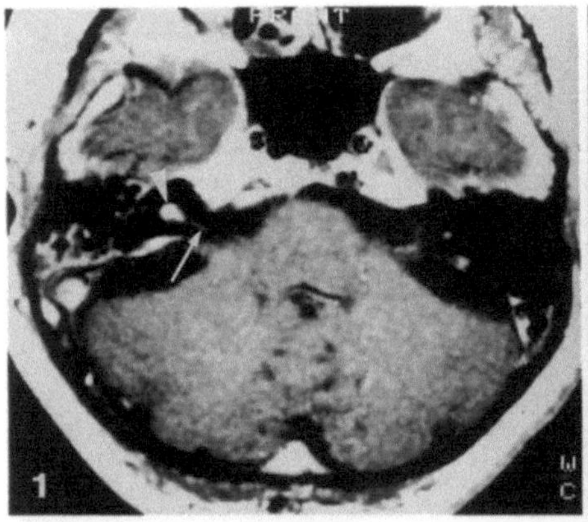

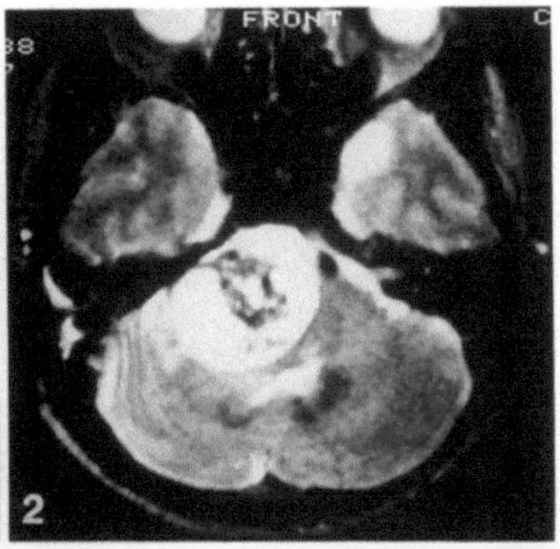

Fig. 1. Small acoustic neuroma. Axial T1-weighted image (T1WI) with gadolinium-DTPA discloses a small enhancing tumour *(arrowhead)* in the lateral part of the right internal auditory canal, continuous with the vestibular nerve *(arrow)*

Fig. 2. Large acoustic neuroma. Axial T2-weighted image (T2WI) reveals a hyperintense tumour with a central hypointense area, representing haemosiderin deposits

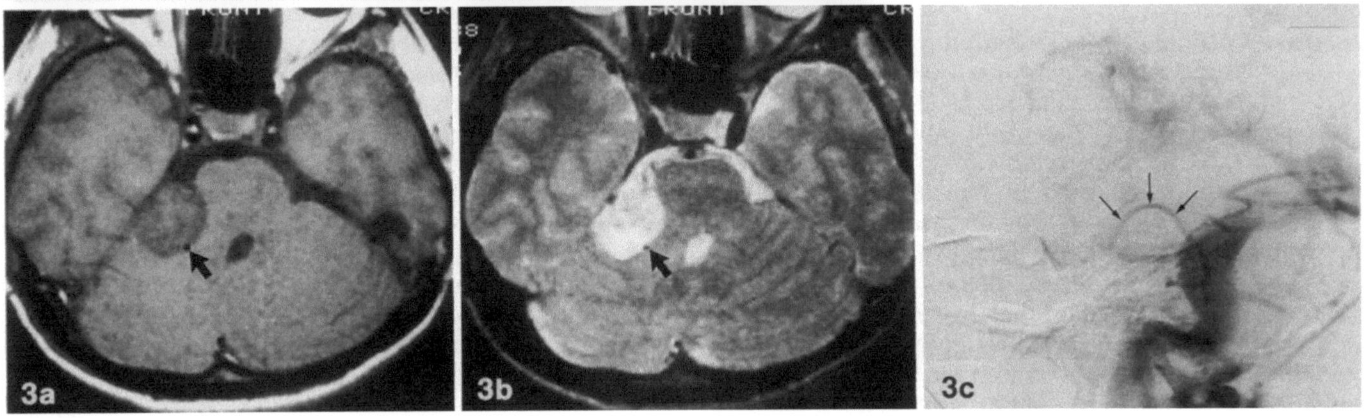

Fig. 3 a–c. Large acoustic neuroma. **a** Axial T1WI shows hypo- to isointense tumour in the right cerebellopontine angle. **b** On a T2WI the tumour appears hyperintense. Signal void is noted at its periphery, representing a vascular structure (*arrows* in both **a** and **b**) **c** Lateral view of venous phase of vertebral angiogram shows "abnormal vein" *(arrows)* around the tumour corresponding to the signal void demonstrated on MRI

generative features, such as cystic change, vascular change and haemorrhage are occasionally observed on histological examination of neuromas [5, 6]. Heterogeneity of the tumours on MRI is thought to result from these degenerative changes. There have been few reports of haemorrhage in acoustic neuroma on diagnostic imaging. In our series, hypointensity on T2WI representing haemosiderin deposits was demonstrated in 4 large neuromas. Haemoglobin degradation products can easily be detected by virtue of their magnetic susceptibility, so that detection of haemorrhage in larger acoustic neuromas will probably be more frequent using MRI. Signal void was noted at the periphery of 8 tumours which corresponded to displaced veins seen on vertebral angiography, described as "abnormal veins" in earlier angiographic studies [7]. Although similar findings were also observed in cases of meningioma, peripheral signal void seems to be one of the differential diagnostic points in cerebellopontine angle tumours [2].

References

1. Valvassori GE, Morales FG, Palacios E (1988) MR of normal and abnormal internal auditory canal. AJNR 9: 115–119
2. Press GA, Hesselink JR (1988) MR imaging of cerebellopontine angle and internal auditory canal lesions at 1.5 T. AJNR 9: 241–251
3. Daniels DL, Millen SV, Meyer GA (1984) MR detection of tumor in the internal auditory canal. AJNR 8: 249–252
4. Curati WL, Graif M, Kingsley DPE (1986) Acoustic neuromas: Gd-DTPA enhancement in MR imaging. Radiology 158: 447–451
5. Okazaki H (1989) Fundamentals of neuropathology. Igaku-Shoin, Tokyo
6. Kasantikul V, Netsky MG, Glasscock ME (1988) Acoustic neurilemmoma: clinico-anatomical study of 103 patients. J Neurosurg 52: 28–35
7. Takahashi M, Okudera T, Tomonaga M (1971) Angiographic diagnosis of acoustic neurinomas: analysis of 30 lesions. Neuroradiology 2: 191–200

K. Ishii
Department of Radiology
School of Medicine
Tohoku University
1-1, Seiryo-machi, Aoba-ku
Sendai, 980 Japan

Neuroradiology (1991) 33 [Suppl]: 309–310

Neuro radiology
© Springer-Verlag 1991

Meningeal enhancement within the internal auditory canal caused by cerebellopontine angle meningiomas: 1.5T MRI with gadolinium-DTPA

S. Aoki, Y. Sasaki, T. Machida, T. Okubo, and H. Tanioka

Department of Radiology, Faculty of Medicine, University of Tokyo, Tokyo, Japan

Summary. We retrospectively studied six patients with cerebellopontine angle (CPA) meningiomas who showed enhancement within the internal auditory canal (IAC) on gadolinium-DTPA-enhanced MRI at 1.5T. In three patients, intracanalicular enhancement took the form of fine linear enhancement, along the walls, while in the others enhancement was observed diffusely within the canal. Enhancement within the IAC might be observed in patients with CPA meningiomas with or without invasion and high resolution MRI was helpful to separate meningeal spaces from the nerve complex within the IAC and to demonstrate the meningeal origin of enhancement by meningiomas.

Key words: Posterior fossa meningioma – Internal auditory canal – Gadolinium-DTPA – Acoustic neuroma – Magnetic resonance imaging

Contrast-enhanced MRI has been reported to be extremely sensitive to meningeal abnormalities [1–3]. Normal meningeal enhancement is fine linear enhancement in short segments [1] and enhancement is increased by meningeal abnormalities, such as meningiomas [2, 3].

Patients and methods

We reviewed six patients with surgically proven cerebellopontine angle (CPA) meningiomas associated with enhancement in the internal auditory canal (IAC) on gadolinium (Gd)-DTPA-enhanced MRI (Table 1).

Patients were examined on 1.5T MR imagers (Siemens). Short TR/TE sequences (SE 500–600/17–34) before and after intravenous administration of Gd-DTPA with 2- to 5-mm section/thickness were performed routinely in the transverse and coronal planes. Contiguous thin section (2 mm) spin echo sequences were performed in one patient (case 6) using an ear coil.

Operation reports were reviewed for all patients. A CT air-cisternogram was available for one patient (case 6).

Results

All tumours were CPA dural-based masses showing homogeneous enhancement (Table 1). In three patients, intracanalicular enhancement was observed as fine linear enhancement only along the walls (Figs. 1, 2). In the others, separation of the nerve complex and enhancing dura mater was impossible and enhancement was observed diffusely within the canal.

Abnormal dural enhancement was always observed in other sites adjacent to the masses: tentorium(3/6), cli-

Table 1. Patients and findings

Case	Age (years)/sex	Size cm	Operative findings	IAC enlarged on CT, MRI	Meningeal enhancement
1	37F	2.5	Intact seventh/eighth CN, no IAC involvement, attached at anterior porus	–	IAC clivus, petrous bone
2	47M	1.5	Intact seventh/eighth CN, no IAC involvement, attached at anterior porus	–	Wall of IAC near porus acousticus
3	53F	3	Invasion of meatus, attached at tentorium	–	IAC tentorium, petrous bone jugular foramen
4	56M	5	Displaced seventh/eighth CN, involved fifth CN, attached at tentorium	+	IAC tentorium, clivus
5	59M	3.5	Displaced fifth CN, attached at tentorium	–	Wall of IAC tentorium, clivus petrous bone
6	70F	1.5	Intact seventh/eighth CN, attached near jugular foramen	–	Wall of IAC clivus, petrous bone jugular foramen

IAC, Internal auditory canal; CN, cranial nerve(s)

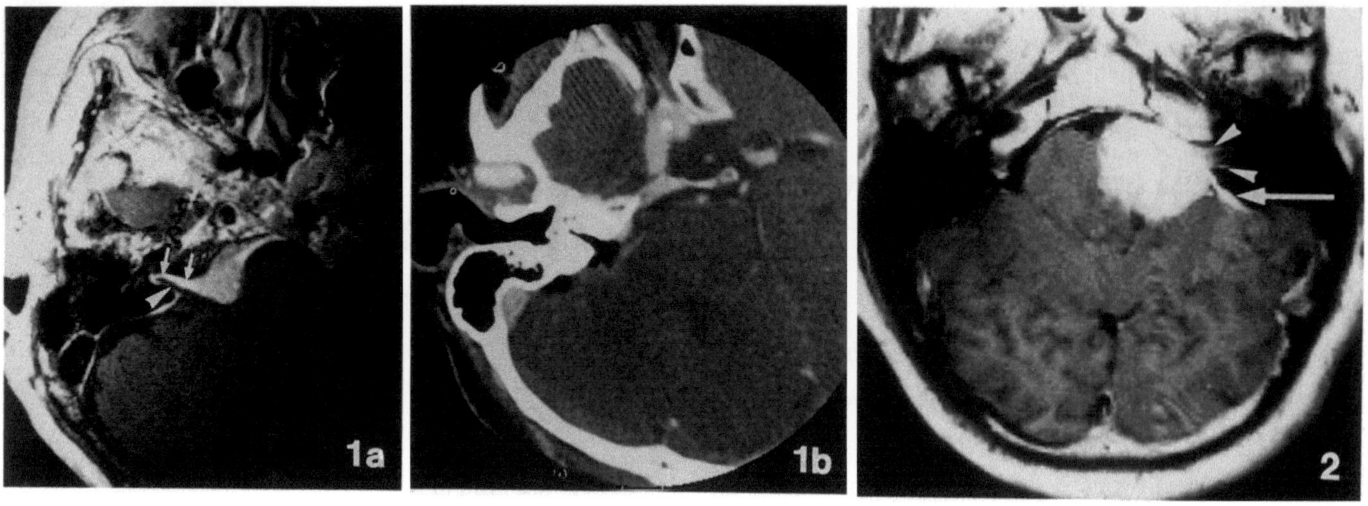

Fig. 1 a, b. A 70-year-old woman with a 1.5-cm cerebellopontine angle (CPA) meningioma. **a** Gadolinium (Gd)-DTPA-enhanced short TR/TE (600/22) axial MRI using an ear-coil with 2-mm slice thickness. Meningeal enhancement along the wall of the internal auditory canal (IAC) is clearly demonstrated *(arrows)*. Note the normal nerve complex, seen as a defect in the enhancement within the IAC *(arrowhead)*. **b** Air-CT cisternogram in left lateral decubitus position shows air filling within the right IAC

Fig. 2. A 59-year-old man with a 3.5-cm tentorial meningioma. Gd-DTPA-enhanced short TR/TE (500/17) axial MRI. The tentorial meningioma extends into the CPA. Meningeal enhancement is seen along the IAC *(arrow heads)* and the posterior surface of the petrous bone *(arrow)*

vus(4/6), petrous bone(6/6) and jugular foramen(2/6) (Table 1; Figs. 1, 2).

Operative findings are summarised in Table 1. Air-CT cisternography of one patient showed good filling of the IAC (case 6, Fig. 1).

Discussion

Meningiomas and acoustic neuromas are the two major CPA tumours. Differential diagnosis between these two using MRI has been reported [4–5]. Enhancement within the IAC is usually considered a sign of acoustic neuroma [4]. However, MRI is so sensitive to meningeal abnormalities that meningeal enhancement due to meningiomas may be observed within the IAC.

The IAC is lined by the meninges (dura and arachnoid mater). The subarachnoid space, containing cerebrospinal fluid (CSF) extends into the canal. The tubular CSF space is well seen on gas or positive contrast cisternography. Dural or meningeal inflammatory processes are well-recognised causes of non-neoplastic filling defects on cisternograms.

Thickening and enhancement of the dura mater surrounding meningiomas have been reported by Wilms et al. [2], who found tumour invasion of the dura mater in one case. Borovich and Doron [6] reported very frequent tiny meningotheliomatous cell nodules on the dura mater distant from globoid meningiomas, and Wilms et al. [2] suggested that these changes were the cause of diffuse dural enhancement. However, dural enhancement surrounding meningiomas without invasion has also been reported. Tokumaru et al. [3] found markedly increased collagen tissue, vascularity and dilated vessels, but no obvious direct tumour invasion of the enhanced dura mater adjacent to convexity meningiomas in all their cases.

We postulate therefore that intracanalicular enhancement associated with CPA meningiomas observed on contrast-enhanced MRI may be reactive or represent diffuse invasion. We postulate that MRI is so sensitive to the changes in the meninges that fine linear enhancement adjacent to meningiomas is probably due to reactive changes in the meninges.

References

1. Sze G, Soletsky S, Bronen R, Krol G (1989) MR imaging of the cranial meninges with emphasis on contrast enhancement and meningeal carcinomatosis. AJNR 10: 965–975
2. Wilms G, Lammens M, Marchal G (1989) Thickening of dura surrounding meningiomas. MR features. J Comput Assist Tomogr 13: 763–768
3. Tokumaru A, O'Uchi T, Eguchi T (1990) Prominent dural enhancement adjacent to meningioma on Gd-DTPA-enhanced MR imaging: histopathologic correlation. Radiology 175: 431–433
4. Stack JP, Ramsden RT, Antoun NM, Lye RH, Isherwood I, Jenkins JPR (1988) Magnetic resonance imaging of acoustic neuromas: the role of gadolinium-DTPA. Br J Radiol 61: 800–805
5. Curati WL, Graif M, Kingsley DPE, Niensdorf HP, Young IR (1986) Acoustic neuromas: Gd-DTPA enhancement in MR imaging. Radiology 158: 447–451
6. Borovich B, Doron Y (1986) Recurrence of meningiomas: role played by regional multicentricity. J Neurosurg 64: 58–63

Dr. S. Aoki
Department of Radiology
Faculty of Medicine
University of Tokyo
7-3-1 Hongo, Bunkyo-Ku
Tokyo 113, Japan

Neuroradiology (1991) 33 [Suppl]: 311–312

Neuro radiology
© Springer-Verlag 1991

MRI of spontaneously ruptured dermoids in the middle cranial fossa

T. Ohkubo, Y. Sasaki, S. Aoki, T. Machida, and T. Kokubo

Department of Radiology, Faculty of Medicine, University of Tokyo, Tokyo, Japan

Summary. MRI of four patients with spontaneously ruptured middle cranial fossa dermoids was reviewed. In all patients, MRI clearly demonstrated the primary tumour, and T1-weighted images showed high signal areas with fat-fluid levels in the ventricles(3/4) and/or high signal spots in the cerebrospinal fluid (CSF) spaces(4/4). Signal intensity of these areas decreased as images became more heavily T2-weighted, in accordance with the known MRI characteristics of fat. MRI was very sensitive for detection of small fat droplets within CSF and for demonstrating their exact distribution, especially on T1-weighted images.

Key words: Magnetic resonance imaging – Intracranial dermoid – Ruptured dermoid

Neuroradiological aspects of spontaneous rupture of pearly tumours (dermoids, epidermoids, teratomas) have been reported using conventional methods [1–3] and CT [2–8]. However, there has been only one report concerning MRI [9].

MRI has unique potential to demonstrate fat as hyperintense material within the hypointense cerebrospinal fluid (CSF) on T1-weighted images. Direct sagittal and coronal plane MRI has made it possible to see the exact distribution of the leaked materials in the CSF spaces.

Patients and methods

We reviewed MR images of intracranial dermoids with free fat within the ventricles and/or subarachnoid space. Four had no history of surgical procedures and were considered to represent spontaneous rupture. All were located in the middle cranial fossa. Histological confirmation was obtained in two.

Patients were examined using superconductive MR imagers (Table 1) with spin-echo techniques with slice thickness of 5–10 mm. T1-weighted (SE 400–600/15–35) and T2-weighted images (SE 2000–3000/60–120) were obtained in all cases in at least two different planes.

The patients' age, sex and clinical indications for MRI are summarised in Table 1.

Results

MRI showed the extra-axial origin of the primary tumours with fatty contents (hyperintense on T1- and hypointense on T2-weighted images). All were mainly hyperintense on T1-weighted images, but some irregularly iso- to hypointense elements were detected within them.

Small high intensity globules were demonstrated in the subarachnoid space on T1-weighted images (Table 1). Tiny globules seen on T1-weighted images were difficult to detect on T2-weighted images, but relatively large ones (more than 3–5 mm) showed chemical shift artefact and this was helpful to distinguish the high signal of fat from that of flowing blood on T1-weighted images in some locations.

Fat-fluid levels were recognized in the frontal horns of the lateral ventricles(3/4), and chemical shift artefact was identified in three. Protrusion of the fatty material in the cistern into the choroidal fissure, in continuity with fat in the temporal horn was observed in one case (case 3, Fig. 1-b). One case showed dilatation of the lateral ventricles.

Discussion

An epidermoid (epidermoid cyst) consists of a thin connective tissue capsule lined by stratified squamous keratinised epithelium. A dermoid includes structures of the

Table 1. Four patients with ruptured dermoids

Case no.	Age (years)/sex	Indication for MRI (Tesla)	Operation	Distribution of fat	Hydrocephalus
1	19F	(0.35T)	–	Left sylvian fissure, left ambient cistern	–
2	37M	Headache after mild trauma (1.5T)	–	Both frontal horns, fourth ventricle, basal cisterns	+
3	49M	Fat in the CSF on CT (0.5T)	+	Right temporal horn, basal cisterns, interhemispheric fissure, right lateral ventricle	–
4	50M	Tonic seizure (0.5T)	+	Interhemispheric fissure, right frontal, temporal, parietal subarachnoid space, quadrigeminal, superior cerebellar cisterns, right frontal horn	–

CSF, Cerebrospinal fluid

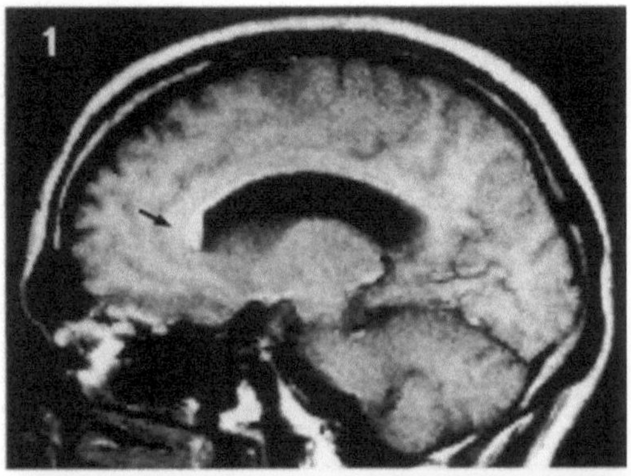

Fig. 1. A 50-year-old man with a surgically verified right middle cranial fossa dermoid (case 4). A sagittal T1-weighted image (SE 300/30) shows a high signal area with fat-fluid level *(arrow)*

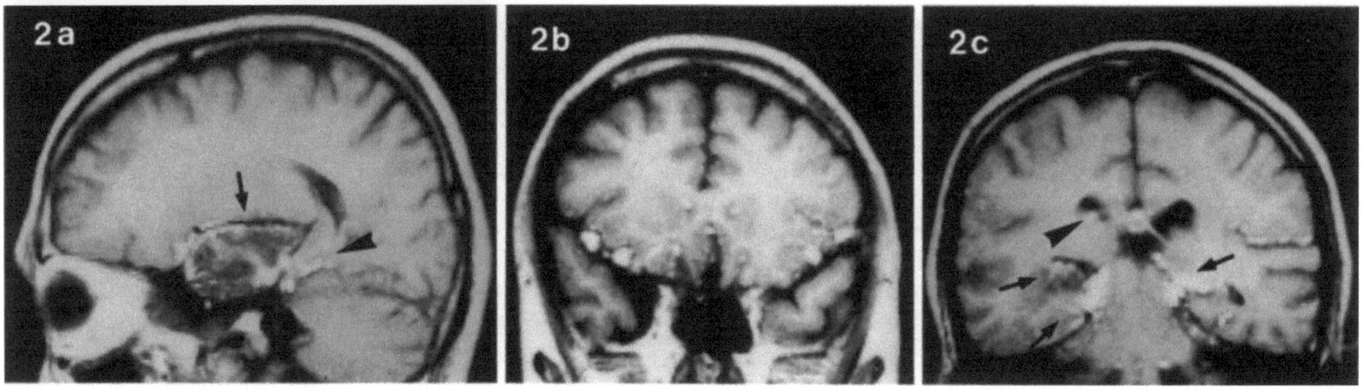

Fig. 2 a–c. A 49-year-old man with a proven right middle fossa dermoid (case 3). **a** A sagittal T1-weighted image (SE 500/22 at 0.5T) shows a mixed intensity mass at the medial end of the sphenoid ridge *(arrow)*. High intensity material protrudes posteriorly *(arrowhead)*. **b** A coronal T1-weighted image (SE 500/22) shows high signal globules in the inferior frontal sulci. **c** A coronal T1-weighted image (SE 500/22) shows high signal area on both sides of the midbrain *(arrows)*. On the right, a high signal area extends from the mildly dilated right temporal to the cistern, through the choroidal fissure. Note a high signal globule in the body of the right lateral ventricle *(arrowhead)*

dermis: hair follicles, sweat and sebaceous glands, in addition to the epithelium of an epidermoid [10]. These tumours are known to contain fat.

Laster et al. [4] reported two cases of ruptured epidermoid and speculated about possible pathways into the ventricles, suggesting that in one of their cases migration might be a result of the patient's position and CSF pulsation. However, other authors [3] reported finding a direct communication with the ventricles at surgery [1, 3].

In our case 3, MRI demonstrated the possible route taken by the fatty material into the ventricle, through the choroidal fissure, which has not been described by previous authors. Between the temporal horn and choroidal fissure, there is only a thin epithelium, continuous with the free margin of fimbria of the hippocampus [11]. Presumably, a relatively large middle cranial fossa dermoid compressing the choroidal fissure could rupture into the temporal horn by tearing this thin structure. Sagittal and coronal images were very useful in making this observation (Fig. 1).

The appearances of these ruptured tumours are almost pathognomonic on MRI. A possible differential diagnosis might be residual fatty contrast medium (such as iodophendylate) after myelography, but the presence of a primary tumour and plan skull films or CT would easily exclude this possibility.

References

1. Maravilla KR (1977) Intraventricular fat-fluid level secondary to rupture of an intracranial dermoid cyst. AJR 128: 500–501
2. Cornell SH, Graf CJ, Dolan KD (1977) Fat-fluid level in intracranial epidermoid cyst. AJR 128: 502–503
3. Fawcitt RA, Isherwood I (1976) Radiodiagnosis of intracranial pearly tumors with particular reference to the value of computed tomography. Neuroradiology 11: 235–242
4. Laster DW, Moody DM, Ball MR (1977) Epidermoid tumors with intraventricular and subarachnoid fat: report of two cases. AJR 128: 504–507
5. Amendola MA, Garfinkle WB, Ostrum BJ (1978) Preoperative diagnosis of a ruptured intracranial dermoid cyst by computerized tomography. J Neurosurg 48: 1035–1037
6. Healy JF, Brahme FJ, Rosenkrantz H (1980) Dermoid cysts and their complications as manifested by computed cranial tomography. Comput Tomogr 4: 111–115
7. Mikhael MA (1982) Transient spasm of carotid siphon complicating ruptured cranial dermoid cyst. Radiology 144: 824
8. Hamer J (1980) Diagnosis by computerized tomography of intradural dermoid with spontaneous rupture of the cyst. Acta Neurochir (Wien) 51: 219–226
9. Hahn FJ, Ong E, McComb RD (1986) MR imaging of ruptured intracranial dermoid. J Comput Assist Tomogr 10: 888–889
10. Russell DS, Rubinstein LJ (1977) Pathology of tumors of the nervous system, 4th edn. Williams and Wilkins, Baltimore, pp 24–32
11. Carpenter MB (1985) Olfactory pathways, hippocampal formation, and amygdala. In: Core textbook of neuroanatomy, 3rd edn. Williams and Wilkins, Baltimore, pp 323–347

Dr. T. Ohkubo
Department of Radiology
Faculty of Medicine
University of Tokyo
7-3-1, Hongo, Bunkyo-Ku, Tokyo 113, Japan

Neuroradiology (1991) 33 [Suppl]: 313–314

Neuro-radiology

© Springer-Verlag 1991

P-31 chemical shift imaging of human brain tumours

M. Sasahira[1], K. Uchimura[1], T. Asakura[1], K. Terada[2], and T. Fujimoto[3]

[1] Department of Neurosurgery, University of Kagoshima, Kagoshima, Japan
Departments of [2] Neurosurgery and [3] Psychiatry, Fujimoto Hospital, Miyakonojo, Japan

Summary. Sixteen patients with brain tumours were examined by P-31 chemical shift imaging (CSI) using the spectroscopic imaging by dephasing amplitude changing (SIDAC) method and four-dimensional Fourier transform multivoxel spectroscopy (4DFT-MVS). P-31 CSI was carried out with a whole-body MRI system operating at 2.0 T. A series of 64 chemical shift images with a 0.9 ppm chemical shift resolution and a $20 \times 20 \times 70$ mm spatial resolution were obtained by SIDAC. P-31 spectra of $8 \times 8 \times 1$ or $8 \times 8 \times 4$ voxels and P-31 CSI were obtained by MVS. The brain tumours were seen as high signal intensity in phosphomonoester images and low signal intensity in phosphocreatine images. P-31 spectra changed after chemoradiotherapy. Localised phosphorus metabolism of brain tumours was thus seen by P-31 CSI as metabolite maps.

Key words: Brain tumour – Astrocytoma – Glioblastoma – Meningioma – P-31 chemical shift imaging

---

P-31 NMR spectroscopy has been used to examine biochemistry and monitor therapy in large experimental and human studies [1, 2]. In this paper we describe the usefulness of P-31 chemical shift imaging (CSI) using the spectroscopic imaging by dephasing amplitude changing (SIDAC) method and four-dimensional Fourier transform multivoxel spectroscopy (4DFT-MVS) in the investigation of human brain tumours [3].

Materials and methods

P-31 CSI was carried out in a 2.0 T superconducting MRI system (Asahi Super 200).
SIDAC method. A series of 64 spectroscopic images with a 0.9 ppm chemical shift resolution and a $20 \times 20 \times 70$ mm spatial resolution was collected in 1 h.
4DFT-MVS. The scan matrices were $8 \times 8 \times 1$ or $8 \times 8 \times 4$. The voxel size was $3.2 \times 3.2 \times 7$ cm or $3.2 \times 3.2 \times 4$ cm. Chemical shift resolution was 0.453 ppm. The total acquisition time was about 1 h.

Sixteen patients with brain tumours were included in this study. Repeat studies were performed in 2 patients, a total of 18 P-31 CSI being performed. Eighteen P-31 CSI were performed by the SIDAC method and the remaining 3 were performed by 4DFT-MVS.

Results

The brain tumours were seen as areas of high signal intensity in phosphomonoester (PME) images and low signal intensity in phosphocreatine (PCr) images. Residual tumours after chemoradiotherapy were seen as low signal intensity in all P-31 images. Intensity of P-31 signal had returned to normal in a case of malignant lymphoma, which showed a good response to chemoradiotherapy.

Discussion

In recent years there has been considerable interest in techniques for localising high resolution spectra in human brain tumours [1, 2, 4, 5]. P-31 MRS has yielded variable pictures of the metabolism of brain tumours. In general, the tumour spectra often show a relatively low level of PCr and a high level of PME. We have studied P-31 MRS using P-31 CSI techniques [6, 7]. Most brain tumours were seen as high signal intensity in PME images and low signal intensity in PCr images.

Spectral changes with therapeutic response have also been documented [5, 8–10]. These spectral changes occurred prior to any changes on X-ray CT, or MRI in some clinical studies [5, 8]. In our study, residual tumours following chemoradiotherapy were seen as low signal intensity in all P-31 images. Intensity of P-31 signal had returned to normal in a case of malignant lymphoma, which showed good response to the chemoradiotherapy. Decreased intensity of all P-31 images in the residual tumours was due to hypometabolism after the chemoradiotherapy.

In conclusion, P-31 CSI will be a useful tool for the investigation of localised phosphorus metabolism.

References

1. Botomley PA (1989) Human in vivo NMR spectroscopy in diagnostic medicine: clinical tool or resarch probe? Radiology 170: 1–15
2. Glickson JD (1989) Clinical NMR spectroscopy of tumors. Current status and future directions. Invest Radiol 24: 1011–1016
3. Miyazaki T (1989) Techniques of multinuclear MR imaging and volume selective spectroscopy. Innervision Jpn 4: 28–32

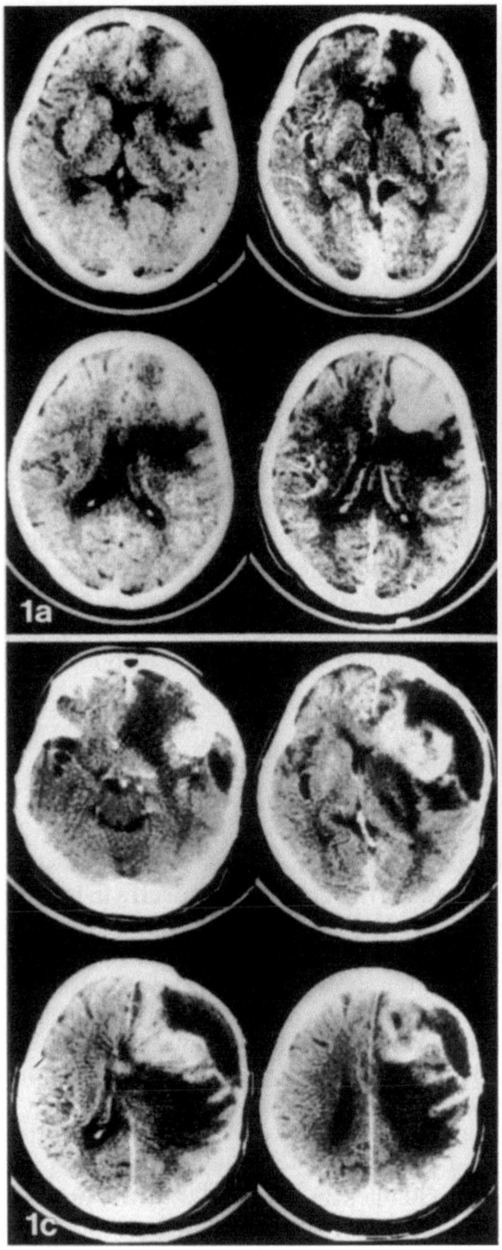

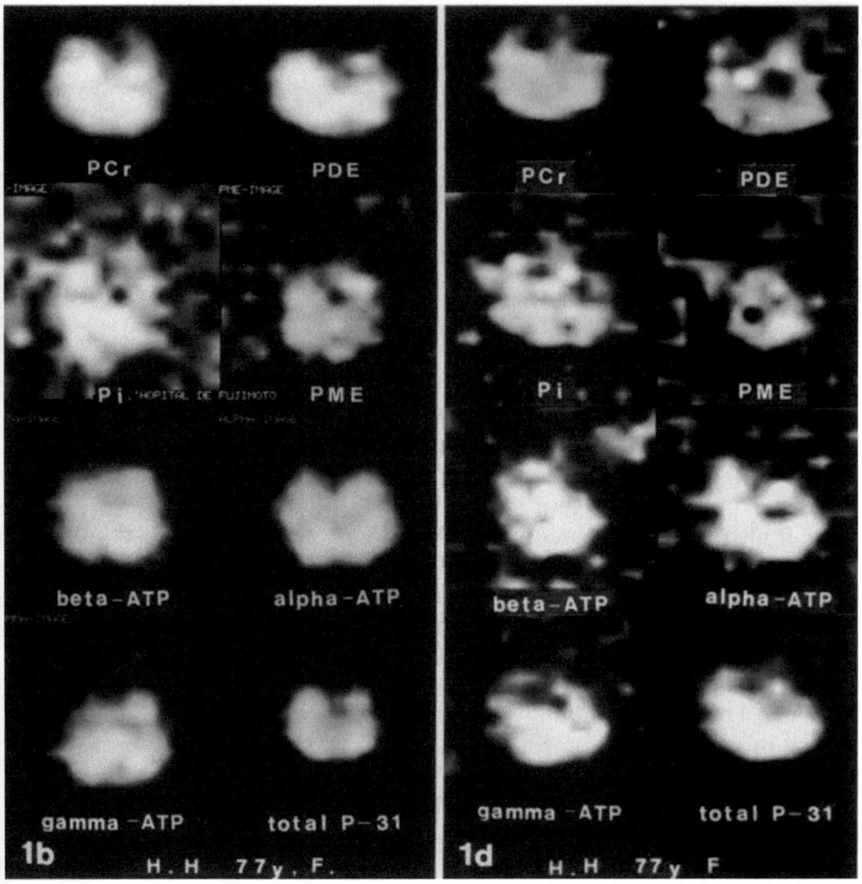

Fig. 1 a–d. Astrocytoma grade III. **a** Plain and enhanced CT. **b** P-31 chemical shift imaging (CSI). Tumour was seen as low signal intensity area in phosphocreatine (PCr) image and high signal intensity area in phosphomonoesters (PME) image. **c** CT after radiotherapy. **d** P-31 CSI after radiotherapy. A low signal area consistent with tumour was noted on PCr, PDE, Pi, PME, ATP and total phosphate images

4. Segebarth CM, Baleriauk DF, Arnold DL (1987) MR image-guided P-31 MR spectroscopy in the evaluation of brain tumor treatment. Radiology 165: 215–219
5. Heindel W, Bunke J, Glathe S (1988) Combined ^{1}H-MR imaging and localized ^{31}P spectroscopy of intracranial tumors in 43 patients. J Comput Assist Tomogr 12: 907–916
6. Asakura R, Sasahira M, Uchimura K (1989) Chemical shift imaging. J Med Imaging Jpn 9: 942–952
7. Lenkinski RE, Holland GA, Allman T (1988) Integrated MR imaging and spectroscopy with chemical shift imaging of P-31 at 1.5 T: initial clinical experience. Radiology 169: 201–206
8. Arnold DL, Shoubridge EA, Feindel W (1987) Metabolic changes in cerebral gliomas within hours of treatment with intra-arterial BCNU demonstrated by phosphorus magnetic resonance spectroscopy. Can J Neurol Sci 14: 570–575
9. Semmler W, Gademann G, Baumann PB (1988) Monitoring human tumor response to therapy by means of P-31 spectroscopy. Radiology 166: 533–539
10. Ross BD, Tropp J, Derby KA (1989) Metabolic response of glioblastoma to adoptive immunotherapy: detection by phosphorus MR spectroscopy. J Comput Assist Tomogr 13: 189–193

Dr. M. Sasahira
Department of Neurosurgery
Akune Shimin Hospital
4531, Akasegawa, Akune-shi
Kagoshima-ken, 899-16, Japan

Neuroradiology (1991) 33 [Suppl]: 315–316

Neuro-radiology
© Springer-Verlag 1991

Pineal region choroid plexus carcinoma: MRI, CT, and pathology correlation

J. M. Sullivan[1], F. J. Hahn[2], J. R. McConnell[2], and P. Y. Hahn[3]

Departments of [1] Neurology, [2] Radiology, and [3] College of Medicine, University of Nebraska, Omaha, Nebraska, USA

Summary. A 30-year-old woman experienced severe headaches, hearing loss, incoordination, vertigo, and diplopia for 1 year and amenorrhea for 4 months leading to concurrent CT and MRI. These revealed a pineal choroid plexus neoplasm causing compression of the tectum and obstruction of the aqueduct of Sylvius, with obstructive hydrocephalus. These findings allowed a correlation between CT and MRI explaining the patient's symptoms and providing a precise surgical/anatomic approach with good clinical result.

Key words: Pineal recess – Choroid plexus – Carcinoma – Papilloma

---

Choroid plexus papilloma is a rare neoplasm arising from the cells covering the cerebral choroid plexus and accounts for less then 1% of all primary intracranial tumors. The malignant counterpart, choroid plexus carcinoma (CPC), is even more rare. Choroid plexus papillomas in infants usually occur in the lateral ventricle whereas in adults most originate in the fourth ventricle. The pattern is not entirely comparable in patients with CPC. Regardless of the patient's age, CPCs originate from the lateral ventricle (90%), fourth ventricle (6%), and third ventricle (4%). Two cases of CPC have been reported in the third ventricle [1–2]. However, no cases have been reported in its suprapineal recess. Most patients present with symptoms of hydrocephalus. Multiple local recurrences and distant metastases are more common in CPCs.

Case report

A 30-year-old white woman presented with a 1-year history of severe headache, hearing loss, incoordination, vertigo, diplopia and a 4-month history of amenorrhea. Neurologic examination revealed chronic papilledema, left lateral strabismus, upward gaze paralysis, decreased gross hearing acuity, right deviation of the tongue and uvula, and ataxia. Muscle strength was within normal limits.

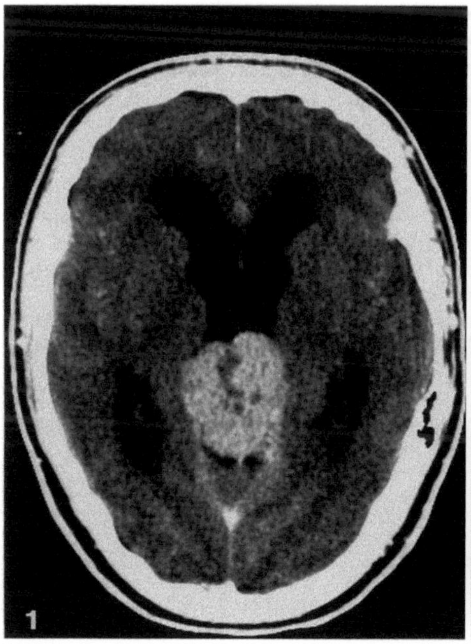

Fig. 1. CT reveals a large contrast-enhancing mass in the pineal region, associated with moderate obstructive hydrocephalus

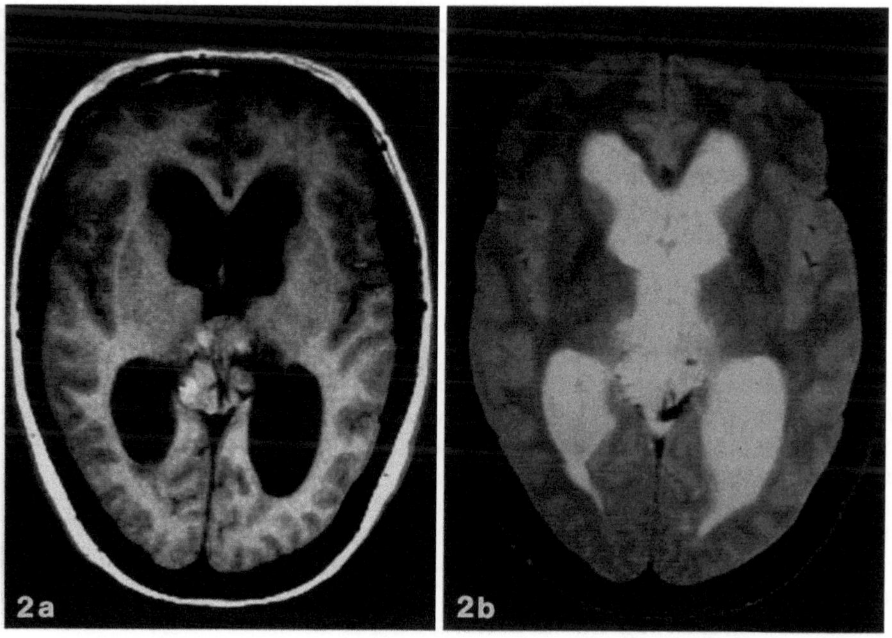

Fig. 2 a, b. MRI shows a large lobulated mass in the pineal region which is generally isodense, with hyperintense spots on T1-weighting and hyperintense on T2-weighting

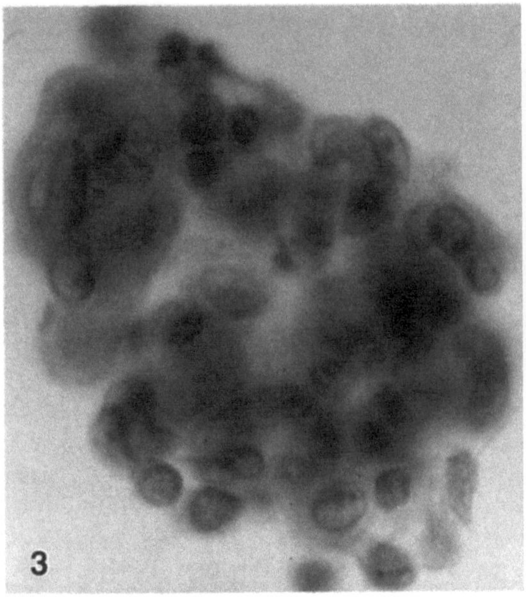

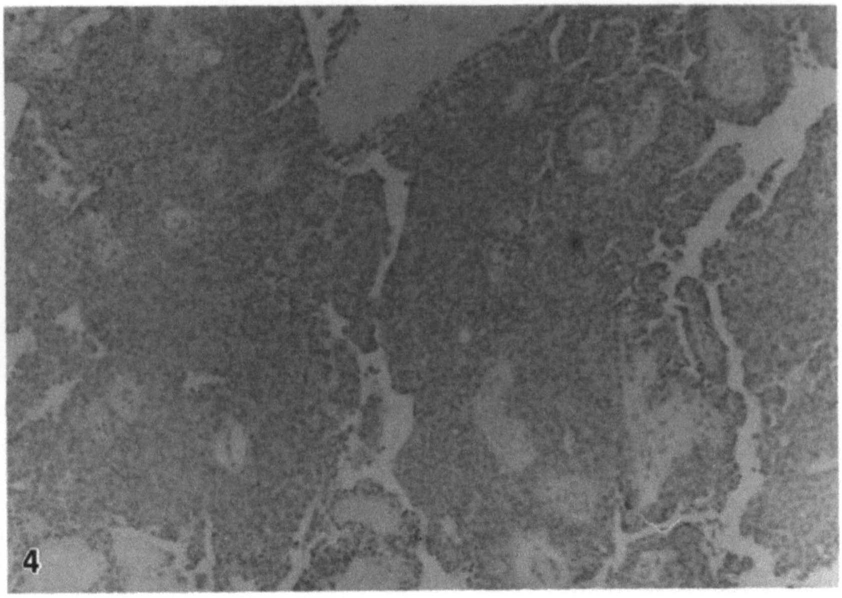

Fig. 3. Cells of choroid plexus carcinoma in cerebrospinal fluid (Papanicolaou stain)

Fig. 4. Neoplasm showing papillary architecture altered by solid sheets of cells

CT revealed a large, contrast-enhancing neoplasm ($6.0 \times 3.5 \times 5.0$ cm) in the pineal region extending down to the quadrigeminal cistern. The tumor contained multiple small cystic areas of varying size and small punctate areas of calcification. Apparent compression of the tectum and obstruction of the aqueduct by the tumor with obstructive hydrocephalus were shown (Fig. 1).

MRI showed a large neoplasm in the pineal region which displayed mixed signal intensity in both T1- and T2-weighted images. The tumor caused compression of the tectum and obstructive hydrocephalus, with diffuse interstitial edema and tonsillar herniation (Fig. 2a, b).

On the 2nd hospital day a ventricular shunt was placed. Cells of CPC were identified in the cerebrospinal fluid with a Papanicolaou stain (Fig. 3) [3].

Histopathology

The neoplasm had a papillary architecture which is altered focally by solid sheets of cells. Stratified layers of cells gave way to large sheets of neoplasm. Distinct cytoplasmic boundaries were identified. Nuclei were fairly uniform with an oval contour, fine chromatin, and distinct nucleoli. The mitotic rate was variable but approached one per high power field in some areas: Small foci of necrosis were scattered throughout the neoplasm (Fig. 4) [4]. Immunoperoxidase studies were performed to identify specific neoplastic cells. Diffuse expression of keratin and carcinoembryonic antigen in the neoplastic cells was present. Neuron specific encase was widespread. Glial fibrillary acidic protein (GFAP) was expressed focally within the tumor as small clusters of cells with elongated processes. These cells constituted a small percentage of the total tumor volume. S100 was expressed in small clusters of astrocytic cells throughout the tumor similar to the distribution of GFAP. Additional neoplastic cells throughout the tumor showed positive staining for S100 protein. Normal choroid plexus epithelium was positive for S100 but negative for keratin and GFAP. The following immunoperoxidase reactions were negative: epithelial membrane antigen, alpha-fetoprotein, human chorionic gonadotropin, thyroglobulin, and muscle specific actin.

Discussion

CPC is a rare neoplasm originating in the lining cells of the cerebral choroid plexus. This invasive and anaplastic neoplasm retains a local papillary structure. Review of the literature disclosed 25 documented cases of CPC. All cases of CPC in infants were located in the fourth ventricle. Only one adult neoplasm originated in the third ventricle. The choroid plexus carcinoma in this case probably originated in the suprapineal recess of the third ventricle presenting as a pineal neoplasm. CPC is hyperdense on enhanced CT and shows marked enhancement after intravenous contrast medium.

References

1. Boyd MC, Steinbok P (1987) Choroid plexus tumors: diagnosis and management. J Neurosurg 66: 800–805
2. Broad RW, Allen PB (1984) Third ventricle choroid plexus carcinoma. Can J Neurol Sci 11: 461–465
3. Kim K, Greenblatt SH, Robinson MG (1985) Choroid plexus carcinoma. Report of a case with cytopathology and differential diagnosis. Acta Cytol 29: 846–849
4. McComb RD, Burger PC (1983) Choroid plexus carcinoma. Report of a case with immunohistochemical and ultrastructural observation. Cancer 51: 470–475

Dr. J. M. Sullivan
Department of Neurology
University of Nebraska
600 South 42nd Street
Omaha, Nebraska 68198
USA

Neuroradiology (1991) 33 [Suppl]: 317–318

Neuro radiology

© Springer-Verlag 1991

Epidermoid cyst with variable contents shown on CT and MRI

W. C. Shen and C. F. Yang

Department of Radiology, Taichung Veterans General Hospital, Taichung, Taiwan, Republic of China

Summary. We report an epidermoid cyst which contained at least three kinds of material. One part of the lesion was of low density (25 HU) on CT, hypointense on T1-weighted images and hyperintense on T2-weighted images. This was a typical pearly tumour. Another part was of high density (96 HU) on CT and very low signal intensity on T2-weighted MR images. This contained viscous brown fluid, which was found microscopically to be haemosiderin. The third portion was calcification (400 HU) in the posterior wall. This epidermoid cyst arose from the third ventricle, a very rare location for such a lesion.

Key words: Epidermoid cyst – Computed tomography – Magnetic resonance imaging – Brain neoplasm – Pearly tumour.

Most epidermoid cysts are of homogeneously low density on CT [1], although hyperdense cysts have been reported [2–5]. In addition, most epidermoid cysts show homogeneous low signal intensity on T1-weighted MRI (T1WI) and hyperintensity on T2-weighted images (T2WI) [6–9], although hypointensity on T2WI has also been reported in rare cases [6]. Usually, the low density epidermoid cyst on CT corresponds to the common finding of T1WI low and T2WI high signal intensity on MRI. However, the MRI characteristics of epidermoid cysts hyperdense on CT have not been reported. We report an unusual epidermoid cyst arising from the third ventricle which had several components, demonstrated as different densities and signal intensities on CT and MRI respectively.

Case report

A 51-year-old female complained of right limb weakness for 6 months, and tremor of the right hand and bitemporal headache for 2 years. Physical examination revealed a right facial palsy of central type, and decreased muscle power of the right limbs. CT disclosed an irregular lesion lying between the lateral ventricles (Fig. 1 a, b), with three densities: 25, 96, 400 HU. CT 1.5 years previously at another hospital was reviewed and no change was found. MRI was performed 1.5 months after CT, and revealed variable signal intensities in the lesion on T1WI and T2WI, with very low signal intensity on T2WI corresponding to the dense portion on CT and hyperintensity corresponding to the low density portion.

At craniotomy the cyst was found to arise from the third ventricle, extruding superiorly and encroaching on both lateral ventricles. The right side of the tumour was cystic, containing brown, viscous fluid and the left side was a typical pearly tumour with pale, soft and solid contents. There was calcification in the posterior wall of the tumour.

Pathological examination showed squamous epithelium in the capsule and an epidermoid cyst was diagnosed. The contents on the right side were haemosiderin deposits mixed with keratinous material, and there was keratinous material and cholesterol in the soft tissue taken from the left side of the tumour. Calcification in the capsule was also noted microscopically.

Discussion

Most epidermoid cysts are of low density on CT, hypointense on T1WI, and hyperintense on T2-weighted MR images [6–9]. Grossly, such cysts are solid, soft, pearly, and contain waxy, pliable material rich in cholesterol and keratin [6–10]. They typically have prolonged T1 and T2 relaxation times, and although they invariably contain cholesterol, they rarely produce high signal on T1WI, except when they contain lipid mixed with triglycerides [10]. In contrast to some craniopharyngiomas, since epidermoids contain solid cholesterol, absence of hydrolysed cholesterol may contribute to prolongation of T1 [7]. In our case, the left side of the cyst, which was pearly in appearance and contained keratinous material with solid cholesterol, had these MR characteristics. Another rare type of epidermoid cyst hyperdense on CT always contains brown, viscous fluid [2–5]. The high density was assumed to result from calcification of keratinised debris [2], iron-containing pigment, such as ferrocalcium or haemosiderin [2–4] or high protein [5]. The signal intensities on MRI of epidermoid cysts hyperdense on CT has not previously been reported. In our case, the portion on the right side, of high density on CT and very low signal intensity on T2WI was this type of epidermoid cyst, since its cystic nature and brown, viscous contents were confirmed surgically, and haemosiderin mixed with keratinous material was revealed pathologically. The haemosiderin can explain the very low signal intensity on T2WI, because haemosiderin produces a selective T2 relaxation enhancement [11].

Microscopically, the capsule of epidermoids is stratified squamous epithelium, and may contain calcification, seen as thin, curvilinear or nodular densities on CT [5]. In our case the calcification in the posterior part of the cyst was obvious on CT but not seen on MRI.

Intracranial epidermoid cysts are most common in the cerebellopontine angle and parasellar area [12, 13], but rare in the ventricles or cerebral hemispheres. If they occur in the ventricle, the fourth ventricle is the most com-

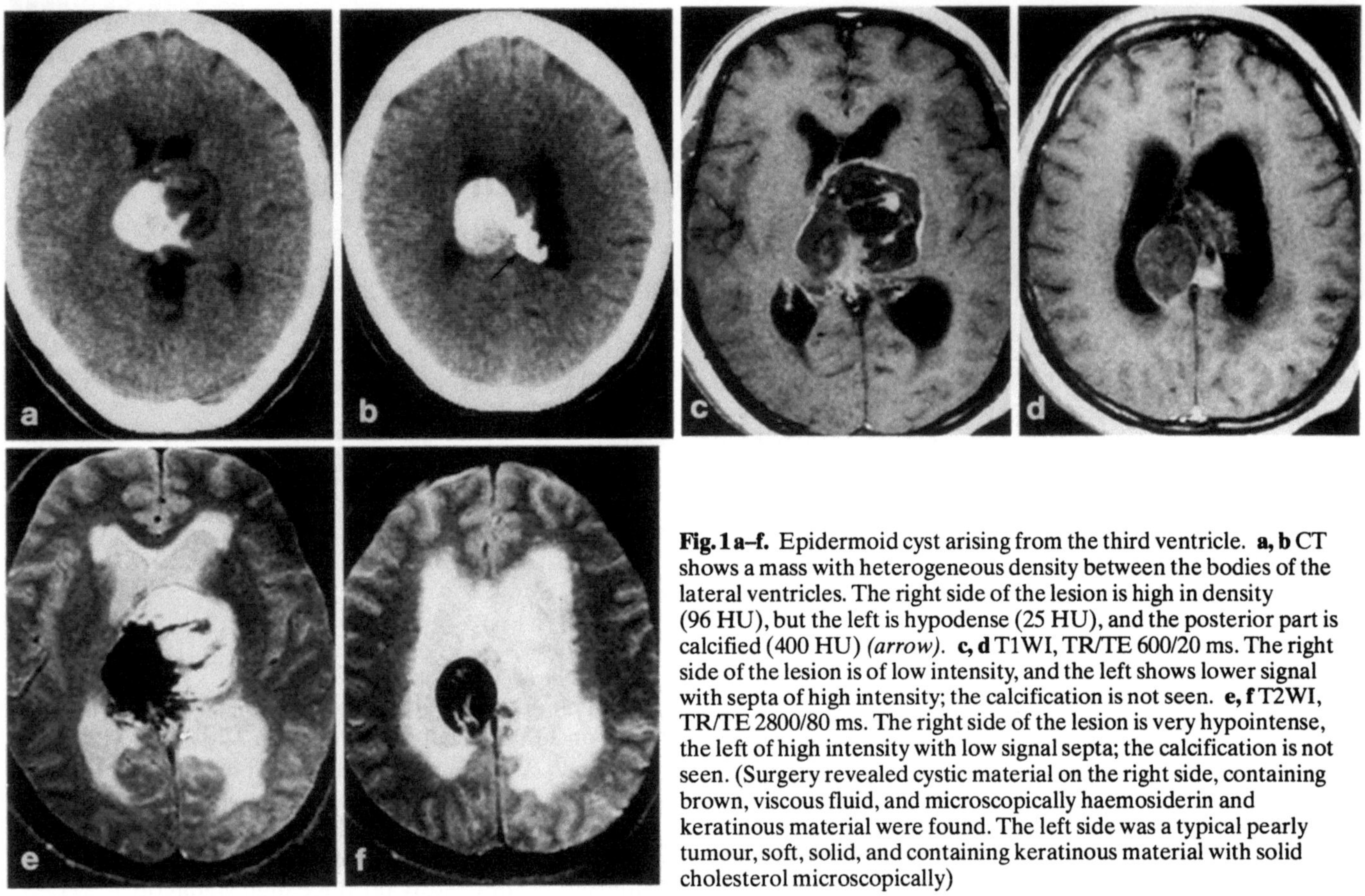

Fig. 1 a–f. Epidermoid cyst arising from the third ventricle. **a, b** CT shows a mass with heterogeneous density between the bodies of the lateral ventricles. The right side of the lesion is high in density (96 HU), but the left is hypodense (25 HU), and the posterior part is calcified (400 HU) *(arrow)*. **c, d** T1WI, TR/TE 600/20 ms. The right side of the lesion is of low intensity, and the left shows lower signal with septa of high intensity; the calcification is not seen. **e, f** T2WI, TR/TE 2800/80 ms. The right side of the lesion is very hypointense, the left of high intensity with low signal septa; the calcification is not seen. (Surgery revealed cystic material on the right side, containing brown, viscous fluid, and microscopically haemosiderin and keratinous material were found. The left side was a typical pearly tumour, soft, solid, and containing keratinous material with solid cholesterol microscopically)

mon site. A cyst arising from the third ventricle, as in our case, is very rare: few cases have been reported [13].

References

1. Davis KR, Roberson GH, Taveras JM, New PF, Trevor R (1976) Diagnosis of epidermoid tumor by computed tomography. Radiology 119: 347–353
2. Braun IF, Naidich TP, Leeds NE, Koslow M, Zimmerman HM, Chase NE (1977) Dense intracranial epidermoid tumors. Radiology 122: 717–719
3. Hasegama H, Bitoh S, Nakata M, Fujiwara M, Yasuda H (1980) Intracranial epidermoid mimicking meningioma. Surg Neurol 15: 372–374
4. Dunn RC, Archer CA, Rapport RL, Looi LM (1981) Unusual CT-dense posterior fossa epidermoid cyst, case report. J Neurosurg 55: 654–656
5. Nagshima C, Takahama M, Sakaguchi A (1981) Dense cerebellopontine epidermoid cyst. Surg Neurol 17: 172–177
6. Vion-Dury J, Vincentelli F, Jiddane M, Bunnen YV, Rumeau C, Grisoli F (1987) MR imaging of epidermoid cysts. Neuroradiology 29: 333–338
7. Yuh WTC, Barloon TJ, Jacoby CG, Shultz DH (1988) MR of fourth-ventricular epidermoid tumors. AJNR 9: 794–796
8. Steffey DJ, Fillipp GJ, Spera T, Gabrielsen TO (1988) MR imaging of primary epidermoid tumors. J Comput Assist Tomogr 12: 438–440
9. Tampieri D, Melanson D, Ethier R (1989) MR imaging of epidermoid cysts. AJNR 10: 351–356
10. Horowitz B, Chari MV, James R, Bryan RN (1990) MR of intracranial epidermoid tumors: correlation of in vivo imaging with in vitro ^{13}C spectroscopy. AJNR 11: 299–302
11. Gomori JM, Grossman RI, Hackney DB, Goldberg HI, Zimmerman RA, Bilaniuk LT (1987) Variable appearance of subacute intracranial hematomas in high-field spin-echo MR. AJNR 8: 1019–1026
12. Netsky MG (1988) Epidermoid tumors, review of the literature. Surg Neurol 29: 477–483
13. Rubin G, Scienza R, Pasqualin A, Rosta L, Pian RD (1989) Craniocerebral epidermoids and dermoids. Acta Neurochir (Wien) 97: 1–16

Dr. W. C. Shen
Department of Radiology
Taichung Veterans General Hospital
Taichung, 40705
Taiwan, Republic of China

Neuroradiology (1991) 33 [Suppl]: 319–321

Neuro radiology

© Springer-Verlag 1991

Intraarterial ACNU chemotherapy in malignant cerebral gliomas: preliminary results

C. Piana[1], U. Pasquini[1], M. De Nicola[1], F. Bevilacqua[1], F. Menichelli[1], U. Salvolini[1], F. Pauri[2], F. Rychlicki[2], A. Paccapelo[3], F. Sturba[3], M. Bonsignori[3], and V. Abbasciano[4]

[1] Neuroradiology Service, [2] Neurosurgical Department, [3] Medical Oncology Department,
[4] Ophthalmological Department, General Regional Hospital, Ancona, Italy

Summary. The authors report their experience with intra-arterial chemotherapy (ACNU) in 20 patients with malignant gliomas of the central nervous system. They describe their methodology and emphasise the absence of important complications. At the moment, intra-arterial chemotherapy seems to be one of the most interesting of the new methods used to treat malignant brain tumours, but wider experience is needed for better assessment of the results.

Key words: Intra-arterial chemotherapy – Malignant glioma – Central nervous system

Prognosis of malignant cerebral gliomas still remains poor despite combined use of the traditional therapies (surgery, chemotherapy, radiotherapy).

Therefore, any trial devoted to improving the clinical course of this disease must be carefully evaluated.

The aim of our work is to report our experience in the treatment of cerebral malignant gliomas using intra-arterial ACNU monotherapy.

ACNU (Nimustin) is a nitrosourea with a strong antimitotic effect both *in vivo* and *in vitro* on neurogenic cells [1]. Nevertheless, intravenous administration cannot produce therapeutic concentrations without also producing toxic effects [2, 3].

Therefore, selective intra-arterial drug administration using catheterisation of the extracerebral feeding arteries is to preferred [4, 5].

Materials and methods

Our therapeutic protocol consists of 100 mg/m^2 ACNU administered intra-arterially every 6 weeks for four consecutive cycles.

Intra-arterial administration is carried out by Seldinger catheterisation of the extracranial arteries without blood-brain barrier disruption.

Our trial began in July 1988 and includes 20 patients with malignant cerebral gliomas, 16 verified histologically by surgical partial excision or stereotactic biopsy, and 4 diagnosed on clinical and radiological criteria. Every patient is carefully studied from clinical, laboratory and neuroradiological points of view (by CT, MRI and angiography) before and after every intra-arterial infusion of ACNU.

Preliminary results

The vessels used for the treatment were: in 18 cases the internal carotid artery alone; in 1 case, both internal carotid arteries; in the last case, the internal carotid and the ipsilateral vertebral arteries.

Repeat CT studies carried out between treatment cycles have shown that in 10 of 20 cases the morphological features of the lesion underwent a change: an increase in the hypodense and necrotic component with minor perilesional oedema.

In 8 cases a reduction in lesion size occurred: in 1 case after the second cycle of therapy, in the others after the third cycle. In 1 case, at the end of the treatment, CT revealed a hypodense lesion resembling an infarct, with clear margins, in the occipital lobe contralateral to the tumour. This lesion was believed to be unrelated to the treatment because it appeared 6 months after the end of the therapeutic cycle. Angiographic follow-up demonstrated a notable reduction in the pathological blush in 4 of 5 cases with previous evident hypervascularisation.

Ten of 20 patients showed neurological improvement after the second cycle of therapy.

After the third cycle 5 patients gave signs of cognitive deterioration, due in four to further growth of the tumour as demonstrated by CT.

No complications were observed in the ophthalmological examinations. Repeated examinations of the blood showed transitory grade I–II leukopenia in only 10 cases, and 1 case of platelet reduction grade I (grades given according to the WHO international classification). NMR carried out in 5 patients only, before and after a cycle of therapy did not show any substantial signal changes in white or grey matter.

Discussion

The small number of our patients and the brief observation period do not allow conclusive observations, especially in relation to the survival rate.

Nevertheless our observations agree with the most recent reports [4, 5] that suggest an improvement in the results of the treatment of malignant cerebral gliomas using

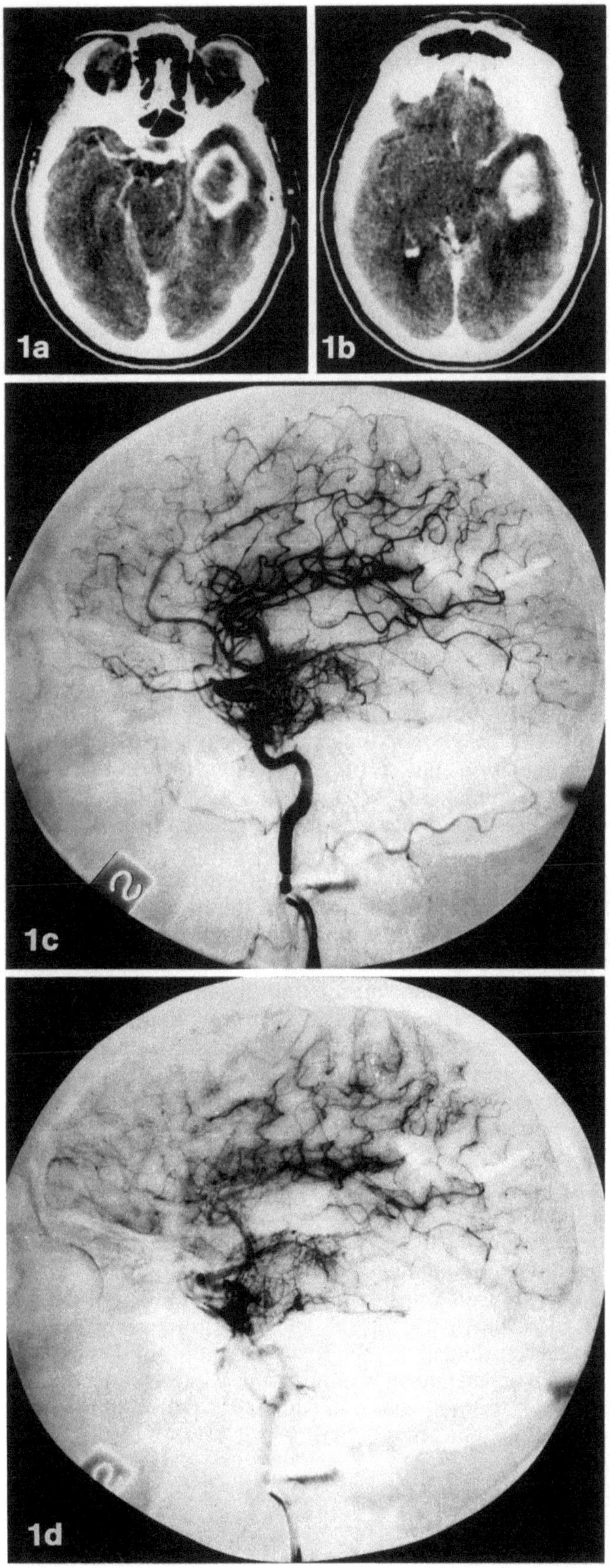

Fig. 1 a–d. Female, 59 years, with left temporal glioma. Before endoarterial ACNU chemotherapy. Physical examination: intracranial hypertension, stupor, hemiparesis; CT: left temporal expanding lesion with oedema; angiography: left temporal tumour stain

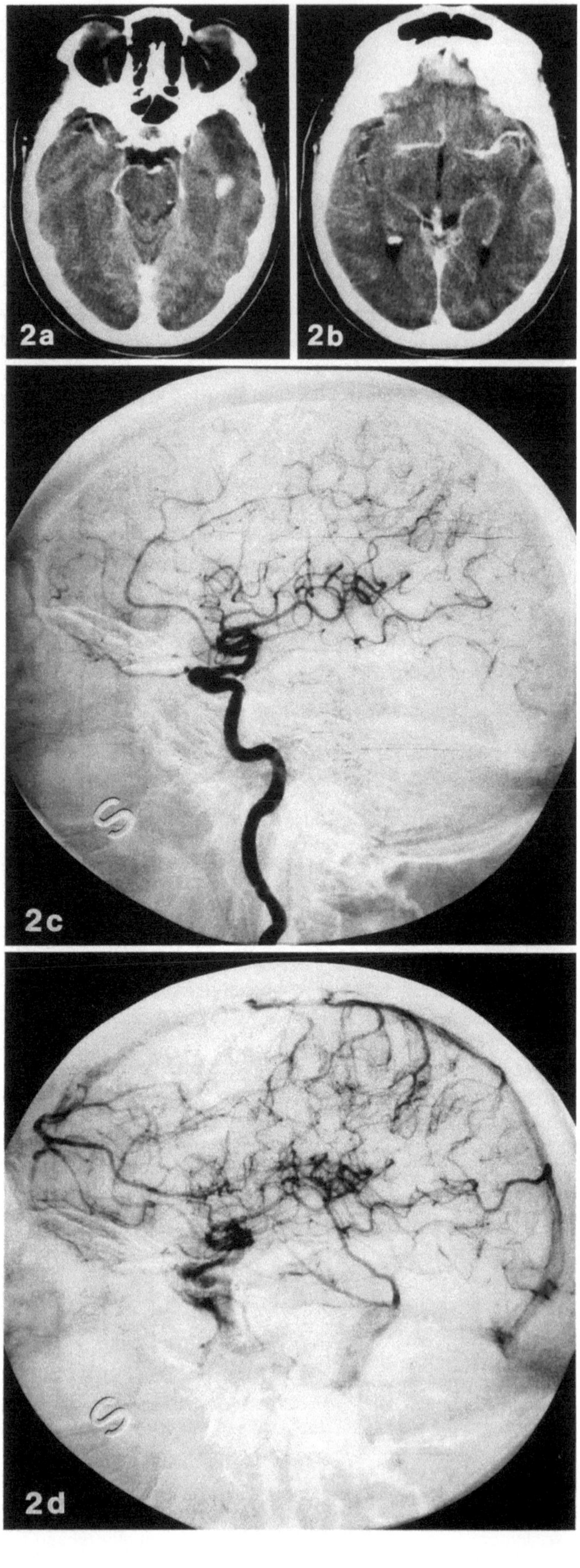

Fig. 2 a–d. Same patient after endoarterial ACNU chemotherapy. Physical examination: normal; CT: major reduction in the space-occupying lesion; angiography: disappearance of the tumour stain

intra-arterial chemotherapy in comparison with the traditional therapy.

Furthermore, the absence of severe side effects of the therapy, together with the encouraging preliminary results, leads us to continue the trial.

References

1. Bamberg M, Budach V, Stuschke M, Gerhard L (1988) Preliminary experimental results with the nitrosourea derivative ACNU in the treatment of malignant gliomas. Radiother Oncol 12: 25–29
2. Papavero L, Loew F, Jaksche H (1987) Intracarotid infusion of ACNU and BCNU as adjuvant therapy of malignant gliomas. Clinical aspects and critical considerations. Acta Neurochir (Wien) 85: 128–137
3. Walker MD, Alexander E, Hunt WE (1978) Evaluation of ACNU and/or radiotherapy in the treatment of anaplastic gliomas. J Neurosurg 49: 333–343
4. Chiras J, Dormont D, Fauchon F, Debussche C, Bories J (1988) Chimiotherapie intra-artérielle des gliomes malins. J Neuroradiol 15: 31–48
5. Chiras J, Fauchon F (1989) Traitement médical des gliomes malins inopérables. Chimiothérapie intra-artérielle non hypersélèctive par HECNU suivie de radiothérapie conventionelle. Rev Neurol (Paris) 145: 829–837

Dr. Ugo Pasquini
Neuroradiologia
Ospedale Generale Regionale
60020 Torrette-Ancona, Italy

Neuroradiology (1991) 33 [Suppl]: 322–323

Neuro radiology
© Springer-Verlag 1991

MRI in meningiomas – more than just a diagnostic tool?

W. Schima[1], D. Wimberger[1,2], L. Prayer[1], J. Kramer[1], E. Schindler[3], and H. Imhof[1]

[1] Departments of Radiodiagnosis and MR-Institute,
Departments of [2] Neurology and [3] Neurosurgery, University of Vienna, Austria

Summary. The ability of MRI to detect invasion of venous sinuses and meningeal thickening suggestive of neoplastic infiltration was determined by review of 42 examinations (37 patients) with meningiomas. The preoperative reports were compared with intraoperative findings in 22 operated cases. MRI detected 12 of 13 sinuses found surgically to be involved; in 1 case MRI was falsely positive. MRI evidence of meningeal thickening does not necessarily indicate neoplastic infiltration of the dura mater, because reactive changes are sometimes present surrounding the tumour.

Key words: Intracranial tumour, magnetic resonance imaging – Meningioma – Meningeal thickening – Venous sinus involvement

Prognosis of meningiomas depends mainly on the completeness of resection. Even small tumour residua affecting the meninges carry the risk of recurrence. Frequently, macro- or microscopic tumour involvement of the surrounding dura mater can be found [1]. Two facts are of interest preoperatively: the extent of meningeal spread and possible involvement of adjacent venous sinuses. The ability of MRI to show there features has not been studied previously.

Patients and methods

Of 37 patients (12 men, 25 women; 16–79 years, mean 55 years) 22 were operated upon after MRI studies; 8 patients were first examined after the first operation, and 7 patients were not operated upon (42 examinations in total). MRI examination: 1.5 T superconducting system, slice orientation appropriate to the localisation of the lesion, images in at least two perpendicular planes, slice thickness: 3–5 mm, 50% intersection gap. T1-weighted (700 ms/15 ms) and T2-weighted (2500 ms/15 ms, 70 ms) SE sequences, 0.1 mmol gadolinium-DTPA/kg body weight.

The MRI studies were assessed according to the following criteria: (1) evidence of lesion (+ localisation); (2) delineation, as judged by space-occupying effect and/or different signal intensities and/or contrast enhancement; (3) venous sinus involvement, evidenced by abnormal contrast enhancement, and/or encasement or displacement of vessels (cavernous sinus), or flow changes; (4) meningeal thickening: contrast enhancement extending more than 5 mm beyond the tumour margins.

Results

Thirty-three patients had one tumour, 2 had two tumours, and 2 suffered from meningiomatosis. The tumours were evident on precontrast scans in 37 (100%), and delineated in 26 (70%). There was evidence of sinus involvement in 17 (47%) (Table 1; Figs. 1, 2). In 1 patient invasion of the venous confluence was overlooked, since it showed high signal on precontrast scans. Meningeal enhancement was found in 20 of 42 examinations (48%) (Table 2; Figs. 2, 3).

Discussion

Although all the meningiomas were readily identified on precontrast images, delineation of the entire tumour was possible in only 70%. Contrast enhanced-MRI is the most sensitive technique for detection and delineation of the tumour [2]. For demonstration of invasion of a venous sinus MRI is superior to angiography, because it shows the anatomical relations of the tumour to the sinus [3]. In the case of cavernous sinus involvement MRI shows not only narrowing and displacement, but also encasement of the intracavernous portion of the carotid artery [4]. However, this last observation may be misleading, as the lateral wall of the sinus cannot be delineated. Invasion may therefore be incorrectly diagnosed. Meningeal thickening, demonstrated on the postcontrast images of preoperative studies, may be indicative of neoplastic infiltration [5]. In

Table 1. Sinus involvement

	MRI	Operation		No operation
		True positive	False positive	
Cavernous sinus	11	6	1[a]	4
Sigmoid sinus	2	2	0	0
Superior sagittal sinus	4	4	0	0
	17	12	1	4

[a] In this patient MRI revealed encasement of the carotid artery and invasion of the cavernous sinus was assumed. At operation the sinus was found not to be infiltrated

Table 2. Meningeal enhancement

		Preoperative	Postoperative
Meningeal enhancement ($n = 20$)	True positive	5	0
	False positive	4	0
	No operation	2	9
		11	9
		Preoperative	Postoperative
No meningeal enhancement ($n = 22$)	True negative	11	0
	False negative	0	0
	No operation	6	5
		17	5

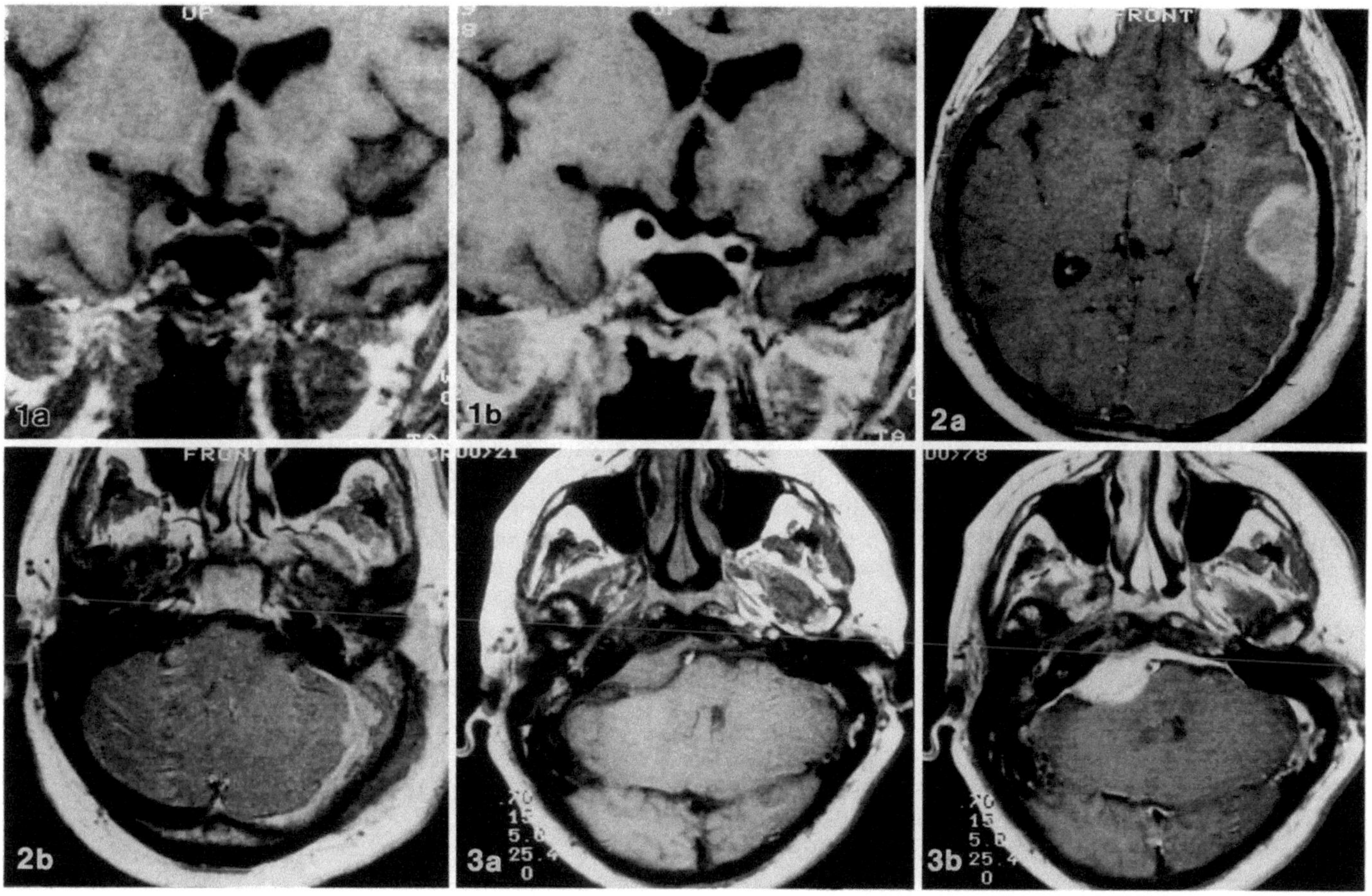

Fig. 1 a, b. 60-year-old man, suffering from double vision. **a** T1-weighted coronal MRI: there is a space-occupying lesion in the right cavernous sinus, bulging its lateral wall; encasement and shifting of the internal carotid artery. **b** T1-weighted coronal MRI with intravenous gadolinium adds no further information; meningioma and cavernous sinus both enhance

Fig. 2 a, b. 40-year-old man with aphasia. **a** T1-weighted axial MRI with gadolinium: there is a tumour in the left temporal region, compressing the lateral ventricle; widespread meningeal thickening is seen surrounding the lesion. **b** T1-weighted axial MRI with gadolinium: abnormal enhancement is seen in the left sigmoid and transverse sinuses; (compare with the signal void in the right sided sinuses)

Fig. 3 a, b. 60-year-old man with multiple cranial nerve palsies on the right. **a** T1-weighted axial MRI: an isointense tumour extends from the tentorium to the pontine cistern. **b** After intravenous gadolinium, meningeal thickening around the tumour becomes visible

postoperative examinations a high percentage of patients show localised or diffuse meningeal enhancement, probably representing reactive changes [6]. Even in preoperative studies meningeal enhancement is sometimes due to proliferation of connective tissue and hypervascularity, as we found in 4 cases [7].

We conclude that MRI is useful for answering questions concerning involvement of the venous sinuses and meninges, which allow assessment of operability and the likelihood of radical removal.

Acknowledgement. This work was supported in part by the Ludwig-Boltzmann-Institut of Radiophysical Tumour Diagnosis.

References

1. Borovich B, Doron Y (1986) Recurrence of intracranial meningiomas: the role played by regional multicentricity. J Neurosurg 64: 58–63
2. Schoerner W, Schubeus P, Henkes H, Rottacker C, Hamm B, Felix R (1990) Intracranial meningiomas: comparison of plain and contrast-enhanced examinations in CT and MRI. Neuroradiology 32: 12–18
3. Spagnoli MV, Goldberg HI, Grossman RI, Bilaniuk LI, Gomori JM, Hackney DB, Zimmerman DB (1986) Intracranial meningiomas: high-field MR imaging. Radiology 161: 369–375
4. Young SC, Grossman RI, Goldberg HI, Spagnoli MV, Hackney DB, Zimmerman RA, Bilaniuk LT (1988) MR of vascular encasement in parasellar masses: comparison with angiography and MRI. AJNR 9: 35–38
5. Wilms G, Lammens M, Marchal G, Van Calenbergh F, Plets C, Van Fraeyenhoven L, Baert AL (1989) Thickening of dura surrounding meningiomas: MR features. J Comput Assist Tomogr 13: 763–768
6. Burke JW, Podrasky AE, Bradley WG (1990) Meninges: benign postoperative changes on MR images. Radiology 174: 99–102
7. Tokumaru A, O'uchi T, Eguchi T, Kawamoto S, Kokubo T, Suzuki M, Kameda T (1990) Prominent meningeal enhancement adjacent to meningiomas on Gd-DTPA-enhanced MR images: histopathologic correlation. Radiology 175: 431–433

Dr. Wolfgang Schima
Department of Radiodiagnosis
University of Vienna
Alserstrasse 4
A-1090 Vienna, Austria

Neuroradiology (1991) 33 [Suppl]: 324–325

Neuro-radiology
© Springer-Verlag 1991

The radiological diagnosis of epidermoid tumours

G. L. V. Tatler and B. E. Kendall

The National Hospital for Nervous Diseases, Queen Square, London, UK

Summary. The diagnosis of epidermoid/dermoid tumour was made by imaging in 160 cases over a period of 20 years. Diagnosis in the earlier cases was usually by angiography and pneumoencephalography. CT improved specific diagnosis to 84% and with MRI confirmation of the diagnosis, a conservative approach to management became a reasonable alternative to biopsy in many cases.

Key words: Epidermoid – Dermoid – Computed tomography – Magnetic resonance imaging

Epidermoids and dermoids account for between 0.2% and 1.0% of all intracranial tumours [1]. They are benign slow-growing masses which can frequently be managed conservatively if a diagnosis can be established, preferably without resorting to biopsy.

Materials and methods

All cases where a radiological diagnosis of epidermoid/dermoid was made over the past 20 years were included in the series (Table 1). Cases misdiagnosed radiologically but proven histologically to be epidermoid/dermoid were also studied. The radiology of every patient was reviewed.

Results

Histology was obtained in 106 cases and epidermoid or dermoid was confirmed in 89. Radiological diagnosis in the proven cases was based on the demonstration of a lobulated extra-axial mass in one of the sites of predilection [1]. A different pathology was found in 17 cases, i.e. schwannoma 4, arachnoid cyst 3, and 1 case each of chordoma, craniopharyngioma, enterogenous cyst, oligodendroglioma, granuloma, plasmacytoma, benign osteoblastoma, ependymoma, encephalitis, and equivocal changes suggestive of glioma. In a further 32 patients follow-up studies for up to 8 years have shown a benign clinical course and slow progression of an extra-axial mass entirely consistent with the radiological diagnosis.

Table 1. Distribution of epidermoid/dermoid tumours (some tumours involved more than one region)

Cerebellopontine angle	37
Pontine cistern	14
Quadrigeminal cistern	4
Chiasmatic cistern	12
Parasellar region	15
Middle fossa subarachnoid space	16
Sylvian fissure	5
Ventricles	18
Cranial diploe	7

CT [2] and MRI [3, 4] features of histologically proven dermoid/epidermoid tumours are listed in Tables 2 and 3. False negative diagnoses were made on CT in cases with unusual features (isodensity or hyperdensity relative to brain, and enhancement, usually peripherally, in the rim). MRI, characterised by signal of cerebrospinal fluid (CSF) intensity on T1-weighted images and high signal, usually higher than that of brain and CSF on moderately to intermediately T2-weighted sequences, has reduced the frequency of misdiagnosis in otherwise unusual cases.

Table 2. Histologically proven epidermoid/dermoid tumours

CT features	Radiological diagnosis		
	Correct	Other	Total
Fat to CSF density	8	0	8
CSF density	35	7	42
CSF to brain density	17	2	19
Brain density	3	3	6
Above brain density	2	4	6
Calcification	11	4	15
Contrast enhancement	8	6	14
Bone changes	13	5	18

CSF, Cerebrospinal fluid

Table 3. MRI features of histologically proven epidermoid/dermoid tumours

Signal	T1-weighted sequences		
	Inversion recovery	SE400–600	
Equal to CSF	10	2	
Slightly higher than CSF		2	
Equal to brain		1	
Higher than CSF and brain		1	
Total	10	6	
Signal	**T2-weighted sequences**		
	moderately	intermediately	heavily
Equal to CSF		1	2
Higher than CSF, less than brain	1		
Higher than CSF, equal to brain		1	
Higher than CSF and brain	1	8	
Total	2	10	2

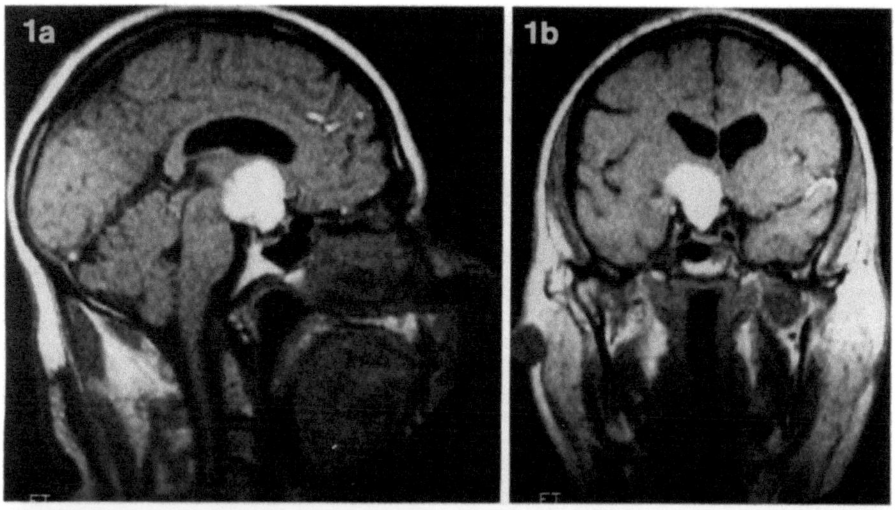

Fig. 1a, b. Dermoid tumour. **a** Sagittal TE26/440, **b** TE26/560 MRI. Mixed signal: mainly very high, higher than cerebrospinal fluid (CSF) and brain but some parts similar to brain. Highest intensity element represents fat, some of which is free in the cerebral sulci

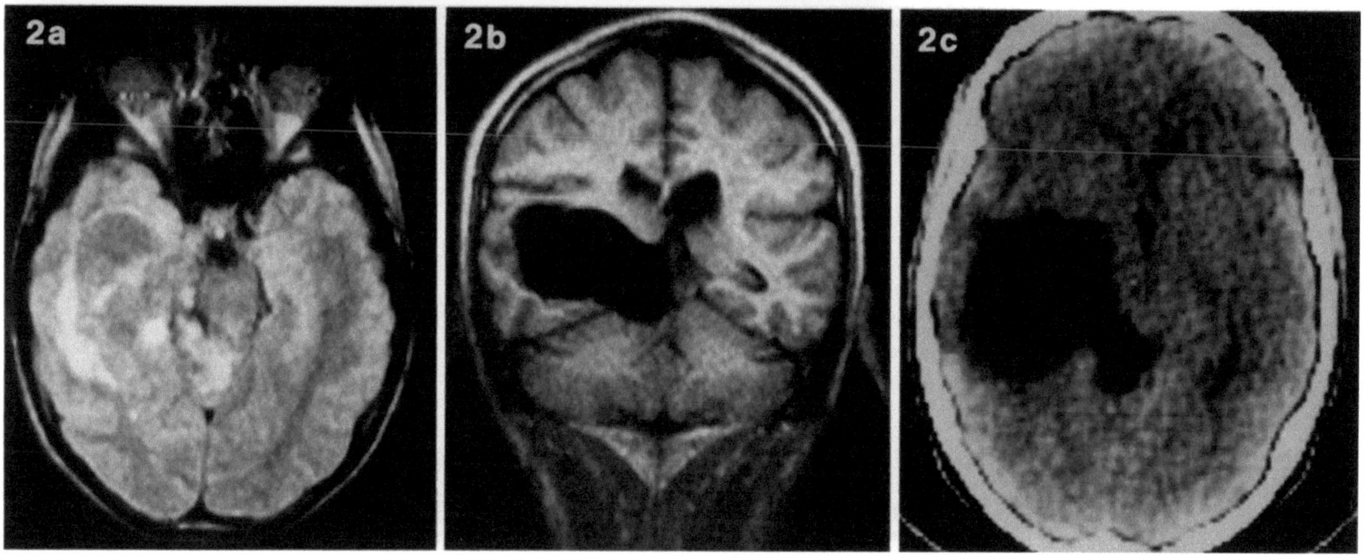

Fig. 2a–c. Epidermoid tumour. **a** Axial TE80/2000 MRI. Inhomogeneous signal, higher than CSF and brain with region of lower signal of CSF in temporal horn. **b** Coronal IR5000 with signal of CSF intensity. **c** CT: density slightly higher than CSF

Discussion

It is apparent that although skull radiographs, angiograms and air studies [5, 6] provided a positive diagnosis in about 50% of these tumours, biopsy was necessary in most cases to distinguish more aggressive lesions.

Diagnosis was markedly improved by CT, but unusual features such as the presence of isodense or hyperdense substance, contrast enhancement, sometimes within a nodule but more often in the rim of the lesion, and areas of calcification, confused the diagnosis of epidermoid/dermoid tumours in about 20%.

MRI, characterised by low signal (CSF intensity) on T1-weighted sequences, and signals usually of high intensity on T2-weighted images has further increased the accuracy of specific diagnosis to a point where conservative management is the elective method in many cases.

Table 4. Histologically proven epidermoid/dermoid tumours

	Radiological diagnosis			
	Definite	Possible	Other diagnosis	Total
Pre CT/MRI	4 (19%)	7 (33%)	10 (48%)	21
Post CT/MRI	45 (66%)	12 (18%)	11 (16%)	68
Total	49	19	21	89

References

1. Russell DS, Rubinstein LJ (eds) (1989) Pathology of tumours of the nervous system, 5th edn. Arnold, London pp 693
2. Davis KR, Roberson GH, Taveras JM, New PFJ, Trevor R (1989) Diagnosis of epidermoid tumor by computed tomography. Radiology 119: 347–353
3. Savader SJ, Murtagh FR, Savader BL, Martinez CR (1989) Magnetic resonance imaging of intracranial epidermoid tumours. Clin Radiol 40: 282–285
4. Gentry LR, Jacoby CG, Turski PA, Houston LW, Strother CM, Sackett JF (1987) Cerebellopontine angle-petromastoid mass lesions: comparative study of diagnosis with MR imaging and CT. Radiology 162: 513–520
5. Long JL, Kier EL, Schechter MM (1973) The radiology of epidermoid tumors of the cerebellopontine angle. Neuroradiology 6: 188–192
6. Dee RH, Kishore PRS, Young HF (1980) Radiological evaluation of cerebello-pontine angle epidermoid tumor. Surg Neurol 13: 293–296

Dr. G. L. V. Tatler
Lysholm Radiological Department
The National Hospital for Nervous Diseases
Queen Square
London WC1N 3BG, UK

Neuroradiology (1991) 33 [Suppl]: 326–327

Neuro-radiology
© Springer-Verlag 1991

Intratumoural haemorrhage as the presenting feature of primitive neuroectodermal tumour: a delayed sequel to cranial irradiation

A. C. Rovira, M. Rovira, F. Romero, A. Ortega, B. Ibarra, and A. Vivas

Neuroradiological and Anatomopathological Services, Hospital del Valle de Hebrón de la Seguridad Social, Barcelona, Spain
Centro Radiológico Computarizado, Barcelona, Spain

Summary. An 11-year-old girl developed a primitive neuroectodermal tumour (PNET) 9 years after receiving prophylactic cranial radiation to a total of 2,400 cGy and intrathecal methotrexate for lymphoblastic leukaemia. This is the second case of radiation-induced PNET to be reported. In addition to the rarity of this tumour, its rapid development is of interest: CT of the brain performed 6 months prior to the onset of symptoms had been normal.

Key words: Radiation-induced tumour – Primitive neuroectodermal tumour

Case report

An 11-year-old girl had been diagnosed as having acute lymphoblastic leukaemia at the age of 2 years. She received multiagent chemotherapy, 2,400 cGy prophylactic cranial irradiation and intrathecal methotrexate. She was believed to be in remission. Several follow-up CT studies were normal. Six months after the last of these (Fig. 1), she was admitted because of acutely raised intracranial pressure with headache, vomiting and progressive drowsiness. CT revealed an intracerebral haematoma in the right frontotemporal region with oedema and mass effect, displacing midline structures (Fig. 2). Slight contrast enhancement was observed in the periphery of the lesion. During hospitalisation a left hemiparesis developed which persisted. As a tumour was suspected, biopsy was performed. Histological examination showed non-specific inflammatory tissue with no evidence of neoplasia or infection.

Four months later, she developed bifrontal headaches, which failed to respond to conventional treatment. CT then showed a tumour with cystic and haemorrhagic areas and irregular contrast enhancement, in the same frontotemporal region (Fig. 3). The tumour was surgically removed. Biopsy, and light microscopy of tumour tissue revealed predominantly small undifferentiated cells in sheets. These cells exhibited round or oval hyperchromatic nuclei and little or no visible cytoplasm. There were some larger cells with a more obvious eosinophilic perikaryon which in some cases had a tapered end. Mitotic figures were conspicuous. The tumour had areas of necrosis and numerous small blood vessels with scanty connective tissue (Fig. 4). Chemotherapy was started but the patient died 6 months later.

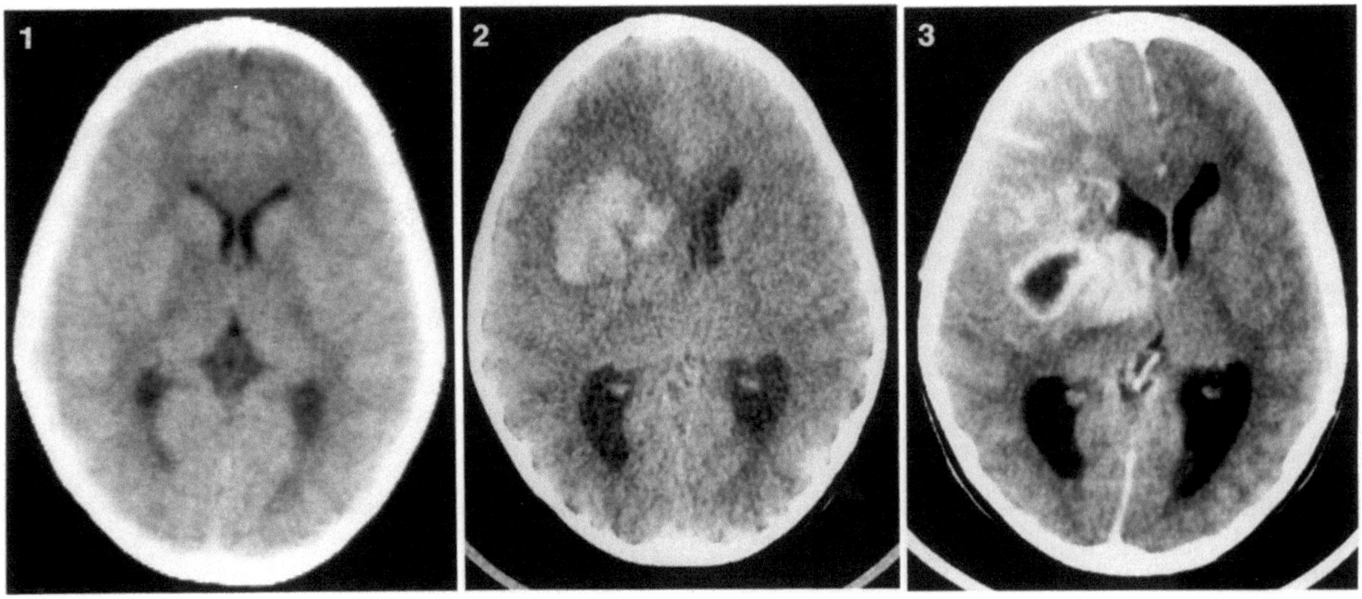

Fig. 1. Normal CT, July 1988

Fig. 2. Frontotemporal haematoma, December 1988

Fig. 3. Cystic and solid tumour with irregular contrast enhancement, April 1989

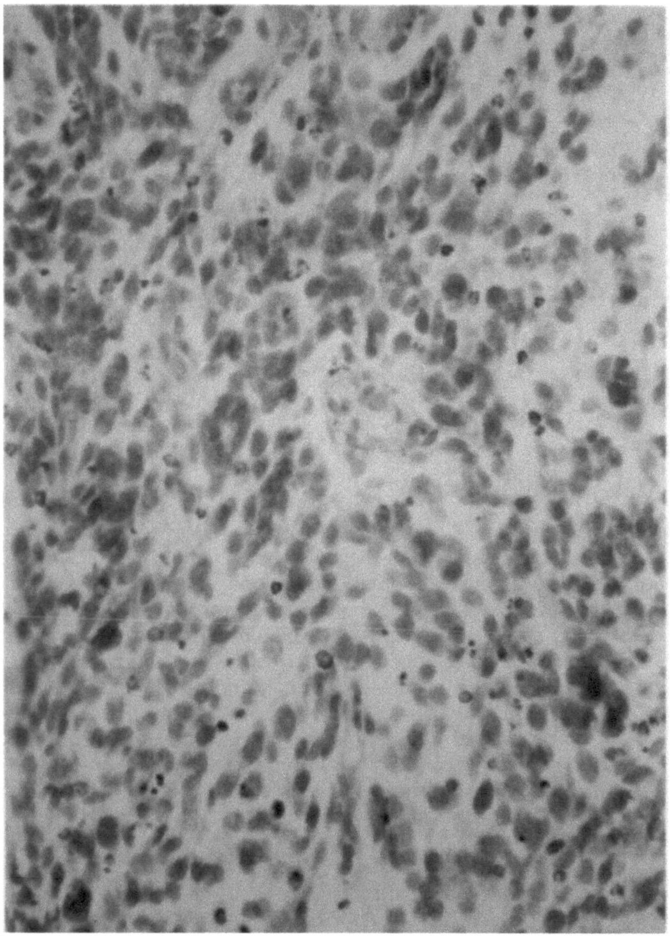

Fig. 4. Small undifferentiated cells in sheets with hyperchromatic nuclei and little or no visible cytoplasm

Discussion

CT findings in cases of primitive neuroectodermal tumour (PNET) are suggestive of the diagnosis, but are non-specific. These tumours are frequently large and have both cystic and solid components, [1] as occurred in our case. Calcification may be present but was absent from our patient. Haemorrhage into the tumour has been described [2, 3], and was the presenting syndrome in this case. Rapid growth is characteristic of these tumours, as shown in this patient, whose CT was normal 6 months prior to the haemorrhage. This neoplasm corresponds to the previously described PNET of the brain [4, 5], which was added to the WHO classification in 1985 [6]. Some neuropathologists consider this controversial term an evasion [7] but it does indicate that the tumour has no distinguishing features which permit identification of its cells as belonging to recognizable differentiated categories.

PNET was diagnosed 9 years after the patient was treated with whole-brain irradiation and intrathecal methotrexate for her leukaemia. The tumour met the criteria for defining a neoplasm as radiation-induced, namely; a long quiescent latent period, location within the irradiated area and a tumour distinctly different from the lesion for which the patient was irradiated [8]. No case of PNET was described in a recent review by Shapiro et al. [8] of 37 cases of central nervous system radiation-induced tumours. Only one case of radiation-induced PNET has been reported previously [9]. In addition to the rarity of this tumour, our case is of interest because of the rapid development of the tumour as demonstrated by a normal CT scan 6 months prior to the onset of symptoms.

References

1. Kingsley DP (1984) Radiological features of the neuroectodermal tumors of childhood. Neuroradiology 26
2. Figueroa RE (1989) MR findings on primitive neuroectodermal tumors. J Comput Assist Tomogr 13: 773–778
3. Zimmerman RA (1989) CT of primary and secondary craniocerebral neuroblastoma. AJNR 135: 1239–1242
4. Hart MN (1963) Primitive neuroectodermal tumors of the brain in children. Cancer 32: 890–897
5. Becker LE (1983) Primitive neuroectodermal tumors of the central nervous system. Hum Pathol 16: 538–550
6. Rocke LB (1985) Classification of brain tumors for childhood. Cancer 56: 1869–1886
7. Fields WS (1989) Primary brain tumors. A review of histologic classification. Springer, Berlin Heidelberg New York
8. Shapiro S (1989) Radiation-induced intracranial malignant gliomas. J Neurosurg 71: 77–82
9. Banasch ES (1988) Primitive neuroectodermal tumor presenting as a delayed sequela to cranial irradiation and intrathecal methotrexate. Pediatr Neurol 4: 375–378

Dr. A. C. Rovira
Muntaner 535
08022 Barcelona, Spain

Neuroradiology (1991) 33 [Suppl]: 328–330

Neuro-radiology
© Springer-Verlag 1991

Primary CNS lymphomas: correlation of CT and MRI with neuropathological findings

U. Salvolini[1], M. Scarpelli[2], L. Chiaramoni[3], N. Foschi[3], M. Maricotti[3], L. Salvolini[1], R. Rossi[4], G. M. Mariuzzi[2], and F. Angeleri[3]

Departments of [1] Neuroradiology, [2] Pathology, and [3] Neurology, Local Health Authority no. 12, University of Ancona, Ancona, Italy
[4] Department of Radiology, I. N. R. C. A., Ancona, Italy

Summary. Nine primary malignant lymphomas of the central nervous system in non-AIDS patients were studied. Neuroradiological and histological appearances and immunophenotyping are reported. No correlation was found between the radiological appearances and the histological classification.

Key words: Brain lymphomas – Computed tomography scan – Magnetic resonance imaging – Histopathology – Immunophenotyping

Although primary intracerebral malignant lymphomas (PIML) are rare, comprising less than 1% of all brain tumours and 1.6% of extranodal non-Hodgkin's lymphomas, their frequency has trebled in the last decade. The CT appearances have been well described: they are isodense or hyperdense with marked enhancement after intravenous contrast medium and involve central brain structures more frequently than other central nervous system (CNS) tumours. Histological types in the CNS are identical to those elsewhere. The presence of many different classifications has obscured the precise relationship between histological type, radiological appearances and prognosis. The aim of this report was to study, in a series of PIML, how these tumours progressed on serial neuroradiological examinations and to analyse the relationship between CT appearances and histological type.

Materials and methods

Nine consecutive primary brain lymphomas arising in non-AIDS patients have been included in the study. All had multiple CT studies which were examined for: number of lesions present when seen for the first time, tumour contact with ependymal layer, precontrast density, enhancement pattern. Three patients also underwent MRI. In one case the MRI was performed both in vivo and after death. The diagnosis was made by open or stereotaxic biopsy in all patients but one, adopting the Kiel classification. For practical purposes, the tumours were classified according to the three diagnostic categories of the working formulation (WF): low, intermediate, high grade. Immunophenotyping was performed by means of a series of monoclonal antibodies (Clonab-Biotest).

Results

Neuroradiological findings

In all patients a single discrete tumour was documented on admission CT. In three patients the lesion was located in the cortex/white matter of the temporal lobe and in the remaining six it was seen as a subependymal lesion in the posterior fossa (2 patients) or in the hemispheres, involving the basal ganglia, thalamus and hypothalamus. All the lesions were hypodense and showed marked enhancement (inhomogeneous in 2 patients) after contrast medium; they were very well defined with a hypodense halo. On serial CT all patients showed progression to a multiple lesion pattern. Partial regression was observed following therapy. MRI T1-weighted images showed lesions slightly hypointense and difficult to detect; long TR studies revealed inhomogeneous hyperintense lesions in the sub-

Table 1. Clinical and neuroradiological findings

Patient no.	Age (years)	Sex	Surgery	Lesion location	Duration of neuro-radiological follow-up	No. of lesions when first observed
1	55	M	Stereotaxic	Basal ganglia	1 Year	Single
2	69	F	–	Temporal	2 Years	Single
3	58	M	Stereotaxic	Hypothalamus	3 Months	Single
4	54	M	Stereotaxic	Paraventricular	1 Year	Single
5	59	M	Open	Cerebellum	3 Months	Single
6	57	M	Open	Temporal	1.5 Years	Single
7	48	M	Open	Cerebellum	1 Month	Single
8	61	F	Open	Temporal/occipital	2 Months	Single
9	54	M	Open	Thalamus	1 Year	Single

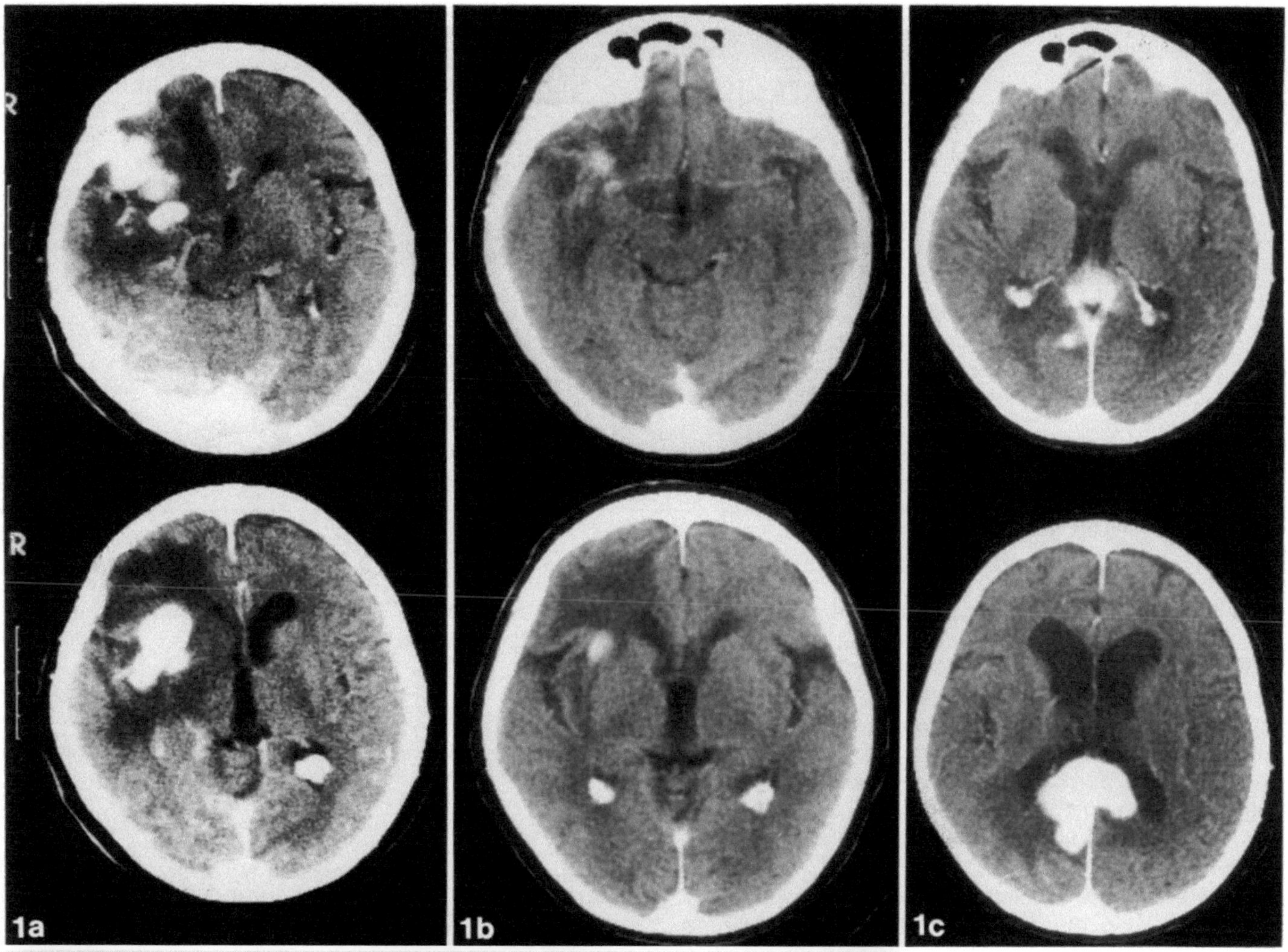

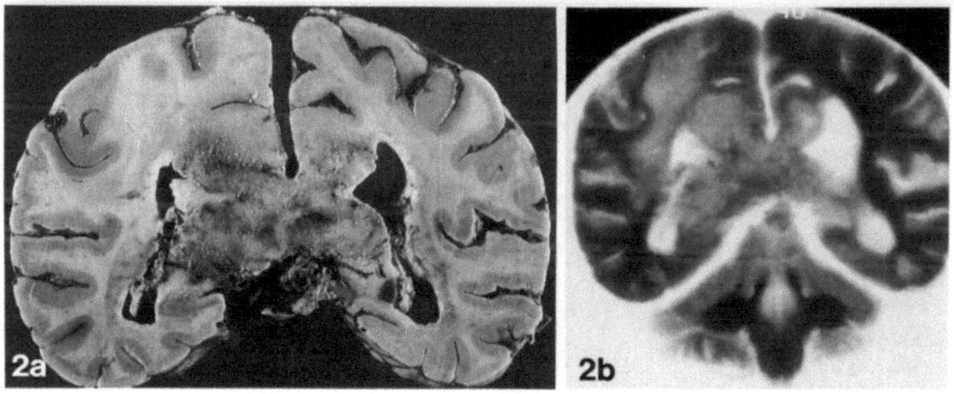

Fig. 1 a–c. Patient 2, serial CT: **a** right frontotemporal nodular lesions with hypodense halo; **b** 20 days later after therapy (marked reduction in size); **c** 2 years later (nodular mass in the region of the corpus callosum)

Fig. 2 a, b. Patient 2, gross and MRI appearance. **a** Tumour in the splenium of the corpus callosum. **b** Postmortem MRI of the brain

ependymal white matter. Difficulties arose in distinguishing tumour from oedema. The clinical and neuroradiological findings are summarized in Table 1. The serial CT images, and neuropathological findings in case 2 are shown as an example (Figs. 1, 2).

Histopathological findings

The results of classification and immunophenotyping are summarized in Table 2. There were two lymphoblastic lymphomas, three immunoblastic, one lymphoplasmacytoid polymorphic and the remainder were classified as centroblastic-centrocytic. According to the WF, five were of high grade and the remainder of intermediate grade.

Discussion

According to different authors [1, 2], brain lymphomas in non-AIDS patients are predominantly large, solitary masses progressing to a multifocal pattern in a variable period of time. They frequently involve the deep midline

Table 2. Histological findings

Patient no.	Classification	WF (grade)	Clonab antibodies							
			ML	MT1	MT2	MB1	MB2	LN1	LN2	LN3
1	Lymphoblastic	High	–	–	–	–	+/–	–	–	+/–
2	Lymphoplasma-cytoid polymorphic	Intermediate	+/–	–	+	–	–	+	–	–
3	Lymphoblastic	High	–	–	–	–	–	–	–	–
4	Centroblastic-centrocytic	Intermediate	+	+	–	+	+	–	+	+
5	Immunoblastic	High	+/–	+/–	–	–	+	–	–	–
6	Centroblastic-centrocytic	Intermediate	–	–	–	–	+	–	+/–	+
7	Centroblastic-centrocytic	Intermediate	+ (R)	+ (R)	–	–	+	+/–	–	–
8	Immunoblastic	High	–	–	–	–	+	+/–	–	–
9	Immunoblastic	High	+ (R)	+ (R)	–	+/–	+	–	+/–	+

WF, Working formulation; R, reactive cells

structures, this being the preferred site in some published series [3]. This pattern was found in our patients, with single masses being seen for the first time shortly after the onset of symptoms; the midline structures were involved in six of them. The neuroradiological investigations are often inconclusive even though contrast enhancement can be observed in more than 90% of the lesions according to Hocberg and Miller [4], and was in fact observed in all our cases. T1- and T2-weighted MRI studies have shown few advantages over CT in differentiating PIML from other neoplastic and non-neoplastic lesions [1]. As to the histological classification, we observed no low grade lymphomas but only intermediate grade (3 centroblastic-centrocytic, 1 lymphoplasmacytoid polymorphic) and high grade (3 immunoblastic, 2 lymphoblastic). This distribution of the histological types has also been observed by others, the high grade lymphomas prevailing in most series [5]. As for the immunophenotyping results, only a few studies have been published in which monoclonal antibodies reactive with paraffin-embedded tissue have been used [6]. In our hands this panel of antibodies gave good results even though in some cases the stain was rather pale and difficult to interpret; one case was completely negative, perhaps due to poor fixation. No correlation was found between neuroradiological findings and histology, nor between histological type and duration of the radiological follow-up. In particular, no relationship was found between histological type and precontrast tumour density or propensity to contact ependyma. These findings are in agreement with those of others [7] even though a longer survival time (mean, 2 years) has been reported in low-grade lymphoplasmacytoid tumours [8].

References

1. Schwaighofer BW, Hesselink JR, Press GA, Wolf RL, Healy ME, Berthoty DP (1989) Primary intracranial CNS lymphoma: MR manifestations. AJNR 10: 725–729
2. Poon T, Matoso L, Tchertkoff V, Weitzner I, Gade M (1989) CT features of primary cerebral lymphoma in AIDS and non-AIDS patients. J Comput Assist Tomogr 13: 6–9
3. Bonnin JM, Garcia JH (1987) Primary malignant non-Hodgkin's lymphoma of the central nervous system. Pathol Annu 22: 353–375
4. Hocberg FH, Miller DC (1988) Primary central nervous system lymphoma. J Neurosurg 68: 835–853
5. Merkel KHH, Hansmann ML (1986) Primary non-Hodgkin's lymphomas of the central nervous system. Pathol Res Pract 181: 430–433
6. Murphy JK, O'Brien CS, Ironside JW (1989) Morphologic and immunophenotypic characterization of primary brain lymphomas using paraffin-embedded tissue. Histopathology 15: 449–460
7. Jack CR, O'Neill BP, Banks PM, Reese DF (1988) Central nervous system lymphoma: histologic types and CT appearance. Radiology 167: 211–215
8. Allegranza A, Mariani C, Giardini R, Brambilla MC, Boeri R (1984) Primary malignant lymphomas of the central nervous system: a histological and immunohistological study of 12 cases. Histopathology 8: 781–791

U. Salvolini
Neuroradiologia
Ospedale Nuovo di Torrette
I-60020 Torrette
Ancona, Italy

Neuroradiology (1991) 33 [Suppl]: 331–332

Neuro radiology
© Springer-Verlag 1991

CT and MRI scans in thoracic intradural disc herniation

H. J. Robertson, R. M. Menoni, C. N. Aprill, and R. D. Smith

Departments of Radiology and Neurosurgery, Charity Hospital of New Orleans and
Louisiana State University and Tulane University Schools of Medicine, New Orleans, Louisiana, USA

Summary. Thoracic intradural disc herniation is rare and difficult to diagnose clinically and radiologically. Axial CT myelography and MRI may show a typical complex intrathecal mass consisting of the spinal cord displaced by the disc fragment and one or more adjacent bands extending to the anterior dural surface. Calcified disc fragments may be more easily detectable by CT than by MRI.

Key words: Disc herniation – Thoracic – Intradural – Computed tomography – Magnetic resonance imaging

Symptomatic thoracic intervertebral disc herniation is uncommon and difficult to diagnose clinically [1]. Referred pain may simulate gall bladder disease, peptic ulcer, pancreatitis or cardiac ischemia. Findings may suggest spinal cord tumor, herpes zoster or multiple sclerosis [2]. Thoracic intradural disc herniation is rare and often presents with myelopathy. Radiological studies, particularly CT myelography and MRI are essential in the diagnosis of intradural thoracic disc herniation.

Case reports

Case 1

A 68-year-old woman with rheumatoid arthritis had onset of bilateral lower extremity weakness and paresthesiae progressing to paraplegia with urinary retention. She had leg weakness with absent reflexes and diminished leg vibration and position sensation. There was a lower thoracic scoliosis with localized spinal tenderness. T11 and T12 laminectomies were performed with removal of extra- and intradural disc fragments. Postoperatively pain was relieved and the patient was continent and walking with assistance (Fig. 1 A–D).

Case 2

A 63-year-old female had thoracic and low back pain after a fall. The pain persisted after L4–5 discectomy. An extradural disc herniation was detected at T9–10 level by MRI and was removed via costotransversectomy. CT myelography and MRI later showed a calcified intradural disc fragment at T9–10 level. The fragment was removed by anterolateral thoracotomy approach. Postoperatively there was persistent pain in the lower thoracic and lumbar spine and legs (Fig. 2 A–D).

Discussion

Fewer than 1% of all surgical procedures for herniated disc are thoracic [1]. Two autopsy studies have shown, however, that some thoracic disc herniation is common, occurring in 15%–63% of individuals [3]. Seventy-five percent of disc herniations occur below T8 level, with 25% at T11–12 disc level. Ninety percent of patients have a prolonged history, associated with antecedent trauma in only 20% [2]. Chest pain with weakness and sensory deficit in the legs are common presenting symptoms. Decreased leg reflexes and vibration sense and localized spinal tenderness are frequent physical findings [2, 4, 5].

The herniation of disc material into the subdural space is believed to occur after adhesion formation between the posterior spinal ligament and the adjacent anterior dural surface [6]. Only 11 case reports of thoracic intradural disc herniation are found in the medical literature [3–12]. The intradural disc fragment may be sealed within the meninges by scar and can be overlooked unless detected by preoperative radiological studies.

Thoracic spine radiographs in thoracic disc herniation may show a narrow disc space, disc calcification or vacuum phenomenon and scoliosis. Calcification within the spinal canal is common in thoracic disc herniation but is found also in meningioma and osteochondroma [9, 13]. Myelography shows an anterior extradural defect at the intervertebral disc level. The severely displaced spinal cord and adjacent disc fragment may simulate intradural extramedullary tumor in the event of intradural disc herniation. CT after myelography provides the most useful specific diagnostic demonstration of intradural disc herniation. In addition to the extradural disc herniation there is a complex intrathecal mass outlined by the contrast medium. There are one or more bands of tissue between the anterior thecal surface and the posteriorly displaced spinal cord and intradural disc fragment. Such bands are probably due to ventral nerve roots, disc fragments and adhesive fibrous bands.

Similar findings occur on axial MRI but a calcified disc fragment can be overlooked on T1-weighted images where calcium and spinal fluid have similar signal intensities. Multisequence MRI with sagittal and axial T1- and T2-weighted images is necessary for identification of intradural calcified disc fragments [14].

References

1. Hochman MS, Pena C, Ramirez R (1980) Calcified herniated thoracic disc diagnosed by computerized tomography. J Neurosurg 52: 722–723
2. Arce CA, Dohrmann GJ (1985) Herniated thoracic disks. Neurol Clin 3: 383–392

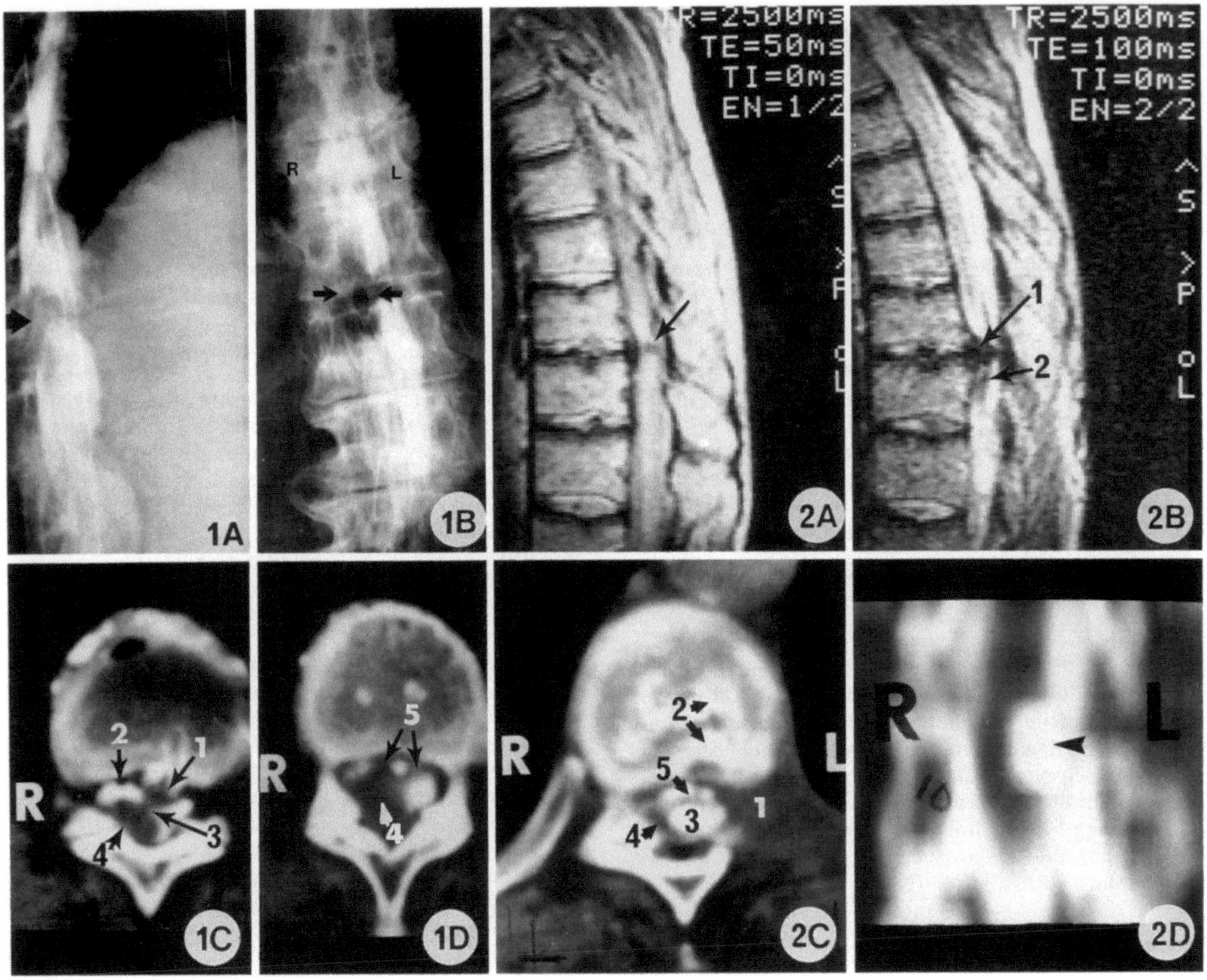

Fig. 1 A–D. Case 1. **A** Metrizamide myelogram with an apparent posterior intradural mass *(arrow)*. **B** Widened conus medullaris *(arrows)* with an oval herniated disc fragment outlined by intradural metrizamide. **C, D** CT post myelogram showing: (1) extradural disc herniation adjacent to spondylosis; (2) extradural gas bubble extruded from disc nucleus; (3) neck of the intradural disc fragment; (4) apparent intradural extramedullary mass from displaced spinal cord and intradural disc fragment; (5) attached complex bands

Fig. 2 A–D. Case 2. **A** MR1 sagittal spin density image with low signal intensity intradural calcified disc fragment *(arrow)*. **B** Sagittal T2-weighted image with: extradural and intradural disc herniation; displaced spinal cord. **C** CT scan post Omnipaque myelogram showing: (1) edema and scar from left costotransversectomy; (2) T9–10 disc calcifications; (3) large intradural calcified disc fragment; (4) displaced spinal cord; (5) complex bands. **D** Computer coronal reformatted image showing the large oval-shaped calcified intradural disc fragment *(arrow)*

3. Tovi D, Strang RR (1960) Thoracic intervertebral disk protrusions. Acta Chir Scand [Suppl] 267: 1–41
4. Love JG, Schorn VG (1965) Thoracic-disc protrusions. JAMA 191: 91–95
5. Benson MKD, Byrnes DP (1975) The clinical syndromes and surgical treatment of thoracic intervertebral disc prolapse. J Bone Joint Surg [Br] 57: 471–477
6. Chowdary UM (1987) Intradural thoracic disc protrusion. Spine 12: 718–719
7. Fisher RG (1965) Protrusions of thoracic disc. The factor of herniation through the dura mater. J Neurosurg 22: 591–593
8. Jefferson A (1975) The treatment of thoracic intervertebral disc protrusions. Clin Neurol Neurosurg 78: 1–9
9. McAllister VL, Sage MR (1976) The radiology of thoracic disc protrusion. Clin Radiol 27: 291–299
10. Patterson RH, Arbit E (1978) A surgical approach through the pedicle to protruded thoracic discs. J Neurosurg 48: 768–772
11. Besel R von, Pothe H (1980) Intradurale Sequestrierung von Diskusprolapsen. Beitr Orthop Traumatol 27: 107–111
12. Wang A, Zamani AA (1986) Intradural herniation of thoracic disc: CT metrizamide myelography. Comput Radiol 10: 115–118
13. Baker HL Jr, Love JG, Uihlein A (1965) Roentgenologic features of protruded thoracic intervertebral disks. Radiology 84: 1059–1065
14. Ross JS, Perez-Reyes N, Masaryk RTJ, Bohlman H, Modic MT (1987) Thoracic disk herniation: MR imaging. Radiology 165: 511–515

Dr. Hugh J. Robertson
Department of Radiology
Louisiana State University School of Medicine
1542 Tulane Avenue
New Orleans, LA 70112, USA

Neuroradiology (1991) 33 [Suppl]: 333–334

Neuro radiology
© Springer-Verlag 1991

Intramedullary change on MRI in cervical spondylotic myelopathy: clinical significance

D. C. Reutens[1], J. S. Adler[2], M. S. Khangure[2], and J. W. Dunne[1]

[1] Department of Neurology, Royal Perth Hospital, Perth, Western Australia
[2] Magnetic Resonance Imaging Unit, QE II Medical Centre, Perth, Western Australia

Summary. The clinical, radiological and electrophysiological features of 15 patients with intramedullary high signal intensity on spin-echo T2-weighted MRI scans and cervical spondylotic myelopathy were reviewed. Intramedullary change was present at the site of maximum cord deformity. A further examination was performed at a median interval of 7 months after surgical decompression in 10 patients. In 8, little or no improvement in symptoms had occurred. Signs of myelopathy persisted in all patients. Abnormal central somatosensory conduction was present in all patients so studied after operation. Of nine postoperative studies, seven showed persistent intramedullary change. In 2 patients the T2 changes had resolved; symptoms had not improved in 1 and sensory disturbance persisted in the other. These results suggest that the response to decompressive surgery is likely to be incomplete in patients with intramedullary change.

Key words: Cervical spondylosis – Myelopathy – Magnetic resonance imaging

Cervical spondylotic myelopathy (CSM) is a common disabling condition. Only some patients benefit from decompressive surgery and reliable predictors of surgical response would be invaluable, particularly in the elderly, high-risk surgical candidate.

Although irreversible pathological changes in the spinal cord correlate with reduction in the ratio of anteroposterior to transverse cord diameter [1], the measurement of cord dimensions on CT seems to be of limited value in predicting surgical outcome [2]. Reports of intramedullary change on T2-weighted MRI in CSM prompted this study of its clinical and prognostic significance.

Patients and methods

Ten males and 5 females, aged from 40 to 85 years, with CSM and intramedullary change on T2-weighted MRI were included in the study. A detailed clinical assessment was performed and their medical records reviewed. MRI was undertaken on a 1.5T system using a standard spin-echo technique. All images were obtained using a 200-mm field of view on a 256 × 256 matrix (slice thickness 4 or 5 mm). T2 sequences were obtained with cardiac gating, flow compensation, a TR of 2 s and TE of 25 and 100 ms (two measurements).

Clinical and MRI examinations were repeated at a median interval of 7 months after surgical decompression; somatosensory evoked potential examination was performed in 4 patients.

Results

The clinical features at presentation are detailed in Table 1. The average duration of symptoms was 20 months (range, 2 weeks to 6 years). Nine patients reported impairment of activities of daily living with upper limb functional disability in 7, mild impairment of mobility in 5 and severe limitation in 2, who required wheelchairs.

High signal was present on T2 images at 18 disc levels in 15 patients (Table 2). It occurred most commonly at C4–5 and C3–4 levels and corresponded with the site of maximal cord flattening.

Cervical laminectomy was performed in 8 patients and anterior decompression and fusion in 2. Symptoms persisted after operation in 9 patients; 6 reported no improvement. Signs of myelopathy were present in all 10 patients; pyramidal tract signs in 9 and lower limb sensory disturbance in 1. Six patients reported persistent functional dis-

Table 1. Clinical data at preoperative examination

Symptoms	No. of patients		
Neck pain		7	
Lhermitte's phenomenon		6	
Upper limb symptoms	Sensory 13		Motor 9
Radicular pain		4	
Lower limb symptoms	Sensory 8		Motor 5
Gait disturbance		12	
Sphincteric symptoms		5	
Neurological signs			
Upper limbs			
Spasticity		6	
Weakness		13	
Radicular sensory loss		2	
Lower limbs			
Spastic paraparesis		9	
Hyper-reflexia only		6	
Gait abnormality		5	
Sensory abnormality		7	

Table 2. Level of intramedullary high signal and cord flattening

Level	Cord indentation (Mean AP cord diameter)	Intramedullary high signal
C 2–3.	1	–
C 3–4.	10 (7 mm)	7
C 4–5.	13 (6.5 mm)	9
C 5–6.	12 (6.3 mm)	2
C 6–7.	5	–

AP, Anteroposterior

ability and, in the 4 patients studied postoperatively, central somatosensory conduction was abnormal.

One patient refused postoperative MRI examination. In the remaining 9, adequate decompression was confirmed. High-signal intensity on T2 images was present in 7 cases. Of the 2 patients with resolution of the intramedullary change, 1 had gained no relief from surgery. Sensory disturbance in the lower limbs persisted in the other.

Discussion

Increasingly used in the investigation of cervical myelopathy, MRI provides accurate anatomical images, often eliminating the need for myelograms and CT [3]. Intramedullary high signal on T2-weighted MRI, corresponding to the level of cord compression in CSM is well described [4–8]. Although its pathophysiological basis has not been clarified, it probably reflects cord ischaemia or gliosis, sometimes with associated oedema.

In this study, the presence of intramedullary high signal was associated with an incomplete response to surgery when patients were assessed several months after operation. Takahashi et al. [7] noted that the frequency of this finding was proportional to the clinical and radiological severity of cord compression and also correlated with a poor response to surgery. Similarly, Mehalic et al. [8] found that patients with a mild or moderate abnormality on preoperative T2-weighted image responded poorly to surgery. Those with an intense T2 signal seemed to fare better; the MRI appearance presumably related to an active and reversible process such as inflammation or oedema.

The results of our pilot study are only tentative as only a small number of patients, without a comparison group free of T2 changes, was studied. Further prospective analysis of the correlation between preoperative MRI appearance and response to surgical or conservative treatment in CSM is required. Consideration of the relative intensity of increased T2 signal, subtypes of T2 changes suggestive of cystic necrosis [6] and cord dimension may increase prognostic accuracy. Gradient-echo imaging in the axial plane at the affected level would provide such information with reasonable spatial resolution and without requiring excessive examination time.

References

1. Ogino H, Tada K, Okada K, Yonenobu K, Yamamoto T, Ono K, Namiki H (1983) Canal diameter, anteroposterior compression ratio and spondylotic myelopathy of the cervical spine. Spine 8: 1–15
2. Yu YL, du Boulay GH, Stevens JM, Kendall BE (1986) Computed tomography in cervical spondylotic myelopathy and radiculopathy: visualisation of structures, myelographic comparison, cord measurements and clinical utility. Neuroradiology 28: 221–236
3. Masaryk TJ, Modic MT, Geisinger MA, Standefer J, Hardy RW, Boumphrey F, Duchesneau PM (1986) Cervical myelopathy: a comparison of magnetic resonance and myelography. J Comput Assist Tomogr 10: 184–194
4. Takahashi M, Sakamoto Y, Miyawaki M, Bussaka H (1987) Increased MR signal intensity secondary to chronic cervical cord compression. Neuroradiology 29: 550–556
5. Ramanauskas WL, Wilner HI, Meter JJ, Lazo A, Kelly JK (1989) MR imaging of compressive myelomalacia. J Comput Assist Tomogr 13: 399–404
6. Al-Mefty O, Harkey LH, Middleton TH, Smith RR, Fox JL (1988) Myelopathic cervical spondylotic lesions demonstrated by magnetic resonance imaging. J Neurosurg 68: 217–222
7. Takahashi M, Yamashita Y, Sakamoto Y, Kojima R (1989) Chronic cervical cord compression: clinical significance of increased signal intensity on MR images. Radiology 173: 219–224
8. Mehalic TF, Pezzuti RT, Applebaum BI (1990) Magnetic resonance imaging and cervical spondylotic myelopathy. Neurosurgery 26: 217–227

M. S. Khangure
Magnetic Resonance Imaging Unit
QE II Medical Centre
Perth, 6009 Western Australia

Neuroradiology (1991) 33 [Suppl]: 335–336

Neuro radiology
© Springer-Verlag 1991

Accuracy of MRI in cervical disc herniation

J. Assheuer[1], E. Volle[2], W. Köning[3], and J.-P. Hedde[2]

[1] MRI Unit, Cologne-Mülheim,
[2] Division of Neuroradiology and [3] Department of Neurosurgery, Cologne-Merheim, Federal Republic of Germany

Summary. Sixty-four patients were examined by MRI for cervical myelopathy and radiculopathy. Magnetic resonance images, if the correct sequences were used, gave accurate results as judged by surgical findings, but tended to overestimate the degree of abnormality.

Key words: Cervical disc herniation – MRI

From 1988 to 1989, 64 patients were examined by MRI for cervical radiculopathy or myelopathy. Sixteen have undergone surgical treatment. The purpose of this investigation was to compare the reliability of MRI with the surgical findings with emphasis on the posterior longitudinal ligament.

Materials and methods

A 1.0 T Picker Vista 2055 HP MR Imager was employed using a surface coil. Field-gradient echo sequences with phase contrast (TR 400–600, TE 10) were used for all patients.

Spin echo T1-weighted SE (500–700, TE 20) and T2-weighted (TR 1600/60) sequences were employed on 40 patients. Short time inversion recovery STIR (TR 1600 TI 125) sequences were used on 14 patients.

Slice thicknesses of 2–3.5 mm were chosen for sagittal, transverse and coronal planes. Field of view of 27 cm and matrix of 256 × 256 were standard, with 2 to 4 averages.

Discussion

The accuracy of MRI diagnosis in cervical disc disease is mainly dependent on the chosen acquisition parameters. There is no standard sequence for all different pathological changes.

For fibrous tissues PS sequences with phase contrast give more signal than SE sequences [1]. Difficulties still exist in distinguishing between structures such as dura mater, epidural veins, fatty tissue, posterior longitudinal ligament and annulus fibrosus.

The epidural venous plexus is highlighted due to slow blood flow or stagnant blood [2].

The medial band of high intensity can also be due to changes in the water content [3].

In the transverse section the interruption of the small retrodiscal band with intermediate signal (PS) is a reliable sign for perforation of the posterior longitudinal ligament.

The condition of the posterior longitudinal ligament was correctly described in 6 of 7 patients with surgically proven sequestration.

One false negative result was due to poor image quality caused by motion artefacts.

Overestimation of protrusion (2 protrusions converted to herniation, 1 protrusion converted to sequestra-

Table 1. Patients examined

	No.	Radicular symptoms	Cord symptoms	Surgical treatment
Males	43	40	3	12[a]
Females	21	19	2	4
Total	64	59	5	16

Mean age females: 48.1
Mean age males: 50.7
[a] Two males had operations at two levels

Table 2. Localisation of disc disease for all patients and for the 16 operated ones (MRI findings)

	C3–4		C4–5		C5–6		C6–7		C7–T1	
	a	b	a	b	a	b	a	b	a	b
Bulging	2	1	1	0	2	1	3	0	0	0
Protrusion	6	3	7	0	16	5	12	3	0	0
Herniation	0	0	4	1	14	4	7	1	1	1
Sequestration	2	2	1	0	8	2	14	5	1	1
Total	10	6	13	1	40	12	36	0	2	2

76% of disc lesions were found at the C5–6 and C6–7 levels, 50% of sequestrations were located at the C6–7 level.
[a] All patients
[b] Operated patients

Table 3. Accompanying pathological changes related to the different disc diseases at the same level (MRI findings)

	Bulging		Protrusion		Herniation		Sequestration	
	a	b	a	b	a	b	a	b
Perforation of posterior longitudinal ligament					5		14	3
Impingement	1	1	20	7	14	1	4	4
Compression					12	2	22	7
Osteophyte	1	1	36	8	24	4	24	5

85% of pathological changes are combined spondylotic and discogenic
[a] All patients
[b] Operated patients

Table 4. Localisation of perforation of the posterior longitudinal ligament for all patients and for the 16 operated ones (MRI findings)

	C3–4 a	C3–4 b	C4–5 a	C4–5 b	C5–6 a	C5–6 b	C6–7 a	C6–7 b	C7–T1 a	C7–T1 b
Perforation of posterior longitudinal ligament	1	1	0	0	7	0	10	2	1	0

90% of perforations are located at the C5-6 and C6-7 levels.
[a] All patients
[b] Operated patients

Table 5. Comparison of MRI diagnosis and surgical findings

Surgical findings	No.	MRI finding	No.
Protrusion	1	Protrusion + osteophyte	1
Protrusion + osteophyte	8	Protrusion + osteophyte	4
		Herniation + osteophyte	2
		Sequestration + osteophyte	1
		Osteophyte	1
Sequestration	4	Sequestration	3
		Sequestration + osteophyte	1
Sequestration + osteophyte	3	Sequestration + osteophyte	2
		Sequestration	1
Osteophyte	2	Osteophyte	2
Total	18	Total	18

Excellent correlation between surgical findings an MRI diagnosis. MRI seems to overestimate the lesions slightly

tion) is probably due to difficult discrimination between annulus tissue and thickened epidural fibrous tissue and/or false slice selection.

It is known that X-ray procedures are more suitable for description of spondylotic disorders.

Combination of both methods, MRI and plain X-ray, will give sufficient information in diagnosis of degenerative disc disease [4].

Conclusions

MRI is the method of choice for investigation of cervical disc disease. The relevant lesion is detected more easily than with other imaging modalities. Perforations of the posterior longitudinal ligament can be detected. MRI leads one to overestimate lesions.

References

1. Assheuer J, Lenz G, Gottschlich KW, Schulitz KP (1987) Fett-/Wassertrennung im Kernspintomogramm. Fortschr Röntgenstr 147: 58–63
2. Flannigan BD, Lufkin RB, McGlade C, Winter J, Batzdorf U, Wilson G, Rauschning W, Bradley WG Jr (1987) MR imaging of cervical spine. Neurovascular anatomy. AJR 148: 785–790
3. McCarron RF, Wimpee MW, Hudkins PG, Laros GS (1987) The inflammatory effect of nucleus pulposus. Spine 12: 760–764
4. Larsson EM, Holtas S, Cronqvist S, Brandt L (1989) Comparison of myelography, CT myelography and magnetic resonance imaging in cervical spondylosis and disc herniation. Acta Radiol 30: 233–239

Dr. Josef Assheuer
MRI-Unit
Department of Neurosurgery
Genovevastrasse 24
W-5000 Köln-Merheim
Federal Republic of Germany

Neuroradiology (1991) 33 [Suppl]: 337–339

Neuro-radiology
© Springer-Verlag 1991

Comparison of MRI, CT and myelography in the diagnosis of lumbar disc disease

K. Yoshizumi[1], Y. Sakamoto[1], Y. Korogi[1], J. Shinzato[1], H. Bussaka[1], T. Sakae[2], and M. Takahashi[1]

[1] Department of Radiology, Kumamoto University School of Medicine, Kumamoto, Japan
[2] Kumamoto Orthopaedic Hospital, Kumamoto, Japan

Summary. The records of 96 herniated lumbar discs of 94 patients were retrospectively analysed as to the diagnostic accuracy of MRI, myelography and CT myelography. Myelography and CT myelography were able to show certain associated findings, especially nerve root compression, but overall diagnostic accuracy of MRI was better than that of myelography and CT myelography.

Key words: Herniated disc – Magnetic resonance imaging – Computed tomography – Myelography

Because of its numerous advantages, MRI has been used widely for the diagnosis of lumbar disc disease. Since myelography and CT myelography (CTM) have also been used in conjuction with MRI, the comparative value of MRI, CTM and myelography has been assessed in the diagnosis of lumbar disc disease.

Materials and methods

MRI was performed on two 0.5T superconductive MRI units (Philips, Gyroscan T5 and S5). Spin echo (SE) pulse sequences TR 400 ms/TE 30 ms for T1-weighted images and TR 1400–2100 ms/TE 30–100 ms for proton- and T2-weighted images. Surface coils were used with a slice thickness of 6 mm or 8 mm with a gap of 1.8 or 0.8 mm, respectively. Both sagittal and transverse views were obtained with SE techniques and transverse views were occasionally obtained using the gradient-echo technique.

Myelography was performed in a routine manner with lumbar injection of nonionic contrast medium. CTM followed 1–3 h after myelography.

In 94 patients the images and records of 96 lesions, which were surgically proven to be lumbar disc herniations, were retrospectively analysed as to the presence of protruded disc material, loss of epidural fat, dural sac compression, nerve root compression and other associated disc and ligamentous changes on MRI, myelography and CTM.

The criteria used for MRI, myelography and CTM were as described by Maravilla et al. [1] and Fagerlund and Thelander [2].

Results

Positive findings

MRI, myelography and CTM provided equal diagnostic information in 51 cases, whereas myelography and CTM yielded information additional to that given by MRI in 29 cases. MRI showed more information than myelography and CTM in 12 cases (Table 1).

MRI was sensitive to some pathological changes, especially protrusion of the disc, loss of the epidural fat and dural sac compression (Fig. 1). Myelography and CTM were useful for nerve root compression, demonstration of a herniated disc margin and a calcified disc.

Since 2 patients with severe pain could not lie still, MR images failed to show the lesion, due to motion artefacts. Three migrated discs were shown better by sagittal MR images than by other procedures.

Discrepancies between the diagnoses of MRI, myelography and CTM

False-negative diagnoses with MRI were encountered less frequently than false-negative diagnoses with CTM and myelography.

Table 1. Summary of demonstration of findings by MRI versus myelography and CT myelography (CTM)

1. MRI, myelography and CTM yielded equal information	51 cases
2. Myelography and CTM yielded additional information	29 cases
root compression	15
herniated disc margin	8
calcified disc	4
MRI failed due to motion artefact	2
3. MRI yielded additional information	12 cases
identified disc herniation missed on both myelography and CTM	6
suggestive root compression missed on myelography or CTM	2
estimated true herniated disc extension	3
herniated disc margin	1
	Total 92 cases

Table 2. Comparison of diagnostic accuracy between MRI and myelography, and between MRI and CT myelography

		Normal disc	Bulging disc	Herniated disc	Total
MRI	Normal disc	0[a]/0[b]	0/0	0/ 0	0/ 0
	Bulging disc	0/1	2/1	1/ 1	3/ 3
	Herniated disc	4/0	11/8	76/83	91/91
	Total	4/1	13/9	77/84	94/94

[a] MRI vs myelography
[b] MRI vs CT myelography

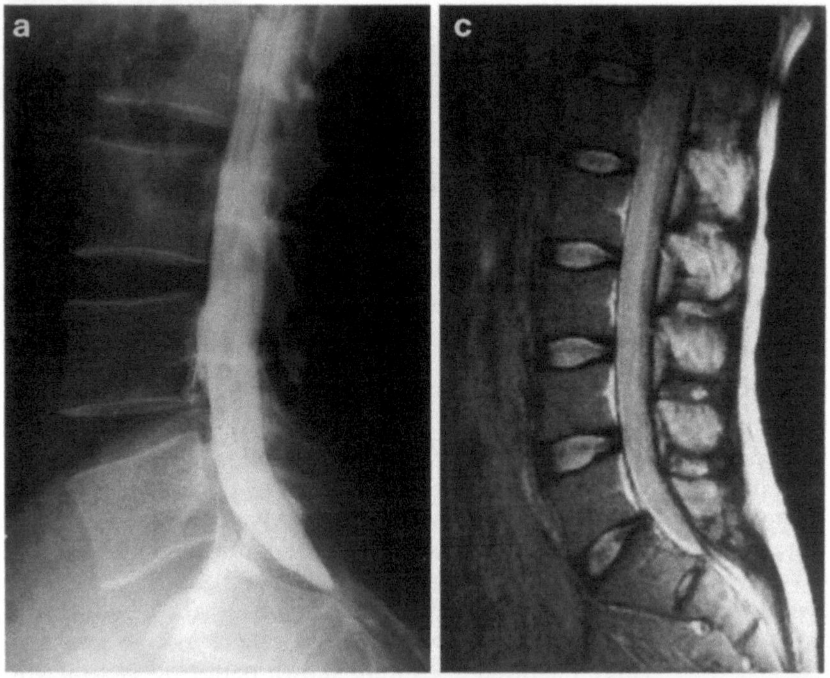

Fig. 1 a–d. A 42-year-old male with right sciatica. **a** Myelogram, lateral projection. No abnormal findings were noted on any films. **b** CT myelogram, L5–S1 level. Bulging is seen with displacement of the right S1 nerve root. No definite herniation is observed. **c** T2-weighted image, sagittal view. There is a small protrusion of disc material at L5–S1. **d** T2-weighted image, transverse view. Very small focal disc herniation is identified, slightly to the right of the midline displacing the right S1 nerve root *(arrow)*

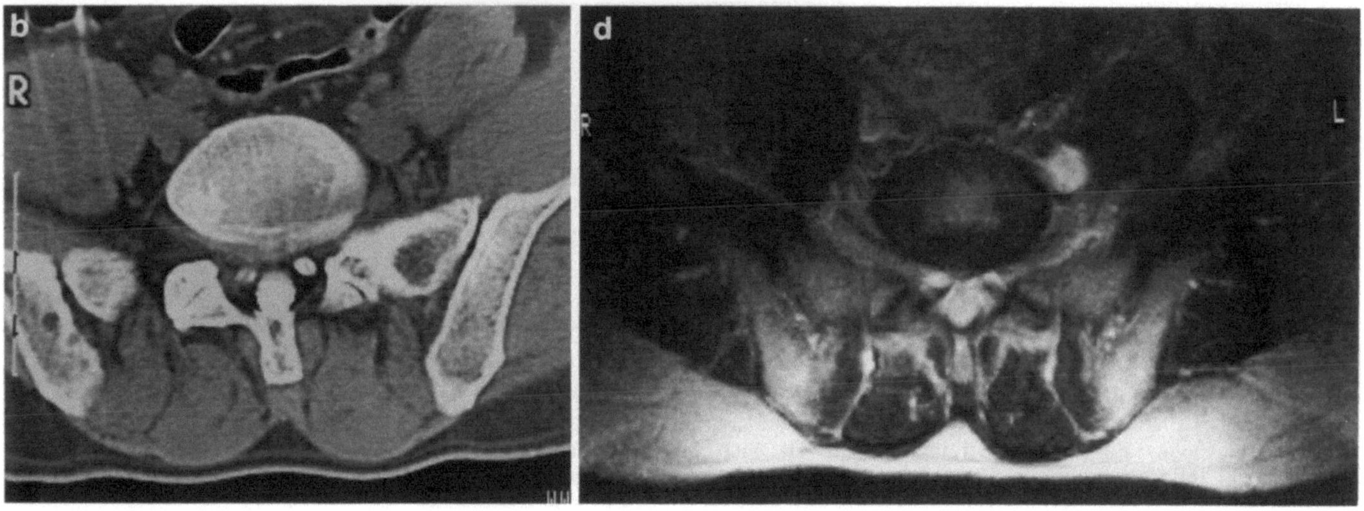

When diagnostic accuracy was compared between MRI and myelography, herniated disc was correctly diagnosed by MRI more often than myelography, which provided findings interpreted as normal or bulging discs in some cases (Table 2).

CTM also had a similar tendency, but 9 cases were diagnosed as a disc bulge by CTM. There were only 3 cases diagnosed as a bulging disc by MRI (Table 2).

Discussion

The advantages of MRI in lumbar disc disease are numerous, including good contrast resolution, direct multiplanar imaging and absence of ionizing radiation. In addition, sagittal MR images directly delinate protruded discs. Because of these advantages, it has been proposed that MRI should replace, rather than supplement, myelography [3], while several authors have reported that the sensitivity of MRI for the diagnosis of herniated discs is equivalent to or better than that of myelography and CTM [1, 3–5]. In our study, MRI was more accurate for the diagnosis of herniated discs than myelography and CTM. False-negative diagnoses were least frequent with MRI.

We studied surgically proven cases only. Therefore, there were no false-positive cases. However, Boden et al. [6] reported frequent false-positive MRI diagnoses, associated with high sensitivity for herniated discs. Our study also showed subtle findings such as root compression and small herniated discs were occasionally missed by MRI, because its spatial resolution was inferior to that of CT. The use of thinner sections and the elimination of the interslice gap will improve the accuracy of MRI in defining herniated discs.

Myelography and CTM can demonstrate detail such as nerve root compression and calcification of disc material; however, MRI demonstrated herniated disc and disc extension to better advantage. The overall diagnostic accuracy was better for MRI than for myelography and CTM.

MRI should be the initial examination for the diagnosis of lumbar disc disease, and other modalities may not always be necessary, except when there is lack of correlation between the clinical and imaging findings.

References

1. Maravilla KR, Lesh P, Weinreb JC, Selby DK, Mooney V (1985) Magnetic resonance imaging of the lumbar spine with CT correlation. AJNR 6: 237–245
2. Fagerlund MKJ, Thelander UE (1989) Comparison of myelography and computed tomography in establishing lumbar disc herniation. Acta Radiol 30: 241–246
3. Weisz GM, Lamond TS, Kitchener PN (1988) Spinal imaging: will MRI replace myelography? Spine 13: 65–68
4. Modic MT, Masaryk T, Boumphrey F, Goormastic M, Bell G (1986) Lumbar herniated disk disease and canal stenosis: prospective evaluation by surface coil MR, CT and myelography. AJR 147: 757–765
5. Lukin RR, Gaskill MF, Wiot JG (1988) Lumbar herniated disk and related topics. Semin Roentgenol 23: 100–105
6. Boden SD, Davis DO, Dina TS, Patronas NJ, Wiesel SW (1990) Abnormal magnetic-resonance scans of the lumbar spine in asymptomatic subjects: a prospective investigation. J Bone Joint Surg [Am] 72: 403–408

K. Yoshizumi
Department of Radiology
Kumamoto University School of Medicine
Kumamoto, Japan

Neuroradiology (1991) 33 [Suppl]: 340–341

Neuro radiology
© Springer-Verlag 1991

The value of MRI in ossification of the posterior longitudinal ligament

H. Bussaka[1], K. Yoshizumi[1], Y. Sakamoto[1], Y. Korogi[1], J. Shinzato[1], K. Ito[1], Y. Yamashita[1], T. Sakae[2], and M. Takahashi[1]

[1] Department of Radiology, Kumamoto University School of Medicine, Kumamoto, Japan
[2] Kumamoto Orthopaedic Hospital, Kumamoto, Japan

Summary. One hundred and thirty-seven patients with ossification of the posterior longitudinal ligament (OPLL) were studied with MRI. The detectability of OPLL was greater on T2-weighted images than T1- or proton-density-weighted images. Intermediate or high signal was considered to be bone marrow produced in the ossification. Cord compression was often associated with high signal intensity. Disc degeneration was also frequently associated with OPLL. MRI was valuable in investigation of OPLL.

Key words: Ossification of the posterior longitudinal ligament – Magnetic resonance imaging – Cord compression

Ossification of the posterior longitudinal ligament (OPLL) is a frequent cause of spinal cord compression in Orientals: the incidence is reported to be 2.4% in Orientals and 0.16% in non-Orientals [1, 2].

We studied the detectability of and radiological findings in OPLL with MRI.

Patients and methods

One hundred and thirty-seven patients (105 men and 32 women, aged 19–76 years, mean 56.7 years) with OPLL diagnosed by CT and plain films were studied by MRI between June 1986 and December 1989. Cervical OPLL was divided into two types on plain radiography according to Seki's classification [3].

MRI was performed on a 0.5 T superconductive unit (Philips Gyroscan S5) in 88 patients and on a 0.22 T resistive unit (Toshiba MRT-22A) in 57. Images were obtained with spin-echo technique using 400–500/30–40 (TR ms/TE ms) sequences) for T1-weighted images, 1600–2000/40–50 sequences for proton-density-weighted images and 1600–2000/80–100 sequences for T2-weighted images. Slice thickness was 5 mm.

Compromise of the dural sac and the degree of cord compression were classified into four degrees on the basis of findings seen on T2-weighted images. The thickness (distance from the posterior edge of the vertebral body to the posterior edge of the main portion of the OPLL) was measured on axial CT and compared with MRI findings.

Results

Detectability

OPLL was recognised as increased distance between the posterior edge of the vertebral bone marrow and the spinal cord. The detectability of OPLL in each location and type is shown in Tables 1 and 2. T2-weighted images were superior for detecting the ossification. The continuous type was more easily recognised than the segmental type.

Table 1. Detectability of ossification of the posterior longitudinal ligament (OPLL) (0.5 T unit)

Pulse sequences	Cervical		Thoracic	Lumbar
	continuous $n = 32$	segmental $n = 48$	$n = 5$	$n = 3$
T1WSE sagittal	22 (68.8%)	18 (37.5%)	3	1
PDWSE sagittal	27 (84.4%)	31 (64.6%)	4	1
T2WSE sagittal	28 (87.5%)	33 (68.8%)	4	1
T2WSE axial	27 (84.4%)	34 (70.8%)	2	2

T1WSE, T1-weighted spin echo; PDWSE, proton-density-weighted spin echo; T2WSE, T2-weighted spin echo

Table 2. Detectability of OPLL (0.22 T unit)[a]

Pulse sequences	Cervical		Thoracic	Lumbar
	continuous $n = 27$	segmental $n = 27$	$n = 1$	$n = 2$
T1SE sagittal	18 (66.7%)	4 (14.8%)	0	0
PDWSE sagittal	22 (81.5%)	7 (25.9%)	1	0
T2WSE sagittal	21 (77.8%)	9 (33.3%)	1	0
T2WSE axial	14 (51.9%)	6 (22.2%)	0	0

[a] Three cases of cervical OPLL were studied with both units

Table 3. MRI findings in OPLL

MRI findings	Cervical		Thoracic	Lumbar
	continuous $n = 51$	segmental $n = 70$	$n = 6$	$n = 5$
Signal in ossification	31 (60.8%)	19 (27.1%)	1	1
Degree of cord compression				
0	3	15	3	1
1	18	32	1	3
2	16	9	2	1
3	10	13	0	0
Postoperative	4	1	0	0
High signal in cord on T2WSE	18 (35.3%)	20 (28.6%)	1	1
Disc degeneration				
None	20	25	4	0
mild	14	24	1	2
severe	17	21	1	3

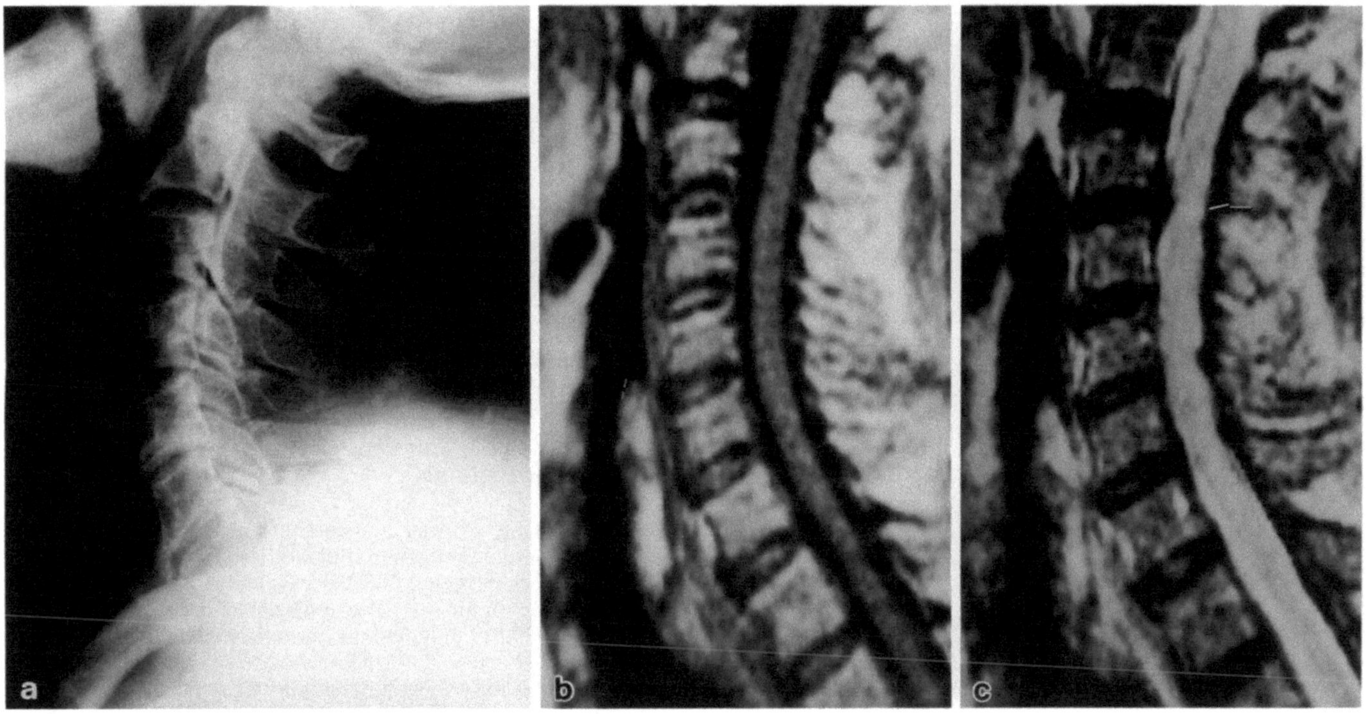

Fig. 1 a–c. A 75-year-old male with incomplete paralysis after a fall several weeks ago. **a** Lateral cervical spine. There is ossification of the posterior longitudinal ligament (OPLL) from C2 to C4. Increased distance is noted between the vertebral body and OPLL. **b** T1-weighted image. There is minimally increased distance from C2 to the upper portion of C4, but no definite cord compression. **c** T2-weighted image. There is high signal intensity within the spinal cord at C3–4 level with marked cord compression *(arrow)*

The average thickness of ossification positively detected on MRI was 5.41 ± 1.76 mm (mean ± SD), while the thickness was 2.80 ± 1.01 mm for cases undetected on MRI. Ossification of more than 3.2 mm was detected on T2-weighted images in 91.4%. Although images from the 0.5 T unit were superior to those from the 0.22 T unit, there was no apparent difference in OPLL detectability between them.

MRI appearance

MRI findings in OPLL are summarised in Table 3. Intermediate or high signal in ossification, considered to be bone marrow within the ossification, was observed in 60.8% or 31 cases of continuous cervical OPLL and 27.1% or 19 cases of segmental type.

Cord abnormality

Cord compression was more severe in the continuous type. Eighteen patients with continuous OPLL and 20 with segmental OPLL with cord compression showed increased signal in the cord on T2-weighted images (Fig. 1), associated with severe myelopathy.

Associated MRI findings

Disc degeneration was frequently associated with cervical OPLL. The degree of degeneration was almost equal in segmental and continuous types. Lumbar OPLL was also associated with lumbar disc disease.

Discussion

Although OPLL is not visualised on MRI, dural sac compression is clearly demonstrated on T2-weighted images. Signal is frequently observed within the continuous type of OPLL, and is considered to arise from bone marrow. The degree and the location of spinal cord compression are directly visualised, and high signal intensity on T2-weighted images correlates with the degree of myelopathy [4]. Cervical disc degeneration is frequently associated with cervical OPLL, and cervical disc herniation and spondylosis should be considered as the differential diagnosis.

References

1. Tsuyama N, Terayama K, Ohtani K (1981) The ossification of the posterior longitudinal ligament of the spine (OPLL). J Jpn Orthop Assoc 55: 425–440
2. Tsuyama N (1984) Ossification of the posterior longitudinal ligament of the spine. Clin Orthop 184: 71–84
3. Seki H (1974) Clinical study of 185 cases of ossification of posterior longitudinal ligament. Seikeigeka 25: 704–710
4. Takahashi M, Sakamoto Y, Miyawaki M (1987) Increased MR signal intensity secondary to chronic cervical cord compression. Neuroradiology 29: 550–556

Dr. H. Bussaka, Kumamoto University School of Medicine
1-1-1 Honjo, Kumamoto 860, Japan

Neuroradiology (1991) 33 [Suppl]: 342–344

Neuro radiology
© Springer-Verlag 1991

Failed back surgery syndrome: justification for reoperation based on clinical and CT/MRI findings

S. Trattnig[1], R. Stiglbauer[2], T. Czech[3], E. Schindler[3], and H. Imhof[2]

[1] Division of Diagnostic Radiology, 2nd Department of Medicine, [2] Central Institute of Radiodiagnosis,
[3] Clinics of Neurosurgery, University of Vienna, Vienna, Austria

Summary. The "failed back surgery syndrome" includes a variety of symptoms following disc surgery. In a prospective study 18 patients who met the criteria of the American Association of Neurological Surgeons (AANS) and American Academy of Orthopedic Surgeons (AAOS) for repeated lumbar spine surgery were examined by MRI and CT (before and after intravenous contrast medium). The findings were then compared with those at microsurgery. MRI produced correct diagnoses in 17 cases, CT in 13 cases. Recurrent disc herniation was responsible for the symptoms in 4 cases, epidural scar formation in 2. In 12 cases there was herniated disc material as well as epidural scar; disc material was preponderant 9 times, scar formation in 3 instances. Thus, MRI with i.v. gadolinium-DTPA appears to be most useful for the selection of patients who will benefit from repeated lumbar spine surgery, and superior to patient selection based upon the criteria of the AANS and AAOS.

Key words: Gadolinium – Magnetic resonance imaging – Contrast media – Spine – Intervertebral discs

The failed back surgery syndrome is characterized by intractable pain and/or varying degrees of neurological deficit after lumbar disc surgery. A prevalence of 10–40% of this syndrome has been reported [1–3]. In addition to bony stenosis and arachnoiditis, two of the more common causes of persistent symptoms are epidural fibrosis and recurrent or persistent disc herniation [1, 4]. Since reoperation on scar without disc material leads to poor surgical results, the differentiation of epidural fibrosis from herniated disc is essential [2, 3, 5]. We have included in this study only patients who met the criteria of the American Association of Neurological Surgeons (AANS) and the American Academy of Orthopedic Surgeons (AAOS) for justification of surgery prior to original operation [6] and who met these criteria completely prior to the second or third operation, with neurological deficits at the same lumbar level and side. The aim of our study was to compare the foregoing clinical criteria for reoperation with analysis of CT and MRI with iv contrast medium and with surgical findings.

Patients and methods

Eighteen patients (10 male, 8 female), ranging in age from 19 to 71 years (mean, 42 years), were studied. They met the criteria of the AANS and AAOS: monoradicular pain and monoradicular reflex, sensory and/or motor loss. The radicular pain and neurological deficit corresponded to typical nerve root compression at the same lumbar segment and on the same side as before operation. This was the justification for a second operation in 15 patients and a third operation in 3. The interval from previous surgery varied from 3 months to 23 years (mean, 3.5 years). The operated lumbar segments were L5-S1 in 9 patients, L4–5 in 8, and L3–4 in 1 patient. CT examinations were performed with a third-generation scanner (Somatom DR 3, Siemens, Matrix 512/512, scanning time 4.5 s). After a scout view, 2-mm-thick transverse contiguous sections were obtained through the level of the previously resected disc from posterior arch to posterior arch, angled to the disc, before and after injection of non-ionic contrast media (Iopamidol 300, Gerot) at a dose of 1 mg/kg body weight. MRI was performed with a 1.5T superconducting unit (Magnetom 63, Siemens, Matrix: 256/256) using an oval surface coil. The first sections were obtained using a T1-weighted spin-echo sequence [repetition time (TR) ms/echo time (TE) ms = 700/15] with four excitations in the sagittal plane in 3-mm sections from intervertebral foramen to intervertebral foramen and in the transverse plane through the operated level. After injection of gadolinium (Gd), T1-weighted sequences in the sagittal/parasagittal and axial/paraxial planes were performed.

Table 1. Comparison of surgical (histological) diagnosis with CT and MRI findings ($n = 18$)

	Disc	Epidural fibrosis	Disc and epidural fibrosis
Surgical diagnosis	4	2	12
CT = MRI	3	1	8
CT > MRI	1	0	0
CT < MRI	0	1	4

Table 2. Patients with both disc and epidural fibrosis

	a) Disc > epidural fibrosis	b) epidural fibrosis > disc
Surgical diagnosis	9	3
CT = MRI	4	1
CT > MRI	0	0
CT < MRI	5	2

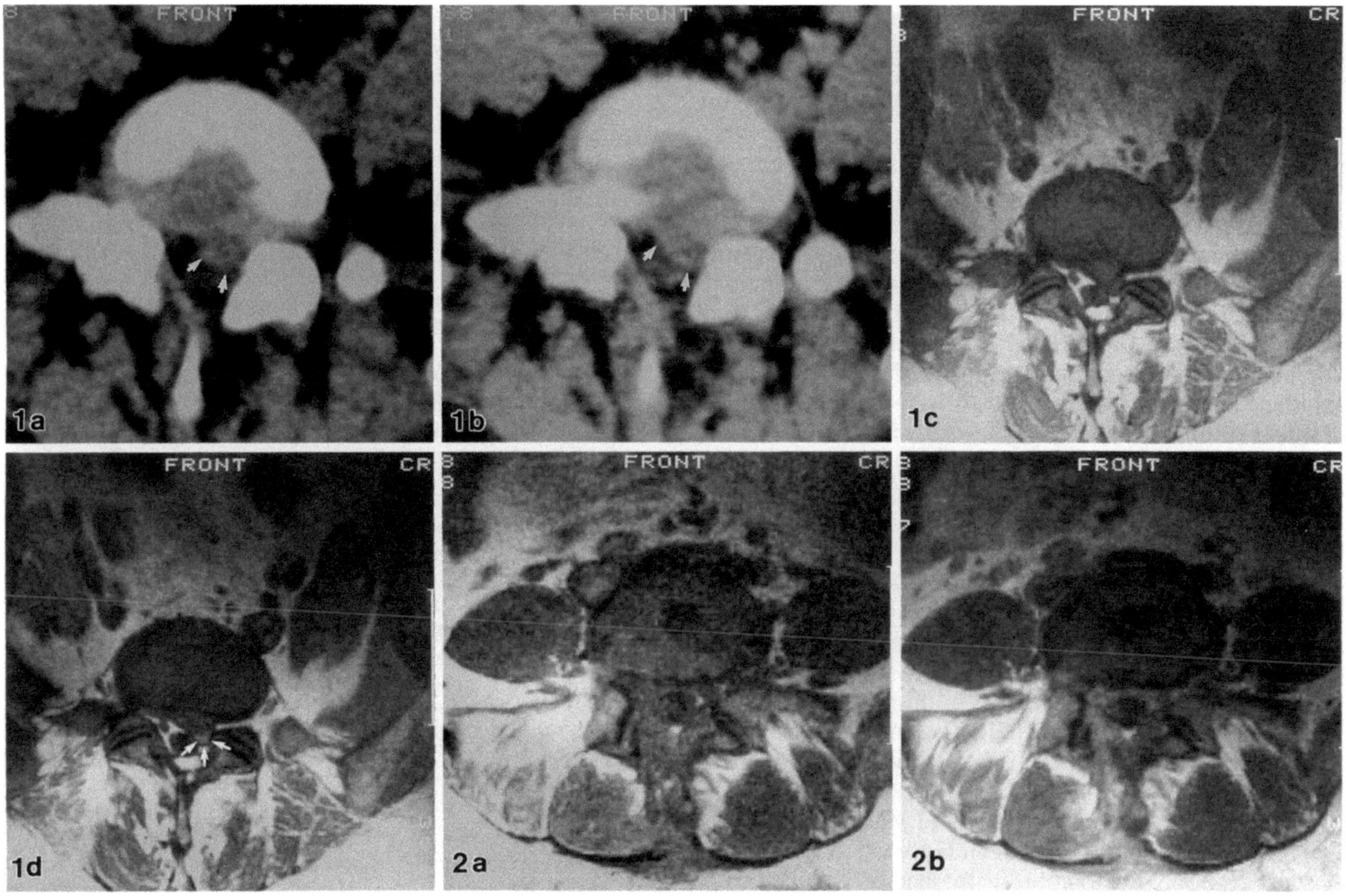

Fig. 1 a–d. A 36-year-old female patient with a left S1 radiculopathy who underwent laminectomy and discectomy at the L5–S1 level 18 months previously. **a** High-resolution CT shows nodular, hyperdense epidural soft tissue contiguous with the L5-S1 intervertebral disc *(arrows)*. **b** On post-contrast CT the abnormal epidural tissue shows no contrast enhancement. CT diagnosis: recurrent or persistent disc at L5–S1. **c** MRI demonstrates a large amount of pathological soft tissue contiguous with the disc, with little mass effect. **d** MRI after injection of Gd-DTPA shows a central non-enhancing mass surrounded by irregular peripheral enhancement *(arrows)*. MRI diagnosis: recurrent disc and scar. Surgical diagnosis: disc and scar

Fig. 2 a, b. A 40-year-old woman with a right L5 radiculopathy who underwent laminectomy and discectomy at L4–5 3 months previously. **a** MRI shows a large band or semicircle of pathological soft tissue with obliteration of the epidural fat. There is no mass effect. **b** after injection of Gd-DTPA there is intense homogeneous enhancement of the abnormal epidural soft tissue. Surgical diagnosis: epidural fibrosis

The major diagnostic criterion used to distinguish scar from disc was the presence or absence of enhancement within abnormal epidural soft tissue on post-contrast images. We subdivided our findings into four groups: (a) abnormal epidural soft tissue that did not enhance was classified as disc; (b) abnormal epidural soft tissue that did enhance was classified as scar (regardless of the presence of mass effect or contiguity to the disc space); (c) a non-enhancing mass surrounded by irregular peripheral enhancement was classified as disc surrounded by scar (disc > scar); (d) a non-enhancing mass intermixed with and surrounded by enhancement was classified as disc incorporated in scar (scar > disc).

All patients underwent a second (or third) operation and the gross surgical and histological findings were compared with CT and MRI diagnoses.

Results

Table 1 lists the 18 patients who were operated on again at one lumbar level and correlates the CT and MRI findings with the gross surgical and histological findings. Final histological diagnoses were disc ($n = 4$), disc and scar ($n = 12$) and scar ($n = 2$). The diagnoses based on post-contrast MRI were identical in all but 1 case, in which scar was diagnosed because of homogeneous enhancement. At surgery marked distension of the venous plexus was found, which possibly concealed a small sequestred disc. CT findings agreed with histological findings in 13 of 18 patients. The surgical and histological findings in patients with both disc and scar are listed in Table 2 with respect to prominence of one or other component and correlation with CT and MRI diagnoses. The findings from post-contrast MRI agreed with the surgical findings in all cases of this group.

Discussion

We selected a group of patients with complaints of continued pain following surgery for disc herniation and whose physical examination was typical of nerve root compression, as it was prior to the original operation. This selection was expected to increase the likelihood of recurrent or persistent disc herniation with nerve root compression. This was partially confirmed by the operative findings of disc herniation in 4 cases and mixed disc herniation and epidural scar in 12. However, there were also 2 patients with epidural scars alone and 3 with predominant scar. Reoperation on scar unaccompanied by significant disc material generally leads to a poor surgical result, since fibrosis often recurs after reoperation [2, 5]. Thus, although all patients met with the clinical criteria approved by the AANS and the AAOS for selection of surgery, patients with epidural scar should ideally have been excluded. Therefore, preoperative differentiation of epidural scar from herniated disc is crucial. Unenhanced spinal CT has been used to assess morphological features, location, mass effect or traction on the thecal space and density. However, CT density criteria have proved less reliable in postoperative patients [7]. With the use of intravenous contrast medium accuracy of 67%–100% has been reported [7–9]; scar demonstrates homogeneous enhancement after administration of contrast material. In our study, CT with contrast medium was effective in 56%, the majority of false diagnoses resulting from missing one component in patients with both disc and fibrosis or in an incorrect assessment of the relative importance of these components (Fig. 1 a, b).

Unenhanced MRI with T1- and T2-weighted images in sagittal and axial planes has been reported to have an accuracy of 80%, comparable with that of enhanced CT [10–12].

Our study demonstrates that the use of Gd-DTPA increases the accuracy of the differentiation between epidural fibrosis and disc herniation. Accurate delineation even of the amount and location of epidural fibrosis compared with that of disc material in patients with mixed histological findings is possible. These results agree with these of a recent study by Hueftle et al. [13], who reported 100% accuracy in the detection of the character of abnormal epidural soft tissue in 17 patients using enhanced MRI. The major criterion in our study was the presence of enhancement on post-contrast T1-weighted spin echo images (Figs. 1 c, d, 2 a, b).

MR imaging with i.v. Gd-DTPA is the method of choice for selection of patients for repeat back surgery, because even though all our patients met the AANS and AAOS criteria for justification of surgery, several patients with epidural scar or prodominant fibrosis were found, who would probably not benefit from repeat lumbar spine surgery.

References

1. Burton CV, Kirkaldy-Willis WH, Yong-Hing K, Heitthoff KB (1981) Causes of failure of surgery on the lumbar spine. Clin Orthop 157: 191–199
2. Finnegan WJ, Fenlin JM, Marvel JP, Nardini RJ, Rothman RH (1979) Results of surgical intervention in the symptomatic multiply-operated back patient. J Bone Joint Surg [Am] 61: 1077–1082
3. Law JD, Lehman RAW, Kirsch WM (1978) Reoperation after lumbar intervertebral disk surgery. J Neurosurg 48: 259–263
4. Greenwood J Jr, Mc Guire T, Kimbell F (1952) Study of causes of failure in the herniated intervertebral disk operation: an analysis of sixty-seven reoperation cases. J Neurosurg 9: 15–20
5. Hardy RW Jr (1982) Repeat operation for lumbar disk disease. In: Hardy RW Jr (ed) Seminars in neurological surgery-lumbar disk disease. Raven, New York, pp 193–202
6. White AA, Gordon SL (eds) (1982) The American Academy of Orthopaedic Surgeons Symposium on Idiopathic Low Back Pain. Mosby, St. Louis
7. Braun IF, Hoffmann JC Jr, Davis PC, Landman JA, Tindall GT (1985) Contrast enhancement in CT differentiation between recurrent disk herniation and postoperative scar: prospective study. AJNR 6: 607–612
8. Schubiger O, Valavanis A (1982) CT-differentiation between recurrent disk herniation and postoperative scar formation: the value of contrast enhancement. Neuroradiology 22: 251–254
9. Teplick JG, Haskin ME (1984) Intravenous contrast-enhanced CT of the postoperative lumbar spine: improved identification of recurrent disk herniation, scar, arachnoiditis and diskitis. AJNR 5: 373–383
10. Bundschuh CV, Modic MT, Ross JS, Masaryk TJ, Bohlmann H (1988) Epidural fibrosis and recurrent disk herniation in the lumbar spine: assessment with magnetic resonance. AJNR 9: 169–178
11. Mikhael MA, Ciric IS, Kudrna JC, Hindo WA (1985) Recognition of lumbar disk disease with magnetic resonance imaging. Comput Radiol 9: 213–222
12. Modic MT, Masaryk TJ, Paushter D (1986) Magnetic resonance imaging of the spine. Radiol Clin North Am 24: 229–245
13. Hueftle MG, Modic MT, Ross JS, Masaryk TJ, Carter JR, Wilber RG, Bohlmann HH, Steinberg PM, Delamarter RB (1988) Lumbar spine: postoperative MR-imaging with Gd-DTPA. Radiology 167: 817–824

Dr. Siegfried Trattnig
2nd Department of Medicine
Division of Diagnostic Radiology
Garnisongasse 13
A-1090 Vienna, Austria

Neuroradiology (1991) 33 [Suppl]: 345–346

Neuro radiology
© Springer-Verlag 1991

Is there a familial component in early disc failure?

A. D. North[2], G. P. Wilde[2], R. W. Kerslake[1], R. C. Mulholland[2], and B. S. Worthington[1]

[1] Department of Radiology, Queens Medical Centre, Nottingham, UK
[2] Spinal Research Unit, Harlow Wood Hospital, Near Mansfield, Nottingham, UK

Summary. Patients with adolescent disc prolapse have a tendency to multiple level disc degeneration. This has led to the suggestion of a disc degeneration diathesis and that this may be familial. The first degree relatives of 15 patients with adolescent disc prolapse had the degenerative state of their discs assessed using MRI. These were compared with an age-/sex-matched control group. The first degree relatives had a significantly higher degenerative score than the controls. This difference was most significant at the lumbosacral disc. We believe this is further evidence for a familial component to adolescent disc failure.

Key words: Spine – Disc lumbar – Disc prolapse – Disc degeneration – Disc adolescent

Adolescent disc prolapse before the age of 20 years is a rare but well recognised clinical entity, representing 1%–2.5% of all cases of disc prolapse [1]. Clinically, adolescent disc prolapse is characterised by a greater incidence of paravertebral muscle spasm and severity of leg pain [2]. The results of conservative therapy are said to be poor [3] but treatment by either formal surgery [4, 5] or chemonucleolysis [6] generally gives good results.

Gibson et al. [7] investigated the lumbar intervertebral discs of 20 patients with adolescent disc failure, using MRI, to assess the quality of the discs. They found that, compared to an age-sex-matched control group, the patients tended to have multiple level disc degeneration. This led them to suggest that there may be a constitutional predisposition, or diathesis, to disc failure and that this might be familial. Varlotta [8] interviewed the parents of 63 adolescent disc patients regarding their back pain status. They found double the incidence of significant back pain in these parents compared with a control group. Porter [9] investigated the relatives of patients, of all ages, with disc herniation and found four times as many relatives with back pain in the herniation group as in the control group.

Until recently the ability to assess the state of degeneration of the intervertebral disc has been limited: plain radiographs give poor information, discography is invasive and its use in screening asymptomatic controls unjustifiable. MRI has revolutionised our ability to assess the disc, having the advantages of giving qualitative information about the disc without invasion or radiation. Gibson et al. [10] have shown the information gained to be comparable to discography.

We have assessed the lumbar discs of the first degree relatives of 15 adolescent disc patients and compared these with a group of asymptomatic age- and sex-matched controls.

Patients and methods

Fifteen patients with adolescent disc prolapse, proven at open fenestration discectomy, were identified. The first degree relatives of these patients ($n = 45$, 1 defaulter) underwent MRI of their lumbar spines, along with an age- and sex-matched group of volunteer controls, without previous history of significant back pain or sciatica. The scans were carried out on an 0.15 T resistive system using a short T1 inversion recovery or STIR sequence (TR 1100 ms, TI 100 ms) [11]. The discs were scored in the midsagittal plane (Figs. 1, 2). Each of the lumbar discs were given a degenerative score on a 0–4 scale (0 = normal signal, 4 = complete degeneration) after Gibson et al. [10]. All scans were read blind by a radiologist conversant with grading intervertebral disc degeneration. Comparison between the two groups was made using the Mann-Whitney U test for non-parametric data.

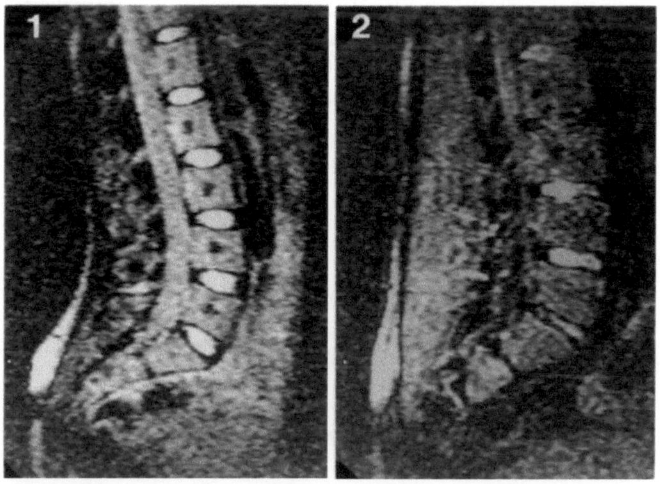

Fig. 1. MRI scan of the lumbar spine showing normal signal from all discs (TR 1100 ms, TI 100 ms)

Fig. 2. MRI scan of the lumbar spine showing various degrees of disc degeneration at L1–2, L2–3 and L5–S1 (TR 1100 ms, TI 100 ms)

Table 1. Degenerative scores for lumbar discs in relatives and controls

	Relatives	Controls	*P*
L1/2	0.93	0.36	0.05 > *P* > 0.02
L2/3	0.4	0.2	*P* > 0.01
L3/4	0.44	0.13	0.02 > *P* > 0.01
L4/5	1.46	0.51	0.0. > *P* > 0.001
L5/S1	2.51	0.58	*P* > 0.001

Results

Mean scores for each intervertebral level are shown in Table 1.

As would be expected the L4–5 and L5–S1 intervertebral discs were the most degenerate in both groups, these discs being the most prone to failure [12]. The results suggest that the first degree relatives of patients with adolescent disc failure have higher levels of disc degeneration than a similar group of controls. The difference is more pronounced in the lower lumbar discs, being maximal at L5–S1.

Discussion

Adolescent disc failure is comparatively rare and presents before other mechanical influences on the spine (heavy manual labour, prolonged driving etc.) become important factors. Patients with adolescent disc failure also have a tendency to multiple level failure and it has therefore been suggested that there may be an underlying disc failure diathesis [7] and that this diathesis is familial. The above results indicate that at all lumbar intervertebral levels there is increased degeneration in the first degree relatives of adolescent disc patients when compared with a normal control group.

The difference between the two groups is more marked in the caudal discs which suggests therefore that, if there is an underlying diathesis, then it makes the intervertebral discs more susceptible to mechanical injury and subsequent failure.

In summary, the first relatives of adolescent disc patients have an increased incidence of lumbar intervertebral disc degeneration compared with matched controls. This gives increasing credence to the theory that adolescent disc failure may have a familial element.

Acknowledgements. The authors would like to thank Mrs. P. Tulsa for her secretarial help, Dr. J. Pearson for his statistical advice and Mr. S. Chipperfield for his help with MRI scanning. We are also grateful for the financial support of the Medical Research Council and the Department of Health and Social Security.

References

1. Love JG (1947) The disc factor in low back pain with and without sciatica. J Bone Joint Surg 29: 438–447
2. Bulos S (1973) Herniated intervertebral lumbar disc in the teenager. J Bone Joint Surg [Br] 55: 273–278
3. Grobler LJ, Simmons EH, Barrington TW (1979) Intervertebral disc herniation in the adolescent. Spine 4: 267–277
4. Bradford DS, Garcia A (1969) Herniations of the lumbar intervertebral disc in children and adolescents. JAMA 210: 2045–2051
5. Webb HJ, Kennedy RLJ (1954) Protruded lumbar intervertebral discs in children. JAMA 1153–1155
6. Lorenz M, McCulloch J (1985) Chemonucleolysis for herniated nucleus pulposus in adolescents. J Bone Joint Surg [Am] 67: 1402–1404
7. Gibson MJ, Szypryt EP, Buckley JH, Worthington BS, Mulholland RC (1987) Magnetic resonance imaging of adolescent disc herniation. J Bone Joint Surg [Br] 69: 699–703
8. Varlotta GP (1988) Familial predisposition for adolescent disc displacement (abstract). International Society for the Study of the Lumbar Spine, Miami
9. Porter RW (1968) Familial aspects of disc protrusion (abstract). International Society for the Study of the Lumbar Spine, Dallas
10. Gibson MJ, Buckley J, Mawhinney R, Mulholland RC, Worthington BS (1986) Magnetic resonance imaging and discography in the diagnosis of disc degeneration. J Bone Joint Surg [Br] 68: 369–373
11. Bydder GM, Young IR (1985) Clinical use of the inversion recovery sequence. J Comput Assist Tomogr 9: 659–675
12. Kortelainen P, Puranen J, Koivisto E, Lahde S (1983) Symptoms and signs of sciatica and their relation to the localisation of the lumbar disc herniation. Spine 10: 88–92

Prof. B. S. Worthington
Department of Radiology
University Hospital
Queens Medical Centre
Nottingham
NG7 2UH, UK

Neuroradiology (1991) 33 [Suppl]: 347–348

Neuroradiology

© Springer-Verlag 1991

Thoracic intervertebral disc herniation: diagnostic value of MRI and CT

S. Wieslander[1], J. Præstholm[2], H. Videbæk[2], V. Hennild[2], O. Osgaard[3], and O. Henriksen[1]

[1] Danish Research Centre for Magnetic Resonance, Departments of [2] Neuroradiology and [3] Neurosurgery, Hvidovre University Hospital, Copenhagen, Denmark

Summary. Eight consecutive patients with thoracic intervertebral disc herniation presented protean manifestations mimicking vertebral, medullary and visceral disorders. MRI with sagittal overviews of the thoracic spine was found to be a reliable screening procedure. Calcification was present in all cases and made CT ideal for visualization of the structure of the herniation before operation.

Key words: Thoracic disc herniation – Computed tomography – Magnetic resonance imaging

Thoracic intervertebral disc herniation (TIDH) is an uncommon disease which has been reported to appear with a frequency of one patient per million population per annum [1]. The advent of water-soluble contrast medium myelography and whole-body CT [2, 3] and MRI [4, 5] greatly facilitated diagnosis.

Patients and methods

From June 1985 to February 1990 eight patients with sensory, motor and visceral symptoms have been diagnosed in our imaging departments as suffering from TIDH. Myelography was performed in seven patients using 12.5 ml iohexol 300 mg I/ml, CT myelography in six patients with a Siemens Somatom DRG, and MRI in four patients with a Siemens Magnetom 1.5 T using an oval surface coil.

A summary of the diagnostic imaging findings in our eight patients with TIDH is given in Table 1.

Case reports

Case 1

A 44-year-old male experienced back pain during weight bearing and developed weakness of both legs. Two weeks later he was admitted with a diagnosis of cauda equina syndrome with retention of urine. Neurological examination showed severe paraparesis and bilateral Babinski sign. Anaesthesia with an upper limit at dermatome T11 was present. A calcified nucleus pulposus of the eighth thoracic disc and a calcareous hernial canal and prolapse with compression of the dural sac were demonstrated. At operation a soft prolapse was removed.

Case 2

A 28-year-old female was admitted to the urological department with attacks of colic in the right lower abdomen for 24 h. Laboratory examinations of urine and intravenous pyelography were normal. At a subsequent neurological examination an area of hypaesthesia was

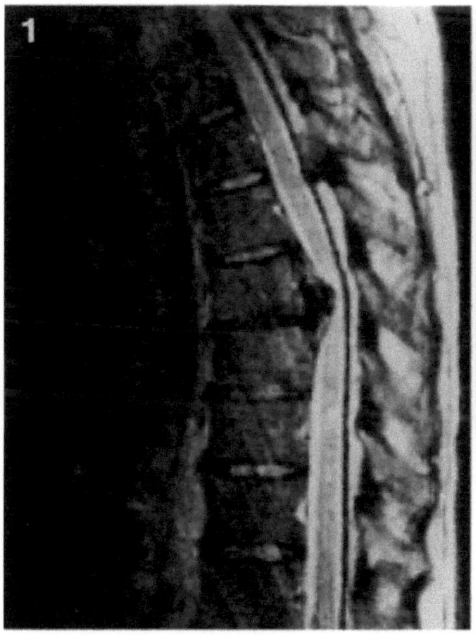

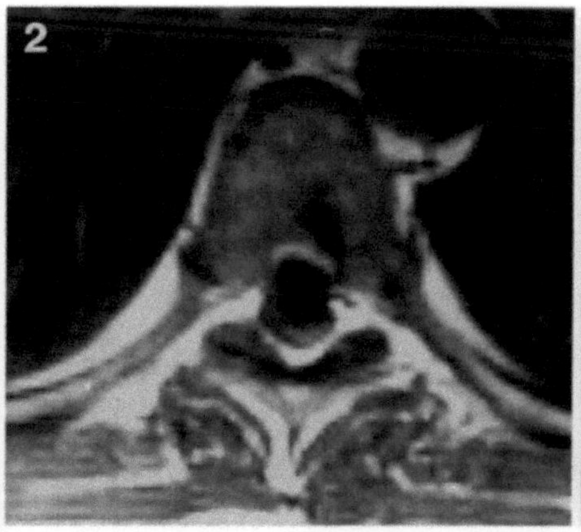

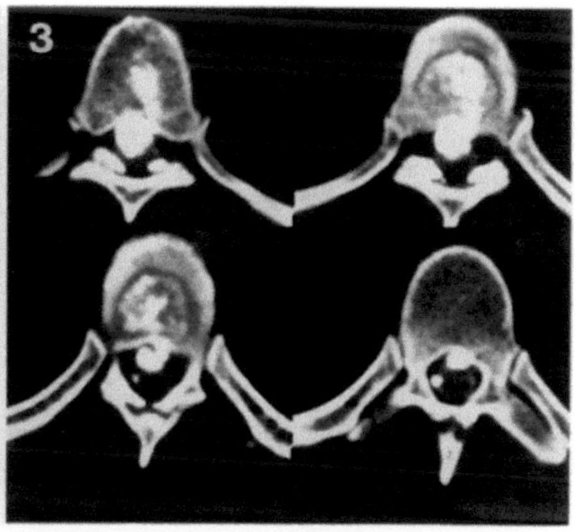

Fig. 1. Case 3. MRI midsagittal image at 1.5 T. This T2-weighted image (SE 1800/90) demonstrates reduced hight of the T7–8 intervertebral space and hypointensity of corresponding disc, which is protruding and compressing the spinal cord

Fig. 2. Case 3. MRI axial image at 1.5 T. This T1-weighted image (SE 500/17) demonstrates a hypointense nucleus pulposus T7–8, which is not separated from a hypointense herniation compressing the isointense spinal cord

Fig. 3. Case 3. CT demonstrates a calcified nucleus pulposus T7–8 in continuity with a calcareous hernial canal and prolapse, (125 V, 520 mAs, window w/c: 800/350)

Table 1. Radiological findings in eight patients with thoracic intervertebral disc herniation on MRI ($n = 4$) and CT ($n = 6$)

Narrow intervertebral disc	5/8
Calcified nucleus pulposus	8/8
Calcareous hernial canal on CT	6/6
Calcareous prolapse	7/8
Compression of spinal cord	6/8
Low intensity disc on MRI (TR = 1800, TE = 90)	4/4

found in dermatome T12. A calcified nucleus pulposus of the 12th thoracic disc, a calcareous hernial canal and a right-sided lateral prolapse with dislocation of the dural sac were demonstrated. At operation a free prolapse measuring $2 \times 1 \times 0.5$ cm was removed. The colic disappeared within 1 week of operation.

Case 3

A 46-year-old male with gait difficulty for 18 months developed weakness of the right leg. A spastic paresis of the right leg and ataxia were found. Dysaesthesia of the left leg was present with an upper limit in dermatome T11. MRI and CT myelography showed a calcified seventh thoracic disc, a calcareous hernial canal and prolapse with compression of the dural sac (Figs. 1–3). Operation has so far been postponed because of risk of damaging the spinal cord.

Discussion

TIDH is a rare disease which may mimic a wide variety of diseases from multiple sclerosis and spinal cord tumour [6] to urological and gastrointestinal colic, and cauda equina syndrome [7]. It is important to remember potentially curable disease as a differential diagnosis. MRI using the easily obtained sagittal sections is a noninvasive and reliable screening procedure for demonstrating the condition of the intervertebral discs and the spinal cord (Fig. 1). Myelography may be avoided. In all our patients with TIDH there was calcareous material in the nucleus pulposus and in seven of eight cases also in the prolapse. This finding of calcareous material makes CT ideal for detailed visualization of the internal structure of the herniation before the often technically difficult operation [8].

References

1. Carson J, Gumpert J, Jefferson A (1971) Diagnosis and treatment of thoracic intervertebral disc protrusions. J Neurol Neurosurg Psychiatry 34: 68–77
2. Ciapetta P, Celli P, Delfini R, Cantore GP (1982) Computed tomography in the diagnosis of thoracic disk protrusions with technical suggestions. Zbl Neurochir 43: 77–84
3. Bury RW, Powell T (1989) Prolapsed thoracic intervertebral disc: the importance of CT assisted myelography. Clin Radiol 40: 416–421
4. Tadmor R, New PFJ, Shoukimas G, Edelman RR, Brady TJ (1986) Magnetic resonance imaging of the thoracic spinal cord and spine with surface coils. Acta Radiol Diagn [Suppl] (Stockh) 369: 475–480
5. Blumenkopf B (1988) Thoracic intervertebral disc herniations: diagnostic value of magnetic resonance imaging. Neurosurgery 23: 36–40
6. Roosen N, Dietrich U, Nicola N, Irlich G, Gahlen D, Stork W (1987) MR-imaging of calcified herniated thoracic disk. J Comput Assist Tomogr 11: 733–735
7. Love JG, Schorn VG (1965) Thoracic-disk protrusions. JAMA 191: 627–631
8. Arce CA, Dohrmann GJ (1985) Thoracic disc herniation. Improved diagnosis with computed tomographic scanning and a review of the litterature. Surg Neurol 23: 356–361

Dr. S. Wieslander
Department of Diagnostic Radiology 334
Hvidovre University Hospital
DK-2650 Hvidovre, Denmark

Neuroradiology (1991) 33 [Suppl]: 349–351

Neuro radiology
© Springer-Verlag 1991

MRI in the diagnosis of spinal infections

F. Briganti, F. Caranci, V. Giugliano, A. Manto, G. la Tessa, R. Elefante, and F. Smaltino

Department of Radiology and Neuroradiology, Second Faculty of Medicine, University of Naples, Naples, Italy

Summary. We have reviewed 40 cases of spinal infection studied by MRI. Signal intensity features have been assessed in the acute and/or chronic stages. In chronic tuberculous spondylitis signal intensity on T1-weighted images is higher than in other spinal infections and this may be considered specific. Gadolinium-DTPA administered intravenously in 6 patients provided better definition of paravertebral and epidural abscesses, and contributed to the differentiation from neoplastic vertebral lesions.

Key words: Spine – Magnetic resonance imaging – Spondylodiscitis

Spinal infections represent 2% of all cases of osteomyelitis. Early diagnosis is necessary to avoid neurological damage, but is difficult due to a long latent stage (2–8 weeks), and mild and often non-specific symptoms.

The aim of this study is to assess the sensibility and specificity of MRI in this disease, its accuracy in showing changes in the disc space and vertebral body and involvement of the spinal canal and the paravertebral soft tissues, and finally the improvements in diagnosis afforded by gadolinium (Gd)-DTPA.

Patients and Methods

Forty patients whose ages ranged between 10 and 75 years with inflammatory lesions of the intervertebral discs and vertebral bodies have been studied by MRI between June 1987 and April 1990; there were 19 women and 21 men. The inflammatory lesions were acute in 15 patients (5 Staphylococcal, 3 *Brucella*, 3 *Salmonella*, 4 tuberculous). Chronic lesions were observed in 25 cases (13 tuberculous, 5 *Brucella*, 7 unknown aetiology). MRI was performed using a 0.5 T superconductive unit in 34 patients and a 1 T superconductive unit in 6. The patients were imaged with T1-weighted and T2-weighted sequences in sagittal, axial and coronal planes.

In 6 patients T1-weighted images were also obtained after intravenous injection of Gd–DTPA (0.1 mmol/kg).

Results

Patients were classified into two groups based on the stage of the infection.

In the *acute stage* (15 patients) the MR signal abnormalities were not specifically related to the aetiology. In fact, in staphylococcal spondylitis or in spondylitis due to *Brucella, Salmonella* and *Mycobacterium tuberculosis,* the inflammatory lesions were characterised by long T1 and T2 relaxation times and the signal intensities were homogeneous. In patients with tuberculous spondylitis MR showed an epidural abscess, defining its relation to the thecal sac and the nervous structures. Gd-DTPA was administered in 2 patients with *Salmonella* spondylitis and in 1 patient with *Brucella* spondylitis. The paramagnetic contrast medium produced homogeneous enhancement of the involved disc and vertebral bodies on T1-weighted images (Fig. 1).

In the *chronic stage* (25 patients) signal abnormalities were more varied. In *Brucella* infection and in spondylitis of unknown aetiology, the involved vertebral bodies and discs showed inhomogeneous prolongation of T1 and T2 relaxation times. In tuberculous infections (13 patients), the lesions showed slight T1 shortening (Fig. 2). An abscess, with soft tissue and spinal canal involvement, was observed in 7 of these cases.

Gd-DTPA administration, performed in 3 cases of tuberculous spondylitis, produced smooth enhancement of the lesions in the vertebrae and discs and peripheral enhancement of the associated epidural abscess (Fig. 3).

Discussion

MRI allows very early recognition of infections of the vertebrae and discs, and shows the relationship between the lesion and the intraspinal structures and any involvement of the spinal cord [1, 2].

In the *acute stage* of pyogenic, *Salmonella* and *Brucella* spondylitis T1-weighted images show homogeneous low signal intensity in the involved disc space and vertebral bodies; the lesions show high signal intensity in T2-weighted images. This high signal intensity is probably due to increased water content within the inflammatory leukocytes and to local ischaemia. In acute tuberculous spondylitis the preferential localisation is in the anterior part of the thoracic vertebral bodies [3].

In the *chronic stage* signal abnormalities are more varied, and related to the aetiology. In tuberculous spondylitis T1-weighted images show a slightly increased signal intensity, which may prove specific for the disease [3]. MRI also plays a key role in the diagnosis of epidural abscess, precisely defining the extension [3]. It is very important to detect epidural abscess because it can produce paraplegia or bowel and bladder symptoms, sometimes

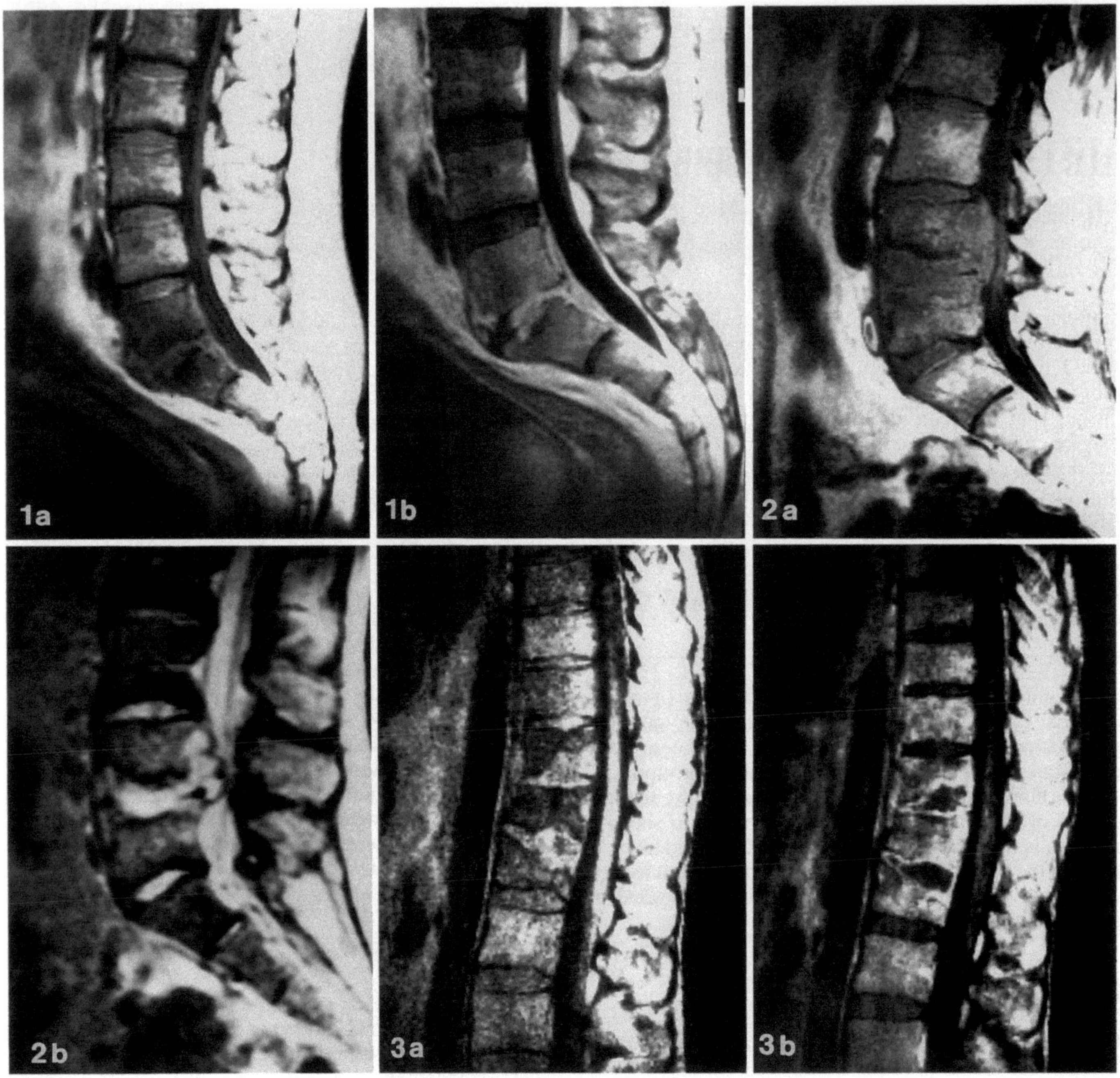

Fig. 1a, b. *Salmonella spondylitis. Acute stage.* **a** Sagittal PS 500/20 shows a decreased signal intensity at L5–S1. **b** Sagittal PS 500/20 after Gd-DTPA shows enhancement of lesion

Fig. 2a, b. *Tuberculous spondylitis. Chronic stage.* **a** Sagittal PS 500/20 shows an inflammatory lesion at L4–L5, involving the spinal canal and characterized by slightly increased signal intensity. **b** Sagittal SE 2500/90 image delineates the posterior extension of lesion

Fig. 3a, b. *Tuberculous spondylitis. Chronic stage.* **a** Sagittal PS 450/28 images shows multiple hyperintense lesions in the thoracic spine. **b** Sagittal PS 450/28 image shows peripheral enhancement of the lesions after intravenous administration of Gd-DTPA

very quickly. MRI usually shows the abscess as a high signal intensity area located in the anterior epidural space, in contiguity with the involved disc and extending superiorly and inferiorly. This area is separated from the thecal sac by a thin line of low signal, probably representing the meninges. MRI is useful in the differential diagnosis between inflammatory vertebral lesions and postoperative changes, degenerative diseases and metastatic lesions. Metastases do not show the low signal intensity area on T1-weighted images, involving the vertebral bodies and disc; moreover, the disc space is not involved [2, 4].

Differential diagnosis is more difficult in the early stages, when the disc space is not involved, and in tuberculous spondylitis, which is very similar to extradural neoplasms, showing lack of involvement of the disc space, involvement of multiple vertebral bodies and the presence of paravertebral masses. Intravenous administration of Gd-DTPA allows better definition of inflammatory lesions, which show homogeneous enhancement in the acute stage, and inhomogeneous enhancement in the chronic stage. The paramagnetic contrast medium gives better delineation of the epidural abscess and enables differentiation from neoplastic lesions, which do not generally show enhancement [5].

References

1. Sharif HS, Aideyan OA, Clark DC, Madkour MM, Aabed MY, Mattsson TA, Al-Deeb SM, Moutaery KR (1989) Brucellar and tuberculous spondylitis: comparative imaging features. Radiology 171: 419–425
2. Modic MT, Feiglin DH, Piraino DW, Boumfrey F, Weinstein M, Duchesneau PM, Rehm S (1985) Vertebral osteomyelitis: assessment using MR. Radiology 157: 157–166
3. Smith AS, Weinstein MA, Mizushima A, Coughlin B, Heyden SP, Lakin MM, Lanzieri CF (1989) MR imaging characteristics of tuberculous vs vertebral osteomyelitis. AJR 153: 399–405
4. Bruns J, Maas S (1989) Advantages of diagnosing bacterial spondylitis with magnetic resonance imaging. Arch Orthop Trauma Surg 108: 30–35
5. Roos A de, van Persijn van Meerten EL, Bloem JL, Bluemm RG (1986) MRI of tuberculous spondylitis. AJR 146: 79–82

Dr. F. Briganti
Department of Radiology and Neuroradiology
Second Faculty of Medicine
Via S. Pansini, 5 Naples, Italy

Neuroradiology (1991) 33 [Suppl]: 352–353

Neuro
radiology
© Springer-Verlag 1991

MR discography: a comparison with CT discography

I. Anatomical experimental basis

N. M. Szeverenyi, S. Yu, S. C. Buckingham, J. J. Moro, and A. E. Rosenbaum

Department of Radiology, MR Research Laboratory, SUNY Health Science Center, Syracuse, New York, USA

Summary. Gadopentetate dimeglumine was demonstrated to be an effective contrast agent for use in MR discography. A combined agent was developed consisting of a mixture of 0.5 mM gadopentetate dimeglumine, iohexol 300 mg I/ml, and 0.06% Fast green dye. Examination of the lumbar discs in two cadaver spines injected with 1–2 ml of this mixture enabled characterization of the disc with MRI, CT and cryomicrotomy in the same specimen. Images from each of the three modalities were obtained in identical sections for axial and sagittal planes. These images display excellent correspondence in the distribution of injected agent. MR T1-weighted images appear to give sharper, more compact representations of the contrast agent as well as details of the annulus and nucleus which were not observed on CT.

Key words: MR discography – Gadopentetate dimeglumine – Intervertebral disc

MRI, CT, or film-screen/CT myelography sometimes fail to explain the source of a patient's back pain. Discography, and more recently CT discography have been used to localize the level of the patient's discogenic pain through the direct injection of contrast medium into the suspect discs' nuclei. This technique, since its inception by Lindblom [1] and Hirsch [2], has provided morphological-physiological correlation using injections of either saline or iodinated contrast media (currently, a non-ionic iodinated medium). With the excellent soft tissue imaging capability of MRI, particularly relating to the detection of water content in discs, it was hoped that MRI would obviate the need for discography. In most instances it has, but some reports [3–5] still describe cases of normal MRI examinations with abnormal discography.

Since MRI has become the premier imaging technique for the examination of disc disease, could this modality also be used when discography is indicated? It would seem that an MRI relaxation agent could be employed, in manner analogous to the injection of iodinated media in the X-ray examination. If such a technique were possible, one would retain the benefits of MRI and still have the possibility of obtaining discographic information. The additional experience gained through MR discography would enhance the radiologist's skills in interpreting the unenhanced MR image.

Contrast media for MRI are formulated from compounds containing unpaired electrons. These paramagnetic substances cause a reduction of T1 and T2 relaxation times of water in tissue with increasing contrast medium concentration. Gadopentetate dimeglumine (Gd-DTPA) is widely used clinically as an intravenous MRI contrast medium and is available under the trade name Magnevist. Undiluted Magnevist, a 500 mM solution of Gd-DTPA, is unsuitable as a MR discogram agent due to the very short T2 relaxation times it induces. In appropriate dilutions with water, however, Gd-DTPA provides strong T1 relaxation while not shortening T2 relaxation significantly compared with TE.

Method

Dilutions of Magnevist were made with iohexol solutions generating a contrast medium that would appear on both T1-weighted MR images and CT images of the same specimen. Although the nuclear spin relaxation behavior of Gd-DTPA solutions is known [3, 4], the effect of iohexol (Omnipaque) on the system was not known. To investigate the relaxation behavior of such a mixture, a phantom was constructed consisting of an array of vials having three iohexol concentrations (180, 240 and 300 mg I/ml) to which a range of gadopentetate concentrations (0, 0.15, 0.25, 0.37, 0.50, 1.0, 1.5, and 2.5 mM) was added. This phantom was imaged alongside the spine using a routine T1-weighted spin-echo imaging sequence (400/10). A direct comparison of signal intensity relative to the spine was afforded and the solution producing the highest intensity was identified for use in the following experiments. Water relaxation was not significantly affected by iohexol concentration, and all Omnipaque solutions performed well with Magnevist diluted 1:1000. Fast green, an organic dye, was added as a third component to this mixture allowing visualization of the injected material on anatomical sections.

Injections of this mixture of contrast media and dye were made into the discs of cadaver lumbar spines. The spines had been dissected, retaining an approximately 10-cm diameter cylinder of tissue and refrigerated until used. The contrast medium (1–2 ml) was injected into the nucleus pulposus of individual discs using two 21 gauge needles from bilateral approaches, anterolateral to the intervertebral disc. MR images were obtained at 1.5 T on a Siemens Magnetom 63SP imager or at 2.0 T on a G. E. CSI research system. Two excitations/256 phase encoding steps were averaged with a field of vision of 15 cm for axial images and 20 cm for sagittal images. Slice thickness was 3 mm on the clinical instrument and 2 mm on the research instrument.

Following MRI, each spine was quickly frozen in liquid nitrogen to prevent further diffusion of contrast medium. CT images were obtained in axial and direct sagittal planes with a Siemens Hi-Q scanner

(190 mA, 133 kVp, time 2.7 s). Frozen spines were subsequently sectioned in axial or sagittal planes using a LKB Model 2258 cryomicrotome. Color photographs were obtained at levels corresponding to the MR and CT images as the cryomicrotome sectioning progressed. There was close correspondence between the CT, MR and anatomical images.

Results and discussion

MR discography using Gd-DTPA was found to be effective and has advantages over CT discography in that abnormal tracking of contrast medium is more accurately defined, with better visualization of the architecture of the intervertebral tissue. One can observe differentiation of nucleus pulposus and the annulus as well as the hyperintensity of the contrast material on MRI. The contrast medium and surrounding soft tissue are both optimally visualized on the same image and MRI additionally provides *direct* high resolution multiplanar imaging capabilities.

It is most likely Gd-DTPA will be less toxic (irritating) than iodinated agents for discography (if intravenous experiences are paralleled). A single injection of the combined contrast medium affords the option of either MR or CT imaging. Using gadopentetate for MR discography can act as an aid in the interpretation of unenhanced MRI, much in the same way as contrast medium has aided our understanding of unenhanced MR images of brain.

References

1. Lindblom K (1948) Diagnostic puncture of intervertebral discs in sciatica. Acta Orthop Scand 17: 231–239
2. Hirsch C (1948) An attempt to diagnose the level of a disc lesion clinically by disc puncture. Acta Orthop Scand 18: 132–139
3. Zucherman J, Derby R, Hsu K (1988) Normal magnetic resonance imaging with abnormal discography. Spine 13: 1355–1359
4. Kornberg M (1985) Discography and magnetic resonance imaging in the diagnosis of lumbar disc disruption. Spine 14: 1368–1372
5. Yu S, Haughton VM, Sether LA, Wagner M (1989) Comparison of MR and discography in detecting radial tears of the annulus. AJNR 10: 1077–1081

Dr. Nikolaus M. Szeverenyi
Department of Radiology
MR Research Laboratory
Suny Health Science Center at Syracuse
750 E. Adams Street
Syracuse, NY 13210, USA

Neuroradiology (1991) 33 [Suppl]: 354–355

Neuro radiology

© Springer-Verlag 1991

Subdural haematoma caused by aneurysm rupture: CT findings and incidence

W. K. Chong

Department of Imaging, Monash Medical Centre, Clayton, Victoria, Australia

Summary. One hundred and four consecutive patients presenting with subdural haematoma (SDH) for treatment were reviewed. The proportion of SDH caused by aneurysm rupture was 3.7% (4/104).

Key words: Subdural haematoma – Aneurysm, rupture – Subarachnoid haemorrhage

Between 0.5% and 11% of ruptured aneurysms and angiomas are complicated by subdural haematoma (SDH) [1, 2]. However, there are few, if any, recent reports of the reverse, i. e. the proportion of SDH caused by aneurysm rupture. Walton [1] cited three references up to 1951 which reported incidences of 1%–8%. A retrospective study and literature review was conducted to determine if there are any distinguishing features on CT of SDH caused by aneurysm rupture.

Methods and results

One hundred and four consecutive patients with SDH treated at Prince Henry's Campus were reviewed. Most CT studies were performed without intravenous contrast medium on either a second- or current-generation high resolution scanner. Cerebral angiograms were performed on clinical grounds and CT findings. All findings were confirmed at surgery or autopsy. Four patients had aneurysm rupture as the cause of the SDH. No angiomas were found. The aneurysms all arose from the carotid system. One patients was suspected of aneurysm rupture on CT and clinical grounds and had surgery without angiogram (Fig. 1). The other 3 patients' angiograms were positive for aneurysms (Figs. 2–4). None of the 4 SDH were traumatic. The proportion of SDH caused by aneurysm rupture was therefore 3.7% (4/104).

CT features of SDH caused by aneurysm rupture

1. All were acute (high attenuation) and nontraumatic.
2. The SDH either overlay the aneurysms with remote extension (cases 1, 3), or were entirely remote from them (cases 2, 4).
3. The SDH were usually on the same side as the aneurysms. However, an anterior communicating aneurysm may be opacified only via the carotid artery on the opposite side to the SDH (case 2).
4. The SDH may be the only finding (cases 1, 2).

CT features suggesting aneurysm rupture

1. Subarachnoid blood which may be diffuse (case 3) or localized around the aneurysm (case 4).
2. Intracerebral haematoma overlying the aneurysm (cases 3, 4).
3. Unusual site of SDH, eg, parasellar (case 1).
4. Aneurysm itself may be seen (case 3).

In one case, (no. 2), none of these features was present.

Discussion

Reported findings are similar to ours [2, 3]. Additional features include bilateral SDH from circle of Willis aneurysms, and convexity SDH from posterior inferior cerebellar aneurysms [1]. Cavernous carotid aneurysm rupture may cause temporal fossa SDH without subarachnoid blood [4]. Posterior communicating and callosomarginal aneurysms may both cause interhemispheric SDH [5, 6].

Ninety-five percent of aneurysms causing SDH arose from the carotid system, and the remainder from the vertebrobasilar circulation [1, 2]. The aneurysms are usually congenital, occasionally atherosclerotic and rarely mycotic [1].

In conclusion, there may or may not be CT features to suggest underlying aneurysm rupture. Localized subarachnoid blood and intracerebral clot are reliable localizing signs to tailor the angiogram. The SDH may occasionally be on the opposite side to the carotid artery which fills the aneurysm.

References

1. Clarke E, Walton J (1953) Subdural haematoma complicating intracranial aneurysm and angioma. Brain 76: 378–404
2. Barton E, Tudor J (1982) Subdural haematoma in association with intracranial aneurysm. Neuroradiology 23: 157–160
3. Eggers FM, Tomsick TA, Larking RR, Chambers AA (1982) Recognition of subdural hematoma secondary to ruptured aneurysm by computed tomography. Comput Tomogr 6: 309–313
4. Hodes JE, Fletcher WA, Goodman DF, Hoyt WF (1988) Rupture of cavernous carotid artery aneurysm causing subdural hematoma and death. Case report. J Neurosurg 69: 617–619
5. Fein JM, Rovit RL (1970) Interhemispheric subdural haematoma secondary to haemorrhage from a calloso-marginal artery aneurysm. Neuroradiology 1: 183–186
6. Friedman MB, Brant-Zawadzki M (1983) Interhemispheric subdural hematoma from ruptured aneurysm. Comput Radiol 7: 129–134

Dr. W. K. Chong
Department of Imaging Monash Medical Centre
Locked Bag 29
Clayton, Victoria 3168, Australia

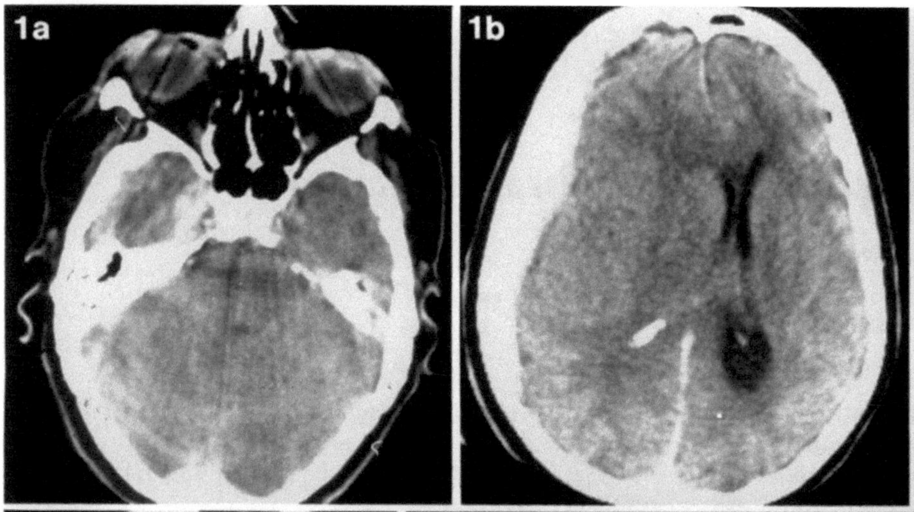

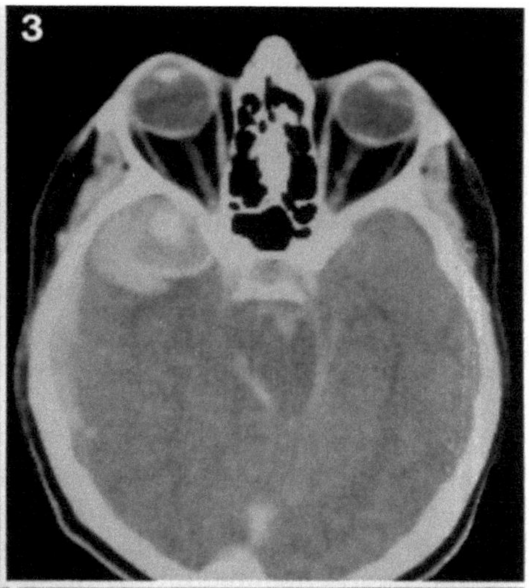

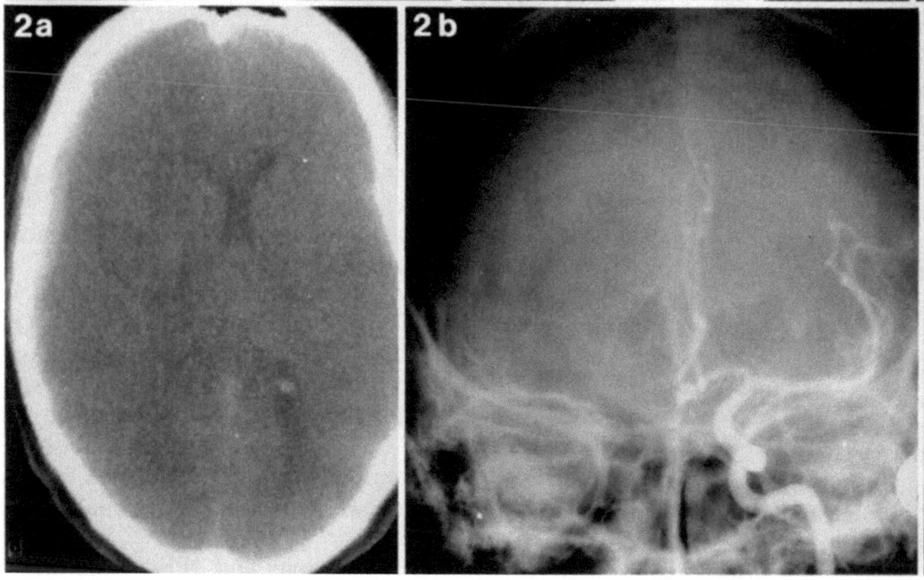

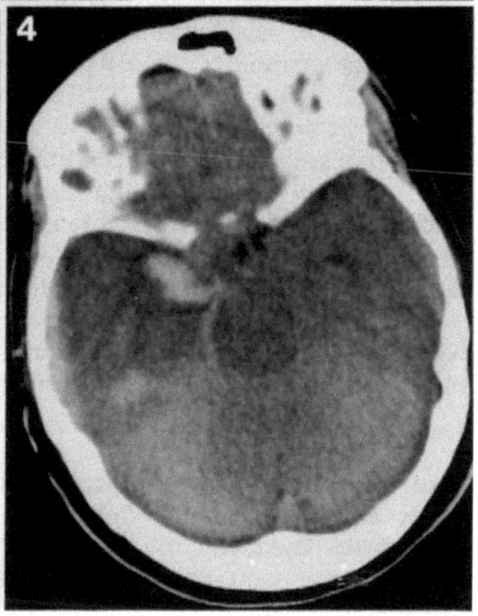

Fig. 1 a, b. Case 1. Unenhanced CT showed acute right parasellar and hemispheric subdural haematoma (SDH). No subarachnoid or intracerebral blood was seen. Right internal carotid/posterior communicating artery aneurysm found

Fig. 2 a, b. Case 2. Unenhanced CT showed a shallow right frontal/parietal SDH without subarachnoid blood. Anterior communicating artery aneurysm filled only from the left carotid artery

Fig. 3. Case 3. Enhanced CT showed an acute right temporal SDH, intracerebral haematoma, extensive subarachnoid blood and a giant aneurysm of the right middle cerebral artery with luminal enhancement and peripheral thrombus

Fig. 4. Case 4. Unenhanced CT showed a right temporal lobe haematoma, right ambient cistern blood and right temporal SDH extending into the frontal region. Right internal carotid/posterior communicating artery aneurysm found

Neuroradiology (1991) 33 [Suppl]: 356–357

Neuro-radiology
© Springer-Verlag 1991

^{31}P-chemical shift imaging of human cerebral infarction

K. Uchimura[1], M. Sasahira[1], T. Asakura[1], K. Terada[2], and T. Fujimoto[3]

[1] Department of Neurosurgery, Faculty of Medicine, Kagoshima University, Kagoshima, Japan
Departments of [2] Neurosurgery and [3] Psychiatry, Fujimoto Hospital, Miyazaki, Japan

Summary. Twenty patients with cerebral infarcts were investigated with phosphorus chemical shift imaging (^{31}P-CSI) using a 2.0 T MRI and spectroscopy system to monitor the energy metabolism in the infarcted brain. All patients were also examined with *N*-isopropyl-*p*-^{123}I-iodoamphetamine (^{123}I-IMP) single photon emission CT (SPECT) and X-ray CT. ^{31}P-CSI in acute cerebral infarction demonstrated increased inorganic phosphate (Pi) and decreased phosphocreatine (PCr) and ATP in a region almost identical to the region of hypoperfusion visualized in ^{123}I-IMP SPECT early images, but larger than the region of low density on X-ray CT. In chronic infarcts, Pi, PCr and ATP were all reduced.

Key words: ^{31}P-chemical shift imaging – ^{31}P-MR spectroscopy – Cerebral infarcts – Energy metabolism

Phosphorus magnetic resonance spectroscopy (^{31}P-MRS) is now employed in many kinds of clinical investigation. Phosphorus chemical shift imaging (^{31}P-CSI), presently under development, can yield chemical shift images and MR spectra of volumes of interest. ^{31}P-CSI reveals the distribution of high-energy phosphate metabolites in the human brain. We studied energy metabolism of patients with cerebral infarction using ^{31}P-CSI.

Patients and methods

Twenty patients with cerebral infarction, aged 37–85 years, were studied between 1 h and 132 days after onset of infarction. ^{31}P-CSI was performed using the method of spectroscopic imaging by dephasing amplitude changing (SIDAC) and 4-dimensional Fourier transform (4DFT). ^{31}P-CSI was obtained in a 2.0 T superconducting MRI system (Asahi Super 200). Using the SIDAC technique, ^{31}P-CSI was obtained in scan times of 68 min at 20 mm $\times$ 20 mm $\times$ 70 mm spatial resolution and 0.90 ppm chemical shift resolution. Using the 4DFT technique, ^{31}P-CSI was obtained in scan times of 60 min at 32 mm $\times$ 32 mm $\times$ 70 mm spatial resolution and 0.45 ppm chemical shift resolution. All patients were also examined with *N*-isopropyl-*p*-^{123}I-iodoamphetamine (^{123}I-IMP), single photon emission CT (SPECT) and X-ray CT.

Results

^{31}P-CSI after acute cerebral infarction demonstrated a region of increased inorganic phosphate (Pi) and decreased phosphocreatine (PCr) and ATP almost identical to a region of hypoperfusion visualized in early ^{123}I-IMP SPECT images but larger than the region of low density on X-ray CT (Fig. 1). In chronic infarcts, Pi, PCr and ATP were all reduced (Fig. 2).

Discussion

^{31}P-CSI and ^{31}P-MRS can detect abnormalities in energy metabolism due to cerebral infarction just after onset. We were therefore able to study hyperacute cerebral infarction 1 h after the ischaemic insult [1].

^{31}P-CSI after acute cerebral infarction showed a marked increase in Pi and a decrease in PCr and ATP. In chronic cerebral infarction it revealed a decrease in Pi, PCr, and ATP; the total ^{31}P-NMR signal was therefore reduced. These results agree with those of previous reports [2, 3] and are consistent with a reduction in the number of metabolically active brain cells and/or a decrease in cellular functional activity [2].

Positron emission tomography and SPECT are more sensitive than X-ray CT for detecting ischaemic lesions [4, 5]. In our cases, ^{31}P-CSI findings were almost as marked, or more so, than ^{123}I-IMP SPECT findings, and very much more so than those of X-ray CT, because ^{31}P-CSI can image regions of energy metabolism disturbance caused by transneuronal depression or selective neuronal loss [5].

In conclusion, ^{31}P-CSI is very useful for noninvasive monitoring of human cerebral infarction.

References

1. Sasahira M, Uchimura K, Yatsushiro K, Fujimoto T, Asakura T (1990) Early detection of cerebral infarction by ^{31}P spectroscopic imaging. Neuroradiology 32: 43–46
2. Bottomley PA, Drayer BP, Smith LS (1986) Chronic adult cerebral infarction studied by phosphorus NMR spectroscopy. Radiology 160: 763–766
3. Uchimura K, Sasahira M, Okada A, Fujimoto T, Yatsushiro K, Asakura T (1989) ^{31}P-chemical shift imaging of human cerebral infarctions. Prog CT 11: 525–533
4. Heiss WD, Herholz K, Böcher-Schwarz HG, Pawlik G, Wienhard K, Steinbrich W, Friedmann G (1986) PET, CT, and MR imaging in cerebrovascular disease. J Comput Assist Tomogr 10: 903–911

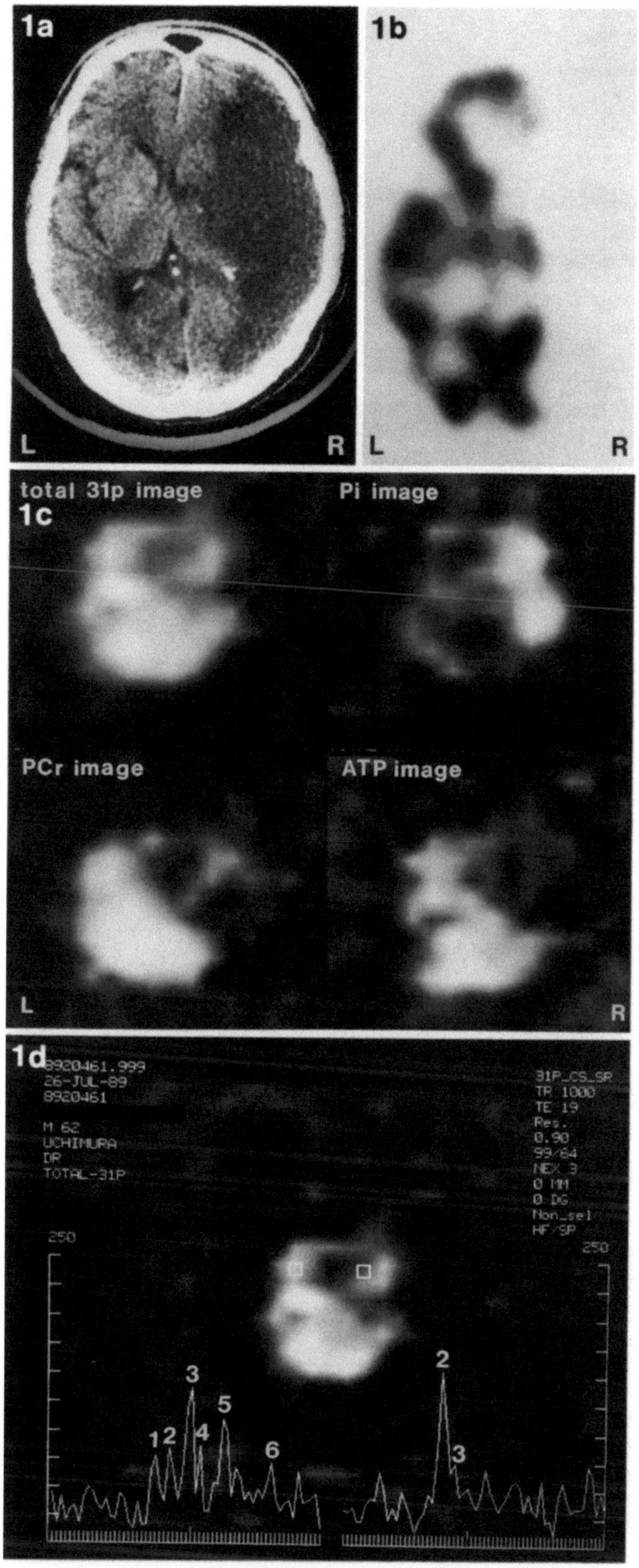

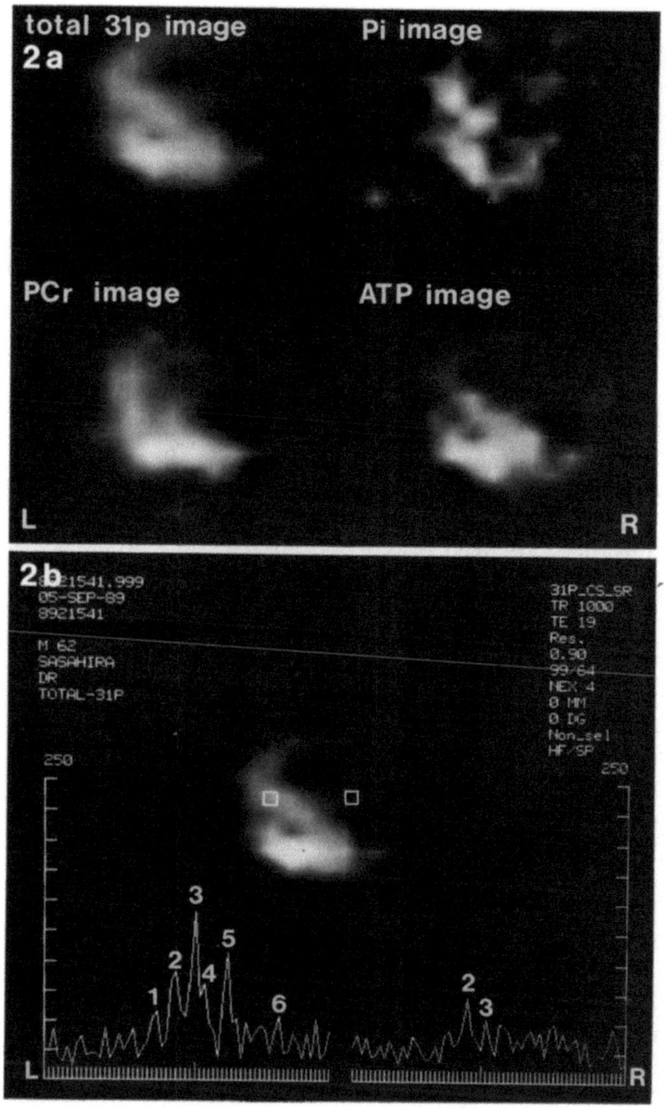

Fig. 1a–d. A 62-year-old male with acute cerebral infarction: **a** X-ray CT; **b** early ^{123}I-IMP single photon emission CT image; **c** ^{31}P-chemical shift images (^{31}P-CSIs) obtained 19 h after onset using the spectroscopic imaging by dephasing amplitude changing (SIDAC) method. The inorganic phosphorus (Pi) image had a high signal, while phosphocreatine (PCr) and ATP images had low signals in the right cerebral hemisphere; **d** ^{31}P-MR spectra of volumes of interest chosen from the total ^{31}P image, one in the infarcted hemisphere and another centred on the homologous region of the opposite hemisphere. The spectrum of the infarct (right side) showed an increase of Pi and a decrease of PCr and ATP. Peak assignments: 1, phosphomonoesters (PME); 2, Pi and phosphodiesters (PDE); 3, PCr; 4, 5, 6, γ, α, β-ATP

Fig. 2a, b. The same patients: ^{31}P-CSI obtained 42 days after onset using the SIDAC method. All ^{31}P-metabolites were reduced in the infarct. Peak assignments: 1, PME; 2, Pi and PDE; 3, PCr; 4, 5, 6, γ, α, β-ATP

5. Raynaud C, Rancurel G, Tzourio N, Soucy JP, Baron JC, Pappata S, Cambon H, Mazoyer B, Lassen NA, Cabanis E, Majdalani A, Bourdoiseau M, Ricard S, Bourguignon M, Syrota A (1989) SPECT analysis of recent cerebral infarction. Stroke 20: 192–204

Dr. Koichi Uchimura
Department of Neurosurgery, Faculty of Medicine
Kagoshima University
1208-1 Usuki-cho, Kagoshima City
Japan 890

Neuroradiology (1991) 33 [Suppl]: 358–359

Neuroradiology
© Springer-Verlag 1991

^{31}P chemical shift imaging of hypertensive intracerebral haematoma

M. Sasahira[1], K. Uchimura[1], T. Asakura[1], K. Terada[2], and T. Fujimoto[3]

[1] Department of Neurosurgery, University of Kagoshima, Kagoshima, Japan
Departments of [2] Neurosurgery and [3] Psychiatry, Fujimoto Hospital, Miyakonojo, Japan

Summary. Fourteen patients with hypertensive intracerebral haematomas were examined by ^{31}P-chemical shift imaging (^{31}P-CSI) using spectroscopic imaging by dephasing amplitude changing method. ^{31}P-CSI was carried out with a whole-body MRI system operating at 2.0 T. In the acute stage, haematoma and perifocal oedema were seen as a low-signal area of total ^{31}P, phosphocreatine (PCr) and ATP, and a high-signal area of inorganic phosphate (Pi). The area of perifocal oedema showed acute hypoxic metabolism due to the compression by haematoma. In the chronic stage, haematoma was seen as a low-signal area of total ^{31}P, PCr, ATP and Pi, which were almost the same as the low perfusion areas in the early image of ^{123}I-IMP single photon emission. The area of haematoma showed hypometabolism due to the reduction of normal activity or normal function by brain damage. ^{31}P-CSI is a very useful method for the study of localised phosphorus metabolism.

Key words: Hypertensive intracerebral haematoma – ^{31}P-chemical shift imaging – ^{31}P-magnetic resonance spectroscopy – ^{123}I-IMP single photon emission computed tomography

Recent advances in ^{31}P-NMR spectroscopy (MRS) allow a noninvasive study of brain metabolism in vivo. ^{31}P-chemical shift imaging (31P-CSI) is a very useful method for the evaluation of localized phosphorus metabolism [1]. We studied the metabolism of intracerebral haematomas by means of ^{31}P-CSI, using spectroscopic imaging by dephasing amplitude changing method [4].

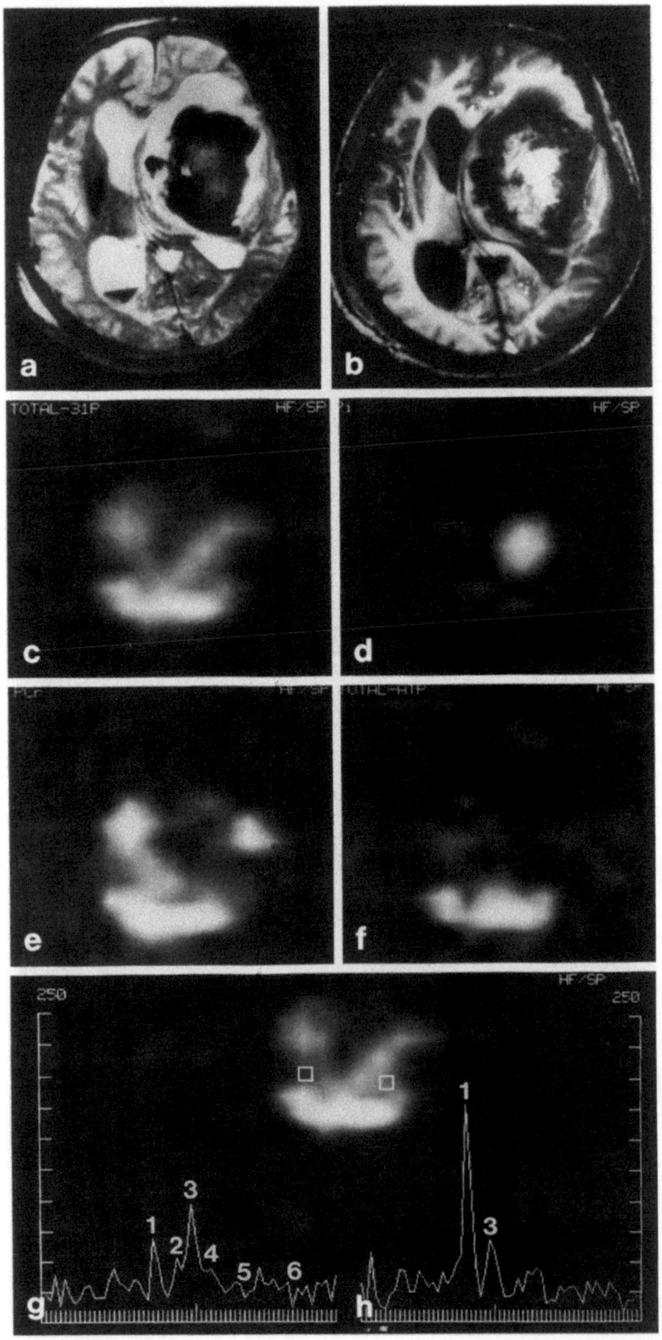

Fig. 1 a–h. Left putaminal haematoma (combined type). **a, b** MRI obtained 38 h after the onset. **c–h** (^{31}P-CSI) ^{31}P-chemical shift imaging was performed 37 h after the onset.
^{1}H MRI: **a** SE, Tr > 2000, Te 82; **b** IR, Tr 2500, Ti 800, Te 14 P-31 CSI: **c** total ^{31}**P** image: **d** inorganic phosphate (Pi) image; **e** phosphocreatine (PCr) image **f** total ATP image P-31 spectrum **g** contralateral hemisphere; **h** area of perifocal oedema 1: PME; 2: PDE; 3: PCr; 4: γ-ATP; 5: α-ATP; 6: β-ATP; 7: Pi

Materials and methods

^{31}P-CSI was carried out using a 2.0 T superconducting MRI system (Asahi Super 200). A series of 64 spectroscopic images with a 0.9 ppm chemical shift resolution and a 20 × 20 × 70 mm spatial resolution were collected in 1 h.

Fourteen patients with a hypertensive intracerebral haematoma were included in this study. Eight patients had a putaminal haematoma, 4 had a thalamic haematoma and the remaining 2 had a subcortical haematoma. Repeat studies were performed in several patients, a total of 20 ^{31}P-CSI being performed in 14 subjects.

Results

In the acute stage, haematoma and perifocal oedema were seen as a low-signal area of total ^{31}P, phosphocreatine (PCr) and ATP, and a high-signal area of inorganic phosphate (Pi). In the subacute (3 days after onset) and the chronic stages, haematoma was seen as a low-signal area of total ^{31}P, PCr, ATP and Pi (Fig. 1).

Discussion

It is important to know more about cerebral metabolism in intracerebral haematomas. However, so far only a few reports have been published on PET and ^{31}P MRS in intracerebral haematomas [2, 3, 5].

PET studies reveal a punched-out defect in cerebral blood flow (CBF) and oxygen metabolic rate ($CMRO_2$) in and around the area of a haematoma and a considerable decrease in CBF and $CMRO_2$ in the tissues surrounding the haematoma. Patients with a haematoma larger than 4.5 cm maximal diameter reveal a remarkable reduction in the mean CBF, with a significant increase in the oxygen extraction fraction. These findings would indicate that increased intracranial pressure, caused by a large haematoma, has reduced tissue perfusion pressure beyond the lower limit of the autoregulatory function of the cerebral circulation [5].

In spontaneous intracerebral haemorrhage induced in SHR SP rats, the ^{31}P MRS, ATP and PCr peaks decreased and Pi peak increased gradually after the onset, but these changes were mild. In a clinical study of intracerebral haematoma using image selected in vivo spectroscopy, the ^{31}P-spectrum showed each signal to have decreased, while the Pi signal had increased, compared with those from the contralateral hemisphere [3].

In our clinical study, haematoma and perifocal oedema were seen in the acute stage as a low-signal area of total ^{31}P, PCr and ATP, and a high-signal area of Pi. CBF of perifocal oedema at the acute stage was reduced due to compression by the haematoma. Haematoma and perifocal oedema in the subacute and chronic stage were seen as a low-signal area of total ^{31}P, PCr, Pi and ATP images, which was almost entirely consistent with the low perfusion area in early images of ^{123}I-IMP SPECT. The area of haematoma and perifocal oedema at this stage showed hypometabolism due to the reduction of normal activity or normal function, by brain damage.

In conclusion, localized phosphorus metabolite maps were obtained by ^{31}P-CSI and this proved a very useful method for the study of metabolism in and around a haematoma.

References

1. Asakura T, Sasahira M, Uchimura K (1989) Chemical shift imaging. J Med Imag Jpn 9: 942–952
2. Naruse S (1987) Brain metabolism detected by magnetic resonance spectroscopy. Neurosurgeons 6: 99–106
3. Tanaka C, Naruse S, Horikawa Y (1988) Image-guided localized ^{31}P-MRS study of human brain tumors and cerebrovascular disease. Prog CT 10: 539–545
4. Miyazaki T, Yamamoto T, Iriguchi N (1989) Spectroscopic imaging by dephasing amplitude changing (SIDAC). Radiat Med 7: 1–5
5. Uemura K, Shishido F, Higano S (1986) Positron emission tomography in patients with a primary intracerebral hematoma. Acta Radiol (Suppl) Stockh 369: 426–428

Dr. M. Sasshira
Department of Neurosurgery
Akune-Shimin Hospital
4513, Akasegawa, Akune-shi
Kagoshima-ken, 899-16
Japan

Neuroradiology (1991) 33 [Suppl]: 360–361

Neuro-radiology
© Springer-Verlag 1991

The extracranial carotid bifurcation: CT findings correlated with angiography

N. Caputo[1], C. Chiurulla[1], S. Ricci[2], P. G. Cao[3], and E. Signorini[1]

[1] Servizio di Neuroradiologia, Ospedale Generale, Perugia, Italy
[2] Clinica Neurologica and [3] Clinica Chirurgica Università di Perugia, Perugia, Italy

Summary. A group of 51 patients with clinical histories suggesting recent or longstanding ischaemia in the territory supplied by the internal carotid artery were studied by thin-section contrast-enhanced dynamic incremental CT and transfemoral selective common carotid artery angiography . The CT findings were correlated with the angiographic and surgical observations (when available). CT proved to be a reliable diagnostic procedure to demonstrate the vessels in the cervical region and for the direct evaluation of the vessel wall. CT was found to be more accurate than angiography in the assessment of luminal stenosis and in the demonstration of an ulcer in a plaque.

Key words: Computed tomography – Transfemoral selective common carotid artery angiography – Carotid artery, stenosis – Carotid artery, ulceration

Atheroma at the extracranial carotid bifurcation is believed to be the most frequent cause of cerebral ischaemia.Cerebral angiography is the radiological investigation most commonly used to study this region but vessel wall abnormalities can be underestimated or even missed [1–3]. Recently, CT has been proposed as a means of visualizing the extracranial carotid vessels [2–8]. In order to assess the reproducibility of the method for demonstrating carotid plaques and assess luminal stenosis, 51 CT studies of carotid bifurcations were reviewed and the results were compared with the angiographic findings.

Materials and methods

CT studies of 102 extracranial carotid bifurcations were obtained by a series of contiguous axial slices, of 3-mm thickness, from the C5 vertebral body to the C2 vertebral body; the acquisition parameters were: 120 kV, 170 mA, 2 s; 16 cm field of view with 512 × 512 matrix and "soft tissue" reconstruction algorithm. Throughout the scanning period, 100–150 ml of nonionic contrast medium (iopamidol 300) were injected intravenously.

In 88 cases transfemoral selective common carotid angiography was performed and 35 cases underwent carotid endarterectomy. The extracranial carotid arteries at the bifurcation were evaluated on the axial CT images for arterial wall abnormalities, ulceration and the size of the residual lumen.

The luminal stenoses were subdivided on the CT images into three groups: mild (0%–49%), moderate (50%–74%) and severe (75%–99%), as described by Culebras et al. [4]. Similar observations were made on the angiographic films.

Results and discussion

In 51 patients, CT was able to demonstrate the cross-sectional appearance of the distal common carotid artery and the proximal external and internal carotid arteries on both sides. The direct visualization of the vessel wall and its abnormalities offered the possibility of differentiating completely obstructed vessels (14) from both narrowed vessels (86) and enlarged vessels (2), and assessing the radiographic density of the atherosclerotic plaques (Figs. 1, 2).

In 14 vessels there was a homogeneous hypodense plaque without calcification. In other cases there was a mixed-density plaque, 46 with a few calcium deposits and 25 with large calcium deposits (Figs. 3–5).

The degree of focal stenosis, shown by CT, correlated closely with the angiographic findings in 51 of 80 cases. In 23 cases, the severity of the luminal involvement was greater on CT than on angiography. In 6 cases, the degree of stenosis was shown better by angiography than by CT. Comparing the ability of CT and angiography to detect carotid artery ulceration, they were in agreement in 45 cases and CT showed an ulcer not seen on angiography in 29 cases. However, in no case did angiography show an ulcer not seen on CT. Of the 35 cases operated on, in 18 cases the surgical description of the stenotic lesion was available and ulcerated plaques were found in 13. In 9 cases both angiography and CT demonstrated the lesion but in 4 cases CT was positive and angiography negative. No ulceration was found in 5 cases. In 1 case both CT and angiography were correctly negative, in 3 cases both were positive and in 1 case CT was positive and angiography negative.

References

1. Edwards JH, Kricheff II, Riles T, Imparato A (1979) Angiographically undetected ulceration of the carotid bifurcation as a cause of embolic stroke. Radiology 132: 369–373

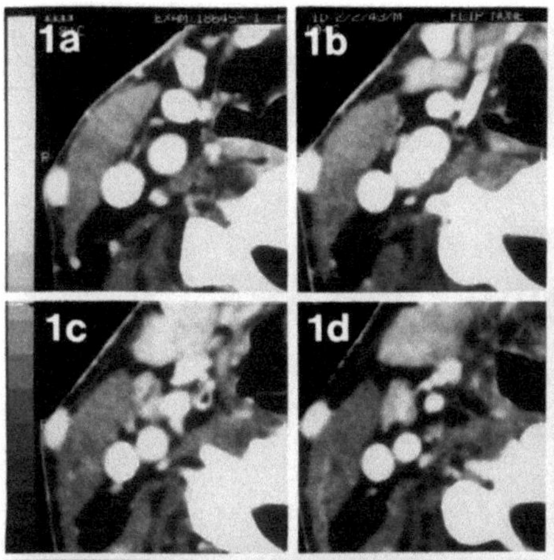

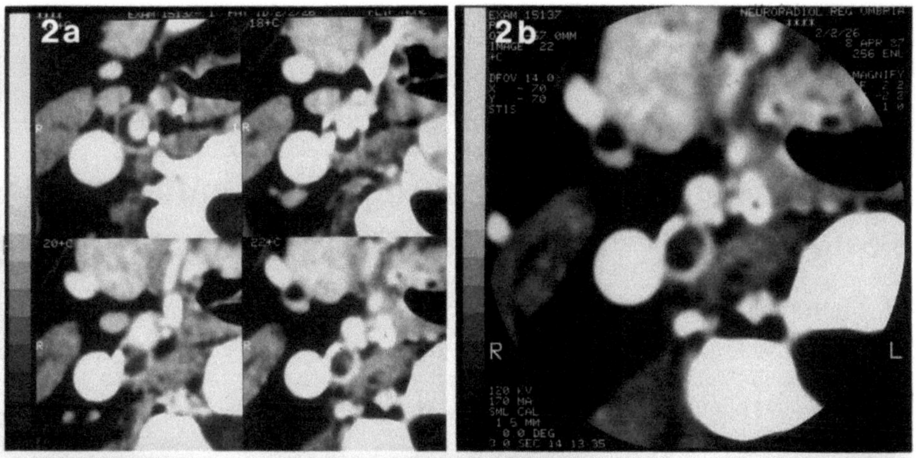

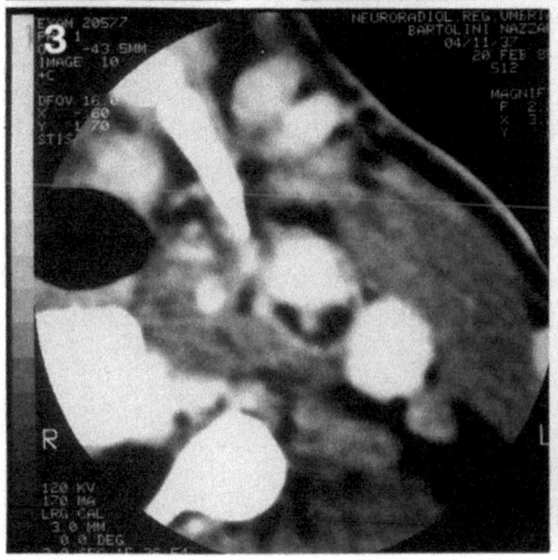

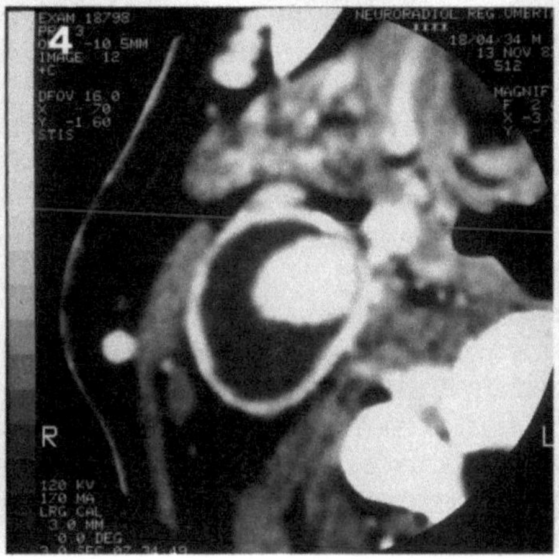

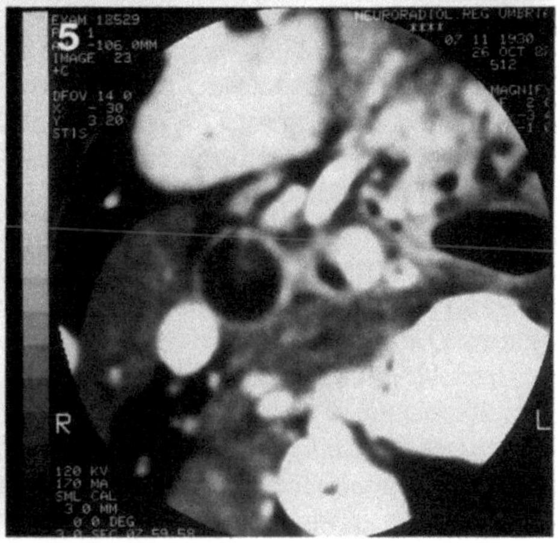

Fig. 1. a, b Normal right carotid bifurcation in the axial plane **a** Common carotid artery, anterior and medial to the internal jugular vein. **b** Normal oval-shaped carotid bifurcation with the origin of the external carotid artery anteromedially and the origin of the internal carotid artery posterolaterally. **c, d** Proximal internal carotid artery anterior and medial to the internal jugular vein and posterior and lateral to the external carotid artery

Fig. 2 a, b. Complete occlusion of the right internal carotid artery at the bifurcation level due to a large mixed plaque with multiple calcium deposits

Fig. 3. Ulcerated plaque in the left distal common carotid artery: the ulceration is the outpouching of contrast medium within the plaque

Fig. 4. Large aneurysm of the proximal right internal carotid artery with an irregular, thin wall and a small peripheral calcium deposit. The vascular lumen is partially occluded by a large organized thrombus

Fig. 5. Right external carotid artery occlusion at the bifurcation level due to a large mixed plaque, also involving the proximal internal carotid artery

2. Heinz ER, Pizer SM, Fuchs EK, Burger P, Drayer BP, Osborne DR (1984) Examination of the extracranial carotid bifurcation by thin-section dynamic CT: direct visualization of intimal atheroma in man (part 1). AJNR 5: 355–359
3. Hodge CJ, Leeson M, Cacayorin E, Petro G, Culebras A, Iliya A (1987) Computed tomography evaluation of extracranial carotid artery disease. Neurosurgery 21: 167–176
4. Culebras A, Magana R, Cacayorin ED (1988) Computed tomography of the cervical carotid artery: significance of the lucent defect. Stroke 19: 723–727
5. Heinz ER, Fuchs J, Osborne D, Drayer B, Yeates A, Fuchs H, Pizer S (1984) Examination of the extracranial carotid bifurcation by thin-section dynamic CT direct visualization of intimal atheroma in man (part 2). AJNR 5: 361–366
6. Leeson MD, Cacayorin ED, Iliya AR, Hodge CJ, Culebras A, Collins GH, Kieffer SA (1985) Atheromatous extracranial carotid arteries: CT evaluation correlated with arteriography and pathologic examination. Radiology 156: 397–402
7. Petro GR, Witwer GA, Cacayorin ED, Hodge CJ, Bredenberg CE, Jastremski MS, Kieffer SA (1986) Spontaneous dissection of the cervical carotid artery: correlation of arteriography, CT, and pathology. AJNR 7: 1053–1058
8. Tress BA, Davis S, Lavain J, Kaye A, Hopper J (1986) Incremental dynamic computed tomography: practical method of imaging the carotid bifurcation. AJNR 7: 49–54

Dr. N. Caputo
Servizio di Neuroradiologia
Ospedale Generale
Perugia, Italy

Neuroradiology (1991) 33 [Suppl]: 362–363

Neuro-radiology
© Springer-Verlag 1991

Cerebral blood flow in cerebral vascular disease: assessment by colour Doppler, transcranial Doppler and SPECT

W. Liboni[1], G. Chianale[2], G. Turco[1], G. Castellano[1], and R. Priulla[3]

[1] Department of Nuclear Medicine, University of Turin, Turin, Italy
[2] Department of Neurology, University of Turin, Turin, Italy
[3] Clinica Pinna Pintor, Turin, Italy

Summary. Since 1988 we have been using SPECT 99Tc-HMPAO, Duplex scanner (DS), colour Doppler imaging (CDI) and transcranial Doppler (TCD) to assess arterial stenosis or occlusion, collateral circulation and blood supply adequacy. In cerebral vascular disease, clinical features do not often predict the presence or degree of vessel lesions, but correlate well with the integrated morphological and functional data about cerebral circulation and perfusion. DS and CDI have a high specificity in detecting atherosclerotic disease (97%). TCD has a high sensitivity for intracranial vascular pathology. SPECT HMPAO is more useful than TCD for imaging brain tissue damage; it shows hypoperfusion in about 70% of transient ischaemic attacks and agrees with the improvement or worsening of the symptoms. These functional images and cerebral artery velocity patterns appear to be important tools in understanding and evaluating brain damage caused by embolism and by haemodynamic failure.

Key words: Cerebral vascular disease – Colour Doppler imaging – Transcranial Doppler – Single photon emission tomography

Stenosis or occlusion of large cerebral vessels can cause a reduction of the cerebral blood flow. Atherosclerotic disease is established as a main source of ischaemic events, including amaurosis fugax, transient ischaemic attacks (TIA) and strokes. Cortical signs and amaurosis fugax, short in duration, often predict severe stenosis or occlusion of the internal carotid artery (ICA); lacunar symptoms are strongly correlated with insignificant or moderate ICA pathology, whereas minor signs such as numbness or weakness are not reliably predictive of the degree of ICA involvment. Cerebral angiography (DSA) is also the method of choice for imaging cerebral vessels and quantifying in vivo the artherosclerotic lesion (ATS). However the clinical and angiographic findings provide clear evidence of pathogenetic mechanisms and distinction of the degree of stenosis, haemodynamic failure, the presence of ulceration and the pathology of intraparenchymal microvessels in some cases only. The Duplex scanner (DS), transcranial Doppler (TCD) and more recently colour Doppler imaging (CDI) are valuable tools in diagnosing and monitoring extracranial ATS and extra-intracranial flow disturbances [1, 2]. Single photon emission tomography (SPECT) following i.v. injection of about 99 MBq of ^{99m}Tc hexamethyl-propylene-amino-oxime (HMPAO) is a very sensitive method for imaging hypoperfused cerebral territories; it is also specific in assessing neuron function. We describe our experience using ultrasound and SPECT in diagnosing the status of vessel haemodynamics and cerebral perfusion correlated with clinical features in cerebral vascular disease [3].

Materials and methods

Forty-three patients have been investigated. Clinical diagnosis of TIA was made in 27, of stroke in 12, of arterovenous malformation (AVM) in 3 and of Alzheimer's disease (DA) in 1. All patients underwent CT and 13 of them MRI. DS (Diasonics 400), TCS (EME TC 264), and SPECT HMPAO (GE 400A connected to computer GE. Star II) were carried out in all patients. Thirteen cases were followed up, 3 patients within 30 days of TIA and 10 patients within 8–12 months of the onset of symptoms. DSA was performed on 15 patients with severe ATS or AVM. CDI (Philips Quantum PV) was carried out in 8 patients.

Results

DS showed a high sensitivity in detecting common carotid and proximal ICA disease. As specifity was 97% in detecting occlusion, we need DSA to properly define very severe stenosis or occlusion. CDI, combining real-time B-mode imaging with semiquantitative colour encoding of the Doppler shift, should increase the accuracy of evaluating occlusion.

TCD was useful in assessing intracranial vascular pathology, both for diagnosis of middle cerebral artery occlusion in the absence of extracranial lesions (1 patient) and for diagnosis of AVM. TCD provided more reliable evaluation of cerebral collateral flow and of the adequacy of supply and the vascular resistance.

HMPAO SPECT provided early information on the perfusion disturbance and neuron function, in comparison with neurological deficit and its evolution: in 3 patients with stroke with partial recovery after ICA occlusion, we observed a disappearance of cerebellar diaschisis and a reduction of the hypoperfused area. In 2 patients with amaurosis fugax and ICA stenosis an improvement was evident in attention and hemispheric perfusion, 1 month after TIA.

Discussion

Our clinical experience points out that the clinical features do not really predict the severity of ATS and the extent of the parenchymal lesion. Among our patients 2 with ICA occlusions had TIA and amaurosis fugax as did 20 patients with insignificant or moderate stenosis. Five patients with AVM and without ICA ATS had stroke. Clinical features and the prognosis are more strongly correlated with collateral supply than with the degree of vessel lesion. For these reasons we believe DS, CDI, TC and HMPAO SPECT are reliable diagnostic tools. They can show and monitor the anatomical and functional condition of cerebral vessels and cells even if CT provides no evidence of a brain tissue lesion.

References

1. Lewis BD, James EM, Welch TJ (1989) Current applications of duplex and color Doppler ultrasound imaging: carotid and peripheral vascular system. Mayo Clin Proc 64: 1147–1157
2. Aaslid R, Lindegaard KF (1986) A transcranial Doppler sonography. Springer, Vienna New York
3. Ell PJ, (1985) Tc 99m labelled radiotracer for the investigation of cerebral vascular disease. Nucl Med Commun 6: 437–441

Dr. W. Liboni
Department of Nuclear Medicine
University of Turin
Turin, Italy

Neuroradiology (1991) 33 [Suppl]: 364–365

Neuro
radiology
© Springer-Verlag 1991

The mechanism of infarction in the territory of the anterior choroidal artery due to embolic occlusion of the internal carotid artery

M. Ueda, S. Hayashi, K. Morinaga, Y. Matsumoto, N. Omiya, J. Mikami, H. Sato, Y. Inoue, and S. Okawara

Okawara Neurosurgical Hospital, Muroran, Japan

Summary. Case 1 was a 69-year-old man and case 2 a 71-year-old woman. The neurological examination in both cases showed left homonymous hemianopia, left facial palsy, left hemiparesis and left hemisensory disturbance. Computed tomography showed infarction in only the territory of the anterior choroidal artery (AChA), and right carotid angiograms showed an occlusion of the internal carotid artery (ICA). The left carotid injection in these cases visualized the right anterior cerebral artery and the right middle cerebral artery via the anterior communicating artery, but the right AChA was not visualized. After comparison of these cases and 15 cases without infarction in the territory of the AChA due to occlusion of the ICA, we offer speculations about the mechanism of infarction in the territory of the AChA.

Key words: Infarction – Anterior choroidal artery – Embolism – Internal carotid artery

Infarction in only the territory of the anterior choroidal artery (AChA) due to occlusion of the ICA is rare. We report two such cases and investigate the mechanism of infarction in the territory of the AChA.

Case reports

Case 1 was a 69-year-old man. He was hospitalized for sudden headache, vomiting and left hemiplegia. At the time of admission, electrocardiogram (ECG) showed atrial fibrillation. The neurological examination revealed right conjugate deviation of the eyes, dysarthria, left facial palsy, left homonymous hemianopia, left hemiplegia and left hemisensory disturbance. Computed tomography (CT) showed no abnormal findings. The right carotid angiogram showed occlusion of the internal carotid artery (ICA) in its cervical segment (Fig. 1 a). The collateral pathways from the right external carotid artery (ECA) and the right posterior communicating artery (PComA) to the right intracranial ICA were not fillied (Fig. 1 b–d). The left carotid injection visualized the right ACA and middle cerebral artery (MCA) via anterior communicating artery (AComA) well, but the right AChA was not visualized (Fig. 1 c). On the 4th day, CT showed infarction in the territory of the right AChA. On the 31st day, the right carotid angiogram showed complete recanalization of the occluded ICA, and the precommunicating segment of the right posterior cerebral artery (PCA) was hypoplastic (Fig. 2). On the 61st day, MRI showed infarction of the right uncus, amygdaloid nucleus, genu and posterior limb of the internal capsule, lateral geniculate body and the tail of the caudate nucleus (Fig. 3). In this case, embolic occlusion of the right ICA was diagnosed by the clinical course and angiographic and ECG findings.

Case 2 was a 71-year-old woman. On admission, ECG showed atrial fibrillation. The neurological examination revealed right conjugate deviation of the eyes, dysarthria, left facial palsy, left homonymous hemianopia, left hemiplegia and left hemisensory disturbance. Right carotid angiograms showed occlusion of the right ICA in the siphon. The collateral pathway from the right ECA to the right intracranial ICA was not supplied. The right ACA and MCA were supplied entirely by the left ICA via flow through the AComA. Vertebral angiography could not be performed. On the 2nd day, CT showed only infarction in the territory of the AChA. In this case, embolic occlusion of the right ICA was diagnosed by the clinical course and ECG findings.

Discussion

Only two cases with infarction in the territory of the AChA due to occlusion of the ICA have been reported because of rich anastomoses between the branches of the AChA and those of the PComA and posterior choroidal arteries (PChA) [1–4]. These anastomoses cannot be demonstrated directly on the angiograms. Among cases with occlusion of the ICA, a comparison was made between the 2 cases with infarction in the territory of the AChA and 15 cases without such infarction (Table 1) as regards:

1. Collateral pathways from the ipsilateral ECA, ipsilateral PComA and AComA to the carotid siphon of the affected ICA.

Table 1. Angiographic findings in 17 cases with and without anterior choroidal artery territory infarction due to occlusion of the internal carotid artery

	With AChA territory infarction		Without AChA territory infarction
	Case 1	Case 2	15 cases
Hypoplasia of ipsilateral P1 segment	+	Not examined	– : 15 cases
Collateral pathway ipsilateral PComA→ICA	–	Not examined	+ : 9 cases, –: 6 cases
Ipsilateral ECA→ICA	–	–	+ : 11 cases, – : 4 cases
Contralateral ICA→AComA→ICA	–	–	– : 15 cases

ICA, Internal carotid artery; ECA, external carotid artery; AChA, anterior choroidal artery; AComA, anterior communicating artery; PComA, posterior communicating artery; P1 segment, precommunicating segment of posterior cerebral artery

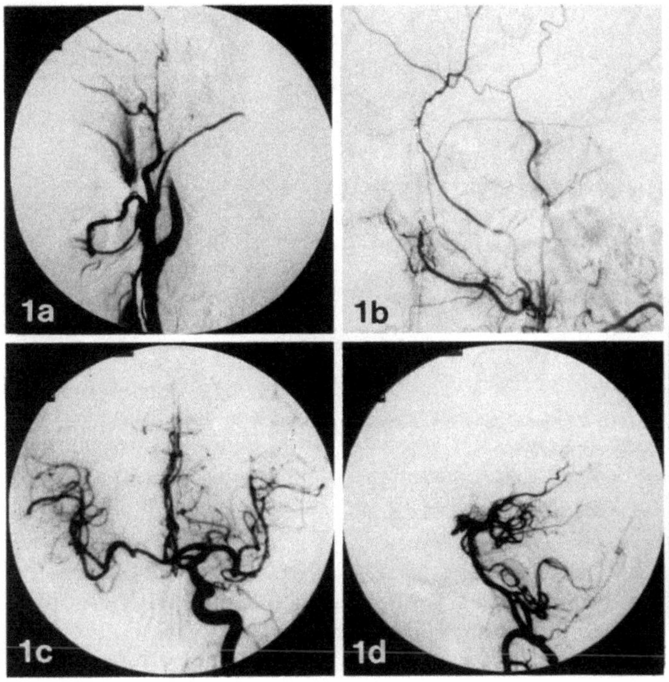

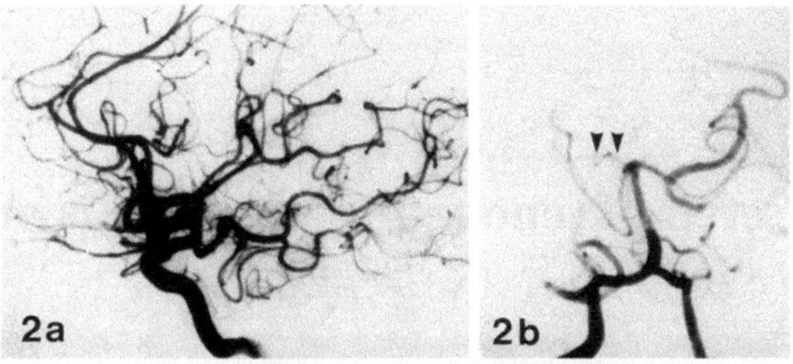

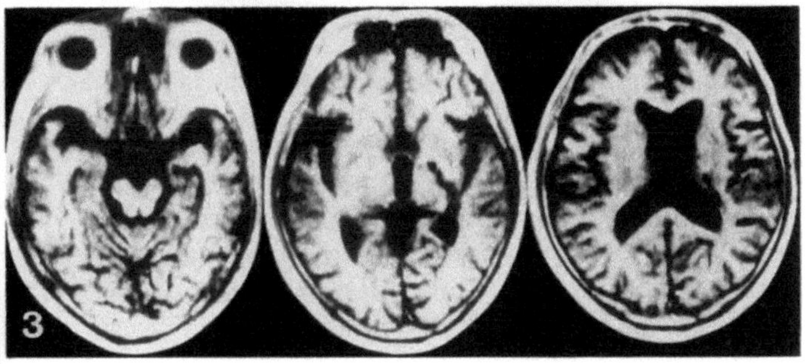

Fig. 1. a, b The right carotid angiograms on admission show occlusion of the internal carotid artery in its cervical segment. **c** The left carotid angiogram demonstrates that the right anterior cerebral artery and middle cerebral artery are supplied entirely by the left internal carotid artery. **d** The left vertebral angiogram shows the poor collateral pathway from the right posterior communicating artery to the right internal carotid artery

Fig. 2. a The right carotid angiogram on the 31st day demonstrates complete recanalization of the internal carotid artery. **b** The right vertebral angiogram shows hypoplasia of the right P1 segment *(arrowhead)*

Fig. 3. T1-weighted magnetic resonance images on the 61st day demonstrate infarction in the territory of the right anterior choroidal artery

2. Hypoplasia of the precommunicating segment of the ipsilateral PCA (ipsilateral P1 segment).

In no cases did angiography show a collateral pathway from the AComA to the carotid siphon of the affected ICA. In the 15 cases without infarction, the ipsilateral P1 segment was not hypoplastic and the collateral pathway from either the ipsilateral ECA or the ipsilateral PComA to the affected ICA was supplied. In these 2 cases collateral pathways from the ipsilateral ECA and ipsilateral PComA to the affected ICA were not supplied. In case 1, the ipsilateral P1 segment was hypoplastic. We thought it likely that the mechanism of infarction in the territory of the AChA was caused not only by the decreased cerebral blood flow in the territory of the AChA consequent to carotid occlusion, but also the poor collateral circulation from the ipsilateral PComA and ipsilateral PChA to the AChA.

References

1. Fisher M, Lingley JF, Blumenfeld A, Felice K (1989) Anterior choroidal artery territory infarction and small-vessel disease. Stroke 20: 1591–1592
2. Goldberg HI (1974) The anterior choroidal artery. In: Newton TH, Potts DG (eds) Radiology of the skull and brain, vol 2. Mosby, St. Louis, pp 1628–1658
3. Rhoton AL Jr, Fujii K, Fradd B (1979) Microsurgical anatomy of the anterior choroidal artery. Surg Neurol 12: 171–187
4. Takahashi S, Kawaya Y, Uemura K (1980) CT findings on anterior choroidal artery occlusion. Jpn J Clin Radiol 25: 575–581

Dr. M. Ueda
Okawara Neurosurgical Hospital
1-5-2, Kotobuki-cho, Muroran 050
Japan

Neuroradiology (1991) 33 [Suppl]: 366–367

Neuroradiology
© Springer-Verlag 1991

Cerebral venous thrombosis – diagnosis and treatment

C. C. Lui[1], S. T. Chen[2], T. Y. Lee[1], and C. C. Tsai[1]

Departments of [1] Diagnostic Radiology and [2] Neurology, Chang Gung Memorial Hospital, Kaohsiung, Taiwan, Republic of China

Summary. Eighteen cases of angiographically verified cerebral venous thrombosis (CVT) were reviewed. The CT findings were not specific except the empty-delta sign (33%). However, in patients whose CT shows multiple haemorrhagic infarcts or diffuse oedema, the possibility of CVT should be kept in mind. Angiography is still the definitive diagnostic tool. Most patients recovered satisfactorily with symptomatic treatment only.

Key words: Cerebral venous thrombosis – Computed tomography – Angiogram – Treatment

Central venous thrombosis (CVT) is not uncommon. The main diagnostic difficulty is the non-specific and protean clinical manifestations [1]. CT findings are mostly non-specific, except the empty-delta and cord signs [2]. Angiography is still necessary, not only to confirm the diagnosis but also to assess prognosis [2–4]. The most controversial point of treatment is the use of anticoagulants.

Materials and methods

During the past 6 years, 18 cases of CVT were diagnosed in our hospital. The diagnosis was considered as proven when angiography showed a partial or complete block of a dural sinus or of cerebral veins. CT (before and after intravenous contrast medium) and angiography were available for all cases. Cavernous sinus thrombosis, and sinus occlusion by tumour involvement were excluded. The clinical manifestations, radiological findings, aetiology, management and outcome of these patients were reviewed retrospectively.

Results

There were 7 males and 11 females, whose ages ranged from 24 to 64 years (average 36 years). Headache was the presenting symptom in 15 (83%) and seizures in 12 (66%); focal weakness was present in 12 (66%), papilloedema in 7 (39%), and impaired consciousness in 7 (39%). The possible aetiologies were: postpartum (3), oral contraceptives (2), paroxysmal nocturnal haemoglobulinuria (2), otitis media (1), dural arteriovenous malformation (1), head injury (1) and unknown (8). CVT was suspected in 2 patients before CT and in 5 patients after CT showed the empty-delta sign. In the remaining cases, the pre-angiographic diagnosis was incorrect.

CT showed a haemorrhagic infarct (Fig. 1 a) in 5 patients, thalamic haemorrhage in 1, focal or multiple low attenuation areas in 3, diffuse oedema in 5, a cord sign in 1, a dense vein sign in 3 (Fig. 2 a), and was normal in 2. Contrast-enhanced CT showed gyral enhancement in 11 and an empty-delta sign (Fig. 3 a) in 6 cases. Angiography showed involvement of the superior sagittal sinus in 15 (Fig. 2 b), straight sinus in 12 (Fig. 1 b), transverse sinus in 5 and cortical veins in 6 patients. Anticonvulsant and/or osmotic agents were used in patients with seizures and/or increased intracranial pressure. Three patients were treated with anticoagulants, 1 of whom developed a fatal intracerebral haemorrhage due to overdosage. All the remaining 17 patients recovered satisfactorily.

Discussion

The true incidence of CVT is not known [5]. The main problem of early diagnosis is that the relatively non-specific and protean clinical manifestations rarely cause the clinician to consider the condition [1]. The diagnosis might be suggested by CT although in 10% of our cases the images were normal [6]. About ten CT findings have been reported to be helpful in the diagnosis of CVT [6]; the most reliable is the empty-delta sign (Fig. 3 a) but this is present in only about 30% of cases [6, 7], although exceptionally high detection rates (60%–70%) have been reported [1, 3]. Moreover, the empty-delta sign is usually not present at the onset of symptoms [8]. In our series, the earliest time of appearance of the empty-delta sign was 6 days after the onset of symptoms, the average being 13 days. Gyral enhancement was common in our series (61%); it had previously been reported in about one third of cases [6]. Haemorrhagic infarction was found in 28% of our cases; it could be differentiated from arterial infarction by its poorly defined, rather rounded configuration, separate haemorrhage and lack of relation to arterial territories [9]. Although angiography is invasive, it is considered the best tool for investigation of CVT, not only to confirm the diagnosis, but also for assessment of collateral circulation, which is said to be of importance to the prognosis (Fig. 2 b). Prognosis has been reported to be poor in patients with focal signs [10], or CT demonstration of haemorrhagic infarct and the empty-delta sign [2], but this was not true in our cases (Fig. 1 a). Because of the wide spectrum of pathological conditions associated with CVT, the treatment is not specific. In our cases, symptomatic treatment was the main measure and most of the patients recovered well. Although some authors recommend early

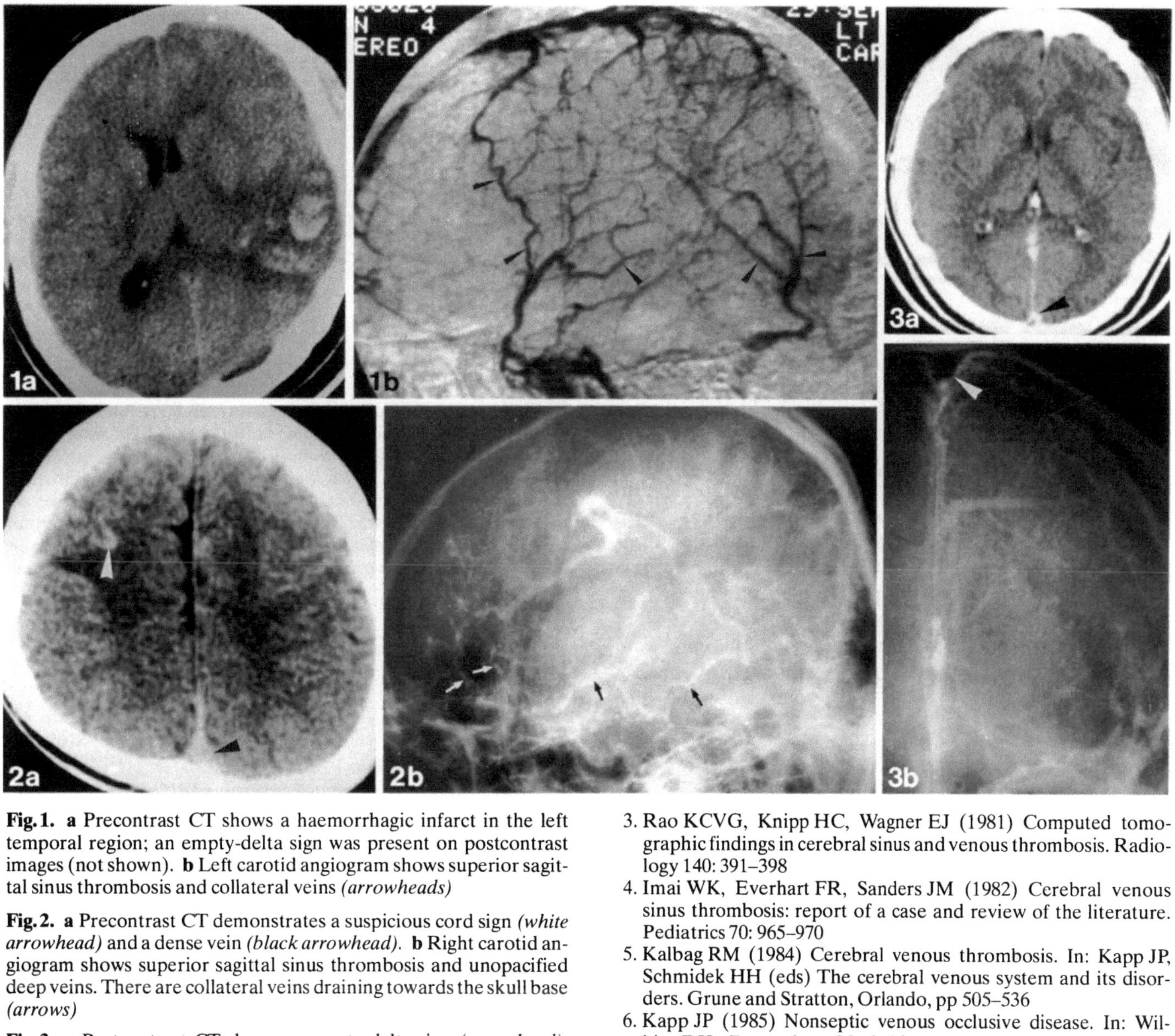

Fig. 1. **a** Precontrast CT shows a haemorrhagic infarct in the left temporal region; an empty-delta sign was present on postcontrast images (not shown). **b** Left carotid angiogram shows superior sagittal sinus thrombosis and collateral veins *(arrowheads)*

Fig. 2. **a** Precontrast CT demonstrates a suspicious cord sign *(white arrowhead)* and a dense vein *(black arrowhead)*. **b** Right carotid angiogram shows superior sagittal sinus thrombosis and unopacified deep veins. There are collateral veins draining towards the skull base *(arrows)*

Fig. 3. **a** Postcontrast CT shows an empty-delta sign *(arrowhead)*. **b** Left carotid angiogram shows corresponding filling defect in the superior sagittal sinus *(arrowhead)*

exhibition of anticoagulants [1, 10], this remains controversial [4].

References

1. Thron A, Wessel K, Linden D, Schroth G, Dichgans J (1986) Superior sagittal sinus thrombosis: neuroradiological evaluation and clinical findings. J Neurol 233: 283–288
2. Virapongse C, Malat J, Sarwar M (1989) Radiology of dural sinus thrombosis. In: Sarwar M, Batnitzky S (eds) Imaging of non-traumatic ischemic and hemorrhagic disorders of the central nervous system. Kluwer, Boston, pp 221–260
3. Rao KCVG, Knipp HC, Wagner EJ (1981) Computed tomographic findings in cerebral sinus and venous thrombosis. Radiology 140: 391–398
4. Imai WK, Everhart FR, Sanders JM (1982) Cerebral venous sinus thrombosis: report of a case and review of the literature. Pediatrics 70: 965–970
5. Kalbag RM (1984) Cerebral venous thrombosis. In: Kapp JP, Schmidek HH (eds) The cerebral venous system and its disorders. Grune and Stratton, Orlando, pp 505–536
6. Kapp JP (1985) Nonseptic venous occlusive disease. In: Wilkins RH, Rengachary SS (eds) Neurosurgery. McGraw-Hill, New York, pp 1300–1307
7. Virapongse C, Cazenave C, Quisling R, Sarwar M, Hunter S (1987) The empty delta sign: frequency and significance in 76 cases of dural sinus thrombosis. Radiology 162: 779–785
8. Shinohara Y, Yoshitoshi M, Yoshii F (1986) Appearance and disappearance of empty delta sign in superior sagittal sinus thrombosis. Stroke 17: 1282–1283
9. Kim KS, Walczak TS (1986) Computed tomography of deep cerebral venous thrombosis. J Comput Assist Tomogr 10: 386–390
10. Bousser MG, Chiras J, Bories J, Castaigne P (1985) Cerebral venous thrombosis – a review of 38 cases. Stroke 16: 199–213

Dr. C. C. Lui
Department of Diagnostic Radiology
Chang Gung Memorial Hospital
123 Ta Pei Rd., Niao Sung Hsiang
Kaohsiung Hsien (83305)
Taiwan, ROC

Neuroradiology (1991) 33 [Suppl]: 368–370

Neuroradiology
© Springer-Verlag 1991

PET in thalamic tumours

T. Ogawa[1], A. Inugami[1], I. Kanno[1], F. Shishido[1], S. Higano[1], H. Fujita[1], K. Uemura[1], K. Mineura[2], and M. Kowada[2]

[1] Department of Radiology and Nuclear Medicine, Research Institute for Brain and Blood Vessels, Akita, Japan
[2] Department of Neurosurgical Service, Akita University School of Medicine, Akita, Japan

Summary. We have studied eight patients with thalamic tumours using positron emission tomography (PET) with ^{15}O-labelled gas and ^{18}F-fluorodeoxyglucose and/or ^{11}C-methionine. PET with ^{11}C-methionine delineated clearly the extension of tumour and provided information for selection of appropriate treatment and evaluation of therapeutic effects on the tumour. PET with ^{18}F-fluorodeoxyglucose displayed malignant tumour as hypermetabolic foci and was useful for deciding the target of stereotactic needle biopsy. Concerning neurological function, hypoperfusion and hypometabolism were observed in the ipsilateral cortex. These results can be interpreted as remote effects via thalamocortical connections.

Key words: Brain neoplasm – Thalamus – Cerebral blood flow – Cerebral metabolism – Positron emission computed tomography

The treatment of thalamic tumours remains controversial. In order to select the appropriate treatment it is necessary to assess the degree of malignancy and extension of the tumour. We have studied these two aspects and also analysed remote effects on cerebral blood flow (CBF) and metabolism resulting from the thalamic tumour, using PET.

Patients and methods

Eight patients with thalamic tumours were studied (Table 1). All tumours were histologically verified except case 7. CBF was studied before treatment using PET with a $C^{15}O_2$ gas steady-state inhalation method in all patients. ^{18}F-fluorodeoxyglucose (^{18}FDG) metabolism and ^{11}C-methionine (^{11}C-Met) uptakes were also studied in five and four patients, respectively. Regional CBF and glucose consumption (CMRGI) at regions of interest placed on the cortical mantle, were obtained. The results were compared with the data from normal controls ($n = 6$).

Results

Qualitative results of PET with ^{18}FDG and ^{11}C-Met are summarized in Table 1. PET with ^{18}FDG (FDG-PET) showed a positive correlation between CMRGI and the degree of malignancy of the tumours. FDG-PET displayed viable and aggressive tumour tissue as hypermetabolic foci (hot spots, Fig. 1). PET with ^{11}C-Met (Met-PET) demarcated the tumour as having markedly higher ^{11}C-Met uptake in comparison with that of surrounding cortex in four patients. The area of high ^{11}C-Met uptake in the tumour tissue was usually larger than the area of the enhancing lesion on CT (Fig. 2a). Remote effects were studied in six patients with unilateral thalamic tumours (Figs 2b, 3). The mean CBF values were significantly lower on the affected side in frontal and temporal lobes and cortical mantle. The mean CBF value in cere-

Table 1. Clinical data and PET findings

Patient no.	Age/sex	Location of tumour	Histology	PET findings	
				^{18}FDG	^{11}C-MET
1	21/M	L thalamus	Astrocytoma grade II	–	ND
2	17/F	R thalamus	Malignant astrocytoma grade III	+	ND
3	53/M	L thalamus	Glioblastoma	ND	+ +
4	79/M	R thalamus	Glioblastoma	ND	+ +
5	67/M	R thalamus	Glioblastoma	ND	+ +
6	11/M	R thalamus L frontal	Glioblastoma	+ +	ND
7	19/M	B thalami	ND (malignant transformation)	+ +	ND
8	72/M	L thalamus	Malignant lymphoma	+ +	+ +

L, Left; R, right; B, bilateral; ND, not done; ^{18}FDG, ^{18}F-fluorodeoxyglucose; ^{11}C-Met, ^{11}C-methionine

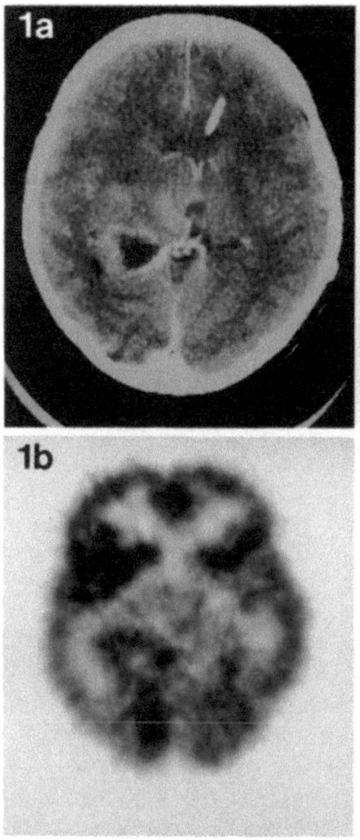

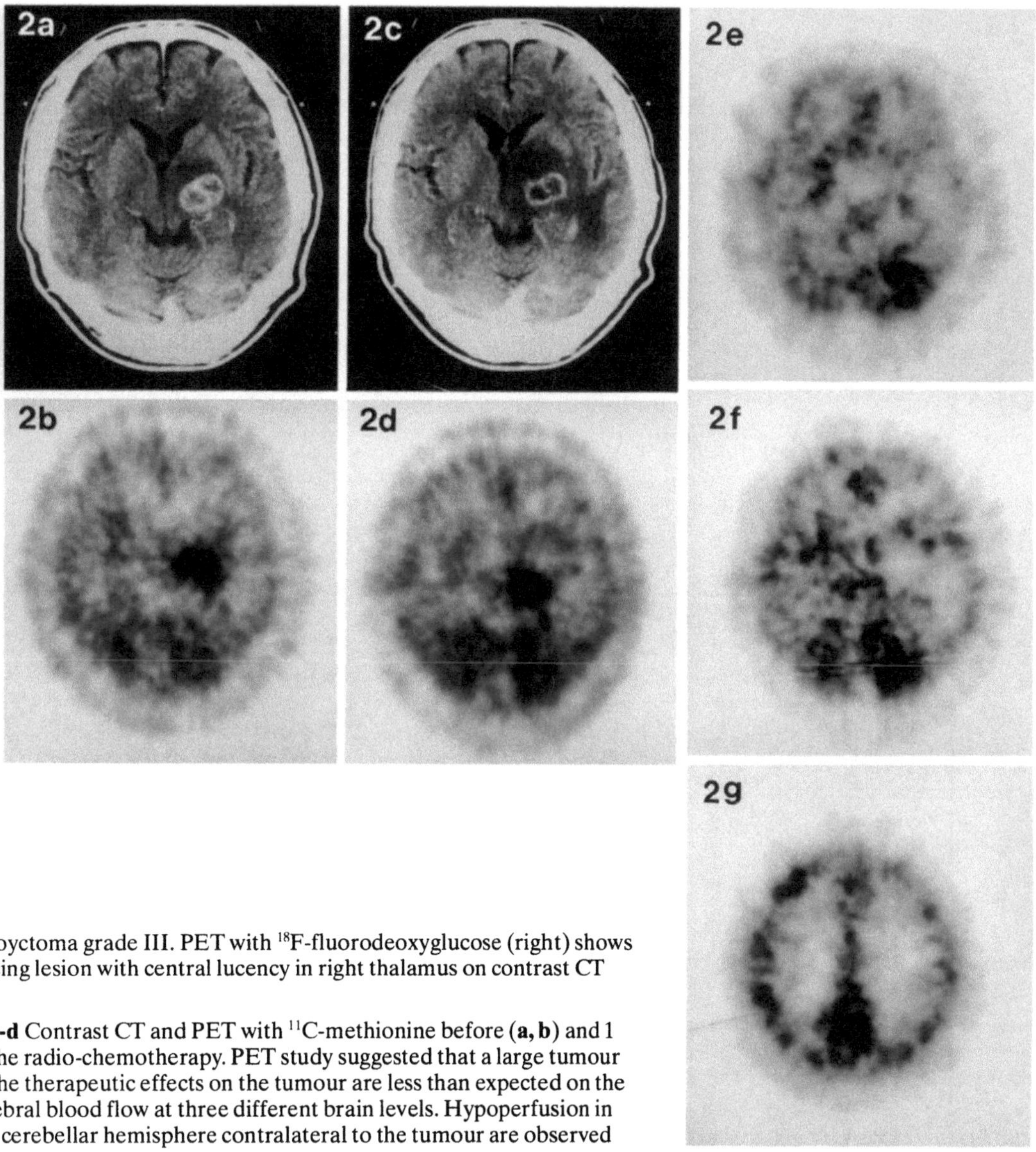

Fig. 1 a, b. Case 2, Malignant astroyctoma grade III. PET with ^{18}F-fluorodeoxyglucose (right) shows hypermetabolic rim of the enhancing lesion with central lucency in right thalamus on contrast CT (left)

Fig. 2 a-f. Case 3, glioblastoma. **a-d** Contrast CT and PET with ^{11}C-methionine before (**a, b**) and 1 month after (**c, d**) completion of the radio-chemotherapy. PET study suggested that a large tumour still remained after the therapy. The therapeutic effects on the tumour are less than expected on the CT. **e-g** Functional images of cerebral blood flow at three different brain levels. Hypoperfusion in the cortical mantle ipsilateral and cerebellar hemisphere contralateral to the tumour are observed

bellar hemispheres was also significantly lower on the unaffected side. Furthermore, the mean CBF values in the frontal, temporal, parietal and occipital lobes, and the cortical mantle in these six patients were significantly lower than in sex- and age-matched controls, on the affected side. The CMRG1 studies gave similar results but the number of patients ($n = 3$) was too small for valid statistical analysis.

Discussion

It was initially shown by Di Chiro et al. [1] using FDG-PET that brain tumours display a positive correlation between the degree of glucose utilization and the grade of malignancy. Malignant brain tumours are made up of heterogenous components such as viable, necrotic and oedematous parts. FDG-PET can display viable and aggressive tumour components as hypermetabolic foci. This technique is useful for deciding the target of stereotactic needle biopsy in deeply located tumours in, for instance, the thalamic region. Mosskin et al. [2] reported that Met-PET was more accurate than the other imaging methods used to assess the extent of viable tumour tissue. Met-PET delineated clearly the extension of the tumours in our series. This technique is useful for deciding the therapeutic strategy and for evaluating its effects. Baron et al. [3] also showed ipsilateral cortical hypoperfusion and hypometabolism associated with thalamic lesions. These may result from remote effects via the thalamocortical connections and, it is suggested, may have resulted in ipsilateral cerebral hemiatrophy in the case with thalamic tumour in childhood.

References

1. Di Chiro G, DeLapaz RL, Brooks RA, Sokoloff L, Kornblith PL, Smith BH, Patronas NJ, Kufta CV, Kessler RM, Johnston GS, Manning RG, Wolf AP (1982) Glucose utilization of cerebral glio-

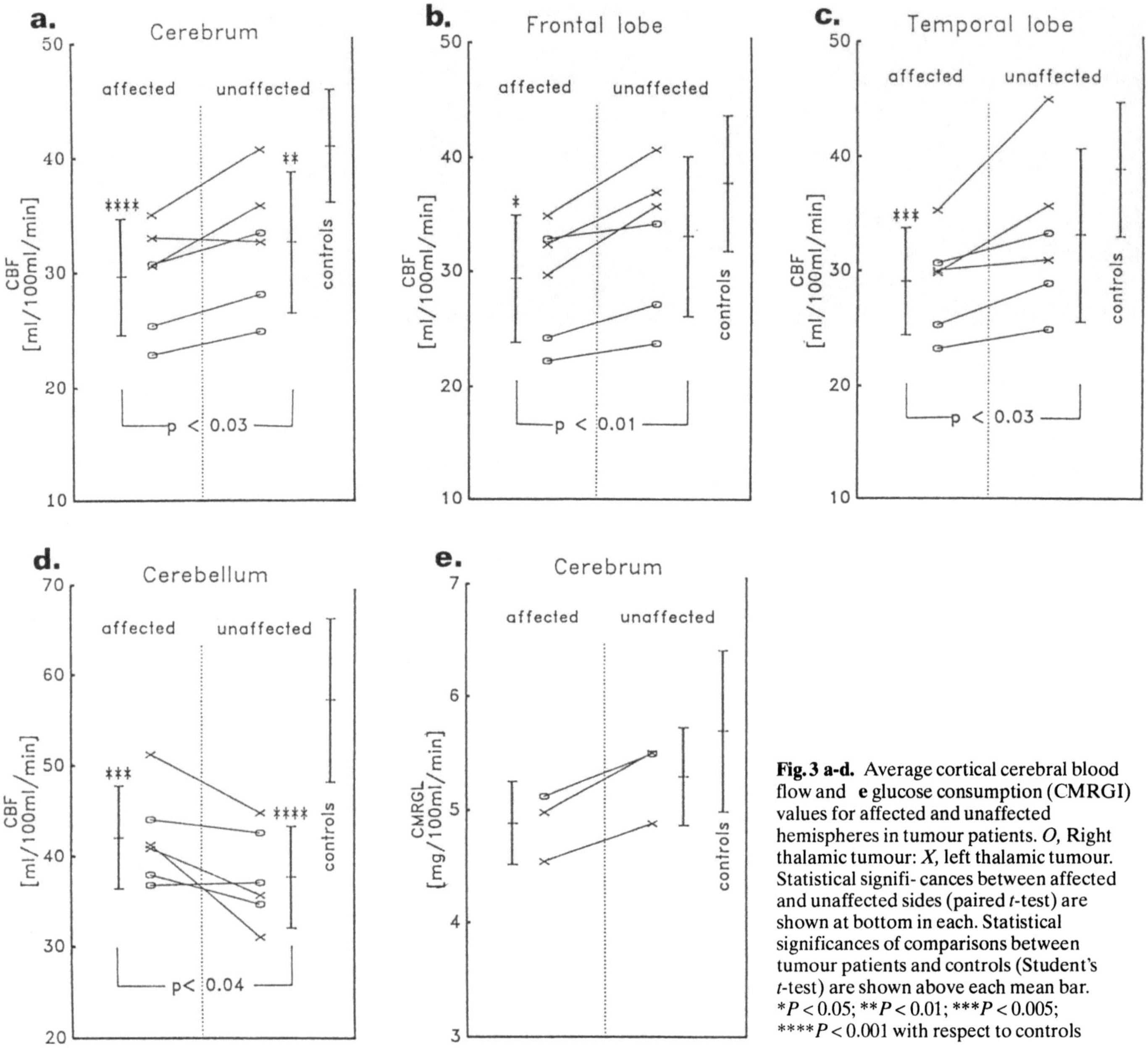

Fig. 3 a-d. Average cortical cerebral blood flow and **e** glucose consumption (CMRGI) values for affected and unaffected hemispheres in tumour patients. *O*, Right thalamic tumour: *X*, left thalamic tumour. Statistical signifi- cances between affected and unaffected sides (paired *t*-test) are shown at bottom in each. Statistical significances of comparisons between tumour patients and controls (Student's *t*-test) are shown above each mean bar. $^{*}P < 0.05$; $^{**}P < 0.01$; $^{***}P < 0.005$; $^{****}P < 0.001$ with respect to controls

mas measured by ^{18}F-fluorodeoxyglucose and positron emission tomography. Neurology 32: 1323–1329

2. Mosskin M, Ericson K, Hindmarsh, Holst H von, Collins VP, Bergström M, Eriksson L, Johnström P (1989) Positron emission tomography compared with magnetic resonance imaging and computed tomography in supratentorial gliomas using multiple stereotactic biopsies as reference. Acta Radiol 30: 225–232
3. Baron JC, D'antona R, Pantano P, Serdaru M, Samson Y, Bousser MG (1986) Effects of thalamic stroke on energy metabolism of the cerebral cortex. A positron tomography study in man. Brain 109: 1243–1259

Dr. Toshihide Ogawa
Department of Radiology and Nuclear Medicine,
Research Institute for Brain and Blood Vessels-Akita,
6–10 Senshu-Kubota-machi,
Akita City, Akita 010, Japan

Neuroradiology (1991) 33 [Suppl]: 371–372

Neuro-
radiology
© Springer-Verlag 1991

MRI in carotid artery occlusion

M. Forsting, J. Scharf, R. v. Kummer, and K. Sartor

Department of Neuroradiology, University of Heidelberg, Heidelberg, Federal Republic of Germany

Summary. The spectrum of neurological deficit associated with occlusion of the internal carotid artery (ICA) is wide and varies from asymptomatic to massive, potentially fatal, cerebral infarction. We prospectively studied 28 patients with Doppler sonographic diagnosis of ICA occlusion, by MRI. Sixty-four percent of patients with transient ischaemic attacks and 57% of asymptomatic patients showed structural lesions in the terminal supply area on the side of the ICA occlusion. We believe that MRI is a useful diagnostic tool to differentiate haemodynamic from embolic stroke mechanisms and to develop criteria for selecting patients, who may benefit from extracranial-intracranial bypass surgery.

Key words: Carotid artery occlusion – Transient ischaemic attack – Haemodynamic stroke – Extracranial-intracranial bypass

Because of uncertainties regarding the pathophysiology of symptomatic internal carotid artery (ICA) occlusion, proper management of this disorder remains controversial [1, 2]. Modern imaging techniques, specifically MRI, detect an increasing number of focal cerebral parenchymal abnormalities in patients with transient ischaemic attacks (TIAs), and raise questions as to the frequency, nature, and clinical significance of such lesions [3]. Since treatment of patients with cerebral parenchymal lesions may differ from treatment of patients without such lesions we wanted to determine by MRI both the frequency and type of these associated lesions in ICA occlusion.

Methods

Twenty-eight patients with a Doppler sonographic diagnosis of ICA occlusion were prospectively studied by MRI on a superconductive 1.0 T system (Picker Vista). Our imaging protocol included axial T1-weighted images (SE 600/20) and both axial and coronal T2-weighted images (SE 2000/80). Slice thickness was 8 mm. Images were reviewed by a neuroradiologist blinded to the clinical data.

Neurologically, 7 patients had completed stroke (group A) and 14 had TIAs (group B). The remaining 7 patients were asymptomatic (group C).

Results

MRI revealed signs of territorial cerebral infarction in all patients of group A. Nine patients (64%) of group B had T2-hyperintense lesions in the subcortical white matter above the level of the corpus callosum classified as low-flow infarcts. Three patients (22%) of this group had lacunar lesions presumably related to TIAs, and 2 patients (14%) had no apparent lesion on MRI. Four asymptomatic patients of group C (57%) also had hyperintense abnormalities in the subcortical white matter that spared the cerebral cortex and basal ganglia. Three patients of this group (47%) had no lesion visible on MRI. Figures 1–6 are examples of lesions classified as low-flow infarcts in asymptomatic patients (Figs. 1, 2) and in patients with TIAs (Figs. 3–6).

Discussion

The spectrum of neurological sequelae of ICA is extremely wide and ranges from absence of any symptoms to massive, potentially fatal, cerebral infarction. Although it is difficult to determine the relative frequency of haemodynamic and thrombo-embolic mechanisms of cerebral ischaemia, most authors agree that in patients with ICA occlusion thrombo-embolic phenomena are probably more frequent [1–4]. In our study, 64% of patients with ICA occlusion who had TIAs and 57% of asymptomatic patients had hyperintense lesions in the subcortical white matter, at or above the level of the corpus callosum, that strictly spared the cerebral cortex and basal ganglia. This lesion pattern is typical of low-flow infarcts in the terminal supply area [5].

The Extracranial-Intracranial Bypass Study Group [6] found worse results in patients with ICA occlusion who had surgery than after medical therapy. While the investigators could not fully explain these findings, they suggested that the external carotid artery and the surgical bypass itself may have acted as a potential route for embolization. Some authors have claimed that the most common cause of stroke in these patients was thrombo-embolic and that the study failed to identify patients with haemodynamic causes of stroke, who might benefit from surgery [1, 7]. We believe also that there exist certain subgroups of patients that may indeed benefit from EC/IC bypass surgery. We further believe that MRI is a suitable diagnostic tool for differentiating haemodynamic from

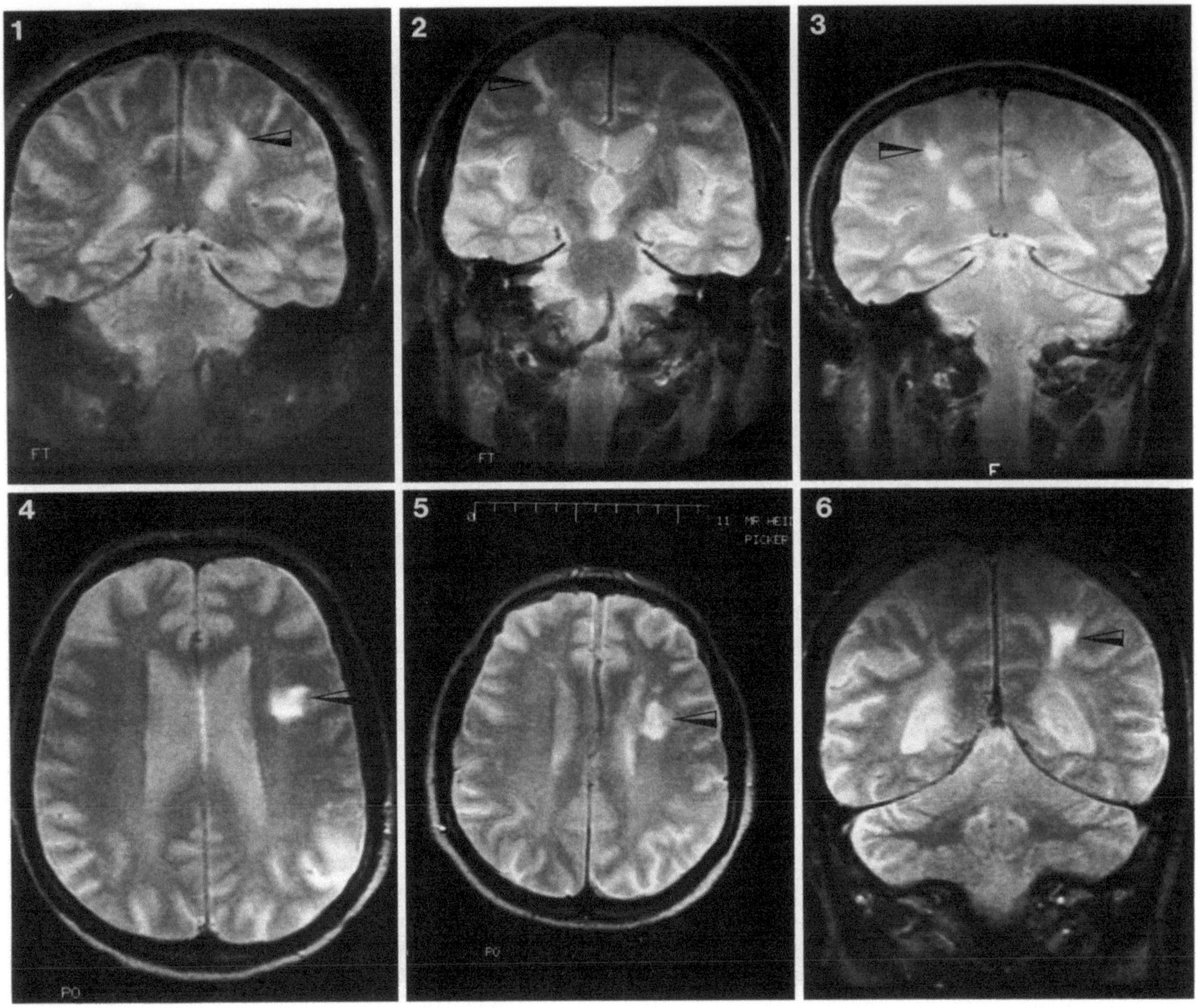

Figs. 1, 2. T2-weighted images of patients with internal carotid artery occlusion and no symptoms.

Figs. 3–6. T2-weighted images of patients who had a history of transient ischaemic attacks. Hyperintense lesions of the white matter *(arrowheads)*, all sparing the cerebral cortex and basal ganglia, were classified as low-flow infarctions in the terminal supply area

embolic stroke and for developing criteria for patient selection.

References

1. Cote R, Caron JC (1989) Management of carotid artery occlusion. Stroke 20: 123–126
2. Ringelstein EB, Zeumer H, Angelou D (1983) The pathogenesis of strokes from internal carotid artery occlusion: diagnostic and therapeutic implications. Stroke 14: 867–875
3. Awad I, Modic M, Little JR, Furlan AJ, Weinstein M (1986) Focal parenchymal lesions in transient ischemic attacks: correlation of computed tomography and magnetic resonance imaging. Stroke 17: 399–403
4. Cote R, Barnett HJM, Taylor DW (1983) Internal carotid occlusion: a prospective study. Stroke 14: 898–902
5. Zeumer H, Ringelstein EB (1987) Computed tomography patterns of brain infarctions as a pathogenetic key. In: Poeck K, Ringelstein EB, Hacke W (eds) New trends in diagnosis and management of stroke. Springer, Berlin Heidelberg New York, pp 75–85
6. EC/IC Bypass Study Group (1985) Failure of extracranial-intracranial arterial bypass to reduce the risk of ischemic stroke. N Engl J Med 313: 1191–1200
7. Day AL, Rhoton AL, Little JR (1986) The extracranial-intracranial bypass study. Surg Neurol 26: 222–226

Dr. Michael Forsting
Department of Neuroradiology
Kopfklinikum der Universität
Im Neuenheimer Feld 400
W-6900 Heidelberg
Federal Republic of Germany

Neuroradiology (1991) 33 [Suppl]: 373–374

Neuro-radiology
© Springer-Verlag 1991

Regional cerebral blood flow in partial seizures as determined by the stable-xenon CT method

A. M. Bidabé[1], D. Gense de Beaufort[1], A. M. Gin[1], A. Rougier[2], and J. M. Caillé[1]

[1] Service de Neuroradiologie, [2] Service de Neurologie, Bordeaux, France

Summary. Regional cerebral blood flow (rCBF) was measured by the stable xenon-enhanced CT method (Xe/CT) in 16 patients with intractable partial seizures. Xe/CT rCBF measures were correlated with results of SPECT rCBF studies and MRI. Xe/CT rCBF method is a useful tool in the investigation of medically refractory partial seizures.

Key words: Stable xenon-enhanced computed tomography – Cerebral blood flow – Intractable partial seizures

Determining the location of cerebral lesions in medically intractable partial seizures (especially deep temporal lesions) is very difficult. Functional imaging [EEG, SEEG, cerebral blood flow (CBF) and metabolism measurement] has added to the information obtained by morphological imagery (CT, MRI).

The purpose of the present study was to measure CBF by CT during stable xenon inhalation [1, 2] (Xe/CT) and to correlate these results with two other investigations: (1) single photon emission tomography after injection of hexamethylpropyleneamideoxide labelled with technetium 99 (SPECT); (2) MRI.

Patients and methods

We studied 16 patients (8 men, 8 women), with a mean age of 28.5 years, meeting the criteria of partial seizures resistant to medical treatment. Fourteen patients were studied during the interictal phase; the other 2 patients had a seizure during the measurement of CBF (cases 12 and 14 in Table 1).

All patients underwent an MRI examination: sagittal T1-weighted and coronal T2-weighted slices with two echoes. CBF was evaluated with SPECT in all patients except 1. The measurement of CBF with Xe/CT is a three-dimensional method that offers excellent spatial resolution [3]. Twelve CT slices were obtained during a 6-min period of inhalation of 32% Xe and oxygen using a Somatom DRH.

The CBF values of regions of interest were compared with the values of the contralateral regions. The percentage of side to side asymmetry was expressed as:

$$\frac{\textit{CBF pathological region} - \textit{CBF controlateral region} \times 100}{\textit{CBF controlateral region}}$$

Results

The results of the different examinations are summarized in Table 1. Nine of 15 patients had abnormal SPECT regional CBF (rCBF) studies, which indicates a sensitivity of 60%. Of 16 patients with Xe/CT rCBF measurements, 12 showed significant focal changes: hypoperfusion during the interictal state and hyperperfusion during status epilepticus (cases 12, 14) (Fig. 1) indicating a sensitivity of 75%.

Table 1. Clinical features and imaging findings

Case no. – Age (years) – Sex	Seizure	Atiology	EEG	MRI	Xe/CT	SPECT
1 – 24 – F	CP	Encephalitis	R. temporal	L. temp. atrophy	↓R temp. pariet.	↓R. temp. pariet
2 – 22 – F	CP, SG	Encephalitis	Bi. spikes	Normal	Normal	↓L. hemisphere
3 – 35 – M	CP	Unknown	L. temporal	Normal	↓L. temp.	Normal
4 – 23 – M	CP, SG	Unknown	R. temporal	Normal	Normal	Normal
5 – 54 – F	CP, SG	Astrocytoma	L. temporal	[a] L. mesial temp.	↓Mesial temp.	/
6 – 20 – F	CP, SG	Unknown	L. temporal	Uncus herniation	Normal	↓L. temp.
7 – 25 – F	SP, SG	Encephalitis	Bi front. slowing	Normal	↓L. frontal occip.	Normal
8 – 25 – M	CP, SG	Birth anoxia	Bi temp. spikes	[a] Temp atrophy	Normal	Normal
9 – 21 – M	CP	Unknown	Diffuse slowing	Normal	↓L. frontal pariet.	↓R. front. temp. ?
10 – 33 – F	CP	Encephalitis	R. temporal	Normal	↓Mesial temp.	Normal
11 – 23 – F	SP, SG	Neonatal disease	R. front.	Normal	↓R. frontal	↓R. frontal
12 – 32 – F	CP	Unknown	Bi temporal	[a] L. mesial temp.	↑L. mesial temp.	↑Normal
13 – 40 – M	CP	Encephalitis	R. parieto temp.	Normal	↓R. temp. pariet.	↓R. temp. pariet.
14 – 26 – M	CP, SG	Unknown	R. fronto temp.	R. centr. semi ov	↑R. front. pariet.	↓L. temp.
15 – 11 – M	CP	Head injury	L. temporal	[a] L. mesial temp.	↓L. mesial temp	↓L. hemisphere
16 – 42 – M	CP	Head injury	Bi temp. spikes	Uncal herniation	↓L. temp.	↓R. frontal ±

SP, Simple partial; CP, complex partial; SG, secondarily generalized; Xe/CT, xenon-enhanced CT

[a] Increased T2-weighted signal intensity

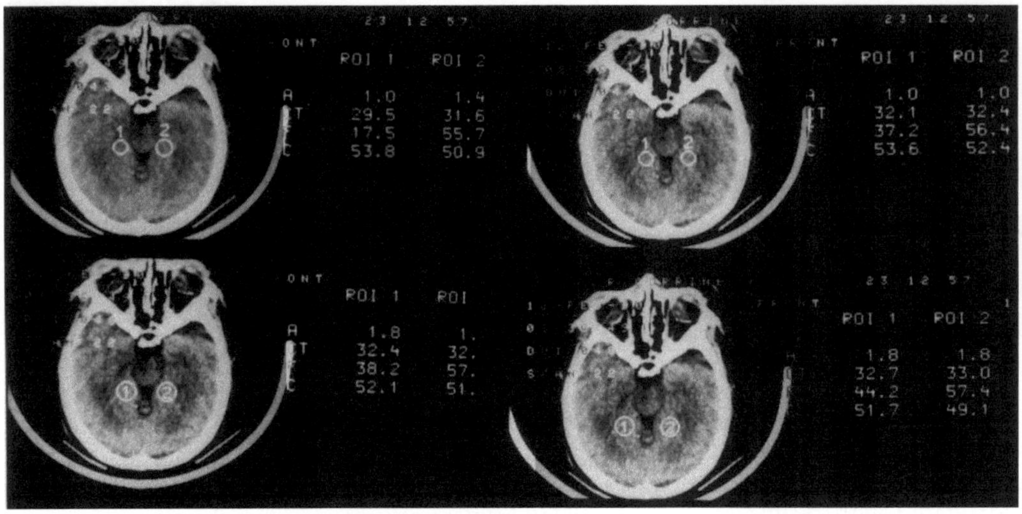

Fig. 1. Case 12: a 32-year-old woman with complex partial seizures for 22 years. rCBF measurement during an active seizure with right twitching, automatism, altered consciousness and postictal amnesia. Increase of rCBF: + 30 + 50% in the left hippocampus and para-hippocampal gyrus

MRI examinations disclosed significant findings in 8 patients, resulting in a sensitivity of 50%.

All subjects had an abnormal EEG but the localization of the abnormal blood flow regions did not always correlate well with the spatial distribution of EEG abnormalities.

Discussion

Many studies have shown the importance of rCBF measurement in the exploration of partial epilepsy [2, 4, 5]. Whatever the method used for the measurement of CBF, with their varying sensitivities, it is clear that during the interictal period the CBF at the epileptogenic focus is decreased, while the blood flow is considerably increased during seizures.

The correlation of the different investigations is illustrated in Tables 2 and 3. Some comments can be made: the normal results obtained with MRI [6–8] do not exclude the presence of microscopic cellular lesions in the area with decreased blood flow. A functional mechanism without underlying pathology could also be responsible for the regional decrease in blood flow, as shown by autoradiographic studies in the model of limbic epilepsy without ultrastructural lesions.

The SPECT gives qualitative information about the CBF in several slices and in the three planes. The Xe/CT study gives quantitative values of blood flow, but at the present time we have only analysed the results on a single slice.

The absence of cross correlation between Tables 2 and 3 leads to the conclusion that each method has some value and none is better than the others in partial seizure patients being evaluated for surgery.

Table 2. Xe/CT cerebral blood flow – SPECT correlations

Results	Patients ($n = 15$)
Both abnormal; good correlation	6
CT abnormal; SPECT normal	3
CT normal; SPECT abnormal	2
Both abnormal; different regions	2
Both normal	2

Table 3. Xe/CT CBF – MRI correlations

Results	Patients ($n = 16$)
Both abnormal; good correlation	6
CT abnormal; MRI normal	6
CT normal; MRI abnormal signal	2
Both normal	2

References

1. Broich K, Elger CE, Hartmann A, Solymosi L, Hufnagel A, Zierz S, Dettmers C, Kalender W (1990) Interictal regional cerebral blood flow with xenon-CCT in patients with refractory complex partial seizures (abstract). International Conference on stable xenon/CT CBF. 8–11 February, Orlando, Florida
2. Fish DR, Lewis TT, Brooks DJ, Zilkha E, Wise RJS, Kendall BE (1987) Regional cerebral blood flow of patients with focal epilepsy studied using xenon enhanced CT brain scanning. J Neurol Neurosurg Psychiatry 50: 1584–1588
3. Drayer BP, Wolfson SK, Reimuth OM, Dujovny M, Boehnke M, Cook EE (1978) Xenon enhanced CT for analysis of cerebral integrity perfusion and blood flow. Stroke 9: 123–130
4. Bonte FJ, Stokely EM, Devous MD, Homan RW (1983) Single-photon tomographic study of regional cerebral blood flow in epilepsy. A priliminary report. Arch Neurol 40
5. Lee BI, Markand ON, Siddiqui AR, Park HM, Mock B, Wellman HH, Worth RM, Edwards MK (1986) Single photon emission computed tomography (SPECT) brain imaging using N,N,N'-trimethyl-N'-(2 hydroxy-3-methyl-5-^{123}I-iodobenzyl)-1,3-propanediamine 2 HCI (HIPDM): intractable complex partial seizures. Neurology 36: 1471–1477
6. Heinz ER, Heinz TR, Radtke R, Darwin R, Drayer BP, Fram E, Djang WT (1989) Efficacy of MR vs CT in epilepsy. AJR 152: 347–352
7. Schömer W, Meencke HJ, Felix R (1987) Temporal-lobe epilepsy: comparison of CT and MT imaging. AJNR 8: 773–781
8. Theodore WH, Dorwart R, Holmes M, Porter RJ, Di Chiro G (1986) Neuroimaging in refractory partial seizures: comparison of PET, CT and MRI. Neurology 36: 750–759

Dr. A. M. Bidabé
Service de Neuroradiologie
CHR, F-33076 Bordeaux, France

Neuroradiology (1991) 33 [Suppl]: 375–376

Neuro radiology

© Springer-Verlag 1991

MR angiographic evaluation of cerebral aneurysms

S. Destian, C. Zee, J. Curran, J. Ahmadi, and H. D. Segall

LA County – USC Medical Center, Los Angeles, California, USA

Summary. To determine whether MR angiography (MRA) could reliably demonstrate cerebral aneurysms in patients with subarachnoid hemorrhage (SAH), five patients with SAH were studied by MRA and conventional angiography. Conventional angiography demonstrated ten aneurysms in the five patients. Eight of the aneurysms were detected by MRA. One aneurysm was not visualized, presumably because of its small size (4 mm), and the other was detected retrospectively, because it was obscured by adjacent vessels. The current limitations of MRA preclude it replacing conventional angiography in the diagnosis of cerebral aneurysms. In the future, with improved resolution and imaging technique, MRA should approach the sensitivity of conventional angiography in patients in whom an aneurysm is suspected.

Key words: Magnetic resonance angiography – Cerebral aneurysms

Conventional angiography has been, and continues to be, the gold standard for the investigation of patients with non-traumatic subarachnoid hemorrhage (SAH). Various techniques for MR angiography (MRA) [1], as well as its clinical applications [2], have been reported in the literature. Since MRA allows us to visualize flow within vessels non-invasively, we compared it with conventional angiography to determine whether MRA could reliably demonstrate the presence of cerebral aneurysms in patients with SAH.

Materials and methods

Five patients with SAH, documented by CT and spinal tap, were studied by MRA and conventional angiography (Table 1). Conventional angiography was performed on a GE biplane unit. MRA was performed with a Philips 1.5 T magnet. Axial images were acquired with a field-echo technique, TR 52 ms/TE 11 ms, and a flip angle of 90°. Slice thickness was 3 mm with a 1-mm overlap. The images were reformatted in 3D. Pre-excitation was used to suppress signal produced by flow in the opposite direction.

Results

Conventional angiography demonstrated ten aneurysms in five patients (Table 1). Eight of the aneurysms were detected by MRA, one was detected retrospectively, and one was not detected.

Patients 1, 2, 3 and 5 accounted for five of the ten aneurysms, ranging in size from 7 to 15 mm. All five aneurysms were well visualized on the MR angiograms. Figure 1 (from patient 2) is representative of these cases.

Of the five aneurysms found in patient 4 (Fig. 2) three (the left middle cerebral, the left posterior communicating, and the basilar tip) were well visualized on the MR angiogram. They measured 6, 4, and 10 mm, respectively. The anterior communicating artery aneurysm, measuring 5 mm, while visible retrospectively, was difficult to diagnose with MRA alone, because it was partially obscured by adjacent vessels. The right posterior communicating artery aneurysm was not detected, most likely because of its small size (3 mm).

Discussion

Ross et al. [3] recently reported that MRA can show aneurysms as small as 3–4 mm. We found that the inferior resolution of MRA, compared with conventional angiography, limits its capacity to demonstrate reliably aneurysms less than 4 mm in size. In addition, since all vessels with flow in the same direction are visualized on the MR angiogram, small aneurysms which are large enough to be detected, i.e., 5 mm, may be obscured by adjacent vessels, despite the fact that the images are reformatted in 3D.

Table 1. Aneurysms seen in five patients with subarachnoid hemorrhage

Patient no.	Age/sex	Conventional angiography	MR angiography
1	40 M	Left internal carotid	Left internal carotid
2	49 F	Left middle cerebral	Left middle cerebral
		Right middle cerebral	Right middle cerebral
3	49 F	Right cavernous carotid	Right cavernous carotid
4	55 F	Anterior communicating	Anterior communicating[a]
		Left middle cerebral	Left middle cerebral
		Left post communicating	Left post communicating
		Right post communicating	Not detected
		Basilar tip	Basilar tip
5	69 M	Basilar tip	Basilar tip

[a] MRI suggestive, but not diagnostic

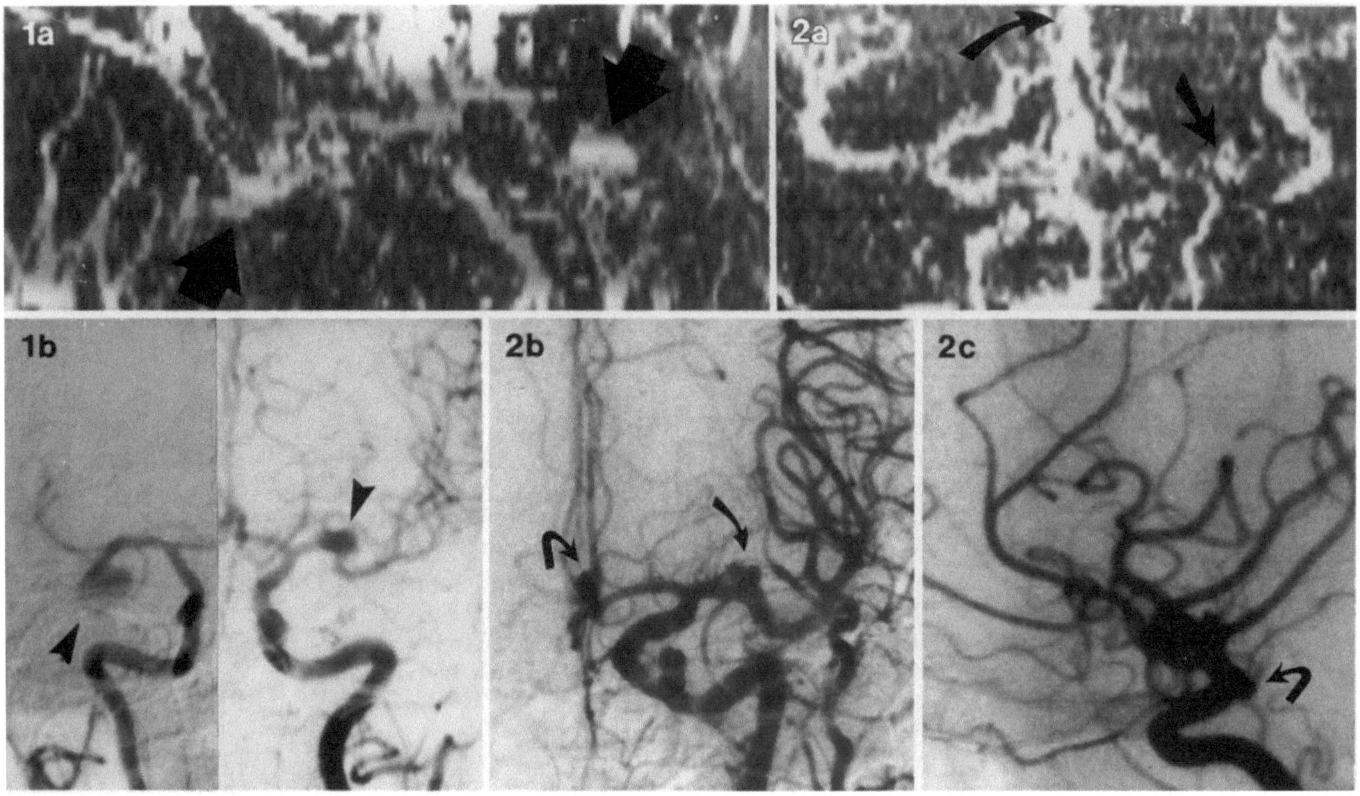

Fig. 1 a, b. Coronal oblique projection from the MR angiogram of patient 2. **a** Bilateral middle cerebral artery aneurysms *(arrows)* at the first bifurcation. **b** Conventional angiography confirms the bilateral aneurysms *(arrowheads)*, larger on the right side

Fig. 2. **a** Coronal projection of the MR angiogram of patient 4 is only suggestive of an anterior communicating artery aneurysm *(curved arrow)*, but demonstrates the left middle cerebral artery aneurysm *(slanted arrow)*. **b** Both aneurysms are well visualized on conventional angiography *(curved arrows)*. **c** A lateral projection from the right carotid artery injection demonstrates a right posterior communicating artery aneurysm *(curved arrow)* which was not detected on the MRA images

Although MRA was able to demonstrate eight of the ten aneurysms in this series, its limitations preclude it's replacing conventional angiography at the present time. For patients with SAH, in whom an aneurysm is suspected, however, it can be used as a guide for conventional angiography in determining the order in which the vessels are to be injected. In the future, we hope that with improved resolution, MRA will approach the sensitivity of conventional angiography in the detection of cerebral aneurysms.

References

1. Ruggieri PM, Laub GA, Masaryk TJ, Modic MT (1989) Intracranial circulation: pulse-sequence considerations in three-dimensional (volume) MR angiography. Radiology 171: 785–791
2. Masaryk TJ, Modic MT, Ross JS (1989) Intracranial circulation: preliminary clinical results with three-dimensional (volume) MR angiography. Radiology 171: 793–799
3. Ross JS, Masaryk TJ, Modic MT (1990) Intracranial aneurysms: evaluation by MR angiography. AJNR 11: 449–456

Dr. Sylvie Destian
LA County – USC Medical Center
1200 North State Street, Box 158
Los Angeles, CA 90033, USA

Neuroradiology (1991) 33 [Suppl]: 377–378

Neuro-radiology

© Springer-Verlag 1991

Embolic middle cerebral artery occlusion responsible for internal borderzone infarction

U. Angeloni[1], L. Bozzao[1], L. M. Fantozzi[1], S. Bastianello[1], G. Brughitta[1], M. Kushner[3], and C. Fieschi[2]

Department of [1] Neurological Sciences, Neuroradiological Section and [2] III Neurologic Clinic, University of Rome "La Sapienza", Rome, Italy, [3] Department of Neurology, University of Pennsylvania, Philadelphia, USA

Summary. We analysed in 36 patients, suffering acute middle cerebral artery (MCA) occlusion, the angiographic findings within 6 h of the ictus, and the chronic CT results at 3 months. Seven developed a pattern of "internal borderzone" infarction on follow-up CT. Angiography showed an MCA occlusion in all, localized at the MCA bifurcation (type III) in 3, involving peripheral MCA branches (type IV) in 3, and beyond the lenticulostriate arteries (type II) in the other. Carotid artery stenosis or occlusion was absent in all 7. These data show that internal borderzone infarcts may result from intracranial MCA branch occlusions alone and need not be associated with haemodynamic alterations due to large vessel extracranial disease.

Key words: Cerebral ischaemia – Borderzone infarction – Watershed – Computed tomography – Cerebral angiography

Watershed cerebral infarcts lie at the borderzone between the vascular territories of two or more major cerebral arteries [1, 2]. These vascular lesions may develop either cortically, along the parenchymal interfaces supplied by the middle cerebral artery (MCA) and anterior cerebral artery or the MCA and the posterior cerebral artery, or in the deep subcortical MCA regions supplied by both MCA medullary branches and lenticulostriate perforators [2–4]. This "deep" watershed territory, called the internal borderzone (IBZ) includes the white matter of the corona radiata and lateral portions of the basal ganglia. Previously, cortical and IBZ watershed infarcts have been associated mainly with haemodynamic stroke due to large vessel disease, such as cervical stenosis or occlusion [1, 2, 5, 6]. These data, obtained from post-mortem series or angiographic studies, came from the chronic phase of stroke alone.

This study, which involved the use of early angiography within 6 h, was designed to assess the significance of MCA occlusion alone in the development of 'cortical' watershed and IBZ infarcts.

Materials and methods

All our patients with acute focal supratentorial neurological deficits were recruited into a superacute multimodal clinical study within 4 h of the onset of their symptoms [7]. We studied 80 patients; early angiography performed within 6 h revealed a MCA occlusion in 47. Eleven patients died before follow-up CT at 3 months. Thus only 36 patients were included in this analysis. A 3-month CT allowed us to define in these patients the late parenchymal damage.

Angiography. MCA occlusions were classified as follows according to a four-point scale [8, 9]: type I, MCA stem occlusion proximal to the origin of the lenticulostriate arteries; type II, MCA trunk occlusion just distal to the origin of the lenticulostriate and proximal to the origin of the temporal pial branches; type III, MCA occlusion distal to the origin of the temporal pial branches; type IV, MCA peripheral MCA occlusion. Collateral blood supply (CBS) was also noted [9, 10].

Computed tomography. A plain CT was performed at 3 months after the stroke. CT findings were classified as: normal, lacunar infarcts, deep MCA territory infarction (involving the structures supplied by the lenticulostriate arteries), superficial MCA territory infarction (involving only the cortical tissue), partial MCA territory infarction (partially involving both the cortical and the subcortical tissue), complete MCA territory infarction (involving both the cortical and the subcortical tissue), IBZ (involving the white matter of the corona radiata, in some cases extending into the adjacent centrum semiovale and occasionally to the lateral putamen).

Results

Angiographic and CT results of our 36 patients are briefly discussed. IBZ infarcts (Fig. 1 a, b) were identified in 7 patients; early angiography showed a type IV MCA occlusion in 3 cases, a type III occlusion in 3 (Fig. 2 a), a type II occlusion in the remaining 1. CBS was always present (Fig. 2 b). No case showed stenosis or occlusion of an intra- or extracranial carotid artery. Complete MCA territory infarcts were found on CT in 5 patients; angiography showed a type I MCA occlusion in all cases with no evidence of CBS. Partial MCA infarcts were observed in 4 patients; angiography showed y type I occlusion in 2 (CBS was present in 1 and absent in the other), a type II in 1 with no evidence of CBS, a type III in 1 with a good CBS. Superficial MCA infarcts were observed in 6 patients; angiography showed a type IV occlusion in 3 with a good CBS in all, a type III in 1 with a good CBS, a type II in 1 with no evidence of CBS and it was normal in the remaining 1. Deep MCA infarcts were observed in 3 patients; angiography showed a type I occlusion in 1 patient with a good CBS and an internal carotid artery (ICA) occlusion (siphon, cervical segment) in 2 also with a good CBS.

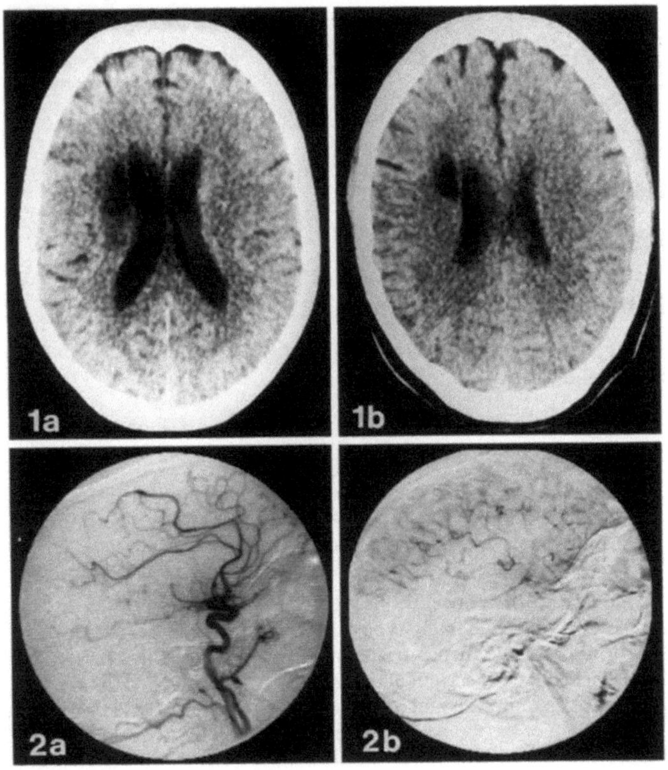

Fig. 1 a, b. CT scan shows an extensive internal borderzone infarct involving the corona radiata

Fig. 2 a, b. The same patient as in Fig. 1. **a** The angiogram in the early phase shows a type III middle cerebral artery occlusion. **b** A good collateral blood supply is noted during the late arterial phase

Lacunar infarcts were observed in 2 cases; angiography showed an ICA occlusion at the bifurcation in 1 with a good CBS, while it was normal in the other.

Follow-up CT was not available for the remaining 9 patients.

Discussion

Pathogenesis of watershed cerebral infarcts has been discussed in previous reports. They suggest an incidence of 10% of all ischaemic infarcts in autopsy series [5]. CT studies reported a higher incidence (40%) for both cortical and IBZ ischaemic lesions. Angiography, performed in these patients, but not in the acute phase of stroke, showed the presence of stenosis or occlusive disease of the carotid artery or siphon, suggesting a haemodynamic pathogenesis for these ischaemic lesions [1]. Systemic hypotension [2], embolization from carotid thrombus or atheroma [11] and thromboarteritis obliterans [12] have been proposed as adjunctive mechanisms for the development of borderzone infarction. We did not find, in our series, any cortical watershed infarcts but only IBZ; they were never associated with stenosis or occlusive pathology of the carotid artery but only with distal MCA branch occlusion. The region involved, located in the deep white matter at the interface between the areas of supply by the superficial MCA and the medullary branches and of the lenticulostriate arteries, may be termed the "terminal" MCA vascular field [13, 14]. So when a distal MCA embolic occlusion developed, no CBS protects these "internal" vascular territories, unlike the superficial regions which may be preserved by a well functioning circulation through leptomeningeal cortical anastomoses, and the deep gray matter which may be saved by a possible unchanged blood flow through the lenticulostriate arteries. Thus it is possible that a local haemodynamic effect could have a role in the pathogenesis of these ischaemic lesions following intracranial MCA branch occlusion.

References

1. Wodarz R (1980) Watershed cerebral infarctions and computed tomography. A topographical study in cases with stenosis or occlusion of the carotid artery. Neuroradiology 19: 245–248
2. Zulch KJ (1961) Über die Entstehung und Lokalisation der Hirninfarkte. Zbl Neurochir 21: 158–178
3. Damasio H (1983) A computed tomography guide to the identification of cerebral vascular territories. Arch Neurol 40: 138–142
4. Zulch KJ (1961) Die Pathogenese von Massenblutung und Erweichung unter besonderer Berücksichtigung klinischer Gesichtspunkte. Acta Neurochir [Suppl] (Wien) 7: 51–117
5. Jorgensen I, Torvik A (1969) Ischemic cerebrovascular disease in an autopsy series. II. Prevalence, location, pathogenesis and clinical course of cerebral infarcts. J Neurol Sci 9: 185–220
6. Torvik A (1984) The pathogenesis of watershed infarcts in the brain. Stroke 15: 221–223
7. Fieschi C, Argentino C, Lenzi GL, Sachetti ML, Toni D, Bozzao L (1989) Clinical and instrumental evaluation of patients with ischemic stroke within the first six hours. J Neurol Sci 91: 311–322
8. Saito I, Segawa H, Shiokawa I, Taniguchi M, Tsutsumi K (1984) Middle cerebral artery occlusion: correlation of computed tomography and angiography with clinical outcome. Stroke 18: 863–868
9. Bozzao L, Fantozzi LM, Bastianello S, Bozzao A, Fieschi C (1989) Early collateral blood supply and late parenchymal brain damage in patients with middle cerebral artery occlusion. Stroke 20: 735–740
10. Mishkin MM, Schreiber MN (1974) Collateral circulation. In: Newton TH, Potts DG (eds) Radiology of the skull and brain, vol 2. Mosby, St. Louis, pp 2344–2374
11. Torvik A, Skullerud K (1982) Watershed infarcts in the brain caused by microemboli. Clin Neuropathol 1: 99–105
12. Lindemberg R, Spatz H (1939) Über die tromboarteritis obliterans der hirngefasse (cerebrale form der V. Wininwater-Buergerschen krankheith). Virchows Arch [A] 305: 531–557
13. Mohr JP (1969) Distal infarction. Neurology 19: 279
14. Caplan L, Babikian V, Helgason C, Hier DB, De Witt D, Patel D, Stein R (1985) Occlusive disease of the middle cerebral artery. Neurology 35: 975–982

Dr. U. Angeloni
Department of Neurological Sciences
Neuroradiological Section
University of Pennsylvania
Philadelphia, Pennsylvania, USA

Neuroradiology (1991) 33 [Suppl]: 379–380

Neuroradiology
© Springer-Verlag 1991

Cerebral lacunes: an image of interterritorial infarction

P. Kalvach, R. Schickerová, and J. Vymazal

Department of Neurology, Postgraduate Medical School, Prague, Czechoslovakia

Summary. Methodological discrepancies in studies of cerebral lacunes make it difficult to unite the viewpoints of pathologists, neuroradiologists and clinicians. Using a neuroradiological approach we defined a lacune as any hypodense CT lesion, less than 2 cm in diameter, presumably of microangiopathic origin. We have studied CT signs of cerebral atrophy, leucoaraiosis and lacunes, and their mutual combination, in 93 patients with clinical and CT evidence of arteriosclerotic encephalopathy – état lacunaire. The position of cerebral lacunes, defined using our own map of cerebrovascular territories, showed a predominant localisation on the borders between individual arterial territories thereby suggesting hypothesis of interterritorial infarction as the pathogenetic mechanism.

Key words: Arteriosclerotic microangiopathy – Interterritorial infarction – Cerebral lacune

The definition of cerebral lacunes is the subject of many differences in individual scientific approach. Traditionally, pathologists define them as small malacic defects, 3–20 mm [1] or 0.5–15 mm [2] in diameter, with the emphasis on the deep location in basal ganglia, with occlusion of a penetrating artery as the aetiology. Clinicians attempt to diagnose lacunar infarcts on clinical symptoms such as Fisher's 21 types of lacunar infarction [3], and disregard the pathologist's premise of necrosed tissue, as well as the location in the basal ganglia. For the purpose of our neuroradiological study we considered a lacune as any hypodense, presumably postischaemic defect less than 2 cm in diameter in patients with clinical and CT evidence of lacunar state.

The purpose of this study was to precisely localise neuroradiologically these lacunes and, using our map of the cerebrovascular territories, arrive at a hypothesis to explain their pathogenesis.

Materials and methods

We reviewed 93 patients, age range 41–81 years (mean 66.9), who had been clinically diagnosed as having the lacunar state and in whom there were at least two of the following criteria on CT: (1) atrophy (periventricular and cortical); (2) periventricular lucencies as a sign of subcortical arteriosclerotic encephalopathy; (3) cerebral lacunes. For the purpose of our neuroradiological study, we considered a lacune as any hypodense, presumably postischaemic, defect of less than 2 cm in diameter. The location of the cerebral lacunes was assessed using our own map of the cerebrovascular territories; we also related the above three criteria to lesions in other parts of the brain.

Results

The periventricular type of cerebral atrophy was found in 71% of patients and cortical in 86%. Diffuse periventricular hypodensities as a sign of subcortical arteriosclerotic encepahlopathy, sometimes called leucoaraiosis, or Binswanger's disease, were present in 76.3% (Fig. 1).

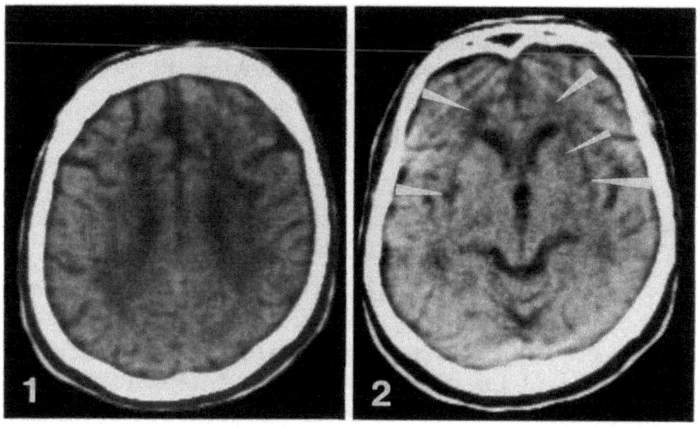

Fig. 1. Periventricular lacunes (leucoaraiosis) as a sign of diffuse lipohyalinosis of small arteries. Subcortical arteriosclerotic encephalopathy

Fig. 2. Cerebral lacunes, localised left and right betwen frontopolar artery and operculofrontal artery beds and between insular branches and anterolateral central arteries, right also between anteromedial central arteries and anterolateral central arteries *(arrows)*

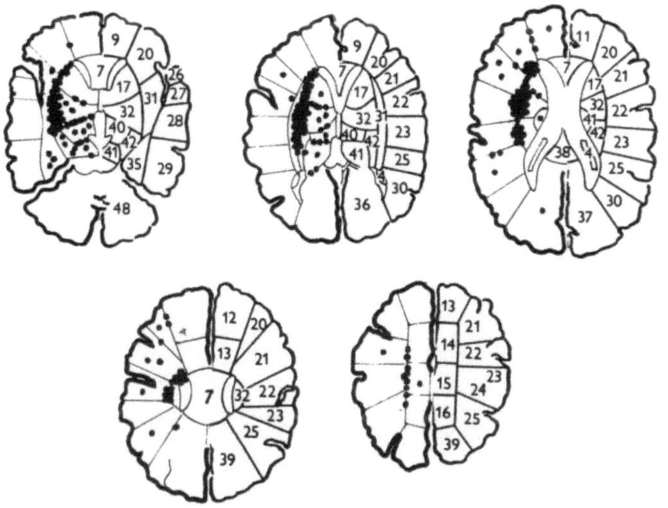

Fig. 3. Position of all lacunes found, presented in the left part of the diagram. Predominant location on the boundaries of arterial territories. Only 15.5% inside the territories

Table 1. Localisation of cerebral lacunes and their relevance to overall boundaries between anterior, middle and posterior cerebral arteries and to overall boundaries between perforating and superficial arteries. These two types of boundary partly overlap

n =	220	(100%)		
Interterritorial	186	(84.5%)		
	boundaries between		80 anterior, middle, posterior cerebral arteries	(47.3%)
	boundaries between		133 perforating and superficial	(71.5%)
Territorial	34	(15.5%)		

Cerebral lacunes were found in 89.0% of patients, with an overall incidence of 220 in 93 patients. An attempt to find if any of these features have a common aetiology brought a negative results.

The great majority of these 220 cerebral lacunes were situated on the borders of individual arterial territories (Fig. 2, Table 1), predominantly between the insular branches of the middle cerebral artery and the perforating arteries of the basal ganglia, or between the peripheral part of the perforating arteries and superficial arterial beds in the cerebral hemispheres (Fig. 3).

Discussion

The CT approach to study of cerebral lacunes does not take into consideration microdefects in basal ganglia, sometimes called Virchow-Robin spaces in pathological analyses [4–6]. On the other hand CT discloses micro-infarcts that have not yet necrosed. The prerequisite for our suggestion of a predominant location of cerebral lacunes on the boundaries of individual arterial territories is to use a fine map of these districts, that of the peripheral beds of the circle of Willis branches, and not just to consider the major anterior, middle and posterior cerebral arteries. Our observation, that most lacunes are small water-shed infarctions, leads to the hypothesis that they are due to general lipohyalinosis of small vessels, where the limited perfusion gives rise to the lesion only under generally deteriorating conditions such as decreased heart output, blood hyperviscosity, decreased elasticity or high aggregability of erythrocytes, decreased oxygen saturation and so on. Distant causes, such as internal carotid stenosis, are also possible deteriorating factors. The predilection of these tissues to develop an ischaemic lesion has also been stressed in experimental studies [7].

References

1. Fisher CM (1982) Lacunar strokes and infarcts: a review. Neurology 32: 871–876
2. Weisberg LA (1982) Lacunar infarcts. Clinical and computed tomographic correlations. Arch Neurol 39: 37–40
3. Bamford JM, Warlow CP (1988) Evolution and testing of the lacunar hypothesis. Stroke 19: 1074–1081
4. Braffman BH, Zimmerman RA, Trojanowski JQ, Gonatas KN, Hickey WF, Schlaepfer WW (1988) Brain MR: pathologic correlation with gross and histopathology. I, II. AJNR 9: 621–636
5. Mohr JP (1982) Lacunes. Stroke 13: 3–11
6. Miller VT (1983) Lacunar stroke. A reassessment. Arch Neurol 40: 129–134
7. Brierly JB (1979) Ischemic necrosis along brain arterial boundary zones. In: Fahn S, Davis JN, Rowland LP (eds) Advances in neurology. Raven Press, New York

Dr. P. Kalvach
Department of Neuradiology
Postgraduate Medical School
Videnska 800
140 59 Prague 4, Czechoslovakia

Neuroradiology (1991) 33 [Suppl]: 381–383

Neuro-radiology
© Springer-Verlag 1991

Reperfusion of intracranial arteries in acute stroke after treatment with intravenous plasminogen activator

R. von Kummer[1], M. Forsting[1], W. Hacke[2], and K. Sartor[1]

Departments of [1] Neuradiology and [2] Neurology, University of Heidelberg, Heidelberg, Federal Republic of Germany

Summary. Twenty-six stroke patients with acute occlusions of large intracranial arteries were treated with 70 mg ($n = 12$) and 100 mg ($n = 14$) alteplase within 6 h of the onset of symptoms. The rate of intracerebral haemorrhage (31%) was not higher than with the natural course, and haemorrhages had no influence on clinical outcome except in 2 patients. Reperfusion demonstrated by angiography and transcranial Doppler sonography was observed in 45% of patients at 70 mg and 64% at 100 mg immediately after treatment, and in 55% and 84%, respectively, 24 h later. Perfusion occurred more frequently than might be expected as a result of spontaneous recanalisation and was slightly more common than is seen with locally applied urokinase. Our preliminary data suggest that a controlled trial assessing the efficacy of 100 mg intravenous alteplase in acute thromboembolic stroke may be useful.

Key words: Arterial recanalization – Thrombolysis – Stroke – Plasminogen activator

Recently, new thrombus-selective agents, such as recombinant tissue plasminogen activator (rtPA) have become available and have been successfully used in the treatment of ischaemic heart disease. Encouraged by reports of successful arterial recanalization, associated with favourable clinical outcome, following intra-arterial infusion of streptokinase or urokinase [1–5], we studied the efficacy and safety of intravenous rtPA in patients with acute thromboembolic vertebrobasilar and middle cerebral artery stroke. In this paper we report its efficacy, in terms of reperfusion demonstrated by angiography and transcranial Doppler sonography (TCD), within 6 and 24 h of onset of symptoms.

Patients and methods

In an open, prospective, and non-randomized trial, a total of 26 patients (12 female, 14 male) were treated with i. v. infusion of 70 mg ($n = 12$) or 100 mg ($n = 14$) alteplase (Actilyse) within 6 h of the onset of symptoms. Inclusion criteria were: (1) clinical diagnosis of acute stroke (2) lack of haemorrhage, local brain swelling, or significant hypodensity due to early infarction as documented by CT (3) angiographic demonstration of corresponding occlusion of large intracranial artery or arteries (4) age of patient between 20 and 70 years (5) informed consent given by patient or relatives. Angiography was repeated immediately after 90 min of rtPA infusion. Reperfusion was graded as: (1) no reperfusion or penetration with minimal reperfusion (2) partial reperfusion (3) complete reperfusion. Reperfusion was also assessed 12–24 h after onset of symptoms by a third angiogram or by TCD. Heparin was given as a bolus of 5,000 IU simultaneously with rtPA and continued at 1,000 IU/h. All patients remained under intensive care for at least 3 days.

Results

Occlusion of vertebrobasilar ateries

The 5 patients with occlusion of the basilar artery ($n = 4$) or of both vertebral arteries ($n = 1$) were treated with 70 mg only. In 2 partial perfusion was achieved within 6 h of the onset of symptoms, and in 1 TCD revealed complete reperfusion after 24 h. Three patients died due to extended ischaemic brain-stem infarction, whereas 1 patient remained locked-in. One patient recovered well and showed no neurological deficit at discharge, despite small brain stem infarcts detected by MRI. Because of this outcome, patients with vertebrobasilar occlusion were not further included in this study but treated with intra-arterially and locally applied urokinase.

Occlusion in the internal carotid territory

Internal carotid artery (ICA). Occlusion of the intracranial ICA was revealed in 5 patients, 4 times in combination with middle cerebral artery (MCA) occlusion. Two patients also showed obliteration of the A1 segment of the anterior cerebral artery (ACA). In these 2 patients no reperfusion was achieved. The other 3 patients showed partial ($n = 2$) or complete reperfusion of the ICA within 6 h of the onset of the stroke. In 1, the MCA remained occluded. This patient died from a space-occupying infarction associated with parenchymal and intraventricular haemorrhage of the ipsilateral hemisphere.

MCA trunk. Ten patients had occlusion of the MCA trunk. After rtPA treatment, 4 showed no reperfusion and 5 only partial reperfusion (Fig. 1). In 1, angiography was not repeated for logistic reasons. The day after stroke no reperfusion was observed in 2 patients, partial reperfusion in 2, and complete reperfusion in 6. With CT, ischaemic brain infarctions were detected in the MCA territory, including the striatum, in 9.

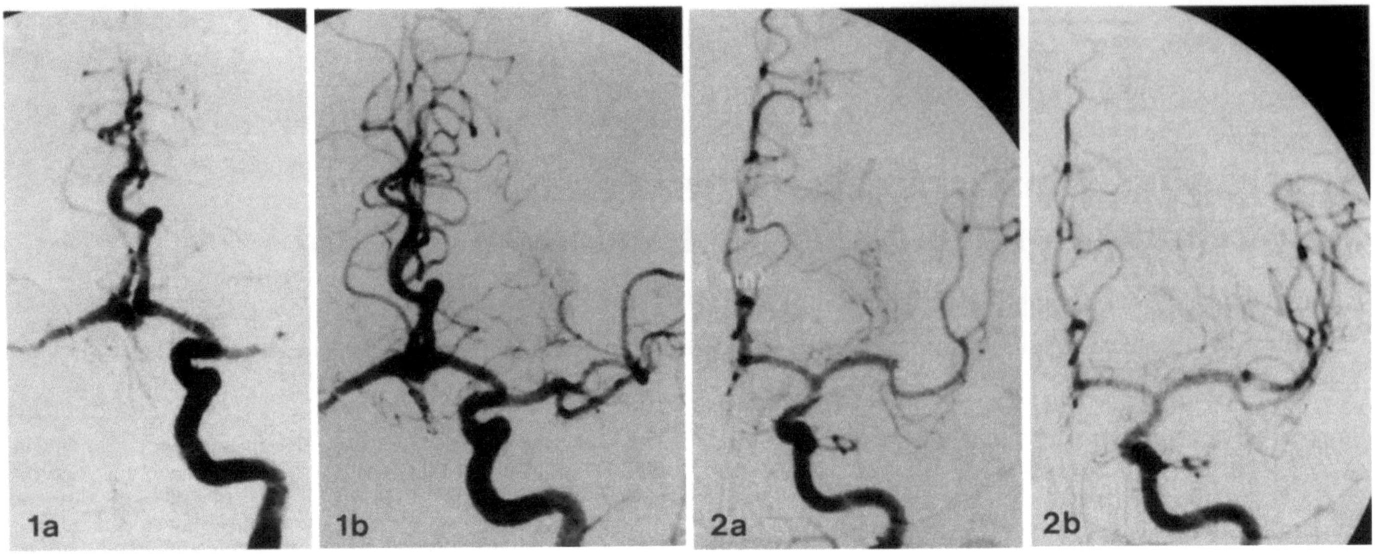

Fig. 1. a Occlusion of the proximal middle cerebral artery (MCA) trunk revealed 4 h after onset of symptoms. **b** Partial (grade 2) reperfusion of left MCA immediately after 100 mg alteplase i.v. asociated with vasodilation and occlusion of distal MCA branches

Fig. 2. a Occlusion of major left MCA branch after 70 mg alteplase i.v. **b** Complete (grade 3) reperfusion at angiography 11 h after treatment

Branches of MCA. In 6 patients MCA branches were occluded at the trifurcation. No reperfusion was observed in 2 patients and partial reperfusion in 4, when angiography was repeated immediately after alteplase infusion. The following day reperfusion was still partial in 3 patients but complete in the other 3 (Fig. 2). The ischaemic infarct was confined to the striatum in 3 patients and in 1 to the insular cortex. In 1, CT revealed a more extensive infarct within the MCA territory. One patient was on aspirin because of coronary artery stenosis and developed disseminated parenchymal haemorrhages in both hemispheres from which she died.

Haemorrhage

Parenchymal haemorrhage occurred in 2 patients, 1 with partial reperfusion of an MCA branch and 1 in whom the MCA remained occluded; both patients had been treated with 100 mg alteplase. In 6 patients, haemorrhagic transformation of the infarct was seen; 5 recovered well. In 4 patients severe bleeding from the puncture site occurred 2–4 days after rtPA treatment, without apparent influence on clinical outcome.

Table 1. Reperfusion within internal carotid artery territory after 70 or 100 mg alteplase i.v., as shown by angiography (6 h) and/or transcranial Doppler sonography (24 h) ($n = 20$)

Interval[a]	Reperfusion		
	None	Partial	Complete
6 h	8	11	1
24 h	4	7	9

[a] Time from onset of symptoms

Reperfusion within ICA territory and dosage of rtPA

Within 6 h of the onset of symptoms, at least partial reperfusion was observed in 3 of 6 patients treated with 70 mg and in 9 of 13 patients treated with 100 mg of rtPA. After 12–24 h, angiography and/or TCD showed the 3 vessels of the 70 mg group still occluded, whereas all vessels except 1 were partially or completely recanalized after 100 mg alteplase (Table 1).

Discussion

Reperfusion after thromboembolic occlusion may result from treatment or spontaneous recanalization. Spontaneous recanalization has been observed angiographically in 27%–59% of patients during the first days following a stroke [6–8]. In our series of 26 patients the recanalization rate was 45% at 70 mg and 64% at 100 mg immediately after alteplase treatment, within 6 h of the onset of symptoms. When reperfusion was assessed later, but within 24 h of the stroke, the recanalization rate was even higher (55% and 86%, respectively). Reocclusion was not observed. We thus consider reperfusion in our patients as mostly alteplase-induced. Reperfusion of the MCA was observed in 56% of patients within 6 h of the stroke and in 88% within 24 h. This recanalization rate is higher than the rate of 45% achieved by intra-arterial urokinase infusion [5], but comparable to results of another study, in which streptokinase or urokinase was applied locally within the carotid territory.

Immediate assessment after alteplase infusion revealed incomplete recanalization of practically all involved vessels, the exception being a short thrombus occluding (and confined to) the distal ICA which was lysed completely. Assessment after 12–24 h, however, showed that late recanalization reduced the number of unperfused vessels from 11 to 7, increasing the number of reperfused arteries from 1 to 10. Apparently, during alteplase infusion, the proximal thrombus was lysed, dislodged, or fragmented, but thrombolysis still occurred in distal branches during the ensuing hours. This may be due to the effect of rtPA being too small in hypoperfused vessels. Intracerebral haemorrhages were observed in 8 patients (31%). One patient with parenchymal bleeding died, possibly in part because of an extended MCA infarction. Disseminated bleeding in both hemisheres, observed in 1 patient pretreated with aspirin, suggested aspirin may be dangerous in combination with rtPA. Apparently, haemorrhagic transformation of the ischaemic infarct did not worsen outcome. The rate of all intracerebral bleeding was higher than with intra-arterial urokinase therapy [4, 5], but lower than that the natural course [9].

In conclusion, our preliminary data suggest that treatment with 100 mg alteplase administered i. v. is safe and effectively produces arterial recanalization within the ICA territory. Efficacy in terms of clinical outcome will be reported soon.

References

1. Zimmermann R, Heuck CC, Harenberg J, Kummer R von, Schmidt-Gayk U, Simon B, Wahl P, Mörl H, Weber PG (1981) Fibrinolytische Therapie einer schweren Arteria-basilaris-Thrombose. Dtsch Med Wochenschr 106: 464–467
2. Zeumer H, Ringelstein EB, Hassel M, Poeck K (1983) Lokale Fibrinolysetherapie bei subtotaler Stenose der A. cerebri media. Dtsch Med Wochenschr 108: 1103–1105
3. Hacke W, Zeumer H, Ferbert A, Brückmann H, Del Zoppo GJ (1988) Intra-arterial thrombolytic therapy improves outcome in patients with acute vertebrobasilar occlusive disease. Stroke 19: 1216–1222
4. Del Zoppo GJ, Ferbert A, Otis S, Brückmann H, Hacke W, Zyroff J, Harker LA, Zeumer H (1988) Local intra-arterial fibrinolytic therapy in acute carotid territory stroke. Stroke 19: 307–313
5. Mori E, Tabuchi M, Yoshida T, Yamadori A (1988) Intracarotid urokinase with thromboembolic occlusion of the middle cerebral artery. Stroke 19: 802–812
6. Bladin PF (1964) A radiologic and pathologic study of embolism of the internal carotid-middle cerebral arterial axis. Radiology 82: 615–625
7. Irino T, Taneda M, Takaku M (1977) Angiographic manifestations in postrecanalized cerebral infarction. Neurology 27: 471–475
8. Mohr JP, Barnett HJM (1978) The Harvard Cooperative Stroke Registry: a prospective registry. Neurology 28: 754–762
9. Hornig CR, Dorndorf W, Agnoli AL (1986) Hemorrhagic cerebral infarction: a prospective study. Stroke 17: 179–185

Dr. R. von Kummer
Abteilung Klinische Neuroradiologie
Neurologische Universitäts-Klinik
Im Neuenheimer Feld 400
W-6900 Heidelberg
Federal Republic of Germany

Neuroradiology (1991) 33 [Suppl]: 384–386

Neuro-radiology
© Springer-Verlag 1991

High field MRI of cranial intraparenchymal haematomas

C. Faubert[1], P. Demaerel[2], and G. Wilms[2]

[1] Neuroradiological Institute, University of Saarland, Homburg-Saar, Federal Republic of Germany
[2] Radiological Department, University Hospitals of Leuven, Leuven, Belgium

Summary. In this study we retrospectively analysed 25 intracranial intraparenchymal haematomas at 1.0 T and 1.5 T using spin-echo technique. T1- and heavily T2-weighted SE sequences were obtained in the axial, coronal, and sagittal planes. The biochemical, microscopic, and macroscopic mechanisms of haematomas are reviewed as well as their effect on signal intensity. Although the evolution is very complex and multifactorial, the haematomas were divided into hyperacute (< 24 h), acute (1–3 days), subacute (4–21 days), chronic (> 3 weeks) and residual stages (> 4 months). MRI is more informative than CT, except in the hyperacute stage.

Key words: Haematoma – Brain – Haemorrhage – Magnetic resonance imaging

Patients and methods

Twenty-five patients with intracranial intraparenchymal haemorrhages were retrospectively studied. Only those patients in whom the onset of the haemorrhage could be clinically verified were chosen. The MR scans were performed on 1.0 T and 1.5 T imagers (Magnetom, Siemens). T1- and heavily T2-weighted images were obtained in the axial, coronal, and sagittal planes. The haematomas were classified into hyperacute (< 24 h), acute (1–3 days), subacute (4–21 days), chronic (> 3 weeks) and residual (> 4 months) stages.

Results

Hyperacute stage (> 24 h)

Here there is intraparenchymal bleeding with entry of plasma and intact red blood cells, producing a local mass effect [1–5]. Oxyhaemoglobin is diamagnetic with one unpaired electron. It is transformed into deoxyhaemoglobin which is paramagnetic with four unpaired electrons. There is not enough deoxyhaemoglobin to induce a signal. The haematomas examined in the first few hours showed no signal. Then, progressively (after 6 h) there was a homogeneous hypointense signal on T1-weighted images and a hyperintense signal on T2-weighted images corresponding to that of the plasma. There was no oedema. CT was consistently more informative than MRI.

Subacute haemorrhage (3–21 days)

There were two phases [6].

Phase with intact red blood cells. Deoxyhaemoglobin is spontaneously oxidised to methaemoglobin. The latter is strongly paramagnetic with five unpaired electrons. Because of the preferentialy higher PO_2 at the periphery this process evolves centripetally. Methaemoglobin is responsible for a reduction in both T1 and T2. We obtained an outer rim of hyperintensity on T1-weighted images with an hypointense central core. On T2-weighted images there was a hypointense homogeneous zone.

Phase with haemolysed red blood cells. Water diffuses in and methaemoglobin becomes uniformly dispersed. The inhomogeneous susceptibility effect disappears. This increases T2. We have not been able to determine when the hyperintense rim on T2-weighted images appears. At 21 days this process was well established (Fig. 1). T1-weighted images were not affected and remained hyperintense. Macrophages remove haemoglobin from the middle of the lesion and deposit haemosiderin and ferritin at the border of the haematoma. Both lower T2 and do not affect T1. We always obtained a hypointense rim on T2-weighted images. MRI was more informative than CT.

Chronic stage (> 3 weeks)

In the majority of cases (Fig. 2) we obtained a homogeneous hyperintense zone on both T1- and T2-weighted images. Atypical images (Fig. 3 a, b) were also obtained with a central hypointense zone on both T1- and T2-weighted images, but the patient shown in Fig. 3 had a tumoral bleed (melanoma) possibly indicating a delayed methaemoglobin formation. The oedema usually started disappearing after 4 weeks but oedema was sometimes seen up to 4 months after haemorrhage (Fig. 2). The ferritin/haemosiderin hypointense rim was always present on T2-weighted images. MRI was more informative than CT.

Residual stage (> 4 months)

Blood residues were detected up to 3 years after haemorrhage. Ferritin and other breakdown products were responsible for a hypointensity on T2-weighted images.

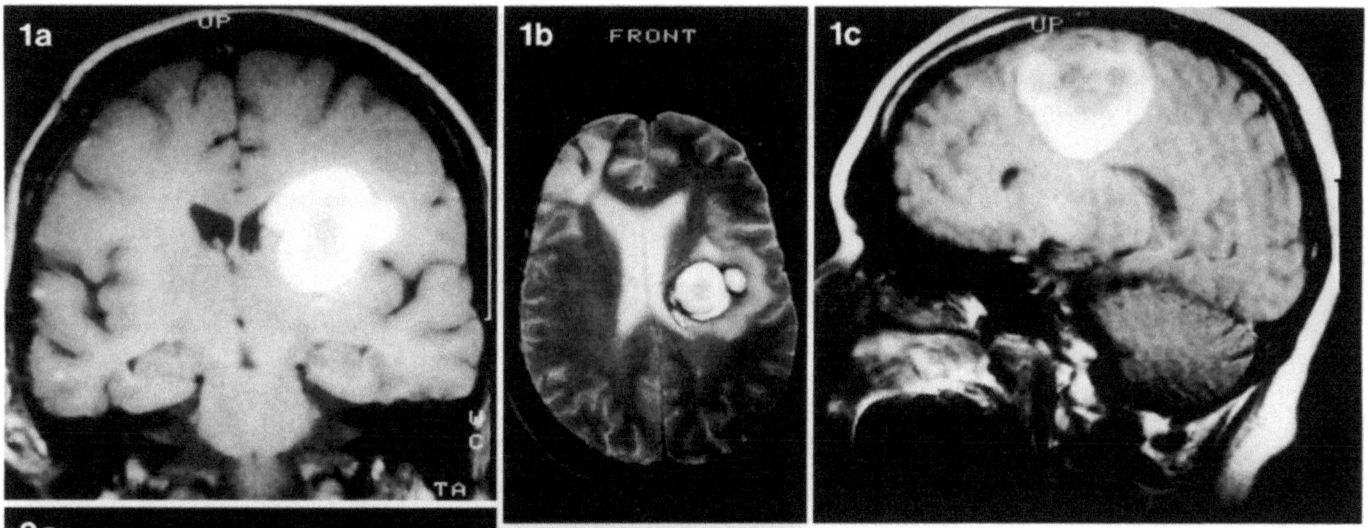

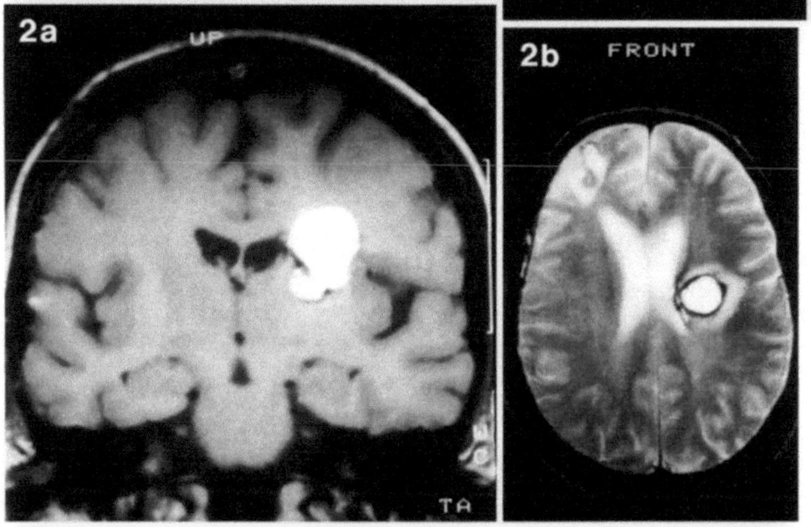

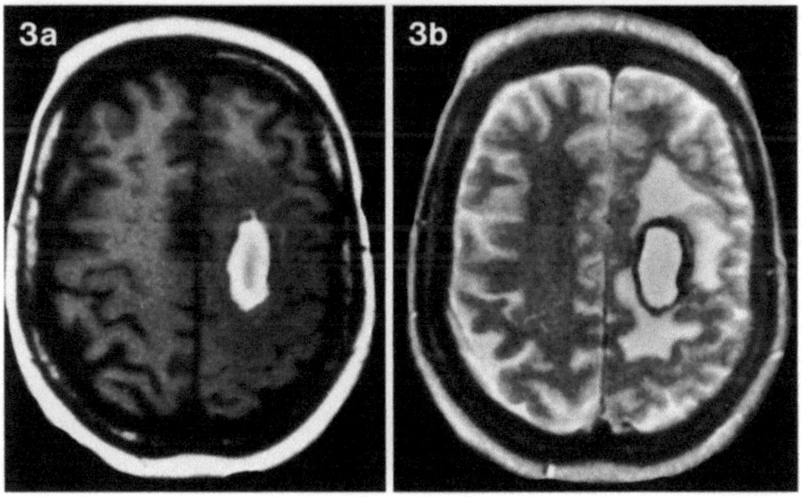

Fig. 1 a–c. A patient at 21 days posthaemorrhage on **a** coronal T1- and **b** axial T2-weighted images. Note the central hypointense zone surrounded by hyperintense peripheral zone. The hypointense haemosiderin/feritin rim is well visualised on T2-weighted image. **c** Ten-day-old left hemispheric bleeding on sagittal T1-weighted image

Fig. 2 a, b. A 4-month-old haematoma. There is a hyperintense zone on both **a** T1- and **b** T2-weighted image. A hypointense rim surrounds the haematoma and the oedema is still present

Fig. 3 a, b. Tumoral bleeding (melanoma). A 2.5-month-old haematoma. **a** T1-weighted image, **b** T2-weighted image. Unusual appearance, notice that there is still a slight hypointense zone on both T1- and T2-weighted images

Perifocal parenchymal alterations were also seen. Calcification was hypointense on both T1- and T2-weighted images. Reactive gliosis and perifocal atrophy were hypo- and hyperintense on T1- and T2-weighted images respectively. If there was no calcification or perifocal atrophy, CT was often normal at this stage while MRI was highly sensitive. MRI was the most reliable imaging method. It often also demonstrated the aetiology of the haemorrhage by showing a tumour or an arteriovenous malformation.

Discussion

Cranial intraparenchymal haematomas are frequent. At the University of Saarland there were 481 cases over a 10-year period. There was a high (40%) mortality, being higher for haemorrhage due to aneurysms than due to angiomas. Starting at the acute stage, MRI is the most reliable imaging modality, thus helping to optimize patient management. A thorough understanding of the mechanisms involved is essential for MRI interpretation of haematomas. There is a complex multifactorial contribution to the signal. There is no absolute classification. MRI appearances depend on the aetiology, the localization, and on local factors. The haematoma formed after an acute aneurysmal rupture might be expected to deoxygenate faster than that due to trauma. On high field MRI, blood pigments and perifocal parenchymal changes provide direct and indirect evidence of haematomas many years after, with a high sensitivity but a low specificity.

References

1. Sipponen JT, Sipponen RE, Sivula A (1983) NMR imaging of intracerebral hemorrhage in the acute and resolving phases. J Comput Assist Tomogr 7: 954–959
2. Zimmerman RD, Deck MDF (1986) Intracranial hematomas: imaging by high field MR. Radiology 159: 565–566
3. Barkovich AJ, Atlas SW (1988) MRI of intracranial hemorrhage. Radiol Clin North Am 26: 801–820
4. Gomori JM, Grossman RI, Goldberg HI (1985) Intracranial hematomas: imaging by high-field MR. Radiology 157: 87–93
5. Gomori JM, Grossman RI (1988) Mechanisms responsible for the MR appearance and evolution of intracranial hemorrhage. Radiographics 3: 427–440
6. Hackey DB, Atlas SW, Grossman RI (1987) Subacute intracranial hemorrhage: contribution of spin density to appearance on spin echo MR images. Radiology 165: 199–202

Dr. C. Faubert
Neuroradiological Institute
University of Saarland
W-665 Homburg-Saar,
Federal Republic of Germany

Neuroradiology (1991) 33 [Suppl]: 387–389

Neuro
radiology
© Springer-Verlag 1991

Three-dimensional MR angiography in the study of intracranial neoplasms

R. Gasparotti, G. F. Gualandi, A. Orlandini, and A. Chiesa

Department of Radiology, Section of Neuroradiology, University of Brescia, Italy

Summary. MR angiography (MRA) was performed in 25 patients with primary intracranial tumours in association with a standard brain spin-echo technique, in order to assess its technical feasibility and its clinical usefulness. MRA findings were compared with those of angiography (digital subtraction or conventional). The results indicate that MRA can accurately depict the mass effect of cerebral neoplasms on major cerebral vessels with a good correlation with angiography; however MRA is still insufficient for precise evaluation of the vascular supply and neovascularisation of tumours.

Key words: Brain neoplasms – Cerebral angiography – Magnetic resonance image processing – Magnetic resonance angiography

Until recently, MR vascular applications have been limited due to technical problems. With the development of flow-sensitive sequences (gradient-echo) and complex algorithmic approaches to image postprocessing, MR angiography (MRA) is becoming a new potential tool for a noninvasive evaluation of the cerebral vasculature [1, 2]. While the first clinical investigations were mainly addressed to the study of peripheral vessels there is still a lack of information on the possibilities of MRA in the study of cerebral neoplasms [3–6].

In order to assess its clinical usefulness a recently developed MR angiographic technique, the so-called time of flight three-dimensional (3D) MRA, was tested on 25 patients with cerebral neoplasm [7, 8]. The purpose of the study was to determine the sensitivity of this technique in depicting the brain vascular changes produced by tumours.

Materials and methods

Twenty-five patients with primary intracranial tumours were studied with MRI (10 gliomas, 10 meningiomas, 3 acoustic neuromas, 2 pituitary macroadenomas). The MRI examinations were performed with a 1.5 T superconducting unit (Helicon, Siemens, Erlangen). T1- and T2-weighted spin-echo images of the brain were obtained in two different planes in order to localise the tumour exactly. MRA was performed after the tumour identification, with an additional examination time of 10–20 min, depending on the vascular anatomy. In all patients angiography [digital subtraction (DSA) or conventional] was available for comparison. MR and DSA or conventional angiography were independently reviewed by two neuroradiologists. The MR angiographic technique, the so called time of flight 3D MRA, consisted of volume acquisitions obtained with gradient-echo sequences (FISP 3D) (TR 50 ms; TE 12 ms; FA 15°–20°; 64 partitions; slice thickness 1.25 mm). Image processing was performed with a ray-tracing algorithm based on maximum intensity projections which allows the reconstruction of the vascular tree in any plane and with any rotation angle from the original data set. In every patient MR angiograms were obtained in three orthogonal planes, with different projection angles, in order to better depict the relationships of the tumour to major intracranial vessels.

Results

The MRA findings are shown in Table 1.

Major intracranial vessel displacement was shown in 20 of 25 patients (80%, Fig. 1). The particular anatomical location of meningiomas allowed a clear visualization of the relationships to the circle of Willis in 9 of 10 cases. In 4 cases of glial tumour, the peripheral location and the small size prevented the identification of the mass effect on the vessels, due to insufficient spatial resolution of MRA. For the same reason the vascular supply of tumours was identified in only 8 of 25 cases. However, in 5 meningiomas MRA demonstrated hypertrophied meningeal vessels (Fig. 2). Neovascularity was clearly visualized in only 6 of 25 cases.

Discussion

The results of the study indicate that time of flight 3D MRA can be routinely integrated with a spin-echo examination of intracranial tumours, without a significant in-

Table 1. Findings from 3D MR angiography

		Size (cm)	Vessel displacement	Vascular supply	Neovascularity
Meningiomas	[a] 9	3–6	9/9	5/9	3/9
	[b] 1	3	–	–	–
Gliomas	[a] 8	2–5	5/8	3/8	3/8
	[b] 2	1–3	1/2	–	–
Acoustic neuromas	3	2–4	2/3	–	–
Macroadenomas	2	2–4	3/3	–	–

[a] Supratentorial
[b] Posterior fossa

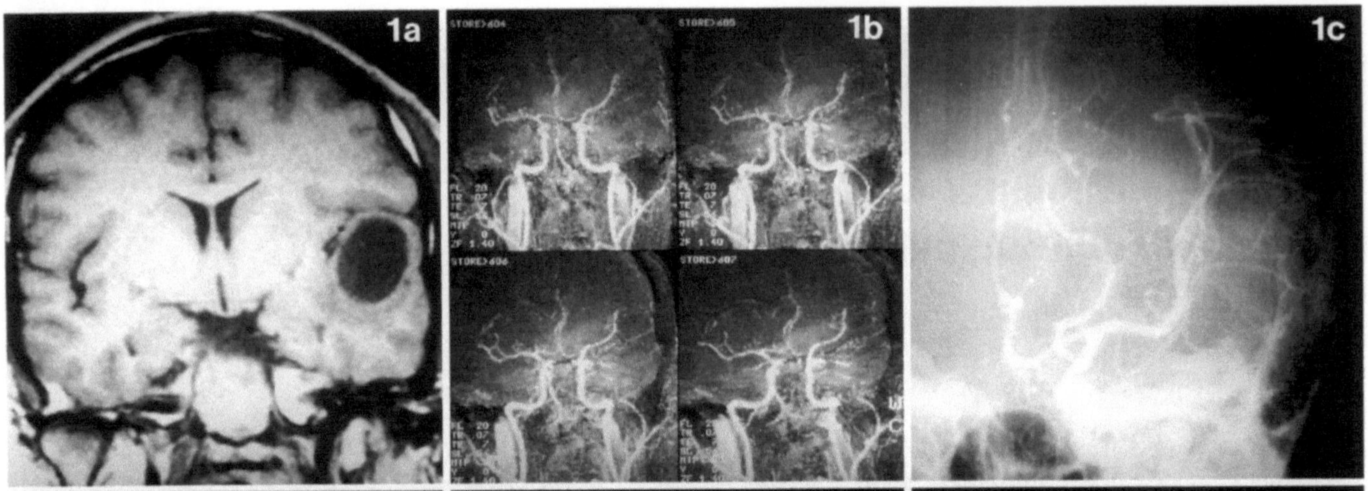

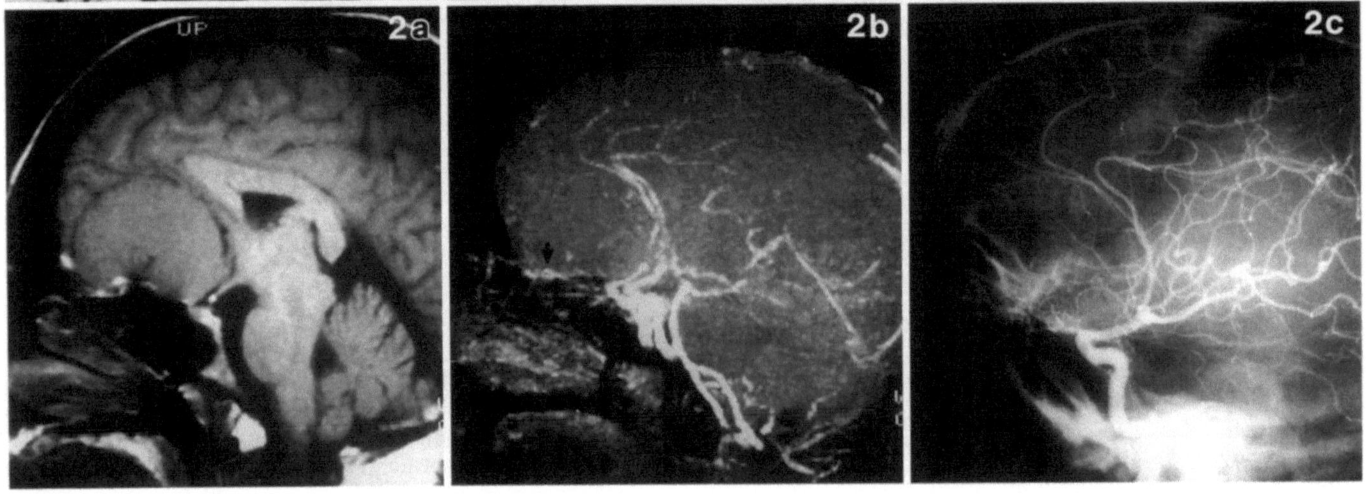

Fig. 1 a–c. Grade III astrocytoma of the left fronto-temporoparietal region. **a** T1-weighted coronal image (SE 600/15). **b** Three-dimensional MR angiography with multiple projections in the coronal plane (rotation angle 0° > 30°). The middle cerebral artery (MCA) is shifted medially and superiorly. **c** The left internal carotid angiogram confirms the MCA displacement produced by the tumour

Fig. 2 a–c. Olfactory groove meningioma. **a** T1-weighted sagittal image (SE 600/15). **b** The MR angiogram demonstrates a mass effect on the anterior cerebral artery. Hypertrophied meningeal vessels can also be recognized *(arrow)*. **c** The left internal carotid angiogram confirms the anterior cerebral artery displacement and the vascular supply originating from ethmoidal arteries

crease in total examination time. With this technique the visualisation of the cerebral vessels is strictly related to at least two different factors: (1) spatial resolution which, at present, is not still comparable with that of DSA; (2) physical properties of blood flow (T1-relaxation time, velocity, acceleration and pulsatility) [7, 8].

The major intracranial vessel displacement produced by tumours can be accurately demonstrated by 3D MRA; moreover the 3D display of the vascular anatomy offers the advantage of following the entire course of a displaced vessel or of a feeding artery by an accurate selection of the projection angles. The ray-tracing algorithm also allows unusual angiographic projections which can be used to better advantage in establishing the tumour relationships with vascular structures. MRA seems to be not so accurate in the visualisation of the vascular supply of brain tumours: supplying vessels can be identified only when their calibre is large enough, as in hypertrophied meningeal vessels supplying meningiomas. Even if further technical development is needed to improve spatial resolution, MRA can play a role in the preoperative investigation of meningiomas; in this case MRA provides clinically useful information on cerebral circulation which can be integrated with information given by spin-echo images, in order to obtain optimal planning of the surgical procedure.

The demonstration of tumour neovascularity is still limited due to both insufficient spatial resolution and low sensitivity of time of flight techniques to slow laminar flow, which is typical of this kind of vessel. As a consequence, the diagnostic usefulness of 3D MRA is reduced in gliomas. In conclusion, time of flight 3D MRA can provide an accurate demonstration of the main vascular changes related to intracranial tumours and can be a complementary source of information in the MR evaluation of the brain.

References

1. Laub GA, Kaiser WA (1988) MR angiography with gradient motion refocusing. J Comput Assist Tomogr 12: 377-382
2. Edelman RR, Wentz KU, Mattle HP, O'Reilly GV, Candia G, Liu C, Zhao B, Kjellberg RN, Davis KR (1989) Intracerebral arte-

riovenous malformations: evaluation with selective MR angiography and venography. Radiology 173: 831–837
3. Alfidi RJ, Masaryk TJ, Haacke EM, Lenz GW, Ross JS, Modic MT, Nelson AD, LiPuma JP, Cohen AM (1987) MR angiography of peripheral, carotid, and coronary arteries. AJR 149: 1097–1109
4. Dumoulin CT, Hart HR (1986) Magnetic resonance angiography. Radiology 161: 717–720
5. Spritzer CE, Blinder RA (1989) Vascular applications of magnetic resonance imaging. Magn Reson Q 5: 205–227
6. Lewin JS, Masaryk TM, Modic MT, Ross JS, Stork EK, Wizniter M (1989) Extracorporeal membrane oxygenation in infants: angiographic and parenchymal evaluation of the brain with MR imaging. Radiology 173: 361–365
7. Masaryk TJ, Modic MT, Ross JS, Ruggieri PM, Laub GA, Lenz GW, Haacke EM, Selman WR, Wizniter M, Harik SI (1989) Intracranial circulation: preliminary clinical results with three-dimensional (volume) MR angiography. Radiology 171: 793–799
8. Ruggieri PM, Laub GA, Masaryk TJ, Modic MT (1989) Intracranial circulation: pulse sequence considerations in three-dimensional (volume) MR angiography. Radiology 171: 785–791

Dr. R. Gasparotti
Sezione di Neuroradiologia
Cattedra di Radiologia, Università di Brescia
Spedali Civili di Brescia
I-25100 Brescia, Italy

Neuroradiology (1991) 33 [Suppl]: 390–391

Neuro-radiology
© Springer-Verlag 1991

Localisation and classification of acute unilateral pontine and mesencephalic infarction with MRI

H. Brückmann, A. Thron, and A. Ferbert

Department of Neuroradiology, Klinikum RWTH, Aachen, Federal Republic of Germany

Summary. We present 24 patients with clinically suspected acute unilateral brain-stem stroke. T2-weighted MRI examinations were performed in all patients. The various infarction patterns of the arterial territories were micro-angiographically studied in 30 brain-stem specimens. Our data indicate: (1) in the paramedian sagittal section, triangular or trapezoid territorial infarcts are orientated with their main axis to the fastigium; this is due to a converging course of the paramedian pontine arteries towards the floor of the fourth ventricle; (2) unilateral midpontine infarcts do not usually extend to the pontine tegmentum; this is due to the convergence of all paramedian pontine arteries to the fastigium and to the fact that the midpontine tegmentum is mainly supplied by the descending and ascending paramedian branches of the upper and lower basilar artery. (3) the sagittal plane is often necessary to differentiate between unilateral territory pontine and lacunar infarction.

Key words: Brain-stem infarction – Microangiography – Magnetic resonance imaging – Classification of infarcts

In order to correlate the infarction patterns of our MRI examinations with arterial territories, microangiographic studies were performed on 30 brain-stem specimens following injection of barium sulphate. Our microangiographic findings were compared with the arterial angio-architecture described by Duvernoy [1].

Methods and results

Microangiography

In 28 patients transverse cross-sections (thickness 4 mm) were cut through the upper pons (Fig. 1).

The intrinsic brain-stem arteries fall into four major groups: (1) the paramedian pontine branches supplying the anteromedial group; they always respect the midline and supply the whole central pontine tegmentum; (2) the short circumferential arteries supplying the anterolateral group; very often they have one common orifice with paramedian pontine arteries; (3) the long circumferential arteries supplying the territory of the lateral group; (4) the posterior group of the pontomesencephalic junction is derived from the collicular arteries (Fig. 1).

In 4 patients paramedian sagittal dissections of the brain-stem were made. The paramedian arteries run at varying angles with the

Fig. 1. Microangiogram. Transverse microangiographic cross-section through the pons at its upper level: *1*, anteromedial group; *2*, anterolateral group; *3*, lateral group; *4*, posterior group

Fig. 2. Microangiogram. Paramedian longitudinal section. Note the paramedian arteries converging to the roof of the fourth ventricle

Fig. 3. T2-weighted MRI in sagittal plane. Typical wedge-shaped anteromedial/anterolateral pontine infarction. Note that the infarction makes contact with the pontine circumference

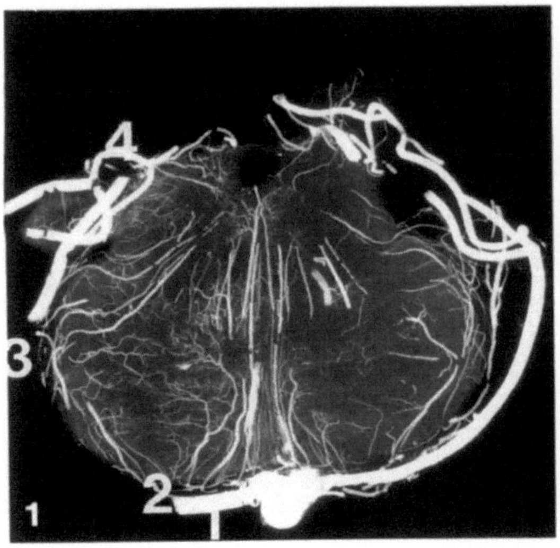

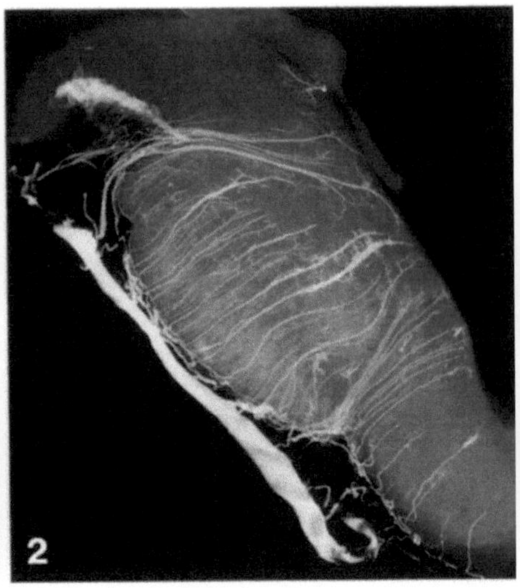

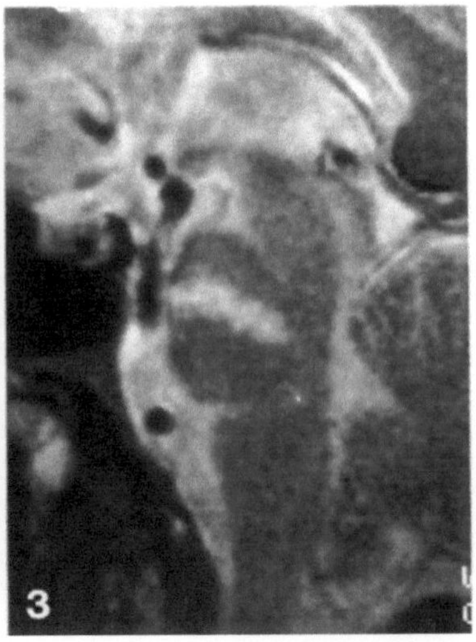

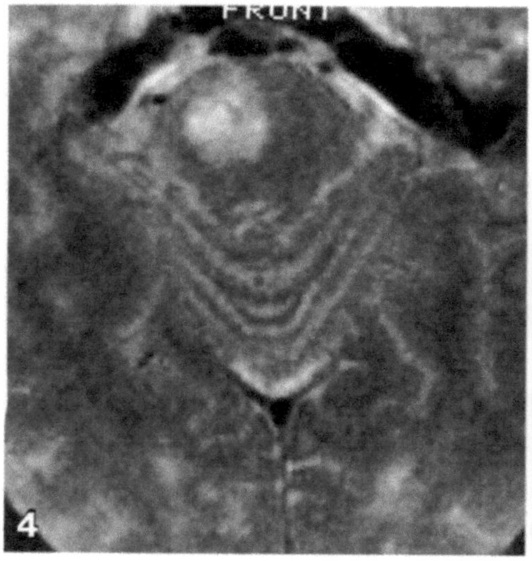

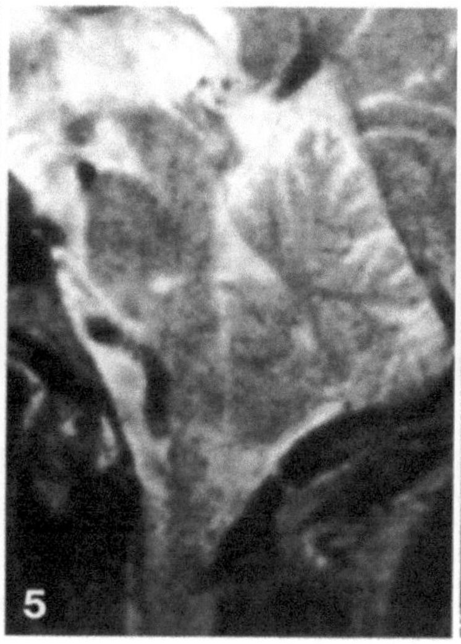

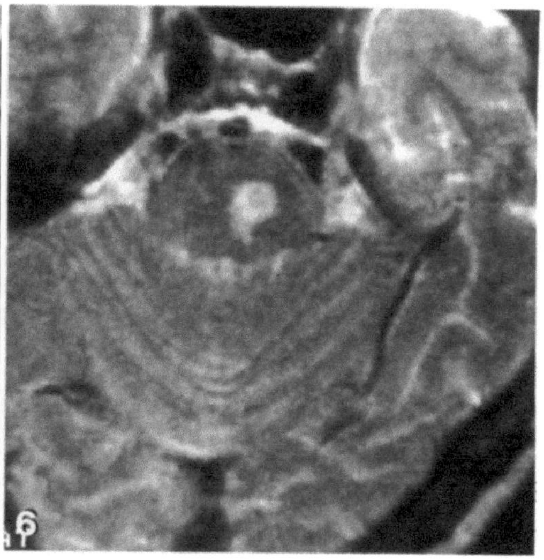

Fig. 4. T2-weighted MRI in axial plane

Figs. 5, 6. T2-weighted MRI of the brain-stem. Hyperintense lacunar infarct, visible at lower pontine level. Note that this lesion lies at the border of the pontine tegmentum

longitudinal axis of the pons and converge to the roof of the fourth ventricle (Fig. 2).

Top of the basilar level. The paramedian pontine branches curve downward caudo-dorsally directed to the floor of the fourth ventricle.

Midbasilar level. The midpontine anteromedial branches show a nearly horizontal course.

Caudal basilar level. The long anteromedial arteries derived from the vertebrobasilar junction run in a ventrodorsal direction inclined rostrally and reach the tegmentum.

MRI examinations

In 24 patients T2-weighted MRI examinations were performed in axial and sagittal planes. MRI findings were localised with respect to the reference sections according to the diagrams of Duvernoy [1]. Six patients showed unilateral single territory brain-stem infarction. In 8 patients infarction was visible in multiple territories. The following results were notable: (1) the infarcts reach the pontine circumference (Fig. 3); (2) the anteromedial/anterolateral infarcts always respect the midline (Fig. 4); (3) the infarcts rarely extend to the tegmentum pontis (Figs. 3, 4); (4) in the sagittal section the infarcts are approximately triangular or trapezoid with the main axis orientated toward the fastigium.

In 10 patients typical lacunar infarctions were differentiated; 8 of the 10 patients had additional white matter lesions due to subcortical arteriosclerotic encephalopathy. Most of these ovoid lesions were situated in the middle third of the basis pontis (Figs. 5, 6).

Discussion

MRI enables differentiation between unilateral pontine infarction due to occlusion of small pontine branches at their origin from the basilar artery and lacunar infarction due to an occlusive microangiopathic lesion within the distal segments of the perforating pontine arteries. The sagittal plane is especially useful for differentiating unilateral pontine infarction.

Reference

1. Duvernoy H (1978) The human brainstem vessels. Springer, Berlin Heidelberg New York

Dr. H. Brückmann
Department of Neuroradiology
Klinikum RWTH
Pauwelsstrasse
W-5100 Aachen, Federal Republic of Germany

Neuroradiology (1991) 33 [Suppl]: 392–393

Neuro radiology
© Springer-Verlag 1991

Preliminary experience of 3D MR angiography in ivestigating cerebrovascular disease

A. M. Wang[1], D. P. Wesolowski[1], A. N. Shetty[6], R. M. Ernstoff[2], R. E. Olson[3], R. A. Ellwood[1], J. Gilroy[2], D. I. Bojrab[4], S. Mounayer[2], S. E. Boodin[3], P. Friedman[3], E. M. Cohn[5], and J. Farah[1]

Departments of [1] Diagnostic Radiology, [2] Neurology, [3] Neurosurgery, [4] Otology, [5] Neuro-ophthalmology, William Beaumont Hospital, Royal Oak, Michigan, USA [6] Siemens Medical Systems, Iselin, New Jersey, USA

Summary. The clinical value of three-dimensional (3D) (volume) time of flight (flow-related enhancement) gradient-echo MR angiography (MRA) was assessed in 40 patients presenting with clinical cerebrovascular disease. Nine had aneurysms, 12 had occlusive vascular disease, 10 had a vascular malformation or fistula and 9 patients had normal studies (2 patients with subarachnoid hemorrhage, 1 patient with unilateral third cranial nerve palsy, 6 patients with headache and migraine). 3D MRA was compared with intra-arterial digital subtraction angiography in all 40 patients and in most correlated closely. The results of this preliminary experience suggest that 3D MRA can adequately define the fast-flowing medium- to large-sized intracranial vessels and detect pathological involvement with reasonable certainty, noninvasively.

Key words: Cerebrovascular disease – Aneurysm – Arteriovenous malformation or fistula – Occlusive vascular disease – Intracranial three-dimensional magnetic resonance angiography

The normal intracranial arteries have rapid blood flow during both systole and diastole but the veins have slow continuous blood flow. Gradient refocussed echo pulse sequence, together with flow compensation and phase-sensitive imaging techniques, produces images in which flowing blood appears much brighter than stationary tissues. Intracranially, motion is primarily due to vascular pulsation. Two techniques that are commonly used to image flowing blood are based on: (1) time of flight (TOF) effect; (2) spin-phase change effects. The technique that was used in our study is a type of TOF effect in which the advantage of flow-related enhancement was utilized. This technique is based on the detection of unsaturated inflowing spins into a saturated 3D volume [1]. Several variations in 3D (volume) gradient-echo MR angiography (MRA) have been recently introduced clinically for investigating cerebrovascular disease noninvasively [2–5]. The object of our study was to assess the clinical utility of noninvasive 3D MRA technique as compared with intra-arterial digital subtraction angiography (DSA) in investigating intracranial vascular pathology.

Materials and methods

The study population consisted of 40 patients with clinically suspected cerebrovascular disease (19 female, 21 male), ranging in age from 16 to 71 years. MRI examinations were performed with a Siemens Magnetom unit operated at 1.0 T with a 6-mT/m gradient capability and a circularly polarized head coil used. A 3D volume gradient-echo MRA was performed in addition to routine spin-echo MRI with 6–24 min extra time. The technique used for 3D MRA was a gradient-echo fast low-angle shot sequence (TR 40–50 ms/ TE 9 ms) with a 15° flip angle.

Gadolinium (Gd) DTPA (gadopentetate dimeglumine) enhancement was utilized in 5 patients. An additional 5 slices of 2D gradient-echo fast low-angle shot imaging sequence (TR 200 ms/ TE 12 ms) with a 40°–50° flip angle and 4-mm thickness 1 slice were used to study the areas of interest. Correlation with intra-arterial DSA was available in all patients.

Results

Most of the 3D MRA studies, showing the arteriovenous malformation, arteriovenous fistula, small aneurysm (Fig. 2), occlusive vascular disease and normal appearances, as well as normal variants, correlated closely with DSA. There were two false negatives (2 patients with small venous angioma which were not seen on 3D MRA, but were visualized on 2D gradient-echo study and 3D MRA with Gd enhancement, Fig. 1), and 1 false-positive (a patient with occlusion of both distal vertebral arteries with excellent retrograde flow to the basilar artery and right posterior cerebral artery through the left posterior communicating artery which was demonstrated by DSA, but the right posterior cerebral artery was not visualized on 3D MRA). One giant aneurysm and 1 thrombosed giant aneurysm were partially visualized on 3D MRA without Gd enhancement but were well demonstrated by 3D MRA with Gd enhancement.

Discussion

The MRA technique used in our study is based on wash-in of unsaturated (fully relaxed) spins, entering an image slice region that partially vacated by the wash-out of saturated spins. These fresh spins, due to their maximum longitudinal magnetization component (not affected by

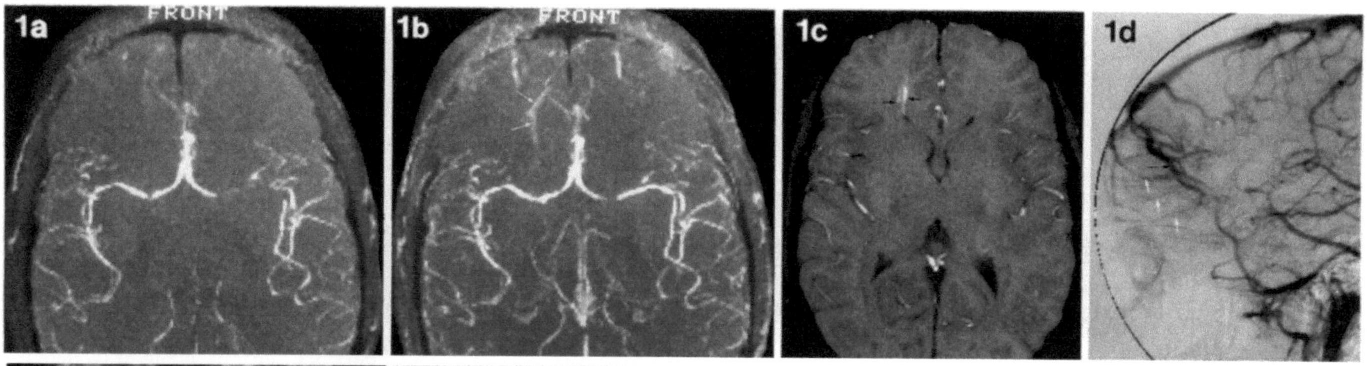

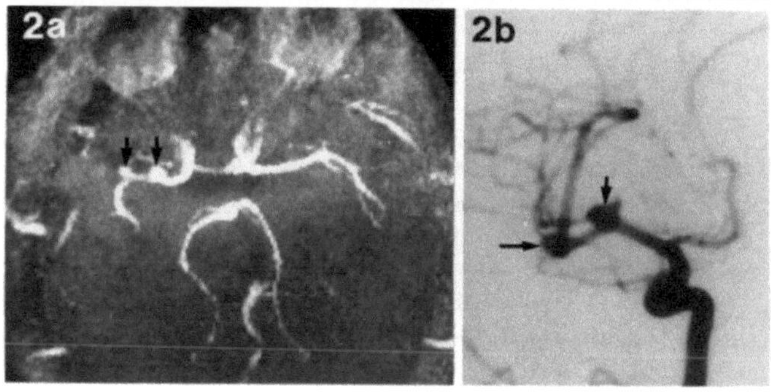

Fig. 1 a–d. A 16-year-old male with a right frontal lobe venous angioma. **a** 3D MR angiography (MRA) without gadolinium (Gd) enhancement fails to demonstrate a venous angioma *(arrows)* which is seen on **b** Gd-enhanced 3D MRA, and **c** 2D FLASH images without Gd. **d** Lateral view of venous phase of right carotid digital subtraction angiography (DSA) shows dilated medullary veins *(white arrows)* draining into the dilated superficial cortical vein *(arrow)*

Fig. 2 a, b. A 36-year-old male with two saccular aneurysms *(arrows)* of right middle cerebral artery demonstrated on **a** 3D MRA and **b** arterial DSA

radiofrequency) give rise to maximal signal. In addition, phase variations due to motion are compensated by using flow compensating gradient. FLASH and FISP (fast imaging with steady precession) 3D MR sequences, frequently used for 3D MRA, include velocity rephasing along the read and slice directions. Since the dephasing is quadratic with respect to TE, motion-related spin dephasing is minimized with short TE. The TR was shortened, compared with T1 relaxation time of the tissue, so that stationary spins are partially saturated to give minimal signal. Although the FISP sequence is better suited for shorter TE, in our study we used the FLASH sequence which gives T1 weighting for surrounding tissue.

A few limitations of this technique need to be stressed. Firstly, slow-flowing lesions such as a giant aneurysm and a venous angioma are poorly visualized on 3D MRA, due to the saturation of the moving spins residing for too long within the excited volume. For the same reason, a large aneurysm may appear smaller on 3D MRA than demonstrated by DSA. Moreover the decreased blood flow in the tightly stenotic arteries resulting from occlusive cerebral vascular disease may be overread as complete occlusion. This situation can be improved with the use of either gadolinium, which decreases the T1-relaxation time, or 2D gradient-echo studies. Particularly in a large thrombosed aneurysm, the residual lumen of the parent vessel and the thrombosed portion of the aneurysm sac, as well as the wall of the thrombosed aneurysm, are better visualized by Gd-enhanced 3D MRA than 3D MRA without GD enhancement. Gd-enhanced 3D MRA may be even better than DSA in identifying its thrombosed portion, as well as the wall of a thrombosed aneurysm.

Secondly, since the volume gradient-echo technique requires at least 20 min acquisition time to cover the entire intracranial vasculature, patient cooperation plays an important role in a satisfactory study. A thin volume slab is needed to avoid the patient's motion artifact or the lesion may be missed or not completely covered by the study. Thirdly, the resolution of 3D MRA is slightly inferior to that of DSA, but it is reasonably valuable clinically for evaluation of medium-to-large-sized intracranial vessels.

In summary, 86.5% of 3D MRA without Gd enhancement and 97.5% of 3D MRA with additional Gd enhancement were considered to be useful for diagnosis in this study. Although the accuracy of the data is limited by the small study population (40 patients), our results suggest that in conjunction with Gd enhancement, 3D MRA holds promise as a noninvasive intracranial vascular screening examination in patients with cerebrovascular disease.

References

1. Laub GA, Kaiser WA (1988) MR angiography with gradient motion refocussing. J Comput Assist Tomogr 12: 377–382
2. Ruggieri PM, Laub GA, Masaryk TJ, Modic MT (1989) Intracranial circulation: pulse-sequence considerations in three-dimensional (volume) MR angiography. Radiology 171: 785–791
3. Masaryk TJ, Modic MT, Ross JS (1989) Intracranial circulation: preliminary clinical results with three-dimensional (volume) MR angiography. Radiology 171: 793–799
4. Ross JS, Masaryk TJ, Modic MT (1990) Intracranial aneurysms: evaluation by MR angiography. AJNR 11: 449–456
5. Marchal G, Bosmans H, Van Fraeyenhoven L (1990) Intracranial vascular lesions: optimization and clinical evaluation of three-dimensional time-of-flight MR angiography. Radiology 175: 443–448

Dr. Ay-Ming Wang
Department of Diagnostic Radiology
William Beaumont Hospital
3601 West Thirteen Mile Road
Royal Oak, MI 48073, USA

Neuroradiology (1991) 33 [Suppl]: 394–396

Neuro radiology
© Springer-Verlag 1991

Percutaneous transluminal angioplasty of the subclavian, vertebral and basilar arteries: technical considerations

R. T. Higashida[1], F. Y. Tsai[2], V. V. Halbach[1], G. B. Hieshima[1], C. F. Dowd[1], and S. L. Barnwell[1]

[1] Departments of Radiology and Neurological Surgery, Interventional Neuroradiology Section, University of California at San Francisco, San Francisco, California, USA
[2] University of Missouri, Kansas City School of Medicine, Truman Medical Center, Kansas City, Missouri, USA

Summary. Percutaneous transluminal angioplasty of brachiocephalic vessels is being performed with increasing frequency. The indications for treatment include symptomatic stenosis refractory to medical therapy. Patients are now being treated for atherosclerotic disease, fibromuscular dysplasia, and arteritis causing critical stenosis of the subclavian, vertebral, and basilar arteries. From a transfemoral or transaxillary approach, the balloon dilatation catheter is guided across the area of stenosis, and inflated once or twice, at 10–12 atmospheres of pressure for 6–10 s, to produce dilatation. To date 130 patients have been treated. Complications included 4 instances of transient cerebral ischemia, 2 stroke and 1 vessel occlusion. This technique can be efficacious for treatment of patients with symptomatic, critical stenosis of the posterior circulation.

Key words: Transluminal angioplasty – Atherosclerotic lesions – Posterior fossa ischemia – Balloon dilatation – Interventional neuroradiology

Percutaneous transluminal angioplasty (PTA) treatment of atherosclerotic lesions was first reported in 1964 [1]. It was not, however, until the early 1980s that the first reports describing PTA of brachiocephalic vessels appeared [2–4]. Over the past 6 years, our group has performed PTA in 132 cases of lesions involving the subclavian, vertebral and basilar arteries. The technique, indications and therapeutic results are described.

Materials and Methods

Since 1984, 130 patients have been treated by balloon dilatation techniques for symptomatic stenosis involving the posterior circulation. The stenosed vessels treated included the subclavian artery in 108 patients, the vertebral artery in 22, and the basilar artery in 2. The indications for treatment included stenoses due to atherosclerosis, vasculitis or fibromuscular dysplasia. The patients presented with symptoms of transient cerebral ischemia, the subclavian steal syndrome, multiple strokes involving the posterior circulation, or brain stem ischemia. All were initially managed by medical therapy, including antiplatelet and/or anticoagulant medication. Only patients who failed to respond to medical therapy were considered for angioplasty [5].

All patients underwent a complete cerebral arteriogram to identify the site and degree of stenosis, the status of the contralateral subclavian and vertebral artery, and collateral blood flow from the anterior circulation. Patients were started on antiplatelet medication (aspirin or dipyridamole) prior to the procedure, and this was continued for 6 months. Anticoagulation during the procedure was by i. v. administration of heparin (72 units/kg).

From a transfemoral or transaxillary approach, an 0.035 in diameter, 260 cm long guidewire was placed across the area of stenosis and into the distal vessel, in cases of subclavian or proximal vertebral artery stenosis. A 7.1 F straight, polyethylene catheter, tapered to 5.0 F, was then guided over the wire to dilate the stenotic segment to 7.1 F. In the distal vertebral and basilar arteries, an

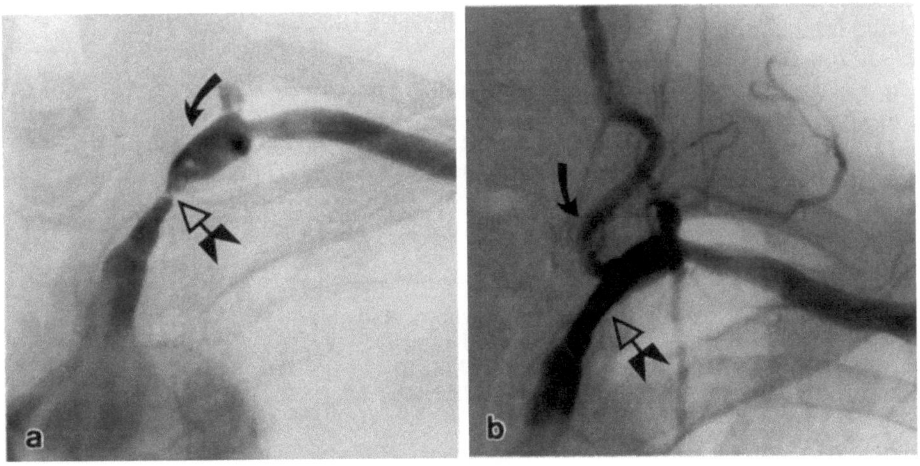

Fig. 1. a Selective subclavian arteriogram demonstrates high-grade stenosis of the proximal left subclavian artery *(arrow)*. This patient presented with the subclavian steal syndrome. Note that the vertebral artery does not fill *(curved arrow)*. **b** Following successful transluminal angioplasty with a 6.0-mm balloon, there is wide patency of the subclavian artery *(arrow)*, and normal antegrade filling of the vertebral artery *(curved arrow)*

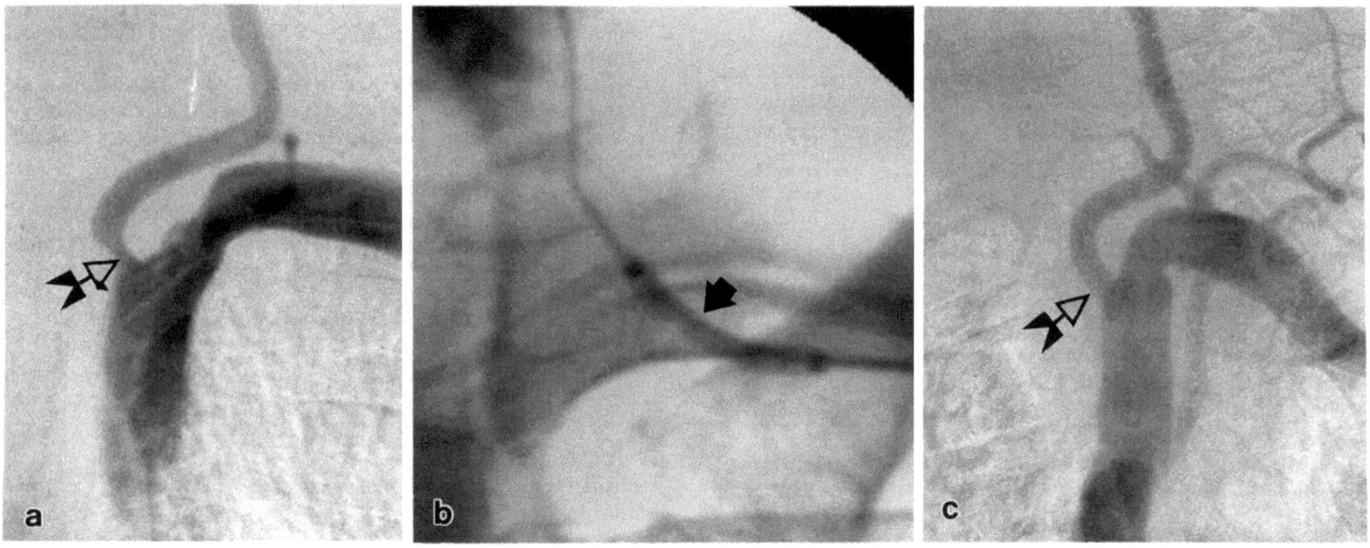

Fig. 2. **a** Selective subclavian artery injection demonstrates a stenosis of the proximal vertebral artery (arrow) in a patient presenting with symptoms of brain stem ischemia. **b** The 4.0-mm angioplasty balloon catheter is across the stenosis and inflated to dilate the lesion. **c** Follow-up angiogram 12 months after dilatation demonstrates wide patency of the vertebral artery, with return to normal luminal diameter

0.018 in guidewire was used, in conjuction with a 3.2 F catheter. The appropriate angioplasty balloon was then selected to match the normal luminal diameter of the vessel to be treated. For the subclavian artery the balloon utilized was between 5 and 8 mm, for the vertebral artery 4–6 mm, and for the basilar artery 2.5–4.0 mm (Fig. 1 a, b). Currently, several types of balloon dilatation catheter are available. Those most commonly used were the Olbert Balloon Dilatation System (Meadox Surgimed); MediTech Balloon Dilatation System (MediTech, Watertown, Mass.); and the Stealth Dilatation Catheter (Target Therapeutics, San Jose, Calif.) for intracranial use. Under fluoroscopic vizualization, the balloon was guided across the stenosis, and then inflated to 10–12 atmospheres of pressure, for 5–10 s, once or twice, to dilate the narrowed segment. The catheter and guidewire were then removed and the patient was examined neurologically. A post angioplasty arteriogram was performed in all cases to assess the degree of luminal enlargement, patency of the vessel, evidence of intimal damage, and to exclude distal embolization of normal branches (Fig. 2 a–c).

Patients were then monitored in the neurosurgical observation unit for 24–48 h and, if stable, discharged on antiplatelet medication. Follow-up studies were performed at 1, 3, and 12 months following treatment by clinical examination and with MRI, CT, Doppler blood flow studies, and/or angiography if clinically indicated.

Results

Of the 132 patients in whom percutaneous balloon angioplasty was attempted, there were only 2 in whom treatment could not be performed due to tortuosity of vessels. Complications included transient cerebral ischemia during or after the procedure, which resolved within 30 min, in 4 patients. There were 2 cases of a posterior fossa stroke. One was probably due to angioplasty of the basilar artery producing occlusion of brain stem perforating vessels. The second stroke occurred following angioplasty of a high grade stenosis of a vertebral artery at the C-1 level. In 1 patient the distal vertebral artery ruptured during angioplasty. In 7 patients (5.3%), retreatment was necessary due to recurrence of stenosis on follow-up studies. All 7 of these patients had atherosclerotic lesions of the subclavian artery [6].

Discussion

Treatment of high-grade stenotic arterial lesions in the head and neck is being performed with increasing frequency by interventional techniques [6, 7]. The mechanism of dilatation is similar to that of balloon angioplasty of other vessels. For atherosclerotic lesions, the balloon mechanically causes stretching and fissuring of the intima and media. This results in fracturing of the plaque and remodelling of the lesion with secondary fibrosis and re-endothelialization at the angioplasty site. Initially, the lesion appears irregular, with evidence of subintimal hemorrhage, fissuring, and tearing of the plaque and vessel. However, over several weeks, the site of injury heals and the luminal diameter may actually increase due to continued retraction of the vessel wall [8, 9].

The diameter of the balloon selected for treatment should correspond to the normal internal diameter of the vessel being treated. Overdistention may cause severe vessel injury, perforation, and/or damage to the normal intima and media around the stenosis [8]. When carrying out angioplasty of the posterior circulation, we keep balloon occlusion time below 10 s to avoid inducing further brain stem ischemia. To date, only 4 patients in our series have experienced transient ischemic symptoms following the procedure. Other potential complications include brain stem stroke, respiratory and cardiac arrest, thromboembolic strokes, vessel occlusion or perforation, intimal dissection leading to delayed occlusion, and occlusion of adjacent normal branches arising from the vessel being treated.

The results of balloon dilatation of high-grade stenotic lesions, refractory to medical therapy, appear favorable. Long term follow-up to assess the efficacy of balloon angioplasty is ongoing. Comparison with surgical results in comparable groups of patients may be needed to further assess this treatment modality [10].

References

1. Dotter CT, Judkins MP (1964) Transluminal treatment of arteriosclerotic obstruction: description of a new technique and preliminary report of its application. Circulation 30: 654–670
2. Kerber CS, Cromwell LD, Leohden OL (1980) Catheter dilatation of proximal carotid stenosis during distal bifurcation endarterectomy. AJNR 1: 348–349
3. Motarjeme A, Keifer JW, Zuska AJ (1982) Percutaneous transluminal angioplasty of the brachiocephalic arteries. AJR 138: 457–462
4. Tsai FY, Matovich V, Hieshima G (1986) Percutaneous transluminal angioplasty of the carotid artery. AJNR 7: 349–358
5. Higashida RT, Hieshima GB, Tsai FY, Bentson JR, Halbach VV (1986) Percutaneous transluminal angioplasty of the subclavian and vertebral arteries. Acta Radiol [Suppl 369]: 124–126
6. Higashida RT, Hieshima BG, Tsai FY (1987) Transluminal angioplasty of the vertebral and basilar artery. AJNR 8: 745–749
7. Théron JG (1987) Angioplasty of supra-aortic arteries. Semin Interven Radiol 4: 331–342
8. Castañeda-Zuñiga WR, Formanek A, Tadavarthy M (1980) The mechanism of balloon angioplasty. Radiology 135: 565–571
9. Zollikofer CL, Salomonowitz E, Sibley R (1984) Transluminal angioplasty evaluated by electron microscopy. Radiology 153: 372–374
10. Jonas S, Hass WK (1979) An approach to the maximal acceptance stroke complication rate after surgery for TIA. Stroke 10: 104

Dr. R. T. Higashida
University of California at San Francisco
Medical Center
505 Parnassus Avenue, L-352
San Francisco, California, USA

Neuroradiology (1991) 33 [Suppl]: 397–398

Neuro-radiology

© Springer-Verlag 1991

Seven years' experience with percutaneous transluminal angioplasty for carotid stenosis

F. Y. Tsai[1], R. Higashida[2], V. Matovich[1], K. Alfieri[1], and S. Kobayashi[3]

[1] University of Missouri-Kansas City School of Medicine, Kansas City, Missouri, USA
[2] University of California-San Francisco Medical Center, San Francisco, California, USA
[3] Nippon Medical College, Tokyo, Japan

Summary. Carotid stenosis is one of the most common causes of a cerebrovascular accident. The treatment of choice has been endarterectomy. Stenoses may occur in any segment of the carotid artery, as well as the most frequent site, the carotid bifurcation. In recent years, percutaneous transluminal angioplasty (PTA) has been used for those lesions which are difficult, or inaccessible to direct surgical intervention [1–15]. We report our 7 years' of experience treating carotid stenosis by PTA.

Key words: Carotid artery – Stenosis – Percutaneous transluminal angioplasty

Materials and methods

Fifty-eight patients who underwent 62 procedures are presented in this report. Patients were followed up every 6 months for 2–5 years. The vessels treated were as follows: common carotid – 37 patients; external carotid – 5 patients; internal carotid and bifurcation – 16 patients.

The preliminary studies included CT and SPECT nuclear brain scans, cerebral angiography and carotid Doppler blood-flow studies. All patients received oral and/or intravenous anticoagulants for 1 week to 10 days prior to the procedure; also 10 mg of oral Decadron was given twice daily for 2 days before the percutaneous transluminal angiography (PTA). All patients were monitored with EEG during the procedure. After the PTA, a tapering dose schedule of prednisolone was given for 1 week and one aspirin daily for 6 months. The size of the balloon catheter was carefully selected according to the true size of the carotid artery to avoid overdilation. Once the 5 F catheter crossed the stenosis, an exchange wire was slowly advanced distally and a short-tipped balloon catheter (Meditech, Watertown, Mass.) replaced the 5 F catheter. After removal of the guide wire, fresh heparinized arterial blood was injected through the inner lumen during inflation of the balloon. After deflating the balloon, a Doppler sonographic angiography examination to determine the residual stenosis, if any, and a conventional angiogram for final confirmation were obtained. It was rarely necessary to perform more than two inflations [10, 11, 14].

Results

Of the 58 patients, 25 had unchanged symptoms and 33 patients experienced improvement immediately after PTA. Among the 25 patients with unchanged symptoms, 6 patients had clinical improvement 6–8 months after PTA. Nineteen of these 25 patients remained unchanged throughout follow-up. Four patients died from cardiac and/or pulmonary disease, unrelated to carotid artery disease, within 2 years of the procedure and 9 patients died within 3 years. Three of the unchanged patients and 1 of the improved patients had early restenosis 1 year after PTA (all in the proximal internal carotid artery) just at the bifurcation. Two patients required endarterectomy 1 year after PTA, due to restenosis, and two patients had a second PTA procedure. No further procedures were performed. Three of the 19 patients with unchanged symptoms had mild restenosis but no symptoms at 3 years. Two of the 33 improved patients had a second procedure 2 months after the initial PTA because of an eccentric lesion.

Discussion

Although the development of PTA in supra-aortic stenosis has been slow because of the fear of distal embolization, the reported morbidity of carotid angioplasty has been very low. The use of PTA of carotid arteries has increased since the initiation of this treatment in 1980 [1–15]. The results have been favorable, but long-term follow-up is still not available. Our report hopes to provide some useful data to fill the gap. Although not all of our patients have had a follow-up angiogram or Doppler blood-flow study to define the long-term results, the clinical follow-up is very favorable. We have had only two patients with symptomatic restenosis requiring surgery and only two additional patients underwent a second PTA. A large number of patients were unchanged in symptoms after PTA and no further symptoms of stroke occurred. We believe these patients benefited from the aspirin treatment and PTA. We have reviewed the literature and, in our own experience, no definite stroke was reported during PTA [1–15]. Although a case report indicated that some fine debris had been collected during intraoperative retrograde balloon angioplasty, no anticoagulant treatment prior to the operation was described in the report [15]. We believe that anticoagulants may play a very important role in avoiding soft plaque break-up and distal dislodgement. Injection of fresh arterial blood during inflation has helped to avoid transient ischemia during inflation of the balloon.

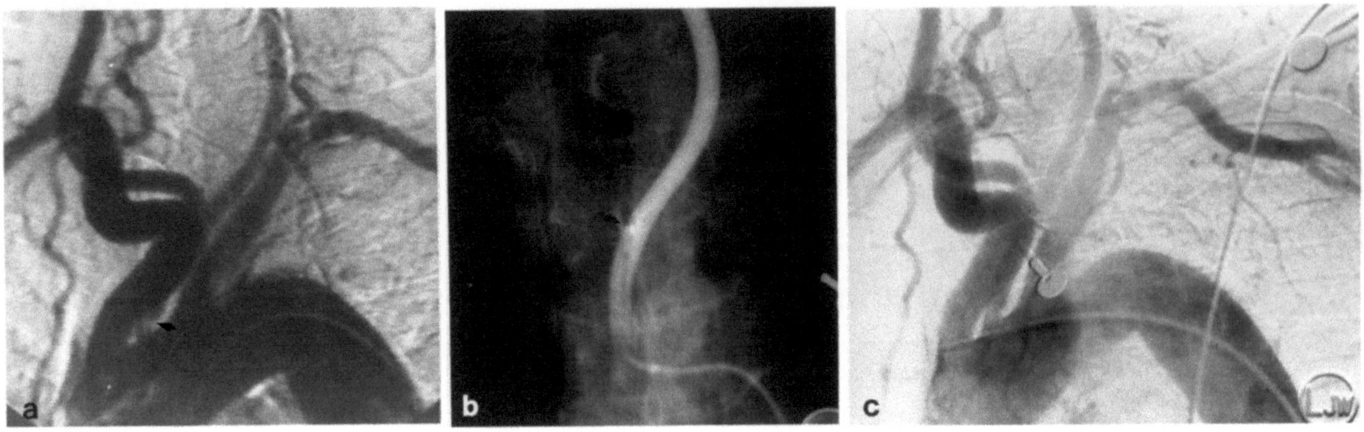

Fig. 1. a Arch angiography showing an isolated stenosis of the proximal left common carotid artery *(arrow)*. **b** Angiography immediately after angioplasty, showing restoration of the carotid lumen with angioplastic catheter in place *(arrow)*. **c** Arch angiography confirming successful dilatation of left common carotid artery

In our experience, multiple vessel disease did not suggest poor results would be seen. On the contrary, the results were very promising and no different from those seen in patients with an isolated lesion. Although our results do not statistically reflect clinically uniform improvement in all patients, the results are quite favorable. Until there is an ideal and perfectly safe surgical technique for treating carotid disease, PTA could be tried for those patients with severe vascular disease, independently or as an adjunct to a surgical procedure. However, the patients must be carefully selected and the risks and benefits weighed before the procedure. Although we do not recommend that PTA should be performed routinely, it may be considered as an alternative procedure for treating the high-risk patient or the surgically inaccessible lesion. We need further experience to determine the role of PTA in carotid stenosis therapy.

References

1. Kerber CW, Cromwell LD, Loehden OL (1980) Catheter dilatation of proximal carotid stenosis during distal bifurcation endarterectomy. AJNR 1: 348–349
2. Mathias K, Mitlermeyer C, Ehsinger H, Neff W (1980) Percutane Katherdilatation von karotis Stenosen. Fortsch Röntgenstr 133: 348–361
3. Motarjeme A, Keifer JW, Zuska AJ (1982) Percutaneous transluminal angioplasty of the brachiocephalic arteries. AJR 138: 457–462
4. Bockenheimer SA, Mathias K (1983) Percutaneous transluminal angioplasty in arteriosclerotic internal carotid artery stenosis. AJNR 4: 791–792
5. Smith RR, Moore TS, Russell WF (1983) Transluminal angioplasty of the cerebral circulation. Clin Neurosurg 31: 117–134
6. Tievsky AL, Druy EM, Mardiat JG (1983) Transluminal angioplasty in postsurgical stenosis of the extracranial carotid artery. AJNR 4: 899–902
7. Vitek JJ (1983) Percutaneous transluminal angioplasty of the carotid artery. AJNR 4: 796–799
8. Wiggli U, Gratzl O (1983) Transluminal angioplasty of stenotic carotid arteries: case reports and protocol. AJNR 4: 793–795
9. Pritz MB, Smolin MF (1984) Treatment of tandem lesions of the extracranial carotid artery. Neurosurgery 15: 233–236
10. Tsai FY, Matovich V, Hieshima G (1986) Percutaneous transluminal angioplasty of the carotid artery. AJNR 7: 349–358
11. Tsai FY, Matovich VB, Hieshima GB, Higashida R (1986) Practical aspects of PTA of the carotid artery. Acta Radiol 369 [Suppl]: 127–130
12. Freitag G, Freitag J, Koch RD, Wagner W (1986) PTA of carotid artery stenoses. Neuroradiology 28: 126–127
13. Higashida RT, Hieshima GB, Tsai TY (1987) Transluminal angioplasty of the vertebral and basilar artery. AJNR 8: 745–749
14. Tsai FY, Hieshima GB, Higashida R (1989) PTA for the treatment of stroke. In: Fisher M (ed) Dekker, New York, pp 203–239
15. DeMonte F, Peerless SJ, Rankin RN (1989) Carotid transluminal angioplasty with evidence of distal embolization. J Neurosurg 70: 138–141

Dr. Fong Y. Tsai
Truman Medical Center
2301 Holmes Road
Kansas City, MO 64108, USA

Neuroradiology (1991) 33 [Suppl]: 399–400

Neuro radiology

© Springer-Verlag 1991

Cerebral digital subtraction angiography via aortic arch injection: accuracy in aneurysm detection

J. E. Gillespie and W. St. C. Forbes

Department of Neuroradiology, Hope Hospital, Salford, UK

Summary. The accuracy of a pancerebral view of the intracranial vasculature in aneurysm detection was assessed by comparison with selective intra-arterial digital subtraction angiography. Of 46 aneurysms present in 87 patients, 31 were demonstrated on the pancerebral view. Aneurysm conspicuity was related to size and orientation. Availability of a lateral-oblique view in addition to an anterior view did not improve the detection rate.

Key words: Aneurysm – Digital subtraction angiography

Patients with suspected cerebrovascular disease commonly undergo digital subtraction angiography (DSA) as part of their overall investigation, using either the intravenous or intra-arterial route. Following visualisation of the extracranial circulation, an anterior view of the intracranial arteries is usually obtained to exclude aneurysms or other significant pathology [1]. Screening of asymptomatic relatives of patients with familial intracranial aneurysms using IV DSA has been advocated [2]. In the context of subarachnoid haemorrhage, IV DSA has been used for preliminary aneurysm localisation, followed by a limited selective intra-arterial study [3].

There is little information in the literature, however, regarding the accuracy of the pancerebral "screening" view in detecting aneurysms, whether obtained by the intravenous or intra-arterial route. We undertook the present study to provide this information.

Method

All examinations were performed on a Siemens Angiotron. Ninety-one patients suspected of having an intracranial aneurysm or arteriovenous malformation were studied, including 61 with proven intracranial haemorrhage. Immediately prior to selective angiography a 5F pig-tail or straight catheter was positioned in the aortic arch; 45 ml 70% Niopam 300 was injected at 25 ml/s by a Med-Rad injection pump. In 62 patients a single anterior view was obtained; 29 patients had both an anterior and an 18°-18° left lateral oblique view. The presence and location of any vascular lesion was noted by the angiographer before proceeding to selective catheterisation.

Results

Four examinations were not of diagnostic quality and excluded from the study. In the remaining 87 patients, 46 aneurysms were demonstrated by selective angiography. Fifteen of these (32.6%) were not identified on the pancerebral view by the angiographer (Table 1). The availability of the lateral-oblique view did not improve the detection rate with 9 out of 28, and 6 out of 18 aneurysms missed on the one- and two-view studies respectively. Posterior communicating artery aneurysms were the most easily missed with half remaining undetected even when the second view was available. Aneurysms escaping detection were those small enough to be obscured by superimposed normal vessels.

With regard to the individual patients, there were 32 true-positive, 37 true-negative, 3 false-positive, 8 false-negative and 7 partially true studies, the latter representing cases with multiple aneurysms in which at least one lesion was visible.

Discussion

Because of their size, medium and large aneurysms were visible in most locations despite vessel superimposition (Figs. 1, 2). Conspicuity of smaller aneurysms was dependent not only upon size, but orientation (Figs. 3, 4). We expected the lateral-oblique view to improve the detection of small posteriorly directed posterior communicating aneurysms in particular, but in practice the carotid siphons usually remained partially obscured. Further projections might have overcome this problem, but were not performed in this study. Despite these limitations, the pancerebral view correctly predicted a normal or abnormal selective angiographic result in 76 of 87 patients.

Table 1. Aneurysm detection on the pancerebral digital subtraction angiography study as compared with selective angiography

Location	Demonstrated	Missed
Anterior cerebral		
Anterior communicating	13	3
Pericallosal	0	1
Middle cerebral	5	2
Internal carotid		
Posterior communicating	6	6
Bifurcation	2	1
Cavernous	0	1
Posterior circulation		
Basilar bifurcation	3	0
Other	2	1

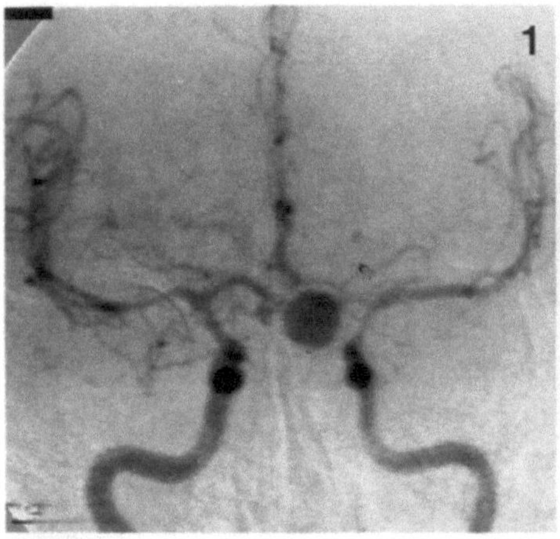

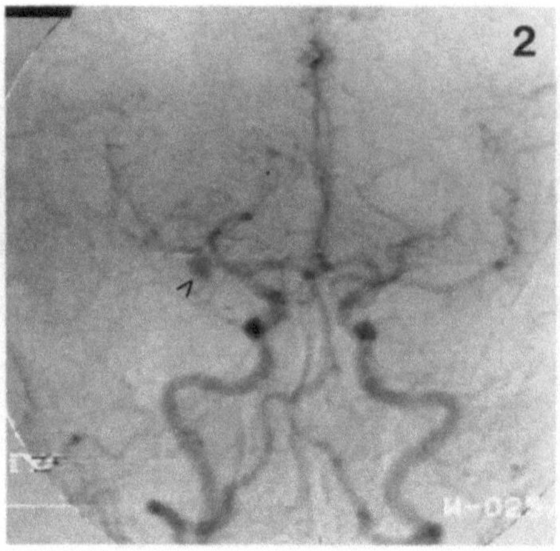

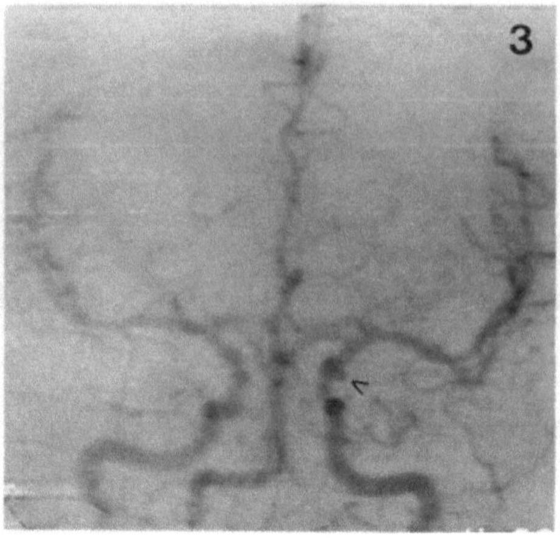

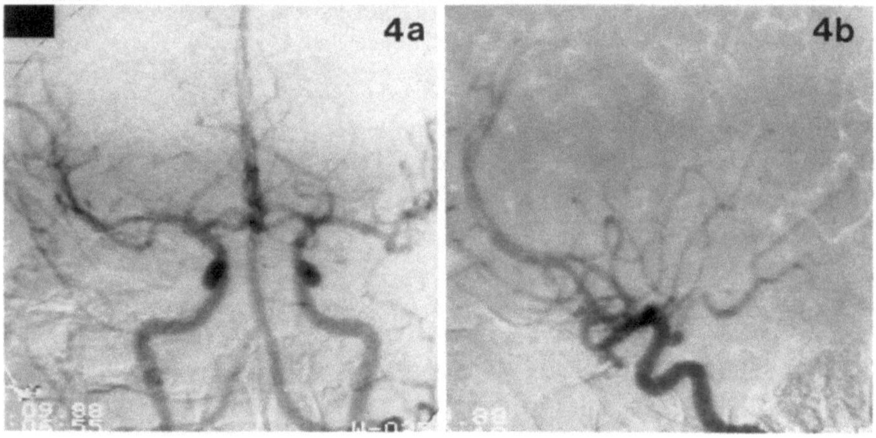

Fig. 1. Anterior pancerebral view showing a large anterior communicating artery aneurysm. Note spasm of the distal left internal carotid and anterior cerebral (A 1) vessels

Fig. 2. Anterior pancerebral view showing a right middle cerebral artery aneurysm with distal spasm

Fig. 3. Anterior pancerebral view. A small left posterior communicating artery aneurysm is just visible as it projects posterolaterally from its internal carotid artery origin

Fig. 4. **a** Anterior pancerebral view regarded as normal. **b** The selective left lateral carotid angiogram demonstrated a small posterior communicating artery aneurysm pointing directly posteriorly. While similar in size to that in Fig. 3, its orientation makes it virtually indiscernible on the pancerebral view

In conclusion, the majority of cerebral aneurysms can be detected on a single anterior pancerebral projection. Small, but potentially significant lesions, however, may not be reliably depicted and this should be borne in mind when using the technique as a screening procedure. This is particularly important with intravenous studies where image quality is more variable.

References

1. Gonzalez CF, Doan HT, Han SS, De Filipp GJ (1986) Extracranial vascular angiography. Radiol Clin North Am 24: 419–451
2. Ter Berg JWM, Overtoom TMD, Ludwig JW, Bijlsma JB, Tulleken CAF, Willemse J (1987) Detection of unruptured familial intracranial aneurysms by intravenous digital subtraction angiography. Neuroradiology 29: 272–276
3. Boone RM (1986) Digital subtraction angiography in neurology. In: Digital subtraction angiography in clinical practice. Philips Medical Systems, Best, The Netherlands, pp 105–111

Dr. J. E. Gillespie
Department of Neuroradiology
Hope Hospital
Eccles Old Road
Salford M6 8HD, UK

Neuroradiology (1991) 33 [Suppl]: 401–403

Neuro-radiology
© Springer-Verlag 1991

The application of vascular endoscopy to intravascular surgery – experimental study

S. Miyachi, M. Negoro, and K. Sugita

Department of Neurosurgery, Nagoya University School of Medicine, Nagoya, Japan

Summary. Improvements in blood elimination and the development of an ultrathin, flexible fibrescope have made it possible to perform intravascular endoscopy safely and effectively. A new endoscopic system was used to occlude experimental aneurysms created in canine carotid arteries. Endoscopy provides valuable information about the aneurysmal orifice and lumen and is helpful in balloon placement and detachment.

Key words: Vascular endoscope – Experimental aneurysm – Balloon occlusion

Intravascular surgery is usually performed using radiofluoroscopic guidance, and results are assessed by angiography. These radiographic methods, however, are limited to defining suspected lesions by morphological changes in the vascular lumen [1, 2]. Vascular endoscopy makes it possible to observe intravascular lesions directly. We used a newly developed vascular endoscope to perform balloon occlusion of experimental aneurysms. Vascular endoscopy is a valuable tool for pre- and postoperative studies of intravascular interventions.

Materials and methods

Endoscope. The vascular fibreoptic endoscope (Model AS-001, Fukuda-Denshi, Tokyo, Japan) used in this study was 0.75 mm in diameter and 205 cm in length. The depth of the field of vision was 2–15 mm and the maximum width was 55°. The endoscope was connected to a video processor system (FCA-8000, Fukuda-Denshi, Tokyo, Japan), and the image displayed on a colour monitor.

Guidance and blood elimination system. A 6-Fr double-lumen balloon occlusion catheter was introduced via the femoral or carotid artery by the Seldinger technique, and the fibrescope was advanced to the tip of the guide catheter. Blood elimination was achieved by balloon inflation and continuous high-pressure saline irrigation.

Experimental aneurysm [3]. Carotid artery aneurysms were created by anastomosing a pouch of jugular vein to the lateral wall of the common carotid arteries of 40 mongrel dogs (weight 12–13 kg). The existence of aneurysms about 8 mm in diameter was confirmed by angiography.

Endoscopic observation. The orifice and internal lumen of the aneurysm were visualized endoscopically. Subsequently balloon placement and detachment were observed directly during aneurysmal occlusion. Balloon placement was studied both angiographically and endoscopically, and endothelialization of the occluded aneurysmal orifice was studied serially.

Results

The extent of the visual field and the optical quality in all cases was excellent. The endoscope showed not only the shape of the aneurysmal orifice and the state of the vascular lumen in detail (e.g. presence of thrombus, scar and even the suture on the anastomosis), but also irregularity of the aneurysmal lumen, which has not been detected angiographically (Fig. 1). Actual balloon placement and the moment of detachment were captured on the video processor and the timing of detachment could be better controlled. Unexpectedly, the tail of the detached balloon was often observed to protrude into the lumen of the parent artery, causing stenosis (Fig. 2). Endoscopy demonstrated the degree of stenosis more accurately than two-dimensional angiography. The surface of the occluding balloon was covered partially by thrombus for several hours after occlusion (Fig. 2). Endothelialization was completed, and the orifice became smooth about 2 months after the procedure.

Discussion

Recent technical advances in glass fibre optics have made the development of a high-quality, flexible, thin fibrescope (less than 1 mm) possible. This endoscope can be inserted into coronary arteries [4–6], extracranial [7] and other peripheral vessels [1, 2, 8, 9] safely with minimal trauma. In vivo blood elimination has been a major problem for vascular endoscopists [1, 2, 8–11]. We have devised a technique which uses a combination of a double-lumen balloon occlusion catheter [5, 7] and a high-pressure saline irrigation system [8], which permits continuous observation. However, when using this method to observe the neurovascular system, the occlusion balloon should be deflated every few minutes to prevent brain ischaemia. During continuous observation, the saline infusion pressure should be equal to the blood pressure after the primary flush to avoid barotrauma.

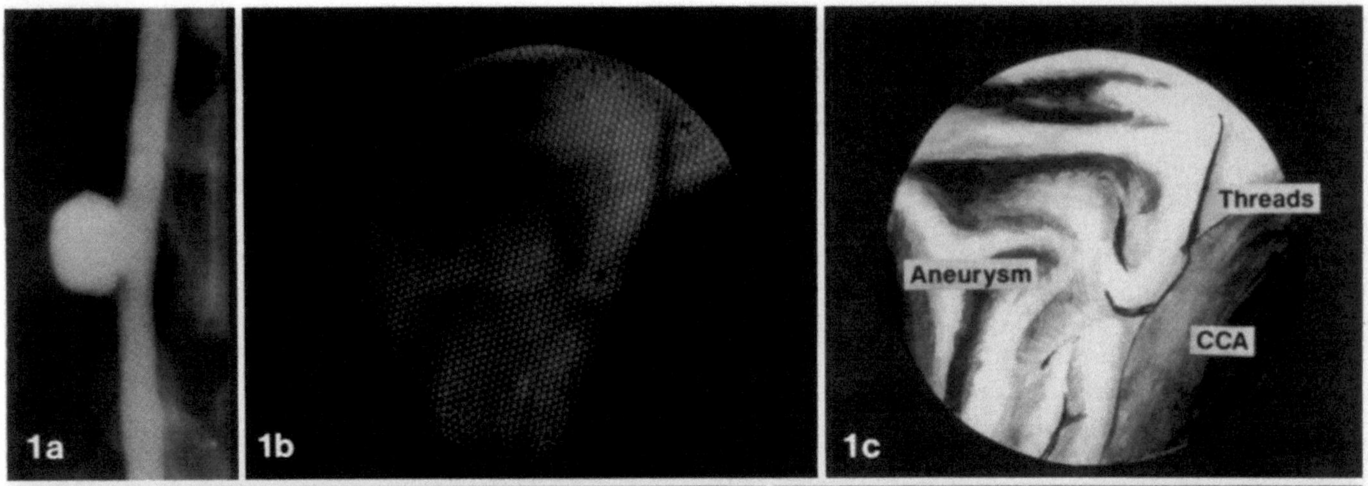

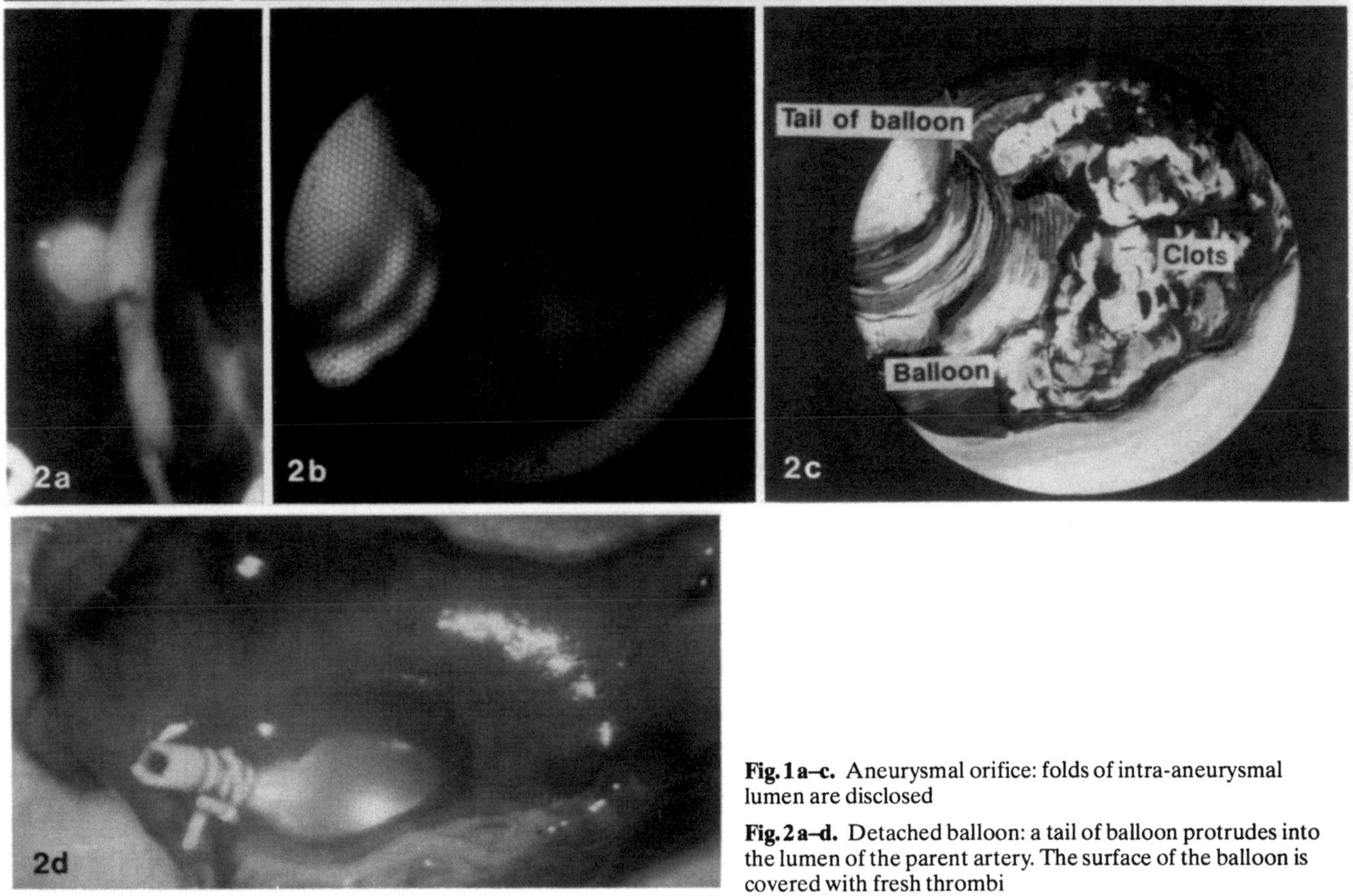

Fig. 1 a–c. Aneurysmal orifice: folds of intra-aneurysmal lumen are disclosed

Fig. 2 a–d. Detached balloon: a tail of balloon protrudes into the lumen of the parent artery. The surface of the balloon is covered with fresh thrombi

Knowing the shape and size of the aneurysmal orifice as well as the intra-aneurysmal features provides valuable information in selecting the most suitable balloon for occlusion and anticipating technical difficulties in balloon placement. The risk of embolic complications caused by intra-aneurysmal thrombi can also be estimated in advance of balloon placement. However, the ability to see into the aneurysm was limited, and a blind spot remained proximally, even when a modified catheter with an angled tip was used. Further improvement in the fibrescope's thickness and flexibility is, therefore, desirable.

Direct visualization of balloon detachment adds precision to a manoeuvre which currently depends only on the operator's "feeling". After detachment, endoscopy provided additional information concerning parent artery stenosis by the balloon and intimal injury with thrombus formation resulting from manipulation. These findings may help to determine additional therapy, such as replacement with a non-detachable balloon catheter or post-operative medical treatment [2]. However, endoscopic appreciation of parent artery stenosis varies according to the angle of view. Endoscopic findings should, therefore, be correlated with angiographic findings in deciding clinical management.

Vascular endoscopy may be applicable to other types of vascular lesion (e.g. vascular occlusive disease, carotid cavernous fistula, and vascular invasion by malignant tumour). Furthermore, endoscopy may be applicable to the other "spaces" in the CNS such as the spinal canal and ventricles.

References

1. Inoue K, Kuwaki K, Takahashi M, Hiramoto J, Tsuno K (1984) Observation of the inner structure of the canine vessels in vivo using a newly developed ultrathin fiberoptic angioscope (in Japanese). Coronary 1: 241–248
2. Nakamoto T, Kato S, Kawai H, Sakuma G, Matsuyama T (1988) Vascular endoscopy (in Japanese). Curr Med 20: 1759–1766
3. German WJ, Black SPW (1954) Experimental production of carotid aneurysms. N Engl J Med 250: 104–106
4. Spears JR, Marais HJ, Serur J, Pomerantzeff O, Geyer RP, Spitzner RS, Weintraub R, Thurer R, Paulin S, Gerstin R, Grossman W (1983) In vivo coronary angioscopy. J Am Coll Cardiol 1: 1311–1314
5. Uchida Y, Masuo M, Tomaru T, Kato S, Sugimoto T (1987) Percutaneous coronary angioscopy in patients with ischemic heart disease. Am Heart J 114: 1216–1222
6. Inoue K, Kuwaki K, Takano E (1987) Angioscopy guided PTCA – experimental study of in vivo canine coronary artery (in Japanese). Coronary 4: 13–18
7. Miyamoto S, Kikuchi H, Nagata I, Yamagata S, Kaneko T, Akiyama Y, Ito K, Kim S, Mitsuno K (1989) The application of vascular endoscope for the extracranial cerebrovascular occlusive disease: the development of the endoscopic system (in Japanese). Neurol Surg 17: 625–628
8. Adachi I, Nakashima N, Takahara Z, Ando T, Fujita T, Manabe H (1983) Clinical application of vascular endoscopy (in Japanese). J Jpn Coll Angiol 23: 223–227
9. Tomaru T, Uchida Y, Kato S, Masuo M, Sugimoto T (1985) Experimental arterial thrombosis and thrombolysis in dogs: a fiberscopic study (in Japanese). J Jpn Coll Angiol 25: 1205–1210
10. Itoh T, Hori M (1983) Vascular endoscopy for major vascular reconstruction: experimental and clinical studies. Surgery 93: 391–396
11. Greenstone SM, Shore JM, Heringtonman EC, Massl TB (1966) Arterial endoscopy (arterioscopy). Arch Surg 93: 811–812

Dr. Shigeru Miyachi
Department of Neurosurgery
Nagoya University School of Medicine
65 Tsurumai-cho
Showa-ku, Nagoya 466, Japan

Neuroradiology (1991) 33 [Suppl]: 404–405

Neuro-radiology
© Springer-Verlag 1991

Lipid imaging to detect myelin breakdown in multiple sclerosis

C. P. Hawkins[1], S. C. R. Williams[2], G. J. Barker[1], B. Youl[1], T. Revesz[3], J. Newcombe[4], A. Brar[4], D. G. MacManus[1], E. P. G. H. du Boulay[1], and W. I. McDonald[1]

[1] (MS NMR Research group) Institute of Neurology, [2] NMR Facility (Department of Chemistry), Queen Mary College
[3] Department of Neuropathology, Maida Vale Hospital, [4] Multiple Sclerosis Society Laboratory, London, UK

Summary. Lipid imaging has been used to study the multiple sclerosis (MS) lesion both in vivo and in vitro. With echo difference imaging (EDI) to detect free lipid, regions of high signal were seen at the periphery of lesions in post-mortem brain slices, and these corresponded histologically with the presence of neutral lipid derived from myelin breakdown in regions of active inflammation. In vivo, regions of high signal on EDI were also seen in MS lesions, and were associated with blood-brain barrier breakdown and inflammation as assessed by gadolinium-DTPA enhancement. NMR spectra from unfixed MS spinal cord suggest that the abnormal EDI signal originates from methylene and methyl protons in the lipids. Thus, it is now possible to detect the two major destructive processes in the MS lesion, demyelination and inflammation. Lipid imaging promises to be useful in monitoring the time course of demyelination and its modification by treatment.

Key words: Demyelination – Lipid – Myelin – Multiple sclerosis – Magnetic resonance imaging

Demyelination is the hallmark of multiple sclerosis (MS), but the question whether it inevitably follows inflammation, or can occur independently of it, remains unanswered because no satisfactory technique has been available to monitor the development and time course of demyelination in vivo. Although normal myelin gives no NMR signal because the protons in it are relatively fixed, a signal should be detectable from the more mobile protons in the free lipid produced by myelin breakdown. A method for lipid imaging has thus been developed, and has been evaluated both in vivo and in vitro. Echo difference imaging (EDI) is effective at low field strength (0.5T) and depends on the relative difference in behaviour of coupled and uncoupled NMR spins when subjected to two sequential 90° radiofrequency pulses (the "90-echo") [1].

Materials and methods

Six post-mortem formalin-fixed brain slices from three MS patients and two control brain slices were studied by EDI in a 0.5T Picker International imager (SE 200/60, 5 mm section thickness, 256 phase encoding increments, pixel size 1 × 1 mm, 50 repetitions). Bottles containing formaldehyde and water (with a T1 relaxation time similar to that of normal-appearing white matter) were included to confirm the subtraction of uncoupled spins. Standard T2-weighted images (SE 1500/120) and calculated images of T1 and T2 relaxation times were used [2]. Subsequent histological sections in the same planes as the MRI sections were stained with oil red 0 to show the presence of neutral lipid. Unfixed spinal cords from three patients with a diagnosis of MS (two at 4.7T and one at 0.5T) and one control unfixed cord were studied (SE 3000/30, 2 mm section thickness, 256 phase encoding increments, pixel size 0.5 × 0.5 mm, 4 repetitions). After careful dissection of the spinal cords from the meninges to remove extraneous lipid, an NMR spectrum was obtained. Four MS patients and two healthy volunteers were studied by EDI in vivo (SE 200/60, 10 mm section thickness, 128 phase encoding increments, pixel size 1 × 1 mm, 32 repetitions). Transverse sections were selected from standard T2-weighted images (SE 1500/60), and when possible (in three patients) MRI was subsequently enhanced with gadolinium (Gd)-DTPA (0.1 mmol/kg, SE 540/40.

Results

In control post-mortem brain slices and spinal cord, and healthy volunteers in vivo EDI showed only a low-grade, uniform signal in the white matter, indicating a low level of coupled spins, which may reflect the presence of amino acids and neurotransmitters. When MS brain slices were studied, regions of high signal on EDI were observed in three sections, usually at the periphery of lesions on T2-weighted images (Fig. 1), and associated with reduced T1 relaxation time compared to that of the adjacent normal-

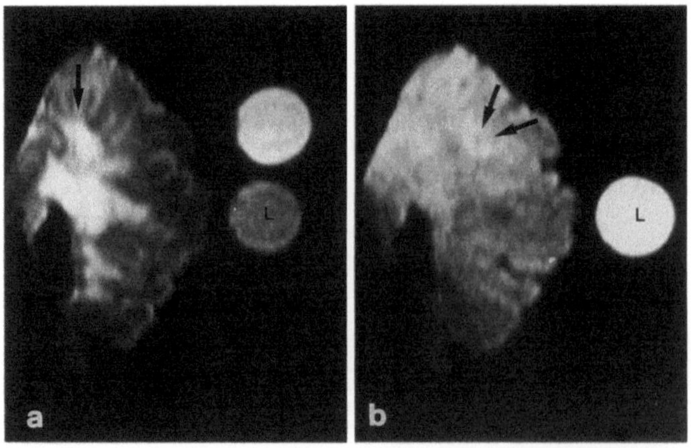

Fig. 1 a, b. MRI of a formalin-fixed multiple sclerosis (MS) brain slice (occipital). **a** (Left) T2-weighted image (SE 1500/120) showing periventricular high signal *(arrow)*. **b** (right) Echo difference imaging (EDI) showing diffuse high signal at the periphery of the lesion with a more focal region of abnormal signal (shown by the *arrows*). Signal from lipid bottle *(L)* is enhanced and the water signal is no longer visible

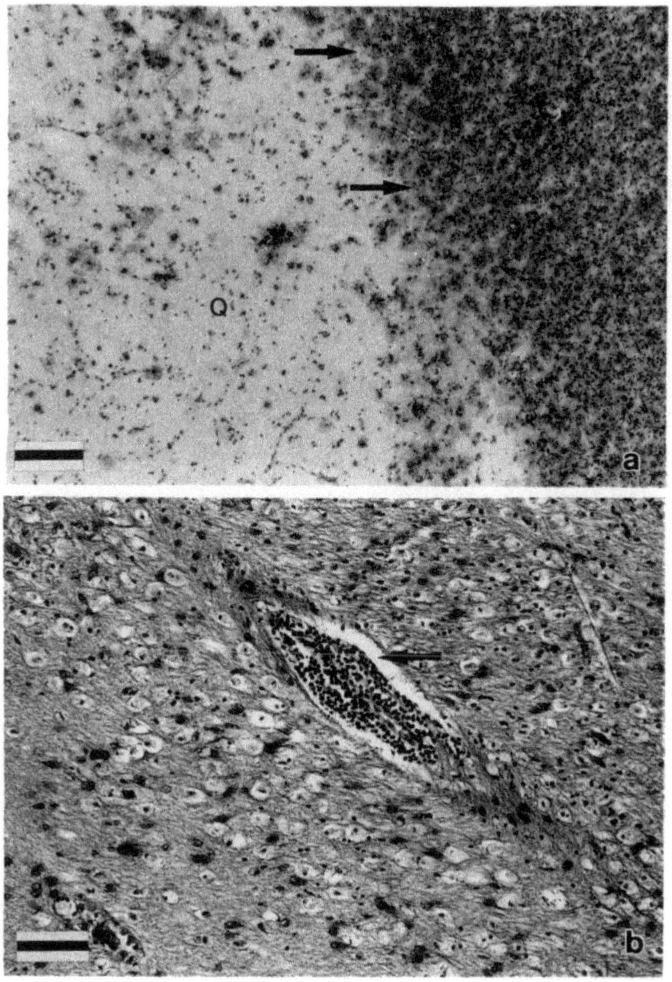

Fig. 2 a, b. Histological sections taken from the focal region of abnormal EDI signal shown by the *arrows* in Fig. 1B. **a** Neutral lipid detected by oil red 0 staining at the periphery of the demyelinated plaque *(Q)*; most of the lipid is within macrophages *(arrows)*. *Bar* = 167 μm. **b** Paraffin-wax section showing corresponding perivascular inflammation (mostly lymphocytes) at the edge of the plaque *(arrow)*. Haematoxylin and eosin. *Bar* = 80 μm

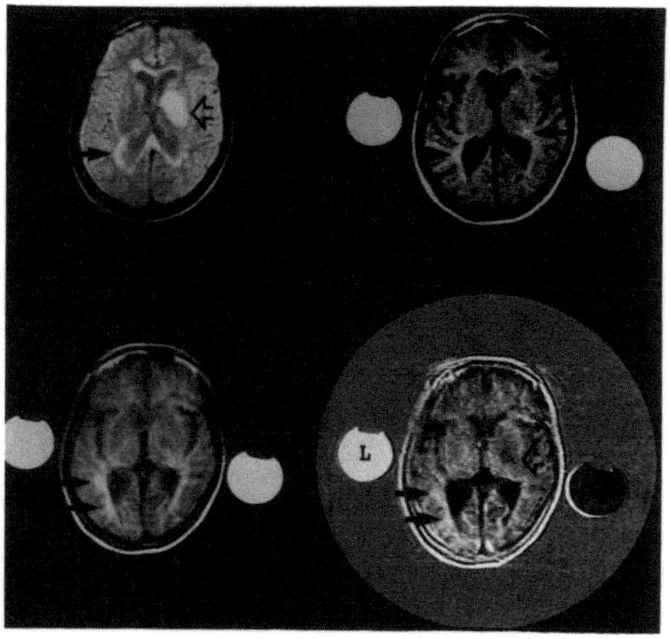

Fig. 3. MRI of a patient with MS. (Top left) T2-weighted image (SE 1500/60) showing a large lesion in the region of the right internal capsule *(large arrow)* and periventricular high signal *(small arrow)*. (Top right) Gd-DTPA-enhanced MRI at the same level; a T1-weighted image (SE 540/40 and 0.1 mmol/kg Gd-DTPA injected) showing areas of enhancement *(arrows)* (Bottom left) "90-echo" (SE 200/60) suggesting a region of abnormal periventricular signal *(arrows)*. (Bottom right) EDI confirming periventricular region of high signal *(arrows)*. Signal from the lipid bottle (*L*) is enhanced and the water signal has cancelled

appearing white matter. Subsequent histological sections showed that regions of high signal on EDI corresponded with the presence of neutral lipid, mostly within macrophages in association with inflammation (Fig. 2). Regions of abnormal EDI signal were seen in unfixed MS spinal cords (two out of three cords studied), which again corresponded with neutral lipid histologically. NMR spectra demonstrated a broad lipid peak (1–2.4 ppm) suggesting that the abnormal EDI signal originates from methylene (CH_2) and methyl (CH_3) protons in the lipids. In vivo, regions of abnormal EDI signal were also seen in relation to MS lesions on standard images (Fig. 3), and were associated with blood-brain barrier breakdown and inflammation as assessed by Gd-DTPA enhancement [3, 4].

Discussion

The EDI method has identified regions of active myelin breakdown in MS with the release of free lipid, associated with inflammation in the lesions as assessed histologically and by Gd-DTPA enhancement in vivo. It should now be possible, using a combination of Gd-DTPA-enhanced MRI and lipid imaging, to determine whether inflammation inevitably leads to demyelination in the evolution of the MS lesion, and whether myelin breakdown can occur in the absence of inflammation in the later stages of the disease. Lipid imaging should be useful in monitoring the effect of different putative treatments on the process of demyelination.

References

1. Hall LD, Norwood TJ, Williams DCR (1988) Coupled-spin-filtered imaging in an inhomogeneous magnetic field. J Mag Reson 79: 363–368
2. Johnson G, Ormerod IEC, Barnes D, Tofts PS, MacManus D (1987) Accuracy and precision in the measurement of relaxation times from nuclear magnetic resonance images. Br J Radiol 60: 143–53
3. Kermode AG, Tofts PS, Thompson AJ, MacManus DG, Rudge P, Kendall BE, Kingsley DPE, Moseley IF, du Boulay EPGH, McDonald WI (1990) Heterogeneity of blood-brain barrier changes in multiple sclerosis: an MRI study. Neurology 40: 229–235
4. Hawkins CP, Munro PMG, MacKenzie F, Kesselring J, Tofts PS, du Boulay EPGH, Landon DN, McDonald WI (1990) Duration and selectivity of blood-brain barrier breakdown in chronic relapsing experimental allergic encephalomyelitis by Gd-DTPA and protein markers, Brain 113: 365–378

Dr. C. P. Hawkins
Institute of Neurology, Queen Square, London, UK

Neuroradiology (1991) 33 [Suppl]: 406–407

Neuro
radiology
© Springer-Verlag 1991

Multiple sclerosis: Indian experience

V. C. Shah, S. B. Desai, O. J. Tavri, and P. Rao

Department of Magnetic Resonance Imaging, Breach Candy Hospital and Research Centre, Bombay, India

Summary. A retrospective analysis of 4,000 consecutive MRI studies carried out in a period of about 1 year revealed classical MR features of multiple sclerosis in 102 patients. The MR images revealed lesions in brain and spinal cord suggesting an entity otherwise thought to be rare in India.

Key words: Multiple sclerosis – Brain – Spinal cord – Plaque – India – Magnetic resonance

Multiple sclerosis is a complex disease with varied classical manifestations and an unpredictable clinical course [1, 2]. The axiom of lesions of the central nervous system separated in time and space aptly describes the clinical presentation of patients with multiple sclerosis. It was believed that multiple sclerosis rarely exists to the east of Suez. However, MRI has disproved this belief conclusively and the myth lies shattered. MRI allows demyelinating plaques to be directly visualized with great sensitivity and precision [3, 4]. We present our initial data on 102 patients with characteristic MR findings in brain and spinal cord with or without supportive positive paraclinical tests and cerebrospinal fluid (CSF) studies.

Materials and methods

A retrospective review of 102 patients with the radiological diagnosis of multiple sclerosis out of a total of 4,000 consecutive patients in a year was carried out. Detailed clinical assessment and routine investigations were performed in all cases.

The criteria for diagnosis of multiple sclerosis were: (1) characteristic clinical presentation, (2) CSF IgG [5], (3) evoked responses, and (4) MR findings.

MR images were obtained with a Siemens Magnetom superconducting magnet operating at 1.0 T. Multiple slice spin echo images were obtained with a short repetition time (TR) usually 0.5–0.75 s and a longer TR of 2.5–3.0 s. Echo delay times (TE) of 17, 23, and 90 ms were used. Axial, coronal and/or sagittal slices were obtained. Slice thickness of 5–8 mm with 0.8–1.6 mm interslice gap and 256 × 256 or 128 × 256 matrix were used. A few patients were also injected with gadolinium-DTPA to study the activity of the plaques.

Results

Multiple sclerosis lesions were identified in all age groups but were predominantly seen in patients in the second to fourth decades (56/90 = 62.22%)

Males and females were almost equally affected. No significant predilection for a particular community or socioeconomic stratum was found.

Patients with multiple sclerosis comprised 2.55% of a total of 4,000 patients studied by MRI and 3.19% of those undergoing MRI of brain and spine. Thirty-one (30%) presented acutely; 71 (70%) presented in a chronic stage and 24 (23%) had a relapsing illness.

Discussion

It is well recognized that MRI is a sensitive technique for detecting the characteristic plaques of multiple sclerosis and a diagnosis of multiple sclerosis can be made on the MR characteristics [1–6]. Although characteristic location of lesions in the deep white matter (78/102 = 76%) predominated in our series (Fig. 1 a, b), other areas like the brain stem (32/102 = 31%) (Fig. 2 a, b), cerebellum (18/102 = 8%) and spinal cord (12/102 = 12%) (Fig. 3) were also involved. We encountered 4 patients (3%) with solitary lesions (Table 1).

There were 4 patients (4%) with brain stem plaques without supratentorial involvement, while in four patients (4%) the plaques were identified solely in the spinal cord, without brain involvement.

The CSF IgG studies were positive in 85 patients (83%), while evoked responses were positive in 81 patients (81%).

It is interesting to note that only 60% of these patients were thought to have multiple sclerosis prior to the MR study (Table 2). In the rest of the 40% of patients initial clinical suspicions included possibilities such as craniovertebral anomaly, spinocerebellar degeneration, cerebral mass lesions, myelopathy, normal pressure hydrocephalus, psychosis etc. MRI in these cases was unquestionably of great help in diagnosing multiple sclerosis.

Table 1. Intracranial demyelinating plaques

Solitary plaque	3	(3%)
Multiple plaques	95	(93%)
Total	98/102	(96%)

Table 2. Initial clinical diagnoses

Multiple sclerosis	61/102 (60%)
Other pathologies	41/102 (40%)

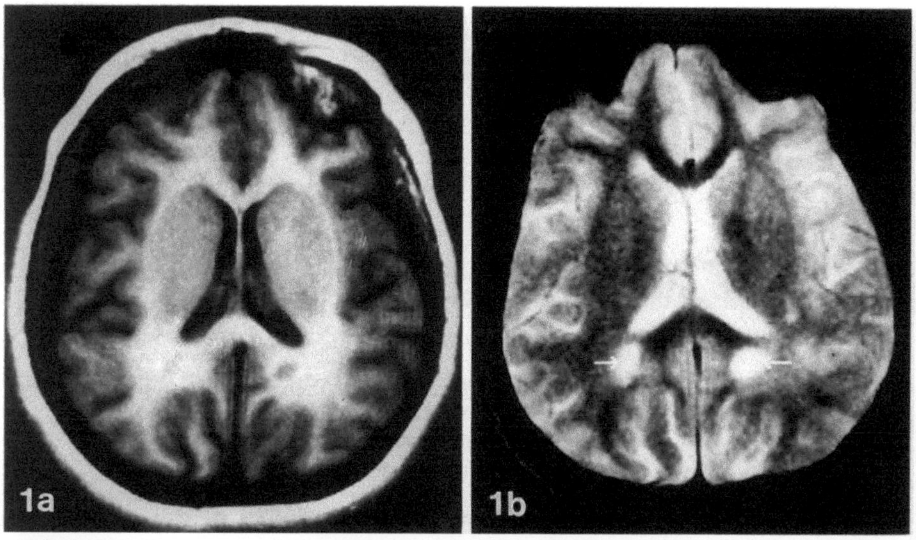

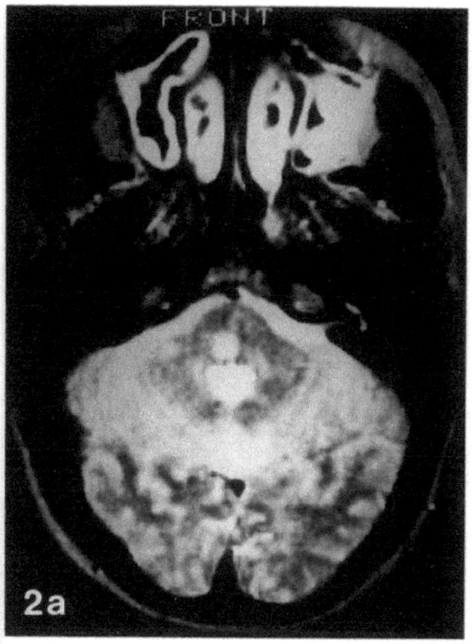

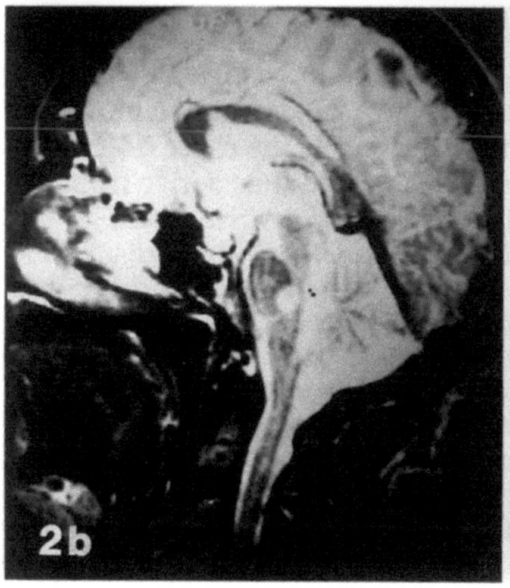

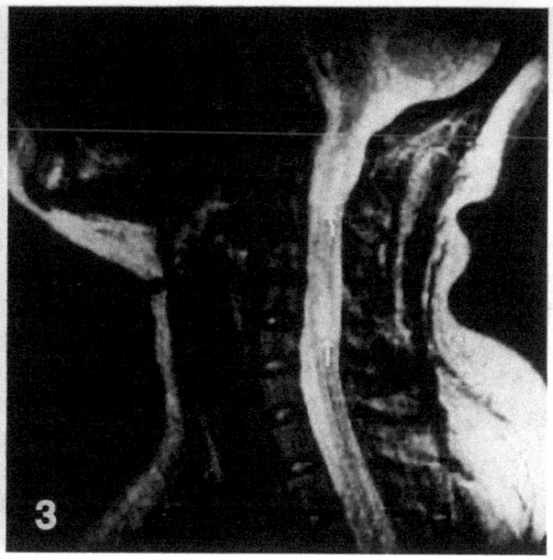

Fig. 1. a Axial T1-weighted image showing classical paraventricular deep white matter hypointense plaques. **b** Axial T2-weighted image reveals bilateral deep white matter hypointense plaques

Fig. 2. a T2-weighted sagittal images reveal a large plaque in the pons. **b** T2-weighted axial image

Fig. 3. T2-weighted sagittal section of cervical spinal cord revealing a longitudinal plaque

Multiple sclerosis is not an uncommon disease in the Indian subcontinent. It is possibly an underdiagnosed clinical entity.

References

1. Edwards MK, Farlow MR, Stevens JC (1986) Multiple sclerosis. MRI and clinical correlation AJNR 7: 595–598
2. Farlow MR, Markand ON, Edwardo MK, Stevens JC (1987) Magnetic resonance imaging in multiple sclerosis – analyses of correlations to peripheral blood and spinal fluid abnormalities. Neurology 37: 1527–1530
3. Hallpike JF, Adams WM, Tourtellotte WW (1986) Multiple sclerosis, Chapman and Hall, London
4. Jackson LA, Leake DR, Schneiders NJ, Rolak LA (1985) MRI in multiple sclerosis – results in 37 cases AJNR 6: 171–176
5. Sheldon JJ, Sidhaothan R, Tobias J, Sheremata WA (1985) MR imaging of multiple sclerosis – comparison with clinical and CT examination in 74 patients. AJNR 6: 683–690
6. Poser CM (1979) Diseases of myelin sheath. In: Houston Meritt H (ed) A text book of neurology, 6th edn. Lea and Febiger, Philadelphia, pp 763–823

Dr. V. C. Shah
Department of Magnetic Resonance Imaging
Breach Candy Hospital
60, B. Desai Road
Bombay-400026, India

Neuroradiology (1991) 33 [Suppl]: 408–409

Neuro radiology

© Springer-Verlag 1991

Differential diagnostic criteria in "plaque-like" MRI findings

S. Cirillo, L. Simonetti, F. Di Salle, F. Spadetta, R. Elefante, and F. Smaltino

Departments of Radiology and Neuroradiology, Faculty of Medicine, University of Naples, Naples, Italy

Summary. A retrospective analysis of 197 multiple sclerosis (MS) and 197 chronic atherosclerotic encephalopathy (CAE) patients' MR images has been performed. Site, number, morphology and distribution of lesions have been examined and provided valuable differential diagnostic criteria concerning symmetry and coexisting supra- and infratentorial localizations.

Key words: Magnetic resonance imaging – Multiple sclerosis

Many pathological changes appear on MRI as "plaque-like" lesions [1], among which the lacunar infarcts of chronic atherosclerotic encephalopathy (CAE) most frequently cause differential diagnostic difficulty [2].

The aim of this study was to identify differential diagnostic criteria between multiple sclerosis (MS) plaque and CAE "plaque-like" lesions dependent on lesion distribution.

Materials and methods

A retrospective analysis of 197 patients with definite of MS, all having abnormal sensory evoked potentials (SEP) and positive IgG findings in cerebrospinal fluid has been performed [3]. These data have been compared to those obtained from a control sample of 197 patients randomly selected from 498 certainly suffering from CAE, aged over 60 and with abnormal duplex ultrasound studies of neck vessels.

Several parameters were examined concerning site, number, morphology and distribution of lesions, such as symmetry and coexisting supra- and infratentorial localizations.

Results and discussion

High signal intensity areas observed in the corpus callosum are strongly specific for MS (Fig. 1). Their frequent detection in the most advanced stages of the disease suggests Wallerian degeneration as the cause of involvement of this structure, which could thus derive from primarily paraventricular or subcortical MS lesions.

The middle cerebellar peduncles (Fig. 2) are a typical localization for MS plaques. In patients with more than 4 years' of symptoms, this preferential localization has been observed in 100%. The localization of "plaque-like" images in temporal lobes (Fig. 3) is another highly specific MS feature, not affected by the stage of the disease, as it can be observed in patients with the first clinically evident attack.

Symmetrical distribution of MS plaques is frequently observed at every stage of the disease. In CAE a symmetrical localization of the lacunar infarcts is not as rare as might be expected. The coexistent supra- and infratentorial distribution, frequent in all stages of the disease, is a reliable distinguishing feature between MS and CAE (73.1% vs 5.6%).

Conclusions

Possibilities of tissue identification by MRI have been thought to be limited by the similar in signal from different lesions. In white matter pathology MRI provides a high sensitivity but a lower specificity because of the difficult

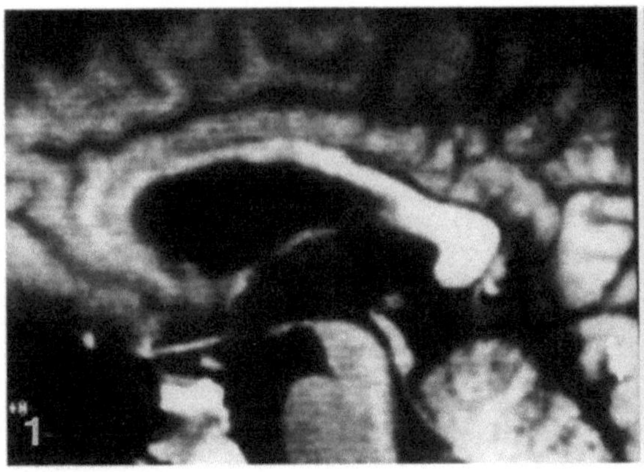

Fig. 1. T1-weighted MR: corpus callosum involvement

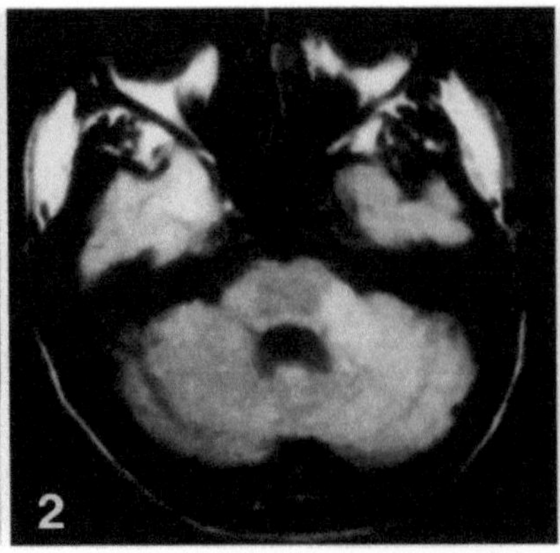

Fig. 2. Proton-density-weighted MR: middle cerebellar peduncule lesion

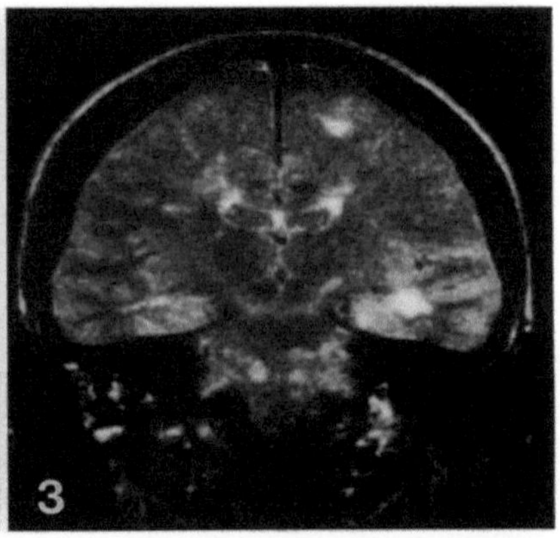

Fig. 3. T2-weighted MR: temporal lobe multiple sclerosis lesions

differential diagnosis. Lesion characterization based on morphological and distribution characteristics can, then, be useful and may provide a complete differential diagnosis.

References

1. Valk J, Knaap van der MS (1989) MRI of myelin, myelination and myelin disorders. Springer, New York Berlin Heidelberg
2. Miller DH (1988) MRI: sensitive and safe in diagnosing multiple sclerosis. MRI Decisions 1: 17–24
3. Uhlenbrock D, Seidel D, Gehen W, Bayer HK, Haan J, Dickmann E, Zeit T (1988) MRI in multiple sclerosis: comparison with clinical, CSF, and visual evoked potential findings. ANJR 9: 59–67

Dr. S. Cirillo
Università degli Studi di Napoli II
Facoltà di Medicina e Chirurgia Scuola di Specializzazione in Radiologia
Via S. Pansini, 5
I-80131 Naples, Italy

Neuroradiology (1991) 33 [Suppl]: 410–412

Neuro radiology
© Springer-Verlag 1991

Gadolinium-DTPA-enhanced MRI of the cranio-cervical region in rheumatoid arthritis

M. Stiskal, A. Neuhold, M. Brainin, C. Platzer, and J. Smolen

Institute of Diagnostic Imaging, Krankenanstalt Rudolfinerhaus, and 2nd Department of Medicine, KA Lainz, Vienna, Austria

Summary. Seventy-one patients with serologically proven polyarthritis were submitted to MRI without and with gadolinium-DTPA enhancement. Correlation of the appearance of the pannus in the cranio-cervical region with duration of disease, clinical and laboratory status showed that the changes followed rules which were understandable in terms of the nature of the pannus and the process of normalization under treatment.

Key words: Rheumatoid arthritis – Magnetic resonance imaging – Gadolinium – Pannus

Rheumatoid arthritis (RA) is an auto-immune disease caused by a chronic inflammatory process of unknown cause. Its characteristics include fibrinoid swelling, central necrosis, epitheloid connective tissue cells, and frequently positive rheumatoid factors.

Progression is characterized by diffuse proliferative synovitis in the joint, hypertrophy of synovial cells, vascular hyperplasia, and lymphocyte, macrophage and plasma cell infiltrates, leading to pannus formation.

One of the most common sites of adult RA is the cervical spine. The aim of the study was to define the importance of MRI for patients with clinically and laboratory confirmed RA, especially to assess the significance of gadolinium (Gd)-DTPA enhancement for the pannus.

Patients and methods

The ages of the 71 patients (62 female, 9 male) ranged from 32 to 82 years (mean age 57 years). All had serologically proven chronic polyarthritis with a duration of 8–33 years (clinical phase II–IV). Neurological problems had been observed in each patient.

MRI was performed with a 0.5 T superaconductive system (Gyroscan S5 Philips) using a head coil. The technique consisted of (SE) sagittal T1-weighted series with a TR:TE of 450:30 ms before and after i.v. injection of Gd-DTPA. In addition sagittal series with gradient echo technique were performed with TR:TE of 555:40 ms, puls. angle 20°. Slice thickness was 5 mm with a 0.5 mm intersection gap. Imaging matrix was 256 × 256.

Results

The patients were categorized according to the morphology and signal intensity of the pannus as seen on unenhanced images ($n = 71$) and further classified by their enhancement status ($n = 23$) into three groups, which were correlated with laboratory tests (C-reactive protein, rheumatoid factors, and sedimentation rate). MRI and laboratory testing were repeated after 2 months of standardized therapy.

Discussion

MRI-morphology reflects the different phases of the inflammatory process (Figs. 1–4) [1–7]. In phase I pannus is isointense or moderately hyperintense in T1- and T2-weighted images. The signal in T1-weighted images is thought mainly to reflect the fat content of the pannus. In phase II the T1-weighted signal intensity of the pannus remains as before, but on T2-weighting it becomes hyperintense, mostly due to increased free water. In phase III the T1-weighted sequences show hypointense changes without notable changes in T2-weighted images reflecting increased fibrosis and early calcification (Table 1). In 12 of the 23 patients with additional Gd-DTPA scans a clear-cut enhancement of the pannus was noted (Table 2). These patients received non-steroid antirheumatic agents, low-dose cortisone and cimetidine in addi-

Table 1. MRI groups in relation to MRI signal intensity

	T1-weighted	T2-weighted
I	Iso-/hyper-	Iso-
II	Iso-/hypo-	Hyper-
III	Hypo-	Hypo-

Table 2. Correlation of MRI groups with enhancement status

	Gd –	Gd +	Total
N	48	–	48
I	2	1	3
II	1	10	11
III	8	1	9
	59	12	71

Gd, Gadolinium

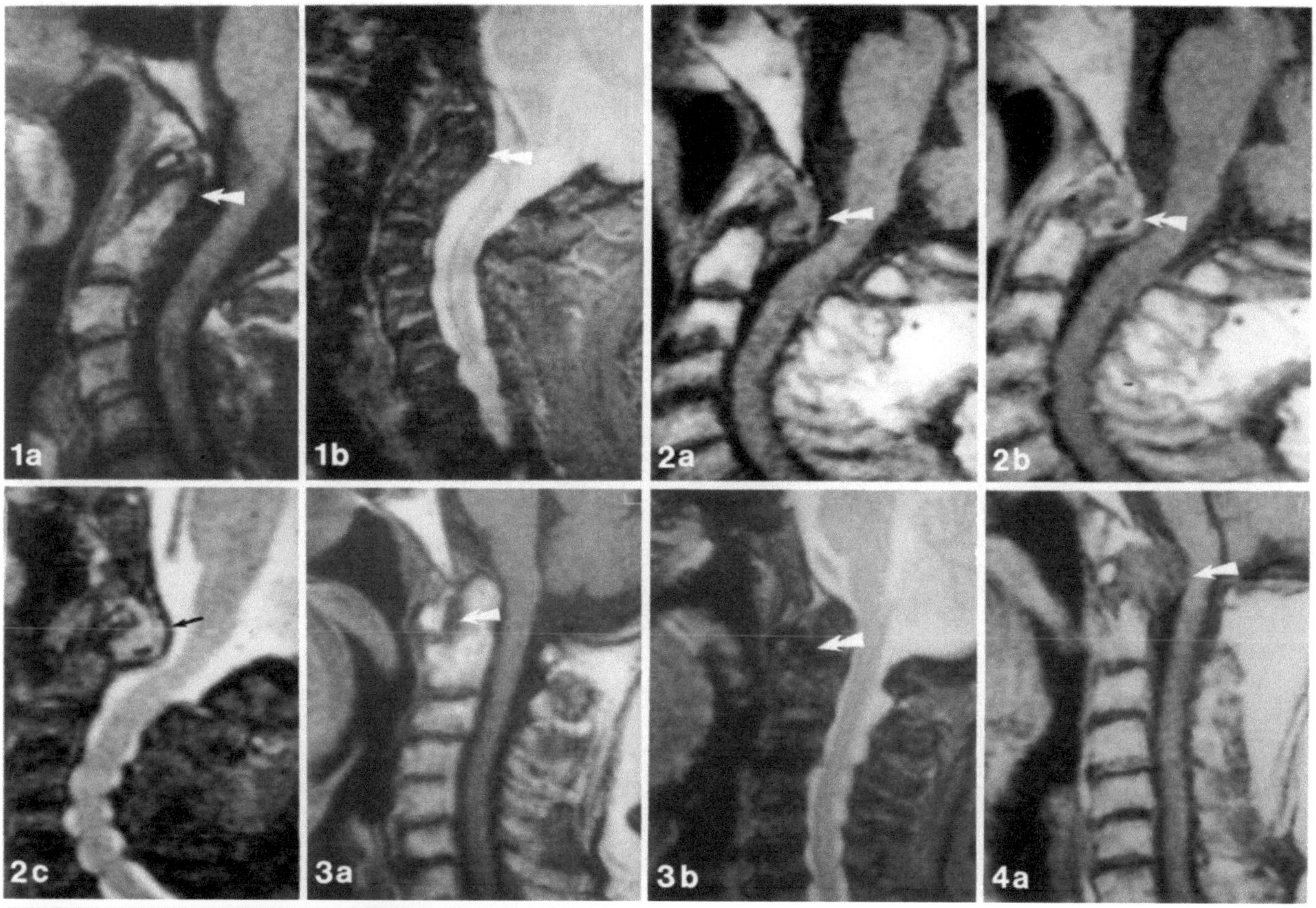

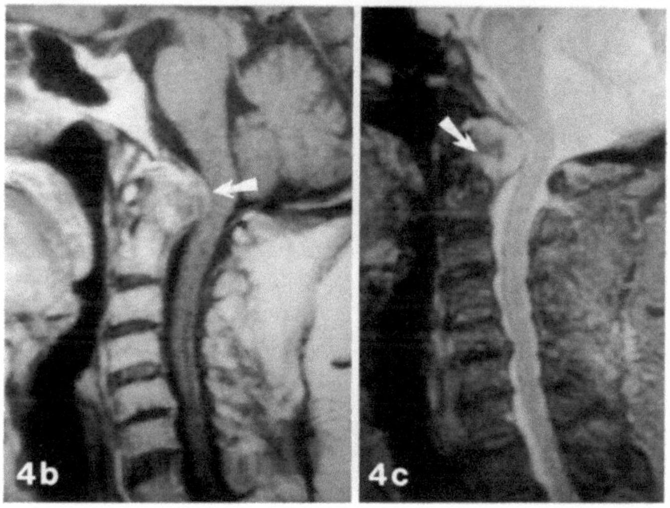

Fig. 1a, b. Type I. **a** T1-weighted image (T1WI), isointense pannus (➧); **b** gradient echo (GE) sagittal isointense pannus; note no signal change (➧)

Fig. 2a–c. Type II. **a** T1WI, sagittal, isointense dorsal pannus formation (➧); **b** T1WI, sagittal plus gadolinium (Gd), clear-cut enhancement of the pannus (➧); **c** GE sagittal, note the high signal intensity of the pannus (➧)

Fig. 3a, b. Type III. **a** T1WI, sagittal, small hypointense ventral pannus formation; **b** GE sagittal, hypointense pannus lesion; note no signal change in relation to T1WI (➧)

Fig. 4a–c. Control group. Initial MRI scan. **a** T1WI, sagittal; **b** T1WI, sagittal + Gd.; **c** GE sagittal. Control MRI scan. **a** T1WI, sagittal; **b** T1WI, sagittal + Gd.; **c** GE sagittal. Note the decrease of signal intensity of pannus on T1WI with Gd-DTPA as well as T2WI comparing the initial MRI scan with the follow-up

tion to basic therapy with salazopyrin and methotrexate. In three patients followed to date decrease of signal intensity of the pannus tissue and normalisation of the laboratory tests have been seen.

Preliminary results show a positive association between enhancing pannus in chronic RA and pathological serology reflecting activity of the disease. In single patients followed to date a decrease of enhancement was seen within 2 months after therapy in accordance with normalization of the laboratory tests.

References

1. Reynolds H, Carter SW, Murtagh FR, Rechtine GR (1987) Cervical rheumatoid arthritis: value of flexion and extension views in imaging. Radiology 164: 215–218
2. Beltran J, Caudill JL, Herman LA, Kantor SM, Hudson PN, Noto AM, Baran AS (1987) Rheumatoid arthritis: MR imaging manifestations. Radiology 165: 153–157
3. Yulish BS, Lieberman JM, Newman AJ, Bryan PJ, Mulopulos GP, Modic MT (1987) Juvenile rheumatoid arthritis: assessment with MR imaging. Radiology 165: 149–152

4. Aisen AM, Martel W, Eellis JH, McCune WJ (1987) Cervical spine involvement in rheumatoid arthritis: MR imaging. Radiology 165: 159–163
5. Bundschuh C, Modic MT, Kearney F, Morris R, Deal C (1988) Rheumatoid arthritis of the cervical spine: surface-coil MR imaging. AJNR 9: 565–571
6. Wolfe BK, O'Keffe D, Mitchell DM, Tchang St. P. K. (1987) Rheumatoid arthritis of the cervical spine: early and progressive radiographic features. Radiology 165: 145–148
7. Pettersson H, Larsson EM, Holtas S, Cronqvist S, Egund N, Zygmunt S, Brattström H (1988) MR imaging of the cervical spine in rheumatoid arthritis. AJNR 9: 573–577

Dr. M. Stiskal
Institute of Diagnostic Imaging
Krankenanstalt Rudolfinerhaus
Vienna, Austria

Neuroradiology (1991) 33 [Suppl]: 413–415

Neuro radiology
© Springer-Verlag 1991

Radiological assessment for transoral surgery in rheumatoid arthritis, using dynamic CT myelography

J. V. Hunter[1], J. Stevens[3], B. E. Kendall[1], R. Moskovich[2], and H. A. Crockard[2]

[1] Lysholm Department of Neuroradiology, The National Hospital for Neurology and Neurosurgery, London, UK
Departments of [2] Neurosurgery and [3] Radiology, The National Hospital for Neurology and Neurosurgery, Maida Vale, London, UK

Summary. A prospective, multidisciplinary study of 78 rheumatoid patients undergoing transoral surgery for relief of cervicomedullary compression was performed. CT myelographic data were correlated with preoperative clinical assessment and postoperative outcome. There was clinical improvement in the majority of patients after surgery. A greater than 50% reduction in cross-sectional area of the cord at the level of maximal compression at the craniocervical junction predicted a high-risk group. Subaxial atrophy of the cervical cord was demonstrated.

Key words: Rheumatoid arthritis – Transoral surgery – Computed myelography – Odontoid translocation – Cervicomedullary compression

The transoral approach, with immediate posterior fixation, for relief of cervicomedullary compression in patients with rheumatoid arthritis possesses advantages over other techniques [1]. Indications for this surgical approach are multifactorial, but one absolute criterion is translocation of the odontoid peg, necessitating partial removal of the dens. This study reports the results of assessment of the degree of translocation and the extent of craniocervical and subaxial compression in patients suffering from rheumatoid arthritis affecting the cervical spine, correlating radiographic measurements with preoperative assessment and postoperative outcome. The main aim of this study was to identify measurable parameters carrying prognostic weight.

Patients and methods

Data were collected from 78 patients, 62 females (mean age 64 years, range 26–82 years) and 16 males (mean age 61 years, range 40–84 years). All suffered from rheumatoid arthritis, with a mean duration of disease of 21.8 years (range 3–60 years). All had clinical features suggesting involvement of the neuraxis at the craniocervical junction. Four measures of disease severity were chosen, namely: (1) daily activity health assessment questionnaire (HAQ); (2) the Ranawat scale (a measure of neurological signs); (3) limb tone; (4) perceived head and neck pain (using a visual analogue scale, range 0–100).

Data from dynamic CT cisternomyelography were analysed [2]. Following the introduction of non-ionic contrast medium 1.5-mm sections were acquired from the base of C2 to the posterior fossa, in flexion and extension, with 5-mm overlapping sections of the subaxial area in the neutral position. All data were evaluated by one experienced radiologist by visual and computer analysis of the image data set. Multiplanar reconstructions were performed to obtain correct projections for measurement. All measurements were made four times to improve statistical confidence. The anteroposterior subarachnoid diameter and cross-sectional area and the anteroposterior sagittal cord diameter and cord cross-sectional area at the level of maximal compression were measured and correlated with pre- and postoperative clinical assessments. Subaxial cord cross-sectional area measurements were assessed in relation to normal values in the literature, and correlated with clinical outcome. Statistical analysis was performed using standard non-parametric methods.

Figure 1 illustrates the projections used for making the various measurements. Figure 2 demonstrates the distance 'b' between the lower endplate of the C2 vertebral body and the palato-occipital line – a measure of translocation [3] 'a + b' is the total length of the peg.

Results

Complete data are available on 49 patients, of whom 20 subsequently died (3 male). There was no difference in the degree of translocation between survivors and those dying; therefore translocation per se is not a suitable measurement for risk stratification ($P > 0.20$). Furthermore, the degree of translocation does not correlate with preoperative clinical impairment (Kendall tau = -0.19, Fig. 3). Comparison of the anteroposterior subarachnoid diameter at the level of maximal compression demonstrated a statistically significant difference between survivors and non-survivors ($P < 0.002$). The subarachnoid cross-sectional area at the same level also showed a statistically significant difference between the two groups ($P < 0.03$). The anteroposterior sagittal cord diameter at the level of maximal compression revealed a statistically significant difference ($P < 0.013$) with a very highly statistically significant difference ($P < 0.008$) in cross-sectional area at the same level between survivors and non-survivors. The mean cord area was 68 $mm^2 \pm 19$ mm^2 in the former and 47 $mm^2 \pm 16$ mm^2 in the latter, compared with an expected lower limit of normal of 90 mm^2 (J. Stevens, unpublished data). At a 'normal' subaxial level (corrected for expected cross-sectional area at that level [4]) there was a statistically significant difference in cord cross-sectional area of the whole group versus normal controls ($P < 0.03$), although

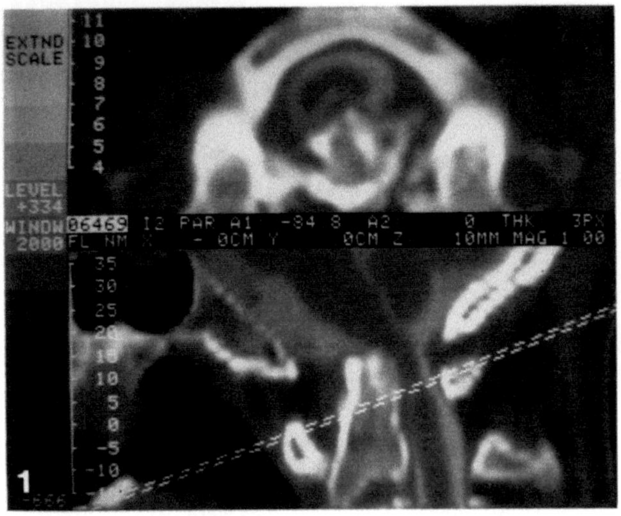

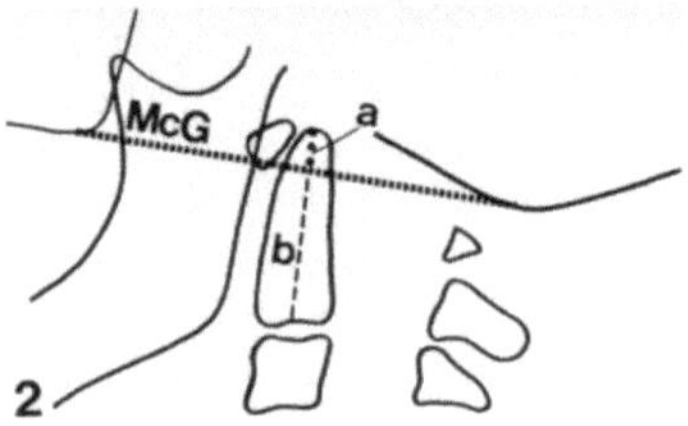

2

Fig. 1. The top image is a transverse axial reconstruction through the level of the C 1 ring prescribed from the lower midline sagittal reconstruction obtained from the original data set

Fig. 2. Representation of the palato-occipital (McGregor's) line *(McG)*. Base of C2 to McG is a measure of translocation. Normal male > 35 mm, normal female > 28 mm. Values below these represent true translocation (vertical subluxation)

Fig. 3. Scatter diagram of relationship between degree of translocation and degree of clinical impairment in 49 patients. Kendall's tau rank test confirms no correlation (tau = − 0.19)

Fig. 4. Representation of the changes in total health assessment questionnaire *(HAQ)* scores before and after surgery. There was a statistically significant difference ($P < 0.03$)

Fig. 5. Representation of the changes in Ranawat scores before and after surgery. There was a very highly statistically significant difference ($P < 0.0001$)

Fig. 6. Representation of the changes in head and neck pain before and after transoral surgery. There was a highly statistically significant difference ($P < 0.005$)

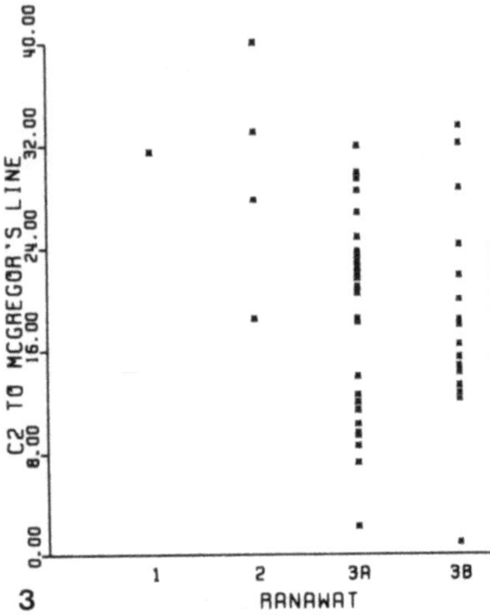

3

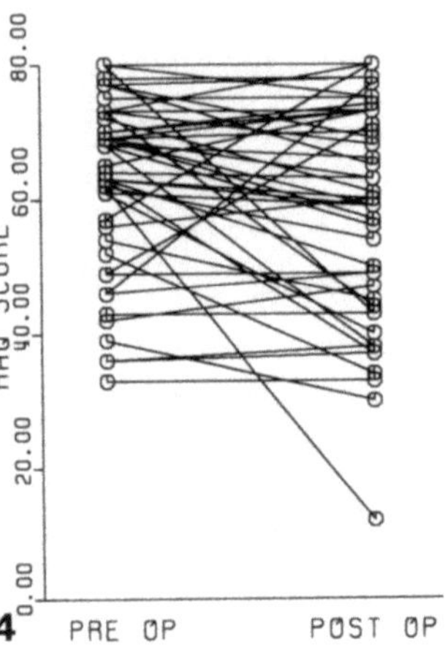

4

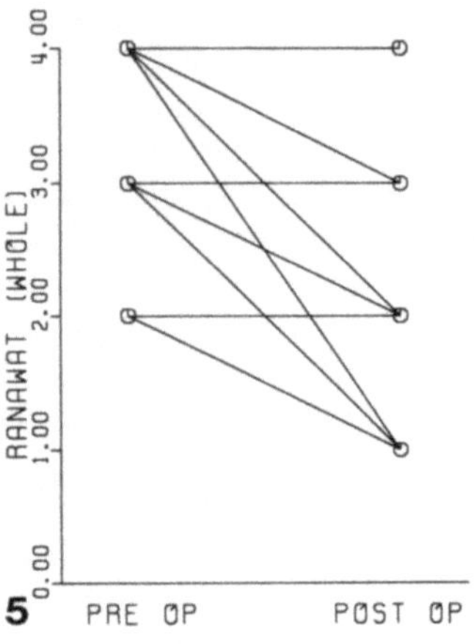

5

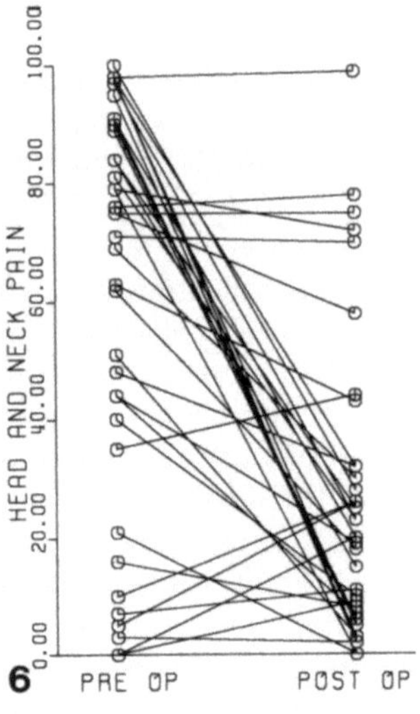

6

there was no difference between ultimate survivors and fatalities ($P > 0.12$).

Using the HAQ, a clear improvement was demonstrated as a result of the operation ($P < 0.03$, Fig. 4), supported by the improvement in Ranawat scores ($P < 0.0001$, Fig. 5), and scale values of head and neck pain ($P < 0.005$, Fig. 6). Of 19 patients with severe lower limb spasticity 12 did not have a successful outcome from surgery.

Discussion

There was improvement in head and neck pain ($P < 0.005$), Ranawat ($P < 0.0001$) and HAQ ($P < 0.03$) scores postoperatively, confirming that transoral surgery with posterior fixation is useful. A 50% or greater reduction in anteroposterior sagittal cord diameter and/or cross-sectional area, *at the level of maximum compression at the craniocervical junction,* appears to predict a poor outcome. There was generalised atrophy of the cervical cord in many of this selected group of patients with active compression of the cord at subaxial levels to account for it. A clinical marker for this high-risk group was lower limb spasticity. Upper limb spasticity did not achieve statistical significance.

This study identifies cord cross-sectional area at the level of maximum cord compression at the craniocervical junction as predicting potential clinical benefit from transoral odontoid peg surgery in this severely affected rheumatoid group. It is hoped that examination of this parameter will allow better stratification of patients into those likely to benefit from salvage surgery and those in whom potential disadvantages outweigh likely benefit.

References

1. Crockard HA (1988) Anterior approaches to lesions of the upper cervical spine. Clin Neurosurg 34: 389–416
2. Stevens JM, Kendall BE, Crockard HA (1986) The spinal cord in rheumatoid arthritis with clinical myelopathy: a computed myelographic study. J Neurol Neurosurg Psychiatry 49: 140–151
3. Redlund-Johnell I (1984) Dislocations of the cervical spine in rheumatoid arthritis. Thesis, Malmo
4. Yuk-Ling Yu (1985) The use of computed tomography in cervical spondylotic myelopathy and radiculopathy. Thesis, Hong Kong

Dr. Jill V. Hunter
Lysholm Department of Neuroradiology
National Hospital for Neurology and Neurosurgery
Queen Square, London, UK

Neuroradiology (1991) 33 [Suppl]: 416–418

Neuro radiology
© Springer-Verlag 1991

Soft tissue masses associated with rheumatoid arthritis of the atlanto-axial joints

B. E. Kendall, J. M. Stevens, and H. A. Crockard

National Hospital for Nervous Diseases, London, UK

Summary. In rheumatoid arthritis of the atlanto-axial joints, a fixed atlanto-dental interval suggests fibrotic rather than florid pannus. Soft tissue (ST) above or behind the dens is more prominent with florid pannus than fibrosis and variation in ST shape with flexion/extension suggests florid pannus and/or fluid. CT density is also influenced by bone-induced artefact to distinguish fluid, florid pannus and fibrosis. On MRI homogeneous low signal in ST on both T1- and T2-weighted sequences distinguishes fibrosis from florid pannus and fluid.

Key words: Rheumatoid arthritis – Atlanto-axial joints

Rheumatoid arthritis (RA) involving the atlanto-axial joints may require surgery for: (1) relief of neuro-axial compression; (2) intractable pain failing to respond to conservative measures; (3) prophylaxis against sudden death due to acute increase in subluxation.

The surgical approach is influenced by: (1) the amount of bone destruction, direction and degree of subluxation, instability and reducibility on flexion and extension; (2) the degree and site of compression of the neuro-axis; (3) the type of compressing tissue, bone and/or abnormal soft tissue (ST).

When compression is due to translocation or is horizontal from the anterior aspect and cannot be reduced by manipulation and traction, a transoral approach for extirpation of the compressing agents, which may be dens and/or a ST mass, together with posterior fixation performed as a single surgical procedure [1], has proved to be a satisfactory method of improving neurological function while incurring a relatively low morbidity in these high-risk patients.

However, the morbidity and mortality are sufficient [2] for preference to be given to the lesser surgical procedure of posterior fixation with or without decompression in appropriate cases. Included are those in which anterior compression is either absent or can be relieved by manipulation and maintained by posterior fixation. Controversy exists regarding the best surgical approach to patients in which the compressing agent is ST behind the dens which persists after manipulation [3, 4]. Reduction in ST after adequate fixation has been clearly demonstrated [4]; the degree to which this occurs and the possibility of predicting it from pre-operative imaging have not been established. The compressing tissue, which cannot be inspected at surgery in cases treated by posterior fixation alone, may be firm and fibrous or soft, maleable and sometimes vascular: compression may also be due to an effusion distending the joint capsule, possibly amenable to percutaneous aspiration or a combination of these features. Absorption could be influenced by such features, the possibility was investigated of pre-operative recognition of the nature of compressing ST using computed myelography (CM) and/or MRI.

Materials and methods

The nature of the compressing agent was noted by the neurosurgeon and verified by histology in 87 patients with RA submitted to transoral surgery for anterior neuro-axial compression. In 16 compression was by bone alone. Imaging studies were available for analysis in 65 of the other 71 cases. These were CMs in 58 and MRIs in 10: T1-weighted sequences in 10, but T2-weighted in only 5. Images were made in flexion and extension in 43 cases and in one position in 22 cases. The images were re-analysed retrospectively for features which might indicate the nature of any ST component at the site of compression. These features included: (1) increased distance between the anterior arch of the atlas and the odontoid peg (ADI) and whether the distance reduced in extension; (2) ST mass posterior to the odontoid peg and whether this mass was reduced by flexion; (3) the shape of the ST, whether smooth or lobulated; (4) calcification in the ST; (5) visible structural components within the ST; (6) electronic density measurements within the ST; (7) signal changes within the ST.

The nature of the compressing agent was unknown to the radiologists at the time of image review.

Table 1. Results of analysis

	Soft tissue		
	Fibrous	Florid	Fluid
ADI reducible	8 (36%)[a]	16 (76%)[a]	
Irreducible	14 (67%)[a]	5 (24%)[a]	
Soft tissue behind/above dens	10 (34%)	16 (47%)	4
Variation with flexion/extension	2 (9%)[a]	17 (81%)[a]	3
Convex	8 (28%)	20 (59%)	5
Lobulated	1 (3%)	7 (21%)	0
Calcification	4 (14%)	7 (21%)	3
MRI signal low	4	0	0
varied	0	5	1

CT density measurements were made unreliable by bone-induced artefact

[a] Of cases with flexion and extension

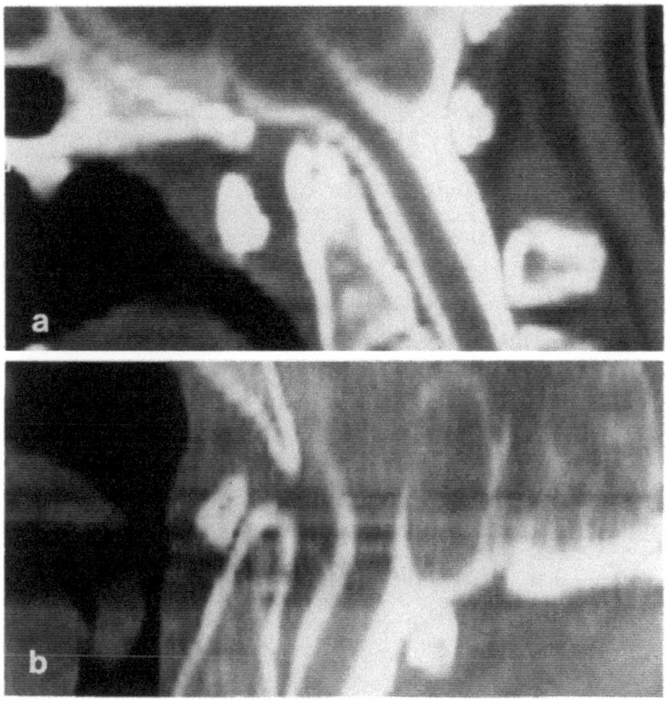

Fig. 1 a, b. Mid-sagittal reformatted images from a computed myelogram in **a** flexion and **b** extension. There is marked atlanto-axial movement and widening of soft tissue thickening posterior to the dens on extension. Typical of soft florid pannus which was found at surgery

Results

The results of the analysis are set out in Table 1.

In 19 patients the ADI was virtually fixed between flexion and extension. In 14 of these the ST appeared fibrous at surgery. Some change in the ADI was present in 24 patients (Fig. 1). In 16 of these soft florid pannus was present, in 2 associated with excess synovial fluid. In 8 fibrous pannus was responsible, in 1 associated with some fluid. In 1 fluid alone was present.

A ST mass behind and/or above the dens which varied in size with flexion (Fig. 1) was present in 19 patients. In 17 it was due to soft florid and 2 to fibrous pannus: in 2 of the former and 1 of the latter there was also some synovial effusion. In 7 cases there was ST behind the dens in flexion; in 3 of these it was due to soft and in two to fibrous pannus and in one there was soft pannus plus fluid.

The ST was lobulated in 8 patients, 6 with florid soft pannus, 1 with fibrous pannus and 1 with soft pannus plus fluid. Flecks of calcification were present in 11 patients; 7 had florid soft and 4 fibrous pannus, in 2 pannus was associated with some fluid and in 1 the mass appeared to be due to fluid alone.

Density measurements were obtained in all patients, but were influenced by bone-induced artefacts and proved not to be useful. The density of fluid, fibrous and soft pannus varied considerably: it could be lower or considerably greater than that of muscle. Variation in density within parts of the ST occurred in patients with fluid and pannus, but was also seen with pannus alone.

Discussion

The natural history of cervical myelopathy in RA is progressive neurological deterioration which is invariably fatal, usually within 1 year of diagnosis [5, 6]. In over 50% this is the consequence of cord compression and in the rest the secondary effects of respiratory insufficiency and the cardiovascular consequences of immobilisation. Conservative treatment such as the use of cervical collars and skull traction devices has only slightly improved prognosis and indeed the use of certain types of skull traction increases the number of complications related to immobilisation, particularly pulmonary embolism.

Reduction of atlanto-axial subluxation and immediate fusion is very satisfactory where cord compression can be relieved [7], but imaging is necessary to check that residual or increased cord compression from ST is avoided. Irreducable, severe anterior compression has been most successfully managed by transoral decompression with immediate posterior fixation [1]. This produces a significant improvement in both Ranawat [8] and health activity questionnaire scores and relieves pain.

Criteria for selection for transoral surgery have until recently been based on dynamic CM on which a clear estimate of the degree of medullary and/or cord compression at the extreme ranges of movement, and of the degree of instability can be made. A recent study [2] was undertaken in order to refine our selection criteria and to identify the higher risk cases. A reduction of greater than 50% in sagittal cord diameter and cross-sectional area at the level of maximum compression correlates with severe lower limb spasticity and a poor outcome from transoral surgery. It may well be that in this subgroup, incomplete relief of ST compression plus posterior fixation is a better alternative if the ST appears likely to regress.

MRI has advantages in examination of the cervical spine in these often deformed and disabled patients. The degree of translocation, subluxation, ST impingement, medullary and/or cord deformity and the relative severity of subaxial disease can all be assessed. Many machines in current use do not allow so precise an assessment of the degree of cord deformity as can be achieved by detailed CM, but this too is possible on the most advanced machines. MRI will also allow assessment of the internal structure of the cord and therefore some estimate of the damage which has already occurred. Gadolinium enhancement was not used in this study. However, active inflammatory pannus enhances and burnt out fibrotic pannus does not, which will be a useful additional criterion in doubtful cases.

Correlation of all these features should allow a more informed estimate of the expectation from the various forms of surgery and a more accurate assessment of prognosis. The wider availability of MRI should aid in the earlier recognition of cervical myelopathy in patients with RA and lead to surgery being performed before irreversible cord damage has occurred.

References

1. Crockard HA, Essigman, Stevens JM, Pozo JL, Ransford AO, Kendall BE (1985) Surgical treatment of cervical cord compression in rheumatoid arthritis. Ann Rheum Dis 44: 809–816
2. Hunter JV, Stevens JM, Kendall BE, Moskovich R, Crockard AC (1990) Radiological assessment for transoral surgery in rheumatoid arthritis using dynamic computed myelography. Neuroradiology (in press)
3. Dvorak J, Grob D, Baumgartner H, Gschwend N, Grauer W, Larsson S (1989) Functional evaluation of the spinal cord by magnetic resonance imaging in patients with rheumatoid arthritis and instability of upper cervical spine. Spine 14: 1057–1064
4. Larsson EM, Holtas S, Zygmunt S (1989) Pre and post-operative MR imaging of the cranio-cervical junction in rheumatoid arthritis. AJNR 10: 89–94
5. Marks JS, Sharp J (1981) Rheumatoid cervical myelopathy. QJ Med 199: 307–319
6. Meijers KAE, Cats A, Kremer HPH, Lugendij KW, Onrlee GJ, Thomeer RTWM (1984) Cervical myelopathy in rheumatoid arthritis. Clin Exp Rheumatol 2: 239–245
7. Boyle AC (1971) The rheumatoid neck. Proc R Soc Med 64: 1161–1165
8. Ranawat (1979) Cervical spine fusion in rheumatoid arthritis. J Bone Joint Surg [Am] 61: 1003–1010

Dr. B. E. Kendall
Radiology Department
National Hospital for Nervous Diseases
Queen Square
London WC1N 3BG, UK

Neuroradiology (1991) 33 [Suppl]: 419–420

Neuro
radiology
© Springer-Verlag 1991

Petrous carotid aneurysms treated by endovascular techniques

V. V. Halbach, R. T. Higashida, G. B. Hieshima, C. F. Dowd, and S. L. Barnwell

Department of Radiology, Neurointerventional Section University of California, San Francisco Hospitals, San Francisco, California, USA

Summary. Aneurysms that arise from the petrous segment of the internal carotid artery are rare, with only 30 cases reported. We report seven additional patients who presented with symptoms due to a petrous carotid aneurysm, all effectively treated by endovascular techniques (6 patients) or surgical ligation (1 patient). In one patient with a saccular aneurysm the aneurysm was thrombosed with preservation of the parent artery. In the remaining six patients, with fusiform aneurysms, proximal occlusion or trapping procedures were performed. In all cases the presenting symptoms were alleviated following aneurysm thrombosis.

Key words: Petrous carotid – Aneurysm – Balloon embolization – Carotid occlusion – Internal carotid aneurysm

Aneurysms arising from the petrous segment of the internal carotid artery can present with cranial nerve dysfunction involving fifth through twelfth nerves, Horner's syndrome, otorrhagia, and epistaxis [1–12]. In our patients the presenting symptoms were as follows: pain (7 patients), and impaired function of the eighth nerve (3 patients), fifth nerve (3 patients), sixth nerve (2 patients), and seventh and third nerve (1 patient each). One patient presented with an embolic event producing transient monocular blindness. The patients' ages ranged from 7 to 62 years with a mean of 30.3 years. Four patients presented before the age of 20 years. One patient had a history of neck trauma 7 years prior to discovery of the aneurysm. Two patients had unexplained hemiatrophy of the body ipsilateral to the aneurysm. All seven patients had MRI or CT documenting intraluminal thrombus within the aneurysm. Six of the seven aneurysms were fusiform.

Six of the patients were treated by the endovascular route. In five patients systemic anticoagulation with heparin was followed by a test occlusion, which was tolerated in all five. Carotid occlusion using detachable balloons was then performed: the aneurysm was trapped in two patients and a proximal occlusion was produced in three. One patient had an aneurysm with a definable neck and a balloon was navigated into the dome of the aneurysm and detached, producing complete thrombosis (Fig. 1). One patient underwent surgical ligation of the internal carotid artery in the neck for treatment of a fusiform aneurysm. All seven patients experienced complete alleviation of their symptoms. One patient with a hypercoagulable state developed one episode of visual loss and was treated with antiplatelet medication, with complete resolution of symptoms.

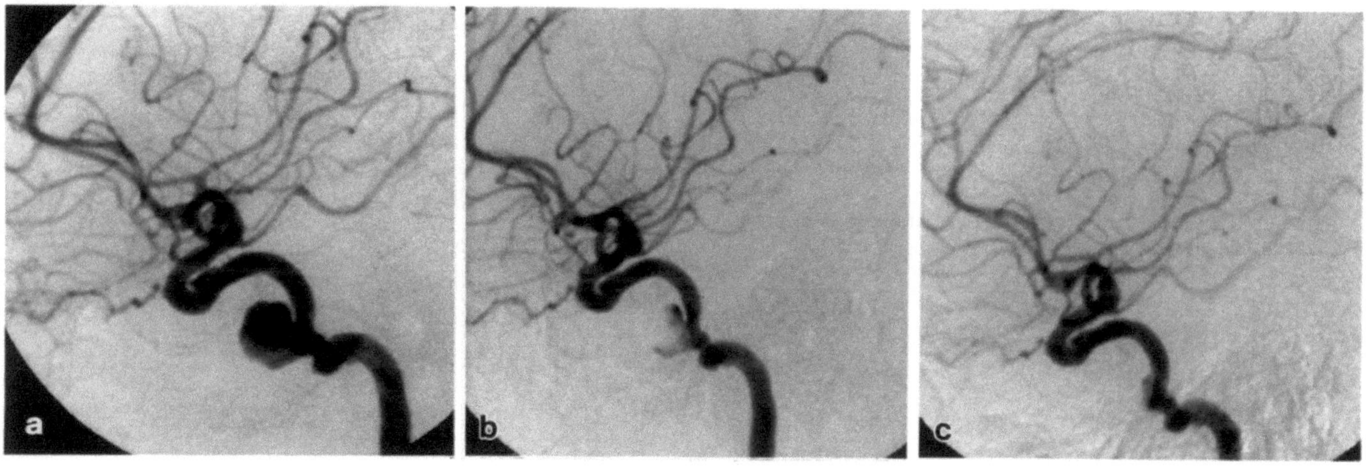

Fig. 1 a–c. A 62-year-old man presented with severe pain related to the fifth nerve ganglion. **a** A left internal carotid angiogram, lateral projection, demonstrates an aneurysm arising from the petrous cavernous junction of the internal carotid artery. The irregularity of the walls suggest intraluminal thrombus. **b** Placement of a silicone balloon within the aneurysm; immediately follwing embolization there is residual filling of the aneurysm. **c** One-week follow-up angiogram demonstrates thrombosis of the dome of the aneurysm

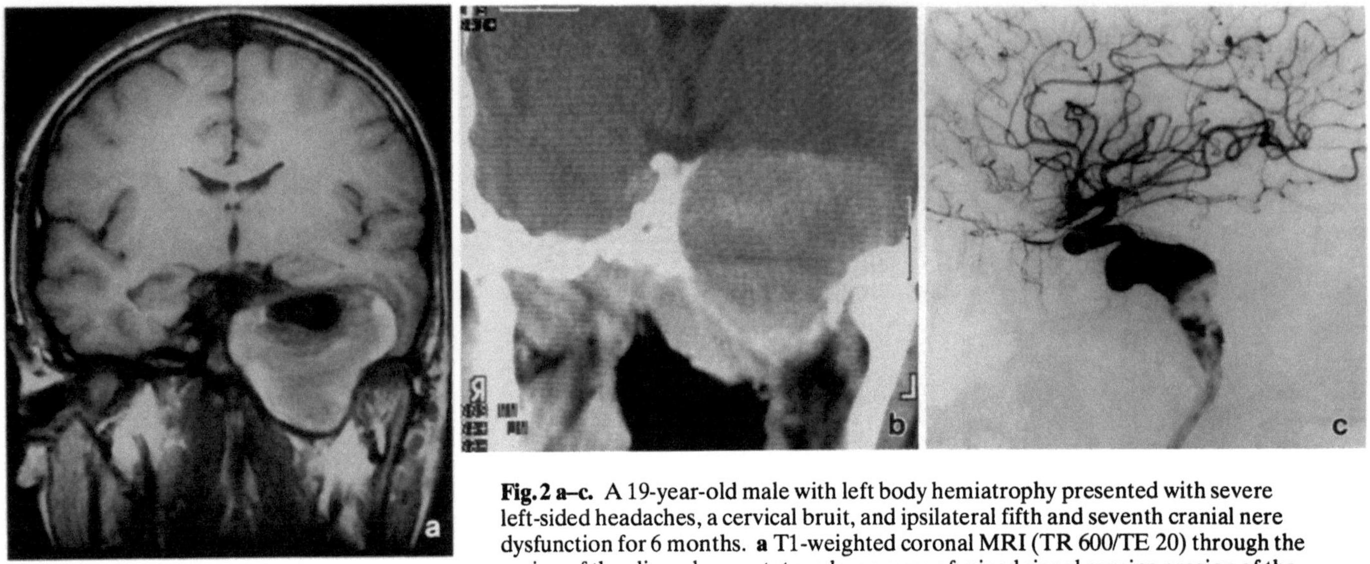

Fig. 2 a–c. A 19-year-old male with left body hemiatrophy presented with severe left-sided headaches, a cervical bruit, and ipsilateral fifth and seventh cranial nere dysfunction for 6 months. **a** T1-weighted coronal MRI (TR 600/TE 20) through the region of the clivus demonstates a large mass of mixed signal causing erosion of the petrous bone. Areas of signal void located superiorly are consistent with flowing blood. **b** Coronal CT demonstates smooth bone erosion involving the sphenoid bone. There is expansion inferiorly into the nasopharynx. **c** A left internal carotid angiogram demonstrates petrous internal carotid aneurysm. Irregular margins correspond to the laminated thrombus

Case reports

Case 1 is a 62-year-old male with severe left-sided headaches and fifth nerve hypersensitivity. An angiogram (Fig. 1 a) and CT revealed a partially thrombosed petrous carotid aneurysm with a well-defined neck. A balloon was navigated into the dome of the aneurysm (Fig. 1 b) and detached. A control angiogram (Fig. 1 c) and CT at 4 months confirmed complete thrombosis of the aneurysm and the patient has had complete resolution of symptoms.

Case 2 is a 19-year-old male with congenital left body hemiatrophy who developed severe left sided headaches, a left seventh nerve palsy and pain in the left fifth nerve distribution. MRI (Fig. 2 a), CT (Fig. 2 b) and an angiogram (Fig. 2 c) revealed a giant, partially thrombosed, left petrous aneurysm. There was no evidence of a collagen deficiency state or phakomatosis. The patient tolerated test occlusion of the left internal carotid artery, which was then surgically interrupted. His symptoms completely resolved over the next 4 months.

References

1. Barrett JH, Lawrence VL (1960) Aneurysm of the internal carotid artery as a complication of mastoidectomy. Arch Otolaryngol 72: 366–368
2. Harrison TH, Odom GL, Kunkle EC (1963) Internal carotid aneurysm arising in the carotid canal. Arch Neurol 8: 112–115
3. Busby DR, Slemmons DH, Miller TF (1968) Fatal epistaxis via carotid aneurysm and eustachian tube. Arch Otolaryngol 87: 293–296
4. Stallings JO, McCabe BF (1969) Congenital middle ear aneurysm of the internal carotid. Arch Otolaryngol 90: 65–69
5. Anderson RD, Liebeskind A, Schechter M (1972) Aneurysms of the internal carotid artery in the carotid canal of the petrous temporal bone. Radiology 102: 639–642
6. Morantz RA, Kirchner F, Kishore P (1976) Aneurysm of the petrous portion of the internal carotid artery. Surg Neurol 6: 313–318
7. Holtzman RN, Parisier SC (1979) Acute spontaneous otorrhagia resulting from a ruptured petrous carotid aneurysm. J Neurosurg 51: 258–261
8. Mofet DA, O'Conner AFF (1980) Bilateral internal carotid aneurysms in the petrous temporal bones. Arch Otolaryngol 106: 172–175
9. Kudo S, Colley DP (1983) Multiple intrapetrous aneurysms of the internal carotid artery. AJNR 4: 1119–1121
10. Berenstein A, Ransohoff J, Kupersmith M, Flamm E, Graeb D (1984) Transvascular treatment of giant aneurysms of the cavernous carotid and vertebral arteries. Functional investigation and embolization. Surg Neurol 21: 3–12
11. Willinsky R, Lasjaunias P, Pruvost P, Boucherat M (1987) Petrous internal carotid aneurysm causing epistaxis: balloon embolization with preservation of the parent vessel. Neuroradiology 29: 570–572
12. Fox AJ, Vinuela F, Pelz PM (1987) Use of detachable balloons for proximal artery occlusion in the treatment of unclippable cerebral aneurysms. J Neurosurg 66: 40–46

Dr. Van V. Halbach
U. C. S. F. Hospitals, L-352
Department of Radiology
505 Parnassus Ave.
San Francisco, California, USA

Neuroradiology (1991) 33 [Suppl]: 421–423

Neuro radiology

© Springer-Verlag 1991

Treatment of intracranial arterial spasm by interventional neurovascular techniques

R. T. Higashida[1], V. V. Halbach[1], S. L. Barnwell[1], C. Dowd[1], B. Dormandy[2], J. Bell[2], and G. B. Hieshima[1]

[1] Departments of Radiology and Neurological Surgery, Interventional Neuroradiology Section, University of California at San Francisco, San Francisco, California, USA

[2] Interventional Therapeutics Corporation, South San Francisco, California, USA

Summary. Patients with symptomatic intracranial arterial spasm are now being treated using interventional neurovascular techniques. From a transfemoral approach, a custom-designed silicone microballoon can be guided through the intracranial circulation and inflated to dilate the spastic vessel(s). In clinical trials, 19 patients, ranging in age from 15 to 73 years, have been treated. A total of 63 vessels have been successfully dilated in the anterior and posterior circulations. Clinical improvement was observed following treatment in 14 patients (73.7%). Complications included 2 instances of vessel rupture and 1 patient suffered delayed intraparenchymal hemorrhage. In patients presenting with symptomatic intracranial vasospasm, unresponsive to medical therapy, treatment by balloon angioplasty may help to improve cerebral perfusion.

Key words: Intracranial vasospasm – Balloon dilatation – Angioplasty of spasm – Subarachnoid hemorrhage – Interventional neuroradiology

Among cerebrovascular disorders, intracranial arterial spasm due to aneurysmal subarachnoid hemorrhage (SAH) remains a leading cause of major morbidity and mortality [1, 2]. Despite recent advances in medical therapy, it is estimated that 20–30% of patients with an acute SAH develop vasospasm leading to stroke or death [3]. Recent advances in interventional therapy have allowed patients with symptomatic vasospasm to be treated by balloon angioplasty in selected cases.

Materials and methods

Our indications for treatment included clinically symptomatic vasospasm, unresponsive to medical therapy, or spasm developing during interventional treatment of an intracranial aneurysm, with neurological decline. A total of 19 patients, 8 males and 11 females, ranging in age from 15 to 73 years (mean 36.5) were treated. The following vessels were dilated: internal carotid artery 16; middle cerebral artery 15; anterior cerebral artery 2; vertebral artery 7; posterior cerebral artery 14; basilar artery 9. In 14 patients (63.7%) spasm was diffuse, affecting multiple vessels, while in 5 (26.3%) the spasm was focal, involving only one vessel.

All procedures were performed in the Interventional Neurovascular Radiology section, using direct fluoroscopic visualization. A complete cerebral arteriogram was performed initially to assess the degree of stenosis, the vessels involved, and collateral circulation. For angioplasty of arterial spasm, a silicone microballoon was developed specifically for use in the intracranial circulation [4]. Uninflated, the balloon measures 0.85 mm × 3.50 mm; it will accept a volume of 0.10 ml, and expand to 7.5 mm × 13.5 mm (Fig. 1). A uniquely blended silicone elastomeric microballoon was chosen because of its properties of malleability, biocompatibility, isotropic expansion, and special conformational structure. This material allows the balloon to conform to the vessel lumen without causing excessive pressure on the arterial wall. The balloon is fixed onto a 2.0 F polyethylene catheter. A guide wire, 0.014 in, can be placed into the catheter to aid navigation into specific vessels [5]. The balloon is guided to the site of spasm, and with gentle inflation and deflation (with pressures between 0.1 and 1.5 atmospheres) dilatation is performed (Fig. 2 a, b).

Following angioplasty an arteriogram was obtained in all cases, to evaluate the change in caliber of the vessels treated, and to determine if there was any structural damage. Patients were monitored by close neurological evaluation throughout the procedure and then observed in the neurosurgical intensive care unit following it (Fig. 3 a–c).

Results

A total of 63 arteries was treated by this balloon dilatation technique. There was angiographic evidence of improved luminal diameter in all cases. Follow-up arteriography, at intervals ranging from 1 day to 2 weeks, demonstrated continued patency of the vessels treated by angioplasty, while the untreated territories continued to remain in spasm. Of the 19 patients treated, 14 showed improvement in their neurological condition (73.7%). The majority of these showed noticeable improvement within minutes to hours of successful dilatation, particularly if the procedure was performed within 24 h of the onset of neurological decline. If treatment was delayed beyond 24 h from the onset of symptoms, improvement was also delayed for 1–5 days. In 5 cases (26.3%), there was no noticeable change in neurological condition, despite angiographic evidence of improved luminal diameter.

Complications included 2 cases of arterial rupture. One, early in our experience, was due to rupture by a latex balloon of the cavernous internal carotid artery, leading to a carotid cavernous sinus fistula. The second case involved rupture of a posterior cerebral artery causing SAH. In one patient, hemorrhage occurred into the basal ganglia re-

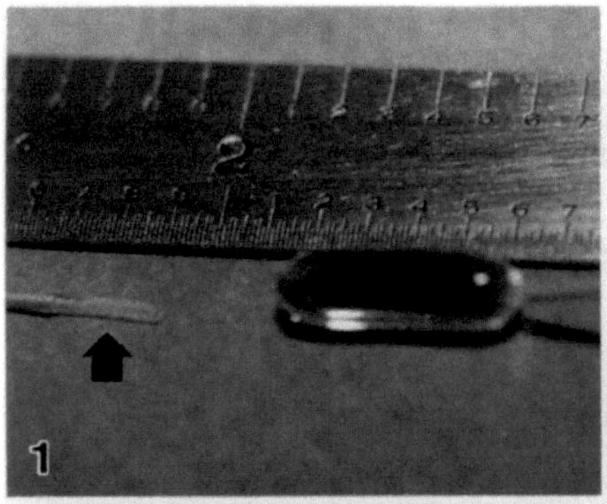

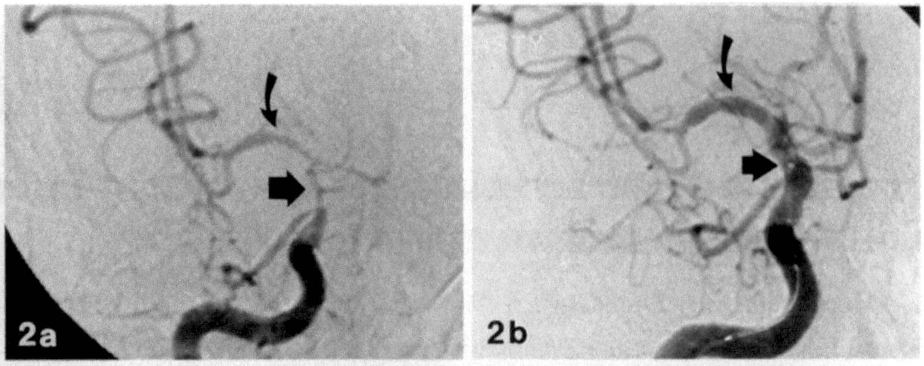

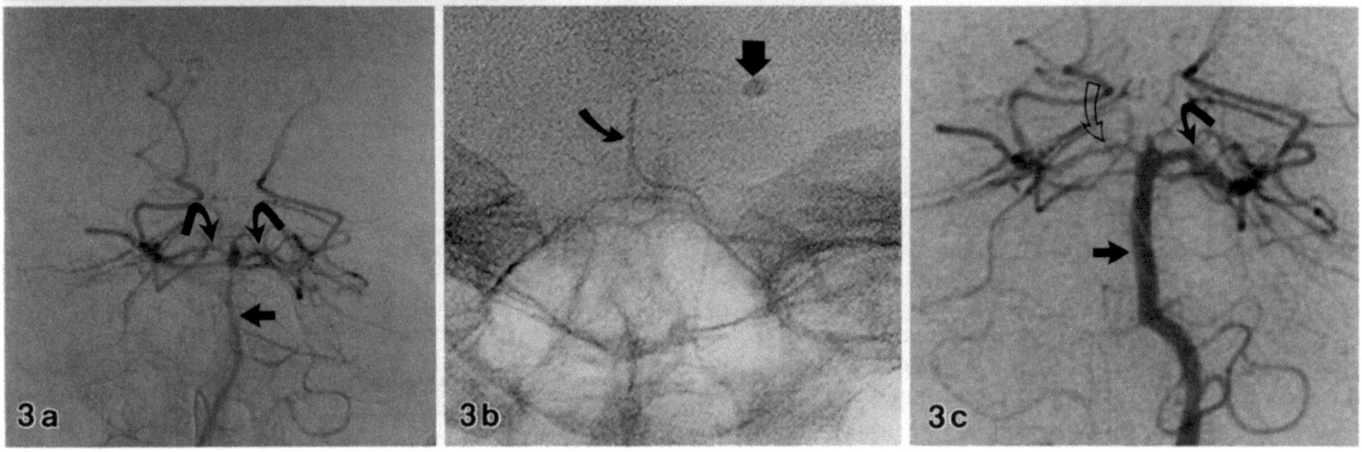

Fig. 1. Silicone balloon used for angioplasty of intracranial arterial spasm. Uninflated *(arrow)* the balloon measures 0.85 mm × 3.50 mm. It will accept a volume of 0.10 ml, and inflate to 3.5 mm × 12.5 mm

Fig. 2. **a** Internal carotid arteriogram demonstrating spasm of the supraclinoid internal carotid *(large arrow)* and middle cerebral arteries *(curved arrow)*. **b** Following successful angioplasty of the internal carotid *(large arrow)* and middle cerebral arteries *(curved arrow)*, there is return of normal luminal diameter, with angiographic evidence of improved cerebral perfusion

Fig. 3. **a** Vertebral arteriogram demonstrating severe spasm of the basilar artery *(straight arrow)* and both posterior cerebral arteries *(curved arrow)*, due to recent subarachnoid hemorrhage. **b** Radiograph demonstrating the angioplasty balloon partially inflated, and attached to the 2.0 F catheter *(curved arrow)* in the left posterior cerebral artery *(large arrow)* **c** Postangioplasty arteriogram demonstrating a return to normal lumen diameter of the entire basilar artery *(straight arrow)*, and the left posterior cerebral artery *(curved arrow)*. The right posterior cerebral artery has not been treated and continues to remain in spasm *(open arrow)*

gion 24 h following angioplasty of the middle cerebral artery and he subsequently died [6].

Discussion

Transluminal angioplasty for atherosclerotic disease was first described in the early 1960s [7]. However, it was not until 1984 that techniques for angioplasty involving the intracranial circulation were first described. At that time, Zubkov et al. [8] reported treatment of 105 vessels in 33 patients, with good results. Since then, two other centers have reported the results of angioplasty for intracranial vasospasm [6, 9].

The mechanism and pathophysiology of cerebral vasospasm are still poorly understood. It has been suggested that spasm is due to muscular contraction of the vessel wall with associated intimal changes leading to hypertrophy and myonecrosis [10, 11]. No pharmacological agent has yet been found that can consistently reverse the effects of spasm due to subarachnoid blood. It is for this reason that balloon dilatation represents an alternative in patients unresponsive to medical therapy.

The process of mechanical balloon dilatation is to expand and dilate the intima, media, and adventia of the vessel. In animal models, this does not seem on histological examination to cause excessive damage to the blood vessel wall, if the balloon does not expand the lumen of the vessel beyond its normal caliber. It is therefore believed that angioplasty of spasm is different from angioplasty in atherosclerotic disease, in which the balloon disrupts and fractures the plaque, involving the intima and media. Indeed, on cerebral arteriograms, both immediate and delayed, following dilatation for spasm, there is no evidence of intimal disruption, hypertrophy, dissection, or other damage to the vessel. The vessel lumen appears to be restored to its normal caliber, whereas untreated adjacent vessels continue to remain in spasm.

In conclusion, we believe that intracranial arterial spasm can be effectively treated by balloon angioplasty techniques in selected cases. Radiographically there is evidence to suggest a restoration to normal luminal diameter following dilatation. In 73.7% of patients treated so far there has been improvement in neurological function. Certainly more extensive research, both clinical and experimental, is needed before this technique becomes an accepted therapeutic alternative for management of patients with symptomatic vasospasm.

References

1. Allcock JM, Drake CG (1965) Ruptured intracranial aneurysms – the role of arterial spasm. J Neurosurg 22: 21–29
2. Ropper AH, Zervas NT (1984) Outcome one year after subarachnoid hemorrhage from cerebral aneurysms. J Neurosurg 60: 909–915
3. Sahs A, Perret GE, Locksley HB, Nishioka H (1969) Intracranial aneurysm and subarachnoid hemorrhage. Lippincott, Philadelphia
4. Higashida RT, Halbach VV, Dormandy B, Bell J, Brant-Zawadski M, Hieshima GB (1990) New microballoon device for transluminal angioplasty of intracranial arterial vasospasm. AJNR 11: 233–238
5. Brothers MF, Holgate RC (1990) Intracranial angioplasty for treatment of vasospasm after subarachnoid hemorrhage: technique and modifications to improve branch access. AJNR 11: 239–248
6. Higashida RT, Halbach VV, Cahan LD (1989) Transluminal angioplasty for treatment of intracranial arterial vasospasm. J Neurosurg 71: 648–653
7. Dotter CT, Judkins MP (1964) Transluminal treatment of arteriosclerotic obstruction: description of a new technique and a preliminary report of its application. Circulation 30: 654–670
8. Zubkov YN, Nikiforov BM, Shustin VA (1984) Balloon catheter technique for dilatation of constricted cerebral arteries after aneurysmal SAH. Acta Neurochir (Wien) 70: 665–679
9. Newell DW, Eskridge JM, Mayberg MR (1989) Angioplasty for the treatment of symptomatic vasospasm following subarachnoid hemorrhage. J Neurosurg 71: 654–660
10. Conway LW, McDonald LW (1972) Structural changes of the intradural arteries following subarachnoid hemorrhage. J Neurosurg 37: 715–723
11. Fein JM, Flor WJ, Cohan SL (1974) Sequential changes of vascular ultrastructure in experimental cerebral vasospasm. Myonecrosis of subarachnoid arteries. J Neurosurg 41: 49–58

Dr. R. T. Higashida
University of California at San Francisco
Medical Center
505 Parnassas Avenue, L-352
San Francisco, California, USA

Neuroradiology (1991) 33 [Suppl]: 424–425

Neuro-radiology
© Springer-Verlag 1991

Endovascular treatment for experimental aneurysm

M. Negoro, K. Terashima, S. Miyachi, T. Handa, and K. Sugita

Department of Neurosurgery, Nagoya University School of Medicine, Nagoya, Japan

Summary. Recent advance of endovascular treatment has brought a significant change in the treatment of cerebral aneurysms. However, there are still unsolved problems in such treatment. In this study we are seeking the definitive method of endovascular therapy. An experimental aneurysm was first produced in the carotid artery of a dog by the venous patch method. Follow-up study of these aneurysms revealed 80% patency rate during a 3-month period. The aneurysm was then treated by detachable latex balloon. Treated aneurysms were studied angiographically and histologically. After 4 weeks the aneurysm lumen was completely covered by epithelial cells. Latex balloon has a satisfactory ability to occlude a large aneurysmal cavity.

Key words: Experimental aneurysm – Detachable balloon

Recently cerebral aneurysm has been treated by the endovascular approach. However, there are still unsolved problems with this treatment, e.g. delayed rupture of an embolized aneurysm. In this study we have tried to find out the reasons for such an undesirable outcome, and also to look for the best materials for embolization.

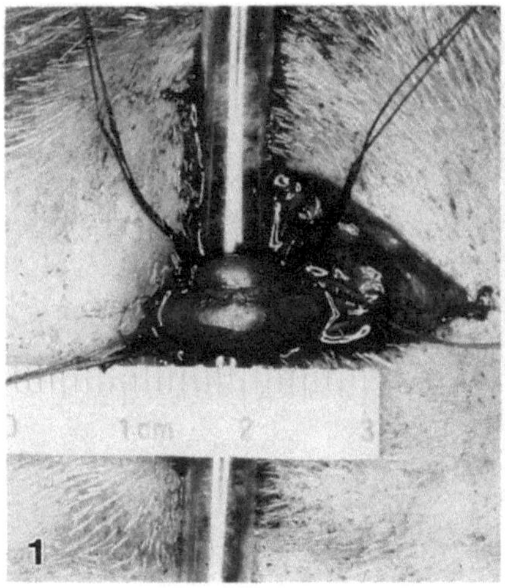

Fig. 1. Anastomosis of the right common carotid artery and jugular vein followed by jugular vein ligation at the proximal and distal ends

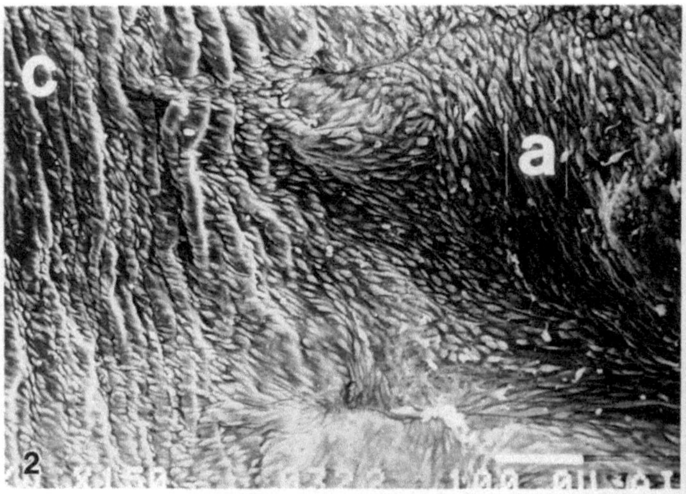

Fig. 2. Scanning electron microscopy of intra-aneurysmal surface. *c*, Carotid artery; *a*, aneurysm

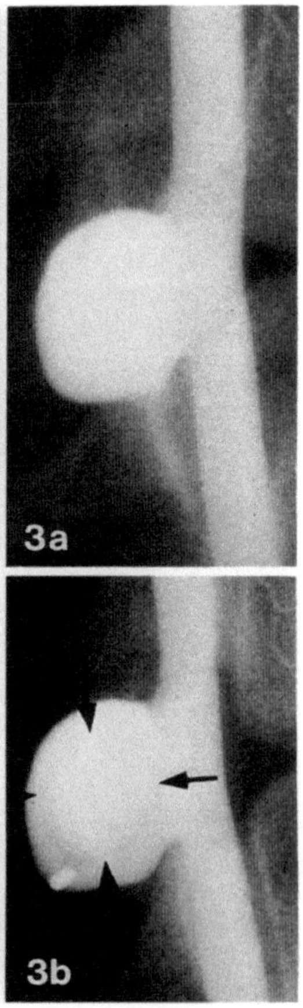

Fig. 3. **a** Pre-embolization; **b** post embolization

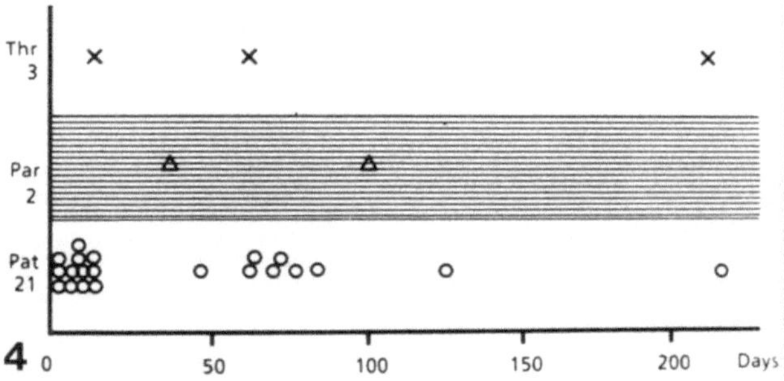

Fig. 4. Angiographic findings (Thr = thrombosed; Par = partially thrombosed; Pat = patent)

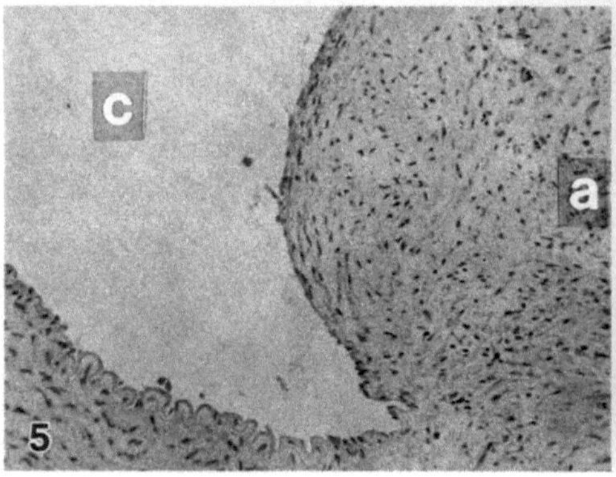

Fig. 5. Histological examination of the aneurysmal orifice

Methods

In 38 mongrel dogs weighing 10–20 kg the right common carotid artery and jugular vein were exposed in the neck. They were anastomosed side to side followed by jugular vein ligation at the proximal and distal ends (Fig. 1). Carotid angiography was performed the same day and repeated weekly. In a control group (without treatment) follow-up angiograms were obtained for 12 months. Their aneurysm patency rate was assessed. For the treated group, endovascular treatment was attempted if the aneurysm was confirmed by the angiogram at 1 week. Follow-up angiography was performed in the same manner.

Histological studies including light and scanning electron microscopy were performed to examine the intimal surface of the aneurysm before and after embolization (Fig. 2). The embolization method consisted of transcatheter detachable latex balloon occlusion of the aneurysm lumen under fluoroscopic control (Fig. 3).

Results

In the control group, 38 animals were operated upon and carotid angiograms were obtained in 26. Carotid aneurysm was successfully made in 21 animals. The patency rate was 81% 4 weeks after the operation (Fig. 4). Histological examination revealed the epithelial covering of the aneurysm's lumen.

In the treated group 10 animals were embolized by detachable balloon. Aneurysms of all treated animals were well occluded by the balloon. Histological examination revealed that the aneurysmal orifice was occluded by a fibrous membrane and covered by the endothelium from the carotid artery. The aneurysm cavity was filled with connective tissue (Fig. 5).

Discussion

The making of experimental aneurysms has been attempted by several investigators. Hypertensive rats were known to show aneurysm formation [1], but were too small to be treated by the endovascular approach.

In a larger animal a surgical method has been applied to make an aneurysm [2, 3]: we have used the venous patch method in dogs [4]. Angiographic and histological study confirmed that this aneurysm may mimic the human cerebral aneurysm and may be used to simulate endovascular treatment.

Our patency rate (81%) is thought to be adequate for the model: spontaneous closure occurred in rare instances.

The latex balloon is able to occlude the aneurysmal cavity permanently and shows no recanalization. Histological study also confirmed that a permanent cure was obtained by this method.

In conclusion, the experimental aneurysm which was made in the dog by a venous patch method can be one of the best models of human cerebral aneurysm. This model is also applicable for the simulation of endovascular treatment. Latex balloon has the ablility to occlude the aneurysm cavity permanently without recanalization.

References

1. Kojima M, Handa H, Hashimoto N, Kim C, Hazama F (1986) Early changes of experimentally induced cerebral aneurysms in rats: scanning electron microscopic study. Stroke 17: 835–841
2. Debrun GM, Varsos V, Liszczak TM, Davis KR, Heros RS, Zervas NT (1984) Obliteration of experimental aneurysms in dogs with isobutyl cyanoacrylate. J Neurosurg 61: 37–43
3. German WJ, Black SPW (1954) Experimental production of carotid aneurysms. N Engl J Med 250: 104–106
4. Keravel Y, Debrun G, Rottan N (1980) Treatment of the experimental aneurysms and carotid jugular fistulas by inflated and detachable balloons. Int J Microsurg 2: 33–38

Dr. Makoto Negoro
Department of Neurosurgery
Nagoya University School of Medicine
Nagoya 466, Japan

Neuroradiology (1991) 33 [Suppl]: 426–427

Neuro radiology
© Springer-Verlag 1991

Hypoplasia of vertebrobasilar arteries

U. Arnold*, R. Lehmann, H.-K. Kursawe, and W. Lückel

Department of Neuroradiology, Clinic for Neurology and Psychiatry, Medicine Section (Charité), Humboldt University, Berlin, Federal Republic of Germany

Summary. The term "hypoplasia of the vertebral artery" often used in clinical practice, is not exactly defined. We studied vertebral angiograms of 160 patients, paying attention to seven defined points, measuring the inner diameter of the vertebrobasilar arteries. The frequency of hypoplasia was recorded. The findings in patients with vertebrobasilar insufficiency (VBI) were correlated with those of other neurological patients. VBI patients had a significantly higher rate of vertebrobasilar hypoplasia and those *with* vertebrobasilar hypoplasia had permanent neurological deficits more frequently than other VBI patients.

Key words: Hypoplasia – Vertebrobasilar arteries – Vertebrobasilar insufficiency

There are few statistically adequate examinations of the calibres of the vertebral (VA) and basilar arteries (BA) [1, 2]. Hypoplasia of VA has not been angiographically defined. We studied vertebral angiograms to discover "normal variances" of diameters of VA and BA.

Materials and methods

From 1984 to 1986 vertebral angiograms (AOT 35 × 35, focus film distance of 110 cm) were studied as regards the diameters of VA and BA. Patients' ages ranged from 18 to 59 years, mean 43 years. The inner diameter was measured at seven defined points (Fig. 1). The left VA was visualised in 127 patients, the right in 62 and both in 7. Patients were in six groups: (1) tumours ($n = 50$); (2) subarachnoid haemorrhage ($n = 39$); (3) other intracranial haematoma ($n = 11$); (4) disturbances of the carotid circulation system ($n = 10$); (5) other neurological diseases ($n = 20$); (6) vertebrobasilar insufficiency (VBI) ($n = 30$).

Criteria for exclusion were: angioma, rare vessel diseases such as fibromuscular dysplasia or collagenosis, BA thrombosis, increased intracranial pressure, local spasm or compression by tumour. Patients with clinical VBI were subdivided into four degrees of severity [3].

Results

The average age of VBI patients was 49 years, and of patients with other neurological diseases 36 years, but there was showed no statistical connection between age and vessel diameter. Vessels of men were larger than those of women but not significantly.

Normal values of vessel calibre were based on their measured diameters in patients with tumours and other neurological diseases because these showed no significant deviation from the total mean value. The vessels were subdivided into five categories of calibre: hypoplastic (1), small (2), normal (3), large (4) and hyperplastic (5). Table 1 shows the calibres at each point of measurement. The diameter of VA decreased from proximal to distal. Altogether 8.4% of VA and 2.6% of BA were hypoplastic. Unilateral hypoplastic or small VA and the combination of two hypoplastic or small VA and BA were significantly more frequent in patients with VBI (Fig. 2).

The next question was the size of the contralateral artery in cases of hypoplastic or small VA (Fig. 3). Figure 4 shows the relation between severity of VBI and vessel diameter.

VBI patients with hypoplastic arteries had permanent neurological deficits more often than VBI patients with small, normal or hyperplastic vessels, but the difference is not significant because of the small numbers.

Discussion

Our results accord with those of Fiegel and Nadjmi [4] in brachiocephalic angiograms; Jung and Kehr [5], Jahn [6] in right vertebral angiograms; Voigt et al. [1] in brachiocephalic and vertebral angiograms, and Akimoto [8] in both projections of vertebral angiograms, all of whom based their "normal" measurements on patients, as we did. Another handicap is that in most cases only one VA was injected, usually the left, and only in 57.7% of cases did contrast medium reflux into the other side. Nevertheless hypoplastic or small VA were found in 21 (70%) in VBI, but in only 52 (40%) of other patients. These facts correlate with findings of Belenkaja [9] and Nothum [10].

In contrast to Toole and Patel [11] we found compensatory dilatation of the contralateral side in only 25% of cases with unilateral hypoplastic VA (Fig. 3).

Table 1. Grading of vertebrobasilar diameter (mm)

Point	Degree						
	1	2	3	4	5	Mean value	Standard deviation
1	< 3.7	< 4.3	4.3–5.4	> 5.4	> 6.0	4.87	0.59
2	< 3.3	< 4.1	4.1–5.6	> 5.6	> 6.3	4.78	0.76
3	< 3.1	< 3.9	3.9–5.6	> 5.6	> 6.5	4.77	0.88
4	< 2.6	< 3.4	3.4–5.0	> 5.0	> 5.9	4.23	0.85
5	< 1.9	< 2.6	2.6–4.1	> 4.1	> 4.9	3.38	0.76
6	< 2.3	< 2.9	2.9–4.4	> 4.4	> 5.0	3.66	0.71
7	< 2.4	< 3.1	3.1–4.3	> 4.3	> 4.9	3.69	0.64

* *Present address:* Klinik für Neurologie und Psychiatrie, Berlin-Lichtenberg, Federal Republic of Germany

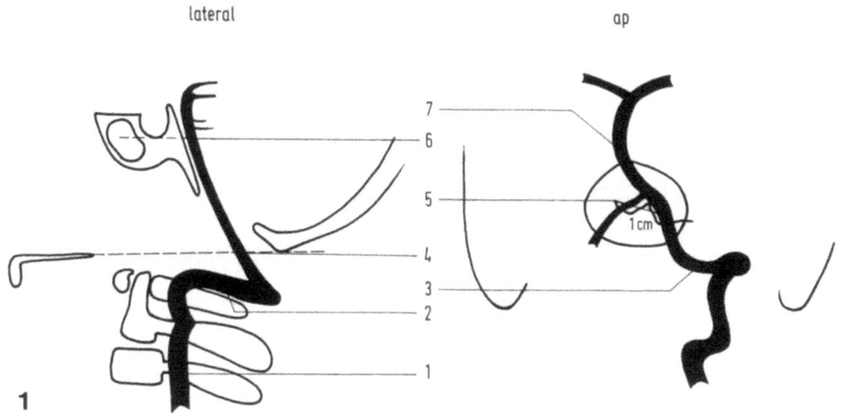

1

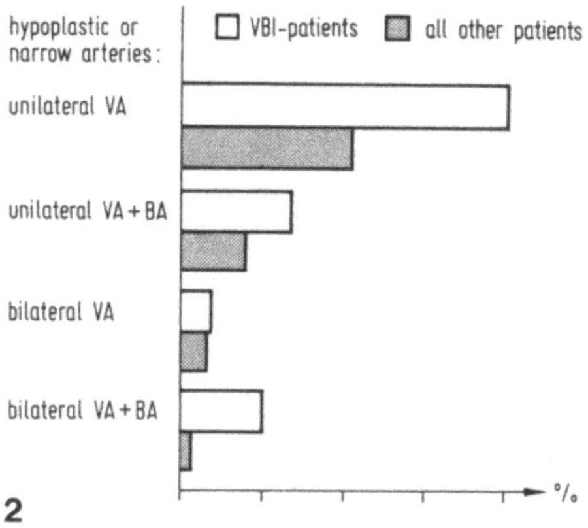

2

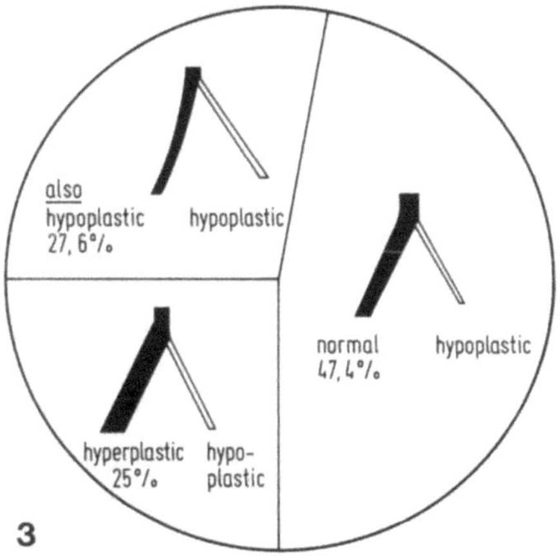

3

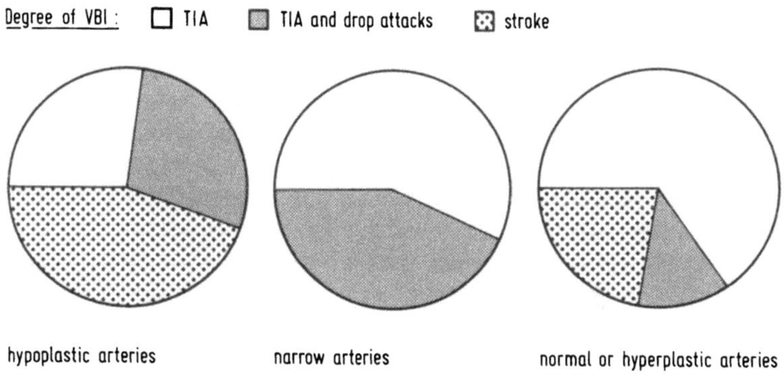

4

Fig. 1. Points of measurement of the inner diameter of the vertebral (VA) and basilar (BA) arteries

Fig. 2. Frequency of vertebrobasilar insufficiency (*VBI*) and other patients with hypoplastic or narrow VA or BA

Fig. 3. Size of contralateral arteries of patients with hypoplastic VA on the side injected

Fig. 4. Neurological deficit of VBI patients in relation to the diameter of VA. *TIA*, Transient ischaemic attack

Not all patients with hypoplasia have VBI; additional features (kinking, coiling, stenoses, blood pressure, blood viscosity, cardiac function etc.) are also important [3, 6, 12]. The choice of medical, operative [2] or interventional therapy such as angioplasty [2, 3, 13] depends upon these factors.

References

1. Blaisdell WF (1969) Joint study of extracranial arterial occlusion. IV. A review of surgical considerations. JAMA 209: 1889–1895
2. Brückmann H (1987) Die Bedeutung der Vertebralisangiographie für die Diagnostik und Therapie der vertebrobasilären Durchblutungsstörungen unter besonderer Berücksichtigung gefäßrekanalisierender Verfahren. Radiologe 27: 495–501
3. Zeumer H, Hauke P (1977) Ergebnisse angiographischer Untersuchungen bei Basilarisinsuffizienz. Dtsch Med Wochenschr 102: 425–428
4. Fiegel A, Nadjmi M (1971) Variationen der Arterien und ihre topometrischen Verhältnisse im retrograden Brachialisangiogramm. Röntgenblätter 24: 73–90
5. Jung A, Kehr P (1972) Das zerviko-enzephale Syndrom bei Arthrosen und nach Traumen der Halswirbelsäule. Manuel Med 10: 97–103
6. Jahn J (1971) Über Verlaufsanomalien im extrakraniellen Abschnitt der Hirnarterien (Tortuosity, Coiling u. Kinking) und ihre klinische Bedeutung für die cerebrovaskuläre Insuffizienz (statistische Korrelationen). Dissertation, Heidelberg
7. Voigt K (1977) Röntgenanatomische Variationsstatistik zur topographischen Beziehung zwischen a. basilaris und Schädelbasisstrukturen. Neuroradiologische Untersuchungen an Vertebralis- und Brachialisangiographien. Arch Psychiatr Nervenkr 215: 376–395
8. Akimoto H (1980) Roentgenological aspect of the basilar artery and its significance in clinical diagnosis (English summary). In: Excerpta Medica, section 8. Neurology and neurosurgery, 50: 1964
9. Belenkaja RM (1970) Cited in: Bragina LK, Koslova EN (1979) Die Bedeutung der Hypoplasie der a. vertebralis für die Durchblutungsstörungen des Gehirns (in Russian). Zh Nevropatol Psikhiatr 79: 1329–1332
10. Nothum U (1975) Über Verlaufsanomalien der Arteria vertebralis, basilaris und ihrer Äste und ihre klinische Bedeutung für die vertebro-basiläre Durchblutungsstörung. Dissertation, Heidelberg
11. Toole JF, Patel AN (1980) Zerebro-vaskuläre Störungen. Springer, Berlin Heidelberg New York
12. Lückel W, Lehmann R (1990) Bilaterale Subklaviaangiographie bei Patienten mit vertebrobasilärer Insuffizienz. Z Klin Med (in press)
13. Courtheoux P (1985) Transcutaneous angioplasty of vertebral artery atheromatous ostial stricture. Neuroradiology 27: 259–264

Dr. U. Arnold
Klinik für Neurologie und Psychiatrie
Berlin-Lichtenberg
Herzbergstraße 79
1130 Berlin, Federal Republic of Germany

Neuroradiology (1991) 33 [Suppl]: 428–429

Neuro-radiology
© Springer-Verlag 1991

Iomeprol in CT of the brain: multicentre phase II study

M. Leonardi[1], C. Del Favero[2], E. Biasizzo[1], G. Fabris[1], A. Lavaroni[1], A. Martegani[2], L. Tufarulo[2], and F. Zappoli[1]

[1] Department of Neuroradiology, H. Civile, Udine, Italy
[2] Department of Neuroradiology, H. Multizenale, Varese, Italy

Summary. The aim of the study was to assess the effectiveness and safety of iomeprol (300 mg I/ml) in CT of the brain. Thirty-one patients were enrolled according to strict inclusion and exclusion criteria necessary for a phase II study. The efficacy was judged to be good in 10 patients and excellent in 21. None of the patients showed clinically significant changes in vital parameters, ECG and EEG tracings or laboratory tests. Among the 31 patients there were no subjective reactions and only 1 patient complained of a side-effect. Taking into account the results of this multicentre trial we can conclude that iomeprol is a good contrast medium with excellent local and systemic tolerability.

Key words: Iomeprol – Water-soluble non-ionic contrast medium – Computed tomography – Brain – Side-effects

Iomeprol (B16880) is a non-ionic water-soluble contrast medium (CM) developed by Bracco Industria Chimica of Milan, Italy. Its chemical structure and physicochemical properties are shown in Fig. 1. Its radio-opacity is due to the presence of a tri-iodinized benzene ring; its water solubility to three side-chains containing highly hydrophylic groups. Preclinical studies revealed its excellent systemic and tissue tolerability in a pharmacokinetic pattern compatible with a two-compartment model, characterised by an apparent distribution volume equivalent to the extracellular space, rapid elimination (almost exclusively through the kidney), no serum protein binding, and no metabolic transformation. A phase I clinical study of 10 patients confirmed excellent toleration of iomeprol as well as its properties. The present paper summarises the results of an open non-controlled phase II study on CT of the brain.

Materials and methods

Thirty-one adult patients (16 males) aged between 18 and 65 years (mean 51 years) were submitted to CT of the brain. Basal assessment (in the 3 days preceding the radiological procedure) included: medical history, complete physical and neurological examination, laboratory tests, and 12-lead ECG and standard EEG recordings. Pregnancy tests were performed in fertile women. All the clinical, laboratory and neurophysiological tests were repeated 24 h after the procedure and at 72 h if altered.

Vital parameters (blood pressure and heart rate) were monitored at entry into the study, before, and 5, 10, 15 and 60 min after the injection. Ninety-five percent confidence intervals were used for statistical analysis. Films were assessed by two different radiologists for technical adequacy and scored for diagnostic quality according to the following scale: 1, inadequate opacification; 2, adequate opacification; 3, good opacification; 4, excellent opacification.

Local tolerability (heat sensation) and systemic adverse reactions that could follow CM administration were carefully recorded. The radiological equipment consisted of a General Electric 8800 and a Siemens Somaton 2. Iomeprol was administered to all patients at a rate of 7–10 ml/s. The mean volume of CM injected in each patient was 88 ml (range 50–100 ml).

Results

On entry into the study the physical and neurological examination was normal in 20 patients while it showed some abnormalities in the other 11; no variations occurred after the radiological procedure in any patient. Haematological and urinary parameters were in the normal range before the radiological procedure; 24-h monitoring showed no significant difference.

As regards blood pressure and heart rate no clinically and/or statistically significant alterations were detected, indicating that iomeprol has no consistent acute or chronic effect on vital parameters. None of the patients showed any changes in their ECG and EEG recordings after the procedure. No heat sensation was noticed by any patient of either centre. In 1 patient only, an adverse reaction was reported: it occurred 10 min after the CM injection, and consisted of some mild wheals and trunk erythema lasting about 1.5 h.

As regards radiographic effectiveness, in both centres there was complete agreement between the two neuroradiologists' judgement. All films were adequate for visualisation and diagnosis. The neuroradiologists judged

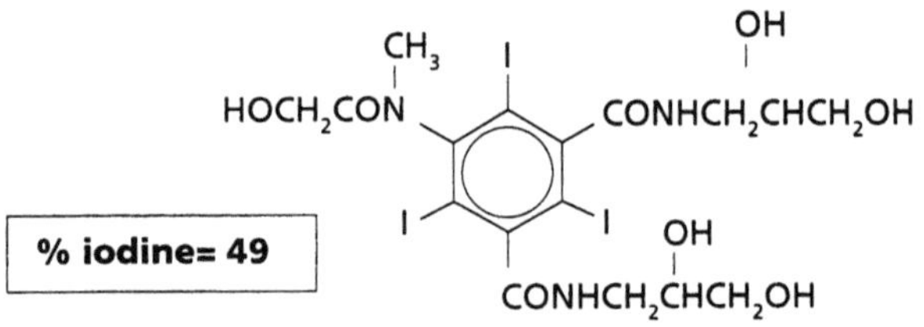

P.M. 777
Osmolality 521±24 mOsmlKg
Viscosity 8.1 mPa·s (20° C) – 4.5 mPa·s (37° C)

Fig. 1. Structural formula and physical characteristics of iomeprol the contrast to be good in 10 (32%) and excellent in 21 (68%) patients. No case of "inadequate" or "adequate" opacification was reported.

Discussion

At an iodine concentration of 300 mg/ml and, at the doses tested, iomeprol has good radiographic efficacy as well as local and systemic tolerability. Neither instrumental nor laboratory findings revealed any clinically and/or statistically significant alteration, confirming therefore that iomeprol is suitable for large-scale clinical trials.

Dr. M. Leonardi
H. Civile Generale Regionale
Via G. Pieri
I-33100 Udine, Italy

Neuroradiology (1991) 33 [Suppl]: 430–431

Neuroradiology
© Springer-Verlag 1991

Delay of tibial F-wave response after lumbar myelography: time course and comparison of two contrast media (iotrolan and iopamidol)

N. Prey, G. Kubina, and P. Stoeter

Elisabethen-Krankenhaus, Ravensburg, Federal Republic of Germany

Summary. In seven patients, the time course of the delay of the tibial F-wave response was examined after lumbar myelography with iopamidol (250 mg I/ml) by recordings before and in 60-min intervals after the examination. The maximum delay was found 3 h after the examination with an average slowing of nerve conduction velocity of 4% and a return to nearly normal values after 5 h. In 36 patients the delay caused by intrathecal iopamidol was compared with that of iotralan (240 mg I/ml). No significant difference was found between the two contrast media. The delay of the tibial F-wave response after lumbar myelography is a reproducible but transient effect without clinical sequelae and may be used as an indicator of "neurotoxicity".

Key words: Delay of tibial F-wave – Lumbar myelography – Iopamidol – Iotrolan – Neurotoxicity

In previous studies, a delay of the tibial F-wave was observed after lumbar myelography with iotrolan [1] and iohexol [2]. This delay was not demonstrated after lumbar puncture alone. It is probably caused by a "neurotoxic" effect of the high concentration of contrast medium (CM) in the lower dural sac around the fibres of the cauda equina. This pool of CM has to be traversed twice by the potential generating the F-wave: after an antidromic excitation of the motor nerve and its alpha motor neuron, the impulse runs back orthodromically to the motor end plate (Fig. 1). For this reason, the delay of the tibial F-wave after lumbar

Fig. 1. Diagramatic representation of F-wave of the tibial nerve. The F-wave is caused by an antidromic excitation of the tibial nerve and its alpha motor neuron. The impulse runs back orthodromically to the motor end plate generating the F-wave potential. Thus, it passes twice through the highly concentrated of contrast medium in the lumbar dural sac

Fig. 2. Time course of F-wave delay. F-wave of the tibial nerve in 60 min intervals after myelography with iopamidol. Transient maximum delay after 3 h

Fig. 3. Comparison of iotrolan and iopamidol. Delay of tibial F-wave shows no significant difference (Wilcoxon-Mann-Whitney U-test, $P > 0.4$)

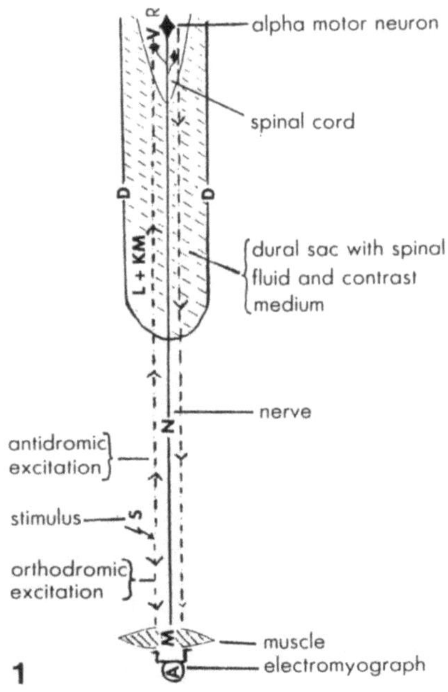

1

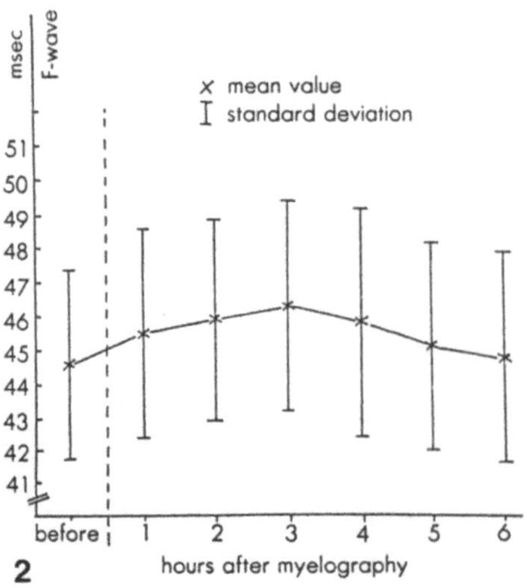

2

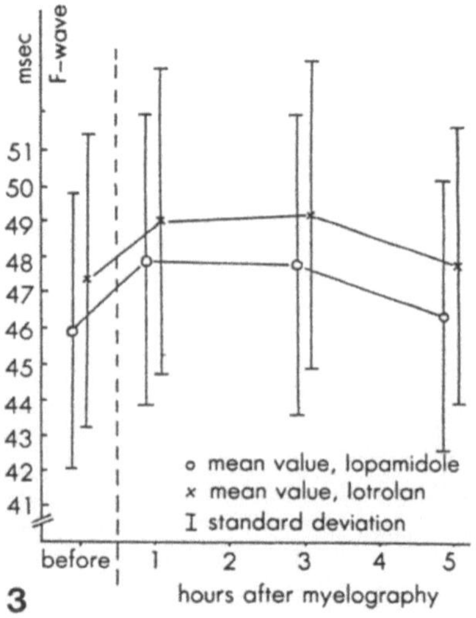

3

myelography is more pronounced than the impairment of the F-wave of the median nerve or the somatosensory evoked potentials [1]. In the present study, the time course of the F-wave delay and the effect of two different CMs were examined.

Patients and methods

For the time course examinations, F-waves of the tibial nerve were recorded before and in 60-min intervals after lumbar myelography with iopamidol (10 ml, 250 mg I/ml) in 7 patients with sciatica. The recording was performed on the non-affected leg. The comparison of iotrolan and iopamidol (240 mg I/ml) was conducted as a double-blind randomized study in 36 patients. The F-waves were recorded before and 1, 3 and 5 h after myelography. The results were compared with the Wilcoxon-Mann-Whitney U-test.

Results

A delay of the tibial F-wave after myelography was observed in every case. Investigation of the time course showed a maximum delay after 3 h with an average slowing of conduction velocity of 4% and a recovery to nearly normal values after 5 h (Fig. 2). Comparison of the F-wave delay after injection of iotrolan and iopamidol showed no significant difference ($P < 0.4$, Fig. 3). No clinical side-effects were observed.

Discussion

Previous studies showing a reproducible delay of the F-wave after lumbar myelography [1] were confirmed by the present study. The impairment of nerve conduction is a transient effect being maximal after 3 h and is observed with monomeric (iopamidol) and dimeric (iotrolan) CM without significant difference. The fact that it was not seen after myelography with metrizamide [2] cannot be explained. Broadbridge et al. [3, 4] found a lengthening of the visual evoked response latency 20 h after myelography with iopamidol and metrizamide, but not with iohexol. These differences could be due to an inappropriate time course of recording.

Because of its reproducibility, the delay of the F-wave may be used as an electrophysiological indicator of "neurotoxicity". However, use of these CM should not be restricted by this effect because it obviously does not cause clinical complaints.

References

1. Prey N, Kubina G, Staudacher T, Stoeter P (1988) Delay of tibial F-wave response after lumbar myeloradiculography. In: Nadjmi M (ed) Imaging of brain metabolism. 15th Congress of the European Society of Neuroradiology. Springer, Berlin Heidelberg New York, pp 233–236
2. Sand T (1988) F-responses after metrizamide and iohexol lumbar myelography. Neuroradiology 30: 534–537
3. Broadbridge AT, Bayliss SG, Firth R, Farrell G (1984) Visual evoked response changes following intrathecal injection of water-soluble contrast media: a possible method of assessing neurotoxicity and a comparison of metrizamide and iopamidol. Clin Radiol 35: 371–373
4. Broadbridge AT, Bayliss SG, Brayshaw CI (1987) The effect of intrathecal iohexol on visual evoked response latency: a comparison including incidence of headache with iopamidol and metrizamide in myeloradiculography. Clin Radiol 38: 71–74

Dr. N. Prey
Elisabethen-Krankenhaus
W-7980 Ravensburg
Federal Republic of Germany

Neuroradiology (1991) 33 [Suppl]: 432–433

Neuro radiology
© Springer-Verlag 1991

Iomeprol in conventional angiography of supra-aortic and cerebral arteries: multicentre phase II study

A. Beltramello, A. Benati, N. Caputo, E. Signorini, C. De Grandi, G. Scialfa, R. Bardo, and G. Belloni

Departments of Neuroradiology of Verona; Perugia; Niguarda Hospital, Milan; Bergamo, Italy

Summary. Iomeprol is a new non-ionic water-soluble contrast medium (CM). The results of an open non-controlled phase II clinical trial carried out in four different Italian centres are reported. The aim of the study was to assess the safety and the efficacy of the 300 mg iodine solution of iomeprol in conventional arteriography of supra-aortic and cerebral arteries. No clinically significant changes of vital signs, laboratory tests and instrumental parameters were observed during and after the procedure in 60 patients (aged 19–63 years) submitted to 191 selective arteriograms (total CM injected ranging between 20 and 125 ml). Contrast effectiveness was scored as good or optimal on 183 occasions, and sufficient in 8. Mild or moderate adverse reactions occurred in 8 patients. According to these results, iomeprol at the tested concentrations and doses proved to be an effective and safe CM for cerebral angiography.

Key words: Iomeprol – Water-soluble non-ionic contrast medium – Cerebral angiography – Side-effects

Iomeprol is a new non-ionic monomeric tri-iodinated water-soluble contrast medium (CM) synthesized in the Research Laboratories of Bracco Industria Chimica, of Milan, Italy. Its physicochemical properties are: molecular weight 777.06, osmolality (300 mg I/ml) 0.52 osmol/kg and viscosity 8.1 mPa/s. Due to these characteristics the product yields more concentrated aqueous solutions, with lower osmolality than other currently available monomeric non-ionic CM. Preclinical studies revealed its excellent systemic and tissue tolerability in a pharmacokinetic pattern compatible with a two-compartment model, characterized by an apparent distribution volume equivalent to the extracellular space, rapid elimination (almost exclusively through the kidney), no serum protein binding, and no metabolic transformation. A phase I clinical study of ten patients in need of urographic examination confirmed the excellent tolerability of iomeprol in doses up to 100 ml of a solution containing 300 mg/ml iodine, as well as its prompt renal elimination and excellent contrasting properties. The present paper summarizes the results of an open non-controlled phase II study.

Materials and methods

Sixty adult patients (38 males) aged between 19 and 63 years (mean 45.2 years) were submitted to conventional arteriography of the supra-aortic and cerebral arteries. Basal assessment (in the 3 days preceding the radiological procedure) included: medical history, complete physical and neurological examinations, laboratory tests, 12-lead ECG and standard EEG recordings. Pregnancy tests were performed in fertile women. All the clinical, laboratory and electrophysiological tests were repeated 24 h after arteriography and at 72 h if alterated. ECG and EEG tracings were recorded throughout the procedure.

Vital parameters (blood pressure and heart rate) were monitored at entry to the study, before, during and after each CM injection and over the next hour (at 5, 10, 15 and 60 min). Ninety-five percent confidence intervals and ANOVA were used for statistical analysis. CM volumes and flow rates were adjusted according to the arterial territory under investigation. Films from each injection were assessed by two different radiologists for technical adequacy and scored for diagnostic quality according to the following scale: 1, inadequate opacification; 2, adequate opacification; 3, good opacification; 4, excellent opacification.

Local tolerability (heat and pain sensations on the side of injection) and systemic adverse reactions that could follow CM administration were carefully recorded. A total of 191 selective cerebral angiograms was performed: iomeprol was administered through 5–6 F catheters by transfemoral approach using an automatic injector. The total CM volume injected varied from 20 ml to 125 ml (mean 60 ml) and the range of injections performed per patient was 1–10.

Results

No change in physical or neurological condition was observed 24 h after iomeprol administration. Post procedural laboratory tests were not statistically different from the basal ones. While no effect on blood pressure and heart rate was detected during the procedure, multiple comparison test according to the Student-Neuman Keuls method showed a statistically significant ($P < 0.05$) increase in systolic blood pressure at 10 min as compared with the basal values in one centre. No relevant ECG and EEG abnormalities were detected during or after the procedures. Patients complained of heat sensation on 174 occasions (11 mild, 51 moderate and 12 severe). Pain occurred after 11 of 191 injections: it was mild, moderate and severe in 1,7 and 3 instances, respectively (Table 1). The severe heat sensations occurred 8 times when the catheter was positioned in a common carotid artery, twice in the internal carotid artery and twice in vertebral arteries. Severe pain sensations were reported after catheter posi-

Table 1. Pain and heat sensations occurring after iomeprol injection

Tolerance	Absent	Mild	Moderate	Severe
Heat sensation	17	110	51	12
Pain sensation	180	1	7	3

12 severe heat sensations: 8 common carotid, 2 internal carotid, 2 vertebral arteries
3 severe pain sensations: common carotid

Table 2. Efficacy of opacification in relation to catheter positioning

Catheter positioning	Insufficient	Sufficient	Good	Excellent
Epi-aortic arteries	–	3	4	16
Common carotid	–	5	66	41
Internal carotid	–	–	7	21
External carotid	–	–	2	1
Vertebral arteries	–	–	8	17
Total	–	8	87	96

tioning in a common carotid artery. Among the 60 patients who underwent the radiological procedure with iomeprol, there was no adverse reaction unequivocally related to the CM. Four patients complained of teichopsia, and 1 of trembling of one side of the body. One patient, 15 min after the last injection, complained of a mild tingling sensation in his hand and face lasting for 20 min. In all cases the reaction spontaneously abated; the investigators excluded any relation to CM administration. One patient complained of mild headache, which was attributed by the investigator to the underlying pathology. In 1 case general discomfort, bradycardia and Jacksonian epilepsy were observed during the catheter positioning: the reaction lasted about 2 min, was moderate and ended after appropriate treatment. The investigators attributed the reaction to a vasovagal reflex trigged by stimulation of the carotid glomus during the positioning of the catheter at the carotid bifurcation. As regards radiographic contrast, in all but one centre there was an almost complete agreement between the two neuroradiologists' judgement. All the images obtained were adequate for radiological diagnosis. The images were scored as adequate in 8 (4%) good in 87 (46%) and excellent in 96 (50%) cases. No case of inadequate opacification was reported (Table 2). In conclusion, iomeprol at the tested concentration and doses proved to be an effective and safe CM for conventional arteriography of supra-aortic and cerebral arteries in adult patients. Image quality was always satisfactory and in all cases radiological diagnosis could be achieved; neither instrumental nor laboratory tests were modified by iomeprol administration; subjective tolerance was good; adverse reactions occurred in only 8 patients and were never related to the CM.

A. Beltramello
Service of Neuroradiology
Verona University Hospital
P. le Stefani 1
Verona, Italy

Neuroradiology (1991) 33 [Suppl]: 434–435

Neuro radiology
© Springer-Verlag 1991

Iomeprol in computed axial tomography of the brain: phase II study in children

P. Minguzzi, R. Ruggiero, G. Carannante, M. C. Buonocore, D. Graziano, and A. Ambrosio

Department of Neurosurgery, Neuroradiological Service, Santobono Hospital, Naples, Italy

Summary. Safety and effectiveness of a new non-ionic contrast medium (CM), iomeprol (300 mg I/ml), were evaluated in children undergoing cranial CT. The results of an open phase II clinical trial are reported. Fifty inpatients (aged 1 month to 14 years) were enrolled and the CM was administered intravenously as a bolus injection (mean total volume between 6 and 90 ml). No clinically important changes in vital parameters or laboratory tests were detected and the mean values after procedure were inside 95% confidence intervals of the preinvestigation mean basal values. Neither ECG nor EEG were modified. Contrast effectiveness was scored as good or excellent on 48 occasions, and adequate on 2. Mild hypotension and tachycardia occurred in 2 patients. These results in paediatric patients confirm the previous data from adults and suggest a good tolerability as well as efficacy of iomeprol.

Key words: Iomeprol – Water-soluble non-ionic contrast medium – Brain – Computed tomography – Side-effects

Iomeprol is a new compound belonging to the class of non-ionic water-soluble contrast media (CM). Its physicochemical properties are: molecular weight 777.06, osmolality (300 mg I/ml) 0.52 osmol/kg and viscosity 8.1 mPa/s at 20 °C. Due to these characteristics the product yields more concentrated aqueous solutions, with lower osmolality than other currently available monomeric non-ionic CM. In vitro and preclinical studies in experimental animals indicated that the new product was well tolerated, produced excellent radiological contrast, and had entirely favourable pharmacodynamic and pharmacokinetic properties. On the strength of such documentation iomeprol was approved for clinical trials in man. A phase I clinical study in healthy volunteers was followed by five multicentre phase II trials in urography, computed axial tomography of the brain and body, angiocardiography, and conventional cerebral, visceral, and peripheral angiography. The results of these studies, involving a total of 300 adult patients, showed that iomeprol was well tolerated and effective in intravascular applications. The present paper summarizes the results of an open non-controlled phase II clinical trial in children carried out in one Italian centre.

Materials and methods

Fifty children (26 males) aged between 1 month and 14 years (Table 1) were subjected to computed axial tomography of the brain. Basal assessment (in the 7 days prior to the radiological procedure) included: medical history, complete physical and neurological examinations, laboratory tests, 12-lead ECG and standard EEG recordings. All the clinical, laboratory and neurophysiological tests were repeated 24 and 72 h after the radiological procedure. Vital parameters (blood pressure, heart rate, and body temperature) were monitored at the entry, before, and after the CM injection (at 1, 30, 60, and 120 min).

Systemic adverse reactions that could follow CM administration were carefully recorded. Ninety-five percent confidence intervals and ANOVA were used at statistical analysis. The CM was administered manually as a bolus intravenous injection; the volumes injected are reported in Table 2 according to age and weight. CT images were evaluated by two different radiologists for technical adequacy and scored for diagnostic quality according to the following scale: 1, inadequate opacification; 2, adequate opacification; 3, good opacification; 4, excellent opacification.

CT numbers were measured before and after CM injection in regions of interest located in grey and white matter and in pathological areas.

Results

No change in physical and neurological condition was observed either 24 or 72 h after iomeprol administration. No clinically important changes in vital parameters and labo-

Table 1. Ages of 50 children studied (26 males)

Subgroup	Age	No. of patients
1	1– 6 months	2
2	7–12 months	6
3	13–23 months	1
4	2– 6 years	23
5	7–10 years	9
6	11–14 years	9

Table 2. Volumes of iomeprol injected according to age and weight

Subgroup	Weight (kg)	Volume (ml)
1	3.6–8	6–20
2	9–12	8–20
3	15	15
4	12–28[a]	6–60[b]
5	25–50	18–60
6	30–50	22–90

[a] 18.83 ± 4.01 (mean ± SD)

[b] 20.04 ± 11.01 (mean ± SD) – bolus injection

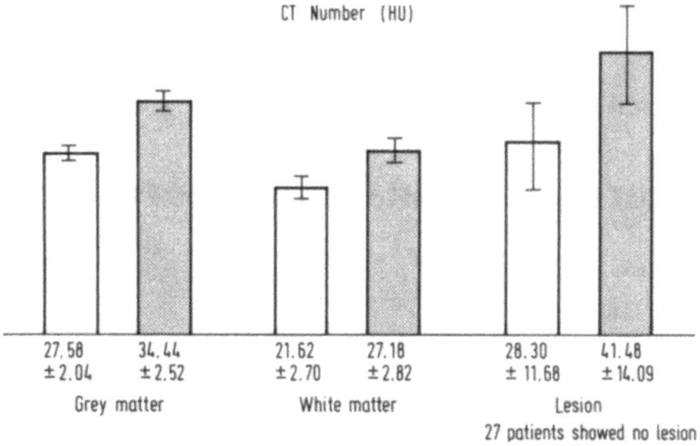

Fig. 1. CT numbers obtained on pre- □ and postinjection ▩ images of grey and white matter and pathological areas

ratory tests were detected and the mean values after the procedure were within 95% confidence intervals of the mean basal values. Neither ECG nor EEG recordings were modified. Two patients complained of mild hypotension and tachycardia which started 1 min after the injection and lasted in the first case 5 min and in the second 30 min. These side-effects were attributed to CM administration. As regards image quality, there was an almost complete agreement between the two neuroradiologists' judgement. All the images obtained were adequate for radiological diagnosis: the images were scored as adequate in 2 (4%) good in 42 (84%) and excellent in 6 (12%) cases. No case of inadequate opacification was reported. CT numbers (Hounsfield units) obtained on pre- and postinjection scans showed contrast enhancement of about 25% in grey matter, 26% in white matter, and 46% in pathological areas (Fig. 1). Lesions were seen only in 23 patients.

Discussion

These results in 50 children confirm the previous data in adults and suggest good toleration of the tested concentration and doses. Image quality was always satisfactory and contrast enhancement allowed in every case accurate demonstation of the pathology.

P. Minguzzi
Medical Department
Bracco Industria Chimica SPA
I-20100 Milan, Italy

Neuroradiology (1991) 33 [Suppl]: 436–437

Neuro-radiology
© Springer-Verlag 1991

Digital subtraction cisternography in cerebrospinal fluid rhinorrhoea and otorrhoea

A. K. Wakhloo[1], M. Schumacher[1], and H. R. Eggert[2]

[1] Section of Neuroradiology, Department of Radiology and
[2] Department of Neurosurgery, University of Freiburg, Freiburg, Federal Republic of Germany

Summary. The study evaluates the ability of digital subtraction cisternography (DSC) to delineate the actual site of dural defect in liquorrhoea. DSC was performed 14 times in 12 patients with cerebrospinal fluid (CSF) rhinorrhoea and 1 patient with otorrhoea: the exact site of a dural lesion could be shown in 7 of 9 cases with active CSF leakage. The investigation was followed by CT cisternography, defining the lesion in the coronal view. In 2 cases the basal subarachnoid space could not be filled sufficiently with contrast medium. DSC performed in a "dry period" (4 cases) did not reveal the site of leakage. In 7 of 8 patients surgery confirmed the site of the lesion. DSC can be recommended in addition to CT cisternography for visualizing the actual site of CSF fistula.

Key words: Cerebrospinal fluid rhinorrhoea – Cerebrospinal fluid otorrhoea – Computed tomographic cisternography – Digital subtraction fluoroscopy – Digital subtraction cisternography

Approximately 80% of cerebrospinal fluid (CSF) fistulae result from trauma to the skull base [1]. Persisting CSF leakage leads to recurrent episodes of meningitis in about 25% of all cases. Exact preoperative localization of the dural defect is essential for successful surgery. CT cisternography has proved to be the most useful method for detecting CSF fistulae [2]. Our study explores the use of digital subtraction cisternography (DSC).

Patients and methods

DSC was performed 14 times in 13 patients (7 men, 6 women, mean age 52 years, range 22–81 years). Twelve patients presented with CSF rhinorrhoea and 1 patient developed CSF otorrhoea after partial petrosectomy for cholesteatoma. At the time of investigation 9 patients showed active leakage. Four had experienced one or more episodes of meningitis. The interval between initial symptoms and diagnosis ranged from 2 weeks to several years. Patients with acute leakage after head injury were excluded.

The patient was placed in the prone position with the head inclined downward 20 ° s, after C1/C2 puncture using a 22-gauge spinal needle. About 8 ml non-ionic contrast medium (200 mg I/ml) was injected intrathecally under real-time digital subtraction fluoroscopy at a rate of 3 pictures/s. None of the sequences exceeded a period of 50 s determined by factors of the DSA unit. In 4 patients who were not actively leaking the CSF pressure was raised by injecting 10 ml saline solution. The passage of contrast medium through the fistula was documented in lateral and in 4 cases in anteroposterior projections. The investigation was followed by CT cisternography in the coronal plane with 2-mm slice thickness. 10 mg i.m. diazepam was administered prophylactically to prevent convulsions.

Results

DSC showed the exact site of CSF leakage in 7 of 9 patients with active rhinorrhoea: in 4 the dural defect was in the cribriform plate; 1 case involved the middle cranial fossa. Two patients showed leakage at the tuberculum sellae. Due to artefacts from the ethmoid cells and superimposition of the frontal cisterns, investigation in the anteroposterior projection did not prove satisfactory even using the digital subtraction technique. CT cisternography did not reveal the site of leakage in more cases but when findings were positive localization in the coronal plane was possible. In 2 cases the frontal subarachnoid space did not fill sufficiently during the 50 s sequence due to haematoma and a case of prefixed chiasm with arachnoid adhesions (Fig. 1). DSC performed in 4 patients without active CSF leakage did not reveal a dural lesion. Attempts to promote leakage by increasing CSF pressure failed.

Altogether, 8 patients were operated upon and rhinorrhoea ceased in all but 1. An elderly woman with a huge partly resected orbital basal cell carcinoma and destruction of the skull base with CSF rhinorrhoea refused

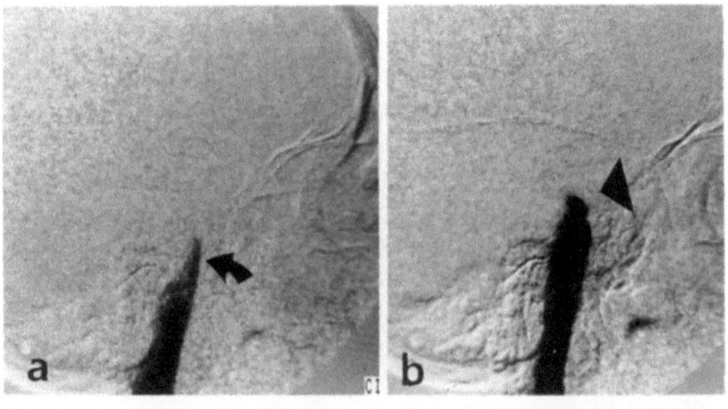

Fig. 1 a, b. Patient with delayed traumatic cerebrospinal fluid (CSF) rhinorrhoea. Digital subtraction cisternography (DSC) in lateral projection. Intrathecally injected contrast medium reaches the pontine cistern *(arrow)* and gradually extends to the interpeduncular cistern *(arrowhead)*. No filling of the chiasmatic cistern or frontal subarachnoid space due to haematoma (surgical finding)

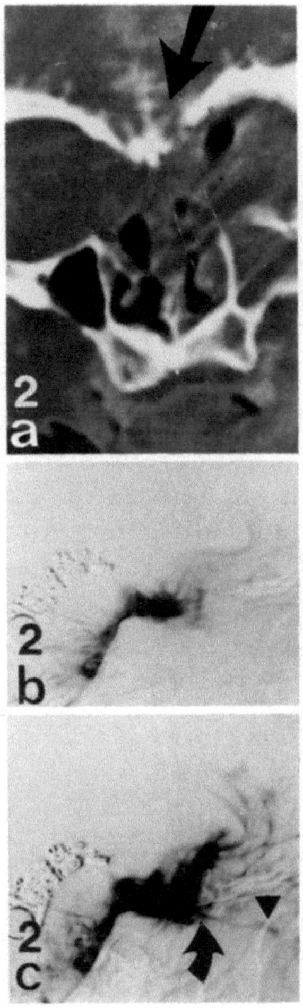

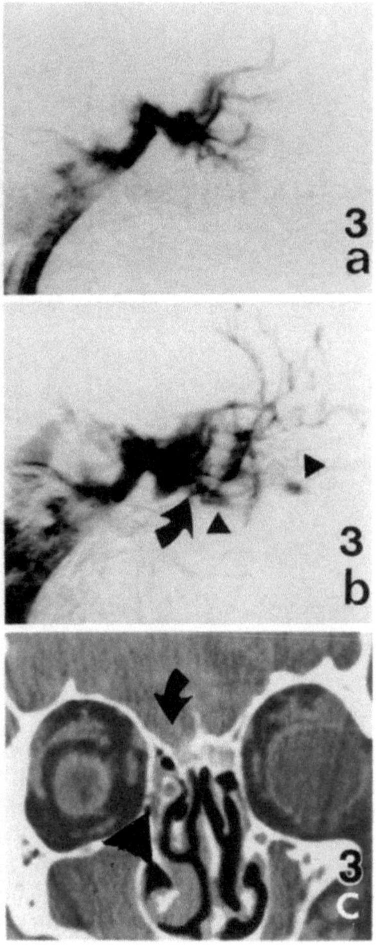

Fig. 2 a–c. Patient with CSF rhinorrhoea after partial resection of an orbital basal cell carcinoma. Coronal CT cisternography (**a**) and DSC in lateral projection (**b, c**) depict the dural and osseous defect in the posterior portion of the cribriform plate (*arrows* in **a, c**). Accumulation of contrast medium within the ethmoidal sinus (*arrowhead* in **c**)

Fig. 3 a–c. Patient presenting with CSF rhinorrhoea due to a meningioma en plaque (surgical finding). DSC (**a, b**) in lateral projection and coronal preoperative CT cisternography (**c**) show dural and osseous defect in the planum sphenoidale (*arrow* in **c**). Leakage of contrast medium at the tuberculum (*arrow* in **b**) and accumulation within the ethmoidal sinus (*arrowheads* in **b, c**)

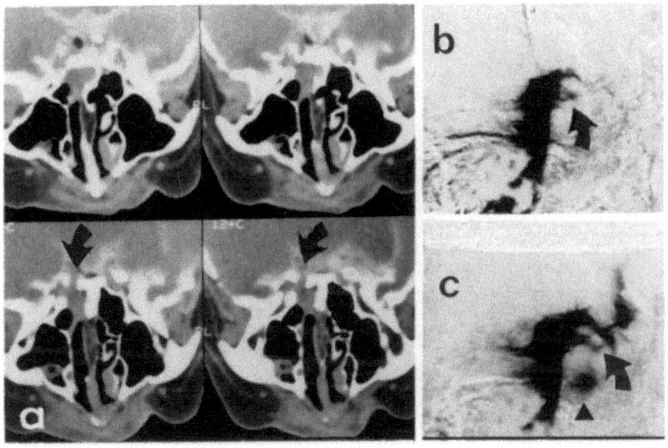

Fig. 4 a–c. Patient with delayed traumatic CSF rhinorrhoea. Semicoronal CT cisternography (**a**) and DSC in lateral projection (**b, c**) reveal a CSF fistula at foramen rotundum *(arrows)* with accumulation of contrast medium within the sphenoid sinus *(arrowhead)*

surgery (Fig. 2). In 2 cases fistulae developed after surgery for anterior fossa meningioma. An endotheliomatous meningioma was found in one case of CSF rhinorrhoea. The tumour was not demonstated by contrast-enhanced preoperative CT (Fig. 3). In 5 cases of traumatic CSF leakage, in only 2 did DSC reveal the site of fistula (Fig. 4). One was a rare case of Meckel's cave fistula with leakage to a hyperplastic sphenoid sinus. CT and MRI in a young patient with recurrent meningitis demonstrated a huge nasal encephalomeningocele. DSC showed the actual site of leakage. Further causes of CSF leakage included hydrocephalus and trans-sphenoidal surgery.

Discussion

The localization of a CSF fistula, especially in "dry periods", when the patient is unaware of leakage, may be quite difficult, but exact delineation of the dural lesion is essential for surgery. Radionuclide cisternography is a reliable method [3]: the side of leakage can usually be detected but the exact point of the fistula is not visible. Plain films may be helpful only in large bone defects. CT cisternography has proved the most precise method for detecting dural and osseous defects. However, being a static investigation, may not indicate whether an osseous defect is responsible for the leakage. This applies particularly to the area of the cribriform plate. Our study confirms the ability of digital subtraction technique to show fistulae, described recently by Takahashi et al. [4] in two cases of traumatic CSF rhinorrhoea.

The exact site of leakage, confirmed surgically could be located in 7 of 9 cases of active leakage. The results were comparable with CT cisternography. DSC performed in the "dry period" did not reveal the defect. Other reasons for negative results were inadequate filling of frontal subarachnoid space.

Being a relatively noninvasive dynamic method with no complications, DSC is recommended in addition to CT cisternography in active CSF rhinorrhoea and otorrhoea.

References

1. Loew F, Pertuiset B, Chaumier EE, Jaksche H (1984) Traumatic, spontaneous and postoperative CSF rhinorrhoea. Adv Tech Stand Neurosurg 11: 169–207
2. Naidich TP, Moran CJ (1980) Precise anatomic localization of atraumatic sphenoethmoidal cerebrospinal fluid rhinorrhea by metrizamide CT cisternography. J Neurosurg 53: 222–228
3. Curnes JT, Vincent LM, Kowalsky RJ, McCartney WH, Staab EV (1985) CSF rhinorrhoea: detection and localization using overpressure cisternography with Tc-99m-DTPA. Radiology 154: 795–799
4. Takahashi T, Mutsuga N, Aoki T, Handa T, Tanoi C, Yoshida J, Kobayash (1988) Localization of dural fistulas using metrizamide digital subtraction fluoroscopic cisternography. J Neurosurg 68: 721–725

Dr. A. K. Wakhloo
Section of Neuroradiology
University of Freiburg
W-7800 Freiburg
Federal Republic of Germany

Neuroradiology (1991) 33 [Suppl]: 438–439

Neuro
radiology
© Springer-Verlag 1991

Digital image management and its use in clinical neuroradiology

K. Miyasaka, S. Terae, S. Abe, and G. Irie

Department of Radiology, Hokkaido University School of Medicine and University Hospital, Sapporo, Japan

Summary. Image quality of the work station is acceptable in neuroimaging, but manipulation of window width and level for brightness is mandatory to CRT diagnosis. Data compression of neuroimages without significant degradation is employed. The Hokkaido University picture archiving communication system and its functions can be acceptable in the management of neuroimages.

Key words: Computer – Image processing – Picture archiving communication system

Medical images have greatly multiplied and now occupy a large amount of hospital space and are not easily accessible for clinical usage and research. Between 5% and 20% are lost within several years. Since 1982, we have tried to manage medical images as digital data using a digital imaging system, optical discs, local area network and computers. Such a digital data management system has recently started clinical service in our hospital although it is still experimental and at present covers only the radiology department and a part of the outpatient clinics. In neuroradiology, the reading of CT and MR images has been increasingly performed at a work station CRT instead of from transparent film. We present the system [so-called Hokkaido University – picture archiving communication system (HU-PACS)] and its preliminary clinical assessment in the neuroradiological field.

Methods

System design (hardware)

The data flow is shown in Fig. 1. Characteristic points of the system are as follows:

1. Local area network (LAN): optical loop LAN of 100 Mbps connected with Eathernet type branch LAN of 10 Mbps.
2. Data storage: optical disc libraries (ODL) of a jukebox type (96 GB × 2) for long-term archives and staging magnetic disc units (MDU, 2.4 GB × 2) for quick data access.
3. Imaging system (date input): all X-rays are to be taken via Fuji Computed Radiology system (CR). Six CR, three CT, one MRI and one film digitiser are now working. CR for angiography will be installed in the next fiscal year.
4. Image display: four image work stations (IWS) with two cathode ray tubes (CRT) monitors in the Radiology Department and 16 image display terminals (IDT) with one monitor for outpatient clinics. Laser printers are also available in HU-PACS.
5. The HU-PACS system is linked with the hospital information system (HIS) via a host computer (ACOS): about 300 ordering terminals are distributed in the HIS. The ACOS manages both image data and HIS including patient administration, laboratory data, prescriptions and so on.
6. Reporting system connecting with HIS: a computerised reporting system is connected with HIS, so that a report can be seen on the ordering terminal although this facility is limited to CT at present.

Management of the system (software)

Data compression. About one-tenth compression for CR and digitised film, and about one-third for CT and MRI are routinely employed.

Prefetching and down loading of images. An old image for reference is transferred beforehand from ODL to MDU for booked patients. A new image is automatically transferred to the referred work station.

Image processing at work station. Functions (software): more than 20 are available in IWS and IDT, including window width and level of grey scale, magnification, frequency enhancement, multidisplay of images and so on.

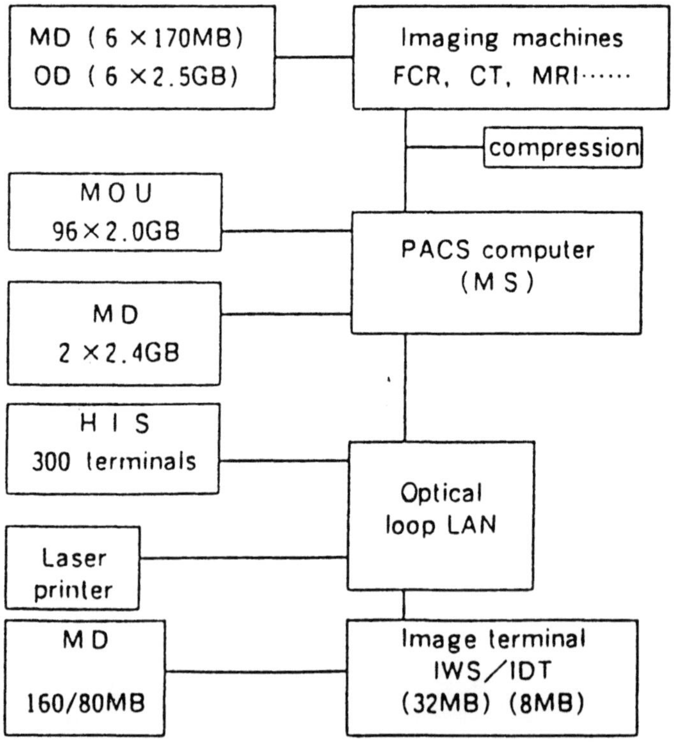

Fig. 1. Data flow of Hokkaido University picture archiving communication system *MOU,* Multioptical disc unit; *MD,* magnetic disc; *OD,* optical disc; *HIS,* hospital information system; *IWS,* image work station; *IDT,* image data terminal

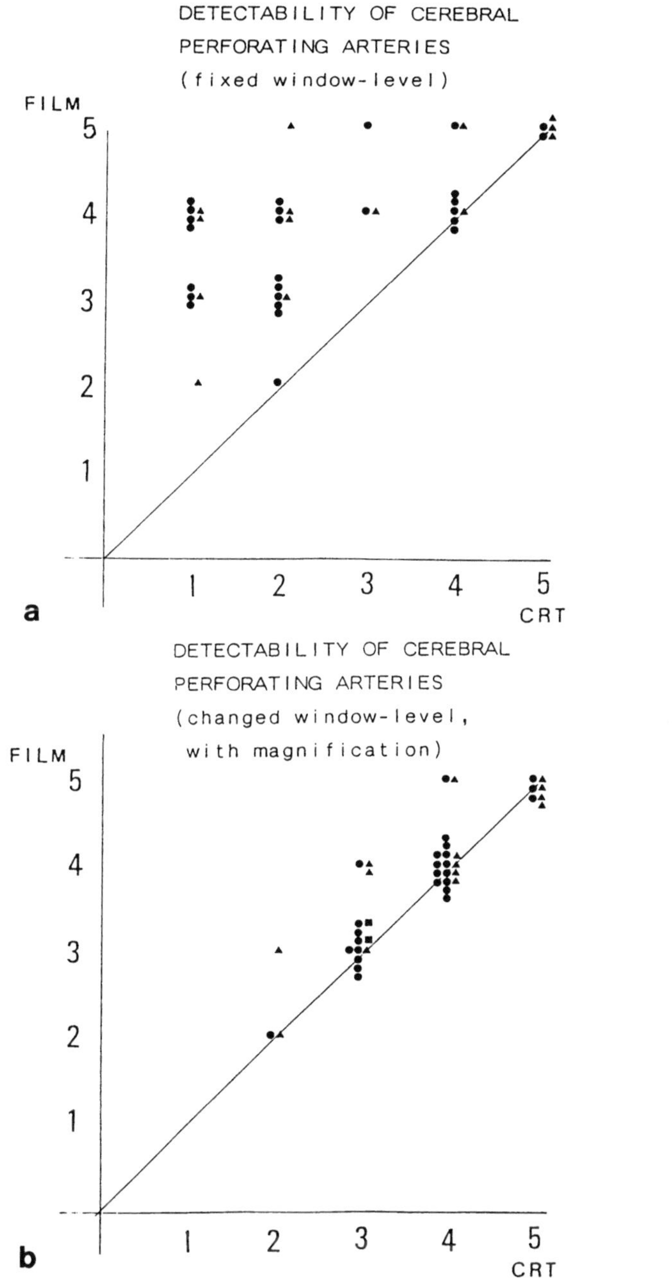

Fig. 2. Visibility of perforating arterie s on CRT compared with conventional film. ●, Lenticulostriate arteries; ▲, thalamo-perforating arteries; 1, not visible; 2, poor; 3, fair; 4, good; 5, excellent

Assessment of the system

Image quality, data access time via LAN and feasibility of the IWS were assessed. Image quality of IWS was evaluated by two neuroradiologists comparing it with conventional transparent film, in terms of detectability of cerebral infarction on CT and visibility of perforating arteries on cerebral angiograms. For evaluation of cerebral angiograms on the CRT, the original film was digitised with computer controlled digitiser (CCD) at 2000 × 2000 × 10 bits, since CR will not be available for angiography until next year. CT data were compressed to about one-third, and angiograms to about one-tenth, so that the effect of data compression could be estimated.

Access time of images was measured since it seemed that LAN and the computer system would be busy during the daytime when most image data were transferred.

Function and manoeuvrability of IWS were also evaluated.

Results and discussion

Image quality

All cerebral infarcts in the selected 40 cases where film display of CT unequivocally showed a lesion (or lesions) were accurately detected on IWS. There was no degradation of images even though one-third data compression was employed.

Visibility of the lenticulostriate and thalamoperforating arteries in 39 carotid and vertebral angiograms was much impaired when window width and level of gray scale of the CRT were fixed (Fig. 2a). Nevertheless, when window width and level were freely changed and magnification of the image was employed if necessary, visibility of these small arteries was significantly improved to reach the degree achieved by conventional film (Fig. 2b). This result indicates that visibility of small arteries is affected by the original film and its picture quality before digitising but not by the quality of IWS. Thus, it is hoped that CR will be adopted for cerebral angiography in CRT diagnosis.

Access time

Access time for an old image stored in the ODL was about 50 s even during busy daytime hours. Access time for a new image from an imaging machine (each modality), through an interface and MDU in the image data base, was about 1.5 min (Fig. 1). These access times will be acceptable in clinical use of HU-PACS.

The software facilities of IWS most commonly used were window width and level presetting, multidisplay of images and magnification.

Dr. Kazuo Miyasaka
Department of Radiology
Hokkaido University School of Medicine N15, W7
Kitaku Sapporo 060, Japan

Neuroradiology (1991) 33 [Suppl]: 440–442

Neuro-radiology
© Springer-Verlag 1991

Vertebral artery dissection proved by follow up

A. Schwartz, M. Mull, and A. Aulich

Department of Neuroradiology, Heinrich Heine University, Düsseldorf, Federal Republic of Germany

Summary. Six cases of dissection of the vertebral artery in the V3 and V4 segment, of spontaneous origin or after minor trauma, were documented by follow up angiography which showed spontaneous recanalisation of the abnormal arterial segment.

Key words: Vertebral artery dissection – Follow up angiography – Spontaneous recanalisation

Compared with the carotid system [1, 2] spontaneous or post-traumatic dissection of the vertebral artery is rare, except in cases of fibromuscular dysplasia.

In contrast with previously published findings of vertebral artery occlusion or aneurysms [3] thought to be of dissecting origin, we present six patients with typical angiographic patterns of spontaneous or post-traumatic dissection, with eccentric stenosis in the V3 and V4 segments of one or both vertebral arteries. The angiographic abnormalities could definitely be discriminated from atherothrombotic changes, especially by follow up angiography.

Case reports

Case 1

A 40-year-old man was admitted to hospital because of recurrent pain in the neck, nausea, hypaesthesia of the right face and atypical disturbances of swallowing and vision. There were signs of a right pontomedullary lesion with paresis of the fifth and ninth cranial nerves, central vestibular nystagmus, contralateral dissociated sensory loss and a Horner's syndrome. Computed tomography showed no focal lesion. On 9 August 1988 right brachial angiography (BAG) (Fig. 1) showed dissection of the V4 segment of the right vertebral artery with pseudoaneurysmal dilatation at the confluence of the vertebral arteries. On 12 August 1988 spontaneous recanalisation of the asymmetrical narrowing of the V4 segment with a persisting pseudoaneurysm was seen. Angiography on 16 March 1989 (Fig. 2, right BAG) showed complete resolution of these abnormalities.

Case 2

A 25-year-old man was admitted because of acute deterioration of a pre-existing brain stem syndrome, beginning in July 1987 with headache of sudden onset and unconsciousness. There was central vestibular nystagmus, right hemiparesis with increased tendon reflexes and bilateral pyramidal signs. Dysmetric movements were noted. Cerebrospinal fluid showed a slight pleocytosis (20 cells/ml), but futher examinations revealed no inflammatory disease. The patient later developed headache, dysarthria, paraparesis and right-sided cerebellar ataxia, right facial and oculomotor palsies and variable disorientation. CT showed hypodensity of the brain stem, right peduncle, right hypothalamus and left thalamus. Angiography on 6 May 1988 and 30 May 1988 (Fig. 3) showed early recanalisation of an occlusion in the left V3 segment and a second tapered narrowing before the confluence. Control angiograms (23 January 1989 and 4 June 1989), demonstrated recanalisation with better contrast in the left posterior inferior cerebellar artery (PICA).

Case 3

A 30-year-old man was admitted with acute right hemianopia and hemihypaesthesia after a kick to the head playing football. There was complete right hemianopia with slow recovery and right hemihypaesthesia without headache or Horner's syndrome. CT showed multiple, well-demarcated lacunar lesions in the territory of the left posterior cerebral artery. Angiography on 8 May 1989 (Fig. 4, right BAG) showed dissection with false aneurysm in the right V4 segment with 50% narrowing of the lumen. On 10 November 1989 (Fig. 4, right vertebral angiogram [VAG]), angiography revealed complete recanalisation and regression of the false aneurysm.

Case 4

A 73-year-old woman was admitted because of sudden left sensorimotor hemiparesis and dysarthria. Three days previously she had an episode of transient bilateral atypical amaurosis. She had bilateral pain in the neck with projection to the vertex. There was bilateral horizontal nystagmus, dysarthria, ataxia of the right limbs and right hemiparesis. Intermittent nausea and diplopia also occurred. CT showed infarction of the right cerebellar hemisphere and upper part of the vermis. Angiography showed eccentric narrowing of the right V4 segment with occlusion of the left vertebral artery and collateral flow from the right to the left PICA. After 4 weeks this typical dissection showed spontaneous recanalisation medication with platelet aggregation inhibitors.

Case 5

A 51-year-old man was admitted with sudden onset dysarthia, left facial nerve palsy and gait disturbance. Clinical examination revealed mild left hemiparesis and arterial hypertension, known for more than 10 years. After admission he developed a new type of headache. CT revealed old, well-demarcated lenticulostriate infarction on the right without definite changes in the posterior cranial fossa. Angiography showed irregular narrowing of the right vertebral artery; small pseudoaneurysms and distal occlusion at the C1 level; the left vertebral artery was patent. After 4 months angiography showed recanalisation of the distal right vertebral artery occlusion.

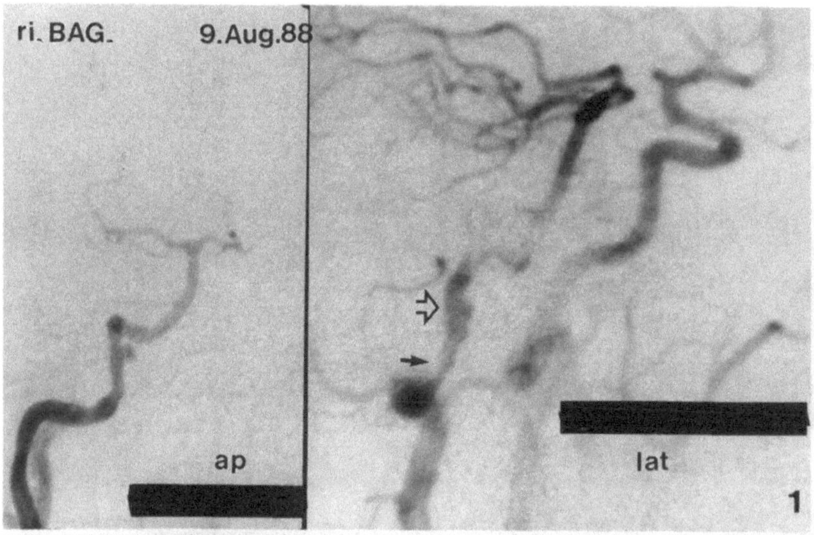

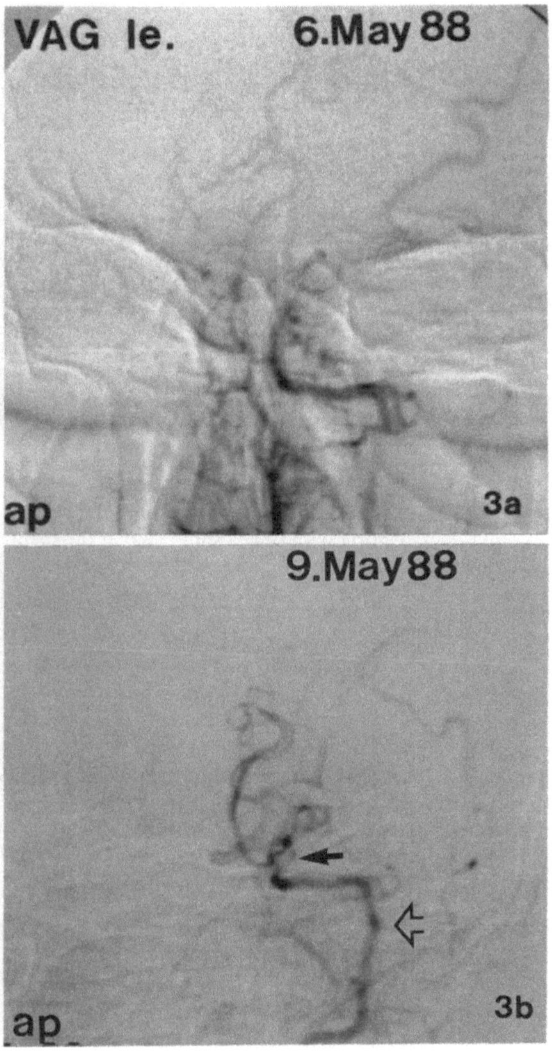

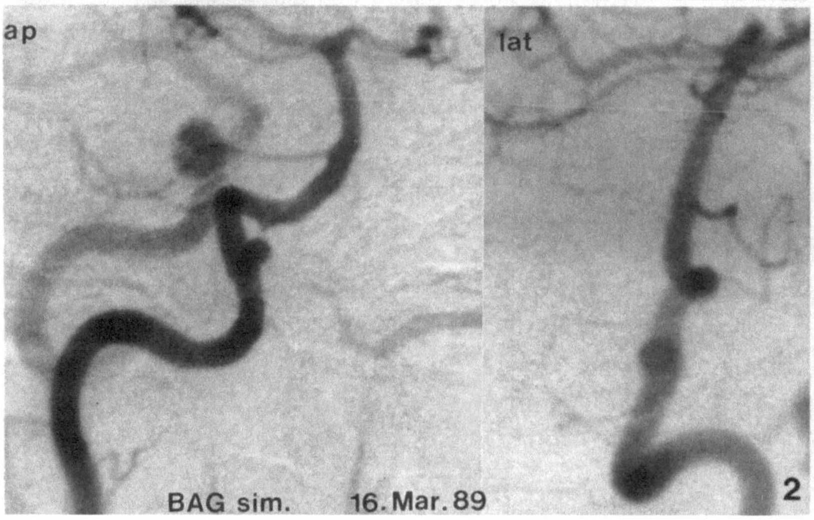

Fig. 1. Right brachial angiogram showing dissection in the V4 segment of the right vertebral artery *(dark arrow)* with pseudoaneurysmal dilatation *(open arrow)* at the confluence of the vertebral arteries

Fig. 2. Spontaneous recanalisation of the asymmetrical narrowing of the V4 segment with a persisting pseudoaneurysm

Fig. 3 a, b. Short-term control angiography of the left vertebral artery reveals early recanalisation of an occlusion in the V3 segment *(open arrow)* and a second tapered narrowing in the following segment before the confluence *(closed arrow)*

Case 6

A 53-year-old woman had transient ischaemic attacks with paraesthesia and hypaesthesia of the left arm and fingers with discrete bradydysdiadochokinesia possibly explained by chronic migraine or known mitral valve proplase. She also described recent neck pain, different from the migraine attacks. On admission her neurological status was normal, as was CT. Left carotid angiogram (CAG) showed an atypical stenosis at the entrance of the left internal carotid artery into the skull base with pseudoaneurysmal dilatation and eccentric narrowing. Vertebral angiography demonstrated that the vertebral arteries were occluded from the origin to the V3 segment with collateralisation by deep cervical arteries to the V3 segment. These changes were thought to represent fibromuscular dyplasia. As expected, the carotid artery changes had resolved on follow up angiograms.

Discussion

In agreement with published data [4–6] we found a preponderance of males in our patients with vertebral artery dissection. None of our patients showed signs of subarachnoid haemorrhage and all had brain stem symptoms or symptoms related to the vertebrobasilar system. In all cases typical changes such as eccentric or tapered narrowing of the lumen irregularity or false aneurysms were shown.

These characteristic signs clearly indicated the cause: other authors were able to confirm dissection only by operation or autopsy. Our patients presented with a typical clinical history [1, 6, 7] and angiography revealed characteristic changes so that the diagnosis could be proved simply by follow up; no operation or autopsy was necessary for confirmation.

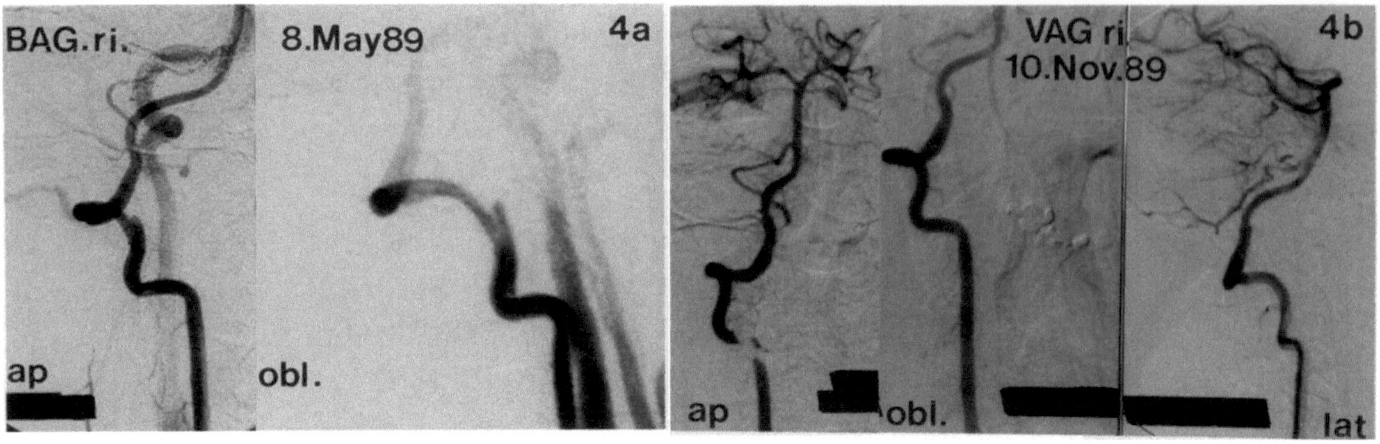

Fig. 4 a, b. Dissection with false aucurysm in the right V4 segment **(a)** and recanalization with only a small step at the distal site of the dissection in the follow-up angiogram **(b)**

References

1. Hennerici M, Steinke W, Rautenberg W (1989) High restistance Doppler flow pattern in extracranial carotid dissection. Arch Neurol 46: 670–676
2. Mokri B, Sundt TM, Houser OW, Sandok BA, Piepgras DG (1986) Spontaneous dissection of the cervical internal carotid artery. Ann Neurol 19: 126–131
3. Chiras J, Marciano S, Molina JV, Touboul J, Poirier B, Bories J (1985) Spontaneous dissecting aneurysm of the extracranial vertebral artery. Neuroradiology 27: 327–333
4. Caplan LR, Baquis GD, Pessin MS, D'Alton J, Adelman LS, DeWitt LD, Ho K, Izukawa O, Kwan ES (1988) Dissection of the intracranial vertebral artery. Neurology 38: 868–877
5. Editorial (1989) Vertebral artery dissection after rapid head turning. AJNR 10: 650
6. Mokri B, Houser OW, Sandok BA, Piepgras DG (1988) Spontaneous dissections of the vertebral arteries. Neurology 38: 880
7. Mokri B, Sundt TM, Houser OW (1979) Spontaneous internal carotid dissection, hemicrania and Horner's syndrome. Arch Neurol 36: 677–680

Priv.-Doz. Dr. A. Schwartz
Neuroradiology-MRI
Heinrich Heine University
W-4000 Düsseldorf 1
Federal Republic of Germany

Neuroradiology (1991) 33 [Suppl]: 443–445

Neuro radiology
© Springer-Verlag 1991

Birefringence as a feature of cerebral microvascular dilatations after cardiopulmonary bypass

M. A. Bell[1, 2], D. M. Moody[1], V. R. Challa[3], W. E. Johnston[4], and D. S. Prough[4]

Departments of [1] Radiology, [2] Anatomy, [3] Pathology, and [4] Anesthesiology, Bowman Gray School of Medicine of the Wake Forest University, Winston-Salem, NC, USA

Summary. Cerebral capillary and arteriolar dilatations have been observed post mortem in humans and dogs following cardiopulmonary bypass. These dilatations often display an unexplained birefringence that facilitates their quick localization and identification.

Key words: Brain, diseases – Brain, microemboli – Brain, vasculature – Cardiac surgery, complications – Cardiopulmonary bypass

Each year in the United States more than 300,000 patients undergo cardiac surgery involving cardiopulmonary bypass (CPB). Of these patients, at least 24% show moderate-to-severe intellectual dysfunction or neurological deficits after their otherwise successful surgery [1, 2]. We have recently reported a structural alteration in cerebral arterioles and capillaries following CPB that may have a bearing on this neurological and neuropsychological outcome [3]. We have found these alterations in ten humans and eight dogs.

When human and animal brains are examined post mortem with a thick celloidin sectioning technique and a modified Gomori stain for alkaline phosphatase [4], the endothelial distribution of this enzyme produces a maplike picture of the arteriolar and capillary network (venules are unstained). In the post-CBP brains we have prepared in this way, capillaries and arterioles up to 30 µm in diameter showed variable numbers of microdilatations (10–50 µm) that might take the shape of discrete ellipsoids, sometimes conforming to bifurcations (Fig. 1), or continuous sausage-shaped swellings (Fig. 2). We interpret these apparently empty swellings as gaseous emboli, or emboli of a soluble substance such as fat. Present in every immediate post-CPB brain we have examined, these microaneurysmal deformations of the microvasculature may nonetheless be transient: the brains of two patients who died 1 month and 6 years after CPB surgery showed no examples. None were seen in 35 human and six dog brains that were not exposed to CPB (or some comparable manipulation). When the dilatations are present, their numbers vary widely, from a few to as many as an estimated 15.3×10^6 per brain (extrapolated from a count of 1740 in one large 100-µm-thick human basal ganglia section).

At light-microscopic levels the walls of the dilatations look normal, albeit stretched and thin. In polarized light many of them display a distinct birefringence, which can take two forms: it may be confined to the thinned wall, outlining the empty lumen of the dilatation (Figs. 1, 2), or it may fill the lumen, displaying a Maltese cross pattern (Fig. 3). The brightness of birefringence varies in different optical systems; under our microscope less than half the dilatations were seen to be birefringent. The dog brains showed mainly the solid Maltese cross pattern (18% of all dilatations seen in the one example analyzed to date), while the human brains more often displayed empty dilatations with birefringent walls (42% in one example). Birefringent dilatations have also been seen in conventional paraffin and semithin resin sections (Fig. 3).

The source of this birefringence is poorly understood. Congo red stains for amyloid revealed none. It might be speculated that the stretching of the vascular wall reorders the molecular organization of the endothelial membranes so they doubly refract the polarized light. In the instances where the dilatation appears packed with birefringent material, some insoluble embolic material such as glove powder or other particulate debris might be suspected. (Arterial line filters used with the CPB pumps do not remove particles smaller than 25 µm.) Alternatively, a birefringent embolic substance, responsible for all the dilatations, might wash out of most of their lumina, leaving some with a thin adherent birefringent coating and a small number with the birefringent contents intact. The argument can also be made that the birefringence, whether luminal or mural, is an artifact of preparation: Buscaino (metachromatic) bodies, a presumed breakdown product of myelin, collect as round patches of varying diameter in the white matter of brain sections. They are ubiquitous and annoying features of thick celloidin preparations, and can also be detected in some routine haematoxylin and eosin-stained paraffin slides and even in semithin resins. Buscaino bodies large and small, discrete and diffuse, may display varying degrees of birefringence, and they frequently collect in tissue crevices such as ventricles or expanded Virchow-Robin spaces. It is possible that some of this material, while migrating through the tissue during processing, becomes trapped in the dilatations and fills the lumina or leaves a birefringent coating on the walls.

Whatever the reason for or significance of the birefringence, it can be a useful aid in locating the dilatations in a

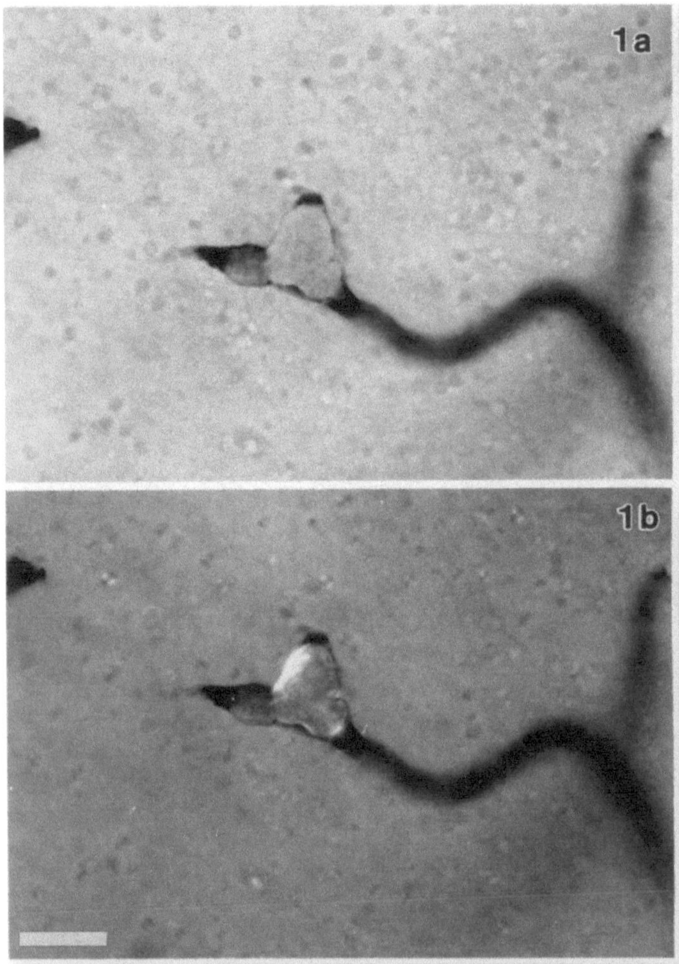

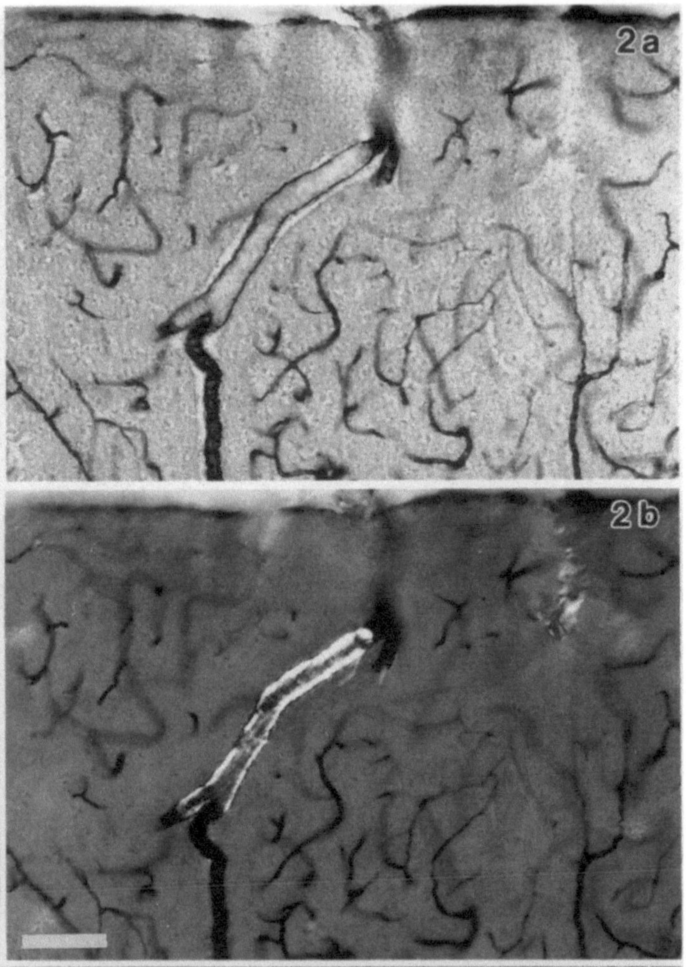

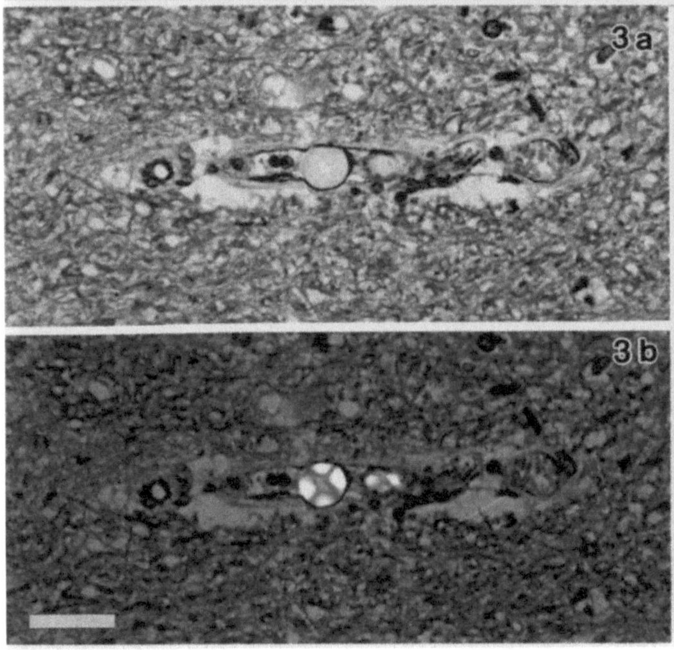

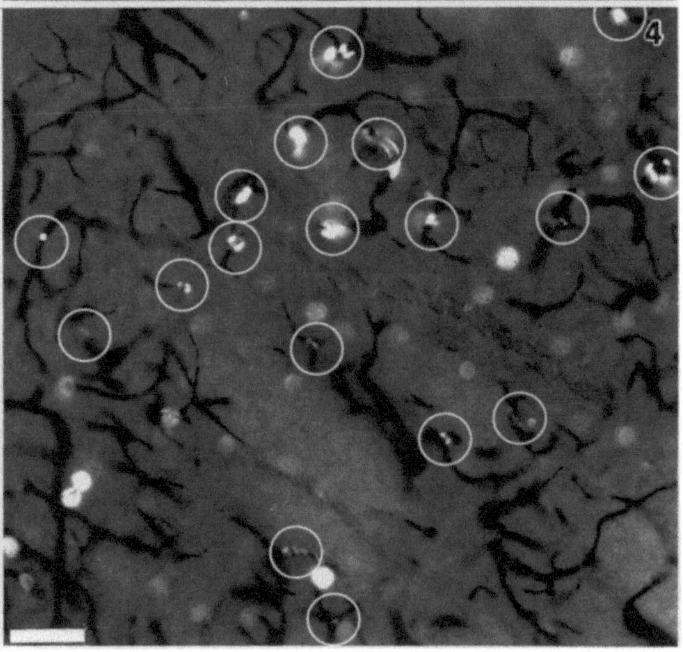

Fig. 1. Human white matter, basal ganglia region, 100-μm celloidin section, alkaline phosphatase stain, without and with crossed polarizing filters. Single empty dilatation, with thinned birefringent wall, extending into capillary bifurcation like a pair of short trousers. *Bar* = 25 μm

Fig. 2. Human frontal cortex, 100-μm celloidin section, alkaline phosphatase stain. Sausage-shaped birefringent dilatation of penetrating arteriole. *Bar* = 100 μ

Fig. 3. Human medulla oblongata, 2-μm resin section, alkaline phosphatase stain and toluidine blue. Dilatation filled with birefringent material displaying Maltese cross. Note (blocked?) blood elements immediately to left in capillary. *Bar* = 25 μm

Fig. 4. Human caudate, 100-μm celloidin section, alkaline phosphatase stain, polarized light. *Circles* mark 18 birefringent dilatations, in and out of focus. Others that are not birefringent are present but not apparent in the field. (Unmarked bright spots are unrelated particles.) In a low power survey, the birefringence aids the quick location of the dilatations and emphasizes the total brain load. *Bar* = 100 μm specimen (Fig. 4). Small shining features stand out clearly when a section is surveyed at low power in polarized light; a check at higher power quickly distinguishes the dilatations from other birefringent debris. It is most useful in the thick specialized vascular preparations described here, but discovered birefringence may call attention to these putative emboli in routine pathological slides as well.

In efforts to characterize the causes of post-CPB neurological and neuropsychological dysfunction, we suggest it is important to screen for these presumed embolic microvascular alterations. The birefringence many of them display makes this screening easier and may eventually provide some clue to the nature of the distending agent.

Acknowledgements. We thank Chris Johnston for technical help and Donna McCain for manuscript preparation. This work was supported by a Jacob K. Javits Neuroscience Investigator Award – NIH Grant NS 20618.

References

1. Shaw PJ, Bates D, Cartlidge NEF, French JM, Heaviside D, Julian DG, Shaw DA (1986) Early intellectual dysfunction following coronary bypass surgery. QJ Med 58: 59–68
2. Smith PLC, Treasure T, Newman SP, Joseph P, Ell PJ, Schneidau A, Harrison MJG (1986) Cerebral consequences of cardiopulmonary bypass. Lancet I: 823–825
3. Moody DM, Bell MA, Challa VR, Johnston WE, Prough DS (1990) Brain microemboli during cardiac surgery or aortography. Ann Neurol (in press)
4. Bell MA, Scarrow WG (1984) Staining for microvascular alkaline phosphatase in thick celloidin sections of nervous tissue: morphometric and pathological applications. Microvasc Res 27: 189–203

Dr. Mary A. Bell
Department of Radiology
Bowman Gray School of Medicine
Winston-Salem, NC 27103, USA

Neuroradiology (1991) 33 [Suppl]: 446–447

Neuro-radiology
© Springer-Verlag 1991

Three-dimensional neuroimaging for brachytherapy of the brain

N. Yoshii[1], H. Samejima[1], T. Mizokami[1], Y. Ushikubo[1], T. Yamazaki[1], N. Inaoka[2], and T. Miyazawa[2]

[1] Department of Neurosurgery, Toho University Omashi Hospital, Tokyo, Japan
[2] Japan IBM, Tokyo, Japan

Summary. For brachytherapy of brain tumours, the exact location of the tumour and the relationship between the tumour and surrounding tissues and ventricles are very important. Three-dimensional neuroimaging using a volume-rendering method has been found very useful for this purpose. The number of introducers for isotope seeds can be determined and the length of seed which should be inserted into each introducer is also determined practically.

Key words: Brachytherapy – Brain tumour – Three-dimensional neuroimaging

Medical three-dimensional imaging is becoming sophisticated and is keeping pace with the rapid development of computer graphics [1, 2]. We report a method we have developed for internal irradiation of brain tumours.

Methods

CT slices 3 mm thick were obtained. On average it took 20 min for the scan and 3–4 h for postprocessing.

A surface rendering method was used. Now, however, three-dimensional imaging of brain tumours is performed, using the volume-rendering method, and the tumour is localized from the image; then internal irradiation is provided by isotope seeds inserted into the tumour.

Results

A brain tumour was partially exposed on the cerebral surface, and the CT image was processed to emphasize the tumour site semiautomatically and colour mapped. After three-dimensional volume data had been constructed from previously processed CT data, volume rendering was carried out. Figure 1 shows the three-dimensional shape of the tumour in the brain by indicating bones and tissues such as brain parenchyma semitransparently and brain tumour opaquely. Figure 2 shows a cross-sectional view perpendicular to the skull. Brain parenchyma is indicated semitransparently and bones and brain tumour part-opaquely.

Figure 3 is an actual CT scan film, where the part surrounded by an annular high-density zone on the right is a tumour. By colour mapping (the second picture process) as shown in Fig. 4, a picture in which different opacity is applied to each part of the tumour is created. Three-dimensional imaging of the tumour is possible as in Fig. 5 a similarly, by the volume rendering method, superimposing each slice of the CT study. The tumour is then cut at any level and the upper part is removed, as shown in Figure 5 b. As any section of tumour can be obtained at any level, the optimal direction for introduction of isotope seeds can be determined and the parallel and perpendicular sections to this direction can be indicated as images. Then the number of introducers for seeds and the appropriate length of isotope seed which should be inserted into each introducer are determined (Figs. 6, 7). For actual application of internal irradiation of the tumour, it is best to insert isotope seeds as parallel to the axis of the tumour as possible because this avoids increasing the number of isotope introducers. The internal irradiation dose is calculated by a distribution computer.

Discussion

Three-dimensional imaging is useful for many purposes in the medical field. As the greater part of the nervous system is overlain by solid bone, imaging the brain and the spinal cord and lesions within the complicated structure of the central nervous system three-dimensionally will be especially useful in diagnosis for both clinical and educational aspects of treatment within a few years. However, at the present time it has limited use because of the very complicated relationships between various brain tissues, blood vessels and ventricles. The surface-rendering method is not particularly useful for these complicated matters. The volume-rendering method is much better for (stereotactic) brachytherapy of brain tumour.

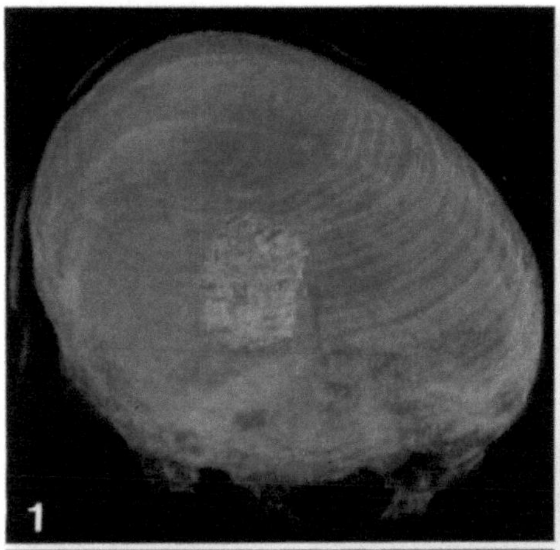

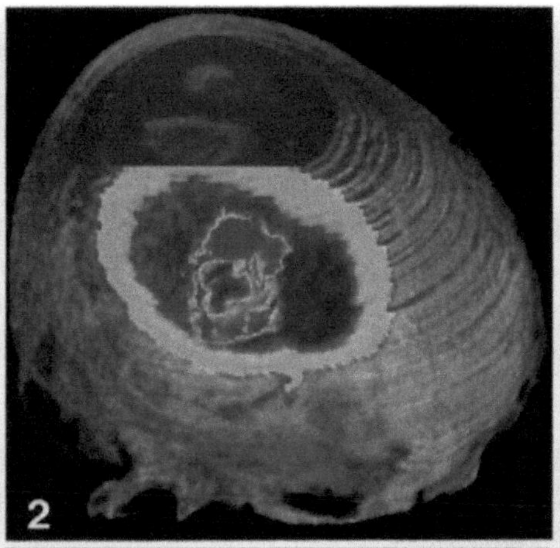

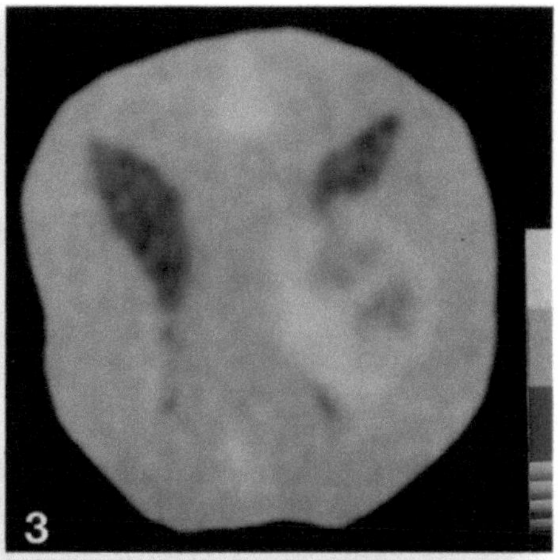

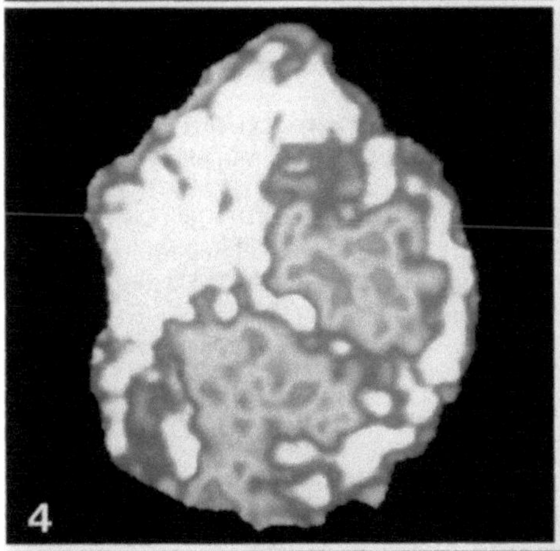

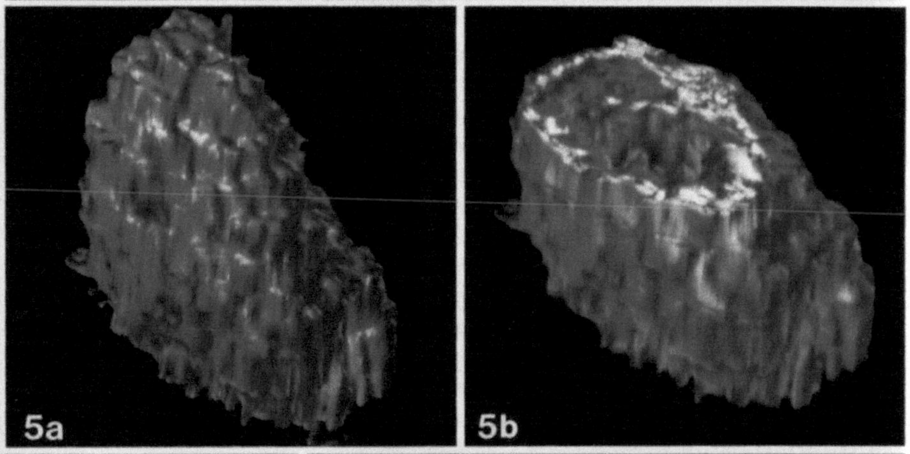

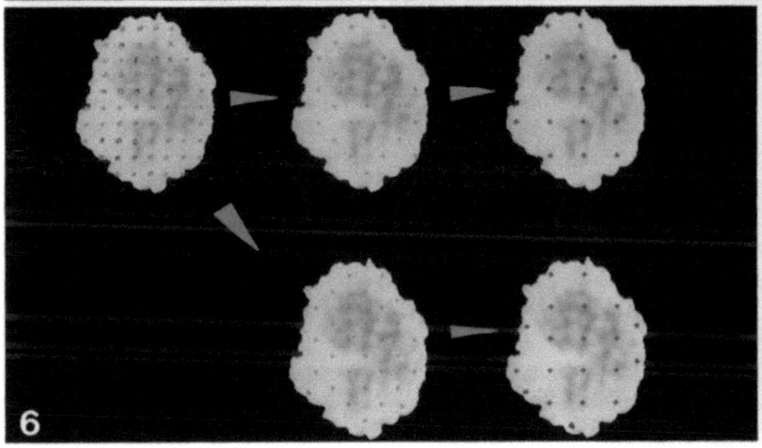

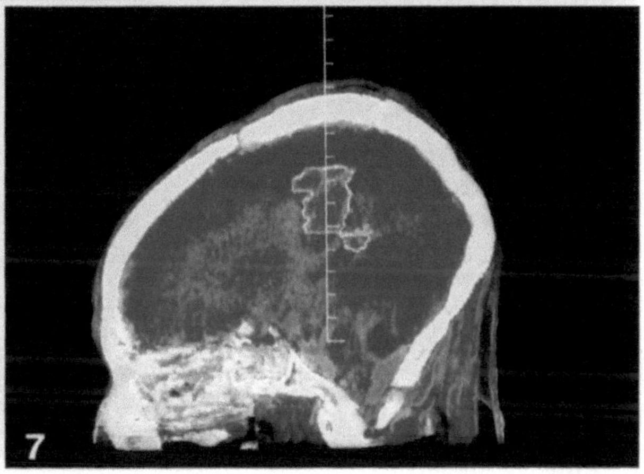

Fig. 1. The overall shape of the tumour

Fig. 2. Cross-sectional view perpendicular to skull

Fig. 3. CT image: annular high density outlines tumour

Fig. 4. Colour map

Fig. 5. (**a**) Three dimensional image, sectioned at chosen level (**b**)

Fig. 6. Number of isotope seeds to be inserted

Fig. 7. Depth of insertion

References

1. Suzuki N (1988) Three dimensional study of brain tissue, blood vessel and ventrical. Diagn Med Imaging 4: 45–49
2. Inaoka N (1990) In: Yoshii N (ed) Medical use of three dimensional neuroimaging, basic neuroradiology – CT, MRI, PET. Nihonigakukan, Tokyo, pp 93–101

Dr. N. Yoshii
Department of Neurosurgery
Toho University
Ohohashi Hospital
Tokyo, Japan

Neuroradiology (1991) 33 [Suppl]: 448–450

Neuro-radiology
© Springer-Verlag 1991

The callosal impingement syndrome of hydrocephalus*

J. R. Jinkins

Neuroradiology Section, The University of Texas Health Science Center at San Antonio, San Antonio, Texas, USA

Summary. Individuals with idiopathic hydrocephalus exhibit a generalized reduction in coordinated motor and cognitive function. A retrospective review of subjects with hydrocephalus was undertaken to study specific MRI correlates of the associated signs and symptoms. Forty adults were studied to elucidate specific clinico-radiologic patterns. The significant change, not described previously, was localized dorsal flattening and thinning of the posterior body of the corpus callosum. The structure responsible for this flattening is the rigid free surface of the falx cerebri, which impinges upon the caudal upwardly expanding corpus callosum and supracallosal hippocampal formation. This mechanical insult could cause variable, incomplete axonal dysfunction resulting initially in a neuroelectrically active bihemispherically radiating commissural and supracallosal forniceal axonopathy. It is postulated that this combined commissuropathy/fornicopathy represents a dynamic partial intra- and inter-hemispheric disconnection accounting, in part, for the complex clinical state associated with hydrocephalus.

Key words: Magnetic resonance imaging – Corpus callosum – Hippocampal formation – Hydrocephalus – Cerebral disconnection syndrome

The signs and symptoms manifested by patients with idiopathic hydrocephalus (HC) seem to imply some specific, progressive pathologic insult in addition to global changes associated with ventricular dilatation with or without increased pressure. A retrospective review was undertaken of subjects judged to have HC to seek discrete abnormalities which might be clues to the pathophysiologic mechanisms underlying the symptoms of HC.

* Symposium Fellowship Award, Honourable Mention

Patients and methods

Forty adults with HC were studied to elucidate specific MRI patterns of abnormality. Spin-echo MRI techniques were utilized with T_1, 500–600/20–40/2 (TR/TE/excitations) and/or T_2-weighted, double echo acquisitions (2000–3000/30–80/1–2) in two or three orthogonal planes. Criteria for HC included dilated lateral ventricles, outwardly expanded cerebral hemispheres, a distended third ventricle, and an elevated corpus callosum (CC) [1, 2].

Results

The morphologic change observed in the majority of these patients, not previously described in HC, was dorsal flattening and/or thinning of the posterior body of the CC (Fig. 1). All but 3 of the 24 individuals (87.5%) with imbalance, gait disturbance, mild memory deficits or dementia, and psychopathologic behaviour showed this, and were classified as group I, symptomatic HC.

Sixteen additional subjects not showing this callosal abnormality were categorized as group II, clinically occult HC. Most presented with nonspecific symptoms, some possibly related to increased intracranial pressure, but not HC per se (i.e., headache, visual impairment, sudden paresis, syncope, seizure).

Discussion

The wide range of signs and symptoms of varying severity associated with HC has never been fully accounted for. The association of many elements of the clinical syndrome

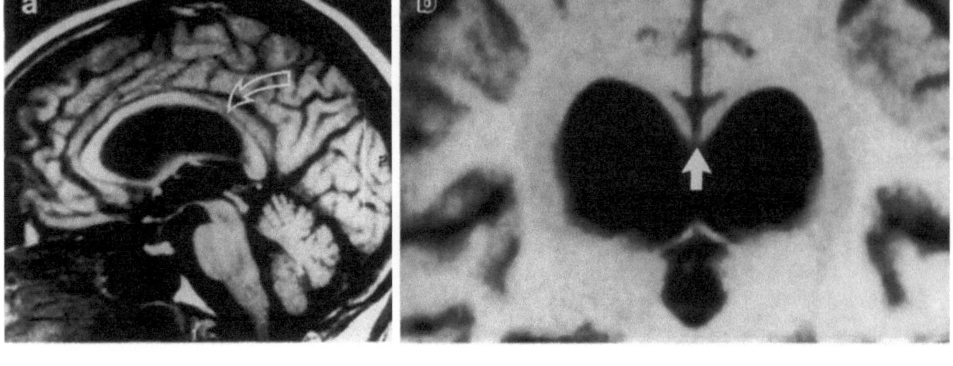

Fig. 1 a, b. Moderate callosal impingement in hydrocephalus. **a** Sagittal T_1-weighted section illustrating the mild curvilinear flattening of the dorsal surface of the posterior body of the corpus callosum (CC) *(arrow)*. **b** Coronal T_1-weighted image illustrating the stretching of the fibers of the CC over the posterior falx with associated extreme thinning and focal loss of callosal signal *(arrow)*

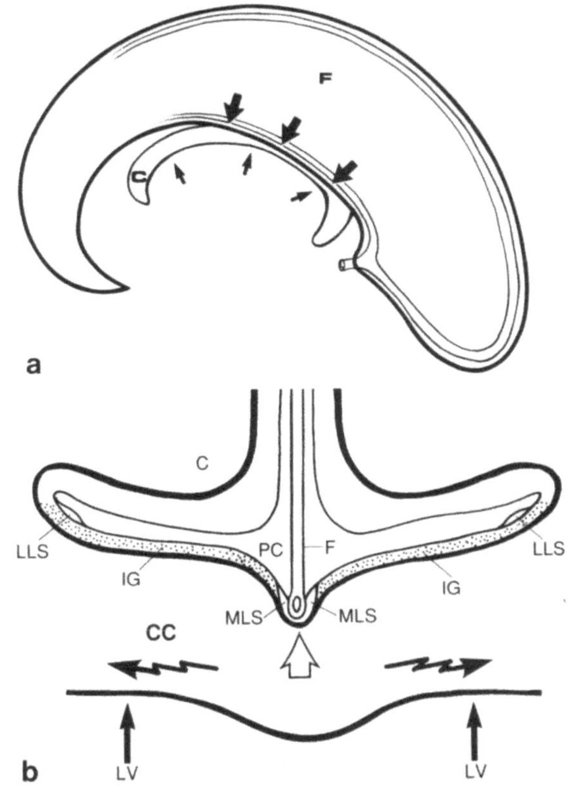

Fig. 2 a, b. Schematic illustration of callosal impingement. **a** Sagittal diagram demonstrating that with callosal impingement in hydrocephalus, there is curvilinear flattening and thinning of the caudal aspect of the dorsal surface of the CC *(arrows)*. **b** Coronal diagram illustrating impingement on callosal structures by the falx cerebri *(F)*. *C*, Cerebrum; *IG*, indusium griseum (stippling); *LLS*, lateral longitudinal striae; *MLS*, medial longitudinal striae; *PC*, pericallosal cistern; *LV*, subcallosal lateral ventricles; *hollow arrow*, region of impingement; *solid arrows*, elevation of CC by dilated lateral ventricles; *projecting arrows*, radiating callosal axonopathy

of HC with dorsal flattening and thinning of the posterior CC would seem to implicate this observation to its genesis. The structure responsible for this change is the rigid free edge of the falx cerebri which impinges caudally on the superiorly displaced CC and supracallosal hippocampal formation (Fig. 2). This mechanical insult might result in neuroelectrically active axonal dysfunction. It is postulated that this radiating callosal/hippocampal commissuropathy and fornicopathy in turn yields, in part, the nebulous clinical state allied with HC because of a dynamic associational, commissural and projectional cerebral disconnection [3, 4].

Experimental evidence suggests that information transferred intra- and interhemispherically from neuron to neuron via commissural, association and projection fibers is not primary neurosensory information, but cortically preprocessed neurophysiologic data. The aberrantly transmitted information in a radiating axonal potential may not be coherently perceived consciously. The clinical syndrome might be generated by interference within neuronal projection fields secondary to a quantitatively and qualitatively varying, asymmetric, bihemispheric neuroelectrical shower of activity emanating from the area of impingement and projected toward cortical and subcortical gray matter. Over time this neuroelectrical bombardment causes possibly permanent gross structural changes with altered neurophysiologic implications [5–12].

Like HC, callosal impingement (CI) may be a progressive condition. As some fibers become non-functional due to prolonged compression, with progression of CI other axons previously unimpinged upon become involved in the pathologic process. Inexorable advancement of temporally variable signs and symptoms may ensue. The varied clinical manifestations may include imbalance, vertigo, abnormal position sense, gait disorders, bizarre somesthetic complaints, loss of supratentorial control over sphincter function, and disorders of cognitive skills such as learning, memory, and psychiatric stability.

Possible factors in the genesis of the CI syndrome include the degree of HC, its temporal course, the size and configuration of the CC, the degree of development of the falx cerebri, differences in patient age and bilateral functional neural organization of the cerebral hemispheres and CC, and concomitant developmental or acquired cerebral disease. The completeness of recovery must depend on timely intervention to arrest the impingement, thereby halting the insidious axonal injury, and avoiding the potentially irreversible effects of prolonged radiation of aberrant callosal and hippocampal neuroelectrical action potentials upon the vulnerable cerebrum. Extrapolation of this impingement theory to other active insults to the CC and pericallosal tissues may aid elucidation of the pathophysiologic mechanisms underlying clinical syndromes accompanying many different nonspecific disease processes affecting these structures.

Acknowledgements. I thank Joanne Murray for the manuscript preparation, Cono Farias for the photographic reproductions, and Nancy Place for the accompanying artwork.

References

1. El Gammal TE, Allen MB, Brooks BS, Mark EK (1987) MR evaluation of hydrocephalus. AJNR 8: 591–597
2. Jack CR, Mokri B, Laws ER, Houser OW, Baker HL, Petersen RC (1987) MR findings in normal-pressure hydrocephalus: significance and comparison with other forms of dementia. J Comput Assist Tomogr 11: 923–931
3. Bogen JE (1985) The callosal syndromes. In: Heilman KM, Valenstein E (eds) Clinical neuropsychology. Oxford University Press, New York, pp 295–338
4. Adams RD, Fisher CM, Hakim S, Ojemann RG, Sweet WH (1965) Symptomatic occult hydrocephalus with "normal" cerebrospinal fluid pressure. A treatable syndrome. N Engl J Med 273: 117–126
5. Rydevik B, Nordborg C (1980) Changes in nerve function and nerve fibre structure induced by acute, graded compression. J Neurol Neurosurg Psychiatry 43: 1070–1082
6. Smith KJ, McDonald WI (1980) Spontaneous and mechanically evoked activity due to central demyelinating lesion. Nature 286: 154–155
7. Chang HT (1953) Cortical response to activity of callosal neurons. J Neurophysiol 16: 117–131

8. Chang HT (1953) Interaction of evoked cortical potentials. J Neurophysiol 16: 133–144
9. Bickford RG, Mulder DW, Dodge HW, Svien HJ, Rome HP (1958) Changes in memory function produced by electrical stimulation of the temporal lobe in man. In: The brain and human behavior. Hafner, New York, pp 227–243
10. Morrell F (1961) Lasting changes in synaptic organization produced by continuous neuronal bombardment. In: DeLafresnaye JF (ed) Brain mechanisms and learning. Blackwell, Oxford, pp 375–392
11. Goddard GV, McIntyre DC, Leech CK (1969) A permanent change in brain function resulting from daily electrical stimulation. Exp Neurol 25: 295–330
12. Brown DG, Goldensohn ES (1973) The electroencephalogram in normal pressure hydrocephalus. Arch Neurol 29: 70–71

Dr. J. Randy Jinkins
Neuroradiology Section
The University of Texas Health Science Center at San Antonio
San Antonio, TX 78284-7800, USA

Neuroradiology (1991) 33 [Suppl]: 451–452

Neuro radiology
© Springer-Verlag 1991

Ultrasonography of the peripheral nerves

P. H. Hoogland

Department of Radiology, Westeinde Hospital, The Hague, The Netherlands

Summary. Visualisation of the peripheral nerve system, one of the last territories to be discovered in neuroradiology, was made possible by recent advances in the technology of ultrasonography. We applied high-resolution ultrasound to the examination of the superficial peripheral nerves, in particular to the ulnar and median nerves in the ulnar sulcus and the carpal tunnel and found an excellent correlation between the ultrasonic and intraoperative appearances of these nerves.

Key words: Peripheral nerve – Ulnar nerve – Median nerve – Compression neuropathy – Ultrasonic diagnosis

The most interesting peripheral nerves from a diagnostic and therapeutic point of view are the ulnar and median nerves at the point where they pass through the ulnar sulcus and the carpal tunnel; there the nerve is most frequently damaged and consequently most operated upon. Methods such as CT and MRI can be used for the examination of the peripheral nerves; CT, however, lacks in soft tissue resolution and experience and availability of MRI are still limited, especially on the subject of the peripheral nerve system. Nevertheless these methods can be of special value for the examination of peripheral nerve tumours [1]. Ultrasound has been used in investigation of peripheral nerve tumours [2–4], but the sonographic appearances aspect of the median and ulnar nerves and their entrapment neuropathy have not yet been described.

Materials and methods

The real-time ultrasound examinations were performed on an Aloka SSD 280 with a small 7.5 MHz linear array transducer, the ulnar nerve directly in contact with the ulnar sulcus, and the median nerve with the help of a standoff pad, both nerves in longitudinal and transverse directions. Experience was gathered with a series of 20 healthy volunteers with examination of 40 ulnar and 40 median nerves. This was followed by the examination of 20 patients with complaints of a carpal tunnel syndrome (CTS) with direct surgical confirmation and of 39 patients with suspected compression neuropathy of the ulnar nerve in the ulnar sulcus with surgical confirmation in 20 patients.

Results

The series of normal volunteers was uniform in the appearances of both the ulnar and of the median nerve. The normal ulnar nerve has a diameter between 2 and 3 mm, is of lower echogenicity and has a smooth aspect, surrounded by the echo of the epineurium with some reflections internally due to the perineurium (Fig. 1). The normal aspect of the median nerve in its passage through the carpal tunnel is similarly smooth with a particular relationship to the tendons of the long flexors of the fingers and the transverse carpal ligament. The median nerve is also of lower echogenicity with a clear reflection of the epineurium (Fig. 2). The most frequently encountered abnormality of the median nerve is the change in diameter due to compression by the retinaculum (Fig. 3). Also, increased echolucency of the nerve due to oedematous swelling is clearly observed. The transverse ligament itself, with its higher echogenicity, is more difficult to delineate, especially the superior border. Of the 20 patients with suspected CTS, 18 patients showed an excellent correlation between the ultrasound examination and the intraoperative appearance of the nerve.

Nine patients showed normal appearances of the median nerve, confirmed by operation; 9 patients showed either compression of the nerve, a thickening of the perineurium or a pseudoneuroma, also confirmed by operation. In 1 patient an artefact was misinterpreted as swelling of the nerve and in another patient a small synovial cyst was missed. The ulnar nerve is as easily demonstrated during its passage through the ulnar sulcus and in all patients it was simple to visualise the exact location of the nerve. Pathological luxation during flexion/extension of the arm was easy to demonstrate on real-time images. The well-known pathological changes of the nerve, i. e. pseudoneuroma, swelling due to oedema, post-traumatic (and post-operative) atrophy and other changes of the morphology of the ulnar nerve were clearly seen (Fig. 4). Twenty patients out of 39 were operated upon; 17 patients showed an excellent correlation between the ultrasound appearance of the nerve and the intraoperative findings. In 10 patients the clinical and neurophysiological findings correlated with the ultrasound examination, however without surgical confirmation. In 4 patients with atypical complaints the clinical, myographic and ultrasound findings were normal and in 5 patients the examination was used for localising and establishing pathological luxation of the ulnar nerve.

Discussion

In our experience the normal peripheral nerve is well depicted by high-resolution ultrasonography and is seen as a longitudinal structure of lower echogenicity surrounded

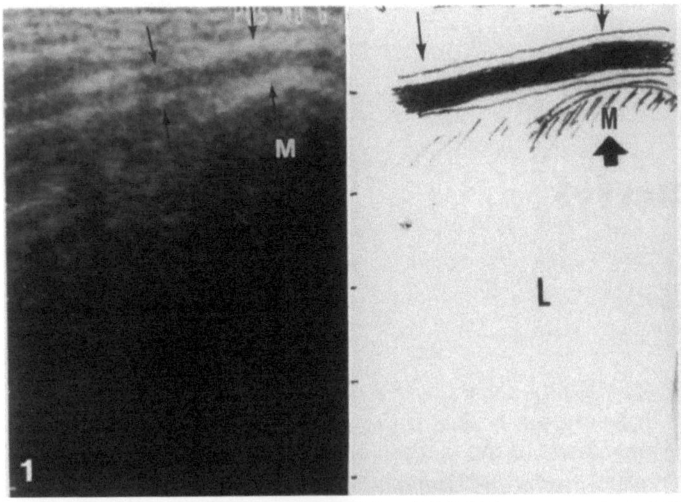

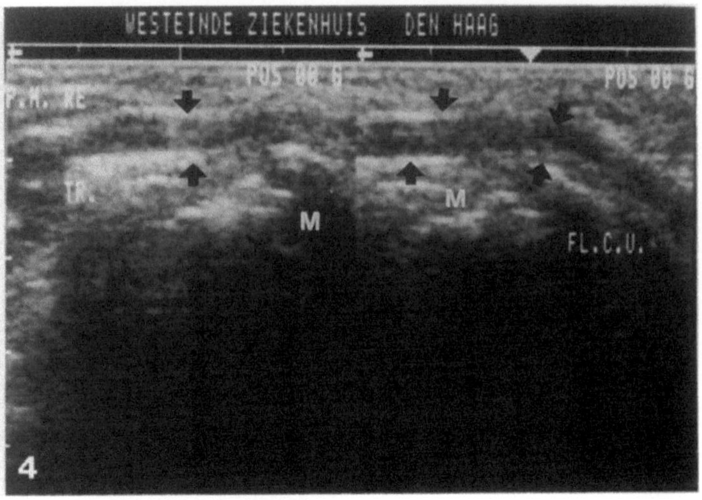

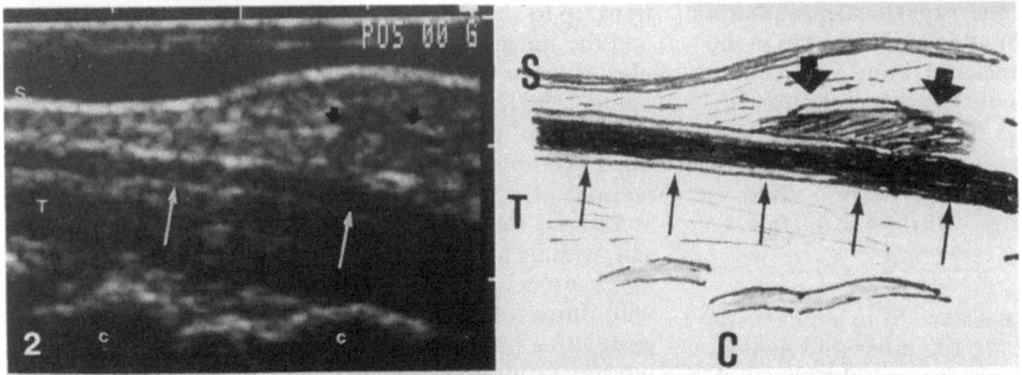

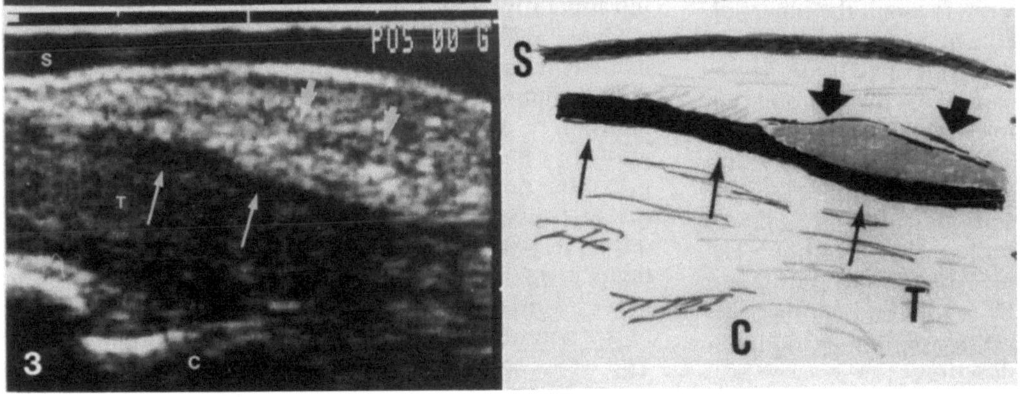

Fig. 1. Normal ulnar nerve (long) →. *M*, Medial condyle ♦

Fig. 2. Normal median nerve (→) passing through carpal tunnel. *S*, Skin; *C*, carpal bones; *T*, tendons; retinaculum (♦)

Fig. 3. Patient with carpal tunnel syndrome compression of median nerve (→) by retinaculum (♦)

Fig. 4. Patient with compression neuropathy of ulnar nerve (♦). Surgical confirmation. *TR*, Triceps; FLCU, Musc. flexor carpi ulnaris

by the epineurium, quite contrary to the opinion of Fornage [4]. The compression neuropathy of the median and ulnar nerves is often a distinct clinical syndrome with, in general, clear clinical and neurophysiological findings. There exist, however, atypical cases, where visualisation of the nerve could be an important factor in the decision on surgical decompression. Other peripheral nerves can be very difficult to demonstrate because of their relation to other soft tissues or bones, and are of less clinical relevance.

In conclusion, the normal and abnormal peripheral nerve, especially the median and ulnar nerves can be visualised by ultrasonography and have typical low echogenicity. Ultrasonography can be a new diagnostic tool in the analysis of entrapment neuropathy of the median and ulnar nerves.

References

1. Fahr LM, Sauser DD (1988) Imaging of peripheral nerve lesions. Orthop Clin North Am 19: 27–41
2. Hughes DG, Wilson DJ (1986) Ultrasound appearances of peripheral nerve tumours. Br J Radiol 59: 1051–1043
3. Hoddick WK, Callen PW, Filly RA, Mahony BS, Edwards MB (1984) Ultrasound evaluation of benign sciatic nerve sheath tumors. J Ultrasound Med 3: 505–507
4. Fornage BD (1988) Peripheral nerves of the extremities: imaging with US. Radiology 167: 179–182

P. H. Hoogland
Dep. of Radiology
Westeinde Hospital
Lijnbaan 32
2512 VA the Hague
The Netherlands

Neuroradiology (1991) 33 [Suppl]: 453–455

Neuro radiology
© Springer-Verlag 1991

A comparison of 100 mm film and intra-arterial digital subtraction angiography in intra-cranial aneurysm angiography

R. J. V. Bartlett[1], G. Brocklehurst[2], and A. E. Pratt[1]

Departments of [1] Radiology and [2] Neurosurgery, Hull Royal Infirmary, Hull, UK

Summary. A prospective study was undertaken to compare the value of intra-arterial digital subtraction angiography and unsubtracted conventional camera film images in the assessment of intracranial aneurysms. Forty patients were investigated. Comparative series of images were obtained under identical circumstances, except for the concentration of contrast media. A number of angiographic features were analysed by three observers independently. There was little difference between the techniques in the overall quality of the investigation and the demonstration of specific diagnostic features. A number of micro-aneurysms were missed, predominantly on the digital images. Two clinically important posterior fossa aneurysms were missed with conventional images.

Key words: Angiography – Digital subtraction – Intracranial aneurysm

In the last few years, digital angiography has become widely available in neuroradiological centres in the United Kingdom. In many institutions conventional film techniques have been abandoned for all aspects of neuroangiography. Nevertheless, there are a number of units where good-quality digital systems are available, but analogue techniques continue to be utilised for aneurysm angiography.

An early comparative trial was reported by Brant-Zawadzki et al. [1] in 1983. They assessed a prototype digital subtraction system in a heterogeneous group of 12 patients, and concluded that intra-arterial digital subtraction angiography was adequate for most, if not all, neuro-applications. Davis and Hoffman [2] reported a larger comparative study utilising a Philips subtraction unit. The majority of their patients had cerebrovascular disease, though it is not clear whether this included a significant number of patients with intracranial aneurysm. Seeger and Carmody [3] stated that conventional angiography was still favoured for studies requiring exquisite vascular detail, such as the investigation of small aneurysms. Foley and Milde [4] also felt that conventional techniques had a role in aneurysm angiography.

In our institution, digital systems have been utilised for all aspects of neuro-angiography. There had been a perception that undue reliance on digital images had led to errors and omissions in the angiographic diagnosis of small aneurysms, and that on occasion this had important clinical consequences. This provided the impetus for the present study.

Patients and methods

Equipment. All images were obtained on a recently installed Philips 'ARC' unit: mounted with a 100-mm cut-film camera and 'DVI-S' digital subtraction system. A 0.6-mm focal spot was used in all occasions. Digital 512^2 matrix is 'compressed' into the circular field of view.

The DVI functions are micro-processor controlled, with anatomically programmed exposures. Selected digital frames were imaged via a Dupont opti-imager, using standard window and enhancement adjustment settings. Exposures for the 100-mm camera were set manually.

Patients. A consecutive group of 40 patients, suspected of harbouring intra-cranial aneurysms, was studied. They were proven or strongly suspected to have subarachnoid haemorrhage, or being investigated for painful third nerve palsy. Patients found to have an arteriovenous malformation were excluded. Other exclusion criteria were: patients under 16 years, known tenuous clinical state, severe spasm shown angiographically, significant renal hepatic or cardiac impairment, any cause for concern by the radiologist during the examination.

All patients were studied under general anaesthesia with intubation. Ventilation was suspended during digital acquisition.

Catheterisation of the common carotid arteries was performed with a Mani-5 catheter from the femoral approach. In 17 patients vertebral arteriography was also performed. Hand injections of 10 ml were used for carotid series, and 7 ml for the vertebrals.

Full strength contrast (iopamidol 300 mg iodine/ml) was used for 100-mm images, and half strength (iopamidol 150 mg iodine/ml) for digital acquisition.

During routine diagnostic arteriography, three of our standard projections of one carotid study were acquired consecutively on both camera-film and digital systems. Conditions were identical other than the strength of contrast medium that was used. The projections were: a 10″ PA continued until the venous phase, a 6″ perorbital arterial phase only, and a 6″ lateral arterial phase only. When appropriate, comparative vertebral images were obtained with a 6″ Townes projection continued until the venous phase. If the first carotid run was suggestive of an aneurysm, comparative images were obtained on that side; if not, the contralateral vessel was utilised. The clinically suspicious side was injected first.

Analysis. Hard copy was retained of the best images, arterial, capillary and venous phase as appropriate. Identification data were removed. This resulted in 80 sets of digital or analogue images. At the conclusion of the trial these were randomised and presented independently to three experienced observers, two neuroradiologists and a neurosurgeon. The observers viewed the images at a single sitting and recorded their findings on a pro forma. Each observer was required to specify a detailed diagnosis for each set of images. Vari-

Table 1. Arteriographic features – mean rating

	Mean rating (1–5)					
	Radiologist A		Surgeon		Radiologist B	
	100 mm	DIG	100 mm	DIG	100 mm	DIG
Confidence of diagnosis	3.8	3.6	3.2	3.5	3.7	3.7
Overall quality of study	3.9	3.3	3.0	3.8	3.0	3.0
Clarity of aneurysm or normal vessels	3.7	3.2	2.8	3.3	3.0	3.3
Clarity of lenticulostriates	4.3	2.8	3.0	3.2	3.0	2.0
Clarity of ophthalmic artery	2.9	3.8	3.3	3.9	2.7	3.1
Clarity of middle cerebral division	3.8	3.4	3.4	4.2	3.0	2.9
Visualisation of cerebral parenchymal blush	1.9	3.1	3.6	4.2	1.3	2.5
Visualisation of cerebral veins and sinuses	3.1	4.2	3.2	4.8	2.3	3.1
Clarity of PICA and AICA	3.1	3.9	2.9	3.9	2.1	2.8
Visualisation of cerebellar veins and sinuses	3.7	4.5	3.1	5.0	2.5	3.2

AICA, Anterior inferior cerebellar artery; DIG, Digital; PICA, Posterior inferior cerebral artery
* Intra-observer difference significant, $P < 0.05$; paired t-test

Table 2. Diagnostic errors for each observer

Patient	Diagnostic errors					
	Radiologist A		Surgeon		Radiologist B	
		Modality		Modality		Modality
S.H.	–		b Micro	DIG	b Micro	DIG and 100
D.O.	–		b Micro	DIG	b Micro and PCA	DIG and 100
J.H.	–		b PICA	100	b PICA	100
E.C.	a Small ACA	100	–		–	
L.L.	–		b Micro	DIG	b Micro	DIG and 100
K.L.	a Micro	DIG	b Micro	DIG	b Micro	DIG and 100
J.M.	–		–		b PICA	100
J.K.	a Second an.	DIG and 100	–		–	

a, False positive; b, false negative; ACA, Anterior cerebral artery; DIG, Digital; PCA, Posterior cerebral artery; PICA, Posterior inferior cerebral artery

ous aspects of the study were rated on a five-point scale, utilising whichever projections were appropriate (Table 1). Specific guidance was given for rating each aspect of the angiogram. A mean value for the rating of each aspect of the study was obtained for each observer (Table 1).

A "true diagnosis" was established from a retrospective review of the complete angiogram and analysis of the operative findings. Errors in the diagnosis established from the trial images by each observer are shown in Table 2.

Results

There were 24 female patients and 16 males, with a mean age of 48 years. Twenty-seven aneurysms were present in 23 patients. These comprised 4 carotid aneurysms, 6 posterior communicating/anterior choroidal aneurysms, 2 anterior communicating aneurysms, 8 middle cerebral aneurysms, 2 Posterior inferior cerebellar artery (PICA) aneurysms, and 5 micro-aneurysms.

Analysis of the images is summarised in Table 1 for each observer. Diagnostic errors are tabulated in Table 2.

Discussion

The spatial resolution of digital systems is considerably inferior to conventional films. A 512^2 matrix with a 10″ field of view permits a best possible resolution of 1 line pair/mm, which in reality is about 0.9 line pairs/mm. This compares with approximately 3.5 line pairs/mm on 100-mm camera film. Best possible digital resolution on a 6″ field is about 1.4 line pairs/mm. This means that there is a four-fold difference in the spatial resolution of the two systems. On digital images, structures smaller than 0.5 mm will only be resolved if they are surrounded by areas of significantly different density, and there will be no resolution of their structure.

One might expect that the detection of small intracranial aneurysms would be the most demanding clinical application for digital equipment. We elected to compare intra-arterial digital images with unsubtracted 100-mm camera film, as this is the practical choice open to us. If a good-quality digital subtraction system is available, it is unlikely that many units would devote the necessary resources to obtaining conventional subtractions.

The circumstances of this trial should favour the digital system. Patient movement has been almost eliminated, ensuring that there was only minimal need for pixel shifting. The comparative views that were selected mainly contain dense overlying bone.

Table 1 demonstrates that there is some variability between the observers. It is likely that this reflects a degree of pre-existing bias. Radiologists preferred the 'crispness' of analogue images for demonstrating fine structures such as the lenticulostriates, but it is remarkable how many of these tiny vessels can be seen on good quality digital images.

The micro-aneurysms which were missed were only 1 or 2 mm in diameter. They were more easily detected on analogue film. The most important 'errors' were the two PICA aneurysms missed on 100-mm film by one or two observers.

In conclusion, radiological visualisation is a complex interaction of spatial and contrast resolution. Under the circumstances of this trial, digital images appear to be clinically very satisfactory. If patient movement were more of a problem, it might be necessary to place greater reliance on analogue images. Current developments of high-resolution digital technology, with 1024^2 matrix and beyond, will produce images of stupendous clarity. It will be necessary to determine whether this actually provides additional important clinical information.

Acknowledgements. We would like to express gratitude to Joy Jackson, Sue Richardson, Sheena Macdonald and Lesley Norrie for radiologic support and enthusiasm, and to Chris Whatling for typing the manuscript.

References

1. Brant-Zawadzki M, Gould R, Norman D, Newton TH, Lane B (1983) Digital subtraction cerebral angiography by intra-arterial injection: comparison with conventional angiography. AJR 140: 347–353
2. Davis PC, Hoffman JC (1983) Work in progress. Intra-arterial digital subtraction angiography: evaluation in 150 patients. Radiology 148: 9–15
3. Seeger JF, Carmody RF (1985) Digital subtraction angiography of the arteries of the head and neck. Radiol Clin North Am 23: 193–210
4. Foley WD, Milde MW (1985) Intra-arterial digital subtraction angiography. Radiol Clin North Am 23: 293–319

R. J. V. Bartlett
X-ray Department
Hull Royal Infirmary
Anlaby Road
Hull HU3 2JZ, UK

Neuroradiology (1991) 33 [Suppl]: 456–458

Neuro-radiology
© Springer-Verlag 1991

Fluid flow measurement in vessels from digital subtraction angiography video recordings

J. N. H. Brunt[1], G. H. du Boulay[2], A. Wallis[2], and D. A. G. Wicks[2]

[1] Department of Medical Biophysics, Stopford Building, University of Manchester, Oxford Road, Manchester, UK
[2] Institute of Neurology, National Hospital for Neurology and Neurosurgery, Queen Square, London, UK

Summary. Measurement of blood flow from Cine-angiograms, using a technique that obtains contrast medium mass values at multitudinous positions along individual vessels and from numerous frames, has been previously reported. We hypothesized that the noise limitations of video recordings could be offset by recording already subtracted angiograms from a digital subtraction angiography (DSA) system, and that the resolution of video was adequate to substitute for film. We recorded validation experiments in which flows, measured using a calibrated electromagnetic flowmeter, passed through tubes of 4–7 mm diameter, during injections of 2–5 ml contrast medium. The video sequences were analysed on a computer system which produced angiographic flow measurements agreeing with the e. m. flows to within 5%. We illustrate the technique using carotid artery DSA. We conclude that accurate flow measurements can be made from DSA video recordings.

Key words: Blood flow velocity – Arteriography – Digital subtraction angiography – Computer-assisted image processing – Computer-assisted image interpretation

Successful measurement of blood flow from angiograms recorded on cine film, using a technique that obtains contrast medium mass values from transverse density profiles at a multitude of positions along vessels and from numerous cine frames, has been previously reported [1, 2]. Video cassette recording (VCR) technology is widely available, convenient and inexpensive. We hypothesized that the poorer signal-to-noise characteristics of VCR (compared with film) could be offset by recording already subtracted angiograms from a digital subtraction angiography (DSA) system, and that the spatial and temporal resolution (in this case, 256×256 pixels and $25\ s^{-1}$) were adequate to utilize the flow measurement technique.

Our initial experiments have been aimed at validating the technique for blood flow measurement in the carotid arteries. The sizes of the phantoms used, and the flows through them, were chosen accordingly. The degree of tortuosity of the carotid arteries is limited and this allowed us to use relatively simple tube configurations in these experiments. More recent experiments, as yet incomplete, relating to blood flow measurement in the cerebral arteries, employ sharply curved and narrow phantoms, together with full three-dimensional calibration.

Materials and methods

Image sequences from a Philips DVI system with the CV option installed were stored on Sony video cassettes using a Sony U-matic VO-5800 VCR. We recorded experiments in which flows ranging between 100 and 1500 $ml \cdot min^{-1}$ passed through straight tubes of 4–7 mm diameter. The flows were measured using a calibrated electromagnetic flowmeter as injections of 2–5 ml contrast medium were introduced. Objects of exactly known dimensions were included in the X-ray field to provide geometrical calibration, and the time calibration was confirmed by imaging a metronome.

The sequences were played back via a second, remotely located Sony VCR and a time base corrector into an image processing system (consisting of a Sun workstation and an AVS-3000 framestore), capable of storing and processing a 64-frame sequence (2.6 s).

We here illustrate the computer processing and analysis using images and data derived from a patients clinical carotid DSA. A sampling area (delineated in Fig. 1 by dots) is positioned over a vessel of interest, and the grey-level image data are sampled within it to produce a new image in which the tortuosity of the vessel is removed with the help of 3D reconstruction. Areas within the "straightened" image are then resampled (boxes over the common and internal carotid arteries), the value from each transverse density profile (corresponding to contrast medium mass per unit vessel length) giving one value in a column or "vector". Each vector, corresponding to a single video frame, or instant of time, is drawn into a "parametric image" representing contrast medium mass as a function of distance along the vessel and of time (Fig. 2). This image is rescaled to represent concentration of contrast medium.

Figure 3 shows an example parametric image, corresponding to a 56-mm length of straightened common and internal carotid arteries and to a time duration of 2 s. The visualization of information has been enhanced by image processing. The instantaneous, local flow velocity can be derived from the inclination of the isoconcentration contour at any point in the image using either a manual algorithm (drawing lines) or by automated algorithms.

Results

Results from the example are shown in Fig. 4. Using two automated algorithms (based respectively on a gradient operator [3] and on a correlation technique [4], reimplemented), instantaneous flow values are plotted over a

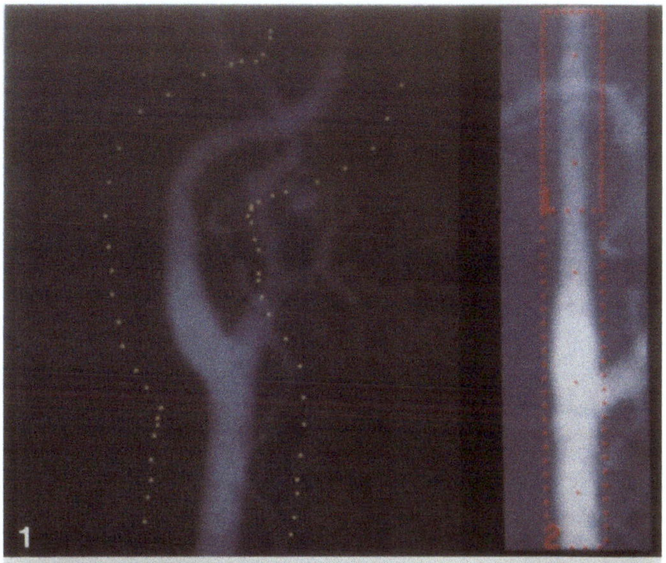

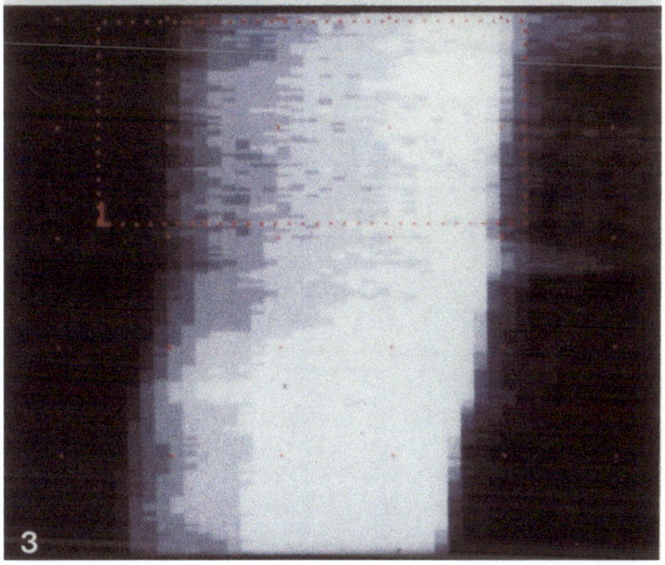

Fig. 1. An area of interest *(dots)* is positioned over a vessel, and the image data are sampled within it to produce a new image exluding vessel tortuosity. Areas within the "straightened" image are then resampled (*boxes* over the common and internal carotid arteries)

Fig. 3. A parametric image (time duration 2 s) from common and internal carotid arteries. Image processing has enhanced visualization of the isoconcentration contours from whose inclination flow velocity can be derived

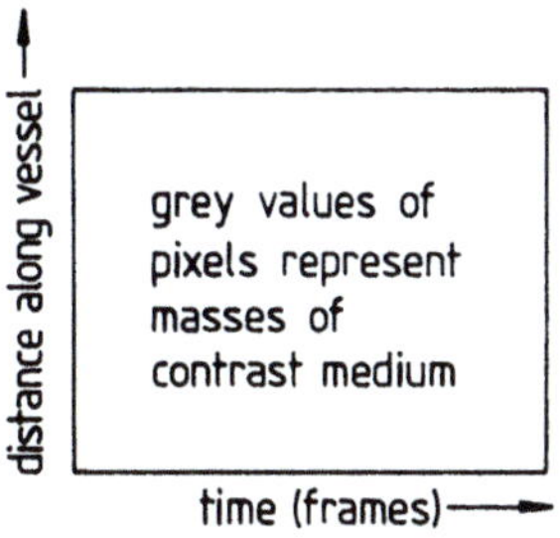

Fig. 2. The information contained in a parametric image

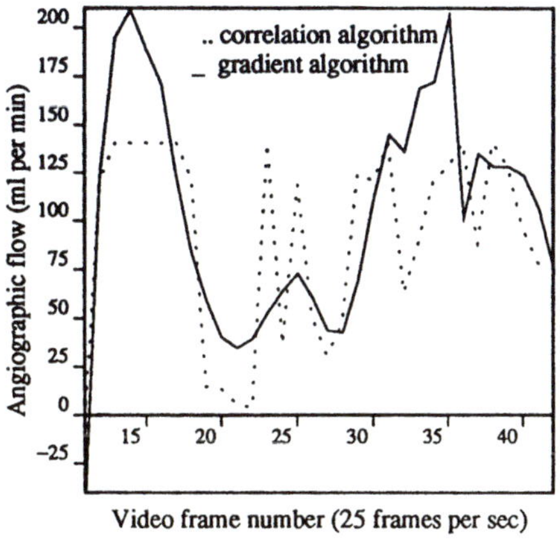

Fig. 4. Using two algorithms, flow values are plotted during 1.3 s (1.6 cardiac cycles) for the distal imaged part of the internal carotid artery, corresponding to the box in Fig. 3. Mean flow measured between the two peaks of the "gradient" graph is 95 ml · min^{-1}

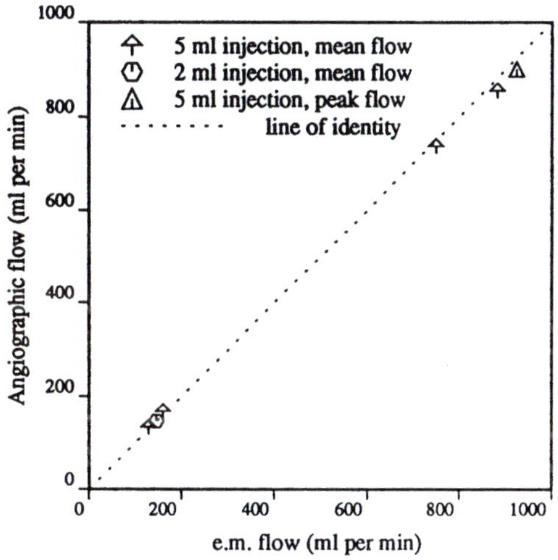

Fig. 5. Results (six values) from the validation experiments

period of 1.3 s (1.6 cardiac cycles) from the distal imaged part of the internal carotid (length 21 mm, mean width 2.9 mm). The corresponding area of the parametric image is shown by the box in Fig. 3. The current implementation of the gradient method is less susceptible to noise. The mean flow measured between the two peaks of the "gradient" graph is 95 ml/min.

The validation experiments indicated that of the three algorithms explored, the gradient-based was the most consistently effective. It produced angiographic flow measurements (Fig. 5) agreeing with e.m. flows to within 5%.

Discussion

We conclude that accurate flow measurements can be made from carotid DSA video recordings. We expect the technique to have sufficient sensitivity to measure flow in the anterior and middle cerebral arteries, but such high precision may not be achieved. It would be directly applicable to peripheral arteries and may be developed for coronary flow measurement.

Acknowledgements. This work follows from earlier work using cineangiograms, done in collaboration with A. C. F. Colchester,

D. J. Hawkes and A. Seifalian. We are grateful to the British Heart Foundation, Philips Medical UK Ltd and Sony (UK) for support.

References

1. Colchester ACF, Hawkes DJ, Brunt JNH, du Boulay GH, Wallis A (1986) Pulsatile blood flow measurements with the aid of 3-D reconstruction from dynamic angiographic recordings. In: Bacharach SL (ed) Information processing in medical imaging. 9. Martinus Nijhoff, Dordrecht, pp 247–265
2. du Boulay GH, Brunt J, Colchester A, Hawkes D, Wallis A, Wicks D (1987) Volume flow measurement of pulsatiale flow by digitised cine angiography. Acta Radiol Suppl (Stockh) 369: 59–62
3. Wicks DAG, Brunt JNH, Colchester ACF, du Boulay GH, Hawkes DJ, Wallis A (1986) A quantitative cineangiographic technique to estimate blood flow in identified vessels (abstract). Proceedings of the 26th Annual Conference Biological Engineering Society, p 60
4. Seifalian AM, Hawkes DJ, Colchester AFC, Hobbs KEF (1989) A new algorithm for deriving pulsatile blood flow waveforms, tested using stimulated dynamic angiographic data. Neuroradiology 31: 263–269

J. N. H. Brunt
Department of Medical Biophysics
Stopford Building
University of Manchester
Oxford Road
Manchester M13 9PT, UK

Neuroradiology (1991) 33 [Suppl]: 459–461

Neuroradiology

© Springer-Verlag 1991

Contrast media and microcirculation: red blood cell aggregation and deformation study

L. Monnier[1], A. Laurent[1], A. Othmane[2], J. Dufaux[2], P. Mills[2], and J. J. Merland[1]

[1] Department of Interventional Neuroradiology, Lariboisière Hospital, Paris, France
[2] Laboratory of Biorheology and Hydrodynamic Physiology, Jussieu, Paris, France

Summary. We studied the effects of six contrast media (iohexol, ioxaglate, iopamidol, ioversol, iotrolan and diatrizoate) on red blood cell (RBC) aggregation and deformation with normal blood from a single donor. RBC aggregation was studied in an erythroaggregometer with various concentrations of contrast media or saline (0%–20%). An apparent decrease of RBC aggregation was observed with most contrast media when concentrations were increased. Similar results were observed with physiological saline, suggesting dilution interference. Thus, we observed what occurred after the dilution was corrected by adding fibrinogen: hyperaggregation was found with all agents when fibrinogen was added to the solution. RBC deformation was quantified after short contact with contrast media (20% vol/vol) by light microscopy. It depends on the nature of the contrast medium. Deformation was always reversible.

Key words: Red blood cell – Contrast media – Microcirculation – Aggregation – Echinocytosis

This work tries to find out if some complications of vascular contrast media can be explained by microcirculation flow modifications related to red blood cell (RBC) hyperaggregation or echinocytosis. If so, are these RBC modifications due to the contrast medium or to its interaction with a specific patient's blood?

Materials and methods

We studied six contrast media (CM), ionic and non-ionic: diatrizoate, iohexol, iopamidol, ioversol, ioxaglate and iotrolan, at 300 mg I/ml, versus normal saline. Solutions were made with normal blood (from a single healthy donor). We used human fibrinogen lyophilized powder (Kabivitrum, Stockholm, Sweden) in solution (15 g/l), to correct for dilution effects. Aggregation was studied at 37°C, with an erythroaggregometer (Sefam-Inserm) and a viscometer (low shear-contraves [1]), measuring respectively the disaggregability threshold γ (s^{-1}) and the viscosity η (cP). The disaggregability shear stress which is the force needed to separate RBC aggregates, is calculated as follows: $\tau = \gamma \cdot \eta$ ($dynes/cm^2$). Deformation was quantified by light microscopy. We measured disaggregability shear stress variations of: (1) blood-CM mixtures with increasing concentrations of CM (0%, 1%, 5%, 10% and 20%, vol/vol) and (2) 20% blood-CM mixtures (vol/vol) with increasing fibrinogen concentrations (2.83, 3.23, 4.13 and 6.23 g/l). We quantified RBC morphology of 20% blood-CM mixtures in contact for 1–10 min using a 5-range echinocytosis RBC morphological classification [2]. The reversibility of deformation was observed on 20% blood-contrast medium mixtures in contact for 30 min, after centrifugation, aspiration of supernatant and reimmersion of RBCs in fresh plasma for 10 min. For each sample we measured pH, viscosity, osmolality and molecular weight.

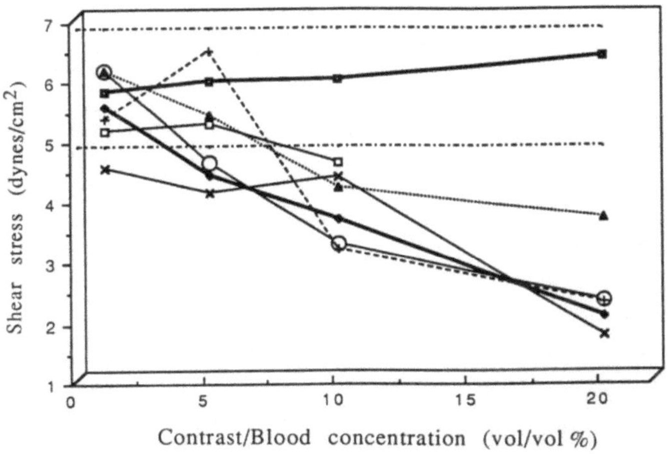

Fig. 1. Effect of contrast media on red blood cell (RBC) aggregation. ○—○, iohexol; ▲---▲, iotrolan; ■—■, ioxaglate; ◆—◆, serum physio; ×—×, iopamidol; + --- +, ioversol; □—□, diatrizoate; -·-·-, normal blood

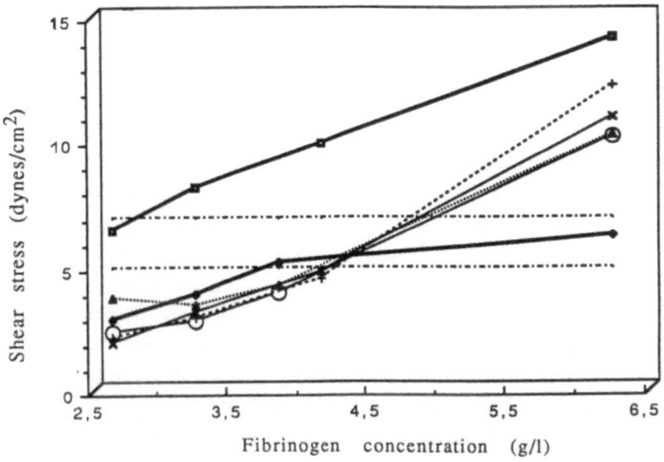

Fig. 2. Disaggregability shear stress of blood-contrast medium mixtures (20% vol/vol) with increasing fibrinogen concentrations. ○—○, iohexol; ▲---▲, iotrolan; ■—■, ioxaglate; ◆—◆, physiological serum; ×—×, iopamidol; + --- +, ioversol; -·-·-, normal blood

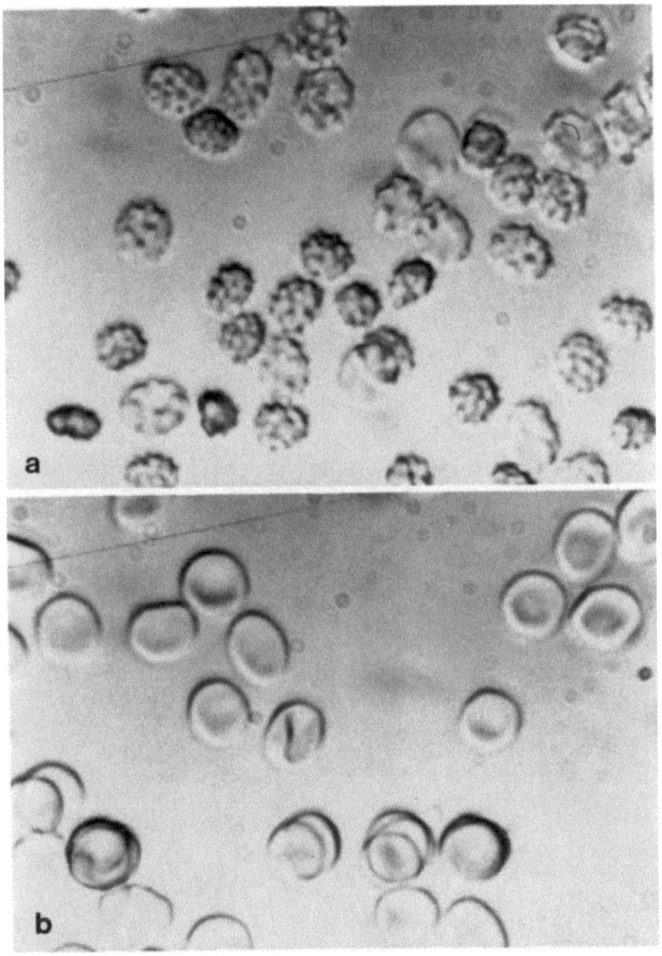

Fig. 3 a, b. Echinocytosis and reversibility study. **a** Microscopic appearances of RBC in a 20% blood-diatrizoate mixture (vol/vol). **b** Reversibility study: microscopic appearances of RBCs observed in Fig. 1 a, after reimmersion in fresh plasma

Statistics. The following were used: randomisation of measurements, SAS North Carolina Institute with GLM procedures, analysis of variance, Student-Neuman-Keuls test.

Results and discussion

Aggregation study (Figs. 1, 2)

An apparent decrease of RBC aggregation was observed with most CM when concentration increased, as described by several authors [3, 4]. However, physiological saline had the same effect. Thus, we suspected a dilution effect of some blood proteins, such as fibrinogen, which are important in RBC aggregation [5, 6]. We corrected this dilution effect by adding fibrinogen to the solutions: RBC aggregation increased more with CM than with saline, regardless of the type of CM. This may be explained by additive or multiplicative effects on RBC membranes. The effect of ioxaglate was not related to dilution. This is not explained by any of its physiological properties (pH, osmolality, viscosity, molecular weight). It could be due to its particular molecular structure (ionic dimer). Diatrizoate could not be tested because of the technical limits of the aggregometer.

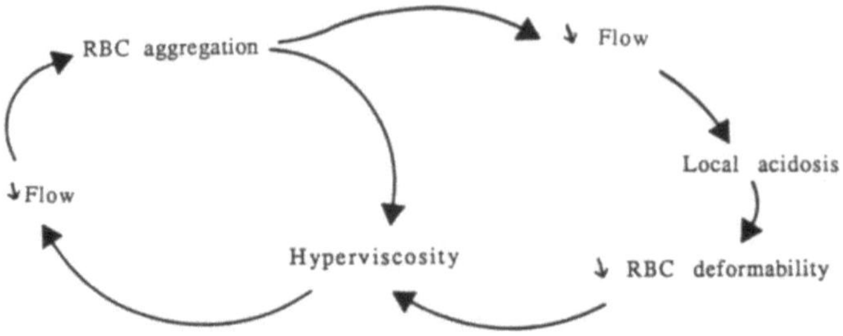

Fig. 4. Haemorheological vicious circle

RBC deformation study (Table 1, Fig. 3 a)

RBC were transformed into echinocytes and stomatocytes with all CM after 1–10 min contact. These deformations were dependant on two mechanisms.

1. *Osmolality* [3, 7]: the most significant deformations were observed with diatrizoate, a hyperosmolar ionic CM.

2. *Chemotoxicity* [8]: iopamidol gave more deformation than similar osmolar agents. The rheological behaviour of these echinocytes is contested. Meiselman [9] described normal deformability of echinocytes at high shear rates. Others believe they are more rigid than discocytes and could thus slow microcirculation [10]. Echinocytosis was reversible (Table 1, Fig. 3 b) with all CM studied, as previously described [3, 7, 11]. In contrast with others who concluded that echinocytosis is innocuous, we believe that conditions of reversibility do not always exist *in vivo* and that echinocytosis may be dangerous.

Hyperaggregation and echinocytosis may slow down the microcirculatory flow. Moreover, echinocytes aggregate more than normal RBC. These two phenomena may result in a haemorheological vicious circle (Fig. 4). This might explain some complications due to CM without angiographic occlusion. For prevention, measurement of fibrinogen levels should be considered before arteriography.

Table 1. Red blood cell deformation in 20% blood-contrast medium mixtures (vol/vol), reversibility study. Disco, Discocytes; Stomato, stomatocytes; Echino, echinocytes

%	Disco	Stomato	Echino I	Echino II	Echino III
Iopamidol	47	1.5	14.5	29.8	7.2
Reversibility	93.5	4	2.5	0	0
Diatrizoate	0	0	1	1	98
Reversibility	98	0	0	2	0
Iohexol	77.7	0	13.2	5.8	3.3
Reversibility	100	0	0	0	0
Ioxaglate	86	1.1	9.6	2.2	1.1
Reversibility	97.2	0	2.8	0	0
Ioversol	71	0	21.5	7.5	0
Reversibility	94.3	2.5	3.2	0	0
Iotrolan	93.5	3	1.7	0.9	0.9

References

1. Dufaux J, Quemada D, Mills P (1980) Determination of rheological properties of red blood cells by Couette viscosimetry. Rev Phys Appl 15: 1367–1374
2. Bessis M (1976) Réinterprétation des frottis sanguins. Masson, Paris
3. Aspelin P, Schmid-Schönbein H (1978) Effect of ionic contrast media on red cell aggregation in vitro. Acta Radiol Diagn 19: 776–784
4. Nguyen P, Potron G, Brodier V, Marcus C, Petitfrere E, Menanteau B (1989) Influence of ionic and non ionic contrast media on erythrocytic aggregation and deformability in vitro and ex vivo. Biorheology 26: 571
5. Merrill EW, Gilliland ER, Lee TS, Salzman EW (1966) Blood rheology: effect of fibrinogen deduced by addition. Circ Res 18: 437–446
6. Wells RE, Gawronski TH, Cox PJ, Perera RD (1964) Influence of fibrinogen on flow properties of erythrocyte suspensions. Am J Physiol 207: 1035–1040
7. Dawson P, Harrison JG, Weisblatt E (1983) Effect of contrast media on red cell filtrability and morphology. Br J Radiol 56: 707–710
8. Brown R, Youmans R, Livanec G, Derrick JR, Bond TP, Guest M (1968) Cinematographic observations of the effects of contrast media on the microcirculation. Vasc Surg 2: 109–115
9. Meiselman JH (1978) Rheology of shape-transformed human cells. Biorheology 15: 225–237
10. Berling C, Bucherer C, Lelievre JC, Lacombe C (1985) Comparison between viscosimetry and filtration. Applications on stored and artificially modified red blood cells. Clin Hemorheol 5: 217–223
11. Lemignon MM, Nain DIT, Ducret M, Bonnemain B, Donadieu AM (1988) Effect of contrast media on whole blood filtrability. An in vitro comparative study of Iohexol, Iopamidol and Ioxaglate on rat blood. Acta Radiol 29: 593–597

Laurence Monnier
Lariboisière Hospital
2, rue A. Paré
75010 Paris, France

Neuroradiology (1991) 33 [Suppl]: 462–463

Neuro radiology
© Springer-Verlag 1991

A note on the cerebral arteries of Perissodactyla: the rete caroticum of *Diceros bicornis*

Dubious nomenclature of the internal carotid artery of horses

G. H. du Boulay

Institute of Zoology, Zoological Society of London, Regents Park, London, UK

Summary. The existence of a rete caroticum is reported in an adult black rhinoceros *(Diceros bicornis)*. Comparison of the arterial supply to the brain in other Perissodactyla, including the horse, suggests that what in them is generally called the "internal carotid" is the homologue of the ascending pharyngeal artery. This has far-reaching physiological implications.

Key words: Rete caroticum – Perissodactyla – *Diceros bicornis*

Since Thomas Willis (1684) [1], a clear distinction has been drawn between even-toed ungulates, all of which have retia carotica, and odd-toed ungulates, which have been thought to have a very different system. The cloven-footed (cattle, deer, antelope, pig, giraffe, hippopotamus) supply their cerebral arteries via complex networks of small arteries lying within the cavernous sinuses where they are bathed by venous blood. These retia are all supplied by branches such as the arteria anastomotica, the ramus anastomoticus or the ascending pharyngeal that originally derive from the external carotid. In many species the rete has been implicated as a heat exchanger in brain temperature regulation [2, 3]. du Boulay et al. [4] showed that, at least in the goat, the rete and branches that supplied it were also capable of autoregulation to favour the brain's blood supply during systemic arterial hypotension.

The theoretical advantage of an extradural method of autoregulation for long-legged, pronograde mammals has been previously propounded [4]. At that time the discovery that the adult black rhinoceros *(Diceros bicornis)* possessed a well-developed rete was also recorded, entirely against the preconception, following Willis [1], that Perissodactyla (odd-toed ungulates, the horse family) supplied their brains, like man via an undivided internal carotid artery.

The radiograph first demonstrating the rete caroticum of the rhinocerus has not been published until now.

Materials and methods

Single adult specimens of *D. bicornis* (black rhinoceros), *Equus caballus* (the horse), *E. burchelli* (zebra), and *Tapirus indicus* (tapir) were obtained as a result of death from natural causes. The heads were amputated and the cut ends of the common carotid arteries identified. Cannulae were tied into these and barium sulphate suspension (Micropaque) injected until adequate radiographs could be obtained showing the situation, branching and bony relationships of the major cerebral vessels. Stereoscopic views were usually used.

The head of *D. bicornis* was then deep frozen and divided in two by a single sagittal saw cut. After thawing, the two halves of the head were dissected by W. R. Cooke and G. H. du Boulay. The brain, with its barium-filled vessels, was subsequently radiographed on its own.

Results

Diceros bicornis

Radiographs. The rete caroticum is a symmetrical, more or less bilobed, very complex collection of interconnected vessels of irregular calibre, averaging about 1.2 mm in diameter. It lies astride the midline, embracing the basisphenoid, and receives its blood supply from two pairs of arteries. The smaller pair runs directly backwards from the facially-directed continuation of the maxillary artery and enters the rete at the anterolateral corners in a way very similar to the arteria anastomotica of, for instance, the goat. Each of the larger pair of supplying arteries is given off from the common carotid just proximal to the large occipital artery. It runs anteriorly, dorsally and medially in a gentle curve to a point immediately ventral to the rete, where it penetrates the skull base and enters the rete at its most lateral margin, two-thirds of the distance from the front of that structure.

Dissection. The vessels of the rete lay, as shown in the radiograph (Fig. 1), surrounded by the cavernous sinus. Anteriorly the vessels extended into the region of the orbital fissure; inferolaterally they lay adjacent to foramen lacerum, through which the larger artery of supply appeared to enter directly into the network. This artery could be followed directly from its origin in the neck; it lay in close proximity to the guttural pouch and then disappeared into the skull base at foramen lacerum. There was no internal carotid artery as seen in most mammals (other than Ungulates and Felidae), in which it enters the carotid canal close to the mastoid bulla and usually gives rise to the more or less well-developed stapedial artery; nor was there any other artery that might be considered the homologue of the ascending pharyngeal.

From the superior surface of the rete, both in the radiographs and on dissection, the paired anterior cerebral arteries, the middle cerebral and, on dissection, at

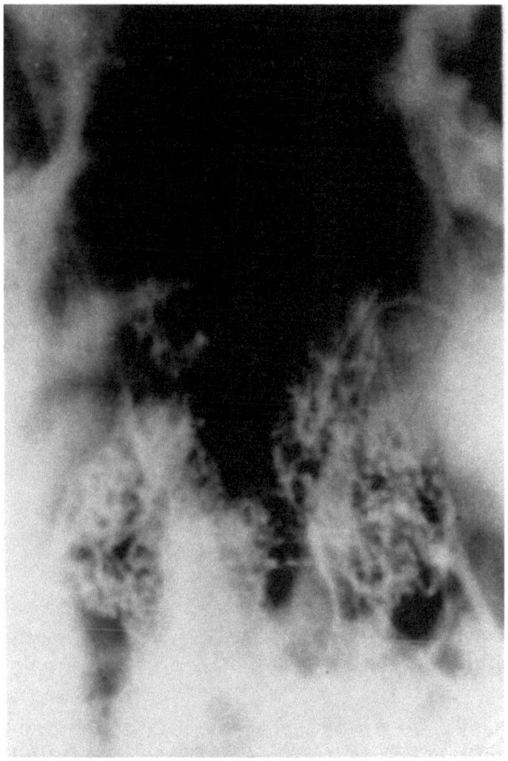

Fig. 1. Ventro-dorsal radiograph of the injected rete caroticum of the adult black rhinoceros

least two pairs of posterior cerebral arteries could be seen arising directly from the rete. There was no intracranial internal carotid artery but the cerebral vessels penetrated the dura directly from their origin in the retial network. Subsequent dissection and radiography of the brain showed in more detail the pial and perforating arteries, generally in line with the description by Garrod [5].

Equus caballus

Radiographs ([6], pp 238–241) show the similarity between horse and rhinoceros in the course of the main artery to the brain and particularly its point of entry into the cranial cavity. The intercarotid artery, an extradural anastomosis between the two brain-supplying arteries has been visualised.

The radiographs show how the occipital arteries (external carotid branches) are interposed between the major neck arteries (common carotid) and the cerebral vertebral arteries. There is little if any possibility of direct cervical vertebral-to-basilar artery blood flow.

Equus burchelli

Radiographs ([6], pp 242–243) show how the main vessel supplying the brain, close to a point where it perforates the fibrocartilaginous skull base, supplies a branch, not as in the horse to the opposite "carotid", but to pierce the dura mater, forming an anastomotic channel to supply the network of vessels on the ventral surface of the brain stem.

Tapirus indicus

Radiographs ([6], pp 244–245) show an arrangement more like the zebra than the horse.

Discussion

The demonstration of an elaborate rete caroticum in two single specimens of *D. bicornis,* one in an embryo [7] and the present adult, though the material is slight, establishes the likelihood that this is the pattern of arterial blood supply in the rhinoceros and unites the odd- and even-toed ungulates in way that might have been, but was not expected. Davies [7] does not seem to have realised the importance of his finding.

The anatomy of what has been thought and spoken of as the "internal carotid" of the horse by generations of zoologists and veterinary surgeons was described by Vaughan in 1892. Every feature, except its size, resembles the ascending pharyngeal artery of man, so familiar to neuroradiologists, including the perforation of the skull base by a meningeal branch. The works of Nanda and Getty [8, 9] on the arteria intercarotica caudalis and the arteria caroticobasilaris of the horse, although they give no consideration to the ascending pharyngeal, do emphasise the importance of dural and transdural anastomotic networks forming pathways to the brain stem, as our radiographs showed in the zebra and the tapir.

The vessel in *E. caballus* commonly called pharyngeal or ascending pharyngeal does not reach the skull base, but pursues a course like other pharyngeal branches of the external carotid artery in *Homo.*

The conclusion that all odd-toed ungulates share with even-toed ungulates the physiological advantages that may be derived from interposing smaller branches of the external carotid between the main arterial trunk of common carotid and the intracranial cerebral vessels seems inescapable.

In addition the rhinoceros possesses what is likely to be a highly developed heat exchanger to aid its brain temperature regulation.

References

1. Willis T (1684) Dr Willis' practice of physick, being the whole medical work of that physician. Translated into English by S. Pordage, London
2. Baker MA, Hayward JN (1967) Carotid rete and brain temperature of cat. Nature 216: 139–141
3. Baker MA, Hayward JN (1968) The influence of the nasal mucosa and the carotid rete upon hypothalamic temperature in sheep. J Physiol (Lond) 198: 561–579
4. du Boulay G, Kendall BE, Crockard A, Sage M, Belloni G (1975) The autoregulatory capability of Galen's rete cerebri and its connections. Neuroradiology 9: 171–181
5. Garrod AG (1878) On the brain of the Sumatran rhinoceros *(Ceratorrhinus sumatrensis).* Proc Zool Soc Lond 10: 411–413
6. du Boulay GH, Verity PM (1973) The cranial arteries of mammals. Heinemann, London
7. Davies J (1952–1953) The anatomy of a twenty-two millimetre embryo of the African Rhinoceros *(Rhinoceros bicornis).* Proc Zool Soc Lond 122: 593–613
8. Nanda BS, Getty R (1975) Arteria intercarotica caudalis and its homologue in the domestic animals. Anat Anz 137: 110–115
9. Nanda BS, Getty R (1975) Presence of the arteria caroticobasilaris in the horse. Anat Anz 137: 116–119

George H. du Boulay M. B., B. S., F. R. C. R.
Institute of Zoology
Regents Park, London, UK

Neuroradiology (1991) 33 [Suppl]: 464–466

Neuro radiology
© Springer-Verlag 1991

Postmortem MRI of brains in vitro: correlation with neuropathological findings

U. Salvolini[1], M. Scarpelli[3], L. Chiaromoni[2], N. Foschi[2], M. Maricotti[2], L. Salvolini[1], G. M. Mariuzzi[3], and F. Angeleri[2]

[1] Department of Neuroradiology, Local Health Authority no. 12,
Departments of [2] Neurology, and [3] Pathology, University of Ancona, Ancona, Italy

Summary. MRI was used for routine examination of postmortem formalin-fixed brains. The correlation of MRI with neuropathological findings allowed us to clarify the nature of brain lesions. MRI was useful for identifying sites for histological examination.

Key words: Magnetic resonance imaging – Neuropathology

MRI has been introduced recently into our university and weekly clinicopathological meetings are organized to discuss the most intriguing cases. We observed a number of lesions difficult to explain on the basis of the neurological history. This prompted us to initiate research to establish correlation between MRI and neuropathological findings. The following three cases were chosen because they represented examples of the most common lesions we encountered.

Materials and methods

The brains were immediately fixed in 10% neutral buffered formalin for 2–3 weeks. Before MRI they were placed in water for 6–12 h. MRI was performed with the specimen placed in a plastic box completely filled with water. A Magnetom Siemens 1.0 T unit with commercial surface and head coils was used. The transverse sections were imaged parallel to a bicommissural plane and the coronal sections parallel to a plane tangential to the floor of the IV ventricle or perpendicular to the bicommissural plane. The examination was performed with spin-echo multisection imaging sequences. Short TR sequences, 450/22 (TR/TE) were obtained in the sagittal plane; long TR sequences, 2000–2500/19–25 (first echo), 90 (second echo), were obtained in the coronal and axial planes. All were obtained with 5-mm slice thickness and a 1-mm gap between slices. The matrix size was 256 × 256. Subsequently the hindbrain was detached from the cerebrum and the hemispheres were cut into slices 1 cm thick. The slices were then imaged again and the most representative were selected for paraffin embedding. The sections were stained with haematoxylin and eosin and Luxol fast blue.

Results

Case 1

MRI. On long TR images small areas of hyperintensity were identified bilaterally at the level of the basal ganglia and left centrum semiovale. One area of increased signal with ill-defined limits was also identified on the right in the precentral gyrus (Fig. 1 a, c).

Neuropathology. The macroscopic examination showed discoloration with no obvious loss of substance in the right posterior frontal lobe and the left centrum semiovale (Fig. 1 b, d).

Microscopically we found ischaemic infarcts characterized by foam cells, reactive astrocytes, microglial hyperplasia and small areas of calcification.

Case 2

MRI. Ventricular enlargement was present, mainly involving the temporal horns and basal cerebrospinal fluid space. Increased signal on long TR/short TE sequence was also detected along the ependyma and subependymal white matter of the frontal horns of the lateral ventricles. Hyperintensity was found in the centrum semiovale and hippocampus.

Neuropathology. The brain was macroscopically normal except for dilatation of the ventricles. There were multiple gaps in the ependyma of the lateral ventricles associated with vacuolization of the underlying brain parenchyma and hyperplasia of the subependymal glia. Lesions were also present bilaterally in the hippocampus, consisting of dilatation of blood vessels and perivascular spaces, loss of neurons and neurofibrillary degeneration.

Case 3

MRI. On long TR MRI inhomogeneous hyperintense foci were found in the subependymal white matter at the corners of the lateral ventricles and in the basal ganglia (Fig. 2 a, c, e).

Neuropathology. The brain was macroscopically normal. The microscopic examination of sections through the mamillary bodies showed multiple gaps in the ependyma associated with reactive gliosis. The perivascular spaces were widened, mainly in the basal ganglia (Fig. 2 b, d, f).

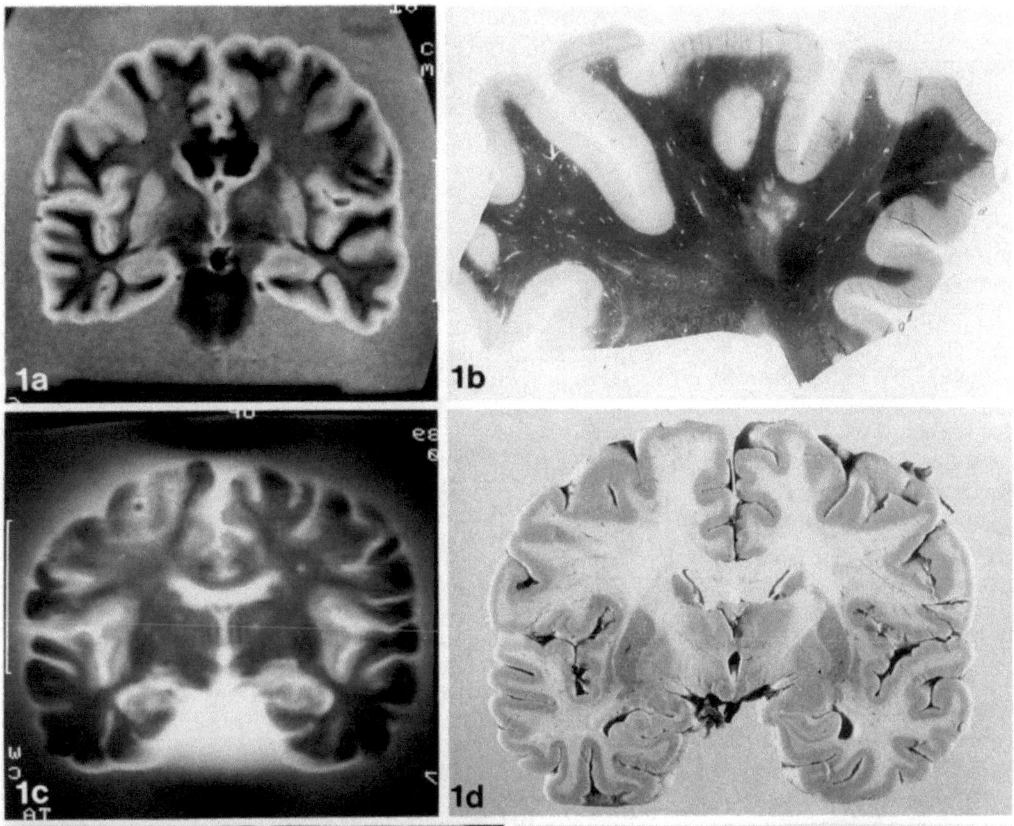

Fig. 1 a–d. Case 1. **a, c** MRI; **b, d** macroscopic examination

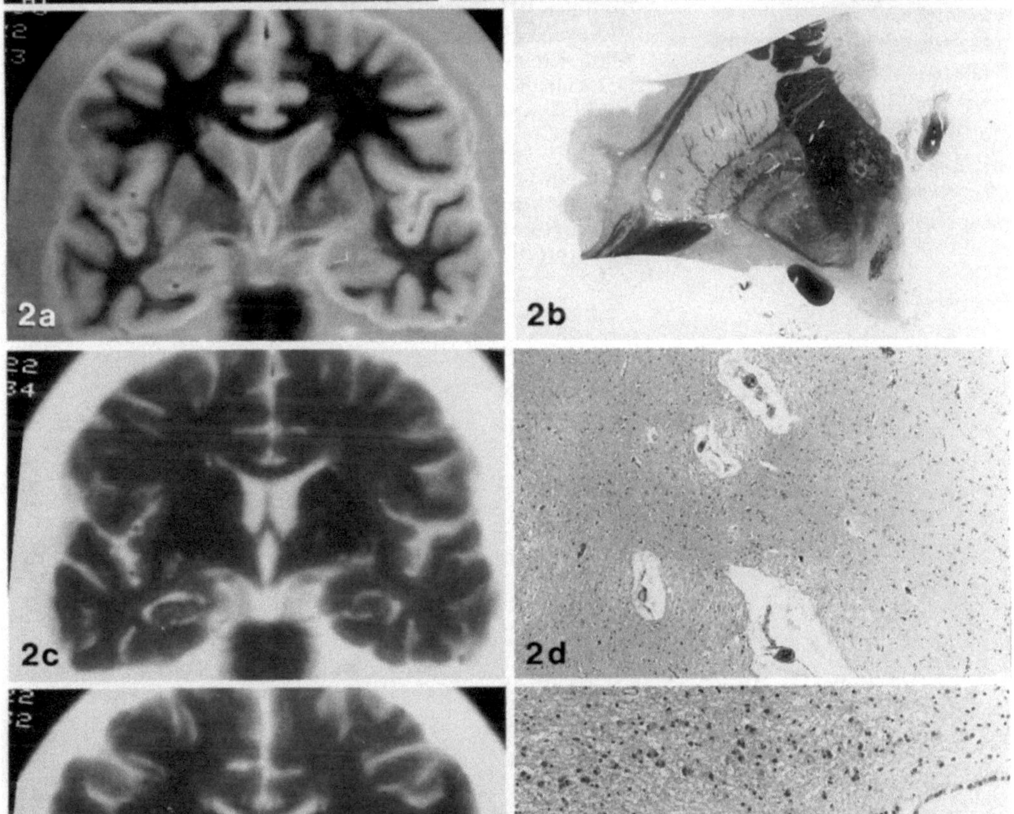

Fig. 2 a–f. Case 3. **a, c, e** MRI; **b, d, f** microscopic sections

Discussion

The lesions we found can be summarized as follows: multiple foci of abnormal high signal in patient 1, confluent periventricular hyperintensity in patient 2 and dilatation of the perivascular spaces in patient 3 [1]. Multiple foci of abnormal high signal are commonly seen in elderly patients. White matter infarction is the lesion most commonly found although atrophy and shrinkage of axons and myelin, with gliosis surrounding thickened tortuous vessels [4] can also be detected. In both cases the changes are due to vascular insufficiency and are common [5] in non-demented patients over 65 years [2, 3]. In our patient the lesion represented multiple infarcts. It is notable that in this patient the lesions were not macroscopically apparent and only a slight discoloration of the white matter made us suspect a lesion apparent on MRI. In our opinion, this finding highlights the usefulness of this method to detect abnormalities which can go unnoticed macroscopically and to indicate the slice to be embedded.

The second lesion we found is represented by confluent periventricular hyperintensity. Zimmerman et al. [6] observed this finding not only in patients with hydrocephalus, demyelinating diseases or other pathologies but also in normal subjects. The underlying lesion can be infarction, gliosis or decrease in myelin and localized breakdown of ependyma [7]. In our patient this finding was present in the absence of any neurological signs and was associated with hydrocephalus. Histologically we found multiple gaps in the ependyma. Patient 3 showed enlarged perivascular spaces mainly in the basal ganglia. Even though, according to Braffman et al. [8], the enlarged perivascular spaces can be distinguished from lacunar infarcts we did not always find it easy to make this distinction, since small cystic infarcts can have the same intensity as the perivascular spaces.

In conclusion MRI of formalin-fixed brains allows us to clarify the nature of lesions commonly encountered in routine work and helps us to discriminate between abnormalities with similar appearances.

References

1. Braffman BH, Zimmerman RA, Troianowski JQ, Gonatas NK, Hickey WF, Schlaepfer WW (1988) Brain MR: pathologic correlation with gross and histopathology. Lacunar infarction and Virchow-Robin spaces. AJNR 9
2. Brant-Zawadzki M, Kucharczyk W (1987) Vascular disease: ischemia. In: Brant-Zawadzki M, Norman D (eds) Magnetic resonance imaging of the central nervous system. Raven, New York, pp 221–234
3. Holland BA (1987) Diseases of white matter. In: Brandt-Zawadzki M, Norman D (eds) Magnetic resonance imaging of the central nervous system. Raven, New York, pp 259–277
4. Kirkpatrick JB, Hayman LA (1987) White-matter lesions in MR imaging of clinically healthy brains of elderly subjects: possible pathologic basis. Radiology 162: 509–511
5. Wisniewski HM, Terry RD (1973) Morphology of the aging brain, human and animal. Prog Brain Res 40: 167–186
6. Zimmerman RD, Fleming CA, Lee BCP, Saint Louis LA, Deck MDF (1986) Periventricular hyperintensity as seen by magnetic resonance: prevalence and significance. AJNR 7: 13–20
7. Sze G, De Armond S, Brant-Zawadzki M (1986) Abnormal MRI foci anterior to the frontal horns: pathologic correlates of an ubiquitous finding (abstract). AJNR 7: 13–20
8. Braffman BH, Zimmerman RA, Trojanowski JQ, Gonatas NK, Hickey WF, Schlaepfer WW (1988) Brain MR: pathologic correlation with gross and histopathology. I. Hyperintense white-matter foci in the elderly. AJNR 9: 629–636

U. Salvolini
Neuroradiologia
Ospedale Nuovo di Torrette
I-60020 Torrette Ancona, Italy

Neuroradiology (1991) 33 [Suppl]: 467–468

Neuro
radiology
© Springer-Verlag 1991

Nondestructive anatomy of CNS: the results of multiplanar reconstruction in MRI

U. Salvolini, L. Salvolini, A. Tartaro, M. De Donatis, and A. Serio

Department of Neuroradiology, General Regional Hospital, Ancona, Villa Serena, Pescara, Italy

Summary. Three-dimensional Fourier transform gradient echo sequences and multiplanar reconstructions are useful tools in anatomical studies. Details of intracranial soft tissues are well shown using suitable planes in the acquisition and reconstruction of the images. The results of this technique in CNS study are discussed.

Key words: Magnetic resonance imaging – Multiplanar reconstruction – Multiplanar reformatting – Central nervous system

The term anatomy itself implies "cutting": a kind of analysis which requires operation of the object by different methods to be able to show the internal structure well.

The methods of classic morphological anatomy are mainly based on analysis of a series of sections or on dissection and erosion. In all cases traditional anatomy uses methods of analysis which destroy the structure of the object and which do not allow other kinds of analysis on the same structure afterwards by different methods. In all cases of analysis involving serial sections, the researcher must be able to reconstruct mentally a structure using the information given by each section: that is why in the past the researcher always referred to the anatomical drawing, which enabled the graphic transcription of the mentally constructed image in a way that allowed it to be shown to others.

Modern neuroradiology is based principally on the methods of morphological analysis by sections (CT, MRI), in other words on methods which emphasise a particular structure, accentuating the contrast in respect to the nearby structures, with the effect of erosion in a wide sense (digital angiography). The analysed object itself is not altered; that is why all different methods of analysis can applied in succession.

The advantages of this anatomical radiology on human beings are notable. Besides overcoming all alterations resulting from cadaveric decomposition, there is, above all, the possibility of analysing the same anatomical specimen in different ways obtaining, one after the other, elements to evaluate differently without destroying the object of the analysis so that one wishes to reconstruct or take apart the object at a later date [1–3].

Results and discussion

In the 3D Fourier transform method, the signal is obtained from all regions within a large volume rather than from a thin plane or narrow line. Therefore, there is an improvement in the signal to noise (s/n) ratio over other methods: it improves with the square root of the number of slices. The thickness of the slice is not limited by the narrowness of the radiofrequency band width or the strength of the gradient as in 2D methods. Very thin slices without interslice gaps are achieved. Very thin contiguous sections (1 mm) show an excellent s/n ratio, even with a medium-power magnet (0.5 T). This technique is therefore particularly useful for a high-resolution morphological study of anatomical details of the skull and spine.

All patients were imaged at 0.5 T on a Toshiba unit. Images were obtained with routine gradient echo pulse sequence with TR = 55 ms, TE = 14 ms, two acquisitions and flip angle between 30 ° and 45 °. Twenty-nine slices, 1 mm thick, were acquired in 13–15 min. The volume ac-

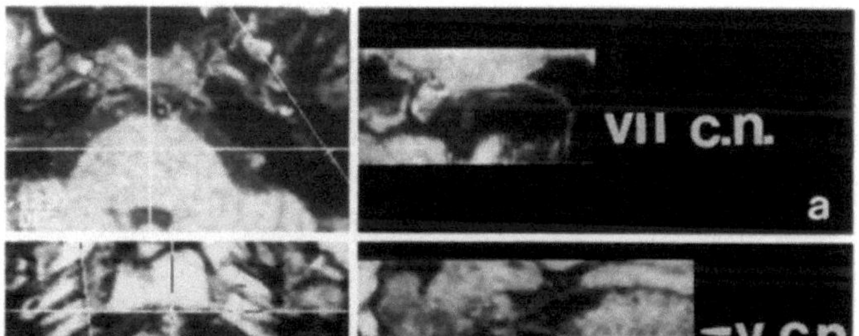

Fig. 1 a–c. Gradient-echo sequence: TR = 55 ms; TE = 14 ms; Flip angle (FA) = 35 °. **a** Para-sagittal reconstruction from axial plane that shows the second and third part of seventh cranial nerve; **b** the fifth and sixth; **c** axial oblique reconstruction showing both fifth cranial newes

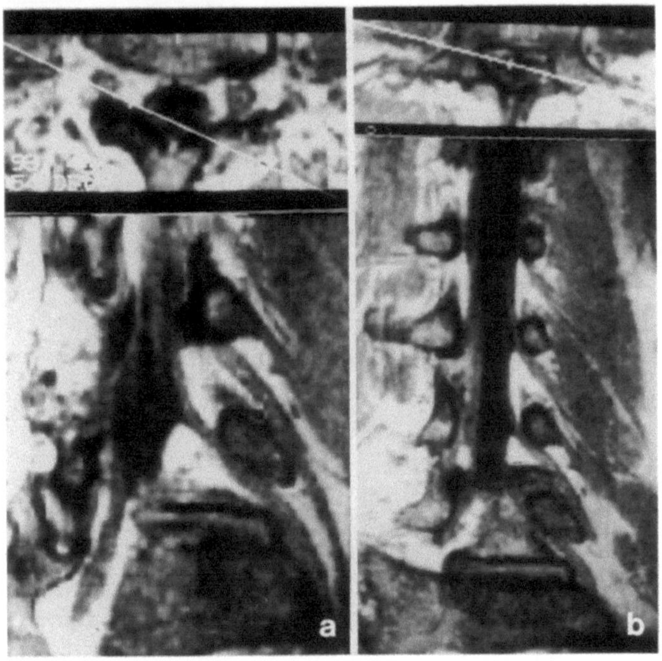

Fig. 2a, b. Gradient-echo sequence: TR = 60 ms; TE = 14 ms; FA = 45 °. Oblique reconstruction of lumbar nerve roots

quisition technique avoids any loss of information among contiguous sections because they happen to be closely contiguous. Such a technique is not only mainly used at brain level for the analysis of the sellar region and chiasmatic pathway, but also for the brain stem and cranial nerves. It is also employed at spinal level.

The best representation of anatomical structure can be obtained by planes oriented according to its spatial development by a successive manipulation of acquired data. The background knowledge of the "classic" anatomy and the results obtained by CT multiplanar reconstruction (MPR) allows the identification of some "nonorthogonal" but "anatomically-oriented" incidences to get a correct MRI representation of anatomical structures, both at brain and spinal level [4, 5].

MPR designates computer retroprocessing of image data obtained in one plane in order to display the same anatomy as if the images had been obtained in other orthogonal or oblique planes. For this procedure the original data must be gathered as contiguous thin sections through the entire volume of anatomical interest (Figs. 1, 2). Selection of an appropriate plane for computer reconstruction requires the physician to recognize significant anatomical landmarks on the initial series of images. Careful choice of the points permits the physician to obtain sections that are "anatomically arranged" in spite of individual variability. Such computer-generated planes can be reproduced time after time to permit accurate assessment of interval change in a single subject, or they can be achieved in different subjects to allow thorough analysis of anatomical variations.

References

1. Salvolini U, Cabanis EA, Iba-Zizen MT, De Nicola M, Hemmy DC (1984) Apport diagnostique de la reconstruction tridimensionelle en scanner RX: coupes et surfaces de l'anatomie cephalique. Ann Chir Plast Esthet 29: 339–357
2. Salvolini U, Menichelli F, Pasquini U, Perugini S, Piana C (1984) La TC ad alta risoluzione con ricostruzioni 3D id sezioni e di superfici: una anatomia in vivo. XXXI Congresso SIRMN 1984. Monduzzi, Florence
3. Salvolini U, Perugini S (1986) La tomodensitometrie: una anatomie in vivo. Radiologie 6: 69–71
4. Frahm J, Haase A, Matthaei D (1986) Technical note. Rapid three-dimensional MRI using the FLASH technique. J Comput Assist Tomogr 10: 663–668
5. Harms SE, Munschler G (1986) Three-dimensional MRI of the knee using surface coils. J Comput Assist Tomogr 10: 773–777

Dr. U. Salvolini
Neuroradiology Department
General Regional Hospital
Ancona, Italy

POSTER SESSION 2

Neuroradiology (1991) 33 [Suppl]: 470–471

Neuro
radiology
© Springer-Verlag 1991

Discography: the decisive factor in the choice of percutaneous or surgical treatment of the herniated lumbar disc

G. Fabris, A. Lavaroni, E. Biasizzo, F. Zappoli, and M. Leonardi

Department of Neuroradiology, Civil Hospital of Udine, Udine, Italy

Summary. Over a period of 4.5 years, 977 discograms were performed on 774 patients, with a complication, septic discitis in only one case. Six hundred and eighty-one patients underwent percutaneous treatment of the herniated lumbar disc [chemonucleolysis or nucleo-aspiration (Onik procedure)], while in the remaining 93 patients the discographic findings contraindicated percutaneous treatment. Discography plays two important roles, one diagnostic and the other decisional. While confirming the clinical and neuroradiological findings of disc herniation, discography verifies the correct positioning of the needle at the centre of the nucleus pulposus and proves decisive in determining the preferential treatment to be undertaken on the basis of morphological, functional and dynamic data.

Key words: Lumbar disc herniation – Discography – Percutaneous treatment

Nine hundred and seventy-seven discograms were performed on 774 patients during the period 20 December 1985 to 17 May 1990.

On the basis of the clinical and neuroradiological findings (plain films, CT or MRI, discography), 681 patients underwent percutaneous treatment of the herniated disc [chemonucleolysis, discal nucleo-aspiration (Onik procedure)]. The discographic findings in the remaining 93 patients contraindicated percutaneous procedures; 35 of these patients underwent surgery. In 977 discograms, there was 1 complication, a septic discitis.

The results of the percutaneous procedures were analysed by means of MacNab's criteria and a check-sheet recording the subjective reactions of the patient. In the first 450 patients treated by chemonucleolysis and followed from 1 to 4.5 years, the results were excellent or good in 85.5% of cases. As regards the first 70 patients treated with the Onik procedure and followed for 1–2 years, excellent or good results were obtained in 70%.

Discussion

Intraoperative discography, performed under fluoroscopic control with a posterolateral extradural approach, represents the last stage of the diagnostic examinations and is decisive in the choice of treatment to be undertaken on the basis of the morphological, functional and dynamic data [1].

The principal morphological information provided by discography consists in its verification of the correct posi-

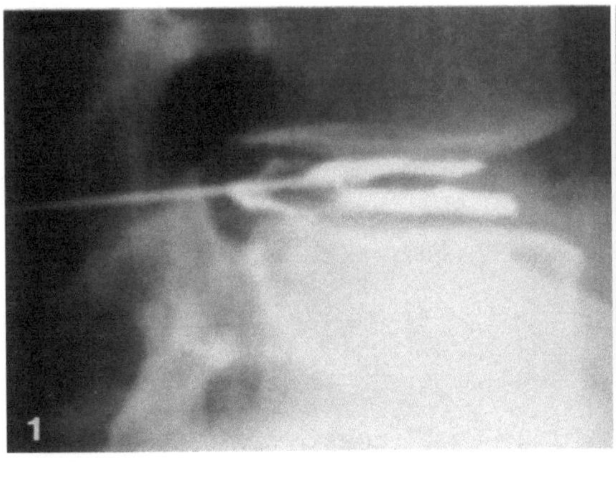

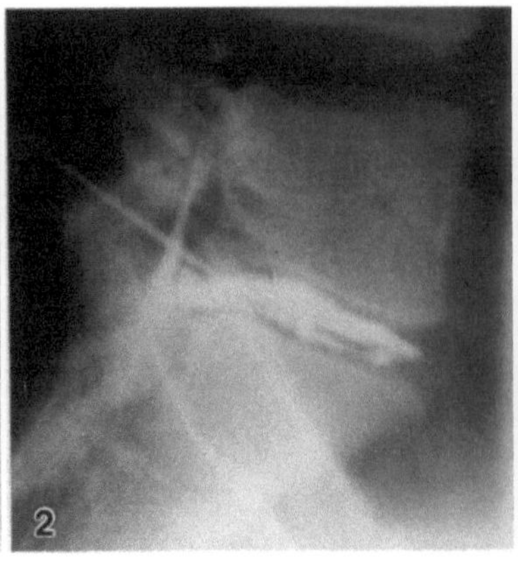

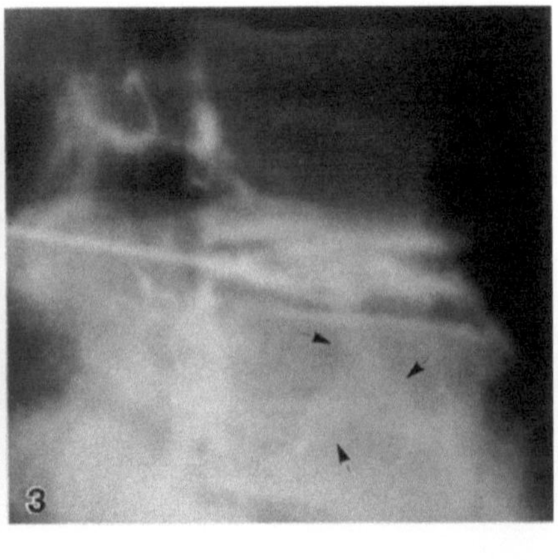

Fig. 1. Discography at L4–5: degenerate, flattened disc; small, contained, subligamentous hernia, which can be treated with automated percutaneous discectomy

Fig. 2. Discography at L5–S1: degenerate, fissured disc; posterolateral epidural leak caused by interruption of the posterior longitudinal ligament (extraligamentous herniation). Good filling of the herniated surface; medium-sized herniation, contiguous with the nucleus pulposus, which can be treated with chemonucleolysis

Fig. 3. Discography at level L4–5: marked posterolateral epidural leak, with seepage of contrast into the vertebral venous rete (vascular leak, *arrows*). This discographic finding contraindicates percutaneous treatment tioning of the needle. Other morphological data include the degree of disc degeneration and the morphological characteristics of the herniation. Discography is able to demonstrate annulus bulging, subligamentous and extra-ligamentous herniation; to delineate the cranial or caudal extension of the hernia, its dimensions and particular features such as annulography, vascular leak, discal incontinence or intradural hernia. The morphological characteristics, filling capacity of the herniated area and size of the hernia provide guidelines for determining the preferential treatment to be undertaken (the decisional role of discography) (Fig. 1–3).

Discography supplies functional details about intradiscal pressure, based on the greater or lesser resistance encountered in injecting the contrast medium. This finding is an important point of reference for chemonucleolysis, as it gives information about the dose of enzyme to be injected. The intradiscal pressure may be more effectively measured through discomanometry.

Discography furthermore supplies data of a dynamic nature, such as the pain response elicited and the pattern of contrast medium diffusion in the epidural space. The pain response is of considerable prognostic value: its presence, in the case of a well-opacified, medium-to-large herniation increases the probability of obtaining good-to-excellent results from therapy to about 97% of cases [1]. In the eventuality of multiple pathology, it also provides valuable, clear-cut evidence of the level to be treated.

Discography is the examination which best demonstrates the integrity, detachment or interruption of the posterior longitudinal ligament: diffusion of the contrast medium in the subligamentous space indicates a contained herniation (the posterior longitudinal ligament is intact); leakage of contrast medium into the epidural space may be slight, due to detachment of the posterior longitudinal ligament (subligamentous hernia, still contained) or medium-to-large, caused by the rupture of the ligament (extraligamentous or exteriorised herniation).

These discographic parameters, together with the pain response and clinical findings, are of fundamental importance in determining the treatment preferred: discal nucleo-aspiration, chemonucleolysis or surgery. In discal nucleo-aspiration, the herniation must be small to medium in size and contained or, at most, with a slight epidural leak [2]. In chemonucleolysis, it is preferable to treat medium-to-large herniations, as long as the latter are contiguous with the gelatinous pulp of the nucleus, independently from the integrity of the posterior longitudinal ligament [1, 3, 4]. Discography takes on a decisive role in demonstrating particular findings: vascular leak, discal incontinence, scanty filling of the herniated area, massive epidural leak, and intradural herniation, all of which require surgical treatment. Non-opacification of a herniation previously identified by CT or MRI raises suspicions of a fragmented or excluded herniation, requiring surgery.

References

1. Troisier O, Cypel D (1986) Discography: an element of decision. Surgery versus chemonucleolysis. Clin Orthop 206: 70–78
2. Onik G, Helms CA (1988) Automated percutaneous lumbar discectomy. Radiology Research and Educational Foundation, San Francisco
3. Fabris G, Penco T, Biasizzo E, Zappoli F, Lavaroni A, Leonardi M (1987) Discography and chemonucleolysis. In: Calabro' A, Leonardi M (eds) Computer aided neuroradiology. CIC, Rome, pp 453–457
4. Menkes CJl, Feldmann JL, Ben Sedrine H, Amor B, Chevrot A, Horreard P, Zenny JC, Pallardy J (1982) Traitement des hernies discales lombaires par chimionucleolyse. Rev Rhum 49: 621–628

Dr. Giuliano Fabris
Servizio di Neuroradiologia
Ospedale Civile
I-33100 Udine, Italy

Neuroradiology (1991) 33 [Suppl]: 472–473

Neuroradiology
© Springer-Verlag 1991

Lumbar percutaneous discectomy: initial experience in 28 cases

C. Faubert[1] and W. Caspar[2]

[1] Neuroradiological Institute and [2] Departement of Neurosurgery, University of Saarland, Homburg-Saar, Federal Republic of Germany

Summary. Since November 1988, 28 patients with lumbar radiculopathy refractory to conservative care and with a radiologically verified contained central or mediolateral disc herniation at L4–5 have had a percutaneous discectomy. A short-term follow-up analysis of at least 2 months taking the clinical, functional and work activity features into account revealed a 64.3% (18/28) satisfactory rate and a 32.1% (10/28) failure rate. Of the latter 28.6% (8/28 patients) required further open surgery. One patient who had only partial resolution of pain turned out to have a sequestered craniad prolapse as revealed by postoperative CT and confirmed by open surgery. There were no major complications. One patient developed a sequestered extraforaminal herniation through the nucleotomy canal 3 weeks after the procedure. One patient bled for 2 min; then the bleeding stopped. There were no major vessel injuries. In terms of undesirable side-effects 1 patient reported local muscular pain, and enhanced nerve root pain after introduction of the trocar sleeve. Open surgery on this patient revealed an inflamed nerve.

Key words: Lumbar disc herniation – Percutaneous discectomy

Since November 1988, percutaneous discectomy has been performed in 28 patients with L5 radiculopathy refractory to conservative care and with a radiologically verified L4–5 disc protrusion. A short-term success rate of 64.3% (18/28) was achieved versus a 35.7% (10/28) failure rate.

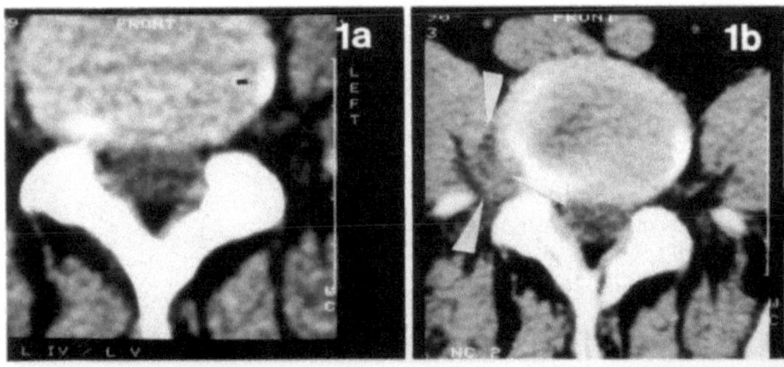

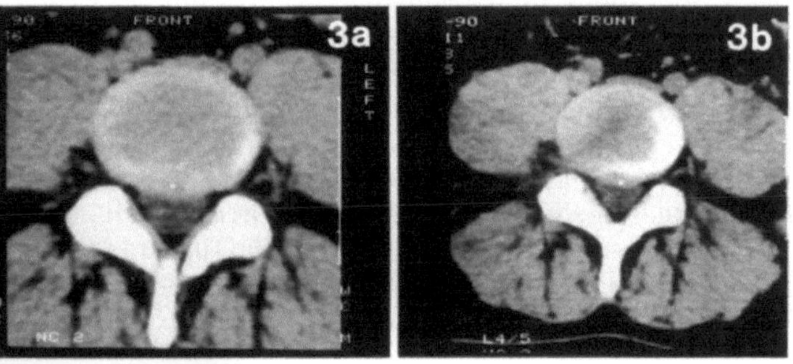

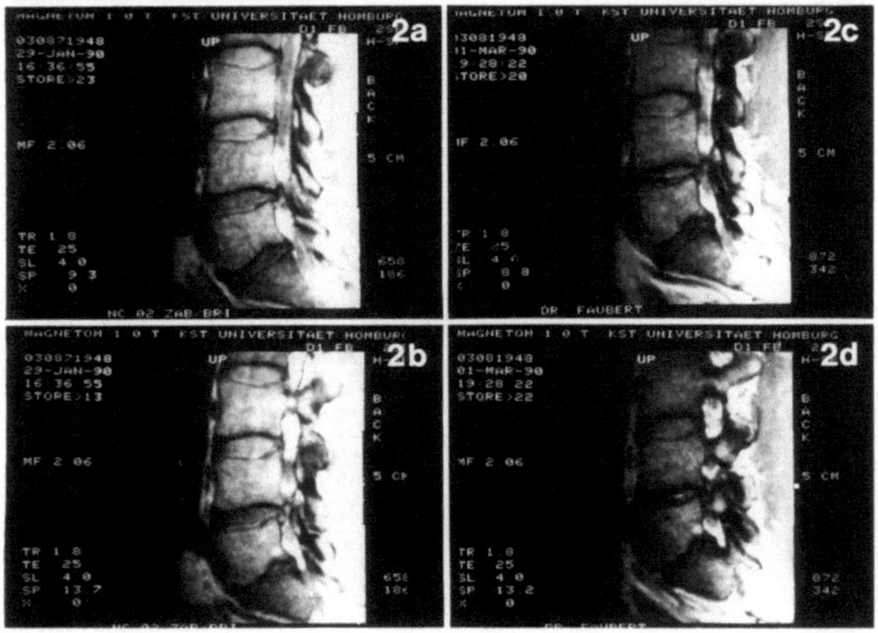

Fig. 1. a Pre- and **b** postoperative L4–5 CT. **b** Note the important surgically verified extraforaminal prolapse *(arrowheads)* through the nucleotomy canal 3 weeks after a percutaneous nucleotomy

Fig. 2. a, b Pre- and **c, d** postoperative (4 weeks) proton density weighted sagittal MRI. Note the significant L4–5 disc space reduction

Fig. 3. a, b. Medial protrusion L4–5. Pre- (**a**) and postoperative (**b**) CT (4 weeks after). Note the nucleotomy canal on the right. The protrusion is unchanged (typical)

Nine patients required further open surgery. Four patients had poor indications because of spinal stenosis, lateralised foraminal herniations, predominance of back pain over leg pain, and all were failures. They were undertaken in a context of patient and medical insistence. If the patients' clinical status remained unchanged or worsened, we did not routinely wait 6 weeks to propose surgery as other authors suggest. There were no major operative complications. The only two minor complications involved 1 patient who experienced acute leg pain after introduction of the trocar sleeve which immediately resolved. Surgery 1 week later revealed an inflamed L5 nerve root. The other had a short period of bleeding for 2 min. The postoperative course was uneventful. One patient initially improved and then 3 weeks later as he climbed into his car developed an extraforaminal prolapse through the nucleotomy canal (Fig. 1). Discography was not performed. One patient came with spinal CT consisting of 4-mm thick slices. He did not respond well and postoperative CT with thin slices showed a sequestered craniad prolapse confirmed by open surgery. There was no correlation between the amount of soft disc material aspirated and regression of leg pain. Some patients (Fig. 2) had disc space narrowing following percutaneous discectomy. Patients under the age of 40 generally respond better. This is due to the higher incidence of spinal degeneration with age.

Discussion

Our 64.3% short-term success rate indicates that percutaneous discectomy in experienced hands and when restricted to the proper patient population is a viable alternative to open surgery as a first-step procedure. The absence of scarring, short hospital stay and early return to full activity are obvious advantageous. Our short-term results compare favourably with those of teams using the automated percutaneous discectomy (so-called "nucleotome"). The latter report for 3031 cases success rates ranging from 61% (Federal Republic of Germany) to 87% (The Netherlands) – an overall success rate of 77%.

The procedure does not influence the results of possible subsequent open surgery. The relative large size of the instrument used allows rapid soft tissue extirpation. It can only be used at the level of L4–5 and above. The relatively large working sleeve was responsible for a nerve root irritation and for an extraforaminal prolapse through the nucleotomy canal. As far as we know this has never been reported before. Just how much material should be aspirated is unclear: more aspiration would probably give fewer recurrences but might lead to disc space narrowing with possible consecutive segmental instability with development of facet joint hypertrophy and mechanical back pain in the long term. Further follow-up studies are necessary. A thorough multimodal radiological work-up is necessary. Lumbar radiographs and CT are compulsory. Sagittal MR images do not replace CT but show the sequestra and the functional state of the disc. Functional myelography may still have its place and can be completed with a myelo-CT. If doubt still exists as to whether the posterior longitudinal ligament is perforated, peroperative discography may be performed. This would show contrast diffusion into the epidural space, in which case the procedure would be contraindicated. Discography increases the risk of infection.

Dr. C. Faubert
Neuroradiological Institute and Department of Neurosurgery
University of Saarland
W-6650 Homburg-Saar, Federal Republic of Germany

Neuroradiology (1991) 33 [Suppl]: 474–475

Neuro radiology
© Springer-Verlag 1991

Nonspondylolytic lateral clefts in the lumbar vertebral arch

J. G. Johansen and F. G. Lilleås

Department of Neuroradiology, Ullevål Hospital, Oslo, Norway

Summary. Besides the rather common cleft in the pars interarticularis there are rare clefts located in the pedicle (retrosomatic cleft) and the lamina (retroisthmic cleft). We reviewed four cases of retrosomatic clefts (one bilateral, three unilateral) and five cases of retroisthmic clefts (all unilateral). Except for one case of retroisthmic cleft, the unilateral clefts were always associated with either contralateral or bilateral spondylolysis. One unilateral retrosomatic cleft was almost healed. We consider the nonspondylolytic clefts to be stress fractures.

Key words: Spine, abnormalities – Spine, fractures – Spine, CT – Spondylolysis

Spondylolysis is a familiar condition with clefts in the pars interarticularis or isthmus. Less common lateral clefts in the neural arch are the retrosomatic cleft in the pedicle [1] and the retroisthmic cleft, which is located in the lamina [2] (Fig. 1). We have encountered several of these rare lesions, and present their features and our impression of their aetiology.

Retrosomatic clefts

There were four cases of pedicular cleft (Table 1, Fig. 2). None was associated with acute spinal injury. In one case (no. 1) the clefts were bilateral. One unilateral cleft (case 2) was associated with bilateral pars defects. In one case (no. 3) the cleft was practically healed (Fig. 3).

Retroisthmic clefts

There were five cases of laminar cleft (Table 1, Fig. 4). None had an acute spinal injury. One case (no. 6) was associated with bilateral pars interarticularis defects. One case (no. 5) was not associated with a pars interarticularis defect, but there were secondary changes in the ipsilateral facet joint probably due to the strain put on it by the loose fragment (Fig. 5).

Discussion

There is no consensus as to the aetiology of retrosomatic and retroisthmic clefts. Spondylolysis, on the other hand, is generally considered to be a stress fracture [3, 4]. Healing of pars interarticularis clefts has been reported [3, 5], but there is usually nonunion because of persistent instability. In unilateral spondylolysis there may be sclerosis and hypertrophy of the contralateral pedicle and pars interarticularis as healing and buttressing reactions to the strain in the unstable arch [6, 7]. A unilateral spondylolysis can progress to be bilateral [6, 8]. It is conceivable that the strain on the contralateral side of the neural arch in unilateral spondylolysis can occasionally lead instead to a stress fracture in the pedicle or lamina.

Most stress fractures in the neural arch occur in the partes interarticulares because they are the weakest parts of the arch. In an experimental study, 74 cadaveric lumbar vertebrae were subjected to a mechanically applied repetitive force [9]. Fifty-three fractured across a pars interarticularis, 5 across a pedicle, and 2 across the pars interarticularis on one side and the pedicle on the other.

Unilateral retrosomatic and retroisthmic clefts are usually associated with contralateral spondylolysis. We also encountered two patients with concomitant bilateral spondylolysis, which demonstrates that a break can occur at more than two places in the neural arch.

Stewart [10] found two vertebral specimens with pedicular clefts showing signs of union in progress. Signs of almost complete healing in one of our cases support the view that the retrosomatic cleft is a stress fracture and is unrelated to the aplastic pedicle [11].

Conclusion

We believe that retrosomatic and retroisthmic clefts are acquired lesions with the same aetiology as spondylolysis.

Table 1. Cleft location and incidence of spondylolysis

Case no.	Sex	Age (years)	Location	Spondylolysis
1	F	44	Pedicle (bilateral)	–
2	M	77	Pedicle (unilateral)	+ (bilateral)
3	F	31	Pedicle (unilateral)	+ (contralateral)
4	M	51	Pedicle (unilateral)	+ (contralateral)
5	M	34	Lamina (unilateral)	–
6	M	28	Lamina (unilateral)	+ (bilateral)
7	M	22	Lamina (unilateral)	+ (contralateral)
8	F	51	Lamina (unilateral)	+ (contralateral)
9	M	50	Lamina (unilateral)	+ (contralateral)

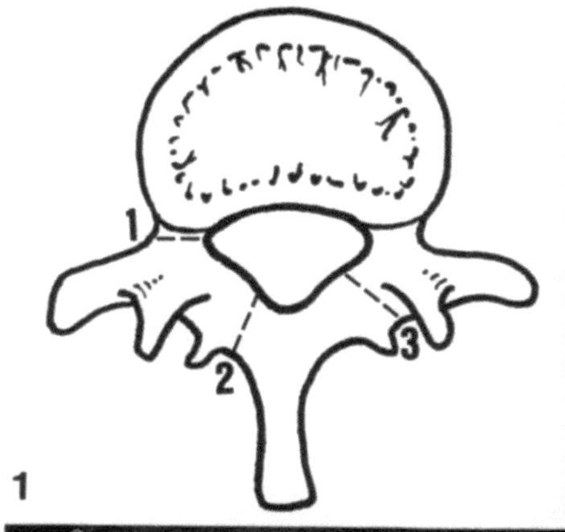

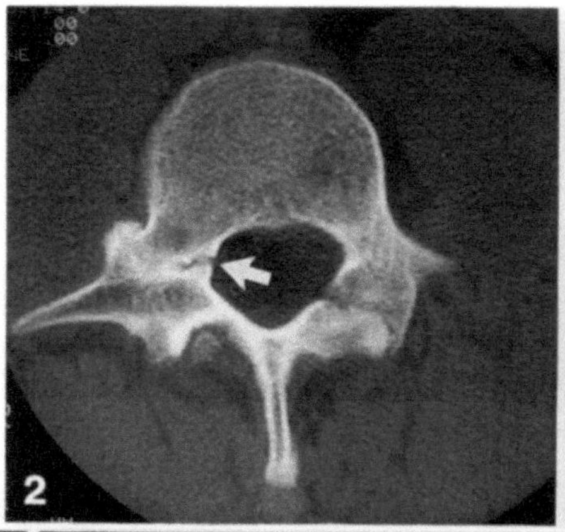

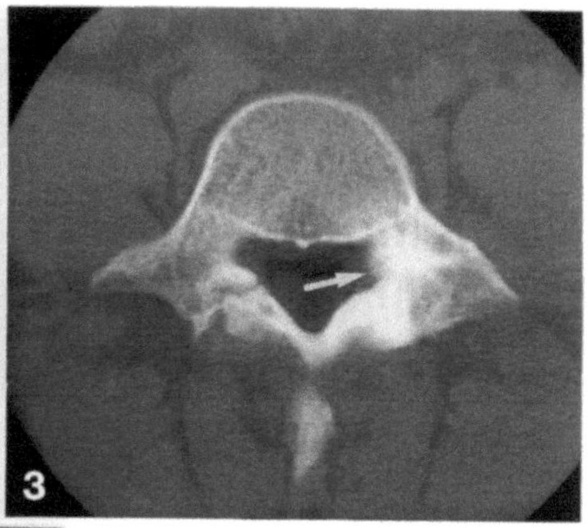

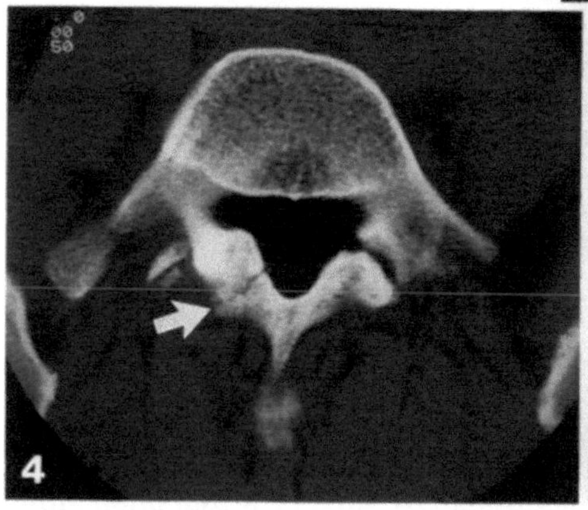

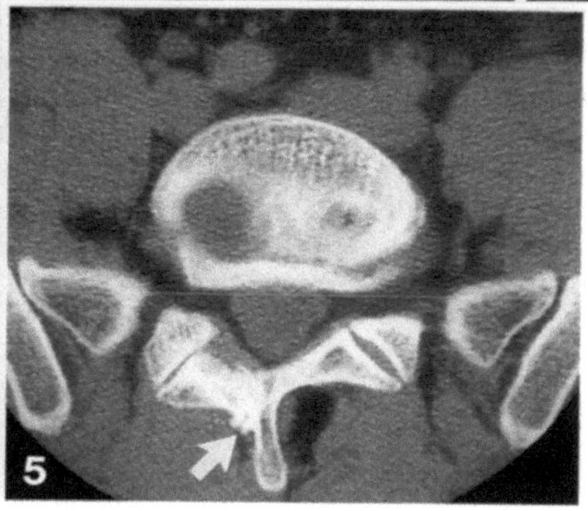

Fig. 1. The retrosomatic cleft *(1)* is in the pedicle, and the retroisthmic cleft *(2)* is located in the lamina. Such unilateral clefts are usually associated with a contralateral cleft in the pars interarticularis *(3)*

Fig. 2. Case 4. There is a retrosomatic cleft *(arrow)* with secondary bone formation on its lateral aspect probably due to instability. Note the contralateral pars interarticularis cleft

Fig. 3. Case 3. This retrosomatic cleft *(arrow)* is barely visible in the medial aspect of the pedicle, which is sclerotic, probably due to healing. There is a contralateral pars interarticularis cleft. There was no interval change at a follow-up examination 2 years later

Fig. 4. Case 9. The retroisthmic cleft *(arrow)* is associated with a contralateral pars interarticularis defect

Fig. 5. Case 5. This retroisthmic cleft *(arrow)* was not associated with spondylolysis. There is secondary bone formation at its edges, and there is narrowing and slight subluxation at the ipsilateral facet joint, indicating a loose fragment

References

1. Johansen JG, McCarty DJ, Haughton VM (1983) Retrosomatic clefts: computed tomographic appearance. Radiology 148: 447–448
2. Johansen JG, Hemminghytt S, Haughton VM (1984) CT appearance of the retroisthmic cleft. AJNR 5: 835–836
3. Wiltse LL, Widell EH Jr, Jackson DW (1975) The aetiology of spondylolisthesis. J Bone Joint Surg [Am] 57: 17–22
4. Cyron BM, Hutton WC, Troup JDG (1976) Spondylolytic fractures. J Bone Joint Surg [Br] 40: 227–239
5. Roche MB (1950) Healing of bilateral fracture of the pars interarticularis of a lumbar neural arch. J Bone Joint Surg [Am] 32: 428–429
6. Sherman FC, Wilkinson R, Hall JE (1977) Reactive sclerosis of a pedicle and spondylolysis in the lumbar spine. J Bone Joint Surg [Am] 59: 49–54
7. Maldague BE, Malghem JJ (1976) Unilateral arch hypertrophy with spinous process tilt: a sign of arch deficiency. Radiology 121: 567–574
8. Fullenlove TM, Wilson JG (1974) Traumatic defects of the pars interarticularis of the lumbar vertebrae. AJR 122: 635–638
9. Cyron BM, Hutton WC (1978) The fatigue strength of the lumbar neural arch in spondylolysis. J Bone Joint Surg [Br] 60: 234–238
10. Stewart TD (1953) The age incidence of neural-arch defects in the Alaskan natives, considered from the standpoint of etiology. J Bone Joint Surg [Am] 35: 937–950
11. Mitzutani M, Yamamuro T, Shikata J (1989) Congenital absence of a lumbar pedicle. Spine 14: 890–891

Dr. J. G. Johansen
Department of Neuroradiology
Ullevål Hospital
0407 Oslo 4
Norway

Neuroradiology (1991) 33 [Suppl]: 476–478

Neuro-radiology
© Springer-Verlag 1991

Possibilities of ultralow magnetic field (0.04 T) in diagnosis of intraspinal tumours

S. Milošević, A. Lovrinčević, D. Stanković, M. Cetinić, and A. Bogdanović

University Medical Centre, Institute of Radiology and Oncology, Sarajevo, Yugoslavia

Summary. The authors have analysed the possibilities and limitations of the ultralow magnetic field in the pathology of intraspinal tumours. The MRI results were compared to clinical data, CT, myelography and CT-myelography. MRI at 0.04 T proved to be superior to the other diagnostic methods in most cases, providing additional imformation about morphology and the precise localization of the lesion.

Key words: Magnetic resonance imaging – Spinal tumours – Ultralow magnetic field

The possibilities of MRI in the investigation of the spinal cord and canal have already been described in numerous reports [1–7]. In recent years advancing technology has provided high field superconducting units capable of producing high quality images. We used a low field (0.04 T), simple unit and tried to evaluate its diagnostic accuracy in assessment of the nature and extent of spinal involvement.

Patients and methods

During the last 12 months we studied ten patients, four woman and six men ranging in age from 19 to 67 years (mean age 42.6), with signs and symptoms suggestive of spinal cord compression. Four underwent myelography, one with lateral cervical puncture; in seven patients CT was performed at the level determined by neurological examination, while two patients underwent CT myelography. In three patients MRI was the initial and final radiological method of examination (excluding standard radiograph of the spine).

MRI scanning was performed on a 0.04 T unit (Magnaview M 110 EH Instrumentarium). All patients had 5–7 mm contiguous sagittal slices using two spin echo sequences (400/40 and 1500/60). In three patients sections were also made in the axial plane (250/40 and 2600/130), as well as in the coronal plane in one case (250/40).

The MR images were compared to available results of other diagnostic methods and to the operative diagnosis; thus MRI was evaluated as a method for detecting the level and extent of the lesion and, if possible its histological nature.

Results

We had three cases of *metastatic involvement of vertebral bodies with extradural spread.* One of these patients (case 7) with already known lung carcinoma showed sudden onset of spinal paraplegia, but the lesion of the spine could be seen neither on standard radiographs, nor on CT. On T2-weighted MR images the level and extent of the lesion were easily found. In the other two patients (cases 2 and 5) the primary tumour was not known and the spinal involvement, detected by MRI, was the first sign of carcinomatous disease. We also had three cases of *extramedullary intradural tumour.* In one (case 6) MRI was the intitial and final diagnostic method and the neurosurgeons decided to operate on the basis of MR findings. MR images (coronal and sagittal) showed a hyperintense extramedullary intradural lesion on the right side thought to be either a *meningioma* or neuroma. At surgery a *psammomatous meningioma* was found at the level and of an extent fully corresponding to MR findings (Fig. 1). In case 3 all radiological methods had given negative results and the patient underwent surgery at the level C4–6 in the belief that *arachnoiditis* was the cause. As the symptoms persisted after surgery, the patient was *referred* to an MR unit which was just starting at that time. MRI showed a hyperintense lesion at C7–T1, extramedullary and intradural in position thought to be either a lipoma or meningioma. At surgery a capillary hemangioma was found in a *juxtamedullary* location. The last patient from this group (case 10) had already been diagnosed by CT, myelography and CT-myelography. However, MRI in the sagittal plane provided aditional information about the upper and lower borders of the tumour (Fig. 2).

We included in this study two cases of *arachnoid pouches* (case 1and 4) because of tumour-like symptoms that they produced. CT and CT-myelography had already shown the nature of the lesion, but its extent was more fully appreciated on sagittal T1-weighted images. The last two cases in our study were intramedullary tumours. One of them (case 8) was a young patient operated on 14 years before for astrocytoma of the posterior fossa. Because of progressive tetraparesis and worsening of the general state, the patient was referred for CT of the brain. A lesion of the brain stem extending to the foramen magnum found at CT was considered to be a recurrent anaplastic astrocytoma. To determine the lower extent of the lesion we made sagittal T1- and T2-weighted images of cervical spine and craniocervical junction. On T2-weighted images a hyperintense lesion was shown spreading from the brain stem to the spinal cord down to C2. The patient is still being treated by irradiation (Fig. 3).

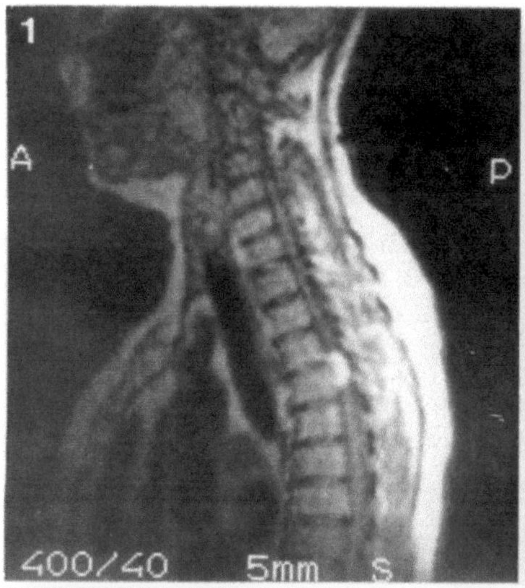

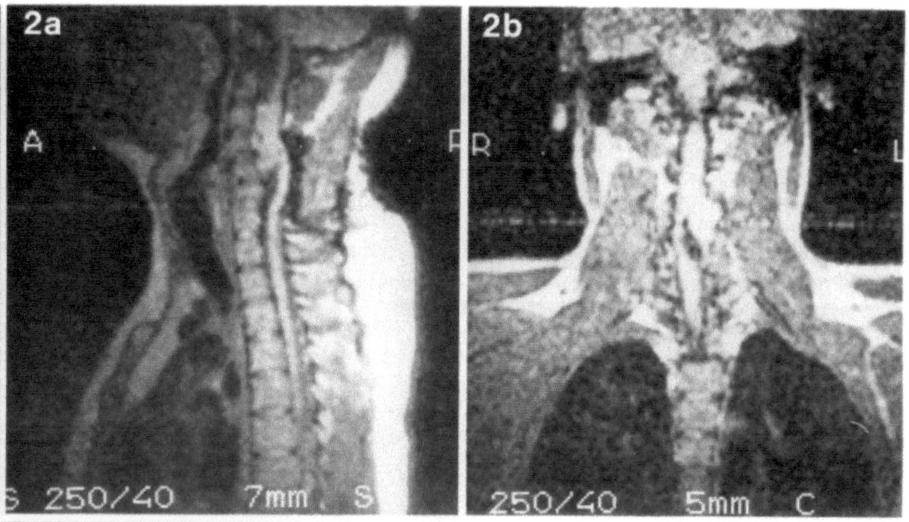

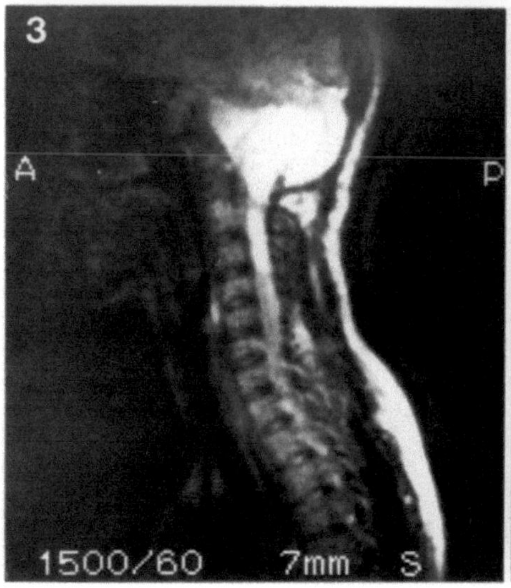

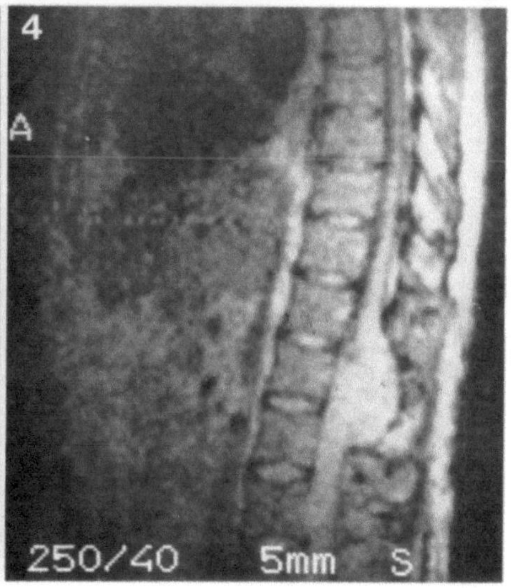

Fig. 1. Case 6. Sagittal T1-weighted image (400/40). Hyperintense extramedullary intradural lesion at T3–4: meningioma

Fig. 2. a, b, Case 10. **a** Sagittal T1-weighted image (250/40). **b** Frontal T1-weighted image (250/40). Extramedullary, intra- and extradural lesion at C3–5: neurinoma

Fig. 3. Case 8. Sagittal T2-weighted image. Intramedullary spread to the C1–2 level. Recurrent anaplastic astrocytoma

Fig. 4. Case 9. Sagittal T1-weighted image (250/40)

In case 9 the tumour was already shown by myelography and CT, but its whole extent was clearly visualized on T1 and T2 sagittal and axial MR slices. It was an intramedullary tumour with extradural and extracanalicular spread at T12. At surgery an infiltrative ependymoma was found (Fig. 4).

Discussion

MRI has already become the imaging modality of choice in the investigation of the spinal canal and its content [5]. The contours of the cord are clearly visualised without the need for intrathecal contrast medium administration. Direct sagittal and coronal imaging is possible without the need for reconstruction from multiple thin slices. Bone artefact is absent in MR images [1].

In this study we tried to show that even the low-field strength unit with relatively limited possibilities may still be adequate for the detection of lesions of spinal cord and canal, to determine their extent and, in some cases, their histological nature. In our cases MRI clearly demonstrated each of ten compressive intraspinal lesions and was superior to CT and CT-myelography which were considered to be negative in three of our patients.

T1-weighted images with relatively short TE (40 ms) in which the cerebrospinal fluid appeared dark were are found most useful. In some cases coronal slices provided useful additional information about the relationship between the tumour and the cord, as well as possible extradural spread. The axial slices gave us some additional information in one case (case 9) where the involvement of paravertebral muscles was clearly seen.

T2-weighted images were useful in cases of metastatic involvement of the vertebral bodies. The increased signal intensity of such bodies was easily seen, as was the extradural involvement. Sometimes T2-weighted images provided a better differentiation between the tumour and surrounding structures in cases where the signal of CSF was more intense than the tumour itself.

Conclusion

Our series is not large enough to allow definite statements about the possibilities of ultralow magnetic field in the diagnosis of intraspinal tumours. However, it shows that this simple and easily available unit may be very useful in the diagnosis of difficult cases.

References

1. Bydder GM, Brown J, Niendorf HP, Young IR (1985) Enhancement of cervical intraspinal tumours in MR imaging with intravenous gadolinium – DTPA. J Comput Assist Tomogr 9: 847–851
2. Di Chiro G, Doppman JL, Dwyer AJ, Patronas NJ Knop RH, Bairamian D, Vermess M, Oldfield EH (1985) Tumours and arteriovenous malformations of the spinal cord: assessment using MR. Radiology 156: 689–697
3. Goy AMC, Pinto RS, Raghavendra BN, Epstein FJ, Kricheff II (1986) Intramedullary spinal cord tumours MR imaging with emphasis on associated cysts. Radiology 161: 381–386
4. Hyman RA, Edwards JH, Vacirca SJ, Stein HL (1985) 0.6 T MR imaging of the cervical spine: multislice and multiecho techniques. AJNR 6: 229–236
5. Manelfe C (1989) Magnetic resonance imaging of the spinal cord. Diagn Intervent Radiol 1: 3–14
6. Scotti G, Scialfa G, Colombo N, Landoni L (1985) MR imaging of intradural extramedullary tumors of the cervical spine. J Comput Assist Tomogr 9: 1037–1041
7. Rubin JM, Aisen AM, DiPietro MA (1986) Ambiguities in MR imaging of tumoral cysts in the spinal cord. J comput Assist Tomogr 10: 395–398

Dr. S. Milošević
University Medical Centre
Institute of Radiology and Oncology
Sarajewo, Jugoslavia

Neuroradiology (1991) 33 [Suppl]: 479–480

Neuroradiology

© Springer-Verlag 1991

Os odontoideum: CT and MRI demonstration of the transverse ligament

J. L. Dietemann, H. Zhu, I. Bricout, S. Athale, C. Romero, G. Zöllner, and A. Wackenheim

Service de Radiologie I, Pavillon Clovis Vincent, Hospices Civils, Strasbourg, France

Summary. It is a matter of controversy whether os odontoideum is acquired or congenital. The ability of high-resolution CT and MRI to demonstrate the transverse ligament provides arguments for a new theory concerning the origin of os odontoideum. Thin axial high-resolution CT and sagittal T1-weighted MRI performed in three patients with os odontoideum demonstrated a short, thick transverse ligament located between the os odontoideum and the body of the axis. Nevertheless from these CT and MRI findings definitive conclusions cannot be reached. The short transverse ligament may be congenital and responsible for separation of the dens, or the os odontoideum may be responsible for hypoplasia of the transverse ligament.

Key words: Spine – Craniovertebral region – Os odontoideum – Magnetic resonance imaging – Computed tomography

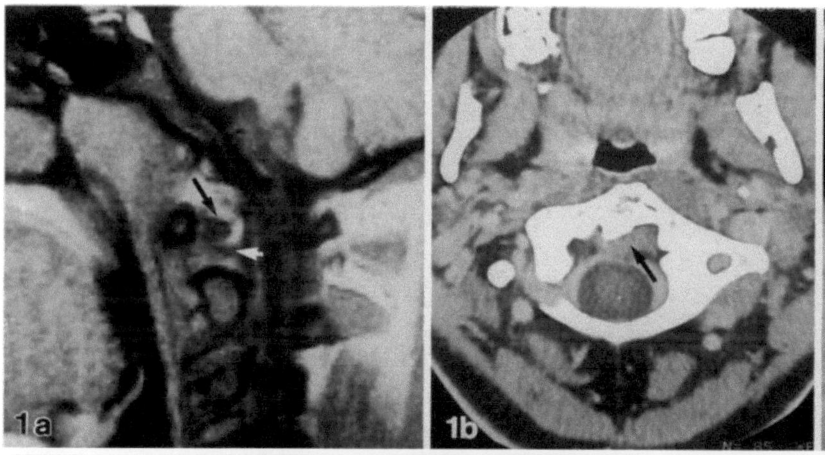

Fig. 1. a, b. Cervical pain in a 35-year-old female. Sagittal T1-weighted section (**a**) through the craniocervical region demonstrates the os odontoideum *(black arrow)* and the transverse ligament located between the os odontoideum and C2 *(white arrow)*. Axial CT (**b**) confirms a short and thick transverse ligament *(arrow)*

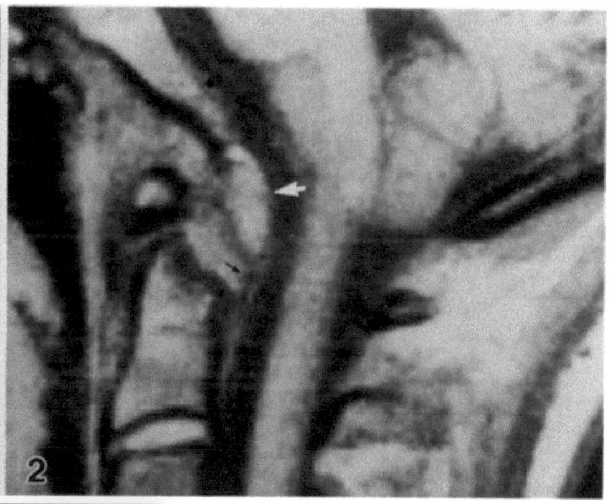

Fig. 2. Cervical pain in a 37-year-old female. Sagittal T1-weighted MRI section through the craniocervical region demonstrates the os odontoideum *(white arrow)* and the transverse ligament located between the os odontoideum and C2 *(black arrow)*

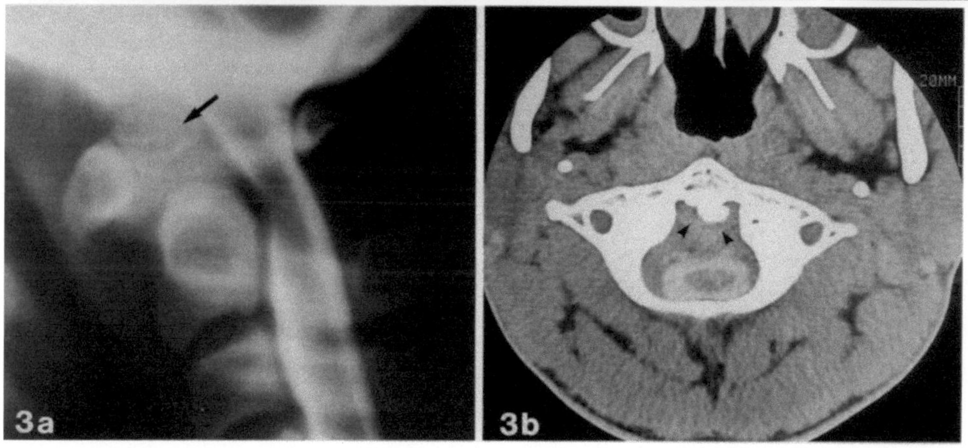

◁

Fig. 3. a, b. Quadriparesis in a 14-year-old boy. Sagittal myelotomogram **(a)** through the craniocervical region demonstrates the os odontoideum *(black arrow)* and narrowing of the spinal canal at the level of C2. Axial myelo-CT **(b)** demonstrates short, thick transverse ligament *(black arrowheads)*

It is a matter of controversy whether the os odontoideum is acquired or congenital. Some authors attest that the abnormality represents an acquired lesion [1], and others have developed the theory of a congenital lesion [2–6]. The possibility of a mixed origin has been emphasised by Wackenheim et al. [7]: a congenitally shortened transverse ligament being responsible for section of the odontoid process.

High-resolution CT allows direct visualisation of the transverse ligament; the ligament may be identified only on 1- or 2-mm-thick slices and appears as a dense structure (90–100 HU) without enhancement after contrast injection. MRI demonstrates the transverse and alar ligaments as a small low-signal area on T1- and T2-weighted sagittal or axial images [1, 7].

In three recent cases of os odontoideum (Figs. 1–3) and in a previous published case [7] we were able to demonstrate by means of MRI and/or CT a short, thick transverse ligament located between the os odontoideum and the body of C2. However, it is impossible to conclude from these findings whether the changes in the transverse ligament are the consequence or the cause of os odontoideum.

References

1. Fielding JW (1974) Os odontoideum: an acquired lesion. J Bone Joint Surg [Am] 56: 187
2. Dietemann JL, Doyon D, Aubin ML (1989) Charnière cervico-occipitale. In: Manelfe C (ed) Imagerie de la moelle et du rachis. Vigot, Paris
3. Minderhoud JM, Braakmann R, Penning L (1969) Os odontoideum – clinical, radiological, and therapeutic aspects. J Neurol Sci 8: 521
4. Morgan MK, Onofrio BM, Bender CE (1989) Familial os odontoideum. Case report. J Neurosurg 70: 636
5. Sherk HH, Dawoud S (1981) Congenital os odentoideum with Klippel-Feil anomaly and fatal atlanto-axial instability. Report of a case. Spine 6: 42–45
6. Wackenheim A (1974) Roentgen diagnosis of the craniovertebral region. Springer, Berlin Heidelberg New York
7. Wackenheim A, Burguet JL, Sick H (1986) Section of the odontoid process by a shortened transverse ligament (a possible etiology for the mobile odontoid). Neuroradiology 28: 281–282

Prof. Jean-Louis Dietemann
Service de Radiologie 1, Pavillon Clovis Vincent
Hospices Civils, Hôpital Central
F-67091 Strasbourg, France

Neuroradiology (1991) 33 [Suppl]: 481–483

Neuro-radiology

© Springer-Verlag 1991

MRI of spinal myelofibrosis

R. J. Foust, R. G. Ramsey, S. Mojtahedi, B. Randall, and S. Verma

Department of Diagnostic Radiology, The University of Chicago, Chicago, IL, USA

Summary. Myelofibrosis is an uncommon clinical entity resulting in fibrosis of the bone marrow that has only been briefly addressed in the MR literature, We were unable to find illustrations of sagittal MR images of the spine in patients with myelofibrosis. We have encountered three patients with myelofibrosis who underwent MR imaging of the spine, which revealed diffuse or patchy decreased signal intensity on T1-weighted images. The appearance of myelofibrosis may be similar to that of such entities as diffuse metastases, sickle cell anemia, and the hypointense marrow in patients with acquired immunodeficiency syndrome. Therefore, the MR appearance must be correlated with the clinical presentation.

Key words: Spine, myelofibrosis – Spine, metastases – Spine, AIDS – Spine, leukemia

Myelofibrosis is an uncommon clinical entity and the MR appearance reveals variable decreased signal intensity in nonspinal marrow-containing spaces; in our experience this MR appearance is similar in the spine.

Case reports

Case 1. A 49-year-old female initially presented with a 5-month history of easy bruising. At the time of initial evaluation the patient had hemoglobin (Hb) 8.8 g; hematocrit (Hct) 25.5; platelets 27,000; there was no hepatosplenomegaly. Two bone marrow biopsies revealed a hypocellular marrow with dysplastic megakaryocytes and dysplastic features compatible with agnogenic myelofibrosis. A core biopsy revealed a hypocellular marrow with dysplastic erythroid hyperplasia consistent with acute nonlymphocytic leukemia – megakaryocytic leukemia – of the M6 type (Fig. 1).

Case 2. An 18-year-old female with a history of 6 months previously having had of a neuroblastoma arising from the right renal area removed. Bone marrow aspiration was attempted three times, but produced no tissue. The fourth attempt revealed abnormal cells consistent with metastatic neuroblastoma. At the time of admission Hb was 14.2, Hct 42.0; there was no hepatosplenomegaly.

Over the next 2 months the patient received a combination of chemotherapy and radiation therapy. The patient then suffered a decrease in platelets as well as a drop in Hb and Hct. The patient was thought to be in clinical remission from her disease and to have marrow suppression and fibrosis secondary to treatment. A spine MRI scan was performed at this time (Fig. 2).

Case 3. A 7-year-old male was originally diagnosed as non-Hodgkin's lymphoma 4.5 years prior to this admission. Initial diagnosis was made by biopsy of a lytic lesion in the femur and a positive bone marrow. Abdomen and thorax were normal. He was treated with chemotherapy and was well and in remission for 2 years.

Five months prior to this admission he presented with decreased strength in his lower extremities. A presacral mass was identified by MRI and a repeat bone marow was positive for non-Hodgkin's lymphoma. The patient was treated with methotrexate, leucovorin and prednisone and received local radiation therapy to the presacral mass. At admission he had Hb 8.8; Hct 35.8; platelets were decreased. The patient did well and was discharged to home care.

The patient was readmitted for follow-up chemotherapy although he was thougt to be in remission and there was no evidence of disease. Repeat MRI revealed a decrease in the size of the presacral mass and the vertebrae revealed changes consistent with myelofibrosis (Fig. 3).

Results

All our cases revealed decreased signal intensity marrow within the vertebral bodies on T1-weighted images. In case 1 this appearance was identified at the time of initial clinical presentation, while in cases 2 and 3 decreased signal intensity appearance developed after chemotherapy. In case 2 the initial clinical presentation was with metastatic neuroblastoma, in case 3 metastatic non-Hodgkin's lymphoma.

Discussion

Myelofibrosis is a myeloproliferative disease that is typified by fibrosis of the bone marrow [1–4]. This stromal reaction of fibrosis results in replacement of the normal hematopoetic tissue with loss of the normal marrow elements. There is fibroblastic proliferation in the bone marrow, marked sclerosis and thickening of individual bone trabecula as well as formation of new trabecula [3, 4]. The combination of these findings results in the areas of diffuse or focal bony sclerosis that may be seen in these patients [5], and causes decreased signal on T1-weighted images.

Myelofibrosis is a descriptive term and has been reported to be caused by the classic type of "idiopathic" or agnogenic myelofibrosis but may also be a result of metastatic carcinoma, leukemia, lymphoma, tuberculosis [6], Gaucher's disease and exposure to toxins [7]. In some reported cases of acute megakaryoblastic leukemia the marrow changes were considered "acute" malignant myelofibrosis [8, 9].

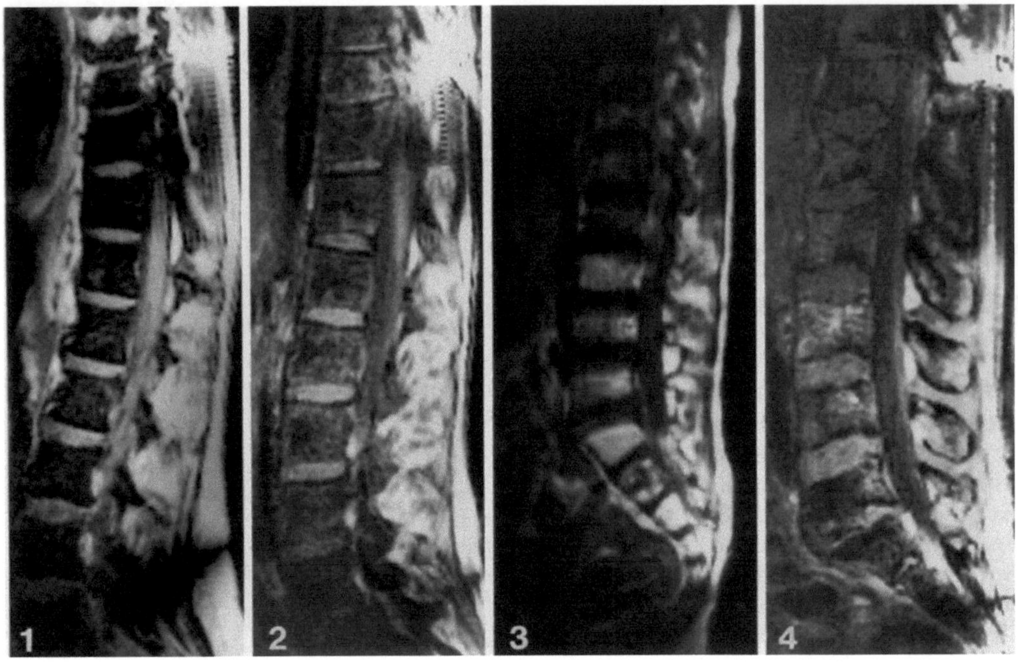

Fig. 1. Myelofibrosis, acute megakaryoblastic leukemia. T1-weighted image reveals diffuse decreased signal intensity of the marrow containing spaces of the spine

Fig. 2. Myelofibrosis secondary to chemotherapy. T1-weighted image reveals generally decreased signal intensity of the spinal marrow spaces

Fig. 3. Myelofibrosis, secondary to radiation and chemotherapy. T1-weighted image reveals mottled decreased signal intensity of the lumbar marrow spaces

Fig. 4. Sickle cell anemia. T1-weighted image reveals diffuse decreased signal intensity of the marrow spaces. There is mild biconvave deformity of the vertebral bodies; there is a degenerated and herniated disc at L4–5

There appear to be four types of myelofibrosis:

1. Agnogenic myelofibrosis with myeloid metaplasia. There is excessive fibroblast proliferation and collagen deposition in the marrow. In association there is myeloid metaplasia, or transformation to marrow producing tissue, in other organs, typically the liver, spleen and lymph nodes. In the absence of an inciting cause this is termed agnogenic myeloid metasplasia. Typically this is a chronic illness and survival in these cases is thought to be approximately 10 years; however, exact times are difficult to ascertain and may be shorter or longer.
2. Myelofibrosis associated with polycythemia vera or chronic granulocytic leukemia as part of the natural history or as a consequence of myelosuppressive therapies.
3. Myelofibrosis and reactive myelofibrosis may also be seen secondary to a wide spectrum of clinical diseases including: severe hemolythic anemia, Hodgkin's disease; various nonhematopoietic neoplasms metastatic to the bone marrow, infections such as tuberculosis, or following bone marrow injury caused by radiation, benzol, fluorine, phosphorus or strontium [6, 7].
4. Acute myelofibrosis, which with its rapidly progressive and fatal clinical course has been shown to be a form of acute megakaryocytic leukemia [8, 9].

In these cases of myelofibrosis bone marrow aspiration frequently results in a dry tap even when the marrow is very cellular; therefore bone biopsy is often necessary. The bone marrow demonstrates areas of bone marrow fibrosis, often with accompanying osteosclerosis.

There have been various reports in the literature of the radiographic bony changes that may be seen with myelofibrosis. These include no radiographic abnormality in the early stages of the disease, diffuse bony sclerosis, osteoporosis, and rarely there may be purely lytic lesions. The skeletal changes have been reviewed in the radiologic literature; however, there has been little mention of this entity in the MR literature [7, 10].

Other diseases may have a similar radiographic and MR appearance. Sickle cell anemia may also present with areas of bone sclerosis. The clinical setting and the typical biconcave appearance of the vertebral bodies allows differentiation between these entities. However, the MR appearance of sickle cell disease of the spine may mimic that of myelofibrosis (Fig. 4) The hypointense MR appearance of sickle cell disease is probably secondary to expansion of the cellular-producing marrow because of the basic underlying disease as well as to multiple microinfarcts.

Conclusion

Myelofibrosis is an uncommon clinical entity that causes diffuse or mottled decreased signal intensity in the spinal bone marrow on T1-weighted images; T2-weighted images have not been helpful. This MR appearance is not pathognomonic and diffuse metastases, sickle cell disease and AIDS may mimic the appearance. Some types of myelofibrosis may actually be examples of acute leukemia. Almost certainly we will identify an increase in the number of cases of myelofibrosis that develop following chemotherapy for other diseases. Advances in chemotherapy are increasing patient longevity and one of the side effects of chemotherapy is unfortunately marrow suppression and resulting myelofibrosis. AIDS is also increasing and therefore the number of cases with an abnormal appearing marrow with decreased signal intensity is also increasing and will therefore be identified more commonly in the future.

As the treatment of these entities is very different, correct diagnosis is important and myelofibrosis should be considered in cases of diffuse or mottled decreased signal intensity on T1-weighted images of spine.

References

1. Lanir A, Aghai JS, Lee RGL, Clouse ME (1986) MR imaging in myelofibrosis. J Comput Assist Tomogr 10: 634–636
2. Berk PD (1988) Myeloproliferative disorders. In: Wyngaarden JB, Smith LH (eds) Cecil textbook of medicine, 18th ed. Saunders, Philadelphia, pp 984–988
3. Jacobsen HG (1959) Agnogenic myeloid metaplasia. Radiology 72: 716–725
4. Leigh TF, Corley CC Jr, Huguley CM Jr, Rogers JV Jr (1959) Myelofibrosis; the general and radiologic findings in 25 proven cases. Am J Roentgenol 82: 183–193
5. Charron D, Rober L, Couty MC, Binet J (1979) Biochemical and histological analysis of bone marrow collagen in myelofibrosis. Br J Haematol 41: 151–161
6. Karasick AU, Karasick D, Schilling J (1982) Acute megakaryoblastic leukemia (acute "malignant" myelofibrosis): an unusual cause of osteosclerosis. Skeletal Radiol 9: 45–56
7. Lanir A, Aghai E, Simon JS, Lee RG (1986) T1 MR imaging im myelofibrosis, J Comput Assist Tomogr 10: 634–636
8. Marino GG, Robinson WL (1989) Acute myelofibrosis: correlation of radiographic, bone scan, and biopsy findings. J Nucl Med 30: 251–254
9. Bennett JM, Catovsky D, Daniel MT (1985) Criteria for the diagnosis of acute leukemia of megakaryocytic lineage (M7). Ann Intern Med 103: 460–462
10. Porter BA, Shields AF, Olson DA (1986) Magnetic resonance imaging of bone marrow disorders. Radiol Clin North Am 24: 269–289

Dr. Ruth G. Ramsey
Department of Diagnostic Radiology- Box 429
The University of Chicago
5841 South Maryland Avenue
Chicago, IL 60637, USA

Neuroradiology (1991) 33 [Suppl]: 484–485

Neuro radiology
© Springer-Verlag 1991

An MRI study of the treatment of lumbar disc protrusion by percutaneous nucleotomy

R. W. Kerslake[1], A. North[2], R. C. Mulholland[2], and B. S. Worthington[1]

Departments of [1] Radiology and [2] Orthopaedics, Queens Medical Centre, University Hospital, Nottingham, UK

Summary. A brief discussion of the results of a prospective study of 30 patients undergoing automated percutaneous nucleotomy (APN) for the treatment of contained protrusions of lumbar intervertebral discs is presented. No significant changes in the disc height, signal intensity or extent of disc protrusion at the levels following APN were seen. APN is an effective method of treatment for selected lumbar disc protrusions, but the mechanism of action is incompletely understood. A more complete account of this work is to be published elsewhere in due course.

Key words: Spine, MRI studies – Spine, intervertebral discs – Spine, surgery

Treatment of lumbar disc herniation by conventional surgical techniques is not always successful and may lead to complications in both the short and long term. Attempts to avoid some of these deficiencies led to the introduction of percutaneous techniques for the treatment of lumbar disc protrusions by Hijikata [1] in 1975. Subsequent refinements resulted in the commercial production of an automated percutaneous device (Nucleotome, Surgical Dynamics) which uses a blunt-tipped 2.8-mm suction-curetting probe [2]. We have prospectively studied a group of 30 patients treated by this technique.

Patients and methods

Thirty patients (21 male, 9 female) with severe back pain and radicular symptoms sufficient to warrent surgical treatment were studied. The patients were aged 19–54 years, mean 33 years. Standard patient selection criteria were followed [2]. Automated percutaneous nucleotomy (APN) was performed at the L4–5 level in 22 patients and at the L5–S1 level in 8 cases; there were no complications.

All patients underwent MRI prior to the study and at 1 month (25 cases), 3months (22 cases) and 12 months (19 cases) using a standard protocol (1.15 T system, lumbar surface coil, 7-mm section thickness, sagittal SE 500/40 and inversion recovery with short inversion time (STIR) sequences, axial SE 500/40 sections). Disc height was measured from a midsagittal SE 500/40 image and expressed as a percentage of normal disc height. Disc signal intensity was assessed on a midsagittal STIR image and graded from 0 (normal) to 4 (complete loss of disc signal). Disc protrusion was graded between 0 (no protrusion) to 3(extensive protrusion). Patients were assessed clinically and by means of pain and functional status charts at the same intervals.

Results

At the final available follow-up, 23 patients (77%) had a successful outcome. Five patients failed within the 1st month after treatment and further follow-up was not available for these. Two further patients failed within 6 months of APN. The mean disc height, disc signal intensity and extent of disc protrusion prior to and following treatment are shown in Table 1. No significant differences have been demonstrated. Disc height was not reduced by more than 20% in any case. Disc signal intensity showed a reduction of more than two grades in only 1 case. The extent of disc protrusion was unchanged in 18 cases (72%); no protrusion resolved completely.

Discussion

Percutaneous techniques for treatment of lumbar disc protrusion avoid the risks of general anaesthesia, delayed bony instability and epidural fibrosis associated with conventional surgery and may result in an earlier return to work [3]. Success rates of the order of 70% may be achieved with both conventional [1] and automated techniques [3, 4] in appropriately selected patient groups and our results accord with these findings.

Morphological changes in the treated disc are notably absent; in particular, the protruded disc does not diminish in size in the majority of cases. Decompression of the nucleus pulposus with subsequent withdrawal of the protrusion back into the disc space would thus not appear to account for the success of this technique. Reduction in intradiscal pressure, which has been documented after

Table 1. Alteration in treated disc prior to and following automated percutaneous nucleotomy

Mean (SD)	Pre	1 Month	3 Months	12 Months
Numberof cases	30	25	22	19
Disc height (% normal)	79.5 (18)	80.76 (16)	79.9 (15)	75 (19)
Disc signal (grade)	2.65 (0.9)	2.79 (0.6)	2.77 (0.7)	2.89 (0.8)
Disc protrusion (grade)	2 (0.6)	2 (0.6)	1.95 (0.6)	1.78 (0.6)

Mean and standard deviation (SD) of pooled data

APN [5], may result in a beneficial alteration in the radial forces transmitted to the annular fibres.

References

1. Hijakata S (1989) Percutaneous nucleotomy. A new concept and 12 years' experience. Clin Orthop 238: 9–23
2. Goldstein TB, Mink JH, Dawson EG (1989) Early experience with automated percutaneous lumbar discectomy in the treatment of lumbar disc herniation. Clin Orthop 238: 77–82
3. North A, Roberts A, Mullholland R (1989) Pressure changes in human cadaveric intervertebral discs during nucleotomy. Book of Abstracts, International Society for the Study of the Lumbar Spine Kyoto, pp 15–16
4. Maroon JC, Onik G, Sternau L (1989) Percutaneous automated discectomy. A new approach to lumbar surgery. Clin Orthop 238: 64–70
5. Onik G, Maroon J, Helms C, Schweigel J, Mooney V, Kahanovitz N, Day A, Morris J, McCulloch JA, Reicher M (1987) Automated percutaneous discectomy: initial patient experience. Radiology 162: 129–132

R. W. Kerslake
MRI Unit
Queens Medical Centre
Nottingham NG7 2UH, UK

Neuroradiology (1991) 33 [Suppl]: 486–487

Neuroradiology
© Springer-Verlag 1991

Comparison of side-effects of myelography performed with 26-gauge and 22-gauge needles

A. G. Wilkinson, R. J. Sellar, and V. G. McDermott

Department of Neuroradiology, Western General Hospital, Edinburgh, UK

Summary. A prospective randomised trial was performed to compare the side-effects caused by the use of 26-gauge and 22-gauge needles for lumbar puncture during myelography in 284 consecutive patients. Use of the finer (26-gauge) needle resulted in a significant reduction in moderate or severe headaches, postural headaches and pain during needle insertion. The incidence of other side-effects following myelography, most commonly back pain and radicular pain or paraesthesiae, was not significantly affected by needle size.

Key words: Myelography – Side-effects – Needle size

Post-lumbar puncture headache is thought to be due to continued leakage of cerebrospinal fluid (CSF) through the defect in the dura mater caused by the spinal needle, and the use of smaller needles has been shown to reduce the incidence of this complication in normal volunteers for lumbar puncture [1]. A feature of the headache is its postural nature, being relieved by lying down [1]. Although several studies comparing side-effects of myelography with different sizes of needles have been performed, results are contradictory. Some authors, including Rolfe and Maguire [2], claim that needle size has no effect while others, including Sand et al. [3, 4], claim a reduction in headache with smaller needles.

Patients and methods

A total of 284 consecutive patients referred to this department for myelography via the lumbar theca were randomised blindly into two groups, a control group in which the lumbar puncture was performed with a 22-gauge needle ($n = 137$) and a study group in which a 26-gauge needle was used ($n = 147$). The 26-gauge needle is advanced down the lumen of a 4-cm 21-gauge needle which has been used for local anaesthesia. The patients were asked to complete a questionnaire on discharge from hospital 24 h after the myelogram. Details of presence and severity of pain during needle insertion and headache following the examination were recorded on a scale of 0 (no pain) to 4 (very severe pain), and the presence of other complaints was recorded. Details of late side-effects were obtained by telephone. Statistical analysis of differences between the two groups was performed using the chi-square test.

Results

The results are summarised in Table 1.

There was a reduction in the total number of headaches from 35.7% (49/137) in the 22-gauge group to 25.2% (37/147) in the 26-gauge group. This just failed to reach statistical significance ($P < 0.05$). However, many of these headaches were considered relatively trivial by the patient and if these were excluded and only headaches in the moderate, severe or very severe categories considered there was a significant reduction from 23.4% (32/137) in the 22-gauge group to 12.9% (19/147) in the 26-gauge group-($P < 0.05$). Postural headaches were significantly reduced from 15.3% (21/137) in the 22-gauge group to 4.8% (7/147) in the 26-gauge group ($P < 0.05$). Other side-effects following myelography, mainly back pain and radicular pain or numbness were slightly lower in the 26-gauge group – 56% (83/147) compared to 64% (89/137) in the 22-gauge group – but the difference was not significant.

Pain during needle insertion was significantly reduced if the moderate, severe and very severe categories were considered – 5.4% (8/147) in the 26-gauge group compared to 18.1% (24/133) in the 22-gauge group ($P < 0.05$) – but failed to reach significance if mild pain was included.

Discussion

Tourtellotte et al. [1] showed that there was a significant reduction in headaches following lumbar puncture if a small (26-gauge) needle was used compared to a larger needle (22-gauge) in a group of healthy volunteers. Persistent CSF leaks have been demonstrated using radioiso-

Table 1. Summary of results

	26-gauge	22-gauge	P value
Time for injection of 10 ml iopamidol	3.2 min	1.2 min	
Total headaches	25.2%	35.7%	$P < 0.05$
Moderate or severe headaches	14.8%	23.4%	$P < 0.05$
Postural headaches	4.8%	15.3%	$P < 0.05$
Moderate or severe pain during needle insertion	5.4%	18.1%	$P < 0.05$
Other side-effects	56%	64%	$P > 0.05$

tope myelography [5]. "Blood patching", the technique of injection of autologous blood into the subdural space, has been claimed to reduce leakage and lower the incidence of post-myelogram headache [6]. Two factors may be responsible for the production of headache following myelography – CSF leakage or the presence of contrast medium in the CSF. The incidence of side-effects using newer low osmolar contrast agents is lower than when metrizamide was used [7]. The incidence of side-effects in our study is broadly similar to that of Tourtellotte et al. [1] in healthy volunteers for lumbar puncture suggesting that CSF leakage is a much more important factor in the production of headache following myelography than the presence of contrast medium in the CSF.

We consider that the use of fine-gauge needles is worthwhile to minimise patient discomfort, in spite of the inconvenience caused by slower injection of contrast medium.

Acknowledgement. We wish to thank Staff Nurses Ann Douglas, Karen Aberdour and Elspeth Findlay for much help in this study.

References

1. Tourtellotte WW, Henderson WG, Tucker RP, Gilland O, Walker JE, Kokman E (1972) A randomised double blind clinical trial comparing the 22 versus 26 gauge needle in the production of the post-lumbar puncture syndrome in normal individuals. Headache 12: 73–78
2. Rolfe EB, Maguire PD (1980) The incidence of headache following various techniques of metrizamide myelography. Br J Radiol 53: 840–844
3. Sand T, Myhr G, Stovner LJ, Dale LG, Tangerud A (1989) Side effects after ambulatory lumbar iohexol myelography. Neuroradiology 31: 49–54
4. Sand T (1989) Which factors affect reported headache incidences after lumbar myelography? A statistical analysis of publications in the literature. Neuroradiology 31: 55–59
5. Leiberman LM, Tourtellotte WW, Newkirk TA (1971) Prolonged post lumbar puncture cerebrospinal fluid leakage from lumbar subarachnoid space demonstrated by radioisotope myelography. Neurology 21: 925–929
6. Gutterman P, Bezier HS (1978) Prophylaxis of post myelogram headaches. J Neurosurg 49: 869–871
7. Elkin CM, Levan AMT, Leeds NE (1986) Tolerance of iohexol, iopamidol and metrizamide in lumbar myelography. Surg Neurol 26: 542–546

R. J. Sellar
Department of Neuroradiology
Western General Hospital
Crewe Road
Edinburgh EH4 2XU, UK

Neuroradiology (1991) 33 [Suppl]: 488–489

Neuro-radiology
© Springer-Verlag 1991

Measurement of dynamic factors in the medulla oblongata in the adult Chiari malformation

J. M. Stevens, B. E. Kendall, A. G. Clifton, and A. Ananthapavan

The National Hospitals for Neurology and Neurosurgery, London, UK

Summary. The cross-sectional area of the medulla oblongata was measured at four specified levels on high-definition computed cisternograms made with the head flexed and extended in 8 patients with pure cerebellar ectopia and eye movement disorders, and in 30 normal controls. The level of maximal variation in area measurements was shifted from the cervical flexure in controls to just below the pontomedullary junction in patients with cerebellar ectopia, which was interpreted as indicating abnormal tractional forces generated near the pontomedullary junction due to relative tethering of the neural axis at the foramen magnum in these patients.

Key words: Medulla oblongata – Adult Chiari malformation

The clinical features attributed to the adult Chiari malformation are protean. The frequency of disturbances of oculovestibular and vestibulospinal reflexes is high in most series, often exceeding 60% [1]. The commonest type of Chiari malformation in adults is said to be pure cerebellar tonsillar ectopia, the medulla oblongata being normal in both length and position [2]. The high incidence of persistent eye movement disorders and truncal ataxia is not explained readily by tonsillar ectopia alone [3].

It was decided to use existing computed myelographic data to explore the efffect of head position on the cross-sectional area of the neural axis at and above the foramen magnum to see if dynamic data might suggest an answer to the above paradox.

Patients and methods

All patients had been examined on a GE8800 scanner, where 1.5-mm contiguous slices had been made from the level of the pons to the base of C2 with the head both flexed and extended. Water-soluble intrathecal contrast medium had been given by lumbar puncture prior to each study. The measuring procedure was carried out at a viewing console. True axial reformatted images were prescribed from midsagittal reformatted images at the levels shown in Fig. 1, and area measurements were made by outlining irregular regions of interest with a light pen, repeated 4 or 5 times at each level to increase confidence in the final figures obtained.

There were eight patients with typical adult Chiari malformation, in whom the cerebellar tonsils descended 8–22 mm below the foramen magnum. In each, the medulla oblongata showed no kink, there was no basilar invagination according to standard criteria, and the pontomedullary junction lay above the lower half of the clivus. All patients had nystagmus (in six mainly of down-beating type), four were ataxic and five had syringomyelia. Thirty cases rheumatoid arthritis and minimal or absent atlantoaxial subluxation and no spinal cord compression were used as controls.

Results

The processed data are displayed in Figs. 2 and 3. Patient numbers in the Chiari group were small and the statistical scatter rather wide, precluding definitive analysis. Nevertheless interesting trends were discernible.

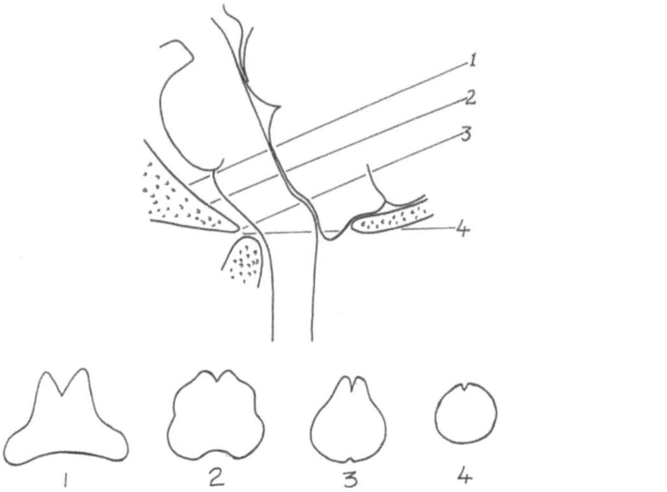

Fig. 1. The levels, orientation and cross-sectional appearances of axial reformatted images

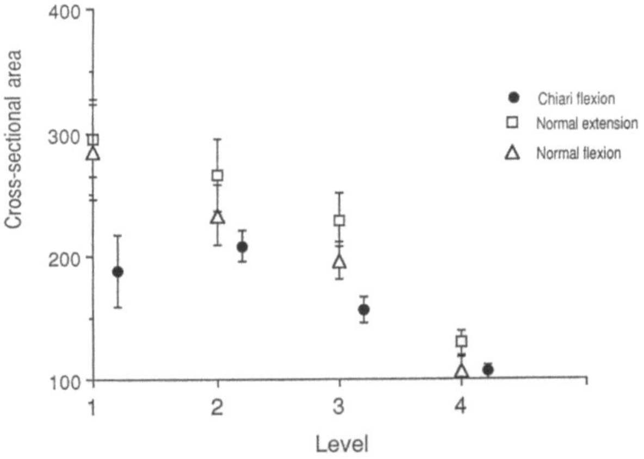

Fig. 2. Cross-sectional area, ranges and means

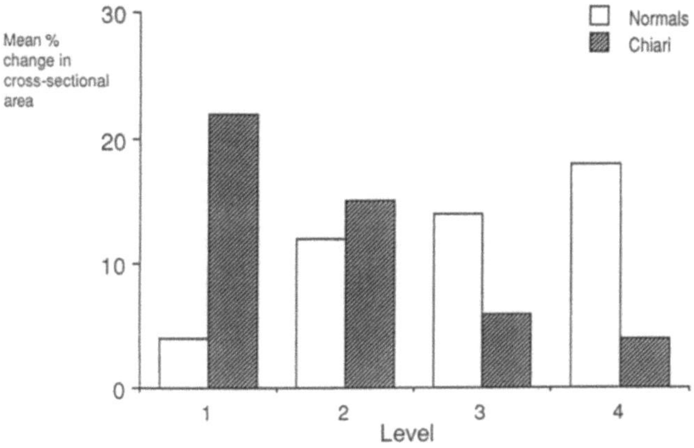

Fig. 3. Mean percentage change in cross-sectional area

Discussion

Cross-sectional area measurements generally carry a smaller relative error than sagittal and transverse linear measures [4]. We have previously estimated the error on our equipment as being between 8% and 12% [4] provided the principles laid down by Seibert et al. [5] were adhered to.

Changes in cross-sectional area of the neural axis between flexion and extension, in the absence of compression, are brought about by axial traction (flexion) and axial compression (extension). In the spinal cord and medulla oblongata there is evidence that levels showing maximal area change are subjected to the greatest changes in axial forces and, in particular, the greatest axial traction on flexion [5].

In the normal controls maximum changes in cross-sectional area occurred at the cervical flexure of the neural axis, which was the fulcrum at which forward bending in flexion occurred. In the Chiari patients the level of maximal area change lay cranial to the cervical flexure, and in all cases was at a point between the pontomedullary junction and the upper pole of the olive. Also the cross-sectional areas of the medulla oblongata at each level were lower than in the normal controls.

These results suggest that in some patients with pure cerebellar ectopia increased tractional forces may be generated in the uppermost part of the medulla oblongata. In this region are located the greater part of the inferior vestibular nucleus, and medial to it the premotor centre important for initiating vertical eye movements, the nucleus praepositus hypoglossi. This observation may explain the recurring dysfunction that develops in controlled movement programmes involving these nuclei.

There are several reasons why the tractional forces associated with head flexion may be shifted cranially in patients with the adult Chiari malformation. The fulcrum of flexion movement may be altered by the presence of a short or flattened clivus, as has been described in 30%–40% [6]. The medulla may be elongated and the pontomedullary junction abnormally low relative to the foramen magnum, as has been reported either alone or in combination with the above in up to 50% [7]. The neural axis may be tethered at the foramen magnum, either by the cerebellar tonsils or arachnoiditis. Although clear evidence of medullary compression and arachnoiditis was absent, the selection criteria determined that this last mechanism was the only appropriate explanation in our eight cases.

It was concluded that abnormal tractional forces generated in the upper medulla oblongata in some patients with Chiari malformation may explain the ataxias and eye movement disorders commonly seen in this condition. This mechanism may operate as well as, or in lieu of, abnormal responses to otolith mediated reflexes in which the flocculonodular lobe and medial part of the cerebellar tonsils (paraflocculus) are involved [8].

References

1. Serva W (1985) Correlation of clinical and radiological features in the adult Chiari malformation. Thesis, University of London
2. Naidich T, McLone DG, Harwood-Nash DC (1982) Malformations of the cranio-cervical junction. In: Newton TH, Potts DG (eds) Modern neuroradiology, vol 1. Computed tomography of the spine and spinal cord, chapter 18. Clavadal Press, San Anselmo, Calif
3. Brodel A (1981) Neurological anatomy in relation to clinical medicine, 3rd edn. Oxford University Press, London
4. Yu YL (1985) Computer assisted tomography in cervical spondylotic myelopathy and radiculopathy. Thesis, University of Hong Kong, Appendix 1, pp 186–203
5. Seibert CE, Barnes JE, Dreisbach SN, Swanson WB, Heck JR (1981) Accurate CT measurements of the spinal cord using metrizamide: physical factors. AJNR 2: 75–78
6. Schadi W, Metcalfe RA, Butler P (1987) The incidence of craniocervical bony anomalies in the adult Chiari malformation. J Neurol Sci 82: 193–203
7. Mohr PD, Strang FA, Sambrook MA, Boddie HG (1976) The clinical and surgical features in 40 patients with primary cerebellar ectopia (adult Chiari malformation). Q J Med 46: 85–96
8. Halmagyi GM, Rudge P, Gresty MA, Sanders MD (1983) Downbeating nystagmus. A review of 62 cases. Arch Neurol 40: 777–784

J. M. Stevens
The National Hospitals for Neurology and Neurosurgery
Maida Vale
London W9, UK

Neuroradiology (1991) 33 [Suppl]: 490–491

Neuro
radiology
© Springer-Verlag 1991

CT investigation of the craniovertebral junction: a three-dimensional study

J. Martos, I. Nagy, and G. Deák

Department of Neuroradiology, National Institute of Neurosurgery, Budapest, Hungary

Summary. The advantages of three-dimensional CT reconstruction in developmental disorders of the craniovertebral junction are demonstrated in a group of seven patients selected from 14 examinations carried out with a programme developed by the authors.

Key words: Three-dimensional computed tomography – Craniospinal pathology

The great importance of CT in assessment of the craniovertebral junction reflects its ability to provide information about the bony structures. Nevertheless, investigating this rather complicated region, one may encounter difficulties using conventional, axial CT images. To overcome these problems two (2D)- and three-dimensional (3D) reconstruction techniques are suggested.

Case reports

Case 1

A 49-year-old man presented with pain localised to the cervico-occipital region radiating into the arms for more than 20 years. Over the last 2–3 years progressive weakness of the upper extremities had developed. CT with 3D images revealed a complex anomaly of the craniovertebral junction (Fig. 1).

Case 2

A 50-year-old woman had frequent episodes of light-headedness lasting only a few seconds, induced by moving her head, for 5 years. CT showed considerable asymmetry of the craniovertebral junction (Fig. 2).

Case 3

A 42-year-old woman experienced vertigo when moving her head. Her complaints worsened for 2 months. CT investigation showed basilar impression, with marked invagination of

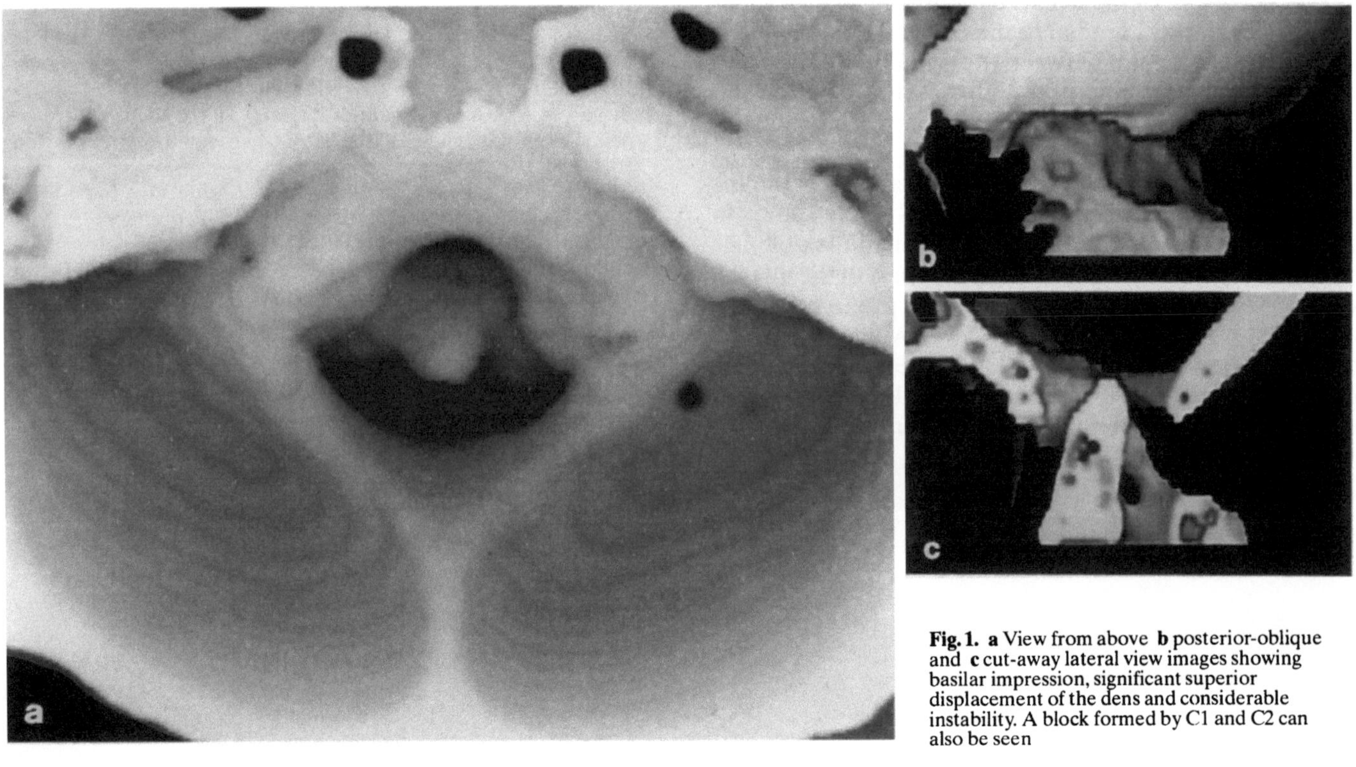

Fig. 1. **a** View from above **b** posterior-oblique and **c** cut-away lateral view images showing basilar impression, significant superior displacement of the dens and considerable instability. A block formed by C1 and C2 can also be seen

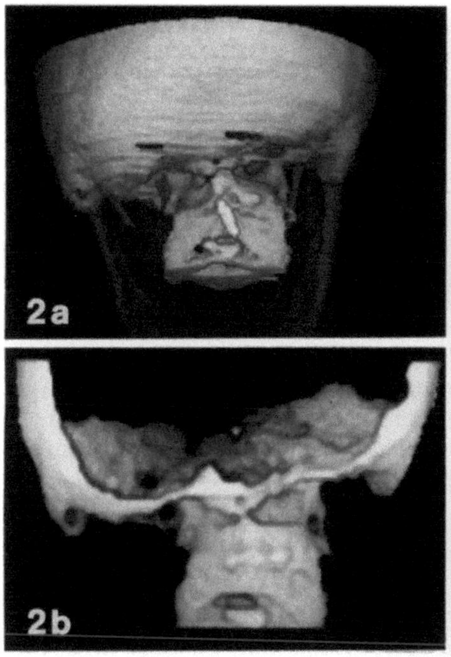

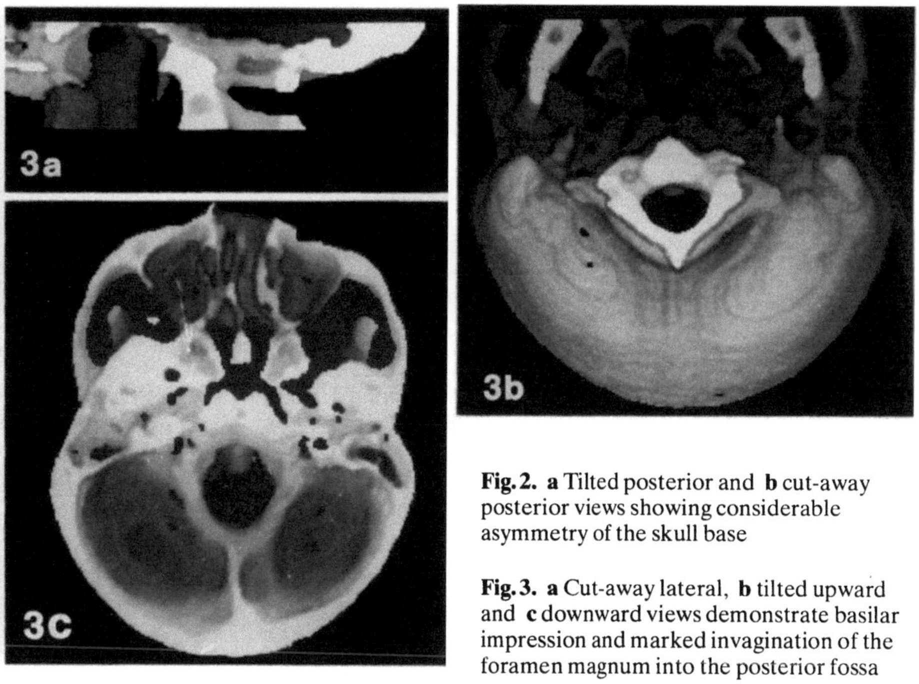

Fig. 2. **a** Tilted posterior and **b** cut-away posterior views showing considerable asymmetry of the skull base

Fig. 3. **a** Cut-away lateral, **b** tilted upward and **c** downward views demonstrate basilar impression and marked invagination of the foramen magnum into the posterior fossa

the bone forming the foramen magnum into the posterior fossa (Fig. 3).

Discussion

When using conventional CT, perception of the third dimension depends on the ability of the radiologist to reconstruct mentally. By means of 3D images one can improve appreciation of the shape and size of abnormalities and enable discussion with surgeons on the basis of a common visible image of the 3D relationships [1, 2].

On the basis of our experience in 14 cases our conclusion is that 3D examination of the craniovertebral junction is of considerable use in planning possible surgical treatment and in determining the functional state of the bony structures.

In craniovertebral disorders high quality images are obtained only by using 1-mm-thick contiguous sections, but 3D images reconstructed from 2-mm-thick sections serve for overall orientation.

A CT study with 3D reconstructions carried out by an on-the-scanner programme may take from less than 1 h to several hours. Despite that fact, we recommend its use because of the information gained, which may be of value in accurate diagnosis and treatment planning [3].

References

1. Zonneveld FW, Akkerveeken JC van der, Koorneef L, Vaandrager JM, Horst CM van der (1987) Three-dimensional imaging and manipulation of CT data. II. clinical applications in orthopaedic and craniofacial surgery. Medicamundi 32: 10–21
2. Herman GT (1988) Three-dimensional imaging in medicine. A response to a critique by surgeons. Scand J Plast Reconstr Surg Hand Surg 22: 61–71
3. Gillespie JE, Isherwood I (1986) Three-dimensional anatomical images from computed tomographic scans. Br J Radiol 59: 289–292

Dr. J. Martos
Department of Neuroradiology
National Institute of Neurosurgery
Budapest, Hungary

Neuroradiology (1991) 33 [Suppl]: 492–494

Neuro radiology
© Springer-Verlag 1991

The occult intrasacral meningocoele

I. Muras[1], F. A. Cioffi[2], A. Punzo[2], and F. P. Bernini[1]

Departments of [1]Neuroradiology and [2]Neurosurgery, First Faculty of Medicine, University of Naples, Naples, Italy

Summary. Extradural meningeal diverticula occurring in the sacral region and arising as a protrusion of the arachnoid mater through a congenitally weak place in the dura mater have been called sacral meningocoeles. Six cases of this rare and potentially progressive lesion are reported. The terminology of the condition is discussed; its pathogenesis and clinical picture are reviewed. Although the diagnosis may be established at myelography, this lesion can be well seen on CT and MRI. It is never too late to offer surgery for this lesion; radical excision should be carried out as soon as possible, before irreversible nerve root changes occur.

Key words: Intrasacral meningocoele – Myelography – Computed tomography – Magnetic resonance imaging

Occult intrasacral meningocoele [1] is a rare lesion; less than 50 cases have been reported in the literature [2]. The authors feel that some of the reported cases were not true meningocoeles. Our experience with the management of this potentially progressive lesion in six patients forms the basis of the present study (Table).

Discussion

The term "meningocoele" is habitually used to describe a protrusion of the meninges through a cranial or vertebral defect [3, 4]. According to Tarlov [4], however, to call meningocoeles meningeal diverticula is, strictly speaking, accurate. The occult intrasacral meningocoele may arise as a congenital diverticulum of the dura mater or as a protrusion of the arachnoid mater through a congenitally weak place or defect in the dura mater, habitually at the end of the thecal sac, resulting from failure of fusion of mesenchymal structures surrounding the neural tube [4–7]. Its cavity is continuous with the lower subarachnoid

Table 1. Case reports

Age, sex	Clinical picture	Plain X-ray films	Myelography (M) computed tomography (CT) magnetic resonance imaging (MRI)	Surgical treatment
44 m	Urinary incontinence Pain in the saddle area Flaccid paraparesis	Erosion of the vertebral bodies with widening of the spinal canal (S 2–S 4)	M: Multiloculated contrast-medium filled cavity with narrow neck at the lower end of the thecal sac	Excision of the meningocoele after ligature of neck Persistant mild paraparesis
26 f	Low back pain radiating into the left leg	Scalloping of the vertebral bodies. Widening of the sacral canal (S 2–S 3) with sclerotic wall	M: Contrast-medium-filled expansion of the subarachnoid space linked by a narrow isthmus to a normal tapering thecal sac	Resection of the meningocoele after ligature of neck Good recovery
33 m	Sphincter disturbances Hypoaesthesia of the sacral dermatomes	Scalloping of the vertebral bodies Erosion of the sacral bone Widening of the lumbosacral canal (L 3–S 3)	CT: Hypodense fluid collection within a widened multiloculated spinal canal M: As case 1	Ligature of neck Partial removal of the walls of the meningocoele Good recovery
50 f	Sphincter disturbances Hypoaesthesia in the saddle area Flaccid paraparesis	Erosion of the vertebral bodies. Widening of the lumbosacral canal (L 5–S 3)	CT: Enlargement of the sacral canal filled by a homogeneous hypodense mass MRI: The mass shows the same CSF intensity signal pattern in different weighted images	Ligature of neck Almost complete removal of the wall Weakness of lower extremities
40 m	Low back pain radiating into the right leg Sensory deficit in the saddle area		MRI: Erosion of S 2 vertebral body. Expanding lesion with CSF intensity signal pattern in the different weighted images	Excision of the meningocoele after ligature of neck Good recovery
46 m	Urinary incontinence Anaesthesia sacral dermatomes Cramps in the toes		MRI: Erosion S 1–3 vertebral bodies. Expanding lesion with CSF intensity signal pattern in different weighted images M: As case 2	Excision of the meningocoele after ligature of neck Immediate p. o. control: urinary disturbance sacral hypoaesthesia

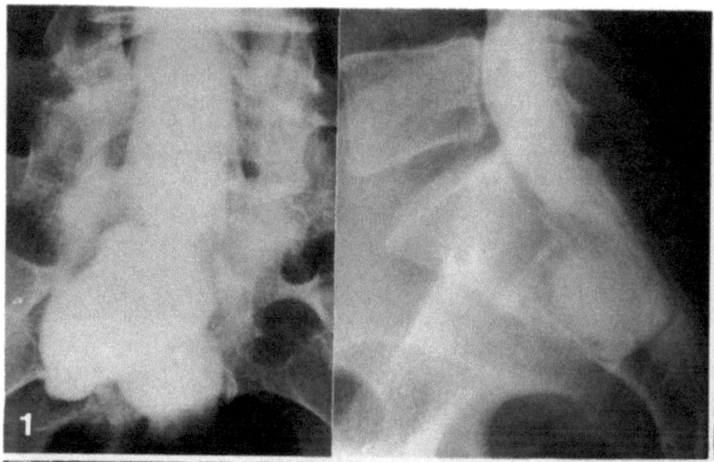

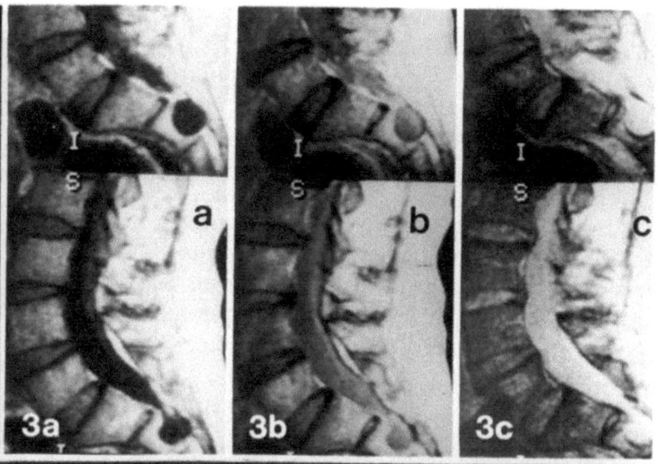

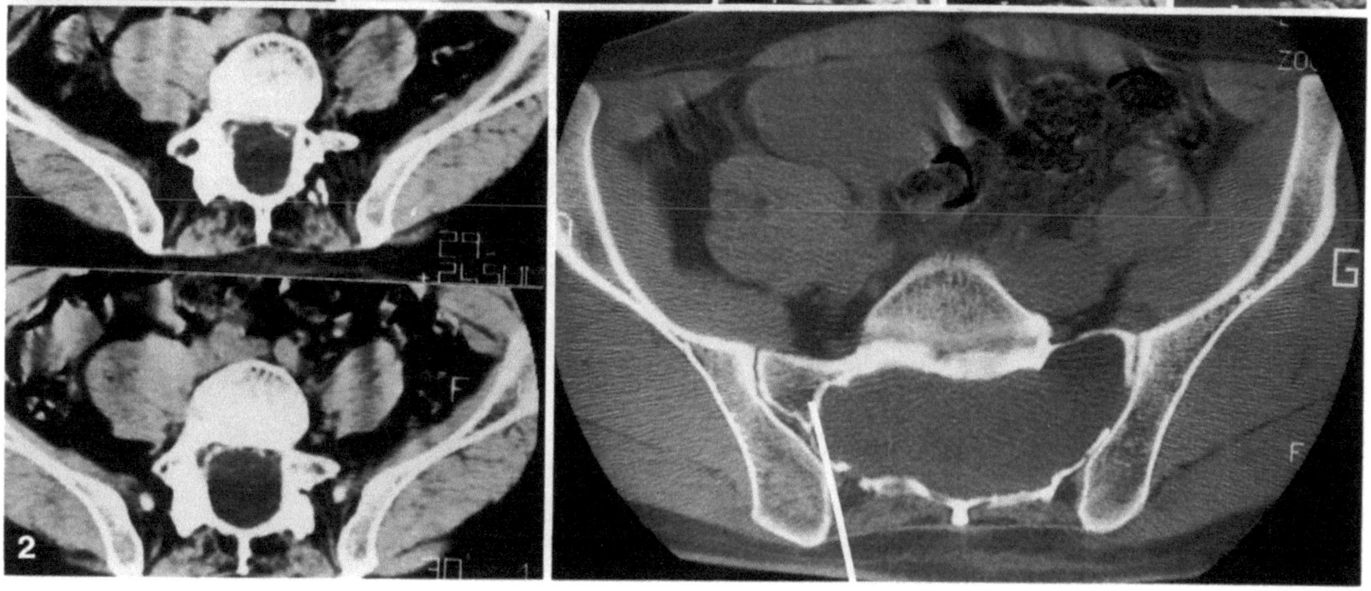

Fig. 1. Case 1. Myelography. The water-soluble contrast medium fills, through a narrow neck at the lower end of a normally tapering thecal sac, a multiloculated intrasacral cavity at S 2–3, bulging to the right. Erosion of the vertebral bodies with widening of the spinal canal

Fig. 2. Case 2. CT of the lumbosacral spine. Scalloping of the vertebral bodies, erosion of the sacral bone with thin sclerotic edges, widening of the lumbosacral canal. The cavity is filled by a homogeneous hypodense mass with the same attenuation values as CSF

Fig. 3 a–c. Case 4. MRI of the lumbosacral spine. A round, low-intensity signal area fills, almost completely, the S 2 vertebral body in T 1-weighted images (**a**). In the proton density (**b**) and T 2-weighted (**c**) images the signal intensity pattern of the lesion is similar to that of lumbar CSF

space through a narrow neck [2, 3, 8, 9]. It may be difficult to distinguish a meningeal diverticulum covered by markedly thinned dura mater from an arachnoid herniation. Histological examination shows a laminated collagenous tissue covered by meningothelial cells, without neural elements [5, 8, 10, 11]. The hydrostatic pressure, pulsations of cerebrospinal fluid (CSF) or the high protein content of the fluid within the cavity tend to dilate the sac with time and produce local erosion of the sacrum [7]. There are different types of meningeal malformation simulating a meningocoele and different aetiological factors may be operative in individual cases [3, 11].

Symptoms may appear at any age, depending on compression by the growing mass of nerve roots [8, 11]. The most common are: disturbances of sphincter function; hypoaesthesia or anaesthesia in the lower sacral dermatomes; low back and sciatic pain that usually become progressively more constant and severe; absence of the ankle jerks and motor impairment related to lumbar or sacral root compression. A few patients complain of headache on straining, due to sudden increase in the intracranial pressure.

Plain X-rays as well as tomography show an enlargement of the sacral canal with thinned, sclerotic wall [2–5, 8]. It is not a specific appearance, since it may be also induced by solid slow-growing tumours. Myelography using water-soluble medium (Fig. 1) is usually diagnostic, showing the size and extent of the sac as well as the diameter of its neck. In some instances, the anatomy of the lesion is more complex; its pedicle may be narrow or the sac may exert pressure upon it, so that the diagnostic reliability of the myelogram may be impaired by the slow filling of the sac, dilution and rapid water-soluble contrast medium resorption. Myelography with oil can be diagnostic, but only after 24–48 h [1, 5, 8]. CT study without contrast medium (Fig. 2) shows the enlargement of the sacral canal with thinning of its wall and vertebral erosion. Densitometry of the mass reveals homogeneously low attenuation values. They are sometimes not equal to water, probably because of a high protein content and a beam-hardening effect. In the densitometric analysis the bladder, which contains urine of about the same attenuation of CSF may be used as a reference value [12]. CT study with intrathecal injection of water-soluble medium may be available to confirm that we are dealing with a meningeal diverticulum, to improve the anatomical demonstration of the lesion and better define its relation to adjacent structures.

MRI has quickly proved to be, in many instances, more sensitive and specific than CT in detection and characterisation of meningocoele. On T1-weighted images (Fig. 3a), a low-intensity signal area contrasting with the high-intensity background signal of the bone marrow demonstrates vertebral erosion. The CSF collection within the meningocoele is identified by comparing its signal intensity pattern to that of subarachnoid CSF in proton density and T2-weighted images (Fig. 3b, c). Although it is never too late to offer surgery for this lesion [3, 13] radical excision should be carried out as soon as possible, before irreversible nerve root changes occur [14]. Whether or not it is possible to ligate the neck and completely remove the sac, care must be taken to avoid injury to the sacral nerve roots and incomplete closure of the fistulous tract [8]. If the sac cannot be dissected free from the nerve roots, occlusion of the fistulous tract and partial removal of the walls result in symptomatic relief. The dural suture must be water-tight to avoid CSF leakage in the postoperative period.

References

1. Enderle C (1932) Meningocele intrasacrale occulto. Riv Neurol 5: 418–423
2. Grivegnee A, Delince P, Ectors P (1981) Comparative aspects of occult intrasacral meningocele with conventional X-ray myelography and CT. Neuroradiology 22: 33–37
3. Florez G, Ucar S (1976) The occult intrasacral meningocele. Neurochirurgia 19: 46–53
4. Tarlov IM (1970) Spinal perineurial and meningeal cysts. J Neurol Neurosurg Psychiatry 33: 833–843
5. Bianchi M, Passerini A, Boeri R (1968) Meningocele occulto sacrale. Minerva Neurochir 12: 184–189
6. Cecotto C, De Vito R (1968) Malformazioni mielo-vertebrali. Minerva Neurochir 12: 1–147
7. Gortvai P (1963) Extradural cysts of the spinal canal. J Neurol Neurosurg Psychiatry 26: 223–230
8. Lamas E, Lobato RD, Amor T (1977) Occult intrasacral meningocele. Surg Neurol 8: 181–184
9. Taveras JM, Wood EH (1964) Diagnostic neuroradiology. Williams and Wilkins, Baltimore
10. Palazzoli A (1963) Rilievi clinici e patogenetici su un caso di meningocele sacrale occulto simulante un'ernia discale. Boll Soc Med Chir 17: 203–225
11. Roma JA, McKenzie T (1970) Occult intrasacral meningocele. J Neurol Neurosurg Psychiatry 33: 493–496
12. Haberbeck Modesto MA, Servadei F (1981) Computed tomography for anterior sacral and intracorporal meningoceles. Neuroradiology 21: 155–158
13. Kak V, Chugh K, Sodhi J (1972) Occult intrasacral meningocele. Neurochirurgie 15: 148–172
14. Pool J (1952) Spinal cord and local signs secondary to occult sacral meningoceles in adult. Bull N Y Acad Med 28: 655–663

I. Muras
Department of Neuroradiology
First Faculty of Medicine
University of Naples
C/O Ospedale CTO
Viala Colli Aminel, 21
I-80131 Naples, Italy

Neuroradiology (1991) 33 [Suppl]: 495–496

Neuro radiology
© Springer-Verlag 1991

Tethered spinal cord: neuroradiological diagnosis in children and adults

N. Mitrović, A. Jašović, M. Perović, and S. Lavrnić

Institute of Oncology and Radiology, Belgrade, Yugoslavia

Summary. A defective closure of the neural tube leads to many different anomalies. The term for all these anomalies – dysraphia – was coined by Lichtenstein in 1940. The worst of these defects is a complete non-closure of the neural tube and the minor and also the most common is spina bifida oculta. Tethered cord is often seen with meningomyelocele but also with spina bifida oculta in only one vertebral body level. The age of diagnosis of the tethered cord varies from under 1 year to 14 years and is very rarely as late as adulthood. The authors analysed myelography and CT findings in four children and two patients of 17 and 20 years and compare these findings. The purpose of this study was to make the precise diagnosis and also make precise planning for therapy, conservative or surgical treatment.

Key words: Tethered spinal cord – Spina bifida – Meningocele

Tethered spinal cord is a congenital anomaly characterised by a low positioned spinal cord conus due to the shortened filum terminale. According to Barson [1] conus level below L2–3 intervertebral space in children older than 5 is abnormal. Patients with a tethered spinal cord consult doctors because of neurological, mostly progressive symptoms such as paresis, muscle atrophy and loss of sensation in the lower extremities with or without pathological reflexes. They often attend an orthopaedic surgeon because of scoliosis or foot deformities or an urologist because of urinary dysfunction and impaired defaecation. Tethered spinal cord symptoms are rare in adults, but when seen they are the same as in children. The appearance of the syndrome in adults (after the growth period), indicates that the pathogenesis of the syndrome cannot be explained just as an embryological disorder. Many symptoms can be explained by ischaemia due to the traction on the spinal cord during the growth period [2, 3]. Early diagnosis and surgery, if indicated, can contribute to the prevention of the progressive and often irreversible neurological defects.

The diagnosis involves standard X-ray examination, myelography and CT myelography [4]. MRI is now a diagnostic method of choice for investigation of a tethered spinal cord syndrome [5].

All the cases of tethered spinal cord that we examined had bony malformations of the lumbosacral area including: incomplete closure of the lumbar and/or sacral spinal canal, block vertebrae and sacral spina bifida oculta of one vertebra. Plain radiographs have a high diagnostic sensitivity but no adequate specific values for the syndrome. Myelographic findings are characterised by: short filum terminale dislocated dorsally in dura and fixed to the periosteum of sacral arches while the conus of the spinal cord is attached at or below the level of L2–3. Tethered cord is often seen with lipomas or with lipomeningocoele. CT myelography enables us to differentiate lipoma from an enlarged and shortened filum terminale.

Patients and methods

Six patients with tethered spinal cord were examined by standard X-ray examinations, conventional myelography and CT myelography. Two children, aged 4 and 6, had undergone an operation, while two children and two adult patients were not operated upon due to their few symptoms and lesser degree of tethered spinal cord. Myelography in children was performed under general anaesthesia and with iodine contrast concentration of 180 mg% and in adults after premedication and with the contrast medium Omnipaque, iodine concentration of 240 mg%.

Discussion

The previously described symptoms dominate the clinical picture in our patients but can vary from severe neurological changes to the abortive (relatively asymptomatic) forms.

The severity of clinical features parallels that of anatomical lesions.

In one patient with abortive form of clinical presentation we suggested a different professional career (the girl was in a professional ballet school), and she still has no need to undergo on operation (Fig. 1).

In two children with significant flaccid paraparesis and incontinence plain films revealed the deformities of the vertebral bodies and spina bifida in one case at two levels and in second patient, at three levels. Myelography showed that the spinal cord was tethered at S1 level (Fig. 2) and that nerve roots coursed less steeply downward, with a small meningocoele. The postoperative

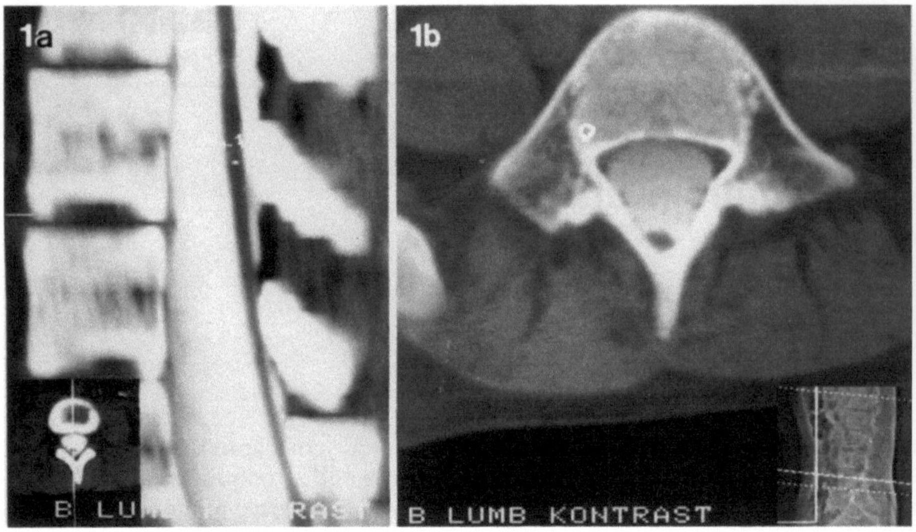

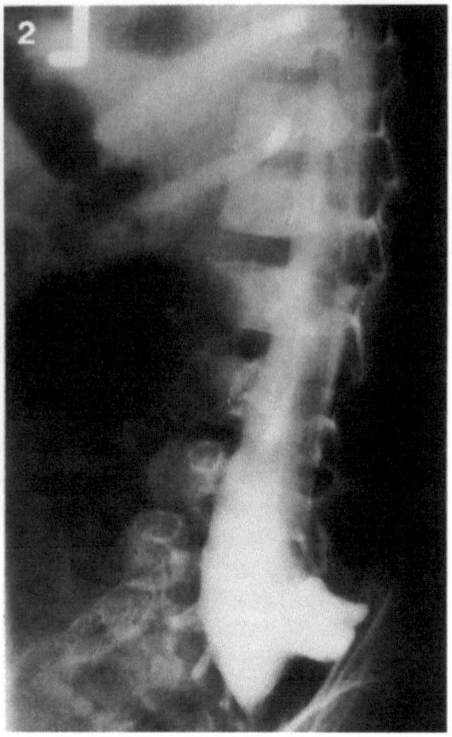

Fig. 1a,b. CT myelography: **a** lateral indirect reconstruction; filum terminale is thickened and dorsally located. It is not possible to precisely locate the level of the conus. **b** Axial cut of the L5 level; thickened filum terminale is fixed to the posterior arch

Fig. 2. Myelography of 3-year-old patient with lipomeningocele. Low conus and abnormal course of nerve roots

course was slow with a partial remission of neurological symptoms.

In our opinion the indications for surgery depend on: (a) severity of clinical features, (b) degree of anatomical changes, (c) age of the patient.

Experience with our patients shows that surgery is not always indicated at the discovery of the disease.

The patients need to be followed-up, if not operated upon.

References

1. Barson AJ (1970) The vertebral level of termination of the spinal cord during normal and abnormal development. J Anat 106: 489–497
2. Hilal SK, Kein HA (1972) Selective spinal angiography in adolescent scoliosis. Radiology 102: 349–359
3. Yamada S, Zinke DE, Sonders D (1981) Pathophysiology of tethered cord syndrome. J Neurosurg 54: 494–503
4. Herix JL, Bakker-Niezen SH, Thijssen HOM, Walder HAD (1989) The tethered spinal cord syndrome: a correlation of radiological features and peroperative findings in 30 patients. Neuroradiology 31: 63–70
5. Rindahl MA, Colletti PM, Zee CS, Tabor P (1989) Magnetic resonance imaging of pediatric spinal dysraphism. Magn Reson Imaging 7: 217–224

Dr. Andja Jašović
Department for Neuroradiology
Institute of Oncology and Radiology
11000 Belgrade, Pasterova 14, Yugoslavia

Neuroradiology (1991) 33 [Suppl]: 497–498

Neuro-radiology
© Springer-Verlag 1991

Magnetic resonance imaging of cervical spinal cord injury and correlation with outcome

T. Nakamura, S. Kadoya, and F. Panggabean

Department of Neurosurgery, Kanazawa Medical University, Uchinada, Japan

Summary. MRI images of cervical spinal cord injury from acute to chronic stages in 20 patients were studied in relation to outcome according Frankel's classification. Sixteen patients showing either normal images or transient (less than 2 months) intramedullary hyperintensity on T2-weighted images recovered well (Frankel's grades D or E, apart from two cases of grade C). Recovery of 4 patients showing persistent hyperintensity (for more than 6 months) on T2-weighted images was poor (Frankel's grades A or B, apart from one case of grade D). These longstanding high-intensity cord lesions on T2-weighted images appeared of low intensity on T1-weighted images, and reflect myelomalacia. Chronological changes on MR images of cervical cord injuries correlate well with functional recovery.

Key words: Magnetic resonance imaging – Spinal cord injuries – Spinal injuries – Spinal cord

---

We previously reported that MRI was very sensitive for detection of the traumatised cord segment in acute spinal cord injury patients [1]. Various pathological processes occurring in spinal cord injury detectable on MRI and their correlation with neurologcial function have been studied from the acute to the chronic stage.

Patients and methods

From April 1985 to March 1990 MRI was performed on 20 patients with cervical cord injury, in the acute to chronic stages, using 0.5 T superconductive and 0.15 resistive units. Patients included in this series were 13 males and 7 females aged 35–66 years. Follow-up period was 4–16 months (average 8.7 months). Neurological function of the injured patients and the degree of their recovery were determined based on Frankel's classification (grade A, complete loss of function; B, sensory function only; C, no useful recovery of motor function; D, useful motor function; E, recovery [2].)

Results

Nine patients having normal MRI in the acute stage showed good recovery (8 patients in Frankel's grade E and one in grade D at the final follow-up examination). Recovery of 7 patients showing intramedullary hyperintensity on T2-weighted images for up to at most 2 months after the injury was variable: five patients ended up as grade D and 2 patients as grade C (Fig. 1). In the remaining 4 patients the traumatised cord showed persistently high intensity on T2-weighted images from the acute to the chronic stage. These lesions were of low intensity on T1-weighted images. Recovery of these patients was poor (Frankel grade A or B, except 1 case in grade D, Fig. 2).

Discussion

Severity of the neurological deficit was reflected in the persistence of a high intensity intramedullary lesion on T2-weighted images. In patients showing transient high intensity cord lesions on T2-weighted images functional recovery was good. These MR abnormalities may represent reversible oedema. In the majority of patients making a poor recovery, with final functional Frankel grades of A or B, the traumatised cord appeared of persistently high intensity on T2-weighted images from the acute to the chronic stage. T1-weighted images of these lesions showed low intensity in the chronic stage. Haemorrhagic necrosis proceeding to myelomalacia may be reflected by these appearances [1, 3, 4]. We conclude that MRI correlates well with neurological deficit in patients with cervical cord injuries, and with their outcome.

References

1. Kadoya S, Nakamura T, Kobayasi S, Yamamoto I (1987) Magnetic resonance imaging of acute spinal cord injury. Report of three cases. Neuroradiology 29: 252–255
2. Frankel HL (1969) The value of postural reduction in the initial management of closed injuries of the spine with paraplegia and tetraplegia. Paraplegia 7: 179–192
3. Kulkarni MV, McArdle CB, Kopanicky D, Miner M, Colter HB, Lee KF, Harris JH (1987) Acute spinal cord injury: MR imaging at 1.5 T. Radiology 164: 837–843
4. Gebarski SS, Maynard FW, Gabrielson TO, Knake JE, Latack JT, Hoff JT (1985) Posttraumatic progressive myelopathy. Clinical and radiological correlation employing MR imaging, delayed CT metrizamide myelography, and intraoperative sonography. Radiology 157: 379–385

Dr. Satoru Kadoya
Department of Neurosurgery
Kanazawa University
Uchinada, Ishikawaken, Japan

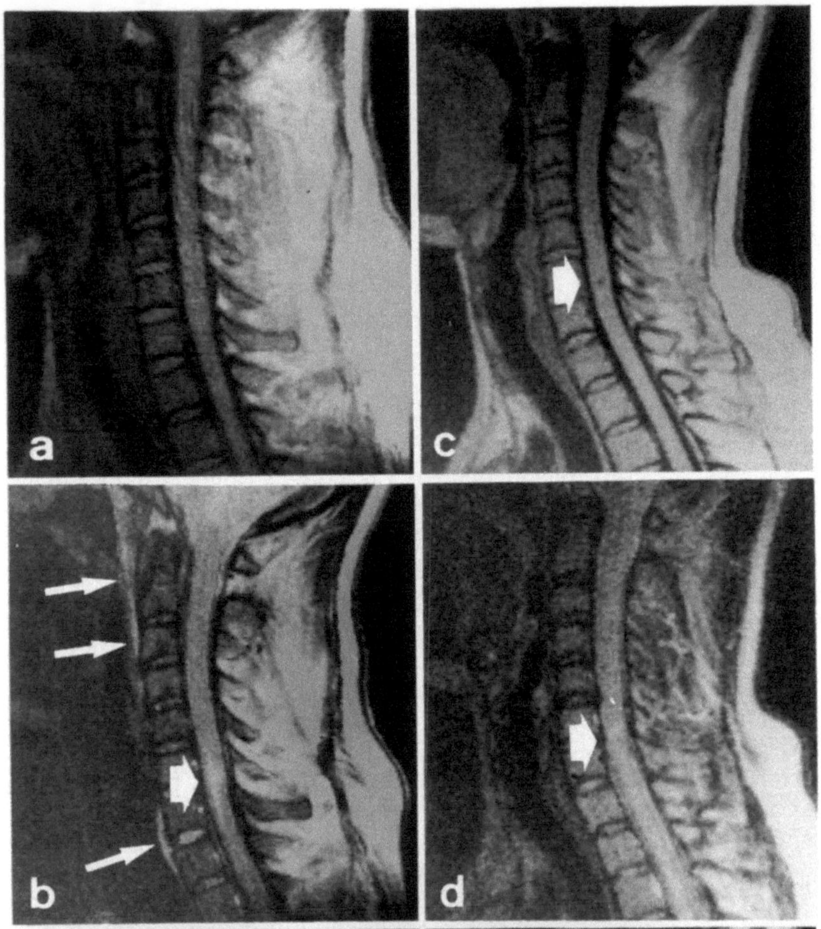

Fig. 1 a–d. MRI of a damaged cervical spinal cord showing good recovery: **a** Sagittal SE 500/40; **b** SE 1800/90 images obtained on the day of a motor vehicle accident. The T1-weighted image appeared normal, but high intensity on the T2-weighted image showed the traumatised cord *(large arrow)* as well as haemorrhage into the prevertebral soft tissues *(small arrow)*. **c** Sagittal SE 500/30 and **d** SE 1800/90 images 4 months after the injury. The high intensity cord lesion on the T2-weighted image has almost disappeared but T1-weighted image shows a small area of low intensity. The neurological function of this patient was initially Frankel's grade C (loss of motor function) and finally was D (useful return of motor function)

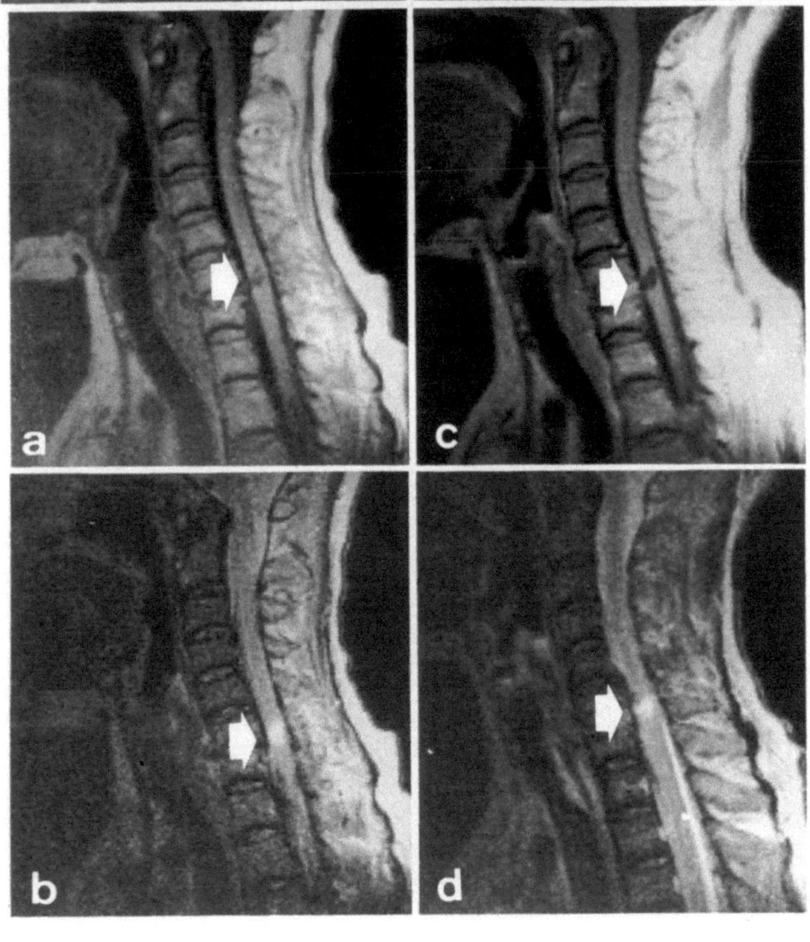

Fig. 2 a–d. MRI of a cervical cord injury showing a complete transverse lesion from acute to chronic stages (the initial and final Frankel's grades were A). **a** Sagittal SE 500/30; **b** 1500/90 images showing the damaged cord segment 1 month after injury. **c** Sagittal SE 500/30; **d** SE 2200/90 images 6 months later. The traumatised cervical cord appears of low intensity on T1-weighted images and high on T2-weighted images *(arrow)*, suggesting myelomalacia

Neuroradiology (1991) 33 [Suppl]: 499–500

Neuroradiology

© Springer-Verlag 1991

Isolated traumatic injuries of the transverse ligament, with rotatory dislocation, detected by functional tomography and computed tomography

J. Kenéz[1], L. Thúróczy[2], and P. Barsi[1]

[1] Neurologic Clinic of Semmelweis Medical University, Budapest, Hungary
[2] National Institute for Traumatology, Department of Neurosurgery, Budapest, Hungary

Summary. Two cases of injury of the transverse ligament were investigated by functional conventional tomography and CT as well as conventional myelotomography and CT myelography. In both cases rotatory dislocation, ligamentous injury and bony disruption of the atlas, indicating ligamentous damage and dural tear with cerebrospinal fluid leakage, were detected. Correct, detailed diagnostic data are essential for proper treatment

Key words: Atlanto-axial region – Transverse ligament – Ligament injury – Rotatory dislocation – Bony disruption – Dural tears

Atlanto-axial traumatic luxations occurring in adults can be divided into anterior, posterior and rotational types. Anterior or posterior luxations are common findings in fractures of the dens and mixed types can be seen in cases of Jefferson fractures of the C1 ring [1]. Traumatic rotational luxation/subluxation can occur without fracture of the surrounding bony structures, due to pure ligamentous injury. The classification of rotational atlas dislocations was given by Fielding and Hawkins [2], following the basic data of Brocher [3], Penning [4], and Wortzman and Dewar [5]. Biomechanical studies of the atlanto-axial complex have indicated that the force necessary to damage the ligaments is always less than that required to fracture the dens [6]. On the other hand, modern CT scanners have proved useful for depicting the ligamentous structures of the atlanto-axial complex [7–9] and previously, functional conventional tomographic studies made it possible to detect chronic ligament damage of the same region. MRI seems to be promising, but we had no possibility to perform such investigations.

In spite of these facts, we did not find well-documented references in the literature dealing with traumatic rotational atlanto-axial dislocations caused by ligamentous damage in adults. We describe two such cases.

Case reports

Case 1

A 36-year-old woman suffered an automobile accident. Shortly afterwards torticollis and a stiff, painful neck developed, but the deformity was always reducible. Repeat plain film studies did not reveal any abnormality. Two years after the accident CT showed rotatory dislocation with remarkable asymmetry between the dens and the C1 ring. This asymmetry could be documented on conventional anteroposterior (a-p) tomograms, and a small isolated bony shadow was seen at the inner border of the left lateral mass of the atlas. On a functional a-p tomogram tilted to the left, this piece of bone separates further (Fig. 1), and on a tomogram tilted to the right, it moved

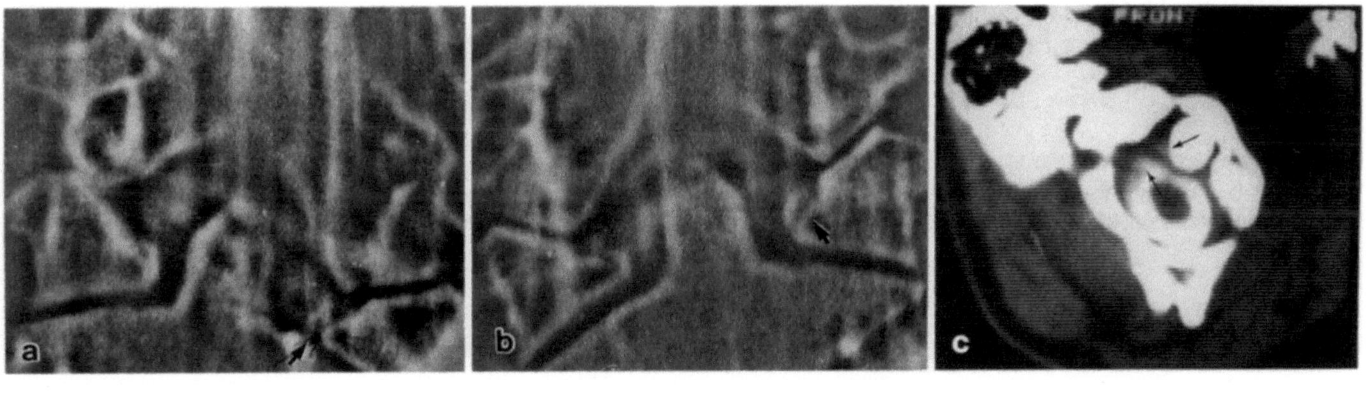

Fig. 1 a–c. Case 1. Anteroposterior tomograms through the dense. A small bony fragment has been detached *(arrows)* from the left lateral mass of C1. It is mobile. **c** CT myelogram. The cerebrospinal fluid space bulges towards the fracture *(lower arrow)*, and a small amount of contrast medium lies in contact with the dens *(upper arrow)*

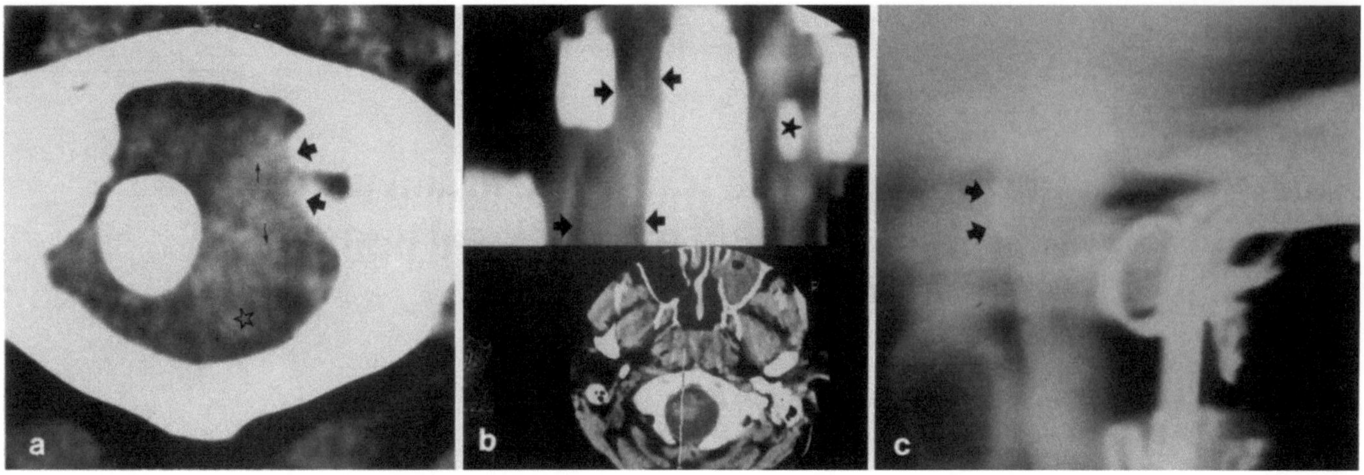

Fig. 2 a–c. Case 2. **a, b** Axial and parasagittal reformatted CT. **a** The dens is displaced posterolaterally. *Small arrows,* Transverse ligament; *larger arrows,* detached bone fragments: *star,* spinal cord. **b** *Asterisk,* Detached fragment; *arrows* space available for spinal cord. **c** Sagittal myelotomogram following surgery: satisfactory alignment. The theca remains irregular at the site of the tear *(arrows)*

back to its place of origin. On CT myelography, bulging of the cerebrospinal fluid (CSF) space was seen, indicating the ligamentous injury, and contrast medium leaked into the dentoligamental articulation, evidence of a dural tear.

Case 2

A 35-year-old man suffered a car accident. Emergency plain films failed to show any abnormality. Over the next 3 months he felt excruciating pain in his neck, preventing him from lying down, so that he slept sitting up. On admission, remarkable torticollis and slight right-sided hemihypaesthesia were noted. On routine plain films and tomograms, an increase in the atlanto-dental distance and a suspected bony fragment were seen. On CT (2 mm), the deformed spinal cord, the swollen, damaged right insertion of the transverse ligament, and the irregular surface of the right atlantal tubercle, from which the bone fragment had been detached *(large arrows)* were demonstrated (Fig. 2). On a reformated image, the deformity of the spinal canal was shown, as was the bony fragment within it.

Because of the presence of this bony fragment, conservative treatment seemed unlikely to succeed; the fragment and the anterior tubercle of atlas were excised via a transoral approach and a modified posterior Crockard fixation was performed. A dural tear with CSF leakage was noted at the damaged right extremity of the transverse ligament. On postoperative myelotomography, satisfactory reconstruction of the spinal canal with a centrally-lying spinal cord and a little pool of contrast medium at the site of the closed dural tear (Fig. 2c) were seen. The patient left hospital fully recovered.

Discussion

We emphasise two important, characteristic patterns of isolated traumatic injuries of the transverse ligament. Firstly, in both cases, little bony flake fractures were demonstrated, which suggests that the weakest part of the transverse ligament is its insertion on the tubercle on the inner surface of the atlas, which is in agreement with the data of Fielding et al. [6] collected from biomechanical studies. Secondly, in both cases, the ligamentous injury caused a dural tear and leakage of CSF into the surrounding structures, which emphasises the need for intrathecal contrast medium.

References

1. Van Gilder JC, Menezes AH, Dolan KD (1987) The craniovertebral junction and its abnormalities. Futura, New York
2. Fielding JW, Hawkins RJ (1977) Atlantoaxial rotatory fixation. J Bone Joint Surg 59: 37–44
3. Brocher JEW (1966) Die Wirbelsäulenleiden und ihre Differentialdiagnose, 4th edn. Thieme, Stuttgart
4. Penning L (1961) Atlantoaxial instability and functional X-ray examination. Medicamundi 7: 113–126
5. Wortzman A, Dewar FP (1968) Rotary fixation of the atlantoaxial joint. Rotational atlantoaxial subluxation. Radiology 90: 479–487
6. Fielding JW, Cochran GB, Lansing JF (1974) Tears of the transverse ligament of the atlas. A clinical and biochemical study. J Bone Joint Surg 56: 1683–1691
7. Burguet JL, Sick H, Dirheimer K, Wackenheim A (1985) CT of the main ligaments of the cervico-occipital hinge. Neuroradiology 27: 112–118
8. Wackenheim A (1974) Roentgen diagnosis of the craniovertebral region. Springer, Berlin Heidelberg New York
9. Daniels DL, Williams AL, Haughton VM (1983) CT of the articulations and the ligaments of the occipito-atlanto-axial region. Radiology 146: 709–716

Dr. J. Kenéz
Semmelweis Medical University
Department of Neurology
Ballassa u. 6
H-1083 Budapest, Hungary

Neuroradiology (1991) 33 [Suppl]: 501–502

Neuro radiology
© Springer-Verlag 1991

Pre-operative MRI assessment for cervical spine surgery in rheumatoid arthritis

H. D. Sinclair[1], B. E, Kendall[2], R. Moskovich[2], M. Corbett[1], M. E. Shipley[1], and H. A. Crockard[2]

[1] Rheumatology Research Department, University College and Middlesex Schools of Medicine, London, UK
[2] National Hospitals for Nervous Diseases, London, UK

Summary. A cervico-medullary angle of less than 135° is a relatively specific (87%) indicator of neurological deficit caused by vertical subluxation of the odontoid peg in rheumatoid arthritis. It is, however, an insensitive (68%) indicator of neurological deficit, since neuraxial compression may also be caused by horizontal atlanto-axial subluxation, retrodental pannus or subaxial subluxation, which do not influence the cervico-medullary angle.

Key words: Rheumatoid arthritis – Cervico-medullary angle – Magnetic resonance imaging

MRI has considerable advantages over CT-myelography (CTM) for assessment of cervico-medullary compression in rheumatoid arthritis (RA), including the direct visualisation of the neuraxis without intrathecal contrast medium, which facilitates repeated examinations in multiple positions. However, precise measurements of the spinal canal and degree of cord compression are more difficult in routine practice with MRI than with CTM. It has been suggested [1] that an angle of less than 135° between the medulla and cord as measured on MRI (cervico-medullary angle) will predict neuraxial compression. The aims of this study were: (1) to determine the range of angulation of the cervico-medullary junction in RA patients; (2) to relate this measurement to clinical evidence of cord compression.

Methods

Thirty-five patients with RA involving the cervical spine were assessed clinically and functionally. Their cervical spines were studied by MRI (Elscint Gyrex 0.5 T) in flexion and extension. The cervico-medullary angle, or the angle between the upper and lower segments of the neuraxis at the site of maximal angulation, was measured on T1-weighted scans (Fig. 1) without reference to neurological status, decision to operate, or choice of surgical technique. The surgical decisions were made independently of the MRI measurements.

Classification of neurological deficit was modified from the method of Ranawat et al. [2], in which grade 1 indicates no deficit; grade 2, subjective weakness, dysaesthesia and hyperreflexia; grade 3, objective weakness and long tract signs in an ambulant patient; grade 4, quadriplegic, or grade 3 but unable to walk.

Functional score was assessed by the Health Assessment Questionnaire (HAQ) [3]: a series of 20 questions relating to activities of daily life, each of which can be scored from 1 to 4. The total pre-operative score for each patient was used as a functional guide.

Results

Thirty-four scans were suitable for measurement. The results are shown in Fig. 2. Seven of the 9 patients with a neuraxial angle less than 135°, but only 4 of the 25 patients with neuraxial angle greater than 135°, needed surgery for medullary compression ($P < 0.01$, χ^2 with Yates' correction). In the former group, medullary compression was always associated with vertical subluxation of the odotoid peg. Severe horizontal atlanto-axial subluxation and/or large amounts of retro-odontoid pannus were significant factors in compression at the cranio-cervical junction in the patients with a neuraxial angle of greater than 135°. Four further patients in the latter group had surgery for subaxial cord compression.

The results for the HAQ are shown in Fig. 3. All 8 patients with a functional score greater than 65 on the HAQ

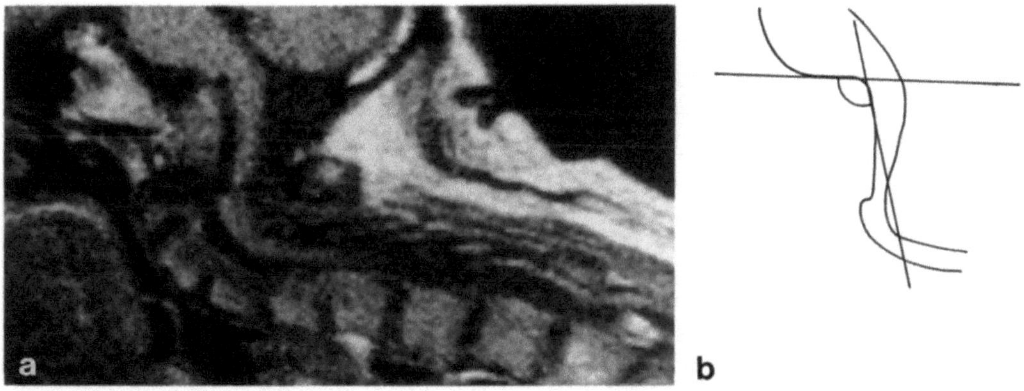

Fig. 1. a Marked translocation of odontoid with angulation of the medulla. Note posterior subluxation of C2 on 3 causing compression of the spinal cord. **b** Angle at site of medullary compression = 104°

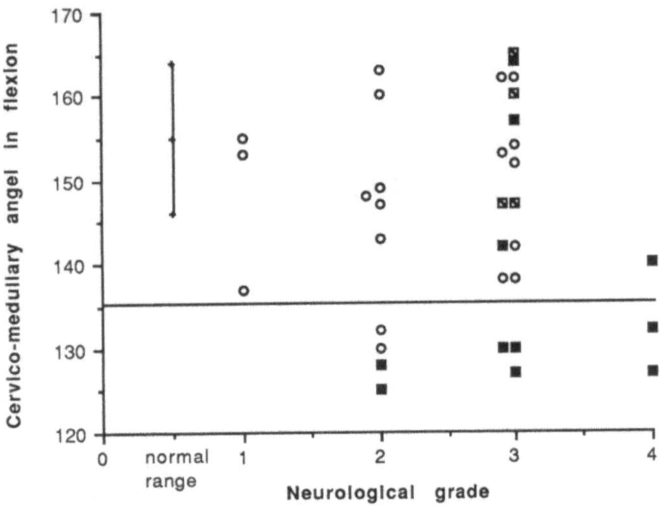

Fig. 2. Cervico-medullary angle: neurological score. ○, No neuraxial compression on MRI; ⧅, subaxial cord compression; ■, medullary compression

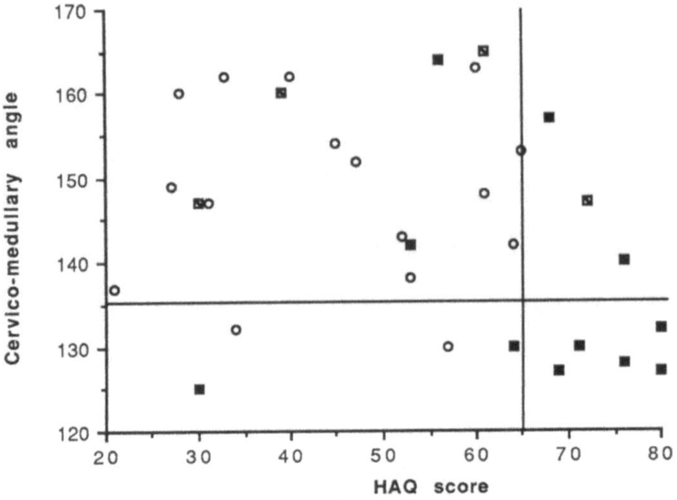

Fig. 3. Cervico-medullary angle: functional score. ○, No neuraxial compression; ⧅, subaxial cord compression; ■, medullary compression

were treated surgically: all of these had an obvious neurological deficit, but 3 had a "normal" neuraxial angle.

Discussion

The neuraxial angle is mainly related to the degree of vertical subluxation of the odontoid peg. In some patients, horizontal atlanto-axial subluxation and/or retrodental pannus contribute significantly to cord compression but do not affect the cervico-medullary angle. A limit of 135° in flexion is a relatively specific (87.5%), but insensitive (68%) means of identifying patients with significant neurological deficit. If the patients treated for medullary compression alone are considered, the sensitivity of this measurement is 80%. Use of the HAQ score will further differentiate those patients in whom surgery is indicated.

Acknowledgements. We would like to thank Charlotte Cornborough, research nurse, Amanda Burls, medical student, the MRI Centre, London and the Appeals Trust, Middlesex Hospital.

References

1. Bundschuh C, Modic MT, Kearney F, Morris R, Deaf C (1988) Rheumatiod arthritis of the cervical spine: surface-coil MR imaging. AJR 151: 181–187
2. Ranawat CS, O'Leary P, Pellicci P, Tsairis P, Marchisello P, Dorr L (1979) Cervical spine fusion in rheumatoid arthritis J Bone Joint Surg [Am] 61: 1003–1010
3. Kirwan JR, Reeback JS (1986) Stanford Health Assessment Questionnaire modified to assess disability in British patients with rheumaotid arthritis. Br J Rheumatol 25: 206–209

Dr. B. E. Kendall
Lysholm Radiological Department
The National Hospital for Nervous Diseases
Queen Square
London WC1, UK

Neuroradiology (1991) 33 [Suppl]: 503–504

Neuro radiology
© Springer-Verlag 1991

MRI of pituitary dwarfism

S. Tazawa[1], S. Takahashi[2], K. Ishii[2], M. Yoshiike[2], K. Matumoto[2], K. Sakamoto[2], and K. Hanew[2]

[1] Radiology Department, Sendai Shakaihoken Hospital, Sendai, Japan
[2] Departments of Radiology and Endocrinology, Tohoku University School of Medicine, Sendai, Japan

Summary. MR images in 52 patients with pituitary dwarfism were reviewed. Pituitary stalk was normal in 20 patients (38%), hypoplastic in 20 (38%), and absent, so-called transection, in 12 (23%). The size of pituitary stalk correlated well with clinical data and other MRI findings. MRI could disclose the morphological basis in patients with pituitary dwarfism.

Key words: Magnetic resonance imaging – Pituitary dwarfism – Pituitary stalk – Transection

Transection of the pituitary stalk and/or development of an ectopic posterior lobe are known to be often present in patients with pituitary dwarfism [1–4]. In this study, we reviewed MR images of pituitary dwarfism to define the frequency of the transection of pituitary stalk and correlation of the MRI findings with clinical data.

Patients and methods

MR images in 52 patients with pituitary dwarfism were reviewed, especially focusing on the state of the stalk.

They were 33 males and 19 females, aged 6–27 (15.1) years. The diagnosis of pituitary dwarfism was made when the patients showed marked retardation of height according to age, poor growth velocity, delay of bone age, low somatomedin C level and absent or subnormal responses in plasma growth hormone (GH) (< 7 ng/ml) to some provocation tests. Replacement therapy of deficient hormones had been given in most patients.

MRI studies were performed on a 1.5-T superconducting unit (Siemens Magnetom). Three-millimetre-thick contiguous T1-weighted images (SE pulse sequence, 500/20) were acquired in both coronal and sagittal planes with 256 × 256 matrix and a 15–20 cm field of vision.

The patients were divided into three groups according to the size of pituitary stalk measured on MR images: group A, normal in 20 patients (38%); group B, hypoplastic in 20 (38%); and group C, absent, so-called transection, in 12 (23%).

The size of pituitary stalk was correlated with clinical data (perinatal abnormality, severity of GH deficiency, other hormonal deficiency, and somatomedin C level) and other MRI findings (the bright posterior lobe, the ectopic lobe, the size of the anterior pituitary lobe and the size of the sella turcica).

Results

Perinatal abnormalities were seen in 30 of 52 patients with pituitary dwarfism; asphyxia in 18, and breech presentation in 16. All patients with a history of one or both of these belonged to group B or C, except 1 (Table 1, Fig. 1).

Severe GH deficiency, multiple-hormone deficiency and decreased level of somatomedin C (< 0.3 unit/ml) were more frequently noted in groups B and C than in group A (Fig. 1).

Ectopic lobe was noted in 23 (72%) patients in groups B and C (Figs. 2, 3), while only in 1 (5%) of group A, although it varied considerably in size, shape and signal intensity. No patient showed both ectopic lobe and bright posterior pituitary lobe. Eight patients had neither and 3 of these had a low antidiuretic hormone (ADH) level (Fig. 1).

Small anterior pituitary lobe (less than 2 mm in height) and small sella turcica (less than 240 mm^3 in volume) were more frequently seen in groups B and C (Figs. 2, 3) than in group A (Fig. 1). The serum GH response to provocation tests did not correlate with the size of the pituitary gland.

There was no significant difference in the features above between groups B and C.

Discussion

It is well known that the stalk is transected and development of an ectopic lobe is seen at the proximal stump above the site of transection corresponding to the median eminence in patients with pituitary dwarfism [2–4]. To our knowledge, however, there has been no report on the frequency of transection of the stalk in these patients. In this study, transection was recognized in 12 of 52

Table 1. Clinical data and MRI findings ($n = 52$)

1. Perinatal abnormality	
asphyxia	18 cases
breech presentation	16
premature baby	7
absent	22
2. Severe growth hormone deficiency	38
3. Multiple-hormone deficiencies	21
4. Somatomedin C unit/ml ($n = 41$)	
~0.3	20
0.3~	21
5. Ectopic lobe	24
6. Bright posterior lobe	20
7. Small anterior lobe	22
8. Small sella turcica (< 240 mm^3)	11

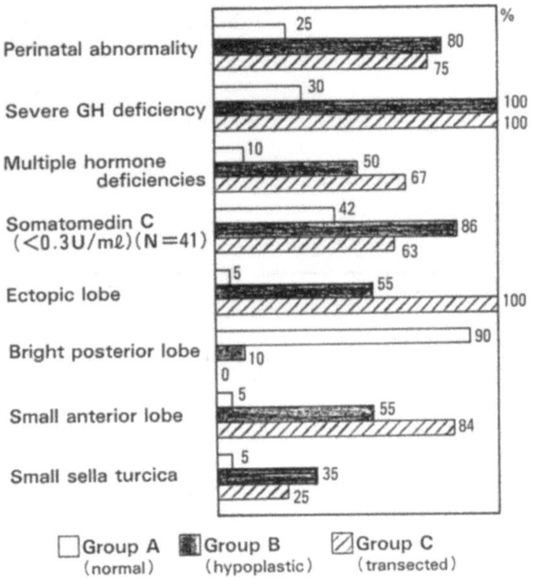

Fig. 1. Clinical data and MRI findings according to the size of the pituitary stalk ($n = 52$)

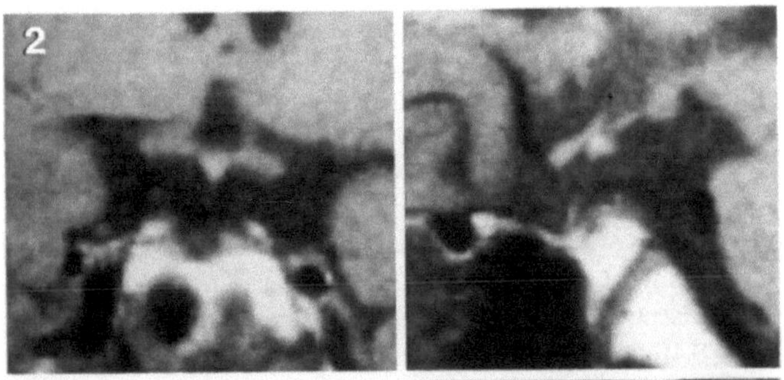

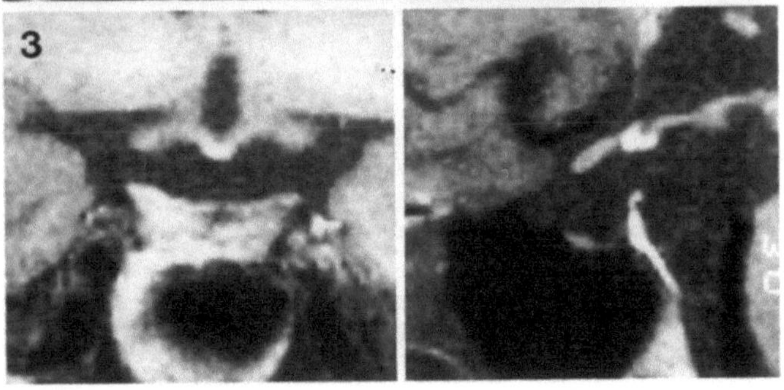

Fig. 2. Group B: hypoplastic pituitary stalk. Ectopic lobe, small anterior pituitary lobe and small sella turcica are seen

Fig. 3. Group C: transected pituitary stalk. Ectopic lobe, small anterior pituitary lobe and small sella turcica are seen

(23%), and hypoplasia in 20 of 52 (38%), normality in 20 of 52 (38%).

Hypothalamic regulation to stimulate anterior pituitary GH secretion begins at 17–18 weeks of gestation. The mechanism of transection of the stalk in pituitary dwarfs is thought to be mechanical trauma, hypoxic stress, or vascular insult to the stalk at delivery, because pituitary dwarfs have been documented to have developed normally in utero and usually achieved normal birth weights [3, 4]. Transection of the stalk might cause obliteration of the hypophyseal portal system, thus resulting in GH deficiency. Panhypopituitarism is rare, however, in pituitary dwarfs in previous reports [1], as well as in our patients. A high frequency of perinatal abnormality noted in our series also supports the presumed mechanism described above.

The posterior lobe has been described as showing a characteristic high signal intensity distinct from that of the anterior lobe on T1-weighted images in 87–100% in healthy subjects [5–7]. Bright posterior lobe has been documented to be absent in patients with diabetes insipidus [6–7]. Fujisawa et al. [2] thought that the high signal intensity was caused by the normal contents of the hypothalamo-hypophyseal tract, including neurosecretory granules with ADH.

Our classification of these patients according to the stalk size correlated well with perinatal abnormality, and severity in GH and other hormone deficiency, in addition to the other MRI findings including ectopic lobe, small anterior lobe etc. Therefore MRI should be of great help in evaluating patients with pituitary dwarfism.

References

1. Inoue Y, Nemoto Y, Fujita K (1986) Pituitary dwarfism: CT evaluation of the pituitary gland. Radiology 159: 171–173
2. Fujisawa I, Kikuchi K, Nishimura K (1987) Transection of the pituitary stalk: development of an ectopic posterior lobe assessed with MR imaging. Radiology 165: 487–489
3. Kikuchi K, Fujisawa I, Momoi T (1988) Hypothalamic-pituitary function in growth hormone-deficient patients with pituitary transection. J Clin Endocrinol Metab 67: 817–823
4. Kelly WM, Kucharczyk W, Kucharczyk J (1988) Posterior pituitary ectopia: an MR feature of pituitary dwarfism. AJNR 9: 453–460
5. Fujisawa I, Asato R, Nishimura K (1987) Anterior and posterior lobes of the pituitary gland: assessment by 1.5T MR imaging. J Comput Assist Tomogr 11: 214–220
6. Fujisawa I, Nishimura K, Asato R (1987) Posterior lobe of the pituitary in diabetes insipidus: MR findings. J Comput Assist Tomogr 11: 221–225
7. Colombo N, Berry I, Kucharczyk J (1987) Posterior pituitary gland: appearance on MR images in normal and pathologic states. Radiology 165: 481–485

Dr. Satoru Tazawa
Radiology Department Sendai Shakaihoken Hospital
3-16-1, Tutumimachi Aobaku, Sendai, Japan (981)

Neuroradiology (1991) 33 [Suppl]: 505–506

Neuro radiology
© Springer-Verlag 1991

MRI findings in children with serious speech disorders

P. O. Hamsten, O. Flodmark, I. Tonnquist, E. Borg, and H. E. Persson

Departments of Neuroradiology, Audiology and Neurophysiology, Karolinska Hospital, Stockholm, Sweden

Summary. Twenty patients in a special school for pupils with speech disorders were examined with neurophysiological and psychodynamic tests and MRI. The neuroradiological showed study one case of corpus callosum agenesis and two of migration disorders.

Key words: Magnetic resonance imaging – Speech disorder

Children with speech disorders have previously been neglected to some extent regarding neuroradiological and neurophysiological examinations in Sweden. Some of them have been studied with CT. EEG has also often been used in the evaluation of brain damage. Patients from all over the country come to Halsboskolan, an educational institute for children with serious language problems, to improve their language use and abilities. During recent years MRI studies have been used to detect anatomical malformations. The patients were also tested for: hearing disability, word perception, intellectual scoring, psychodynamic function, EEG abnormalities, brain electric activity map (BEAM), and auditory brainstem responses (ABR).

Subjects and methods

The subjects were pupils at a Swedish school for children with serious speech problems. Thirty percent of these were eliminated because of severe hearing problems, emotional problems, motor difficulties, and transfer to other schools. In all, 20 children remained, 13 boys and 7 girls (mean age 11 ± 3 years). Thirteen in the group were right-handed.

EEG was recorded both during rest and with photostimulation. Twenty-one electrodes were placed according to the international 10–20 system. Recording was done on a 17-channel machine (Nihon Kohden). The result was classified as normal/pathological or pathological focal/diffuse or epileptogenic/nonepileptogenic. BRA disc electrodes were placed on the vertex and the ipsilateral mastoid bone. Stimuli of 2 kHz sinus wave and a 4 kHz square pulse were applied. Stimulus level was set 75 dB above hearing level (HL). Right and left levels were tested separately.

BEAM was recorded with 17 electrodes placed according to the international 10–20 system. The stimuli were monaurally presented 500 Hz sinus waves 75 dB over HL. Data on the spatial distribution of cortical activity were presented as a coloured picture of the head. The method is still in the experimental stage.

MRI was performed with T1–2 weighted SE and IR acquisitions. Coronal, sagittal and transverse images were obtained with a Siemens Magnetom 0.5 T. The equipment was converted to 1.0 T. After this improvement of quality all the patients in the study with pathology were re-examined. No further information was obtained, but the pictures were of better quality.

Psychological testing included a Reynell receptive and expressive language test and an auditory discrimination test (dichotic listening, short-term memory for sounds).

Results

Nine subjects had pathological EEG findings (1 focal, 1 epileptogen type). Five subjects had pathological ABRs. Five subjects had pathological BEAM. MRI showed partial agenesis of the corpus callosum in one patient (Fig. 1) and migration disorders in two patients. There was a positive correlation between the abnormal EEG and ABR results, a positive but insignificant correlation between average psychological score and pathological EEG, ($P = 0.07$), no significant correlation between BEAM and ABR, and a negative correlation between EEG and BEAM.

Discussion

The prevalence of pathological EEG and, to some degree, also BEAM and ABRs is rather high in this group. The investigation indicates a weak connection between pathological EEG and psychological dysfunction. The pathological findings at MRI examination were few. Earlier studies with pneumoencephalography [1] showed abnormalities in 50% of the cases. Rosenberger and Hier [2] found asymmetry of the brain at CT. Carparulo

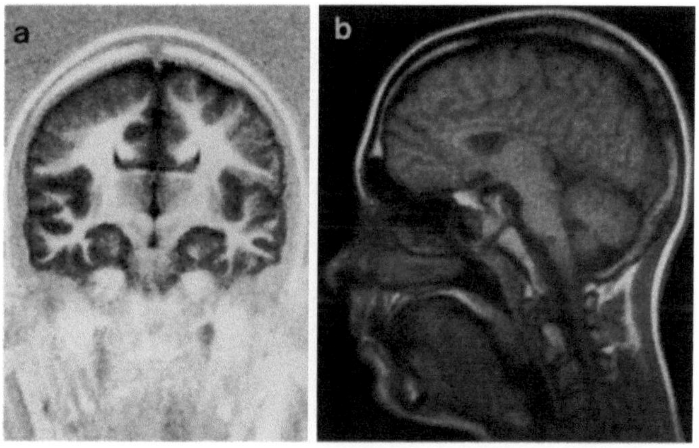

Fig. 1 a, b. MRI acquisitions show partial corpus callosum agenesia

et al. [3] reported 44% abnormal scans. Other investigators have had no over-representation of pathological scans [4, 5].

Conclusion

There are many contradictory results, probably because of the difficulties in defining the sampling and inclusion criteria in the studies. MRI is a good method for detecting anatomical malformations, but these are rather rare among persons in this group. PET and SPECT are probably methods which can give us a further understanding of these patients. Whether there are metabolic disorders among people in this group is unknown. Stereotactic fixation of the head during PET, MRI and CT can make it possible to study these serious speech disorders. Much has to be done for better understanding of these individuals. In conclusion, further studies with more sophisticated methods (for example PET) are needed to gain more knowledge of the basis of these serious speech disorders.

References

1. Dalby M (1977) Diagnose and Ätiologie der Dysfasie; Dysfasie im Kindesalter, Universitets forlag, Oslo, p 3039
2. Rosenberger PB, Hier DB (1980) Cerebral asymmetry and verbal intellectual deficits. Ann Neurol 8: 300–304
3. Carparulo BK, Cohen DJ, Rothman SL, Young JG, Katz JD, Shaywitz SE, Shaywitz (1981) Computed tomographic brain scanning in children with developmental neuropsychiatric disorders. J Am Acad Child Psychiatry 20: 338–357
4. Maccario M, Hefferen SJ, Keblusek SJ, Lipinski KA (1982) Developmental dysphasia and electroencephalographic abnormalies. Dev Med Child Neurol 24: 141–155
5. Harcherich DF, Cohen DJ, Ort S, Paul R, Shaywitz BA, Volkmer FR, Rothman SLG, Leckman JF (1985) Computed tomographic brain scanning in four neuropsychiatric disorders of childhood. Am J Psychiatry 142: 731–734

Dr. Per Olof Hamsten
Departments of Neuroradiology, Audiology and Neurophysiology
Karolinska Hospital
Stockholm, Sweden

Neuroradiology (1991) 33 [Suppl]: 507–508

Neuro-radiology
© Springer-Verlag 1991

MRI findings in Leigh's disease with cytochrome-*c*-oxidase deficiency

M. Savoiardo[1], G. Uziel[2], L. Strada[1], A. Visciani[3], M. Grisoli[1], and G. Wang[1]

Departments of [1] Neuroradiology and [2] Pediatric Neurology, Istituto Nazionale Neurologico "C. Besta", Milan, Italy
[3] Department of Neuroradiology, Ospedale San Raffaele, Milan, Italy

Summary. Of nine patients with subacute necrotizing encephalomyelopathy, six had cytochrome-*c*-oxidase (COX) deficiency. Four of these had very similar distribution of signal abnormalities in brain stem and subthalamic nuclei, without putaminal involvement. The putamen was affected in the other two cases of COX deficiency. White matter of cerebellar or cerebral hemispheres was also affected in COX or other enzyme deficiencies, mimicking a leukodystrophy in one case. Even in patients with the same enzymatic defect the pattern of MRI abnormalities is not homogeneous.

Key words: Leigh's disease – Subacute necrotizing encephalomyelopathy – Brain diseases – Magnetic resonance imaging

Subacute necrotizing encephalomyelopathy (SNE), or Leigh's disease, is a heterogeneous condition which can be diagnosed with certainty only at postmortem examination [1]. Diagnosis in vivo is accepted when there is a combination of appropriate clinical features, lactic acidosis, defects of mitochondrial enzymes and abnormalities on CT or MRI studies in agreement with the variable pathological findings reported [2–6]. Since several mitochondrial enzymes have been associated with SNE, such as pyruvate dehydrogenase complex (PDHC), pyruvate carboxylase, NADH cytochrome b5 reductase, succinate cytochrome-*c*-reductase, NADH dehydrogenase, succinate dehydrogenase and cytochrome-*c*-oxidase (COX), some authors tend to split the variegated clinical picture of SNE according to the different enzymatic deficiencies.

We wish to report nine cases of SNE and to correlate their enzymatic defects with the MRI findings.

Patients and methods

MRI studies performed in nine children (five males, four females) with clinical and laboratory findings compatible with SNE were reviewed. The patients' ages ranged from 7 months to 9 years. All patients presented with a progressive disorder characterized by failure to thrive, hypotonia, and cerebellar signs. Pyramidal signs were often present. Abnormal eye movements and respiratory disturbances tended to develop in the course of the disease. All the patients showed increased levels of blood lactate and pyruvate. In all patients pyruvate dehydrogenase complex and respiratory chain complexes were measured in skeletal muscles and cultured fibroblasts.

MRI studies were performed with a 0.5 T magnet in seven patients, with a 1.5 T unit in two. All patients had sagittal T1-weighted images (w.i.) and transverse SE intermediate and T2-w.i. Often coronal T1- or T2-weighted images were also available.

Results

COX deficiency was demonstrated in six cases (cases 1–6). A defect of succinate cytochrome-*c*-reductase was found in case 7. Case 8 had a defect of the activation of PDHC. In case 9, no enzymatic defects could be demonstrated.

COX deficiency. Patients 1–4 had high signal intensity in intermediate and T2-weighted images in the brain stem with variable involvement of the medulla, of the pontine tegmentum, and midbrain tegmentum and tectum. They all had lesions in the subthalamic area. None of the patients had lesions in the basal ganglia. Minimal periventricular abnormalities were seen. Cases 1 and 2 also had extensive cerebellar white matter abnormalities (Figs. 1, 2a, b). Case 1 also had signal abnormalities in the red nucleus, case 2 in the substantia nigra.

Case 5 had much less prominent lesions in the dorsal brain stem, but had marked abnormalities in the putamina, caudate nuclei, and in the paraventricular white matter of the cerebral hemispheres (Fig. 2c). Posterior corpus callosum and chiasm were also affected.

Case 6 had prominent lesions in the cerebellar white matter and posterior two-thirds of putamina with minimal abnormalities in dorsal brain stem and periventricular white matter of cerebral hemispheres.

In cases 1 and 5, abnormalities were also recognizable in the cervical spinal cord.

Succinate cytochrome-c-reductase deficiency. Case 7 had slightly increased signal intensity in the heads of the caudate nuclei and periaqueductal region. High signal in white matter of cerebral hemispheres was consistent with age (7 months).

PDHC activation defect. Case 8 had only questionable signal abnormalities in the brain stem. Extensive abnormalities were present in the white matter of the cerebral hemispheres (Fig. 3).

Undetermined enzymatic defect. Case 9 had abnormalities in the brain stem, in the white matter of the cerebral hemispheres and, less extensive, of the cerebellum.

Discussion

The first four cases of COX deficiency we observed had a quite uniform MRI pattern of signal abnormalities that raised the hope of identifying a significant correlation be-

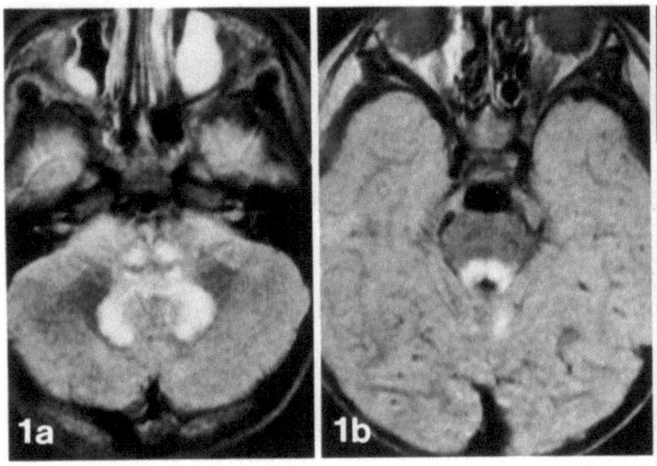

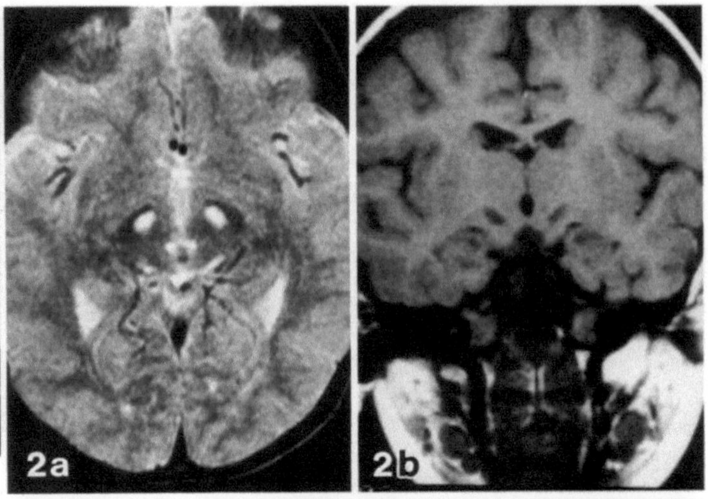

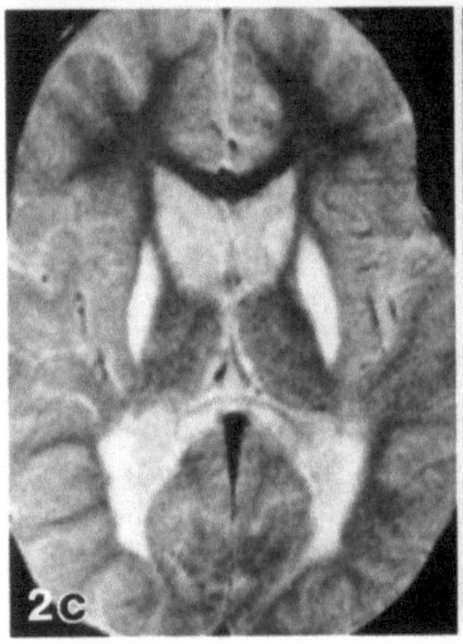

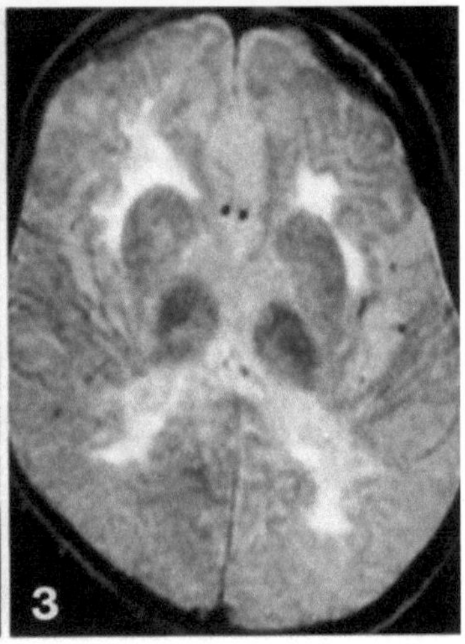

Fig. 1 a, b. Cytochrome-*c*-oxidase (COX) deficiency. **a** Case 2: SE 2100/100. High signal in medulla and deep cerebellar white matter. **b** Case 1: SE 2100/50. Abnormalities in upper pontine tegmentum

Fig. 2 a–c. COX deficiency. **a** Case 2: SE 2100/100. High signal in periaqueductal region and in subthalamic nuclei. **b** Case 4: SE 700/23. Coronal view of subthalamic nuclei lesions. Putamina are normal. **c** Case 5: SE 2100/100. Lesions in putamina, caudate nuclei and posterior periventricular white matter

Fig. 3. Pyruvate dehydrogenase complex activation in a 3-year-old boy (case 8) with diffuse white matter abnormalities mimicking a leukodystrophy

tween distribution of lesions and a single enzymatic defect. However, the fifth and sixth cases of COX deficiency we observed showed a different picture with absence of subthalamic abnormalities and presence of putaminal lesions which were not found in the first four cases. In addition, Medina et al. [6] recently demonstrated putaminal abnormalities in all their three cases of COX deficiency, and subthalamic lesions only in one. These authors suggested that putaminal lesions are a hallmark for the diagnosis of SNE. Our results do not confirm this view. Even in a selected group with COX deficiency there is no uniformity of signal abnormalities. The other three cases which had clinical and laboratory findings compatible with SNE but with different enzymatic defects (cases 7–9) showed even more heterogeneous MRI abnormalities. Case 7 had minimal basal ganglia abnormalities; case 8 mimicked a leukodystrophic process; and case 9 had diffuse white matter abnormalities associated with brain stem and cerebellar lesions, but without basal ganglia involvement.

In conclusion, lesions of the brain stem particularly involving the tegmentum are the most common finding in SNE. Symmetrical lesions in the basal ganglia, particularly in the putamen, or in the subthalamic nucleus or in the cerebellar white matter also strongly suggest the diagnosis of SNE. However, no homogeneous pattern of MRI abnormalities is present even when the same enzymatic defect is found. White matter involvement is rare but can be very extensive and misleading.

References

1. Di Mauro S, Servidei S, Zeviani M, Di Rocco M, De Vivo DC, Di Donato S, Uziel G, Berry K, Hoganson G, Johnsen SD, Johnson PC (1987) Cytochrome c oxidase deficiency in Leigh syndrome. Ann Neurol 22: 498–506
2. Koch TK, Yee MHC, Hutchinson HT, Berg BO (1986) Magnetic resonance imaging in subacute necrotizing encephalomyelopathy (Leigh's disease). Ann Neurol 19: 605–607
3. Davis PC, Hoffman JC Jr, Braun IF, Ahmann P, Krawiecki N (1987) MR of Leigh's disease (subacute necrotizing encephalomyelopathy). AJNR 8: 71–75
4. Kissel JT, Kolkin S, Chakeres D, Boesel C, Weiss K (1987) Magnetic resonance imaging in a case of autopsy-proved adult subacute necrotizing encephalomyelopathy (Leigh's disease). Arch Neurol 44: 563–566
5. Geyer CA, Sartor KJ, Prensky AJ, Abramson CL, Hodges FJ, Gado MH (1988) Leigh disease (subacute necrotizing encephalomyelopathy): CT and MR in five cases. J Comput Assist Tomogr 12: 40–44
6. Medina L, Chi TL, De Vivo DC, Hilal SK (1990) MR findings in patients with subacute necrotizing encephalomyelopathy (Leigh syndrome): correlation with biochemical defect. AJNR 11: 379–384

Dr. M. Savoiardo
Department of Neuroradiology
Istituto Nazionale Neurologico "C. Besta"
Via Celoria 11
I-20133 Milan, Italy

Neuroradiology (1991) 33 [Suppl]: 509–511

Neuro-radiology
© Springer-Verlag 1991

CT and MRI of extra- and subdural effusions

H. Henkes[1], W. Schörner[1], C. Sprung[2], K. Terstegge[2], N. Hosten[1], J. C. Böck[1] and R. Felix[1]

Departments of [1] Radiology and [2] Neurosurgery, Universitätsklinikum Rudolf Virchow, Charlottenburg, Freie Universität Berlin, Berlin, Federal Republic of Germany

Summary. A total of 32 patients with 37 extra- or subdural effusions was studied prospectively by unenhanced and contrast-enhanced cranial CT and MRI. Diagnoses included acute extradural haematoma (1), acute subdural haematoma (3), early subacute subdural haematoma (4), late subacute subdural Haematoma (6), chronic subdural haematoma (9), hygroma (9), empyema (2), residual changes (3). On *long TR/TE* images, 33 fluid collections were hyperintense; 1 acute subdural haematoma, 2 hygromas and 1 residual change demonstrated relatively low signal intensities similar to cerebrospinal fluid. On *short TR/TE* images, 19 effusions were hyper-, 5 iso- and 13 hypointense. The signal intensity of the fluid collections on short TR/TE and long TR/TE images correlated well with characteristics of the effusions such as age and content. The *sensitivity* of MRI in the detection of the lesions was judged equivalent to CT in 8 and superior in 22 effusions. In 7 fluid collections, CT was normal and only MRI allowed precise demonstration. Abnormal contrast enhancement of meningeal structures was detected in 15 cases by means of gadolinium-DTPA-enhanced short TR/TE MRI.

Key words: Magnestic resonance imaging – Gadolinium-DTPA – Intracranial haemorrhage – Chronic subdural haematoma – Hygroma – Empyema

Several papers have been published in recent years, dealing with MRI in investigation of closed head trauma [1], extracerebral haematomas [2–8], hygromas [7] and empyemas [9]. With few exceptions [1, 8] these studies described unenhanced MRI in only a small number of patients.

The purpose of this study was: (1) to determine the MRI appearance of different extra- and subdural fluid collections; (2) to compare the sensitivity of CT and MRI for detecting these effusions; (3) to evaluate the use of intravenously injected gadolinium (Gd)-DTPA as a paramagnetic contrast medium for MRI.

Patients and methods

A total of 32 patients (ages 7–87 years) with 37 intracranial extra-axial fluid collections confirmed by CT was prospectively examined using a 0.5 T Magnetom. Imaging protocol: SE, 1600/30,70 (TR/TE), axial plane; FLASH, 315/14, $\alpha = 90^\circ$, prior to and immediately after intravenous injection of 0.1 mmol Gd-DTPA/kg body weight, axial and coronal planes. Slice thickness: 10mm; 256^2 matrix.

Features studied were: localisation (extra- or subdural), content (haematoma, hygroma, empyema), age (< 1 week acute; > 1 and < 2 weeks early subacute; > 2 weeks and < 1 month late subacute; > 1 month chronic) [5–8], density (CT) and signal intensity (SI) (MRI), relative to the adjacent grey matter; sensitivity of both imaging modalities in the detection of the effusions; presence of meningeal contrast enhancement.

Results

Diagnoses (number of effusions in parentheses) and MRI appearance

Acute extradural (1) *and subdural haematomas* (3): hyperdense and iso- to hyperintense in all three MRI sequences. *Subdural hematomas:* hyperdense [early *subacute* (4)] to hypodense [late *subacute* (6), *chronic* (9)] and "panhyperintense" (i.e. high SI in all applied MRI sequences) (Figs. 1, 2), with the only exception of 3 cases of chronic subdural haematomas with low SI on short TR/TE images. *Hygromas* (9): hypodense and iso- to hypointense on short TR/TE images, hyperintense on long TR/TE images, with varying SI on long TR/short TE images. *Empyemas* (2): hypodense and hyperintense on long TR/TE images; however, one showed characteristics of a haematoma (with high SI on short TR/TE) whilst the other was similar to the hygromas (Fig. 3). *Residual changes* (3) did not show characteristic signal intensity patterns.

Sensitivity of CT and MRI

Equal diagnostic information from CT and MRI: 8 effusions. MRI clearly superior to CT: 22. CT normal, only MRI showing the fluid collection: 7.

Gd-DTPA-enhanced MRI

Contrast enhancement of adjacent meningeal structures was observed in 15 subdural effusions, 1 acute extradural (Fig. 2), 2 acute subdural, 2 early subacute, 1 late subacute and 5 chronic subdural haematomas, 3 hygroma and 1 empyema.

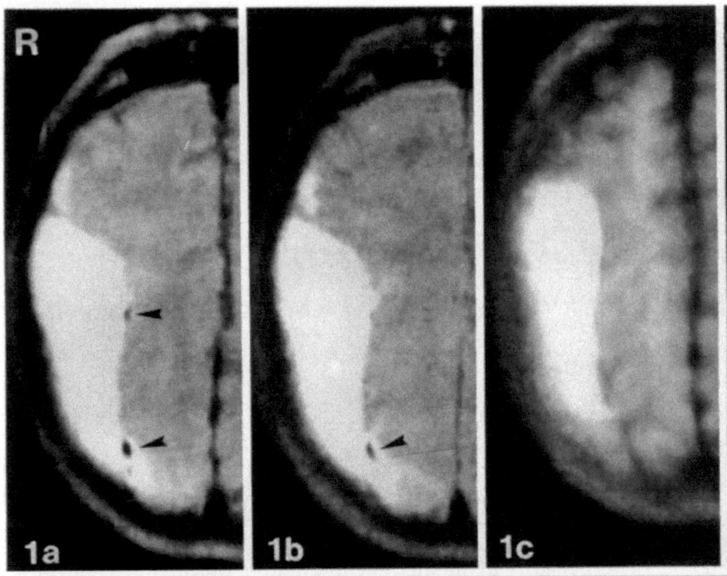

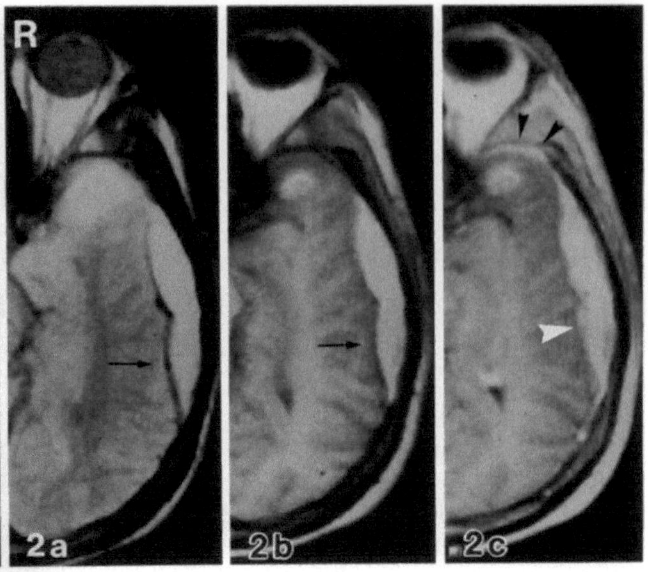

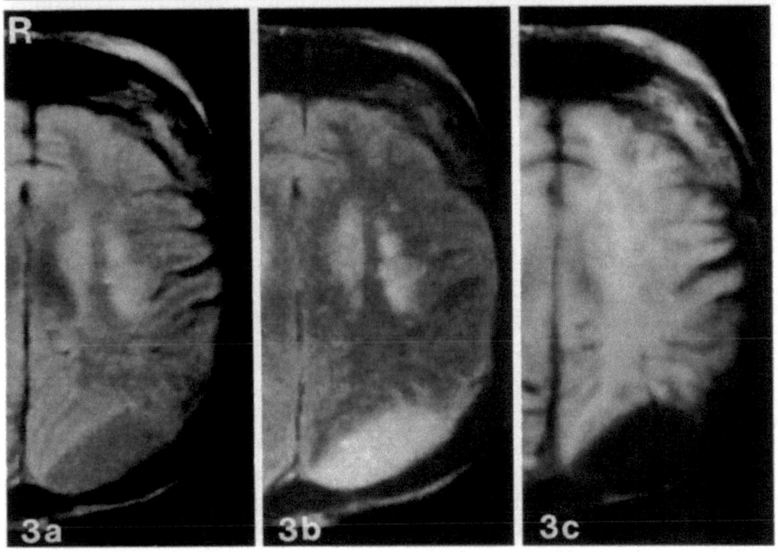

Fig. 3a-c. MRI appearance of a left occipital *empyema* with intermediate signal intensity similar to cerebrospinal fluid on axial long TR/short TE (**a** SE 1600/30), high signal intensity on long TR/TE (**b** SE 1600/70) and low signal intensity on short TR/TE (**c** FLASH 315/14, $\alpha = 90^\circ$) images. (76-year-old female with basal cell carcinoma of the left occiput)

Fig. 1a-c. Typical MRI appearances of a right sided *chronic subdural haematoma* with high signal intensity on axial long TR/short TE (**a** SE 1600/30), long TR/TE (**b** SE 1600/70) as well as on short TR/TE (**c** FLASH 315/14, $\alpha = 90^\circ$) images. Note inward displacement of superficial veins against the brain by the subdural effusion (*black arrowheads* in **a** and **b**) and the biconvex, lentiform shape of the haematoma. This shape is characteristic of unilateral, chronic subdural haematomas in older patients (87-year-old female with recurrent minor head trauma several weeks previously)

Fig. 2a-c. MRI appearance of a left temporal *(sub-)acute extradural haematoma* with high signal intensity on axial long TR/short TE (**a** SE 1600/30), long TR/TE (not shown, SE 1600/70) as well as on short TR/TE (**b** FLASH 315/14, $\alpha = 90^\circ$) images. Between haematoma and adjacent brain tissue, a hypointense rim representing displaced dura mater can be seen on unenhanced images (**a,b** *black arrows*). On gadolinium (Gd)-DTPA-enhanced short TR/TE images (**c** FLASH 315/14, $\alpha = 90^\circ$, after i.v. injection of 0.1 mmol Gd-DTPA/kg body weight), the signal intensity of this rim is significantly increased (**c** *white arrowhead*). Note also meningeal contrast enhancement adjacent to the haemorrhage in the left anterior temporal lobe. (19-year-old male, 4 days after head trauma)

Discussion

MRI appearances

The MRI appearances of intracranial haemorrhage depend mainly on the sequential degradation of haemoglobin to paramagnetic products, e. g. methaemoglobin. Selective T2-relaxation enhancement and proton-electron dipole-dipole proton relaxation enhancement are underlying physical mechanisms [10]. The latter effect and the presence of *dilute* extracellular methaemoglobin results in shortened T1- and T2-relaxation times and increased proton density, which cause the characteristic high SI of early and late subacute and chronic subdural haematomas [6]. Extra-axial empyemas have been described as proteinaceous fluid, hyperintense to cerebrospinal fluid (CSF)and hypointense to white matter on short TR sequences and hyperintense to CSF and brain tissue of long TR sequences [9]. Our case of an empyema with high SI on short TR/TE sequences is probably a secondarily infected subdural haematoma.

Sensitivity

The high sensitivity of MRI in the detection of intracranial extra-axial fluid collections has previously been stressed by several authors [1, 3, 4, 9]. It is due mainly to the lack of bone-hardening artefacts near the skull and related to the high sensitivity of MRI to paramagnetic blood degradation products. However, all effusions in our study which had been missed by CT were small and did not require neurosurgical intervention.

Contrast-enhanced studies

The frequent observation of intense contrast enhancement of meningeal structures can easily be explained by the morphological characteristics of the so-called "neomembranes". They result from cleavage of tissue or fluid within the dural border layer at the dura-arachnoid mater interface followed by a proliferation of the dural border cells. An increased amount of extracellular material and wide extracellular compartments and a dense network of vessels are the ultrastructural features of these neomembranes [11]. These are excellent conditions for the accumulation of contrast media, especially in the absence of a blood-tissue barrier. Contrast enhancement of meningeal structures in chronic extradural haematomas [12] and contrast medium accumulation in chronic subdural haematomas [13] are well known from CT studies. Contrast medium accumulation in hygromas has been found by other authors [14].

MRI is a highly effective imaging modality for the detection and characterisation of intracranial extra-axial fluid collections and it is superior to CT in terms of sensitivity. Contrast enhancement of meningeal structures is a frequent finding in patients with extra- and subdural effusions.

References

1. Gentry LR, Godersky JC, Thompson B, Dunn VD (1988) Prospective comparative study of intermediate-field MR and CT in the evaluation of closed head trauma. AJR 150: 673–682
2. Young IR, Bydder GM, Hall AS, Steiner RE, Worthington BS, Hawkes RC, Holland GN, Moore WS (1983) Extracerebral collections: recognition by NMR imaging. AJNR 4: 833–834
3. Moon KL, Brant-Zawadzki M, Pitts LH, Mills CM (1984) Nuclear magnetic resonance imaging of CT-isodense subdural hematomas. AJNR 5: 319–322
4. Sipponen JT, Sepponen RE, Sivula A (1984) Chronic subdural hematoma: demontration by magnetic resonance. Radiology 150: 79–85
5. Hosoda K, Tamaki N, Masumura M, Matsumoto S, Maeda F (1987) Magnetic resonance images of chronic subdural hematomas. J Neurosurg 67: 677–683
6. Gomori JM, Grossman RI, Hackney DB, Goldberg HI, Zimmerman RA, Bilaniuk LT (1988) Variable appearances of subacute intracranial hematomas on high-field spin-echo MR. AJR 150: 171–178
7. Fobben ES, Grossman RI, Atlas SW, Hackney DB, Goldberg HI, Zimmerman RA, Bilaniuk LT (1989) MR characteristics of subdural hematomas and hygromas at 1.5 T. AJNR 10: 687–693
8. Petersen D, Grodd W, Voigt K (1989) Kernspintomographie (1,5 T) traumatischer extrazerebraler Hämatome. Radiologe 29: 416–422
9. Weingarten K, Zimmerman RD, Becker RD, Heier LA, Haimes AB, Deck MDF (1989) Subdural and epidural empyemas: MR imaging. AJR 152: 615–621
10. Gomori JM, Grossman RI (1988) Mechanisms responsible for the MR appearance and evolution of intracranial hemorrhage. Radiographics 8: 427–440
11. Friede RL, Schachenmayr W (1978) The origin of subdural neomembranes. II. Fine structure of neomembranes. Am J Pathol 92: 69–84
12. Omar MM, Binet EF (1978) Peripheral contrast enhancement in chronic epidural hematomas. J Comput Assist Tomogr 2: 332–335
13. Karasawa H, Tomita S, Suzuki S (1987) Chronic subdural hematomas. Neuroradiology 29: 36–39
14. Stone JL, Lang RGR, Sugar O, Moody RA (1981) Traumatic subdural hygroma. Neurosurgery 8: 542–550

Dr. H. Henkes
Institut für Neuroradiologie
Medizinische Fakultät/Universitätskliniken
W-6650 Homburg/Saar, Federal Republic of Germany

Neuroradiology (1991) 33 [Suppl]: 512–513

Neuro radiology
© Springer-Verlag 1991

CT and MRI of two unusual cases of Sturge-Weber disease

R. Stokmans[1], L. Dom[3], D. Denil[4], L. L. Mortelmans[2], and B. Appel[1]

Departments of [1] Neuroradiology and [2] Radiology Middelheim General Hospital, Antwerp, Belgium
Departments of [3] Neurology and [4] Paediatrics, General Childrens Hospital, Antwerp, Belgium

Summary. Two patients with Sturge-Weber disease (3 and 7 months old) were examined with CT and MRI. Both techniques demonstrated cortical calcification and prominent superficial veins. These cases are unusual because of cutaneous angiomas outside the distribution of the trigeminal nerve in both patients and cortical calcification at an unusually early age (3 months), as well as hypertrophy of hemicranium and hemicortex in one patient.

Key words: Sturge-Weber disease – Angioma – Macrocrania

Sturge-Weber disease is characterised by a congenital facial naevus affecting the first branch of the trigeminal nerve, ipsilateral meningeal venous angioma usually limited to the posterior temporal, parietal and occipital lobes and cortical calcification on the same side becoming radiologically visible after infancy [1–4]. Although calcification has been described in a neonate, its incidence increases with age so that they are most likely to be found after the age of 2 years [1, 2]. Cortical atrophy involves in most cases the entire hemisphere and is generally associated with hypoplasia of the hemicranium. Ipsilateral enlargement of the hemicranium has been reported in this disease [2], but never in association with hypertrophy of the hemicortex.

Case reports

Case 1

Case 1 was a 7-month-old girl with seizures and a left fronto-temporal cutaneous angioma. CT showed microcalcification in an atrophied left occipital lobe (Fig. 1a). After administration of IV contrast medium, enhancement was seen in the same distribution (Fig. 1b), indicating the presence of a leptomeningeal angioma. MRI demonstrated a slight hypointensity of the lesion (Fig. 2), which confirms the CT findings of microcalcification. Hyperintense linear structures, corresponding with stasis in superficial drainage veins, were seen in the same distribution.

Case 2

Case 2 was a 3-month-old girl with convulsions, two right temporo-occipital cutaneous angiomas and a large skull (> p 95 centile). CT demonstrated gyriform cortical calcification in the right parieto-occipital area and hypertrophy of hemicortex and hemicranium (Fig. 3). MRI showed a hypointensity of the affected cortex with gyriform areas of signal void, consistent with calcification (Fig. 4).

Discussion

Sturge-Weber disease is a congenital disorder, marked by angiomatosis of the face and the leptomeninges with cortical calcification and adjacent cerebral hemiatrophy. The facial angioma is usually unilateral and occurs only rarely outside the distribution of the trigeminal nerve. However, both our patients presented angiomatous lesions outside the trigeminal area. The extension of the meningeal angioma can be seen on CT as gyriform superficial contrast enhancement. The exact pathophysiology of this enhancement, however, remains uncertain [3]; it could be due to defects in the blood-brain barrier, congestion in the cerebral veins or cerebral angiomatosis. Cortical calcification underlying the leptomeningeal angiomatosis is the most frequent feature of this disease. It is usually situated posteriorly and appears most often after the age of 2 years. One of our patients showed calcification at an unusually early age (3 months). Ipsilateral cerebral atrophy is often seen and is, in general, associated with a reduced volume of the hemicranium and thickened skull. When associated with an enlarged hemicranium the increased volume is occupied by a dilatated subarachnoid space [2]. One of our patients, however, showed increased volume of the hemicranium associated with an enlargement of the hemicortex. This association has not been reported previously and its aetiology remains unknown. MRI is equal to CT in demonstrating the cortical hemiatrophy but superior to it in revealing abnormalities in the atrophic parenchyma, consisting of abnormal high signal on long-TR, long-TE sequences, probably corresponding to regions of gliosis, demyelination and/or ischaemic damage [4]. In our cases MRI demonstrated slowing of the cerebral blood flow as a hyperintense signal on long-TR, long-TE sequence. This corresponds with certain angiographic findings [4]. CT is superior to MRI in detecting the amount of calcification. On MRI the cortical calcification is thin, serpiginous and hypointense on the long-TR, long-TE sequence.

The presence of cutaneous angiomas outside the distribution of the trigeminal nerve, cortical calcification at the age of 3 months and hypertrophy of hemicortex and hemicranium makes these cases of Sturge-Weber disease

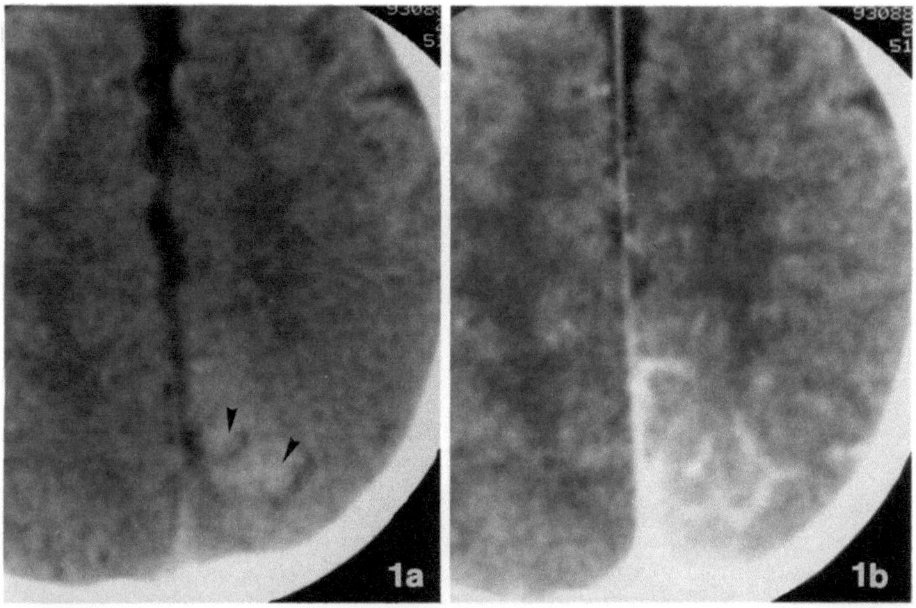

Fig. 1. **a** CT shows slight hyperdensity of the atrophied left occipital cortex: microcalcification *(arrowheads)*. **b** CT with IV contrast infusion: enhancement over the left occipital cortex and visualisation of abnormal vascular structures: meningeal angioma with stasis

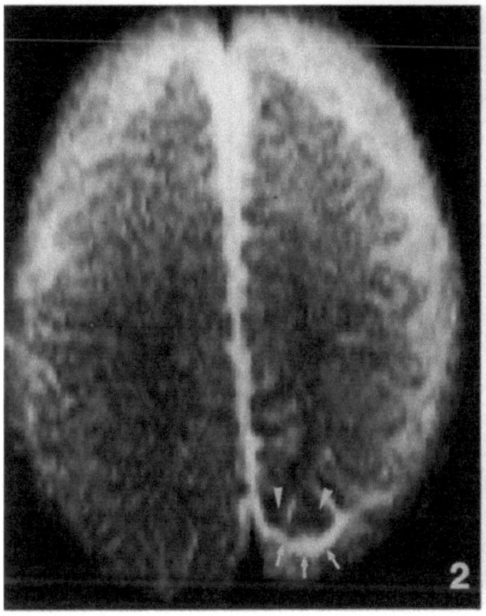

Fig. 2. MRI T2-weighted axial image (TR 1500/TE 120). Hypointensity of the left occipital cortex: microcalcification *(arrowheads)*. Hyperintensity of the vascular structures: stasis of the cerebral blood flow *(arrows)*

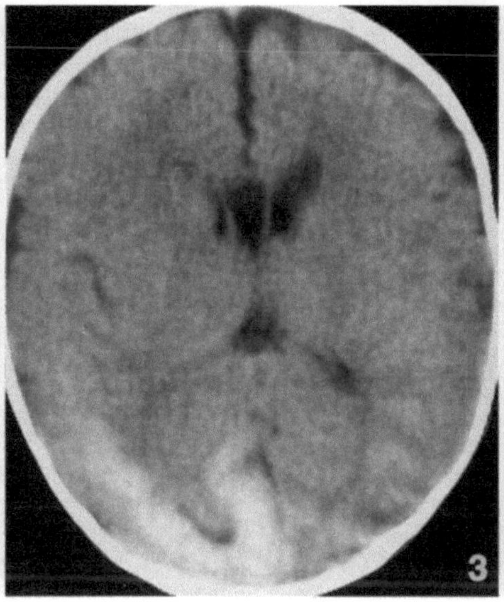

Fig. 3. CT shows hypertrophy of the right hemicortex and gyriform calcification in the right parieto-occipital region

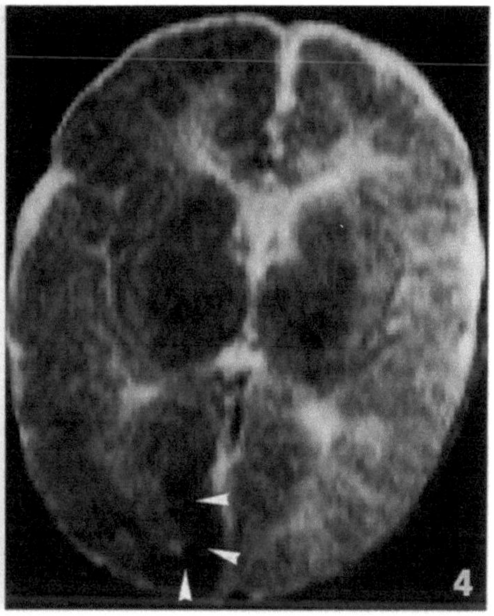

Fig. 4. MRI T2-weighted image (TR 1500/TE 210). Hypointensity of the affected area: calcification *(arrowheads)*

rather atypical. Hemimacrocrania has been reported previously, but never in association with hypertrophy of the hemicortex.

References

1. Alanso A, Taboada D, Ceres L, Beltran J, Olague R, Nogues A (1979) Intracranial calcifications in a neonate with the Sturge-Weber disease and additional problems. Pediatr Radiol 8: 39–41
2. Enzmann DR, Hayward RW, Norman D, Dunn RP (1977) Cranial computed tomographic scan appearance of Sturge-Weber disease: unusual presentation. I. Radiology 122: 721–724
3. Gardeur D, Palmieri A, Mashaly R (1983) Cranial computed tomography in the phakomatoses. Neuroradiology 25: 293–304
4. Braffman BH, Bilaniuk LT, Zimmerman RA (1988) The central nervous system manifestation of the phacomatoses on MR. Radiol Clin North Am 26: 773–801

Dr. R. Stokmans
Department of Neuroradiology
Middelheim General Hospital
Lindendreef 1
B-2020 Antwerp, Belgium

Neuroradiology (1991) 33 [Suppl]: 514–515

Neuro
radiology
© Springer-Verlag 1991

Postoperative or delayed tethering in repaired myelomeningocele patients

F. R. Murtagh, J. Arrington, and L. Love

University Diagnostic Institute, University of South Florida, Tampa, Florida, USA

Summary. Fifty-four patients ages 19 months to 17 years with prior repair of meningocele or myelomeningocele presented with delayed signs and symptoms of recurrent tethering. All were evaluated with MRI of the spine to delineate areas of suspected tethering due to scar tissue formation.

Key words: Myelomeningocele – Delayed tethering – Magnetic resonance imaging

Materials and Methods

MRI was performed on a 1.5T GE Signa or 1.0T Siemens Somatom in at least two planes (sagittal and axial) utilizing only chloral hydrate or nembutal anesthesia. Coronal images were added if there was any suspicion of diastematomyelia. T1-weighted images were utilized exclusively, unless some question of cord tumor arose when T2-weighted images or gadolinium enhancement was added. CT myelography was performed to clarify any questionable areas on MRI or to improve bone detail, particularly in questions of diastematomyelia.

Results

In 32 (60%) of the 54 patients examined, areas of tethering in the previous operative closure site were suggested by the MRI (Figs. 1, 2). Twenty of these underwent surgical exploration and release of scar on the basis of MRI alone. In three patients (6%) syrinx formation was demonstrated.

In an additional 12 patients (22%) demonstration was equivocal and CT myelography was required; 6 (50%) were thought and surgically proven to be tethered.

Discussion

Patients with prior myelomeningocele repair may exhibit late deterioration of function due to tethering of neural tissue by scar tissue in the operative site. MRI is a safe,

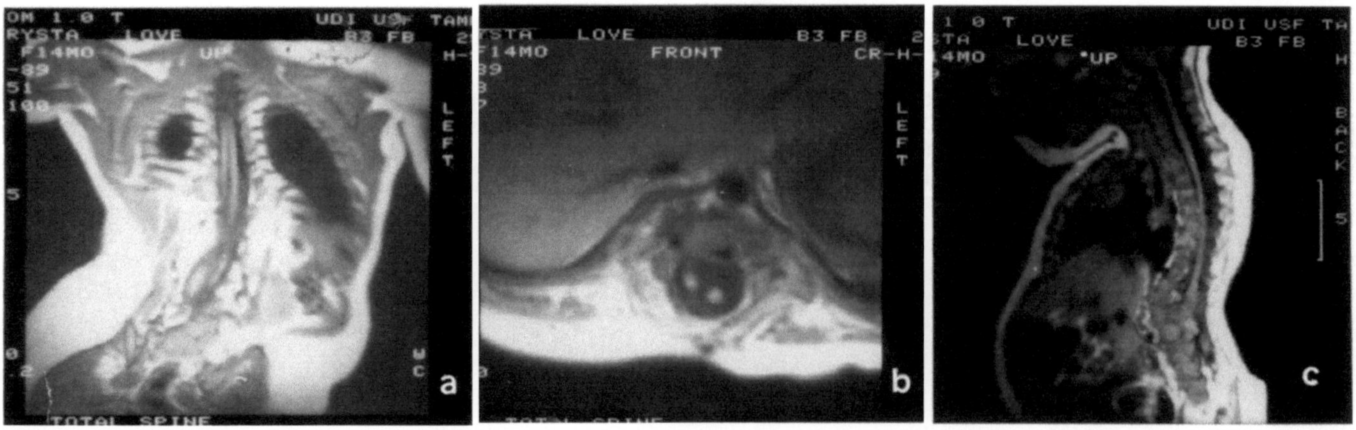

Fig. 1 a–c. A 15-month-old female with previous repair at birth of a large lipomyelomeningocele had increasing deficit and rapidly progressive scoliosis which prompted examination for retethering due to scar. MR images were difficult to obtain because of the extensive bony deformities and scoliosis but did reveal a probable syrinx and two hemicords (**a, b**). Axial MRI in T1-weighted mode demonstrate the two hemicords (**c**). CT was required to better illustrate the bony septum of the diastematomyelia. Surgery addressed the cephalad tethering area at the region of the diastematomyelia and the area of tethering caudally in the region of the two hemicords where scar was noted. Eight-month follow-up showed marked improvement in the patient's symptoms

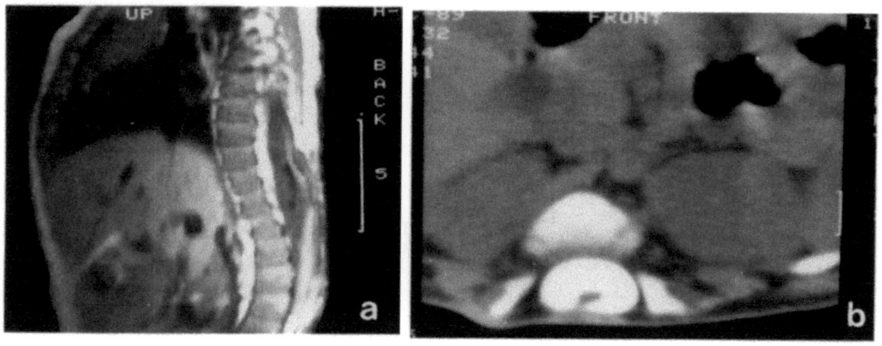

Fig. 2a, b. A 1-year-old male had a previous primary repair of a large lipomyelomeningocele at birth, visualized on plain film when the patient presented with decreasing function. Subsequent MRI demonstrates irregularity of the lower thoracic cord with atrophy. Two areas of tethering were postulated; one at the caudal aspect of the thecal sac including an intradural lipoma and a secondary area of tethering at the thoracolumbar kyphosis which was the site of previous surgical repair. Surgical repair of both lesions had good results

non-invasive study with a high degree of accuracy in depiction of anatomical detail. In our experience, only a small percentage of patients require CT myelography for diagnosis.

At surgery with the operating mciroscope points of fixation are located and sharply dissected. The cord or identifiable neural tissue in cases of tethering is usually attenuated, pale, and non-pulsatile when first exposed; any or all of these features may revert to normal after release.

Dr. F. R. Murtagh
University of South Florida
University Diagnostic Institute
3301 West Oak Drive
Tampa, Florida 33612, USA

Neuroradiology (1991) 33 [Suppl]: 516–517

Neuro radiology
© Springer-Verlag 1991

Paediatric medulloblastoma: atypical CT features at presentation in the SIOP II trial

M. Nelson[1], C. Diebler[2], and W. St. C. Forbes[3]

[1] The General Infirmary, Leeds, UK
[2] Hôpital Foch, 92151 Suresnes, Paris, France
[3] Hope Hospital, Salford, UK

Summary. A review of cranial CT studies of 233 patients for the Second Medulloblastoma Trial of the International Society of Paedriatric Oncology showed "typical" CT appearances in only 30% of patients. The varied appearances encountered are described with particular emphasis on atypical CT features.

Key words: Computed tomography – Medulloblastoma – SIOP II trial

In the literature the typical CT appearences of medulloblastoma are taken to be those of a well-defined, hyperdense enhancing soft tissue mass with surrounding oedema arising in the cerebellar vermis and associated with hydrocephalus [1, 2].

Between January 1984 and December 1988 370 infants and children with a histological diagnosis of medulloblastoma were enrolled in the SIOP II Trial (Second Medulloblastoma Trial of the International Society of Paediatric Oncology). This presentation reviews the radiological findings and illustrates the patterns of disease encountered, with particular emphasis on the rarer CT findings.

Methods

By April 1990 the CT studies at presentation of 233 patients were obtained for review, comprising 136 patients having examinations without and with intravenous contrast enhancement, 77 patients having examinations with contrast enhancement only and 20 patients having examinations without contrast enhancement.

The findings were assessed using the following definitions:

site, defined by the centre of the main tumour mass

size: small lesions were less than the width of the fourth ventricle; medium lesions were less than one third the width of the posterior fossa in diameter

severity of hydrocephalus: mild: ventricular dilatation without an increase in Evans' ratio; moderate: increase in Evans' ratio; severe thinning of the cortical mantle and/or periventricular lucency

soft tissue characteristics: attentuation changes were defined with respect to normal cerebellum. Enhancement was homogeneous if density variation was no greater than in normal brain; enhancement strong if its intensity was comparable with that of vascular structures

tumour margin: well defined if clearly visualised around at least 90% of the margin near the mid part of the tumour mass

cystic change: any clearly defined central or marginal low density area; usually rounded but occasionally linear or angular, called "clefts"

calcification: small if no larger than one quarter the width of the fourth ventricle.

Results

Patients' ages ranged between 5 months and 15 years 10 months (mean ages: males, 7 years 7 months; females, 6 years 10 months). The male: female ratio was 141:77 (65%:35%). Complete data, including tabulated results will be published elsewhere [3].

"Typical" CT appearances were encountered in only 30% of patients. The primary medulloblastoma was usually situated in the inferior vermis, occasionally elsewhere in the posterior fossa (18%). No patient showed a solitary supratentorial mass.

Metastases were seen at presentation in 5% of patients. Their distribution suggests spread through the cerebrospinal fluid. Metastases were usually solitary (7 patients); 2 metastases were present in 3 patients and more than 5 metastases were present in 1.

Most primary tumours were large (71%), medium size and small tumours being encountered in 27% and 2% respectively. In general, hydrocephalus was more severe with larger tumours, though the trend was less marked for non-vermian tumours. Only 1 patient with a small tumour had severe hydrocephalus; 5 patients with large tumours did not show hydrocephalus.

The variable morphology and soft tissue characteristics of the primary tumours are evidenced by the fact that the unenhanced CT showed no high density in 3% and enhancement was absent in 3% of primary tumours; some of these tumours had prominent astrocytic differentiation. In contrast, all the metastatic lesions were solid tumours of high density without cystic change or calcification and showed homogeneous enhancement.

The tumour margins were usually well defined with surrounding oedema. Tumour margins were sufficiently ill defined in 7% of patients as to suggest an infiltrative mode of growth. The primary tumour was broadly based on the pia mater in 2% of patients, superficially suggesting a primary extra-axial lesion. True extra-axial extension was seen in 2% of patients: Local infiltration of the ventricular system was seen in 1%. The correlation between CT assessment of brain stem infiltration and surgical findings was poor.

Cystic change was seen in 59% of primary tumours. Most cysts were centrally situated. Marginal cysts without an enhancing rim, with the appearance of an arachnoid cyst, were present in 5% of patients. The primary tumour was prdominantly cystic with an enhancing rim in 3% of patients. Clefts were observed in 3% of patients and a fluid level was present in 2% of patients. Convincing signs of necrosis were not seen.

Calcification was observed in 21% of primary tumours. Typically there was a central nodular pattern with small or large nodules, single and multiple areas of calcification being equally frequent. Calcification was seen in the margins of solid tumour or tumour cysts in 16% of patients. Non-nodular patterns of calcification were present in 20% of patients.

Discussion

Medulloblastomas with a "typical" CT appearance were surprisingly uncommon. The primary lesions were cystic in 59% of patients, calcified in 22%, cystic and calcified in 15%, ill defined in 7%, not associated with oedema in 5%, not accompained by hydrocephalus in 4%, showed only low density on the unenhanced scan in 3% and showed no enhancement in 3%. The centre of the primary tumour was remote from the vermis in 18% of patients. Metastases were seen at presentation in 5%.

We intend now to correlate the CT appearances at presentation with the surgical and histopathological findings. Data from this series will be analysed using the BRAINS computer-aided advice and interpretation system at Leicester Polytechnic, Leicester, United Kingdom. The development of such expert systems will be facilitated if neuroradiologists and information scientists can establish a set of generally accepted descriptive criteria for CT and other imaging modalities.

References

1. Sandhu A, Kendall B (1987) Computed tomography in the management of medulloblastomas. Neuroradiology 29: 44–52
2. Kazner E, Wende F, Grumme T, Lanksch W, Stochdorph O (eds) (1981) Computed tomography in intracranial tumours – differential diagnosis and clinical aspects. Springer, Berlin Heidelberg New York, pp 148–161
3. Nelson M, Diebler C, Forbes W St C (1990) Paediatric medulloblastoma: atypical CT features at presentation in the SIOP II trial. Full report. Neuroradiology (in press)
4. Teather D, Teather BA, Wills K, Plummer D, du Boulay CH (1991) Computer aid in the interpretation of CT images of the head. Neuroradiology 33 [Suppl]

Dr. M. Nelson
Section of Neuroradiology
The General Infirmary
Great George Street
Leeds LS1 3EX, UK

Neuroradiology (1991) 33 [Suppl]: 518–519

Neuro radiology
© Springer-Verlag 1991

Dynamic MRI of the sellar region

M. Takahashi[1], Y. Sakamoto[1], K. Yoshizumi[1], Y. Korogi[1], J. Shinzato[1], H. Bussaka[1], T. Oguni[1], and Y. Ushio[2]

Departments of [1] Radiology and [2] Neurosurgery, Kumamoto University School of Medicine, Kumamoto, Japan

Summary. Dynamic MRI, following rapid injection of gadolinium-DTPA, demonstrated progressive enhancement of the normal structures of the sellar and parasellar regions, whereas pituitary tumours and other parasellar tumours showed delayed enhancement. It was possible to differentiate the normal pituitary gland and cavernous sinus from tumours arising and invading the pituitary gland and cavernous sinus.

Key words: Pituitary adenoma – Pituitary microadenoma – Parasellar tumour – Dynamic magnetic resonance imaging – Gadolinium-DTPA

Pituitary adenomas have been shown to have slightly different MR enhancement patterns compared with the normal pituitary gland, thus producing slight contrast difference between the adenoma and the normal pituitary gland [1–3].

We have performed dynamic MRI of the sellar and parasellar region in order to differentiate tumours from the normal structures to better advantage.

Patients and methods

The case material included 45 patients: 6 patients who underwent dynamic MRI of the normal sellar area as part of the investigation of intracranial abnormalities of other locations and 39 patients with intrasellar and parasellar lesions.

Dynamic MRI was performed on a 1.5 T superconductive unit, following rapid injection of gadolinium-DTPA in a dose of 0.1 mmol/kg body weight. Serial images of the sellar region were obtained every 20–30 s for 3–5 min using the spin echo technique (TR 200 ms, TE 15 ms). Other parameters included 128 × 256 matrix, 5 mm slice thickness and no averaging.

The images obtained with dynamic MRI were evaluated with generation of time-signal intensity curves for various portions of the intrasellar and parasellar structures and pathology.

Results

Normal structures

The first structures visualized were the cavernous sinus, infundibulum and the posterior pituitary lobe at 30 s, followed by enhancement of the anterior pituitary lobe near the infundibulum at 50 s and the peripheral portion of the anterior pituitary lobe at 80 s (Fig. 1). The dural membrane between the cavernous sinus and the pituitary gland was best demonstrated at 60–180 s. Cranial nerves III, IV, V 1 and VI as well as V 2 were shown better in the early stage of contrast enhancement, usually at about 30–60 s. These structures gradually became difficult to identify as the time elapsed.

Abnormal structures

Many pituitary tumours showed delayed enhancement between 60 s and 200 s, but some tumours showed enhancement earlier than 60 s (Fig. 2). When differential enhancement between the normal pituitary gland and the pituitary tumour was taken, the most prominent difference of enhancement was variable between 30 and 90 s. Most parasellar tumours invading the sella turcica, such as trigeminal neuroma or pharyngeal tumours, showed peak enhancement at 120 s or 180 s.

It was possible to differentiate the postoperative tissue and the recurrent or residual tumour from the normal pituitary gland. The dural membrane between the pituitary gland and the cavernous sinus was well visualized and useful for the diagnosis of tumour invasion into the cavernous sinus.

Dynamic MRI was useful for investigation of sellar and parasellar tumours.

Discussion

It is of great interest that there is a sequential difference in enhancement patterns of the normal as well as the abnormal structures of the sellar and parasellar areas, which can

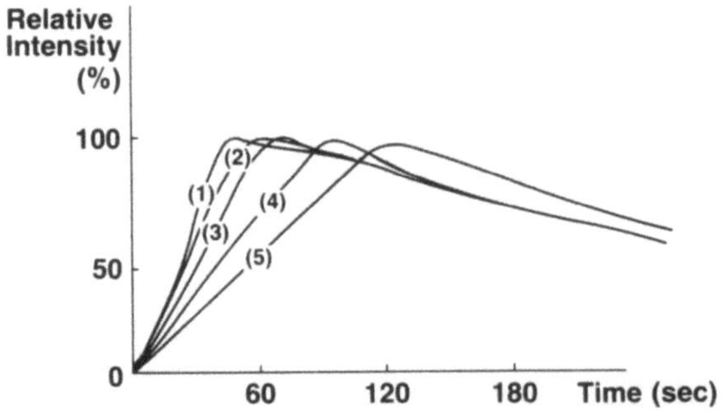

Fig. 1. Sequential contrast enhancement of sellar structures and pituitary adenoma: (1) cavernous sinus; (2) posterior lobe; (3) anterior lobe, proximal portion; (4) anterior lobe, distal portion; (5) pituitary adenoma

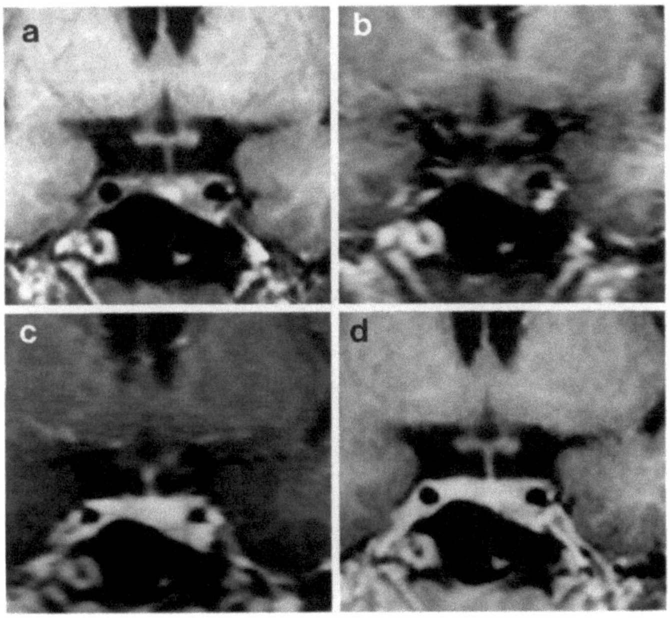

Fig. 2 a–d. A 22-year-old woman with prolactin secreting adenoma. **a** T1-weighted spin echo image; **b** precontrast, dynamic image; **c** 130 s after gadolinium-DTPA injection; **d** T1-weighted SE image with contrast medium

be shown with dynamic MRI, in spite of the fact that the serial imaging is slow, in the range of the every 20–30 s [4].

The blood supply of the structures in the suprasellar, parasellar and sellar areas is responsible for the different patterns described on dynamic MRI. There are two main blood supplies to the pituitary gland [5–7]: the inferior hypophyseal artery from the meningohypophyseal artery and the superior hypophyseal artery directly arising from the supraclinoid portion of the internal carotid artery and the posterior communicating artery. The posterior pituitary lobe is supplied by the inferior hypophyseal artery directly. The superior hypophyseal artery forms an extensive capillary plexus along the infundibulum which drains into the primary pituitary portal system and extends inferiorly for the supply of the anterior pituitary lobe via the secondary portal system.

Therefore, the posterior pituitary lobe and the infundibulum show early enhancement and the anterior pituitary lobe shows gradual enhancement from the junction with the infundibulum to the peripheral portion. The cavernous sinus is enhanced very early probably due to direct blood supply from the capillaries of the internal carotid artery. The normal structures of the cavernous sinus such as cranial nerves and internal carotid artery are shown to better advantage when the cavernous sinus is enhanced at the early stage.

The tumours or other pathological processes arising within the sella turcica and parasellar area are enhanced slightly later than the normal structures [4, 5]. Therefore, differential contrast enhancement is observed between the tumour and the normal structures of the sellar and parasellar regions.

References

1. Dwyer AJ, Frank JA, Doppman JL, Oldfield EH, Kickey AM, Cutler GB, Loriaux DL, Schiable TF (1987) Pituitary adenomas in patients with Cushing disease: initial experience with Gd-DTPA-enhanced MR imaging. Radiology 163: 421–426
2. Davis PC, Hoffman JC Jr, Malko JA, Tindall GT, Takei Y, Avruch L, Braun IF (1987) Gd-DTPA and MR imaging of pituitary adenoma: a preliminary report. AJNR 8: 817–823
3. Newton DR, Dillon WP, Norman D, Newton TH, Wilson CB (1989) Gd-DTPA-enhanced MR imaging of pituitary adenomas. AJNR 10: 949–954
4. Sakamoto Y, Takahashi M, Korogi Y, Bussaka H, Ushio Y (1990) Gd-DTPA dynamic MR imaging of the normal and abnormal pituitary glands. Radiology (in press)
5. Bonneville JF, Cattin F, Moussa-Bacha K, Portha C (1983) Dynamic computed tomography of the pituitary gland: the "tuft sign". Radiology 149: 145–148
6. Treip CS (1984) The hypothalamus and pituitary gland. In: Adams (ed) Greenfield's neuropathology, 4th edn. Arnold, London, pp 748–778
7. Tindall GT, Barrow DL (1986) Disorders of the pituitary, chapter 1. Normal anatomy. Mosby, Saint Louis, pp 1–22

Dr. M. Takahashi
Departments of Radiology
Kumamoto University School of Medicine
Kumamoto, Japan

Neuroradiology (1991) 33 [Suppl]: 520–521

Neuro-
radiology
© Springer-Verlag 1991

Clinical applications of 3D MR angiography using 0.5T MRI

K. Sadamoto[1], H. Miki[2], A. Niida[2], S. Takeda[1], S. Sakaki[3], and K. Hamamoto[4]

Departments of [1]Neurosurgery and [2]Radiology, Washokai Sadamoto Hospital, Matsuyama, Ehime, Japan
Departments of [3]Neurosurgery and [4]Radiology, Ehime University, Shigenobu-cho, Ehime, Japan

Summary. The clinical value of 0.5T three-dimensional (3D) magnetic resonance angiography (MRA) was assessed in 25 patients with intracranial vascular disease; 15 had aneurysms, 8 had arteriovenous malformations (AVMs) and 2 had arterial occlusions. As the result of utilizing 0.5T MRA with optimal parameters, good visualization of main cerebral arteries including the carotid siphon, circle of Willis, second-order branches and intracranial vascular lesions could be obtained. In the diagnosis of cerebral aneurysms, 3D MRA was superior to spin echo (SE) sequence. AVMs and arterial occlusions were equally well appreciated on 3D MRA as on the SE images.

Key words: Aneurysms, cerebral – Arteriovenous malformations, intracranial – Arterial occlusions, cerebral – Cerebral blood vessels – Magnetic resonance imaging

Newly developed 0.5T 3D MR angiography [1–3] was performed in 25 patients with intracranial vascular disease.

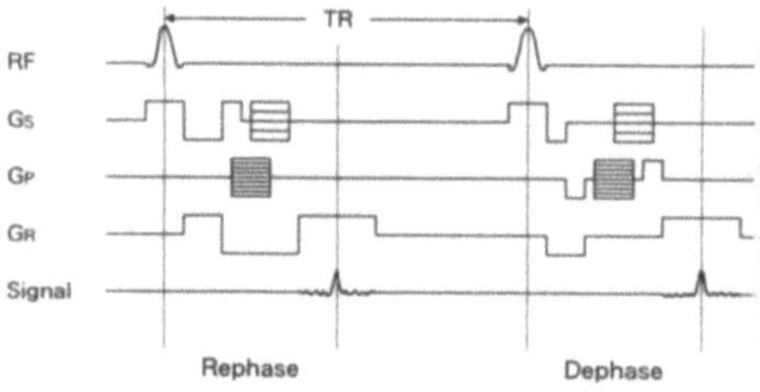

1

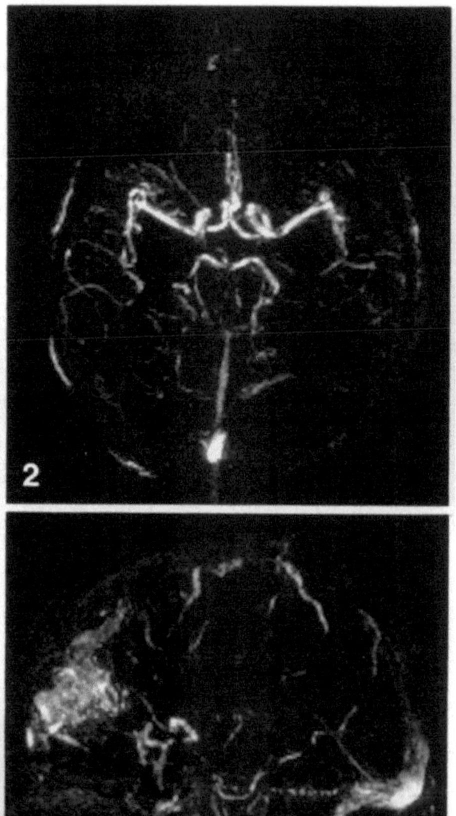

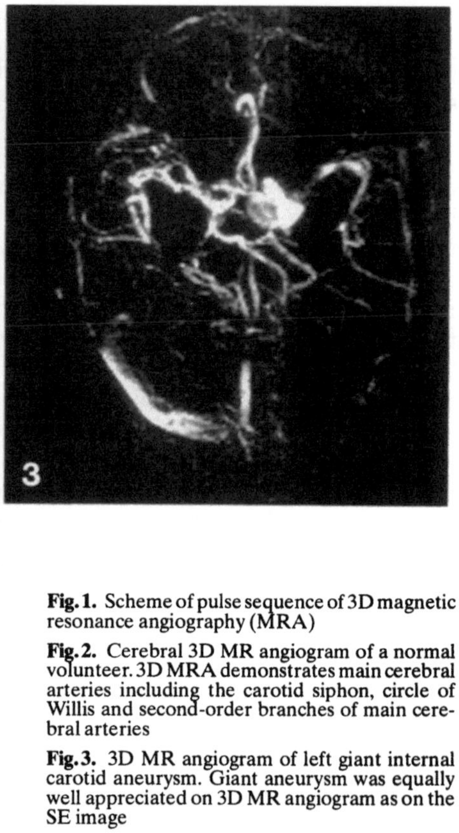

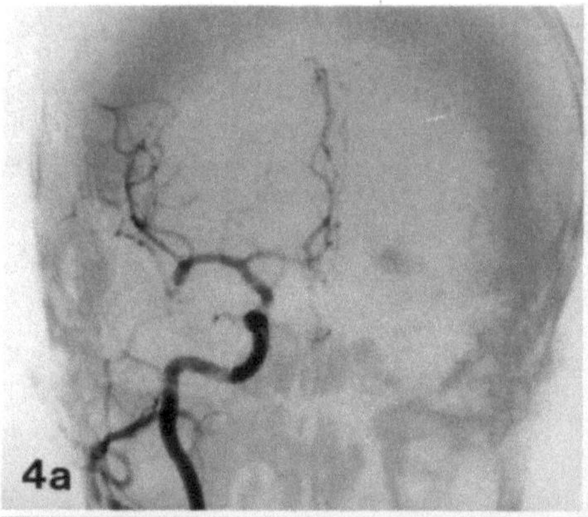

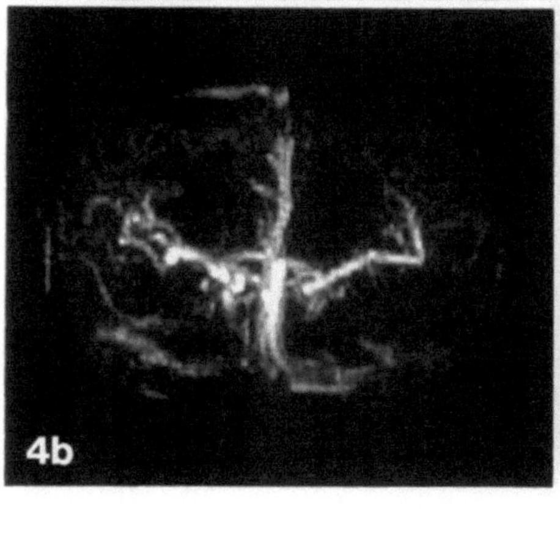

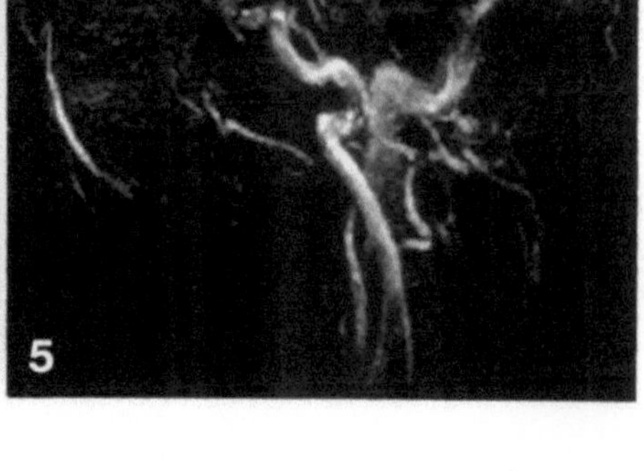

Fig. 1. Scheme of pulse sequence of 3D magnetic resonance angiography (MRA)

Fig. 2. Cerebral 3D MR angiogram of a normal volunteer. 3D MRA demonstrates main cerebral arteries including the carotid siphon, circle of Willis and second-order branches of main cerebral arteries

Fig. 3. 3D MR angiogram of left giant internal carotid aneurysm. Giant aneurysm was equally well appreciated on 3D MR angiogram as on the SE image

Fig. 4 a, b. A case of right middle cerebral artery aneurysm. **a** Right carotid angiogram shows an aneurysm *(arrow)* projecting downward at the bifurcation of right middle cerebral artery. **b** Reconstructed 3D MR angiogram shows the small aneurysm *(arrow)* clearly in the frontal view. The delineation of this aneurysm is difficult in SE images and the axial view of 3D MR angiogram

Fig. 5. 3D MR angiogram of right frontal arteriovenous malformation. A sagittal MR angiogram shows nidus, feeding artery and draining vein in frontal lobe

The purpose of our study was to evaluate the clinical utility of 3D magnetic resonance angiography (MRA) for cerebral aneurysms, arteriovenous malformations (AVMs) and occlusive diseases of cerebral arteries by comparing the images with those produced by spin echo (SE) sequences.

Patients and methods

Fifteen patients with a total of 18 cerebral aneurysms (1 ruptured and 17 unruptured), 8 with AVMs and 2 with middle cerebral artery occlusion were included in this study. Sizes of aneurysms ranged from 3 to 50 mm.

MRI was performed with a 0.5T MRI system (Hitachi G-50). All studies were performed with two signal acquisitions and a 256 × 256 matrix. The SE MRI was performed with multiecho T2-weighted axial pulse sequence. SE images were obtained with a TR of 2000 ms, TEs of 40/80 ms and a 10-mm section thickness.

3D MRA was performed with TRs of 50–60 ms, TEs of 16–18 ms, flip angles of 20–25° and a 256 × 256 × 32 matrix. Imaging volumes ranged in thickness from 64 to 80 mm. In our study, a subtraction technique composed of rephased and dephased sequences was applied (Fig. 1).

Results

As a result of utilizing 0.5T MRA with optimal parameters, good visualization of main cerebral arteries could be obtained, including the carotid siphon, circle of Willis and second-order branches of main cerebral arteries (Fig. 2). Cerebral aneurysms were detected on 3D MRA in 17 cases (94.4%). Only 12 of 18 lesions (66.6%) could be seen on SE images (Fig. 3). 3D MRA was superior to SE sequence in the detection of cerebral aneurysms (Fig. 4). AVMs and occlusions of middle cerebral arteries were equally well appreciated on 3D MRA as on the SE images (Fig. 5).

Discussion

Recently, several groups have proposed the use of 3D MRA [4–6]. All have used high field magnets (almost all of 1.5T MRI). For reasons of cost, performance and future spread of MRI, it is desirable that 3D MRA using midfield magnets should have the same ability. Our newly developed 0.5T 3D MRA has the ability to detect intracranial vascular lesions. We conclude that 0.5T 3D MRA should be the method of choice for screening and follow-up of patients with intracranial vascular disease.

References

1. Miki H, Sadamoto K, Niida A, Hamamoto K (1989) Clinical application of MR angiography. Book of abstracts, 17th International Congress of Radiology, p 880
2. Sano K, Hayakawa K, Yokoyama T, Koizumi H, Miki H, Takeda S, Sadamoto K (1989) Improved three-dimensional MR angiography at 0.5 T. Radiology 173: 473
3. Sadamoto K, Miki H, Takeda S, Hamamoto K, Koizumi H, Sano K, Yokoyama T (1989) Clinical application of angiography using a 0.5-T MRI. International Workshop on Magnetic Resonance Angiography. L'Aquilla, Italy
4. Ruggieri PM, Laub GA, Masaryk TJ, Modic MT (1989) Intracranial circulation: pulse-sequence considerations in three-dimensional (volume) MR angiography. Radiology 171: 785–791
5. Masaryk TJ, Modic MT, Ross JS, Ruggieri PM, Laub GA, Lenz GW, Haacke EM, Selman WR, Wiznitzer M, Harix SI (1989) Intracranial circulation: preliminary clinical results with three-dimensional (volume) MR angiography. Radiology 171: 793–799
6. Marchal G, Bosmans H, Van Fraeyenhoven L, Wilms G, Van Hecke P, Plets C, Baert AL (1990) Intracranial vascular lesions: optimization and clinical evaluation of three-dimensional time-of flight MR angiography. Radiology 175: 443–448

Dr. K. Sadamoto
Department of Neurosurgery
Washokai Sadamoto Hospital
Matsuyama, Ehime, Japan

Neuroradiology (1991) 33 [Suppl]: 522–523

Neuro radiology
© Springer-Verlag 1991

MRI of intracranial tumours: usefulness of multiple echo sequences

M. A. Vaghi[1], M. Grisoli[1], M. G. Bruzzone[1], A. Costa[1], V. Longone[1], A. Allegranza[2], and A. Passerini

Departments of [1] Neuroradiology and [2] Neuropathology, Istituto Nazionale Neurologico "C. Besta", Milan, Italy

Summary. On the basis of the signal pattern in multiple echo sequences, five classes of intracranial tumours are recognized. This classification can provide useful criteria to restrict the number of possible diagnoses, when the classes of tumours are considered according to site, morphology and CT findings. A total of 402 histologically verified intracranial tumours studied with multiple echo sequences were reviewed: 236 cases were studied on a 0.15-T magnetic field scanner and 166 on a 0.5 T.

Key words: Intracranial tumours – Magnetic resonance imaging – Multiple echo sequences

---

MRI is generally known to be more sensitive but less specific than CT in the detection of brain lesions. Multiple echo sequences (MES) can improve MRI specificity [1]. In a previous review of 343 intracranial tumours studied with MES and histologically verified, five classes were recognized [2]. Classes 1, 2 and 3 were defined only on the basis of the signal pattern; the characteristics of classes 4 and 5 are more complex; they were, therefore, defined as glioblastoma model and oligodendroglioma model. Tumours extensively occupied by cysts would no longer fit into these classes and showed a similar pattern independently of the different histology.

The five classes are defined as follows:

Class 1: The T2 values of the tumour decrease more slowly in successive echoes than the T2 values of cerebral spinal fluid (CSF); therefore in MES the signal intensity of the tumour seems to increase progressively in T2-weighted images.

Class 2: The T2 values of the tumour decrease in a shorter time than the T2 values of CSF so that the signal intensity of the tumour seems to decrease progressively in successive T2-weighted images. Class 2 includes two groups: *A* and *B;* in A, the signal intensity of the tumour is higher than the signal intensity of the parenchyma in every echo considered; in B, the tumour shows the same signal intensity as the parenchyma in the last echoes considered. Only the first six echoes were considered because, with our parameters, after the sixth echo image saturation was generally achieved.

Class 3: The tumour has the same signal intensity as the parenchyma in all echoes.

Class 4: "Glioblastoma model", i. e. one or more progressively increasing intensity images (cysts and necrotic or haemorrhagic areas with less hyperintense nodular and/or ring images and surrounding oedema).

Class 5: "Oligodendroglioma model", a confused pattern where tumour tissue, cysts, calcifications and oedema are very difficult to recognize.

Results

All craniopharyngiomas (22/22) and epidermoid tumours (16/16) lay in the first class. Generally craniopharyngiomas showed a bright homogeneous signal from the first echo, while epidermoid tumours in the first echo had a signal only slightly hyperintense in comparison with CSF and showed a typical inhomogeneity. Up to 80% of astrocytomas grade I, II and III lay in the first class (72/91); 16% (15/91) fell in class 2 A and only 4% (4/91) fell in class 2 B. Only 62% of neurinomas were found in the first class and these frequently showed cysts and/or a hypointense component that has been referred to as fibrotic tissue by some authors [3]. The remaining neurinomas fell in class 2 A (10/48) and 2 B (4/48); 4 were cystic tumours.

All medulloblastomas fell into class 2 A (17/17). A mottled non-uniform signal in the late echoes is typical of these tumours. Pituitary adenomas did not show a constant pattern: only up to 53% were contained in class 2 A (16/30): the remaining pituitary adenomas fell in class 1 (4/30), 2 B (5/30) and 3 (2/30). Ten percent (3/30) were cystic. Pituitary adenomas, therefore, sometimes show the same signal intensity as craniopharyngiomas or meningiomas.

All ependymal tumours lay in class 2 B (14/14). Fifty-three percent of meningiomas (28/53) fell into class 2 B, while 36% (19/53) fell in class 3, 10% in class 2 A and 2 cases were not contained in the classification because they were totally calcified.

Up to about 80% of glioblastomas were found in class 4 (48/61), 13% in class 5 (8/61) and 6% in class 2 A (4/61). One showed the pattern of a cystic tumour. Metastases were present in the same classes and at a similar rate as glioblastomas: 75% (21/28) in class 4, 18% (5/28) in class 5 and 7% (2/28) in class 2 A. Metastases and glioblastomas no longer included in classes 4 and 5 were generally difficult to evaluate because small or because studied with low magnetic field.

Eighty-seven percent of oligodendrogliomas were contained in class 5 (21/24), one fell in class 4, one in class 1 and one was cystic.

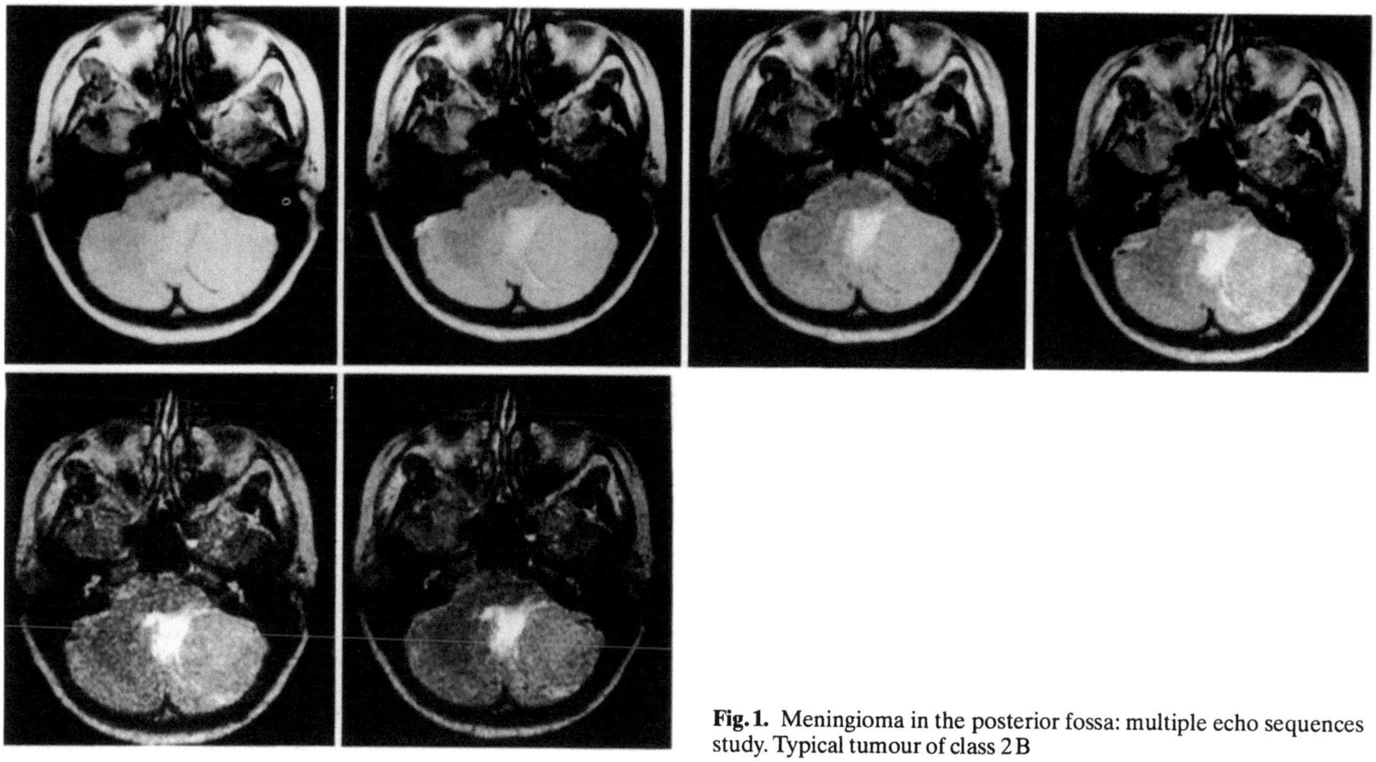

Fig. 1. Meningioma in the posterior fossa: multiple echo sequences study. Typical tumour of class 2 B

Discussion

Most intracranial tumours show a good constancy in signal pattern so that it is possible to recognize some models [4, 5]. In our opinion, and with our technical parameters, the more common brain tumours can be restricted to five classes. While the T1 and T2 values were found to be of very little help in distinguishing the nature of the mass [6], the classification on the basis of MES evaluation may represent progress in improving the specificity of MRI.

Acknowledgements. The authors thank Mrs. Angela Giorgi, Miss Angela Grassi and Mr. Ennio Leporati for technical assistance.

References

1. Harms SE, Siemers PT, Hildenbrand P, Plum G (1986) Multiple spin echo magnetic resonance imaging of the brain. Radiographics 6: 117–134
2. Vaghi MA, Bruzzone MG, Grisoli M, Allegranza A, Longone V, Passerini A (1989) La risonanza magnetica nei tumori cerebrali: classificazione in base al comportamento di segnale nelle sequenze in multieco. Radiol Med 78: 564–577
3. Mayer JS, Kulkarni MV, Yeakley JW (1987) Craniocervical manifestations of neurofibromatosis. MR versus CT studies. J Comput Assist Tomogr 11: 839–844
4. Gado M, Hodges FIII, Sartor K (1987) Principles of interpretation of MR images of the brain. In: Calabro' A, Leonardi M (eds) Computer aided neuroradiology. CIC, Rome, pp 43–60
5. Byrne JV, Kendall BE, Kingsley DPE, Moseley IF (1989) Lesions of the brain stem: assessment by magnetic resonance imaging. Neuroradiology 31: 129–133
6. Just M, Thelen M (1988) Tissue characterization with T1 and T2 and proton density values: results in 160 patients with brain tumors. Radiology 169: 779–785

Dr. M. A. Vaghi
c/o Divisione di Neuroradiologia
Istituto Nazionale Neurologico "C. Besta", via Celoria 11
I-20133 Milan, Italy

Neuroradiology (1991) 33 [Suppl]: 524–526

Neuro radiology
© Springer-Verlag 1991

Three-dimensional FFT FLASH and gadolinium-DTPA of brain tumours: a comparison with postcontrast spin echo sequences

S. Felber[1], G. Birbamer[1], A. Kampel[1], F. Aichner[1], J. Haustein[2], and G. Laub[3]

[1] Department of Magnetic Resonance, University of Innsbruck, Austria
[2] Schering AG, Berlin
[3] Siemens Medical Systems, Erlangen, Federal Republic of Germany

Summary. Twenty patients harbouring intracranial tumours (10 extra-, 10 intra-axial) participated in a comparison between postcontrast spin echo images and a postcontrast 3D fast Fourier transform (FFT) FLASH sequence, including multiplanar reformatted orientations. The relative contrast enhancement produced by gadolinium (Gd)-DTPA was assessed by signal intensity ratios obtained from examination-defined regions of interest. Numerically the relative Gd-DTPA enhancement was higher on spin echo images than FLASH images. This difference is related to the higher spatial resolution, which provides visualization of nonenhancing tumour components and the higher white matter/grey matter contrast inherent in the volume acquisition. The lower relative Gd-DTPA enhancement on the FLASH images did not degrade the diagnostic information in any of the patients, but improved estimation of tumour architecture in most of them. Therefore Gd-DTPA-enhanced 3D FFT FLASH sequences, capable of multiplanar post-processing may replace T1-weighted sequences in future.

Key words: Brain neoplasms – Magnetic resonance imaging – Gradient echo sequences – Gadolinium-DTPA

Three-dimensional (3D) postprocessing of 2D cross-sectional images offers potential advantages in diagnosis of intracranial pathologies [1]. With the advent of 3D fast Fourier transform (FFT) gradient echo sequences acquisition of high resolution 3D data became possible on MRI within reasonable scan times. Short TE is advocated to prevent signal void secondary to susceptibility changes. Together with intermediate flip angles to optimize signal/noise, T1-contrast results [2]. To overcome sensitivity problems in parenchymal diseases the combined use of 3D FLASH sequences with gadolinium (Gd)-DTPA was recently proposed [3, 4].

The purpose of this study was to compare the relative Gd-DTPA enhancement of postcontrast spin echo (SE) images with postcontrast 3D FLASH images in extra- and intra-axial cerebral tumours using signal intensity ratios from defined regions of interest (ROI).

Patients and methods

Twenty patients harbouring intracranial neoplasms with known contrast enhancement on postcontrast CT were selected for the study. All tumours were surgically confirmed at the end of the study. There were 5 meningiomas, 5 neuromas, 5 glioblastomas and 5 recurrent gliomas grade II and III. All patients agreed to the injection of Gd-DTPA and the additional FLASH sequence after the protocol had been explained to them.

The examinations were performed on a 1.5 T Magnetom (Siemens, FRG) using a circular polarized head coil (FOV = 21–25 cm). The examination protocol consisted of a proton density, T2-weighted SE study (TR = 2400/TE = 15/90, slice thickness = 5 mm) followed by a T1-weighted (TR = 550/TE = 15, slice thickness = 4 mm) SE sequence oriented according to tumour location. Then 0.1 mmol/kg/body weight Gd-DTPA was administered intravenously without moving the patient and the T1 SE study repeated without changing any parameter. The examination was terminated by a 3-D FFT FLASH sequence (TR = 40/TE = 5/α = 40) in sagittal orientation. One hundred and twenty-eight contiguous 1- to 1.3-mm thick slices were obtained within 21 min. The resulting voxel dimension was nearly isotropic ($0.19 \times 0.9 \times$ 1–1.2 mm).

For evaluation, the T1-weighted image which best displayed the enhancing lesions was selected. Then an identical orientation was reformatted from the sagittal volume acquisition on an external work station (Kontron). Subsequently ROI were placed within the enhancing lesions, white matter (WM), grey matter (GM) and background noise. The obtained signal intensity values were used to calculate ratios for signal/noise, WM/GM contrast, lesion GM/lesion WM contrast (Figs. 1, 2).

Results

All SE and FLASH studies were of diagnostic quality. Mean signal to noise was 22 (12–36) for the SE T1-weighted images and 13 (8–18) for the reformatted FLASH images. WM to GM contrast was 1.45 ($\pm$0.15) for the FLASH images and 1.2 ($\pm$0.15) for SE images.

Extra-axial tumours had higher Gd-DTPA uptake than intra-axial tumors, on both FLASH and SE sequences. The relative enhancement following Gd-DTPA was higher for SE images than for FLASH images in all patients, the difference was more pronounced as regards tumour-to-WM contrast (Table 1). Qualitative rating of the postcontrast SE and FLASH images by three readers revealed comparable or slightly inferior contrast enhance-

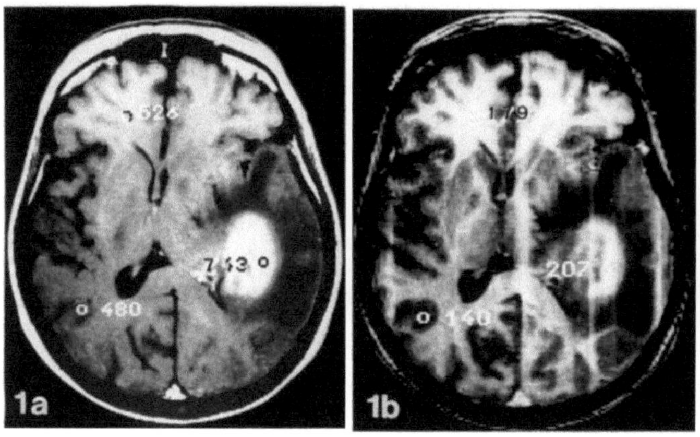

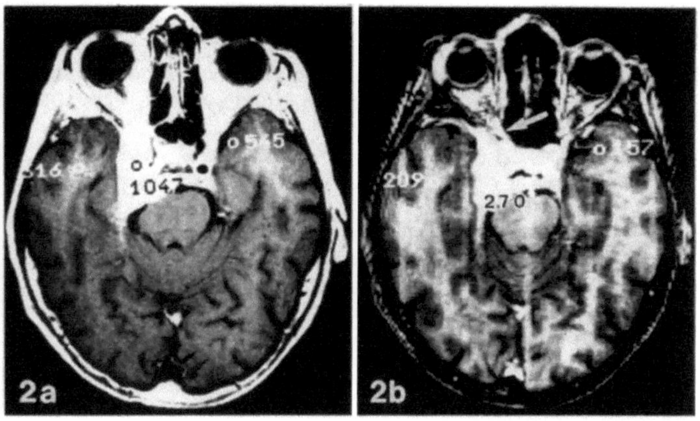

Fig. 1. **a** Left temporal glioblastoma with perifocal oedema and prominent mass effect (T1-weighted spin echo (SE) image 4 mm, tumour/white matter (WN) = 1.4, tumour/grey matter (GM) = 1.6). **b** Axial reconstructed FLASH image (1 mm) shows improved delineation of perifocal oedema. Gadolinium (Gd)-DTPA enhancement is slightly inferior to SE (L/WM = 1.15, L/GM = 1.5)

Fig. 2. **a** Parasellar meningioma in a 63-year-old patient with progressive vision loss. T1-weighted image (SE, 4 mm) revealed higher relative Gd-DTPA enhancement (L/WM = 1.7, L/GM = 1.9) than FLASH (**b**). **b** The reformatted 3-D FFT FLASH image was considered diagnostically superior because the extension of the tumour into the optic canal is better visualized *(straight arrows)*. (L/WM = 1.3, L/GM = 1.7)

ment in 14 patients with the FLASH acquisition; the remaining cases were considered of inferior but diagnostically sufficient enhancement. Diagnostic information considering tumour location, composition and conspicuity was rated superior for FLASH in 12, equal in 6 and inferior in 2 of the patients.

Discussion

High resolution 3D data sets of the entire brain were acquired in 20 patients using a 3D FFT FLASH sequence. Signal/noise of the FLASH images was roughly 50% of the calculated value for SE images, although the slice thickness differed by a factor of 4. These results underline the advantage of 3D FFT sequences which are not limited in respect of RF bandwidth and slice selection gradient strength for the acquisition of very thin slices. Due to its nearly isotropic resolution the 3D volume study could be reformatted in any desired orientation with similar resolution, signal to noise and contrast behaviour as the original sagittal FLASH images. The high spatial resolution was considered to improve diagnostic information about localization of the tumour and also visualization of intratumoural calcification and necrosis in more than 50% of the patients. A further advantage of the volume study was a significantly higher contrast between WM and GM when compared with the SE images. This improvement in T1 contrast is related to a minor degree of partial saturation using limited flip angles as well as to the thin slices which minimized partial volume effects.

Calculation of relative contrast enhancement (rCE) ratios revealed higher relative Gd-DTPA uptake when SE sequences were used. Although diagnostic information was not degraded in any of the patients using FLASH this fact needs further explanation. The rCE ratios for lesion/GM contrast were higher than those of lesion/WM contrast in both SE and FLASH sequences. The difference between both ratios, however, was significantly lower on the SE images because of inherent inferior T1 contrast. Further, the difference in slice thickness has to be taken into consideration. The better resolution of the FLASH images provided visualization of nonenhancing tumour components which were otherwise masked by partial-volume effects on SE images. The numerically inferior contrast enhancement turned out to be an advantage for lesion characterization and delineation. Theoretically, renal filtration of Gd-DTPA might also be considered if postcontrast T1-weighted SE sequences were performed in more than one orientation.

In conclusion, T1-weighted 3D FFT FLASH sequences allow rapid MRI data acquisition of the entire brain, capable of multiplanar and surface postprocessing. This holds further promise for the improvement of surgical and irradiation planning. Gd-DTPA enhancement turned out to be slightly inferior to SE sequences, but this was not disadvantageous as diagnostic information was improved in the majority of patients (Fig. 2b). Our results indicate that Gd-DTPA-enhanced 3D FFT FLASH sequences have the potential to replace T1-weighted SE sequences in future.

Table 1. Relative enhancement of spin echo and FLASH images

	Enhancing lesions/white matter (+/−)	Enhancing lesions/grey matter (+/−)
Extra-axial tumours ($n = 10$)		
Spin echo (4 mm)	1.9 (0.2)	2.1 (0.2)
FLASH (1 mm)	1.4 (0.2)	1.7 (0.2)
Intra-axial tumours ($n = 10$)		
Spin echo (4 mm)	1.5 (0.1)	1.6 (0.2)
FLASH (1 mm)	1.15 (0.1)	1.5 (0.2)

References

1. Aichner F, Mayr U, Degenhart G (1985) Eine neue dreidimensionale Bilddarstellung in der Computertomographie. Fortschr Röntgenstr 142: 395–398
2. Frahm J, Haase A, Matthaei D (1986) Technical note. Rapid threedimensional MR imaging using the FLASH technique. J Comput Assist Tomogr 10: 363–368
3. Runge VM, Wood ML, Kaufmann D, Price AC (1988) Gd-DTPA future applications with advanced imaging techniques. Radiographics 8: 161–179
4. Ross JS, Masaryk TJ, Modic MT (1989) Three-dimensional FLASH imaging: applications with gadolinium-DTPA. J Comput Assist Tomogr 13: 547–552

Dr. S. Felber
Department of Magnetic Resonance
University of Innsbruck
Anichstraße 35, A-6020 Innsbruck, Austria

Neuroradiology (1991) 33 [Suppl]: 527–528

Neuro-radiology
© Springer-Verlag 1991

Comparing MR angiography of craniocervical arteries with intra-arterial digital subtraction angiography

K. Heimberger[1], J. Kramer[2], L. Ehrmann[1], D. Wimberger[1], and H. Imhof[2]

[1] Department of Neuroradiology and [2] Central Institute of Radiodiagnostics (MR-Institute), Vienna University Clinics, Vienna, Austria

Summary. The aim of this study was to explore whether magnetic resonance angiography (MRA) could serve as a substitute for invasive, selective catheter angiography in stenotic disease of craniocervical arteries. MRA was done with the Siemens 1.5T Magnetom. Intra-arterial digital subtraction angiography (IADSA) was performed with the Siemens Angiotron. Thirty-six patients with cerebrovascular accidents or brain tumours were included; up to two regions of interest (ROIs) per side per patient were studied. MR image quality and sensitivity were most affected by patient motion. Spearman's rank correlation *(R)* reveals a highly significant correlation ($R = 0.9$ for internal carotid artery ROIs and $R = 0.6$ for common carotid artery ROIs) of degrees of stenosis in both MRA and IADSA of 132 ROIs of the internal and common carotid arteries. Twelve MRA-ROIs were unusable for various reasons. In spite of good correlation of IADSA grades of stenosis (at an interobserver correlation of 100%), MRA has several pitfalls limiting its use as a preoperative diagnostic tool.

Key words: Magnetic resonance angiography – Digital subtraction angiography – Carotid arteries

Magnetic resonance angiography (MRA) was carried out with the Siemens 1.5T Magnetom, using FISP-3D. (FISP is a gradient field echo sequence in which the magnetisation in the XY plane is refocussed in the phase-encoding direction before each pulse.) The maximum intensity projection method [1] was used for postprocessing; it enables the rotating cinematograph-like visualisation. Intra-arterial digital subtraction angiography (IADSA) was performed with the Siemens Angiotron, using high summation factors. Grades of stenoses were: 0% = grade 0; 1–25% = I; 26–50% = II; 51–75% = III; 76–99% = IV; 100% = V. Two regions of interest (ROIs) per side per patient were studied [distal third of common carotid (CCA) and proximal half of internal carotid arteries (ICA)]. Two persons separately reported on the grades of stenoses, using ruler measurement in axial MR slices at higher grade stenoses. Statistical rank correlation was performed, calculating Spearman's coefficient *R*.

Patients and methods

Thirty-six patients (24 males and 12 females) aged 33–79 years ($\bar{x} = 61.9 \pm 12.1$), suffering from cerebrovascular attacks or brain tumours, were examined by both IADSA and MRA. The time interval between the two examinations was 5 (± 4) days in 31 patients. In the other 5 patients the interval was longer than 14 days.

Results

A total of 144 ROIs were examined; 12 MRA-ROIs were unusable (2 ROIs: operation during interval between examinations; 4 ROIs: malpositioned, outside the volume to be examined, Figs. 1, 2; 6 ROIs: patient motion). In MRA (Tables 1, 2) 30% of IADSA grade I stenoses in ICA-ROIs were underestimated as grade 0; 30% of IADSA grade II stenoses, and 60% of IADSA grade III stenoses (Fig. 3a, b) were overestimated by one grade each. Of 132 evaluable ROIs, 108 were grade correlated

Table 1. DSA/MRA correlation of grades of stenoses: internal carotid artery

	ICA						
DSA\MR	0	I	II	III	IV	V	
0	24						24
I	4	6	1	1	1		13
II		2	5	3			10
III				2	3		5
IV				1	12		13
V					1	2	3
	28	8	6	7	17	2	68

Spearman's rank correlation coefficient ($R = 0.93$; $P < 0.0005$; 99% confidence intervals); 68 ICA-ROIs

Table 2. DSA/MRA correlation of grades of stenoses: common carotid artery

	CCA						
DSA\MR	0	I	II	III	IV	V	
0	55	3					58
I	4	1					5
II			1				1
III							0
IV							0
V						–	0
	59	4	1	0	0	0	64

Spearman's rank correlation coefficient ($R = 0.56$; $P < 0.0005$; 99% confidence intervals); 64 CCA-ROIs

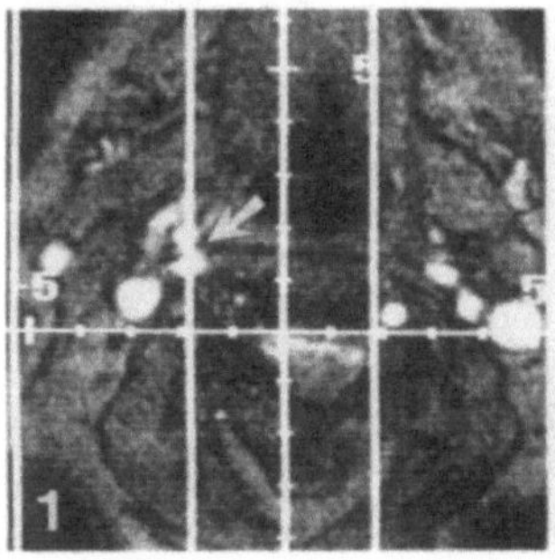

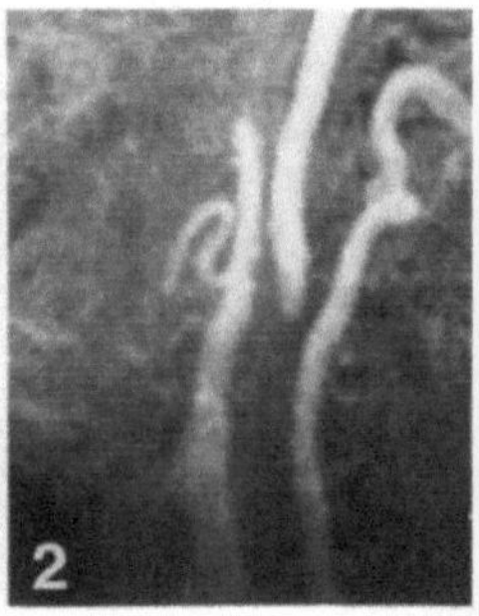

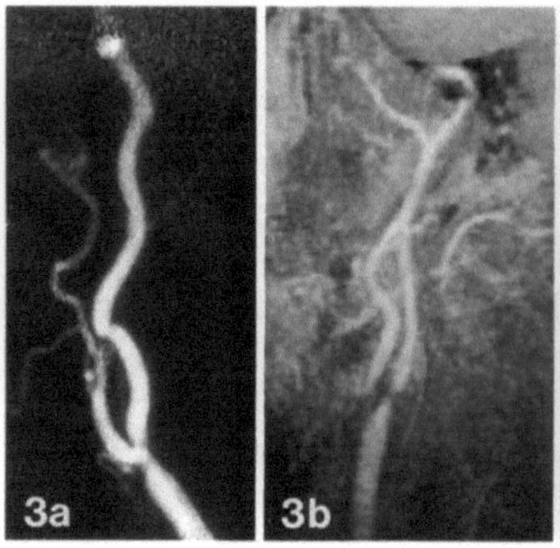

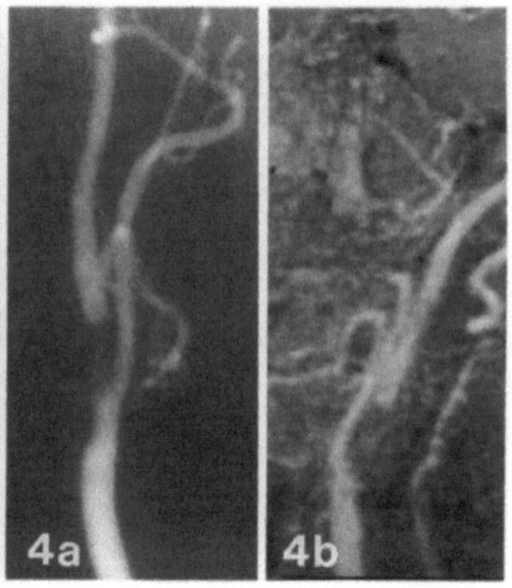

Fig. 1. MR topogram with malpositioned volume to be examined; *arrow* indicates that carotid arteries are positioned partially outside the volume of interest

Fig. 2. Malpositioned region of normal bifurcation, simulating internal carotid artery (ICA) grade IV stenosis

Fig. 3. **a** Intra-arterial DSA of grade III bifurcation stenosis. **b** Magnetic resonance angiography (MRA) of the same region of interest (ROI) as in **a**, overestimating DSA stenosis by one grade because of turbulent flow

Fig. 4. **a** IADSA of ICA grade IV stenosis. **b** MRA of the same ROI as in **a,** showing flow void (high velocity signal loss) at the site of severe stenosis

correctly by MRA, suggesting that the results of selective IADSA are reliable standards. The Spearman rank correlation coefficient, probability, and confidence intervals for ICA- and CCA-ROIs respectively are also shown in Tables 1 and 2.

Discussion

Some reasons for discrepancies of DSA and MRA grades in cases compared are: during a long time interval of 11 days between examinations, the grade IV stenosis had occluded in one patient. Turbulent flow seemed to be the reason for overestimation by MRA of DSA grade III (Fig. 3 a, b). Because of complete visualization of poststenotic flow, none of the DSA grade IV stenoses was misinterpreted as occlusion in MRA. MRA does not outline the vessel's lumen, but images blood flow signals [1, 2]. Therefore MRA may yield imges of *narrow-looking* vessels. DSA 90%-stenoses look like occlusions in MRA (complete loss of signal at the site of severe stenosis, Fig. 4 a, b). They can only be interpreted as MRA grade IV provided the poststenotic vessel is well positioned within the examined volume. The disadvantages of MRA outbalance the advantages (Tables 3, 4). Over- and underestimation of grades of stenoses by MRA (Tables 1, 2, and as reported by Peters [3]) make it difficult for the surgeon to rely upon MRA as a source of preoperative information. It is not probable that increased spatial resolution will help surmount this problem. Cephalad presaturation techniques [4] and axial slices produce additional information on stenoses. However, multiple slices are time consuming. Moreover, complex collateralization can only be recognized with adequate selection of volume and consecutive reporting on 3D rotation in cinematographic mode of MRA. Contrary to good statistical correlation (as shown in Tables 3 and 4, and in the literature [5]), MRA cannot currently serve as a screening method for craniocervical vascular disease.

Table 3. Disadvantages of magnetic resonance angiography (MRA)

Low spatial resolution
Lack of temporal resolution
Movement artefacts
Reduced possibility for differential diagnosis: thrombi/blood flow
Small field of view
Incorrect positioning of volume to be examined

Table 4. Advantages of MRA

Noninvasive method
No contrast media necessary
Independent of examiner's skill
Short time for examination

References

1. Anderson CM, Saloner D, Tsuruda JS, Shapeero LG, Lee RG (1990) Artifacts in maximum intensity projection display of MR angiograms. AJR 154: 623–629
2. Bradley WG (1988) Flow phenomena in MR imaging. AJR 150: 983–994
3. Peters PE, Bongartz G, Drews C (1990) Magnetresonanzangiographie der hirnversorgenden Arterien. Fortschr Röntgenstr 152: 528–533
4. Litt AW, Rusinek H, Simon H, Bennon KR, Weinreb JC (1989) Improving MR angiography of the carotid arteries with spatial presaturation. Radiology 173: 186
5. Masaryk TJ, Ross JS, Masaryk AM, Modic MT, Ruggieri P, Selman W, Harik S (1989) Quantitative comparison of MR angiography and digital subtraction angiography in the evaluation of carotid arterial disease. Radiology 173: 186

Dr. K. Heimberger
Department of Neuroradiology
Vienna University Clinics
Lazarettgasse 14
A-1090 Vienna, Austria

Neuroradiology (1991) 33 [Suppl]: 529–531

Neuro radiology
© Springer-Verlag 1991

Preliminary experiences with a new nonionic gadolinium preparation in patients with intracranial tumors

S. R. Pollei[1], M. Fruin[1], M. Tryhus[1], G. Parker[1], R. Babbel[1], J. M. Jacobs[1], and J. Zielonka[2]

[1] University of Utah Hospitals, Salt Lake City, Utah, USA
[2] Squibb Diagnostics

Summary. This is a preliminary report of the use of a new gadolinium preparation, Gd-HPDO3A for MRI, tried on 12 patients. It has theoretical advantages of lower osmolality, higher LD 50 and greater ligand stability in vitro than Gd-DTPA.

Key words: Magnetic resonance imaging – Contrast enhancement – Gadolinium – Gd-HPDO3A

Several gadolinium preparations [1, 2] have been shown to cause enhancement in neurological diseases [3–5] by decreasing the T1 of tissues where they are deposited. The data summarized here are part of a phase-two clinical trial of a new, zero net charge (low osmolar/nonionic) gadolinium preparation, Gd-HPDO3A (ProHance; Squibb diagnostics). This new gadolinium preparation has theoretical advantages of lower osmolality, higher LD50 and greater ligand stability in vitro over the currently approved Gd agent in the USA, Gd-DTPA.

Patients and methods

Twelve patients with known intracranial lesions were injected with one of four concentrations of Gd-HPDO3A from 0.05 to 0.3 mmol/kg (Table 1). T1 and T2 images were obtained before and T1 images at 3, 15, 30 and 45 min. Patients were monitored by physical examinations, and multiple ECG and laboratory tests (Table 2). No significant adverse effects were noted: one patient complained of a metallic taste and another of transient arm stinging. Postinjection physical examinations and ECGs were unchanged from baseline.

Results

As with previous studies with Gd-DTPA, time-dependent changes in contrast appearance were noted. The low number of patients in each dose group makes it difficult to

Table 1. Patients receiving different doses

Dose (mmol/kg)	0.05	0.1	0.2	0.3
No. of patients	3	3	3	3

Table 2. Monitoring studies

	Preinjection	Postinjection
ECG	Yes	1, 4, 24 h
UA	Yes	1, 4, 24 h
Physical examination	Yes	24 h
Vital signs	Yes	1, 4, 24 h
CBC	Yes	1, 4, 24 h
Electrolytes	Yes	1, 4, 24 h
PT/PTT	Yes	1, 4, 24 h
TIBC/transferrin	Yes	1, 4, 24 h
Serum iron/bilirubin	Yes	1, 2[a], 4, 8[a], 24, 48[a] h
Serum ferritin	Yes	1, 4, 24 h
SMA 20	Yes	1, 4, 24 h

Table 3. Lesion and degree of enhancement

Patient	Dose (mmol/kg)	Site	Diagnosis	Enhancement
1	0.2	Posterior fossa	Astrocytoma	Marked
2	0.3	Sella/suprasellar	Craniopharyngioma	Marked
3	0.05	Pituitary	Adenoma	None/marked
4	0.1	Pituitary	Growth hormone adenoma	Marked
5	0.2	CP angle	Cholesteatoma	Marked
6	0.3	IAC	Acoustic neuroma	Marked
7	0.05	Frontoparietal	Meningioma	Marked
8	0.1	Frontal lobe	Astrocytoma	Marked
9	0.2	Frontal lobe	Glial tumor	Marked
10	0.3	Sphenoid wing/middle fossa	Metastasis	Marked
11	0.05	Pituitary	Adenoma	Slight
12	0.1	Hypothalamus	Glioma	Slight

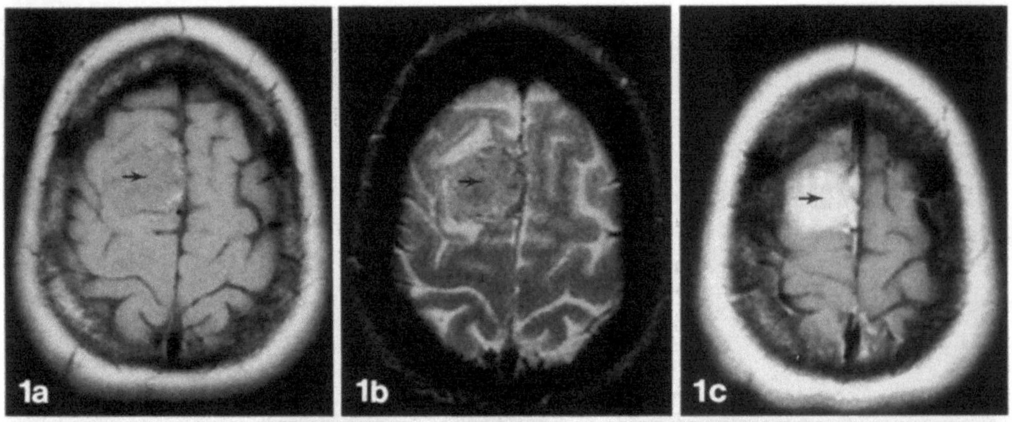

Fig. 1 a–c. Improved conspicuity of lesion. Note the increase in contrast between normal tissue and meningioma *(arrow)* in the enhanced T1 image (**c**) compared to the noncontrast images (**a, b**) where the meningioma is isointense on both T1 and T2.

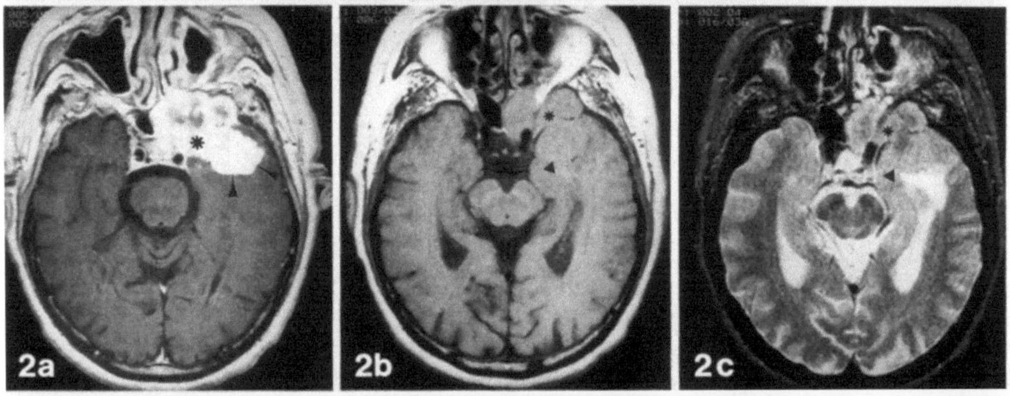

Fig. 2 a–c. Lesion margins. The extension of this skull base lesion *(asterisk)* into the parenchyma of the temporal lobe *(arrowheads)* is better defined on the post-contrast MRI (**a**) than on the noncontrast T1 (**b**) or T2 (**c**) MRI.

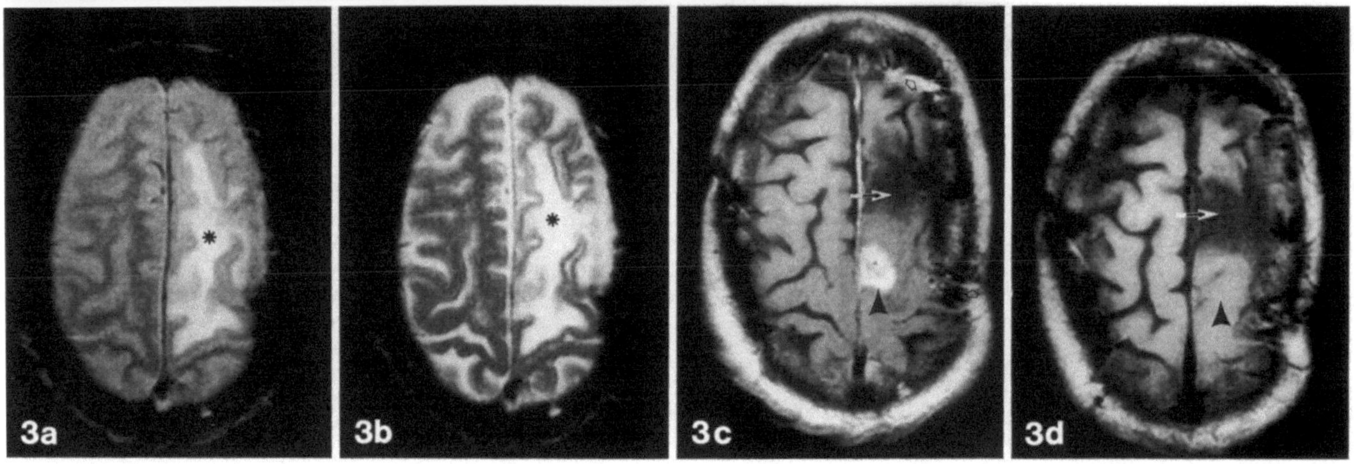

Fig. 3 a–d. Blood-brain barrier leak. Although the large area of edema *(asterisk)* on the proton density (**a**) and T2 image (**b**) marks the overall site of the lesion, the post-contrast study (**c**) better defines the area of blood-brain barrier leak *(arrowhead)* and presumably tumor viability for stereotaxic or open biopsy. The areas of encephalomalacia *(arrows)* and postoperative changes *(open arrow)* are easily differentiated on the post-contrast study. The enhancing lesion is isointense on the noncontrast T1 image (**d**)

draw conclusions about the potential advantage of higher doses in site, degree of enhancement and pathological diagnosis of the 12 patients are displayed in Table 3 it can be seen that lesions other than in the sella/suprasellar region tended to enhance markedly while sella/suprasellar lesions were variable in the amount of enhancement noted. Post-contrast administration improvement in lesion conspicuity is shown in Fig. 1, while better demonstration of lesion borders is well demonstrated in Fig. 2. Gd-HPDO3A's utility in defining the location of a blood barrier leak can be seen in Fig. 3.

Conclusions

1. Gd-HPDO3A has a favorable adverse effects ratio and deserves further study, especially with regard to the utility of higher doses to increase conspicuity of poorly enhancing lesions.
2. Equivalent enhancement with equal dose rates to Gd-DTPA was seen.
3. Gd-HPDO3A, just as other gadolinium agents, shows clinical utility in improving conspicuity, margins and documenting blood brain barrier leaks.

References

1. Hesselink JR, Healy ME, Press GA (1988) Benefits of Gd-DTPA for MR imaging of intracranial abnormalities. J Comput Assist Tomogr 12: 266
2. Parizel PM, Degryse HR, Gheuns J (1989) Gadolinium-DOTA enhanced imaging of intracranial lesions. J Comput Assist Tomogr 13: 378
3. Sze G, Abramson A, Krol G, (1988) Gadolinium-DTPA in the evaluation of intradural, extramedullary spinal disease. AJNR 9: 153
4. Heuftle MG, Modic MT, Ross JS (1988) Lumbar spine: postoperative MR imaging with gadolinium-DTPA. Radiology 167: 817
5. Runge VM, Carollo BR, Wolf CR (1989) Gd-DTPA: a review of clinical indications in central nervous system magnetic resonance imaging. Radiographics 9: 929

Dr. St. Pollei
Department of Radiology 1A71
University of Utah Medical Center
50 N. Medical Drive
Salt Lake City, UT 84132, USA

Neuroradiology (1991) 33 [Suppl]: 532–533

Neuro radiology
© Springer-Verlag 1991

Development of detachable balloons in a variety of shapes: round, spherical, dumbbell and curved types

T. Machida, S. Aoki, Y. Sasaki, and T. Ohkubo

Department of Radiology, Faculty of Medicine, University of Tokyo, Tokyo, Japan

Summary. Currently available detachable balloons are round or spherical. However, intracranial aneurysms are frequently more complex in shape, and two or more balloons may be necessary to embolize them ideally. We developed all-silicone detachable balloons with different shapes and sizes. Our balloons have self-sealing valves (with or without collars) and detach with simple traction. After inflation, round, spherical and our unique dumbbell, "snowman" and curved types are available. Our differently shaped balloons may be useful for embolization of complex aneurysms. In selected cases, we may be able to avoid more complicated procedures, such as the double balloon technique.

Key words: Detachable balloon – Cerebral aneurysms – Intravascular surgery

---

Treatment of vascular lesions such as carotico-cavernous sinus fistulas and giant aneurysms is now being performed with intravascular detachable balloon embolization techniques. However, currently available detachable balloons are round and spherical. We have developed several types of all-Japanese silicone detachable balloon in different sizes and shapes and have started clinical trials.

Structure of balloon (Fig. 1)

The balloon is composed of silicone and contains an internal self-sealing silicone tetracuspid valve. The balloon is attached to a 1.4 to 2.0 F catheter by sliding the catheter through the internal valve and can be detached by applying traction on the catheter. Catheter tips with different diameters are available for different degrees of friction between delivery catheters and balloons. The tetracuspid self-sealing valve is smaller than 0.6 mm and the balloon can easily be placed through a 7 F catheter.

Shapes of balloons

The smallest balloon accepts up to 0.1 ml and balloons which accept up to 0.2, 0.3 and 0.4 ml are available. Several shapes of balloon are currently available, such as round, spherical and dumbbell (Fig. 2). We also have different types of balloon which inflate in different directions, such as from distal to proximal or vice versa, in longer-shaped ones. A "collarless" balloon, which has no valve protrusion after inflation, is also available (Fig. 3).

The attachment portion of the balloon between the catheter has a smooth surface to avoid premature detachment when one withdraws the 2 F ballon catheter system through the 7 F catheter without embolization.

To allow fluoroscopic visualization we can attach a metal marker within the balloon.

Stability of balloons

We have performed in vitro studies to test the stability of the balloon. We immersed balloons filled to capacity with contrast medium (170 mg I/ml) in normal saline and observed them for 1 year and 2 months. The balloons showed no definite change in size or shape.

Because our balloon is made of silicone, it should be filled with contrast medium in 170–250 mgI/ml concentration or with solidification materials. It is well known that balloons may shrink or burst because of diffusion across the semipermeable silicone wall when they are filled with contrast medium in an inappropriate concentration.

A representative case is shown in Fig. 4.

Discussion

Treatment of cerebrovascular diseases by means of the endovascular balloon occlusion technique was described first by Serbinenko [1] in 1974 and later by Debrun et al. [2], Hieshima et al. [3], Taki et al. [4]and others [5, 6]. There are two types of balloon; the one used by Debrun et al. is made of latex and the other used by Hieshima et al. is made of silicone.

Our smallest balloon has now 0.1 ml capacity, and further in size is possible, because our valve is less than 0.6 mm in diameter.

Another unique character of our balloons is that there are different shapes. Although we have only a few clinical trials of this type, a dumbbell-shape balloon might be useful for embolization of complex aneurysms. In selected cases, we might be able to avoid more complicated procedures, such as the double balloon technique.

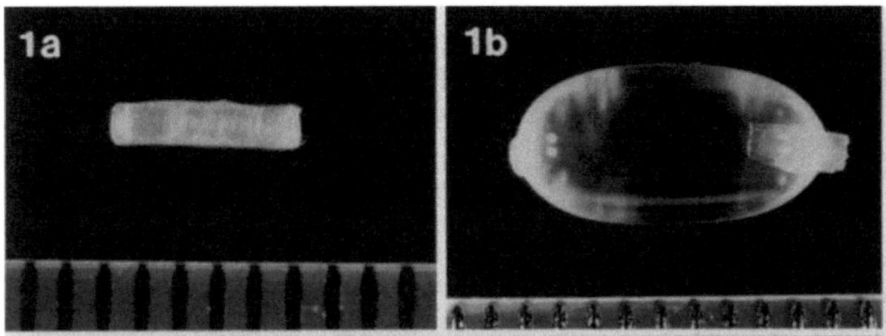

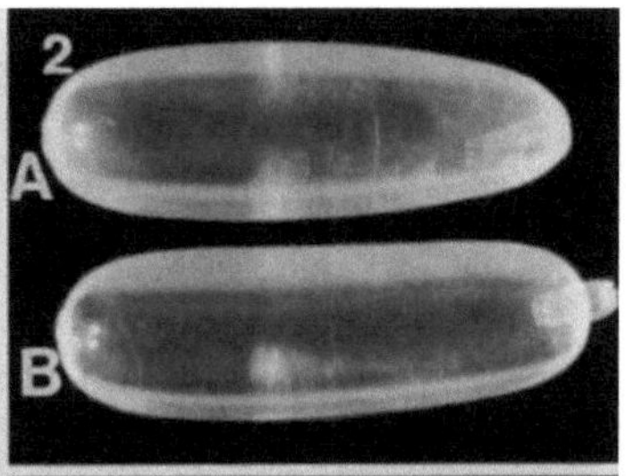

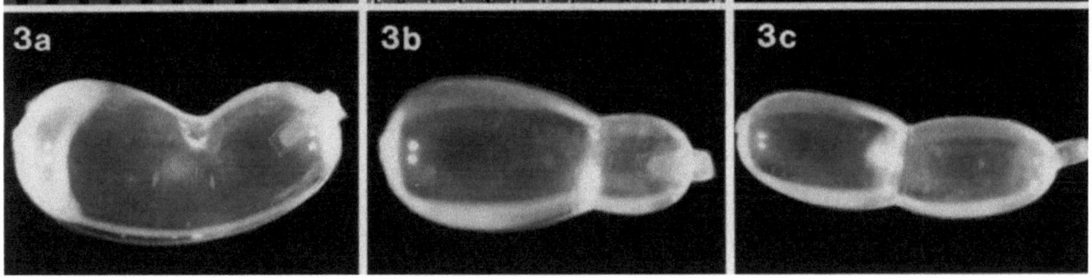

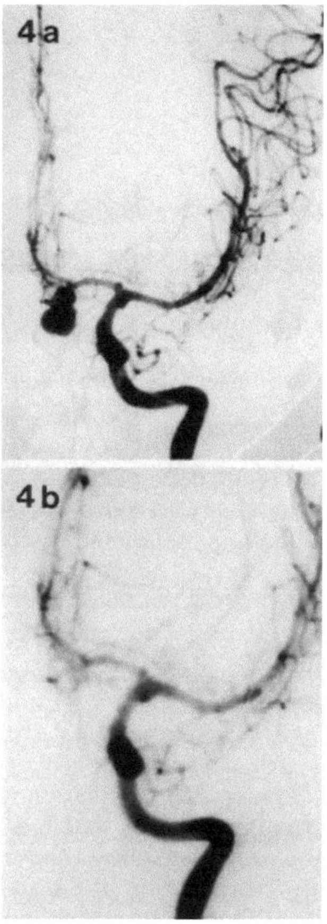

Fig. 1. **a** Uninflated balloon; **b** Inflated balloon

Fig. 2. **a** Collarless balloon; **b** with collar

Fig. 3 a–c. Different balloon shapes. **a** Curved; **b** snowman; **C** dumbbell

Fig. 4 a, b. Anterior communicating aneurysm. **a** Left internal carotid angiogram, AP view (preembolization); **b** Left internal carotid angiogram AP view (DSA, postembolization). The patient was in "grade 4" clinical state. Because the risk of rerupture and the risk involved in operation at that time were both very high, we performed balloon embolization. We successfully embolized a dumbbell-shape anterior communicating aneurysm with our detachable balloon

References

1. Serbinenko FA (1974) Balloon catheterization and occlusion of major cerebral vessels. J Neurosurg 41: 125–145
2. Debrun G, Lacour P, Caron JP, Hurth M, Comoy J, Keravel Y (1978) Detachable balloon and calibrated-leak balloon techniques in the treatment of cerebral vascular lesions. J Neurosurg 49: 635–649
3. Hieshima GB, Grinnell VS, Mehringer CM (1981) A detachable balloon for therapeutic transcatheter occlusions. Radiology 138: 227–228
4. Taki W, Handa H, Yamagata S, Matsuda I, Yonekawa Y, Ikeda Y, Iwata H (1979) Balloon embolization of a giant aneurysm using a newly developed catheter. Surg Neurol 12: 363–365
5. Halbach VV, Hieshima GB, Higashida RT (1987) Treatment of intracranial aneurysms by balloon embolization. Semin Intervent Radiol 4: 261–168
6. Higashida RT, Halbach VV, Cahan LD, Hieshima GB, Konishi Y (1989) Detachable balloon embolization therapy of posterior circulation intracranial aneurysms. J Neurosurg 71: 512–519

Dr. T. Machida
Department of Radiology
Faculty of Medicine
University of Tokyo
Tokyo, Japan

Neuroradiology (1991) 33 [Suppl]: 534–536

Neuro radiology
© Springer-Verlag 1991

Is it possible for a cerebral venous angioma to cause an intraparenchymal haemorrhage?

Y. Ono, N. Kobayashi, M. Toyoda, and Y. Kakinoki

Department of Neuroradiology, Neurological Institute, Tokyo Women's Medical College, Tokyo, Japan

Summary. Review of published cases and 19 reported here reveals an association between bleeding and venous angioma only below the tentorium.

Key words: Venous angioma – Intracranial haemorrhage

The diagnostic and morphological findings of intracranial venous angioma (VA) and associated clinical problems have been reported in recent years. The lesion may appear as either a single enlarged vein with many tributaries or a compact group of such veins on angiography. We have already reported that VA have different characteristics from other angiomas; they may be a compensatory venous drainage system due to maldevelopment or occlusion of the adjacent cortical or deep veins [1]. This hypothesis is supported by some authors. We have doubts that a compensatory venous drainage system may cause haemorrhage or present neurological symptoms. There is also another opinion that VA require operation because they may be neurologically symptomatic or a source of bleeding. We have, therefore, reviewed our 19 cases and the 151 cases previously reported of VA [2–14, 15–38], to try to determine whether they may possibly be a cause of haemorrhage, comparing the angiographic findings of 229 cases of subcortical intracerebral haemorrhage (SICH) or intracerebellar haemorrhage (ICH) in our institute.

Materials and methods

Our series consisted of 10 males and 9 females, ranging from 5 to 58 years old. Cerebral angiography was performed because of epilepsy, headache, tinnitus, vertigo, cerebellar signs, trauma, subarachnoid haemorrhage due to aneurysm rupture and intracerebral haemorrhage due to arteriovenous malformation. In the latter two conditions, full cerebral angiography was carried out. In the cases of epilepsy, EEG findings were compared with sites of VA.

The 151 previously reported angiographically confirmed cases whose symptoms have been discussed consisted of 81 males and 70 females, ranging from 1 to 77 years old.

The angiographic findings of 229 cases of SICH and ICH were reviewed to find any due to VA.

Results

There was no significant difference between our series (group A) and previously reported cases (group B) in sex and age distribution and they cases showed similar frequency and type of symptoms (Table 1). Overall, parenchymal haemorrhage occurred in 13.5% of the 170 cases, but was more frequent in the group of infratentorial VA (31.3%). Subarachnoid haemorrhage was noted in 7 cases of group B, but it was unclear if aneurysms or other vascular lesions were completely ruled out in these cases. Supratentorial neurological symptoms and epilepsy were considered to be incidental to infratentorial VA and infratentorial neurological symptoms (tinnitis and vertigo) were considered to be incidental in cases of supratentorial VA (Table 2). In the cases of epilepsy, coincidence of sites of VA with EEG abnormalities were sought, but only in a few were the EEG reports obtainable. Cases with headaches as the only symptom made up 15.7% of the material, but headaches were common when accompanied by other symptoms, and they are not peculiar to VA. Incidentally found VA were at least 28.8%, and asymptomatic VA may be more frequent if other causes of symptoms are found by careful studies. In our review of angiographic findings of SICH and ICH, we found only 1 haemorrhage caused by VA (0.4%), in which a small ICH coincided with the site of a relatively large VA in the cerebellar hemisphere (Tables 1–3).

Discussion

In our series of SICH and ICH, VA was extremely rare, but present. In our 19 cases, all supratentorial VA were considered to be incidental, but in the infratentorial lesions, there was 1 with ICH and 5 were found associated

Table 1. Main symptoms of venous angioma (VA)

	Group A Our cases		Group B Reported cases	
	ST	IT	ST	IT
Parenchymal haemorrhage	0	1	8	14
Subarachnoid haemorrhage	0	0	5	2
ST-neurological symptoms	0	0	4	0
IT-neurological symptoms	0	5	4	12
Epilepsy	4	0	39	2
Headaches	1	1	22	3
Incidental	6	1	29	7
Total	11	8	111	40
	19		151	

IT, Infratentorial; ST, Supratentorial

Table 2. Symptoms of all VA and percentages

	ST	IT	Total
Parenchymal haemorrhage	8 (6.6%)	15 (31.3%)	23 (13.5%)
Subarachnoid haemorrhage	5 (4.1%)	2 (4.2%)	7 (4.1%)
ST-neurological symptoms	4 (3.3%)	[a]	4 (2.4%)
IT-neurological symptoms	[a]	17 (35.4%)	17 (10.0%)
Epilepsy	43 (35.2%)	[a]	43 (25.3%)
Headache	23 (18.9%)	4 (8.3%)	27 (15.9%)
No definite relation	39 (31.9%)	10 (20.8%)	49 (28.8%)
Total	122 (100%)	48 (100%)	170 (100%)

[a] Calculated in no-definite-relation group

Table 3. Angiographic findings in cases of subcortical intracerebral haemorrhage and intracerebellar haemorrhage

	ST	IT	Total
No abnormal vascularity	104	32	136 (59.5%)
Arteriovenous malformation	52	3	55 (24.0%)
Tumour	20	5	25 (10.9%)
Moyamoya	9	0	9 (3.9%)
Cavernous angioma	1	2	3 (1.3%)
Venous angioma	0	1	1 (0.4%)
Total	186	43	229 (100%)

with infratentorial neurological symptoms. Supra- and infratentorial VA should therefore be discussed separately. Only 3.3% of supratentorial VA and 34.5% of infratentorial VA caused neurological symptoms. Parenchymal haemorrhage was also evidently restricted to the infratentorial lesions. These facts seem not to exclude the possibility that VA may represent a compensatory venous drainage system. But why does VA present with haemorrhage or neurological symptoms and why are they more frequent with the infratentorial VA? VA must be under high pressure to bleed. In our opinion, it may be possible for a large cerebellar VA to be under slightly raised pressure, when the internal jugular vein is directly narrowed due to neck movements. If there are only few veins in the cerebellar hemisphere, except for a large VA, these pressure changes may affect capillary or arterial flow. Then it may also be possible for cerebellar signs or symptoms such as vertebrobasilar insufficiency to appear. Explanations for venous pressure change in VA in the cerebral hemispheres are difficult. VA in the basal ganglia, thalamus or brain stem may show focal mass effect, such as a prominently enlarged vein within the limited area. Careful studies of the exact sites of VA, haematoma and EEG foci are needed and we will extend this study. In our series, no VA coincided with an EEG focus and no supratentorial VA showed haematoma or neurological deficits.

References

1. Saito Y, Kobayashi N (1981) Cerebral venous angiomas. Clinical evaluation and possible etiology. Radiology 139-1: 87–94
2. Constans JP, Dilenge D, Védrenne C (1968) Angiomas veineux cérébraux. Neurochirurgie 14: 641–650
3. Jinnai H, Kondo H, Matsumoto H (1974) Case of bilateral cerebral venous anomaly manifesting signs in the early middle age. Jpn J Clin Radiol 19: 236
4. Scotti LN, Goldman RL, Rao GR (1975) Cerebral venous angioma. Neuroradiology 9: 125–128
5. Wendling LR, Moose JS Jr, Kieffer SA (1976) Interacerebral venous angioma. Radiology 119: 141–147
6. Preissig RS, Preissig SH, Goree JA (1976) Angiographic demonstration of a cerebral venous angioma. Case report. J Neurosurg 44: 628–631
7. Michels LG, Bentson JR, Winter J (1977) Computed tomography of cerebral venous angiomas. J Comput Assist Tomogr 1: 149–154
8. Nishikawa J, Maehara T (1978) CT scan. Cerebral vascular disease. Venous angioma. Igau No Ayumi 104: 137–138
9. Sartor K, Fliedner E, Weber K (1978) Venöse Angiome des Gehirns. Fortschr Geb Roentgenstr Nuklearmed 128: 171–176
10. Fierstien SB, Pribram HW, Hieshima G (1979) Angiography and computed tomography in the evaluation of cerebral venous malformations. Neuroradiology 17: 137–148
11. Solomon EH, Bonstelle CT, Modic MT (1980) Angiographic and computed tomographic correlation in cerebral venous angiomas. J Comput Assist Tomogr 4: 217–221
12. Hammer B, Pohlhammer H (1980) Das venöse Angiom des Gehirns. Radiologe 20: 113–117
13. Pak H, Patel SC, Malik GM (1981) Successful evacuation of a pontine hematoma secondary to rupture of a venous angioma. Surg Neurol 15: 164–167
14. Kasamo S, Kobayashi E, Awa H (1970) A case of cerebral venous angioma as an epileptogenic lesion detected by CT and surgically treated. Neurol Med Chir (Tokyo) 20: 865–873
15. Hacker DA, Latchaw RE, Chou SN (1981) Bilateral cerebellar venous angioma. J Comput Assist Tomogr 5: 424–426
16. Kobayashi K, Nakamura T, Aki T (1981) Two cases of cerebral venous angioma – with special reference to the neuroradiological diagnosis. Neurosurgery 9: 424–431
17. Thron A, Peterson D, Voigt K (1982) Neuroradiologie, Klinik und Pathologie der zerebralen venösen Angiome. Radiologe 22: 389–399
18. Senegor M, Dohrmann G, Wollman RL (1983) Venous angiomas of the posterior fossa should be considered as anomalous venous drainage. Surg Neurol 19: 26–32
19. Olson E, Golmor RL, Richmond B (1984) Cerebral venous angiomas. Radiology 151: 97–104
20. Valvanis A, Wellauer J, Yasargil MG (1983) The radiological diagnosis of cerebral venous angioma: cerebral angiography and computed tomography. Neuroradiology 24: 193–199
21. Nagata K, Kubo T, Fukushima T (1983) Four cases of cerebral venous angioma – with particular reference to the operative indication and the importance of CT diagnosis. Neurosurgery 11: 1201–1208
22. Rothfus WE, Albright AL, Casey KF (1984) Cerebellar venous angioma. "Benign" entity? AJNR 5: 61–66
23. Hatashita S, Hata S, Sato K (1984) Cerebral venous angioma – case report. Neurol Med Chir (Tokyo) 24: 39–41
24. Handa J, Suda K, Sato M (1984) Cerebral venous angioma associated with varix. Surg Neurol 21: 436–440
25. Burke L, Berenberg RA, Kim KS (1984) Choreoballismus: a nonhemorrhagic complication of venous angiomas. Surg Neurol 21: 245–248
26. Agnoli AL, Hildebrandt G (1985) Cerebral venous angiomas. Acta Neurochir (Wien) 78: 4–12
27. Ibayashi S, Sadoshima S, Ogawa K (1986) Cerebral venous angioma of the pons: report of a case with pontine hemorrhage. J Comput Assist Tomogr 10: 377–380
28. Numaguchi Y, Nadell JM, Mizushima A (1984) Cerebral venous angioma and a varix. Surg Neurol 21: 436–440
29. Lim GHK (1987) Venous angioma of the brain: CT and angiographic diagnosis. Australes Radiol 31: 236–240

30. Fontaine S, Sayette V, Gianfelice D (1987) CT, MRI and angiography of venous angiomas: a comparative study. J Can Assoc Radiol 38: 259–263
31. Inoue N, Merubayashi T, Noshi T (1986) Cerebral venous angioma associated with cerebral aneurysm. Report of 2 cases. Neuro Med Chir (Tokyo) 9: 722–727
32. Shiroyama Y, Kurokawa Y, Ueda H (1986) Operated case of cerebral venous angioma with early venous filling on cerebral angiography. Neurosurgery 14: 1355–1360
33. Uchino A, Ohno M (1987) Hematoma in the internal capsule due to venous angioma. A case report. Jpn J Clin Radiol 32: 339–341
34. Harada K, Kobayashi S, Shigemori M (1987) Medullary venous malformation with azygous anterior cerebral artery aneurysm. Neurosurgery 15: 327–333
35. Malik GM, Morgan JK, Boulos RS (1988) Venous angiomas. An underestimated cause of intracranial hemorrhage. Surg Neurol 30: 350–358
36. Ochi M, Futagawa S, Mori H (1987) Cerebral venous angiomas. Jpn J Clin Radiol 32: 681–685
37. Jackson G, Champness P, Sacharias N (1989) Cerebral venous malformations. Australas Radiol 33: 132–139
38. Nakajima K, Takaba H, Tanaka H (1989) Cerebral venous angioma complicated by pontine hemorrhage. Jpn J Assoc Med 78: 688–689

Dr. Y. Ono
Department of Neuroradiology
Neurological Institute
Tokyo Women's Medical College
Tokyo, Japan

Neuroradiology (1991) 33 [Suppl]: 537–538

Neuro-
radiology
© Springer-Verlag 1991

A simple animal model of arteriovenous fistula and aneurysm: in vivo studies of detachable balloon techniques

F.J. Ives[1], H.T. ApSimon[1], and A. Storrie[2]

[1] Department of Diagnostic Radiology, [2] Research Institute, Royal Perth Hospital, Perth, Western Australia

Summary. The technique of manufacture of an "H"-shaped arteriovenous fistula in mongrel dogs is described. This model is useful in testing various techniques of fistula and small aneurysm occlusion.

Key words: Embolisation, therapeutic – Arteriovenous shunt, surgical – Aneurysm – Dogs

The following model was devised in order to gain experience in handling fine flexible catheter and detachable balloon systems required to treat intracranial aneurysm. An "H"-shaped arteriovenous fistula is produced in the neck of mongrel dogs. The size and orientation of the anastomosis are varied to simulate geometrical difficulties which may be encountered in a patient. Closure of the venous end of the fistula with a flow-directed detachable balloon is easily accomplished, leaving a residual sac which may be treated by a detachable balloon, wire coils, electrocoagulation or laser.

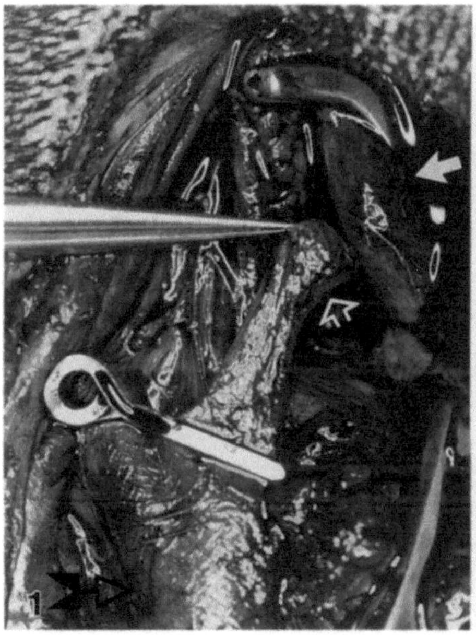

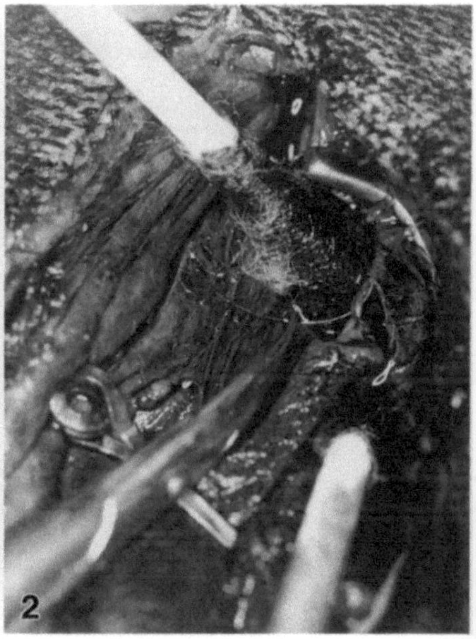

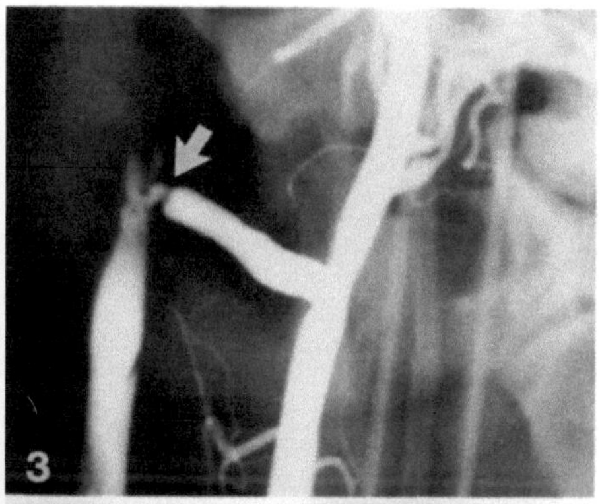

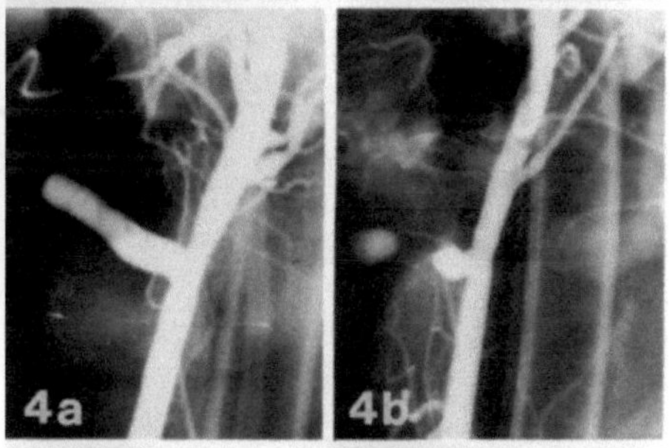

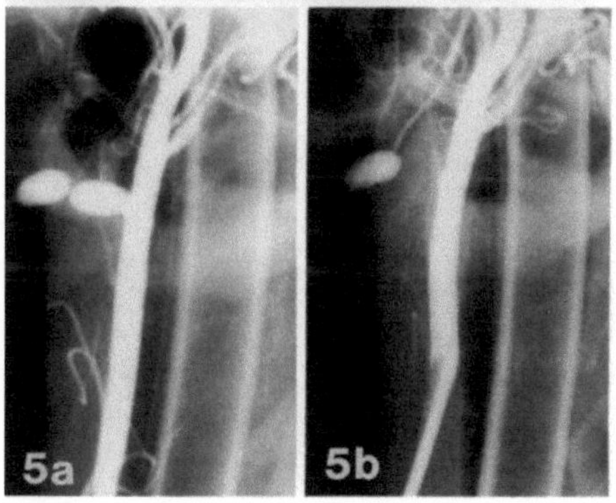

Fig. 1. Surgical photograph shows external jugular vein (▶▷), cut external maxillary vein *(open arrow),* common carotid artery *(white arrow)*

Fig. 2. Anastomosis to small arteriotomy in progress

Fig. 3. Typical fistula appearance at carotid angiography. Note constriction at venous end due to tie *(arrow)*

Fig. 4 a, b. After fistula embolisation (see text)

Fig. 5 a, b. Two week interval between **a** and **b**

Method

Under general anaesthesia the external jugular vein is localised at the level of the thyroid cartilage after shaving the fur. A longitudinal incision medial to the vein, followed by blunt dissection allows exposure of the external maxillary vein and its confluence with the external jugular vein. More medial dissection over the carotid pulsation allows exposure of the common carotid artery. After systemic heparinisation, the arterial clamp is applied and a temporary clip placed at the jugular end of the external maxillary vein. The necessary length of vein is divided after distal ligation (Fig. 1). A small arteriotomy is performed so that the size and position of the orifice along the common carotid artery can be varied. End-to-side vein/artery anastomosis is achieved with approximately ten 8–0 nylon interrupted sutures (Fig. 2). If a narrow-necked aneurysm is desired, the cut end of the vein may need to be cobbled. An operating microscope is useful to assist the anastomosis. The venous end clip is removed, allowing filling of the fistula and testing for anastomotic leak at venous pressure. The arterial clamp can be removed, establishing the high flow fistula. It is necessary to apply a loose 4–0 silk tie at the venous end of the fistula to retain the fistula-closing balloon. Skin closure is achieved with a continous absorbable subcutaneous suture. Two weeks are allowed for wound and anastomosis healing before intervention. No ill effects from this surgery have been noted. Patency of the fistula is easily checked by palpation of the fistula thrill.

Subsequent common carotid arteriography displays a typical fistula appearance (Fig. 3). Closure of the fistula is readily achieved by flow-directed detachable balloon from any desired arterial access point (Fig. 4a). The size of the fistula-closing balloon may be varied to achieve different sizes and shapes of residual sac. It is wise to perform "aneurysm" occlusion at the same session as we observed partial (Fig. 4b) and complete spontaneous sac thrombosis with staged procedures. We routinely use HEMA polymer to fill the balloons. Subsequent serial radiography allows observation of the behaviour of the balloon/polymer embolus with problems such as balloon rupture (Fig. 5), balloon migration and parent vessel thrombosis having been observed. Specimen retrieval and dissection are performed to confirm abnormal behaviour. The apparent loss of embolus in Fig. 5 was due to balloon shell rupture and diffusion of contrast medium, rendering the HEMA cast invisible.

Conclusion

This easily constructed model aneurysm has allowed us to gain confidence using new commercially available and custom made microcatheters and detachable balloon systems, The model is also suitable for gaining experience in other methods of fistula and aneurysm occlusion.

Dr. F. J. Ives
Department of Diagnostic Radiology
Royal Perth Hospital
Perth, Western Australia 6000

Neuroradiology (1991) 33 [Suppl]: 539–541

Neuro radiology
© Springer-Verlag 1991

Polylene threads embolisation as alternative method of treatment of problematic carotid-cavernous fistulae

A. Beltramello, A. Maschio, S. Perini, L. Rosta, E. Piovan, and A. Benati

Service of Neuroradiology, Verona University Hospital, Verona, Italy

Summary. Two peculiar cases of carotid-cavernous fistula (CCF) were embolised with polylene threads. The first was a problematic CCF due to post-traumatic rupture of a persistent trigeminal artery (PTA) in which attempts to enter the PTA with detachable balloons were unsuccessful; the second was a case of congenital CCF fed both by the ophthalmic and maxillary arteries. In both cases intra-arterial navigation with flexible catheters and embolisation with polylene threads of different sizes succeeded in obliterating the fistula while sparing the artery. Follow-up angiograms 6 months after embolisation revealed no recurrence of the fistulae. On the basis of this experience, polylene threads, already used frequently in our department over a long period for preoperative embolisation of intracranial angiomas, can also be considered an efficient, safe and stable form of endovascular treatment for other problematic intracranial arteriovenous fistulae.

Key words: Carotid-cavernous fistulae – Persistent trigeminal artery – Embolisation

Currently available endovascular treatments of carotid-cavernous fistulae (CCF) are well-established procedures: they include transarterial or transvenous (superior ophthalmic vein/inferior petrosal sinus) approaches and embolisation with detachable or non-detachable balloons, glue, coils and other particulate substances [1–3]. Nevertheless, cases may be encountered in which classical procedures are unsuccessful or impossible. In two such cases we used our own embolisation system based on the use of polylene polyfilament 3-0 threads (0.2 mm in diameter), with good results.

Fig. 1 a-f. Case 1. **a** Right post-traumatic carotid-cavernous fistula (CCF). **b** Early right carotid and **c** vertebral angiograms reveal that the fistulous connection with the cavernous sinus is due to a rent in the mid-intracavernous portion of a persistent trigeminal artery *(arrows)*. **d** Right cavernous sinus opacification with a Tracker microcatheter advanced into the cavernous sinus via the trigeminal artery. **e** Embolisation of the cavernous sinus with polylene threads. **f** Control angiogram reveals complete occlusion of the fistula with preservation of internal carotid and trigeminal arteries *(arrows)*

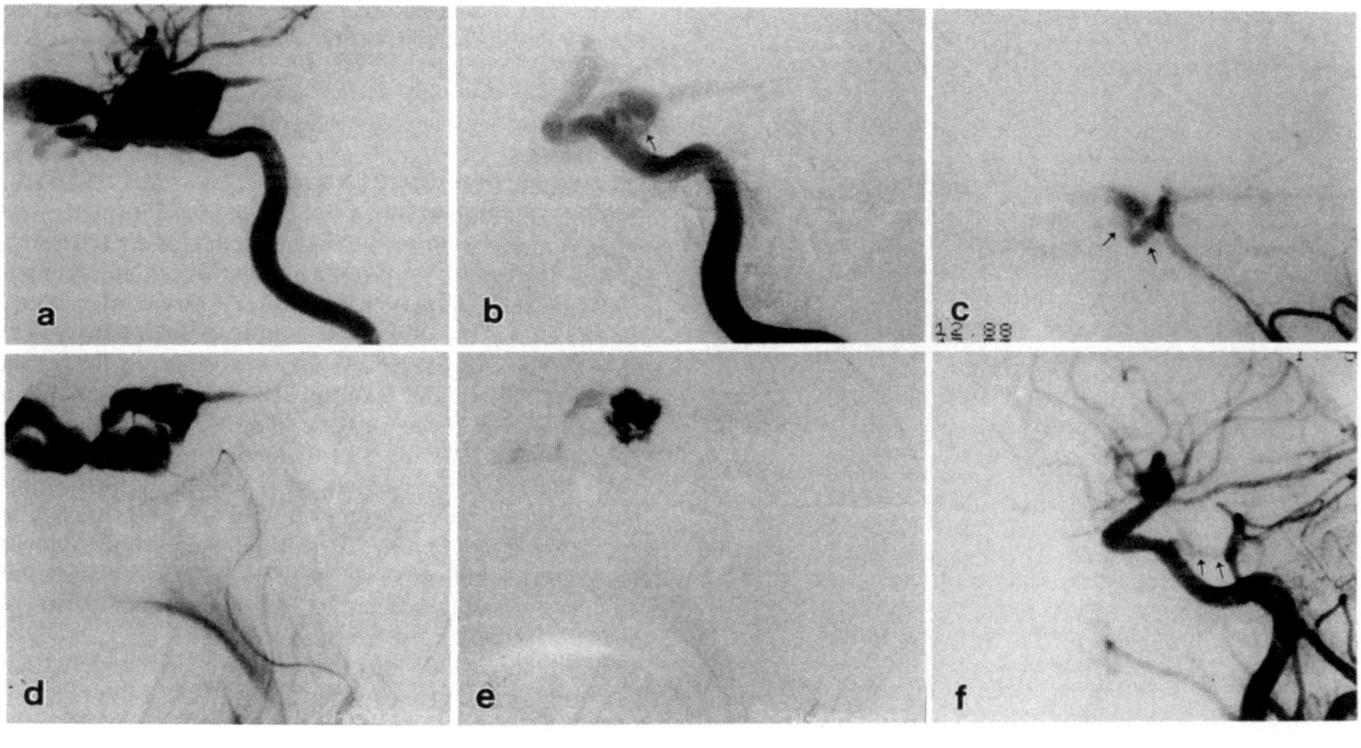

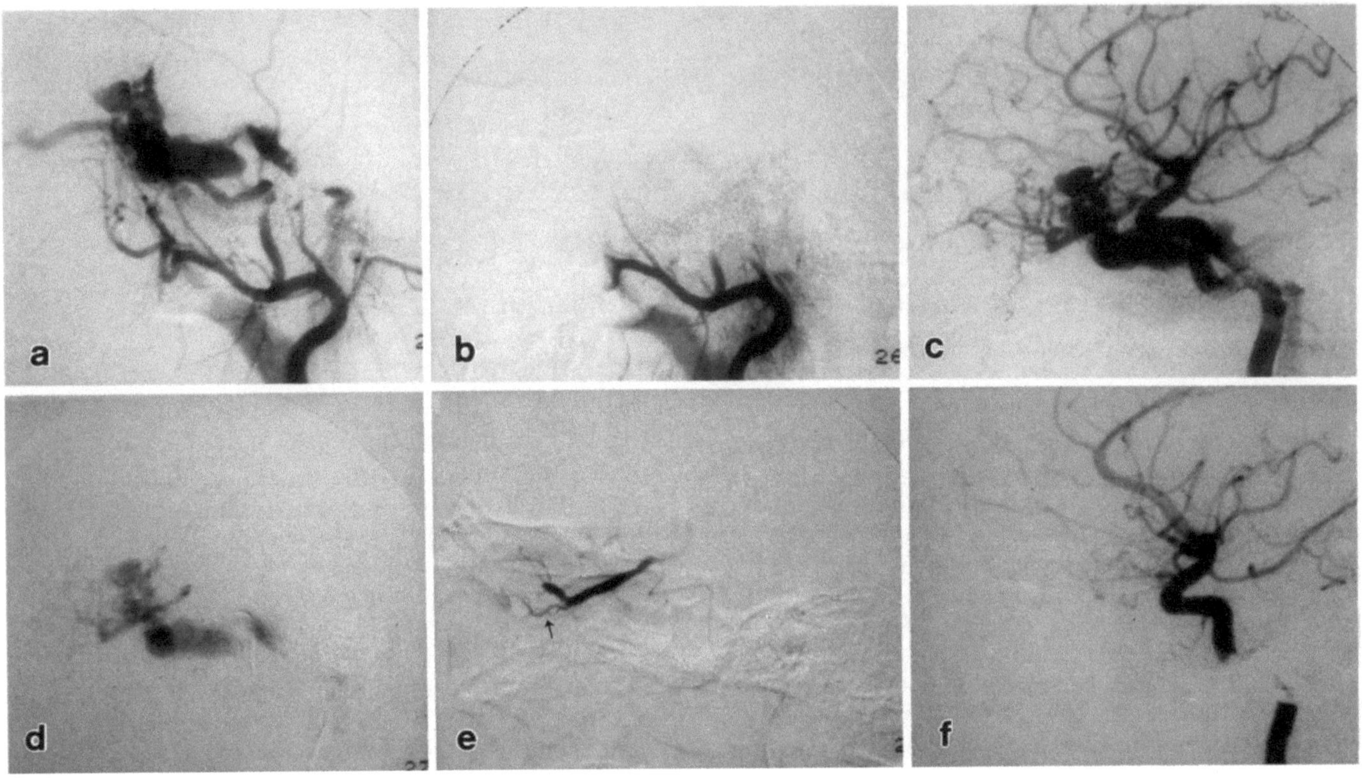

Fig. 2 a–f. Case 2. **a** Left congenital CCF of mixed type: dural supply is by meningeal branches of internal maxillary artery. **b** Embolisation with polyvinyl alcohol. **c** The fistula is fed also by branches of the ophthalmic artery (OA). **d** Superselective left OA angiogram. **e** At the end of the embolisation with polylene threads the ocular complex is visible. **f** Control angiogram reveals complete occlusion of the fistula with preservation of the OA

Case reports

Case 1

A 57-year-old woman was involved in a motor-vehicle accident. She had haemorrhage from her right ear and right sixth and seventh cranial nerve palsies. Twenty days after head injury, she developed marked exophthalmos, conjunctival chemosis, systolic bruit and extraocular muscles palsy of the right eye. Three-vessel angiography revealed the presence of a CCF (Fig. 1 a). Several attempts in two sessions to enter the cavernous sinus with no. 9, 16 and 15 Debrun latex balloons were unsuccessful. During the various phases of the procedure, we realized that the rent was localised in the mid-intracavernous portion of a persistent trigeminal artery (PTA) of the adult type (Fig. 1 b, arrow) so that the uninflated balloon was not able to enter the tear in the artery. Transient occlusion of the internal carotid artery (ICA) near the origin of the PTA did not result in closure of the fistula, fed by the posterior part of the PTA filled by the basilar artery (Fig. 1 c, arrows). A transvenous approach via superior ophthalmic vein failed. Finally, with the help of a tight curved guidewire a Tracker 18 microcatheter was advanced in the PTA and into the cavernous sinus (Fig. 1 d), which was embolised with 21 polylene 3-0 threads 6–20 cm long (Fig. 1 E). The fistula was occluded, the ICA preserved. The result was stable at an angiographic control 6 months later: PTA was still recognisable and very small (Fig. 1 f, arrows).

Case 2

A 15-year-old girl suffered from left proptosis and amaurosis from birth; recent onset of intracranial bruit and worsening exophthalmos was experienced. CT scan and angiography revealed a congenital CCF of mixed type: dural supply was due to meningeal branches of the internal maxillary artery (Fig. 2 a); these pedicles were embolised with polyvinyl alcohol (Fig. 2 b). The fistula was fed also by branches of the ophthalmic artery (OA) (Fig. 2 c). The OA was navigated (Fig. 2 d) and embolised with 1.5–2 mm polylene threads. The ocular complex then became apparent (Fig. 2 e, arrows). The fistula was permanently closed, the OA spared (Fig. 2 f).

Discussion

The frequency rate of a PTA is quoted as from 0.1% to 1%; its presence is linked with a significant association of other vascular malformations such as angiomas and aneurysms. In the adult type, PTA is not a mandatory collateral channel, while in the fetal type the basilar artery is interrupted and the PTA is the only blood supply to the territory normally supplied by its upper portion. In our case 1 the fistula was caused by traumatic rupture of the mid-segment of an adult-type PTA: this occurrence is quite rare and in the reported cases the fistula was always at the junction of the ICA and PTA [4, 5]. In our case 2 embolisation of the ophthalmic artery was possible because of the pre-existing amaurosis; polylene threads worked well: the fistula was closed and a significant improvement in the vascularisation of the eye was obtained, as testified by the opacification of the ocular complex, previously not visible.

Polyfilament polylene threads have been widely used in our department for preoperative embolisation of intracranial angiomas: these agents proved to be efficient, nontoxic and highly biocompatible materials [6]. On the basis of this experience, polylene threads can also be considered an efficient, safe and stable form of endovascular treatment for other problematic intracranial arteriovenous fistulae.

References

1. Benati A, Maschio A, Perini S, Beltramello A (1980) Treatment of post-traumatic carotid-cavernous fistula using a detachable balloon catheter. J Neurosurg 53: 784–786
2. Debrun GM (1983) Treatment of traumatic carotid-cavernous fistula using detachable balloon catheters. AJNR 4: 355–356
3. Halbach VV, Higashida RT, Hieshima GB, Hardin CW, Yang PJ (1988) Transvenous embolization of direct carotid cavernous fistulas. AJNR 9: 741–747
4. Debrun GM, Davis KR, Nauta HJ, Heros RE, Ahn HS (1988) Treatment of carotid cavernous fistulae or cavernous aneurysms associated with persistent trigeminal artery: report of three cases. AJNR 9: 749–755
5. Kerber CW, Manke W (1983) Trigeminal artery to cavernous sinus fistula treated by balloon occlusion. J Neurosurg 58: 611–613
6. Benati A, Beltramello A, Colombari R, Maschio A, Perini S, Da Pian R, Pasqualin A, Scienza R, Rosta L, Piovan E, Scarpa A, Zamboni G (1989) Preoperative embolization of arteriovenous malformations with polylene threads: techniques with wing microcatheter and pathologic results. AJNR 10: 579–586

Dr. A. Beltramello
Service of Neuroradiology
Verona University Hospital
Verona, Italy

Neuroradiology (1991) 33 [Suppl]: 542–544

Neuro-radiology
© Springer-Verlag 1991

Intrinsic lesions of the unenlarged spinal cord: relative utility of spin echo and gradient echo MRI

K. Demarco, D. Seidenwurm, J. Tsuruda, and D. Norman

University of California, San Francisco, California, USA

Summary. The relative efficacy of spin echo versus gradient echo T2-weighted MRI examinations in the depiction of intramedullary lesions in the unenlarged spinal cord was evaluated prospectively. Nineteen patients with cervical myelopathy with normal or compressed cords on sagittal T1-weighted images were studied. Using spin echo images as the reference, nine high signal cord lesions in nine patients were observed. Two were better seen with spin echo and one was better seen with gradient echo. No false-positive lesions were noted on gradient echo. T2-weighted gradient echo sagittal images may replace T2-weighted sagittal images in many cases without significant loss of diagnostic accuracy. The simpler examination is especially useful in the uncooperative patient.

Key words: Spinal cord – Spinal cord abnormality – Magnetic resonance imaging – Multiple sclerosis – Spondylosis

Recent work [1, 2] has suggested the clinical relevance of abnormally high signal on spin echo (SE) T2-weighted magnetic resonance (MR) images within the normal caliber or compressed spinal cord in cervical spondylosis, The depiction of plaques of multiple sclerosis within the unexpanded spinal cord on T2-weighted images frequently correlates with the presence of symptoms referable to the spine [3]. Until now, cardiac gated, flow compensated spin echo images of the cervical spine have been required for the reliable depiction of these lesions. The recent availability of high quality gradient refocussed (GRE) techniques employing gradient based flow compensation (FC) has allowed the production of high quality T2-weighted images with reduced acquisition and set-up time. We undertook a prospective investigation to assess the relative utility of cardiac gated SE T2-weighted images versus GR T2-weighted images in the unenlarged cervical spinal cord in a clinical population of patients referred for imaging of the cervical spine.

Patients and methods

Both SE T2-weighted images and GRE T2-weighted images were obtained in 19 consecutive patients with cervical myelopathy in whom it was clinically feasible to perform an extended MRI examination. Fifteen patients were diagnosed as having spondylytic myelopathy, one had multiple sclerosis, one had systemic lupus erythematosis, one had post-traumatic myelomalacia, and one had transverse myelitis of unknown etiology.

MRI examinations were performed on a 1.5 T imager using commercially available surface coils, cardiac gating apparatus and pulse sequences (General Electric, Milwaukee, Wis, USA) Sagittal SE sequences were performed employing a repetition time (TR) of two R–R intervals which produced a range of TR 1500–2500 ms depending upon the patient's heart rate. Echo time (TE) was 35 and 70 ms. A 256 by 192 matrix and 1 excitation was used. Slice thickness was 3 mm with a 1-mm interslice gap. Sagittal GRE sequences were performed using a flip angle or theta of 20°, TR of 500 ms, TE 15 and 35 ms, 4 excitations and a 256 by 192 matrix. Field of view was 20 cm for all scans and the phase encoding axis was anteroposterior. Gradient based FC was employed in both the SE and GRE sequences. Sagittal SE T1-weighted images and axial three-dimensional Fourier transform volume acquisition GRE completed the clinical examination in each patient.

Scans were reviewed by two observers blinded to the clinical interpretation of the images. Reviewers had the option to reject any scan considered uninterpretable. No attempt was made to blind the observers to the pulse sequence imployed, because neuroradiologists experienced in the interpretaion of clinical MRI scans readily recognize the characteristic appearances and artifacts of the two different iamging techniques. The GRE studies were reviewed first; then the SE images were reviewed. This established the SE examination as the reference. Each abnormal spinal level was assessed for the presence of extradural, intradural-extramedullary or intramedullary disease. The spinal cord was studied for the presence or absence of intramedullary high signal which was graded I–IV (I = normal, II = possible, III = probable, and IV = definite intramedullary high signal). For purposes of analysis grade I and II scans were considered negative and grade III and IV scans were considered positive for intramedullary high signal. Grade I cords were homogeneous and had no areas of increased signal (Fig. 1). Grade II cords had areas of increased cord signal on a single slice or on more than one slice in which an artifact produced equivalent signal variation elsewhere in the image. Grade III cords had areas of increased signal on more than one slice on both the first and second echo image that were somewhat higher in signal than would be accounted for by the greatest variation produced within the cord by artifact (Fig. 2 A, B). Grade IV had elevated signal within the cord on both echoes of more than one slice that was substantially higher than would be accounted for by the greatest artifactual variation (Fig. 2 C, D).

Results

No study was rejected as uninterpretable. Nominal scan duration was comparable for the two sequences, but SE sequences required additional set-up time and variations

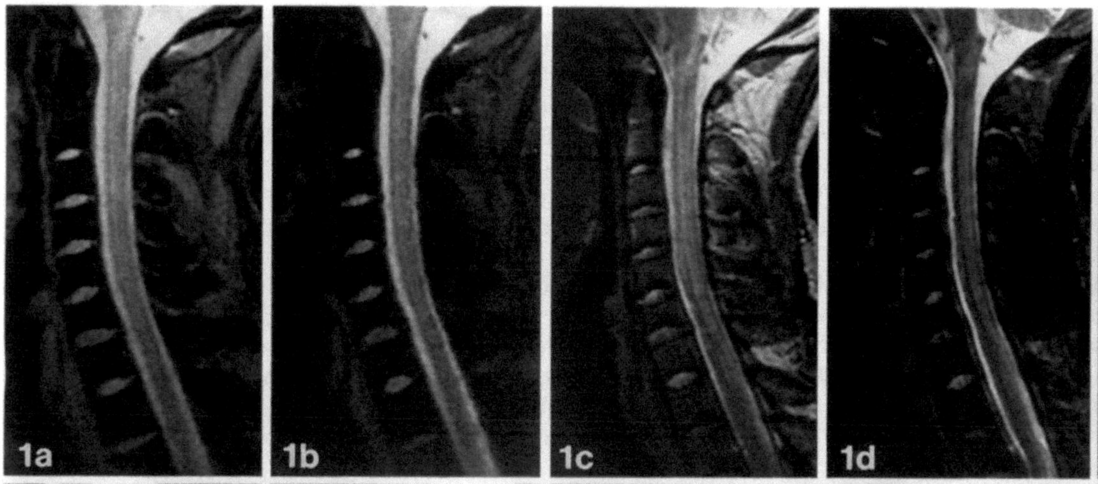

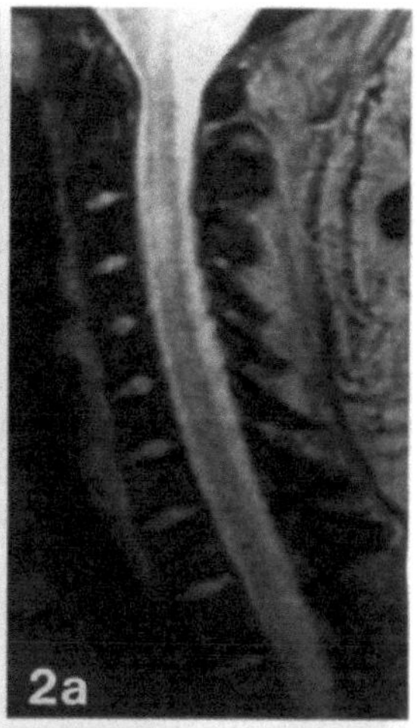

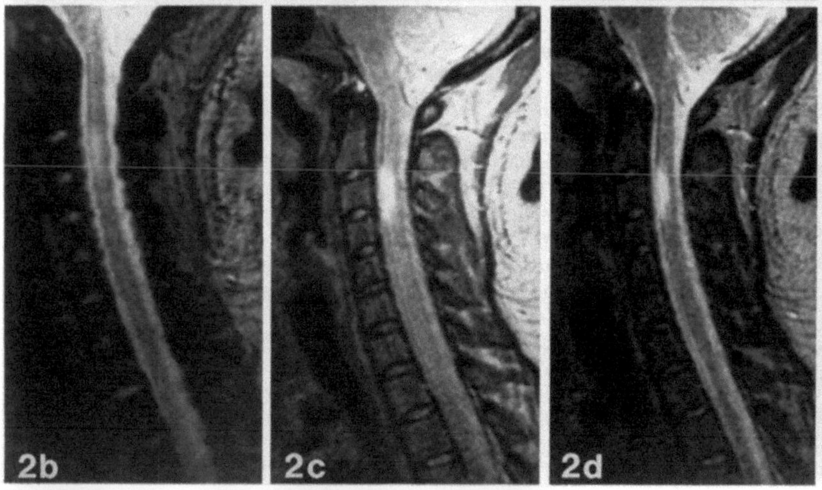

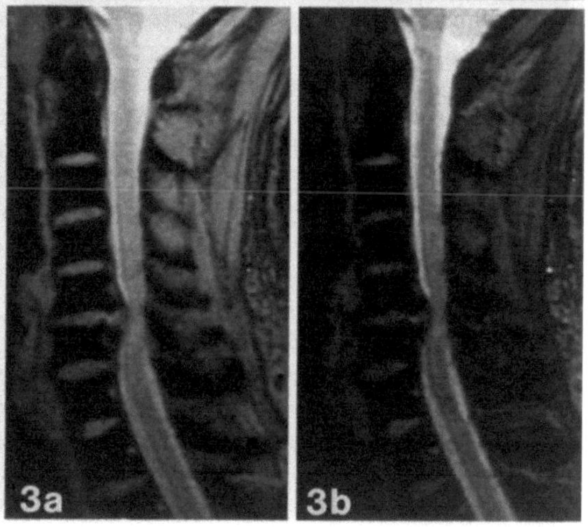

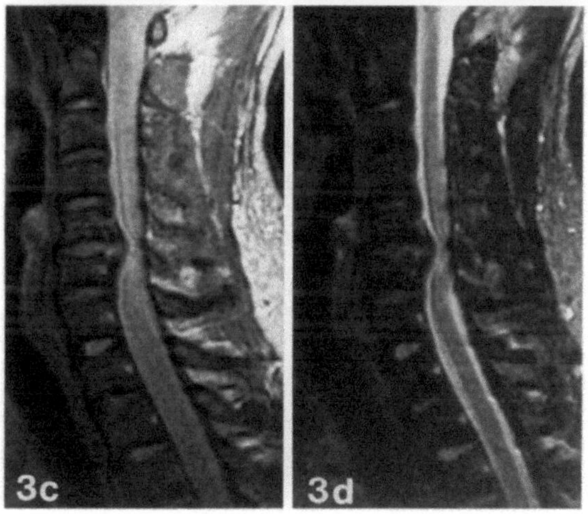

Fig. 1 a–d. Normal. **a, b** First and second echo of GRE sequence demonstrate homogeneous signal intensity within the cord, which is normal in caliber. No compressive lesion is demonstrated. **c, d** First and second echo of SE sequence demonstrate relatively homogeneous signal intensity within the cord. Note the low signal border of the cord due to boundary layer phase dispersion, an artifact noted on cardiac gated scans [9]

Fig. 2 a–d. Multiple sclerosis. **a, b** First and second echo of GRE sequence demonstrate a plaque within the unexpanded cord. This was graded III/IV. **c, d** First and second echo of SE sequence demonstrate a plaque within the unexpanded cord. This was graded IV/IV

Fig. 3 a–d. Degenerative disk disease. **a, b** First and second echo of GRE sequence demonstrate epidural compressive lesion and increased signal within the cord. This was graded III/IV. **c, d** First and second echo of SE sequence demonstrate epidural compressive lesion and increased signal within the cord. This was graded III/IV

in capture of the pulse wave lead to increased scan duration due to "skipped beats." Occasionally, involuntary patient motion distorted the gating signal and also lead to "skipped beats" on the SE sequence.

Thirty-seven abnormal levels in 17 patients were identified. Two examinations were entirely normal. At 27 levels with epidural lesions alone on the SE sequences, grade I, or normal cord signal was identified on the GRE images. Therefore, no false-positive lesions were recognized on the GRE studies. The specifity of the positive finding on the GRE sequence was found to be equivalent to that of the SE sequence.

Nine cord lesions in 9 patients were graded III or IV on the SE sequence, and 8 were graded III or IV on the GRE sequence. Of these 9 lesions, 6 were demonstrated equally well on the two sets of images (Fig. 3). One lesion graded IV on the SE images was graded III on the GRE images. Another lesion graded IV on the GRE images was graded III on the SE images (Fig. 2). These differences were inconsequential, since both grade III and IV scans were considered positive. However, one lesion graded III on SE images had been graded II on the GRE images, leading to a single "missed" lesion in our series.

Discussion

The primary goal in imaging patients with cervical myelopathy is the diagnosis or exclusion of epidural compressive lesions due to cervical spondylosis [4]. This is because cervical spondylosis is the most common specifically remediable cause of cervical myelopathy in the general population. GRE MRI has become the standard method for this purpose [5], providing the screening study and presurgical evaluation in a single setting. Evaluation of intramedullary disease is also a primary goal in imaging the patient with cervical myelopathy. Depiction of the contour of the compressed cord, or elucidation of the nature of an expansile lesion have been the principal contributions of MR [6].

Recent work has focussed attention on the ability of MRI using SE techniques to depict lesions within the unenlarged, non-cavitated spinal cord. These have been noted in compressive myelopathy as well as a variety of vascular and inflammatory conditions [7]. Further investigation of patients with the finding of increased signal within the spinal cord on SE T2-weighted images has lead to the concept that a prognostic significance of this finding may exist, either at presentation or in the postoperative period [1, 2]. However, the data are scanty and our ability to analyze their significance is hampered by the design of the studies reported to date.

Our data suggest that GRE images, which may be superior to SE images in the depiction of spondylytic lesions and disc herniation [8], are equivalent to SE images in the depiction of increased signal lesions within the unexpanded spinal cord. In the context of a clinical protocol for the study of patients with cervical myelopathy, this finding allows us to dispense with the cumbersome and time-consuming gated SE T2-weighted images in the routine evaluation of patients with cervical myelopathy.

Our study may be criticized on several grounds. First the sample size is small, so the data must be considered preliminary. Second, there was no independent reference standard. The methodology we employed could never result in the finding that GRE was superior to SE in the depiction of intrinsic cord lesions, since SE was employed as the reference standard. Since the pathological correlates of increased signal within the compressed spinal cord are largely unknown and cord tissue is not obtained in these patients, this methodological flaw is unavoidable. However, it must be recognized that we may have diagnosed abnormality within the spinal cord when none was present, or failed to diagnose abnormalities which were present. We have no way of estimating the magnitude of these errors. Third, observers were nor blinded to the pulse sequence. Fourth, since MRI instruments differ from manufacturer to manufacturer, and imaging software varies from site to site our conclusions may not be generally applicable.

In conclusion, our data suggest that excellent information regarding intramedullary high signal lesions of the unexpanded spinal cord may be obtained using ungated GRE sequences. This may allow us to dispense with the cardiac gated SE T2-weighted images in the routine evaluation of the cervical spine in myelopathy patients.

References

1. Takahashi M, Yamashita Y, Sakamoto Y, Kojima R (1989) Chronic cervical cord compression: clinical significance of increased signal intensity on MR images. Radiology 173: 219–224
2. Mehalic TF, Pezzuti RT, Appelbaum BI (1990) Magnetic resonance imaging and cervical spondylytic myelopathy. Neurosurgery 26: 217–227
3. De La Paz R (1990) Demyelinating disease of the spinal cord. In: Enzmann D, De La Paz R, Rubin JB (eds) Magnetic resonance of the spine. Mosby, St. Louis
4. Seidenwurm D, (1989) Degenerative disease of the cervical spine. Contemp Diagn Radiol 13: 1–6
5. Van Dyke C, Ross JS, Tkach J (1989) Gradient echo MR imaging of the cervical spine: evaluation of extradural disease. AJNR 10: 627–632
6. Masaryk TJ, Modic MT, Geisinger MT (1986) Cervical myelopathy: a comparison of magnetic resonance and myelopathy. J Comput Assist Tomogr 10: 184–194
7. Katz BH, Quencer RM, Hinks RS (1989) Comparison of gradient-recalled-echo and T-2 weighted spin echo pulse sequences in intramedullary spinal lesions. AJNR 10: 815–822
8. Hedberg MC, Drayer BP, Flom RA (1988) Gradient echo (GRASS) imaging in cervical radioculopathy. AJNR 9:145–151
9. Rubin JB, Enzmann DR, and Wright A (1987) CSF gated MRI of the spine: theory and clinical implemantation. Radiology 173: 784–791

Dr. Kevin Demarco
Post Box 0628
University of California, San Francisco
505 Parnassus Avenue
San Francisco, CA 94143, USA

Neuroradiology (1991) 33 [Suppl]: 545–547

Neuro-radiology

© Springer-Verlag 1991

Pial arteriovenous fistula of the brain

Y. Niimi[1], A. Berenstein[2], I. S. Choi[2], and K. Hirakawa[1]

[1] Department of Neurosurgery, Tokyo Medical and Dental University, Tokyo, Japan
[2] Department of Radiology, New York University Medical Center, New York, USA

Summary. We present 12 cases of arteriovenous fistula between pial arteries and cerebral veins (BAVFs) and have reviewed 34 additional cases in the literature. This type of fistula was frequently associated with venous ectasia and increased cerebrospinal fluid space. These lesions presented with congestive heart failure, macrocephaly, developmental delay, focal neurological deficits, headache or haemorrhage. Haemorrhage occurred in 6 out of 44 (13.6%) cases. This type of fistula should be recognized as a specific entity within the category of brain arteriovenous malformations. BAVFs should be treated either by embolization or surgery early after diagnosis to prevent irreversible deficits.

Key words: Arteriovenous malformation – Arteriovenous fistula – Embolization – Surgery – Cyanoacrylate

Intracranial arteriovenous malformations (AVMs) are usually composed of arterial feeders, nidus and draining veins. Purely fistulous malformations may also occur, most of which drain into dural sinuses or the vein of Galen. Very rarely, purely fistulous malformations between pial arteries and cerebral veins, that is, pial arteriovenous fistulas of the brain (BAVFs) can occur.

Materials and methods

Among more than 500 cases of brain AVM seen at New York University Medical Center between 1978 and 1990, there were 12 cases of BAVF. There were 4 males and 8 females. The age at presentation ranged from newborn to 19 years old. Clinical findings at the time of presentation are shown in Table 1. Loud objective bruit was audible in all 7 patients in whom auscultation findings were recorded. Only 5 out of 12 (41%) patients were neurologically normal at the time of treatment.

Results

CT and/or MRI were available for evaluation in 11 patients. Increased CSF space was found in 8 of these 11 patients. This probably indicated increased venous pressure or disturbance of cerebrospinal fluid (CSF) absorption. At angiography, a single fistula was demonstrated in 2 cases and multiple ones in 10. Venous ectasia was demonstrated in all cases but 1, the only asymptomatic patient. Ventriculoperitoneal shunt alone was performed in 1 case because of the poor condition of the patient. Another patient was treated only medically and was in good condition at 2.5 years follow up. One patient with a single fistula had surgery and was doing well 2 years later. Eight patients underwent endovascular embolization as the sole form of treatment. IBCA or NBCA was used in all patients as the embolic material. A detachable balloon was used in 2 cases in conjunction with acrylic. Complete obliteration of the fistula was obtained in 5 patients with production in 1 case of temporary dyslexia. In 2 patients, more than 80% closure was obtained, compilated 1 case by asymptomatic pulmonary embolism. One patient died of pulmonary embolism during embolization of

Table 1. Clinical presentation of BAVFs

Case no.	Age	Sex	Presentation	Associated findings
1	neonate	F	Klippel-Trenaunay-Weber Syndrome	cardiomegaly
2	4 M	M	Severe CHF	
3	6 D	F	CHF	Bruit
4	18 M	F	Developmental delay	Microcephaly, ataxia, bruit
5	2 D	M	Severe CHF	Hemiparesis, bruit
6	19 Y	F	ICH	Hemiparesis, aphasia, bruit
7	7 D	M	Mild CHF	Macrocephaly, bruit
8	6 D	F	IVH (multiple)	Macrocephaly
9	4 M	F	Macrocephaly	Bruit
10	2 Y	F	ICH	Developmental delay macrocephaly, hemiparesis seizure
11	10 Y	M	IVH	Bruit
12	9 Y	M	Epistaxis	Multiple capillary malformations of the skin AVM of nasal mucosa

Table 2. Treatment of BAVFs

	No. of cases	Complete closure	Mortality
Conservative[a]	8 (2)	–	5 (0)
Surgery (clipping or removal)	19 (1)	18 (1)	1 (0)
Embolization	12 (8)	9 (5)	1 (1)
Embolization and surgery	7 (1)	4 (1)	0 (0)

( ) Our own cases
No information about treatment was recorded in 2 cases from the literature. No permanent procedure-related morbidity was recorded
[a] Include shunt operation only; outcome is unknown on 1 patient

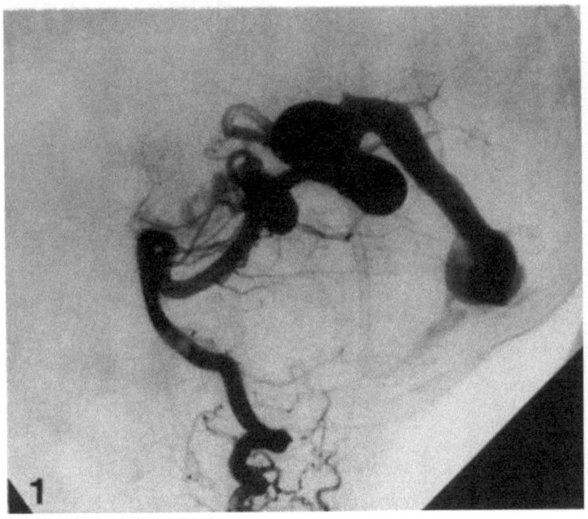

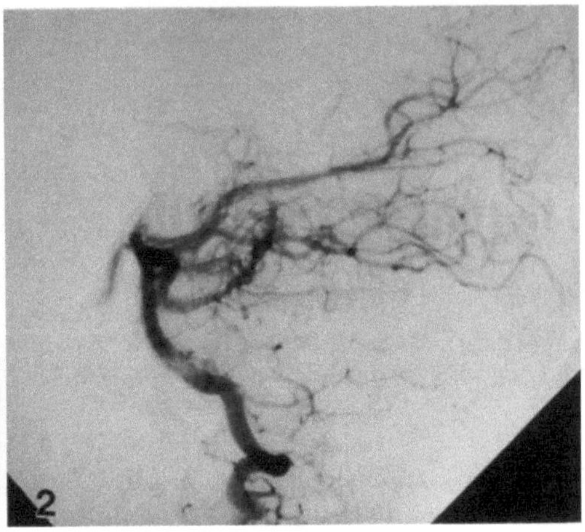

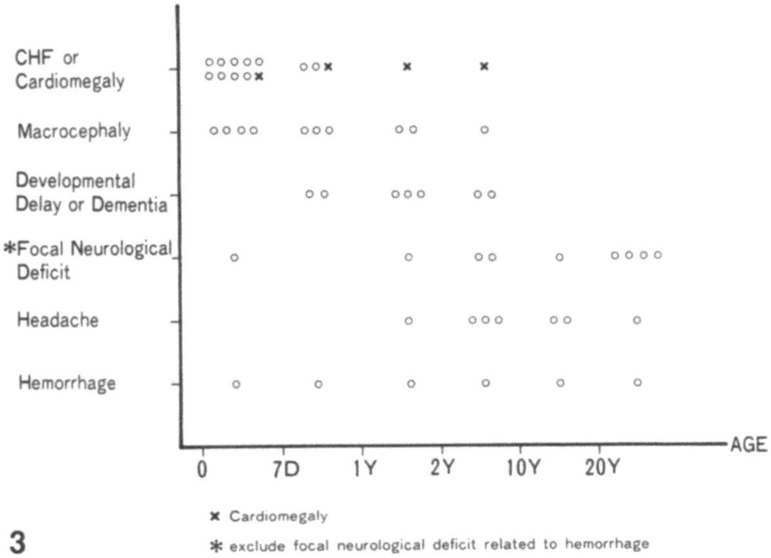

3

Fig. 1. Pre-embolization left vertebral artery angiogram demonstrates a single fistula between the right superior cerebellar artery and the right superior vermian vein

Fig. 2. Post-embolization angiogram shows complete obliteration of the fistula

Fig. 3. Congestive heart failure and macrocephaly are common among neonates. As the age of presentation increases, developmental delay or dementia, focal neurological deficit and headache increase in frequency. Haemorrhage occurs at any age

a large middle cerebral artery fistula. One patient underwent embolization followed by surgical clipping. This resulted in complete closure of the malformation.

Case report

A 4-month-old female presented with enlarging head circumference. She was otherwise neurologically intact. CT demonstrated enlarged subarachnoid space. Vertebral angiogram demonstrated a single fistula between right superior cerebellar artery and superior vermian vein, which then drained into the enlarged vein of Galen (Fig. 1). Complete obliteration of the fistula was obtained by embolization using NBCA (Fig. 2). The patient remained neurologically intact and did not require shunt. The patient was doing well 17 months later.

Discussion

Thirty-four cases of BAVFs have been reported in the literature, on which information about the fistula site by either angiogram or autopsy was available [1–4]. These cases were reviewed and analysed in combination with our own cases.

The patient's sex was recorded in 39 cases. There were 20 (51%) males and 19 (49%) females. The age of presentation was recorded in 43 cases. Single fistula was found in 19 (42%) cases and multiple ones in 26 (58%) cases. Arterial feeders could occur in any vascular territory, but were most common in the middle cerebral artery territory (27 out of 46 feeders: 59%).

Clinical symptoms at the time of presentation were correlated with the age at presentation (Fig. 3). Congestive heart failure and macrocephaly were common during the neonatal period. Developmental delay or dementia was common in infancy. As the age at presentation increased, focal neurological deficits including limb weakness and ataxia increased in number. These features are also seen in patients with vein of Galen fistulas or paediatric dural arteriovenous fistulas (AVFs). However, haemorrhage episodes occured, independent of age, in 6 of 44 (13.6%) cases. Vein of Galen fistulas or pediatric dural AVFs rarely present with haemorrhage.

A summary of the treatment is shown in Table 2. Mortality was high among conservatively treated cases. Most of these cases were very high flow fistulas presenting with severe congestive heart failure early after birth. The rate of complete obliteration of the malformation was high either by embolization or surgery. In addition, most of successfully treated patients also showed improvement or stabilization of their symptoms.

Clinical presentation of BAVFs shares many common features with other types of fistulous malformations, but haemorrhage appears to be more frequent. BAVFs can be treated relatively easily and successfully by embolization of surgery. These patients should be treated soon after diagnosis to prevent irreversible deficits.

References

1. Vinuela F, Drake CG, Fox AJ, Pelz DM (1987) Giant intracranial varices secondary to high flow arteriovenous fistulae, J Neurosurg 66: 198–203
2. Yasargil (1987) Microneurosurgery IIIA. Thieme, New York
3. Halbach VV, Higashida RT, Hieshima GB, Hardin CU, Dowd CF, Barnwell SL (1989) Transarterial occlusion of solitary intracranial arteriovenous fistulas. AJNR 10: 747–752
4. Barnwell SL, Ciricillo SF, Halbach VV, Edwards MS, Cogen PH (1990) Intracerebral arteriovenous fistulas associated with intraparenchymal varix in chilhood: case reports. Neurosurgery 26: 122–125

Dr. Y. Niimi
Department of Neurosurgery
Tokyo Medical and Dental University
1-5-45, Yushima Bunkyo-ku
Tokyo 113, Japan

Neuroradiology (1991) 33 [Suppl]: 548–549

Neuro radiology

© Springer-Verlag 1991

Anterior choroidal artery embolization in cerebral arteriovenous malformations

C. F. Dowd[1], V. V. Halbach[1, 2], S. L. Barnwell[1, 2], R. T. Higashida[1, 2], and G. B. Hieshima[1, 2]

Departments of [1] Radiology and [2] Neurological Surgery, University of California, San Francisco, California, USA

Summary. The anterior choroidal artery (AChA) is commonly recruited to supply arteriovenous malformations (AVMs) in the temporal lobe, basal ganglia, lateral ventricle, and internal capsule. Embolization of this artery is theoretically hazardous due to its supply to eloquent territory, lack of collaterals, and small caliber. However, this procedure can be a beneficial adjunct to surgery or radiation in the treatment of AVMs. We describe our experience in performing particulate embolization of AChA in 15 patients (16 procedures). Significant flow reduction was achieved in 14 patients. There were 4 complications, including permanent hemiparesis in 1 patient.

Key words: Choroidal arteries – Cerebral arteriovenous malformations – Brain hemorrhage – Cerebral blood vessels, therapeutic blockade – Cerebral embolization

---

The anterior choroidal artery (AChA) supplies the internal capsule, basal ganglia, medial temporal lobe, optic pathways, cerebral peduncle, and choroid plexus of the lateral ventricle [1]. This artery may be recruited to supply arteriovenous malformations (AVMs) which involve these structures. Embolization of the AChA can be a beneficial adjunct to surgery or radiation in the treatment of AVMs, but this procedure is theoretically hazardous because of eloquent territory supply, lack of collaterals, small AChA caliber, and abruptly angled AChA origin at the internal carotid artery (ICA). We report our results and complications in performing particulate embolization of the AChA in 15 patients with cerebral AVMs.

Patients and methods

Fifteen patients with cerebral AVMs underwent 16 embolization procedures involving the AChA, using a 3-2.2 F catheter (Target Therapeutics, San Jose, Calif., USA) and systemic anticoagulation. Embolic agents included polyvinyl alcohol particles (Interventional Therapeutics, South San Francisco, Calif., USA; and Pacific Medical Industries, La Mesa, Calif., USA) (15 cases) and platinum coils (Cook, Bloomington Ind., USA) (1 case). The procedure was aborted prior to embolization in 1 patient. Eight patients were embolized in preparation for surgical resection, 6 patients in preparation for radiation, and 1 patient as palliation.

Results

Significant reduction in flow to the AVM was achieved by AChA embolization in 14 patients (15 procedures) (Figs. 1, 2). Four complications included permanent hemiparesis (1 patient), transient mild hemiparesis (1 patient), and arterial perforation without neurological deficit (2 patients). The procedure was aborted prior to embolization in 1 of the patients who suffered a perforation.

Discussion

The microsurgical anatomy of the AChA has been well described [1–3]. Arising most commonly from the supraclinoid ICA, the AChA can be divided into two segments. The *cisternal* segment extends from the AChA origin to the choroidal fissure. Invariably, supply to eloquent territories originates in this segment. Regularly supplied structures include the internal capsule (posterior limb and retrolenticular portion), medial globus pallidus, cerebral peduncle, optic tract, and lateral geniculate body. Occasionally, the caudate tail, amygdala, thalamus, and hypothalamus recieve AChA supply. Infarction in this territory can be devastating, combining the triad of hemiplegia, hemianesthesia, and homonomous hemianopia in its complete form [4, 5]. The *plexal* segment begins anteriorly at the *plexal point,* where it enters the choroidal fissure to penetrate the choroid plexus of the temporal horn. The lateral posterior choroidal artery provides variable collateral supply.

The AChA can be recruited to supply AVMs involving these structures. Surgical access to such feeding arteries would be difficult because of their depth [6, 7]; therein lies the benefit of preoperative AChA embolization. Embolization of this artery could also complement radiosurgery by diminishing arteriovenous shunting, or provide palliation by obliterating a nidus aneurysm. In our series, angiographic decreased flow to the AVM was achieved in all but 1 patient, at the cost of a 25% complication rate (3 transient, 1 permanent complication in 16 procedures).

Careful particulate embolization of the AChA is possible, especially if the catheter tip is placed beyond the plexal point, as adjunctive therapy in the treatment of cerebral AVMs. However, the procedure is hazardous due to difficult catheterization and vascular supply to crucial territories.

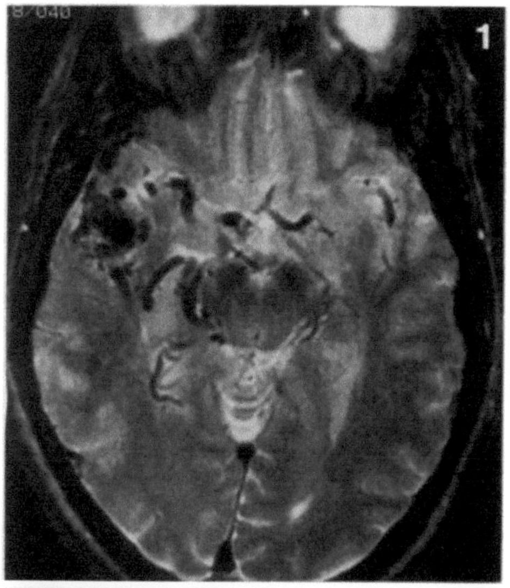

Fig. 1. A 52-year-old man with seizures. Axial SE 2800/80 MRI scan shows an arteriovenous malformation (AVM) in the right temporal lobe

Fig. 2 a–c. Sequential cerebral angiograms in the same patient as Fig. 1, anteroposterior projections. **a** Pre-embolization right internal carotid arteriogram shows right temporal lobe AVM, with anterior choroidal artery supply *(arrows)*. **b** Subselective right anterior choroidal arteriogram, midembolization, shows arteriovenous shunting. Note catheter tip position at the plexal point *(arrow)*. **c** Post polyvinyl alcohol embolization right internal carotid arteriogram shows diminished AVM supply with preservation of anterior choroidal artery *(arrows)*. Several middle cerebral feeding branches to the AVM were also embolized. The AVM was resected safely

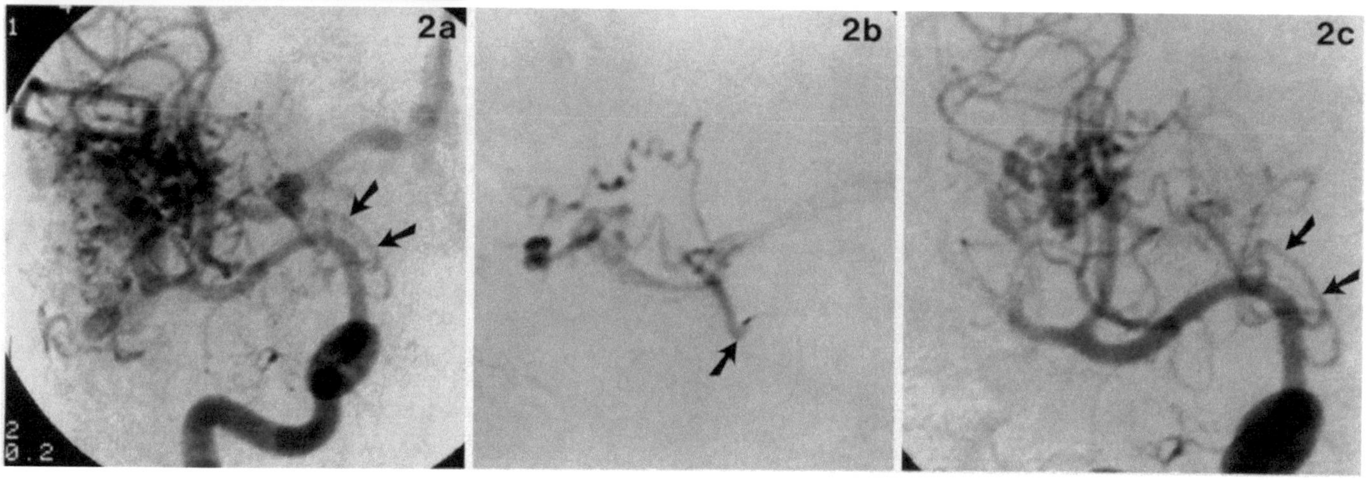

References

1. Rhoton AL, Fujii K, Fradd B (1979) Microsurgical anatomy of the anterior choroidal artery. Surg Neurol 12: 171–187
2. Herman LH, Fernando OU, Gurdjian ES (1966) The anterior choroidal artery: an anatomical study of its area of distribution. Anat Rec 154: 95–101
3. Paroni Sterbini GL, Mossuto Agatiello L, Stocchi A, Solivetti FM (1987) CT of ischemic infarctions in the territory of the anterior choroidal artery: a review of 28 cases. AJNR 8: 229–232
4. Decroix JP, Graveleau P, Masson M, Cambier J (1986) Infarction in the territory of the anterior choroidal artery: a clinical and computerized tomographic study of 16 cases. Brain 109: 1071–1085
5. Helgason CM (1988) A new view of anterior choroidal artery territory infarction. J Neurol 235: 387–391
6. Heros RC (1982) Arteriovenous malformations of the medial temporal lobe: surgical approach and neuroradiological characterization. J Neurosurg 56: 44–52
7. Fujita K, Matsumoto S (1984) Anterior choroidal artery arteriovenous malformation: its clinical manifestations and surgical treatment. Surg Neurol 21: 347–352

Dr. C. F. Dowd
Neuroradiology, L-352
University of California Medical Center
505 Parnassus Avenue
San Francisco, CA 94143-0628, USA

Neuroradiology (1991) 33 [Suppl]: 550–552

Neuro-radiology
© Springer-Verlag 1991

Treatment of dural arteriovenous fistulas involving the transverse and sigmoid sinuses by transvenous embolization: results in 20 patients

V. V. Halbach, R. T. Higashida, C. F. Dowd, S. L. Barnwell, and G. B. Hieshima

Department of Radiology, Neurointerventional Section, University of California, San Francisco, California, USA

Summary. Obliteration of symptomatic dural fistulas involving the sigmoid and transverse sinuses by transvenous embolization has been performed in selected cases at our institution since 1986. We report the results of this new treatment in 20 patients who underwent this procedure.

Key words: Embolization – Dural fistulas – Dural arteriovenous malformations – Transvenous – Coils

Twenty patients with symptomatic dural fistulas involving the transverse or sigmoid sinuses, all with venous occlusive changes, were treated by transvenous embolization. The mean age at the time of treatment was 48.8 years; the fistula occurred on the left in 12, on the right in 8. The transverse sinus was involved in 9, the transverse and sigmoid in 8, and the sigmoid sinus alone in 3. Eleven patients underwent surgical exposure of the involved sinus with direct placement of liquid adhesive or coils into the sinus. The remaining 8 patients underwent the treatment from a transfemoral venous access.

Results

Eleven patients had complete cure: complete angiographic obliteration with resolution of symptoms. Seven patients have had greater than 95% reduction in the fistula, 6 remain symptom free. Two patients, early in the series, had 40% and 50% reduction in fistula size, with modest improvement in symptoms. There were three transient complications, two asymptomatic perforations (sealed immediately with coils), and one temporal lobe hemorrhagic infarct, probably related to the use of epsilon amino caproic acid. The follow-up period ranged from 2 to 38 months with a mean of 20.6 months.

Case report

A 70-year-old female developed unilateral headaches and left-sided bruit. An arteriogram demonstrated a dural fistula involving the left sigmoid sinus supplied primarily from the occipital (Fig. 1 a), posterior auricular, and dural branches of the internal carotid and vertebral arteries. The venous drainage was primarily to dilated cortical veins (Fig. 1 b). A transfemoral venous access was utilized to place a 4.1 Fr microcatheter into the involved sigmoid sinus at the proximal end of the fistula site and a venogram confirmed the drainage to the cortical veins. Embolization of the occipital arterial supply was performed with polyvinyl alcohol particles. Multiple steel coils with Dacron fibers were deposited into the fistula site to produce complete fistula occlusion (Fig. 1 c, d). Twenty-one months following the procedure the patient remains symptom free.

Discussion

Dural fistulas are unusual arteriovenous connections between dural arteries and dural sinuses. The earliest attempts at treatment consisted of feeder artery ligation, which proved ineffective secondary to the recruitment of dural collaterals [1]. Surgical resection of a dural sinus involved with a dural fistula can be performed in many cases but massive hemorrhage can occur secondary to the plethora of small arterial feeders in the region of the fistula site [2]. In addition, surgical resection of a functioning dural sinus can be associated with venous infarction. Transarterial embolization has emerged as an effective treatment of many dural fistulas. Our own results with transarterial embolization have shown that although many patients improve, complete cure can be difficult [3]. Following subtotal occlusion of a dural fistula, recruitment from dural branches that arise from the internal and vertebral artery may occur, which are difficult and often dangerous to embolize [4]. Unlike the dural fistula counterparts in the cavernous sinus region, transverse and sigmoid sinus fistulas can present with severe signs and symptoms including subarachnoid and intracerebral hemorrhage, dementia, stroke, hydrocephalus, and increased intracranial pressure. These severe sequelae are often directly correlated with the venous drainage of the fistula. Patients who exhibit cortical venous drainage from the involved dural sinus having the most severe signs and symptoms. In an attempt to develop a safer technique for the treatment of these high-risk dural fistulas, those which exhibit cortical venous drainage, we have adapted a technique first described by Mullen [5] where thrombogenic material is placed directly involved with

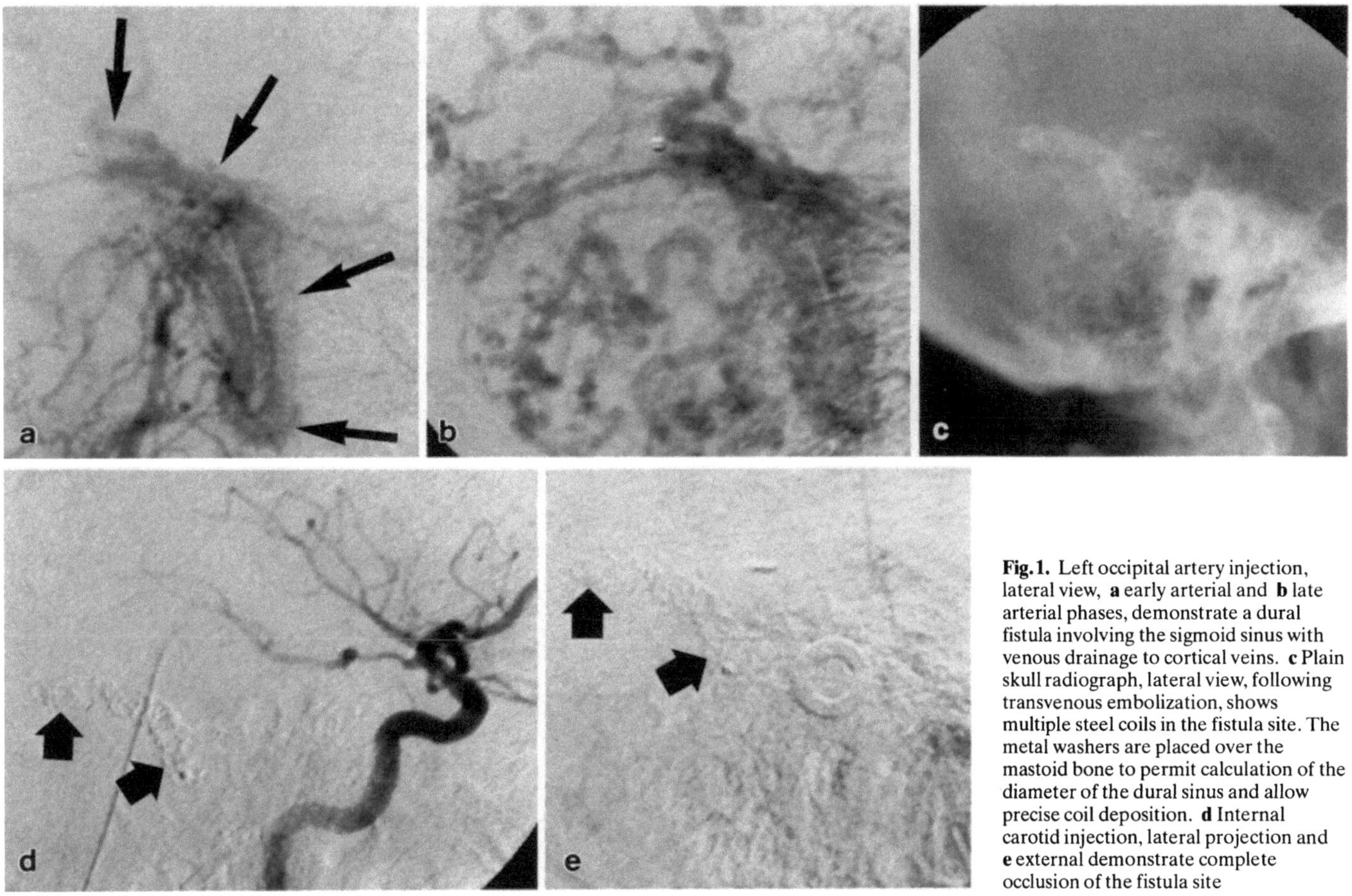

Fig. 1. Left occipital artery injection, lateral view, **a** early arterial and **b** late arterial phases, demonstrate a dural fistula involving the sigmoid sinus with venous drainage to cortical veins. **c** Plain skull radiograph, lateral view, following transvenous embolization, shows multiple steel coils in the fistula site. The metal washers are placed over the mastoid bone to permit calculation of the diameter of the dural sinus and allow precise coil deposition. **d** Internal carotid injection, lateral projection and **e** external demonstrate complete occlusion of the fistula site

the fistula in order to produce thrombosis and occlusion of the fistula site. Our technique utilized small microcatheters placed from a transvenous route, either from a femoral venous access or surgical exposure [6]. Our earliest experience involved isolating a sinus by disconnecting all the draining veins and then injection of liquid adhesives directly into the dural sinus. This technique proved undesirable because it involved the direct exposure of the dural sinus and allowed the passage of the embolic material into unwanted drainage pathways. Platinum and steel coils have emerged as an effective and safer embolic material that can produce the desired occlusion without the risk of migration if appropriately sized and positioned. These can be introduced through a small catheter through a dural sinus puncture away from the fistula site. The advent of more thrombogenic coils available in a variety of sizes and shapes had permitted the treatment of a wide variety of dural fistulas in these locations.

Patient selection is essential as several severe complications can occur that are unique to this form of therapy. If inadequate coils are positioned in the dural sinus then subtotal occlusion can occur. If the segment of sinus is inadequately filled with embolic material then diversion of the remaining dural fistula into cortical veins can occur. Transvenous embolization should only be undertaken if the segment of the sinus to be occluded had venous drainage away from the sinus and the sinus itself is no longer a conduit for cerebral venous drainage. In other words, the arterialized pressure in the sinus must be elevated enough to permit reversal of flow away from the sinus. This segment of sinus is no longer functional and can be removed surgically or obliterated by transvenous embolization. If a functional sinus is resected or occluded then there is the risk of producing a venous infarction.

Conclusion

Patient selection is essential for this new treatment; only patients with cortical drainage and absence of normal antegrade venous drainage should be treated by this technique. Recent development of supple delivery catheters and more thrombogenic coils have allowed increased safety and higher cure rates. Coils have several advantages over other embolic agents. Transvenous embolization is an effective treatment for selected patients with high-risk dural fistulas involving the lateral sinuses.

References

1. Kerber CW, Newton TH (1973) Macro and micro vasculature of the dura matter. Neuroradiology 6: 175–179
2. Sundt TM, Piepgras DG (1983) The surgical approach to arteriovenous malformations of the lateral and sigmoid dural sinuses. J Neurosurg 59: 32–39

3. Halbach VV, Higashida RT, Hieshima GB, Goto K, Norman D, Newton TH (1987) Dural fistulas involving the transverse and sigmoid sinuses. Results in 28 patients. Radiology 163: 443–447
4. Halbach VV, Higashida RT, Hieshima GB, Hardin C (1989) Embolization of branches arising from the cavernous portion of the internal carotid artery. AJNR 10: 143–150
5. Mullan S (1979) Treatment of carotid cavernous fistulas by cavernous sinus thrombosis. J Neurosurg 50: 131–144
6. Halbach VV, Higashida RT, Hieshima GB, Mehringer CM, Hardin C (1989) Transvenous embolization of dural fistulas involving the transverse and sigmoid sinuses. AJNR 10: 385–392

Dr. Van V. Halbach
Department of Radiology, Neurointerventional Section
University of California, San Francisco Hospitals, L-352
505 Parnassus Avenue
San Francisco, CA 94143, USA

Neuroradiology (1991) 33 [Suppl]: 553–554

Neuro-radiology
© Springer-Verlag 1991

NMR follow-up protocol for arteriovenous malformations treated by endovascular techniques and gamma knife

L. Lemme-Plaghos, O. Zamboni, R. Re, and H. Bunge

Buenos Aires Gamma Knife Centre, Clínica del Sol, Buenos Aires, Argentina

Summary. MRI with fast low-angle shots (FLASH) to show flow enhancement phenomena was used in a research protocol to identify evolution of embolised and stereotactically irradiated arteriovenous malformations. Cine-MR with FLASH sequences allows evaluation of pulsatile mass effects, adding a new parameter in the follow-up of these lesions. Experience in the first seven selected cases studied by this new MR protocol is reported.

Key words: Nuclear magnetic resonance – Arteriovenous malformation – Embolization – Radiosurgery

In a series of 20 patients with brain arteriovenous malformations (AVMs) treated sequentially by superselective embolisation and gamma knife radiosurgery, follow-up was by CT, regular NMR and periodic angiograms. Seven underwent research MRI with fast low-angle shot (FLASH) images using a 1.5 T Magneton. Different flip angles, TRs and TEs were used; the flip 10, TR 0.05 sec, TE 13 ms sequences being the best in showing flow enhancement phenomena. All series were obtained with cine-MR, which consists of a movie loop of sequential FLASH images gated to the cardiac cycle, in which flowing blood has high intensity while turbulent flow showed signal loss during systole (Fig. 1). Cine-MR could distinguish haemosiderin from previous bleeding from flowing blood as well as thrombus in draining veins, which demonstrated variable signal intensity not changing during the cardiac cycle (Fig. 2). Pulsatile mass effect in the AVM nidus and draining veins was perfectly assessed in all cases.

Discussion

In patients treated sequentially with embolization and gamma knife radiosurgery, conventional follow-up has the disadvantages of hyperdense artefacts in CT which

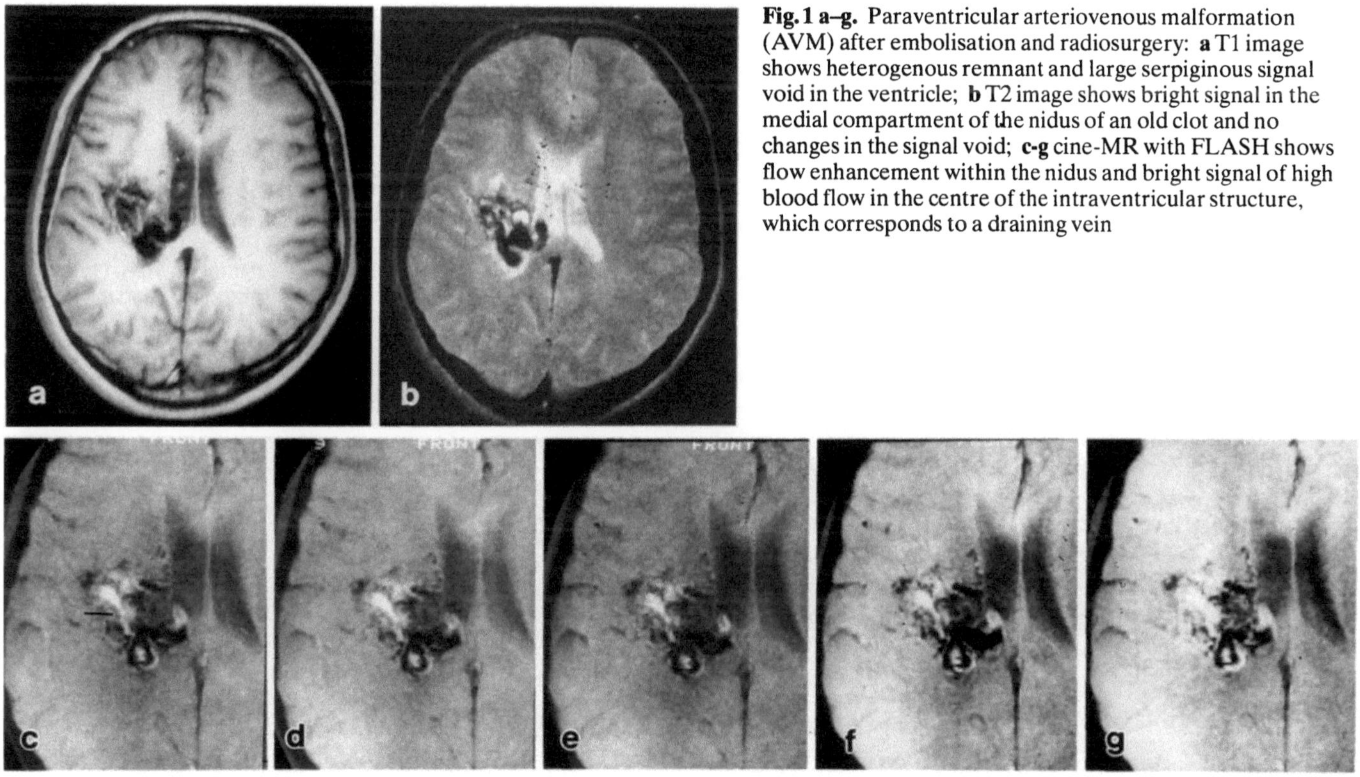

Fig. 1 a–g. Paraventricular arteriovenous malformation (AVM) after embolisation and radiosurgery: **a** T1 image shows heterogenous remnant and large serpiginous signal void in the ventricle; **b** T2 image shows bright signal in the medial compartment of the nidus of an old clot and no changes in the signal void; **c-g** cine-MR with FLASH shows flow enhancement within the nidus and bright signal of high blood flow in the centre of the intraventricular structure, which corresponds to a draining vein

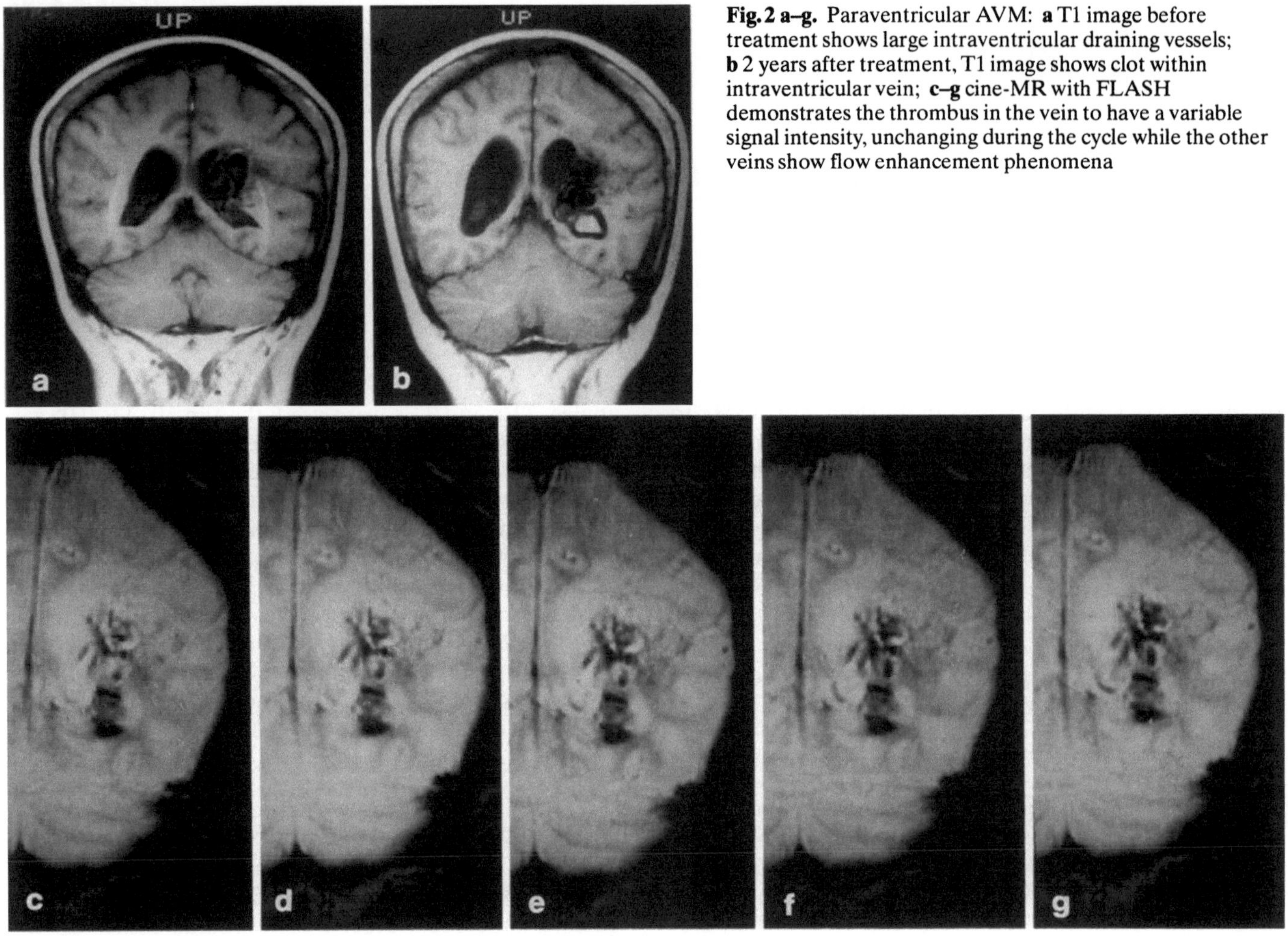

Fig. 2 a–g. Paraventricular AVM: **a** T1 image before treatment shows large intraventricular draining vessels; **b** 2 years after treatment, T1 image shows clot within intraventricular vein; **c–g** cine-MR with FLASH demonstrates the thrombus in the vein to have a variable signal intensity, unchanging during the cycle while the other veins show flow enhancement phenomena

may mask the progressive occlusion of the nidus of the AVM, but standard T1- and T2-weighted images are not enough to identify haemodynamic changes within the area of interest.

Although subtraction angiography remains the only way to assess complete obliteration of the treated AVM, we have found that non-conventional MRI sequences such as FLASH may add useful information about the high flow in remaining pathological vessels, which may be differentiated from haemosiderin and calcification (Fig. 1). Turbulent flow shows other signal characteristics [1] and slow flowing blood may be identified through echo-rephasing phenomena [2], making possible the evaluation of flow changes in all large vessels, an indirect sign of the evolution of the AVM. Cine-MR adds the possibility of evaluating pulsatile mass effect [3] which can provide new indirect evidence of progressive change in the AVM (Fig. 2).

The protocol described fulfils basic requirements of the follow-up of sequentially treated AVMs, although much research is required before it may be established as the definitive examination to replace conventional angiography.

References

1. Needell WM, Maravilla K (1988) MR flow in imaging in vascular malformations using gradient recalled acquisition. AJNR 9: 637–642
2. Kucharczyk W, Brant-Zawadski M, Lemme-Plaghos L (1985) MR technology; effect of even-echo rephasing on calculated T2 values and T2 images. Radiology 157: 95–101
3. Tsueusa JS, Halbach VV, Highashida RT (1988) MR evaluation of large intracranial aneurysm using cine low flip angle gradient refocused imaging. AJNR 9: 4–15

Dr. L. Lemme-Plaghos
Centro de Radiocirugía
Clínica del Sol
Arenales 1468
1061 Buenos Aires
Argentina

Neuroradiology (1991) 33 [Suppl]: 555–557

Neuro
radiology
© Springer-Verlag 1991

Detachable balloon treatment of direct caroticocavernous fistulae

R. Tolun, S. Bahar, and O. Çoban

Department of Neuroradiology, Istanbul University, Istanbul Medical Faculty, Istanbul, Turkey

Summary. Fifteen cases of direct caroticocavernous fistulae (CCFs) were treated with Debrun detachable balloons between 1983 and 1989. Excluding the first 2 cases, when we were still unfamiliar with the technique, balloon detachments were successful in occluding the fistula while preserving flow in the parent artery in 11 of the remaining cases. Only one balloon was detached to occlude the fistula in each case, except one which had two tears. All four patients having neurological complications recovered totally: these were two cases of ocular motor nerve palsy, one case of hemiparesis, and one case of convulsions. Hemiparesis was due to an embolic cortical infarction. Convulsions were due to the breakdown of blood-brain barrier as a result of an excessive amount of iodinated contrast medium injected into the carotid artery of an 8-year-old child, each of whose two tears was occluded by a balloon in the same session. Results in our small series confirm the widely accepted detachable balloon treatment of direct CCFs as the method of choice.

Key words: Caroticocavernous fistula – Contralateral exophthalmos – Detachable balloon – Blood-brain barrier breakdown

Detachable balloon treatment of caroticocavernous fistulae (CCFs), introduced by Serbinenko and pioneered in Europe by Debrun has become the treatment of choice in the last decade [1–3]. We found it worthwhile to report our experience from a developing country on this subject of interventional neuroradiology.

Patients and methods

Between 1983 and 1989, 15 cases of direct CCFs were treated by the detachable balloon system of Debrun, developed for the cervical approach [1].

There were 9 males and 6 females. Three were children aged 8,8 and 10 years. The oldest patient was a 75 year old female.

After the first 3 patients, a 14-gauge catheter needle was preferred instead of the large and stiff introducer. Control angiograms were done in 10 patients, 5–190 days after embolization. Clinical follow-up of the patients was between 1 month and 3 years.

Results

Clinical and angiographic findings, as well as the results of treatment are summarized in Table 1.

Table 1. Clinical and angiographic findings, and treatment results of 15 cases of direct caroticocavernous fistulae

					Symptoms and signs					Angiographic findings												Complications					
Patient no.	Age (years)	Sex	Trauma	Side	Proptosis	Cranial nerve palsy	Visual loss	Bruit	Headache	Fistula site*	CS varix	SOV	IPS	SPS	ICS	PP	SV	PFV	Final treatment	Fistula occluded	Carotid preserved	Cranial nerve palsy	Hemiparesis	Convulsions	Control angiography (days later)	False aneurysm (diameter in mm)	Cure
1	33	M	+	L	+	±	+	+	+	4		+	+		+				S	+	–				–		+
2	8	M	–	L	+	–	–	+		3		+							S	+	–				–		+
3	18	M	+	L	+	3,6	+	+		3		+	+	+	+			+	E	+	+				35	10	+
4	46	M	+	L	+	±	+	+	+	5		+		+	+			+	E	+	+	+			18	5	+
5	38	M	+	L	+	6	–	+		4		+	+						S	+	–				–		+
6	8	F	±	L	+	3,6	+	+		3,5		+	+						E	+	+			+	30	6	+
7	37	F	–	R	+	3,6	–	+	+	3	+		+						E	+	+				7	–	+
8	22	M	+	L	+	3,6	+	+		3		+			+				E	+	+				190	8	+
9	46	F	+	L	+	3,6	+	+	+	5		+	+		+	+			E	?	+				7	–	+
10	75	F	–	R	+	3,6	+	+	+	3		+							E	+	+				–		+
11	20	M	+	R	+	6	+	+		4		+	+	+	+	+	+	+	E	+	+	+			5	7	+
12	32	F	+	R	+	±	–	+		3	+	+	+	+				+	E	+	+				8	3	+
13	28	M	+	R	+	±	–	+		5		+	+	+	+	+			E	+	+				45	4	+
14	10	M	±	L	+	–	–	+		2		+	+						–	–	+				–		–
15	47	F	–	R	+	–	+	+	+	2		+	+		+	+			E	+	+		+		120	12	+

+, Present; –, absent; ±, unclear; ?, temporarily opened; *, segment of the intracavernous carotid artery (1);
CS, cavernous sinus; SOV, superior ophthalmic vein; IPS, inferior petrosal sinus; SPS, superior petrosal sinus; ICS, intercavernous sinus; PP, pterygoid plexus; SV, Sylvian vein; PFV, posterior fossa veins; S, surgery; E, embolization with detachable balloon

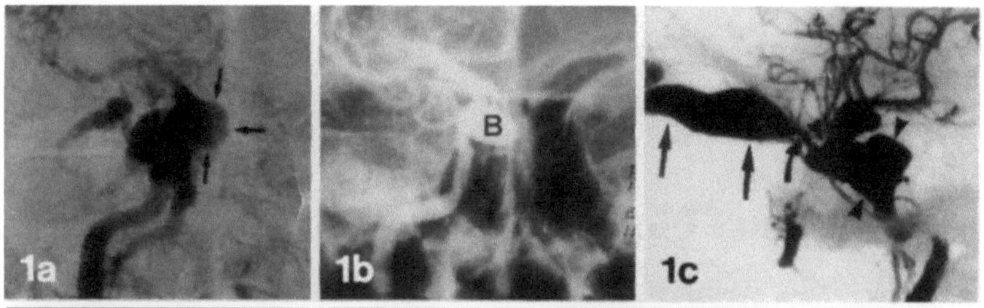

Fig. 1 a, b. Patient 7. **a** Cavernous sinus varix reaching midsellar region. **b** After balloon embolization. Patient 10. Tight stenosis *(curved arrow)* of superior ophthalmic vein *(arrows)*, caroticocavernous fistulae *(arrowheads)*

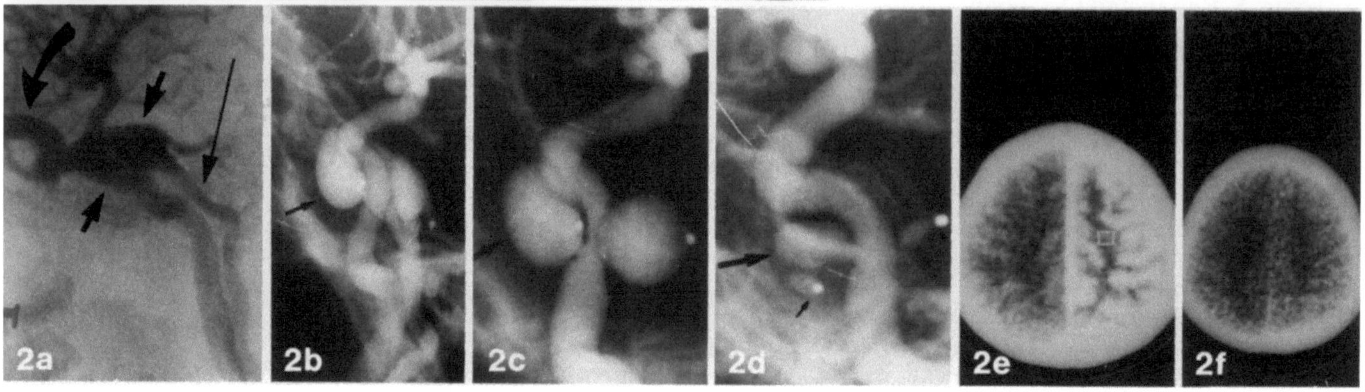

Fig. 2 a–f. Patient 6. **a** Caroticocavernous fistula (CCF; *arrows*), superior ophthalmic vein *(curved arrow)*, inferior petrosal sinus *(long arrow)*. **b** Occlusion of anterior part of CCF with the first balloon *(arrow)*. **c** Total occlusion of the CCF after detachment of the second balloon; and compressed carotid artery. **d** False aneurysm *(arrow)* only at the second fistula site a month later, and deflated *(small arrows)* balloons. **e** CT demonstrating intense gyral enhancement. **f** Contrast-enhanced CT 3 days later

Discussion

The natural history of CCFs is little known [2]. Trauma is known to be the major cause of direct CCFs [1–3]. It may seem peculiar that only 9 out of our 15 cases had definite trauma. Four patients had no history of trauma whatsoever. The remaining 2 children (patients 6,14) had a history of knitting needle injury below the eye ipsilateral to the fistula a few weeks before symptoms began. If they are to be accepted as traumatic cases, minor trauma should be searched for as a possible cause in similar cases. Among the spontaneous cases, symptoms began during pregnancy at the 6th month in patient 7 with arterial hypertension, and while straining in stool in patient 15.

Patient 4 had proptosis contralateral to the fistula side. This is a rarely reported finding of CCFs [3].

Fistula site was almost precisely demonstrated either by vertebral angiography or ipsilateral carotid angiography with ipsilateral carotid compression in both cases.

Patient 12 had a medially projecting cavernous sinus (CS) varix reaching the midsellar region (Fig. 1 a, b). A tight stenosis was present in the superior ophthalmic vein which was the only drainage pathway of the elderly patient 10 (Fig. 1 c). It may be speculated that spontaneous occlusion could have cured this patient.

If we exclude the first two 2 cases which were treated when we were unfamiliar with the system, balloon occlusion of the fistula was successful in 11 of the 13 patients. It was not possible to enter the fistula in patients 5 and 14. The transvenous route failed in patient 5.

One balloon was sufficient to occlude the fistula in all the cases, except patient 6 whose fistula had two tears. Debrun states that 2 of 54 patients had evidence of two rents [1]. In our case with two tears, a girl aged 8 years, each was occluded with a balloon. Although the internal carotid artery was compressed between the two balloons, it was possible to inflate them optimally to occlude the fistula while preserving the carotid flow (Fig. 2 a–d).

Four neurological complications occurred in this series, and all totally recovered. A sixth cranial nerve palsy in patient 11 recovered in 2–3 months. Ocular motor nerve palsies due to treatment were reported in 20% of the 54 cases of Debrun et al. [1].

Patient 6 experienced repeated right-sided convulsions and hemiparesis, which began just after recovering from anaesthesia for the treatment, both clearing totally in 3 days. As will be remembered, this was the only case with two tears.

Occlusion of both tears during the same procedure took 3 h, and about 200 cc iodinated contrast medium were injected into the left carotid artery during this time. We unfortunately somewhat later realized that this was a mistake, although the outcome was positive. Immediate CT showed intense gyral enhancement in the left hemisphere pointing to the presence of blood-brain barrier breakdown due to the injection of excessive contrast medium (Fig. 2 e, f.)

Patient 15 had a cortical infarction leading to left hemiparesis due to breaking off the 2 F Teflon catheter during detachment. The balloon deflated and migrated back into the carotid siphon. Hemiparesis cleared in 20 days, and the CCF was successfully occluded with a balloon.

One other complication, a technical one, occurred in patient 12. A successfully detached balloon deflated totally the next day, and she was symptomatic again. Angiography 45 days later showed occlusion of the anterior part of the CS, and restriction of the previous multiple drainage pathways to only the inferior petrosal sinus. Balloon detachment this time was successful.

Balloon deflations, generally discerned about a week later, occurred within 1–2 months.

False aneurysms with mean diameters of 3–12 mm were observed in 8 of the 10 patients who had control angiograms.

It is generally accepted that spontaneous cures are much more frequent in indirect CCFs than in direct ones. Recently, it has been reported that carotid compression therapy was successful in closure of 17% of direct and 30% of indirect CCFs [2].

Clinical signs and symptoms, and angiographic features associated with increased morbidity and mortality of CCFs are analysed in one large series [2]. Cortical venous drainage, CS varix, epistaxis or declining visual acuity were accepted as features necessitating urgent treatment.

No fatalities occurred in our patients, including the ones who had cavernous sinus varix or cortical venous drainage.

Our results from a small series support the widely accepted detachable balloon treatment of direct CCFs as the method of choice.

References

1. Debrun G, Lacour P, Vinuela F, Fox A, Drake CG, Caron JP (1981) Treatment of 54 traumatic carotid-cavernous fistulas. J Neurosurg 55: 678–692
2. Halbach VV, Hieshima GB, Higashida RT, Reicher M (1987) Carotid cavernous fistulae: indications for urgent treatment. AJNR 8: 627–633
3. Théron J, Olivier A, Melançon D, Ethier R (1985) Left carotico-cavernous fistula with right exophthalmos: treatment by detachable balloon. Neuroradiology 27: 349–353

R. Tolun, M. A.
Istanbul Medical Faculty
Department of Neuradiology
Istanbul, Turkey

Neuroradiology (1991) 33 [Suppl]: 558–559

Neuro radiology
© Springer-Verlag 1991

Embolization therapy and pathological study of intracranial arteriovenous malformations*

L. Feng[1], H. Kewei[2], L. Shushan[1], and D. Guosheng[1]

Departments of [1] Neurosurgery and [2] Neuropathology, The Great Wall Hospital, Beijing, China

Summary. This paper presents 74 embolized cases among the 163 cases of arteriovenous malformation (AVM) treated during the last 3 years in our department. Twenty-six patients were cured or almost cured (15 were operated upon after embolization); 14 regained normal life but still kept a partially reduced AVM; 23 showed marked improvement; 5 showed no change; 6 suffered deterioration, caused in 4 by complications during embolization; 2 died (1 after operation). The causes of AVM bleeding, embolization techniques supportive treatment before and after embolization are discussed.

Key words: Embolization – Arteriovenous malformation – Pathology

In the last 20 years there have been significant advances in the treatment of large arteriovenous malformations (AVMs) due to the developments in microneurosurgery, neuroradiology and neuroanaesthesia [1–3]. The development of interventional neuroradiology and improved techniques of artificial embolization have made a particular contribution to the study on angioarchitecture, haemodynamics and the methods and materials of embolization techniques in AVM [4, 5]. Based on 163 cases of intracranial AVM treated in our department in the last 3 years, this article presents a thorough clinical analysis of 74 cases embolized with IBCA and histomorphological study.

Materials and methods

The study material comprises 163 cases of intracranial AVM treated between April 1986 and December 1989, all diagnosed by cerebral angiography. Embolization was carried out in 74 cases altogether involving 134 sessions. Twenty-two patients underwent operative resection after embolization. The location of AVM in 74 cases was as follows: dural arteriovenous fistula (DAVF) in 10, dural cerebral AVM in 12, aneurysm of Galen in 3, motor area in 11, frontal in 8, temporal in 9, parieto-occipital in 4, corpus callosum in 2, basal ganglia in 8, posterior fossa in 6, intraorbital in 1. The following catheter techniques were employed: (1) calibrated leak balloon catheter [6]; (2) Rufenacht no balloon hyperselective cathetherization [7]; (3) Magic catheter; (4) detachable balloon technique [8]; (5) self-improved catheter by this author. We have modified the above catheters. The materials include (1) 16-gauge needle; (2) 3.6 F catheter; (3) fine steel wire; (4) Pursil catheter. In the manipulation method, a 16-gauge needle is used to puncture the carotid artery; the Pursil catheter, which is coaxially inside the 3.6 F catheter is introduced through the outer tube of the 16-gauge needle. The fine steel wire is threaded into the Pursil catheter, taking case not to let it protrude, to facilitate its movement and is pulled out when the 3.6 F catheter has entered the outer tube of the 16-gauge needle. Then the Pursil catheter is manipulated forwards, led by the 3.6 F catheter and hyperselective catheterization is conducted. The coaxial catheters may have different curve degrees for optimum use. This method is particularly suitable for the basal ganglia, where AVMs are supplied by multiple arteries. Because there is no complicated hydro-pressure driving system and both the travel distance and Pursil catheter are short, the catheter can be used for embolization of several arteries at one go. This means less discarded catheters, an easier approach and reduced cost.

The embolization materials used were mainly IBCA with small amounts of dura mater or Ivalon.

A histopathological study was conducted on the correlation of the vessel wall structure with bleeding. The specimens taken during the 25 AVM operative resections were fixed with 10% formalin, regularly sampled, embedded in wax, H&E stained and observed under an Opton optic microscope coupled with a computerized Kontron image analyser. Of these the 25 cases, 19 had as the main manifestation haemorrhage, 6 headache and epilepsy. The age of the haemorrhage group ranged from 6 to 51, that of the nonhaemorrhage group from 18 to 54, with an average age of 34.8 years.

The image observed under the optical microscope was loaded into the computer and displayed on the monitor screen. A study was conducted on the correlation of the thickness and structure of the vessels with patient age and haemorrhagic state in the haemorrhagic and nonhaemorrhagic groups. All data obtained by computer in this group were subjected to *t*-test and chi-square tests of significance.

Results

Results of computer analysis of vessel walls of the AVM

A total of 229 vessels from 25 cases were examined. The vessel wall thickness in the haemorrhage group was 34.8–103.56 μm, and in the nonhaemorrhage group 61.95–168.29 μm ($t = 4.125$; $P < 0.001$). A regional comparison of the average vessel wall thickness is shown in Table 1.

Table 1. Group comparison of vessel wall thickness

Group (μm)	17–92.75	92.76–168.5	168.6–244.25	244.26–320
Haemorrhage	147 (83.97)	21 (12.14)	4 (2.31)	1 (0.58)
Nonhaemorrhage	18 (32.14)	28 (50.00)	6 (10.71)	4 (7.14)

χ^2 test: $\chi = 65.54$; $P < 0.001$

* Received a Symposium Fellowship Award (Honorable Mention)

Table 2. Angiographic results of embolization

Imaging results	Embolization only (%)	Operation post-embolization (%)	Total (%)
Anatomical cure	12 (16.2)	15 (20.4)	27 (36.6)
Improvement 80%	5 (6.8)	1 (1.3)	6 (8.1)
50–80%	13 (17.6)	4 (5.4)	17 (23.0)
50%	22 (29.7)		22 (29.7)
Death	1 (1.3)	1 (1.3)	2 (2.6)
Total	53 (71.6)	21 (28.4)	74 (100)

Table 3. Complications of embolization

Causes	No.	CNS disturbance	present condition
Perilesion vasospasm	3	Transient weakness	Recovered
Thrombosis	1	Hemiplegia, aphasia	Recovered
Normal branch embolized	1	Diplopia, somnolence	Recovered
Catheter knotted	1	Hemiplegia	Monoplegia
Balloon escape	1	Hemiplegia	Monoplegia
Bled by catheter traction	1	Hemiplegia, aphasia	Recovered
Bled by balloon rupture	3	Coma	1 Monoplegia 1 Vegetative 1 Death

Clinical results of embolization

Out of 74 patients, 26 were cured or almost cured (15 of whom were operated after embolization); 14 cases regained normal life but still with a remnant of AVM; 23 (3 of them were operated on after embolization) showed marked improvement such as epilepsy reduction in 8 cases, muscle power elevation by two grades in 10 cases, intracranial bruit reduction in 5 cases; 5 cases showed no change; 6 cases suffered deterioration, caused in 4 cases by complications during embolization; 2 died (1 after operation). The results of angiography are shown in Table 2, whilst Table 3 lists the complications that occurred.

Discussion

Exploration and revelation of the causes of AVM bleeding

Our results show that AVM vessels lack the integrity of normal arteries and veins. Though malformed vessels are different in size and thickness, each case shows a general trend in the scale of vessel thickness. The test demonstrates that the average thickness in those who have a clinical record of bleeding is 94.01 μm, while that of non-haemorrhagic patients is 151.06 μm ($P < 0.001$). Of the haemorrhagic group 84.97% have a wall thickness below 100 μm, whereas this is true of only 32.4% in the non-haemorrhagic group. This creates a foundation for further histopathological study of AVM bleeding.

Analysis of the treatment effects in this group

Table 3 demonstrates that in the 74 cases of embolization treatment in this group, deep and posterior fossa AVM occupies a higher proportion and poses more difficulties in treatment; yet the rate of anatomic cure is by no means lower than the others. The reasons are as follows:

1. Flexible and skilful application of different catheter techniques to suit various lesion locations can increase the effectiveness of treatment. Different catheters have their own respective merits and disadvantages in the specific spheres of application. To stick to one kind only will definitely bring about restrictions on its use.
2. A meticulous study of the AVM's haemodynamic changes shown on the angiograms should be carried out before and after embolization.
3. The most serious complication is rupture of the nidus by the balloon, which constitutes the main cause of mortality in other groups. Once a rupture occurs, effective rescue measures are vital for the prognosis. Three such cases were seen in this group; 2 were in deep coma with temporary cessation of breathing and heart beat. Emergency intubation was performed and immediate craniotomy, to produce subtemporal decompression as well as ventricular drainage. After positive rescue efforts, 1 patient has recovered to live a basically independent life with slight aphasia and monoplegia; 1 patient is in a vegetative state and 1 has died.
4. Spasm or occlusion of normal arterial supply to the brain can lead to functional disturbance. The measures adopted are as follows: a powerful vasodilatator, papaverine, is immediately injected directly into the artery; on the 1st day back on the ward 30 mg is injected (i.v.) every 15 min; this dose is progressively reduced on the 2nd and 3rd days, and at the same time dextran, nicotinic acid, dexamethasone 40 mg/day, cyto-activator, adenosine triphosphate and cerebrolycin are used to raise the blood pressure and the perfusion pressure and to increase the brain compensation supply to minimise necrosis of nerve cells. Due to this treatment, 4 patients have recovered completely and 2 have been left with monoplegia.

References

1. Sugita K (1985) Microneurosurgical altas, part IV. Arterio-venous malformations. Springer, Berlin Heidelberg New York, pp 36–184
2. Solomon RA, Stein BM (1986) Management of arteriovenous malformations of the brain stem. J Neurosurg 64: 857–864
3. Picard L, Moret J, Lepoire J (1984) Endovascular treatment of intracerebral arteriovenous angiomas: technique, indications and results. J Neuroradiol 11: 9–28
4. Nornes H, Grip A (1980) Hemodynamic aspects of cerebral arteriovenous malformations. J Neurosurg 53: 456–464
5. Lasjaunias P, Manelfe C, Chiu M (1986) Angiographic architecture of intracranial vascular malformations and fistulas: pretherapeutic aspects. Neurosurg Rev 9: 253–263
6. Kerber CW, Bank WO, Cromwell LD (1979) Calibrated leak balloon catheter: a device for arterial exploration and occlusive therapy. AJR 132: 207–212
7. Rufenacht D, Merland JJ (1987) Modifications of a supple catheter avoiding the need of a balloon for flow-guidance hyperselective catheterization and embolization of brain AVM's. In: Valk J (ed) Neuroradiology. Elsevier, Amsterdam, pp 311–314
8. Debrun GM, Viñuela FV, Fox AJ, Kan S (1982) Two different calibrated-leak balloons: experimental work and application in humans. AJNR 3: 407–414

Dr. Ling Feng
Department of Neurosurgery
The Great Wall Hospital
28 Fuxing Road
Beijing 100853, China

Neuroradiology (1991) 33 [Suppl]: 560–561

© Springer-Verlag 1991

Thrombogenicity of arterial catheters depends on catheter type, not base material

A. Laurent[1], R. Eloy[2], and J. J. Merland[1]

[1] Department of Interventional Neuroradiology, Lariboisière Hospital, Paris, France
[2] INSERM 37, Lyon-Bron, France

Summary. To evaluate the thrombogenicity of 5 F angiographic catheters we developed an original in vivo human arterial blood model. Different types of catheter were tested in angiographic conditions. After femoral artery puncture, the test catheter was introduced and blood flow was measured for up to 10 min for catheter thrombosis. Three groups were apparent: group A showed no thrombosis after 10 min; group B showed thrombosis after 7 min; and group C showed thrombosis before 5 min. For all catheters there was no correlation between thrombogenicity and the base material. In fact, the thrombogenicity results from a combination of the base material, technological additives, specific additives, the method of extrusion and the final sterilization process.

Key words: Catheters – Blood compatibility – Thrombogenicity – Embolism – Polymer

Thrombogenicity of arterial catheters is of great interest concerning brain catheterization. In vitro, in vivo and ex vivo models developed for studying blood compatibility have several disadvantages. They generally use animal blood (extrapolation to humans is impossible [1]), venous human blood, or anticoagulated blood, thereby neglecting rheological and physiological conditions. They may include interference by alien materials, or require expensive or complex labelled markers [2, 3]. None of these systems directly tests the thrombogenicity of catheters in flowing human arterial blood in angiographic conditions [4]. The need for a new adapted model led us to create the described original study system based on the principle of the Dudley test [5] developed with animal blood, and secondarily modified by addition of fibrinopeptide A (FPA) measurements [6]. Using our system, we studied the duration of permeability and the generation of FPA and beta-thromboglobulin (BTG) for different types of 5 F catheters.

Materials and methods

In order to develop an appropriate system we listed the following technical requirements: contact of the material with blood only; standardization of the contact surface area and of initial flow; and the possibility of biological sampling. Ethical considerations demanded the use of a minimal quantity of blood (less than 30 ml), an insignificant increase in the duration of angiography (less than 10 min), and no risks for patients. These restrictions were respected with our original test-system (Fig. 1) with which we studied six materials, two polyethylenes (PE1[1], PE2[2]), two polyamides (PA1[1], PA2[3]), one polyurethane (PU[4]) and one polytetrafluoroethylene (PTFE[3]) (Fig. 1).

The surface of all catheters was studied with scanning electronic microscopy (SEM). All test catheders measured 40 cm; an external coaxial valve standardized the flow (3 ml/mn). The study design was approved by our hospital ethics committee. Each type of material was assessed with the blood of three different patients. All patients underwent diagnostic angiography by the femoral route, were older than 18 years, had no infections, inflammatory disease, or blood or coagulation abnormalities, and gave their informed consent. The test material was placed in an introducer for angiography; the samples were taken until thrombosis occurred or up to 10 min if no thrombosis occurred. During the 10-min maximum observation

[1] Guerbet Biomédical, Louvres, France
[2] Balt, Montmorency, France
[3] Cook, Bagnolet, France
[4] Bard, Gentilly, France

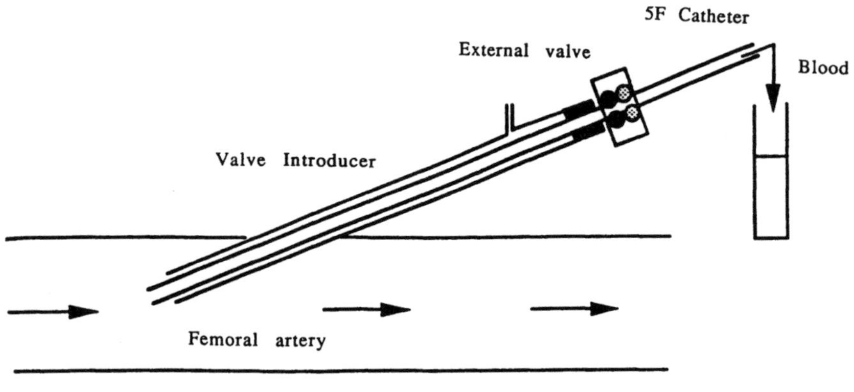

Fig. 1. Schematic drawing of the thrombogenicity test-system. Test material is placed in the valved 5 F introducer. The blood flows through and comes in contact only with the internal lumen of the 5 F catheter

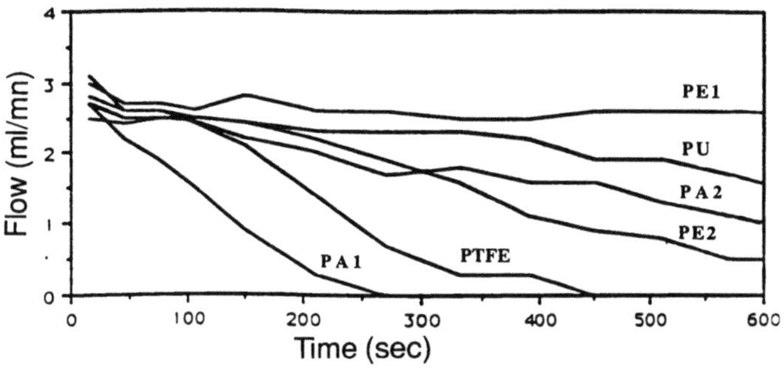

Fig. 2. Mean flow slopes for all materials. *PE1*, Polyethylene no. 1; *PE2*, polyethylene no. 2; *PA1*, polyamide no. 1; *PA2*, polyamide no. 2; *PTFE*, polytetrafluoroethylene; *PU*, polyurethane

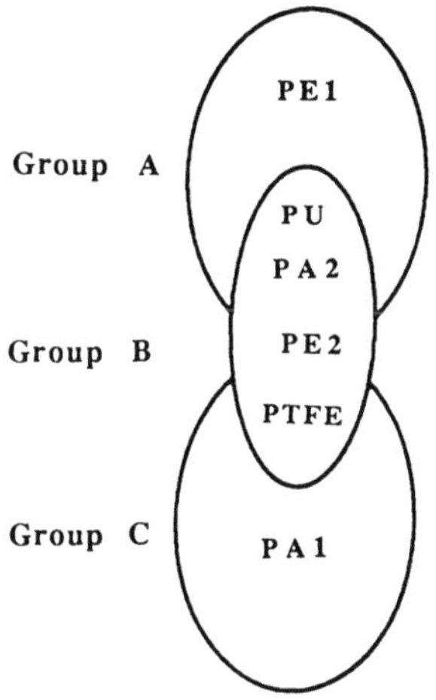

Fig. 3. Statistical groups according to the flow slopes

period, we recorded the flow, the permeability of the tube, and took samples for FPA (marker of thrombin formation) and BTG (marker of platelet activation). Samples were taken alternately for these markers. For each test material we calculated the mean slopes of flow and of the markers. The statistical analysis was with SAS Institute-North Carolina software (General Linear Models procedure).

Results

Mean flow slopes are summarized in Fig. 2. Permeability varied from 3 to over 10 min. Statistical analysis showed several facts: (1) very early (after 4 min, $P = 0.0063$), mean flow rates differ ($P = 0.0022$), as well as the change in flow for all catheters ($p = 0.0001$); (2) 5 F catheters could be divided into three specific groups (Student-Newman-Keuls test: $P < 0.05$): group A (PE2) which shows no flow reduction within the 10 min of observation; group B is representative of most catheters (PA2, PE1, PU, PTFE), which occlude after 7 min; group C (PA1) has a short duration of permeability around 5 mn (Fig. 3); (3) analysis of variance of the PA + PE group showed no correlation between the base material and the permeability. No correlation was found between the surface state revealed by SEM and the thrombogenicity. For most materials there was an inverse relationship between the levels of the FPA and BTG markers and the flow, without contradiction between the flow and the markers.

Discussion

Our system measures the thrombogenicity of 5 F catheters during a 10-min period only. It does not allow us to infer what may occur in longer angiographic procedures. However, it gives a quick and easy evaluation of thrombogenicity for commonly used 5 F catheters in humans. Our results lead us to believe that thrombogenicity is not related to the type of base material, such as PE, PU, PA, etc. ... but only to the manufactured final product. Thrombogenicity of catheters actually comes from many factors including composition of the catheter (base material and mainly the additives: colorants, antioxidants, plastifiers, radio-opacifiers and chemical stabilizers) extrusion conditions, residual products of sterilization, surface state [7].

References

1. Didisheim P, Stropp JQ, Borowick JH, Grabowski EF (1979) Species differences in platelet adhesion to biomaterials. Investigation by a new two stage technique. ASAIO J 2: 124–132
2. Lipton MJ, Doherty PW, Goodwin DA, Bushberg GT, Prager R, Meares CF (1980) Evaluation of catheter thrombogenicity in vivo with indium-labeled platelets. Radiology 135: 191–194
3. O'Connor MK, Brennan SS, Shanik DG (1986) Indium-111-labeled platelet deposition following transfemoral angiography. Radiology 158: 194
4. Baumgartner HR (1973) The role of blood flow in platelet adhesion, fibrin deposition and formation of mural thrombi. Microvasc Res 5: 167
5. Dudley B, Williams JL, Able K, Muller B (1976) Synthesis and characterization of blood compatible surfaces. I Dynamic tube test applied to heparinized surface. Trans Am Soc Artif Intern Organs 22: 538–544
6. Eloy R, Pusireni C, Baguet J, Paul J, Serafini S (1983) Bulk heparinized catheters do not generate fibrinopeptide A in an ex vivo test in dogs. ISAO 7: 88–92
7. Merril EW (1987) Distinctions and correspondences among surfaces contacting blood. Ann NY Acad Sci 516: 196–205

A. Laurent, M. A.
Neuroradiologie
Hôpital Lariboisière
2 rue A. Paré
F-75010 Paris, France

Neuroradiology (1991) 33 [Suppl]: 562–564

Neuro radiology
© Springer-Verlag 1991

Calibrated sphere embolization of craniofacial tumours and arteriovenous malformations

R. Beaujeux[1], A. Laurent[1], J. E. Hodes[1], M. Wassef[2], and J. J. Merland[1]

Departments of [1] Interventional Neuroradiology and [2] Pathology, Lariboisière Hospital, Paris, France

Summary. Clinical study of precisely calibrated microsphere embolization in 56 patients was performed. As well, we compared, in 18 patients, the efficiency of embolization of two ranges of microsphere size, either a narrow range (± 50 µm) of different carefully calibrated sizes or a large range of diameters (± 300 µm). The study was performed in patients with craniofacial tumours or facial arteriovenous malformations (AVMs) correlating the angiographic result, ease of surgery, and the histology. For the 56 patients, embolization with microspheres was easy, efficient, and without aggregate formation. Correlation of angiographic results, ease of surgery, and histology in 18 cases showed that utilization of a precisely calibrated narrow range of microspheres allowed us better to target the desired point of vascular occlusion. Also, with these microspheres, we were better able to control the amount of tumour necrosis and to decrease venous passage in the AVMs.

Key words: Microsphere – Calibration – Embolization – Tumour – Arteriovenous malformation

Microspheres are an embolization material that is more efficient than particulate emboli such as polyvinyl alcohol (PVA) (Fig. 1 A), gelfoam, or pieces of dura mater [1, 2]. These microspheres do not have the disadvantages of irregularly shaped polyhedral particles [3] and are the only existing material that can be reliably calibrated. First, we assessed the feasability of embolization with our carefully calibrated microspheres. Afterwards, we tested the efficiency of embolization with either a narrow range (± 50 µm) of carefully calibrated sizes, or a large range of diameters (± 300 µm). This investigation was performed in patients with facial arteriovenous malformations (AVMs) or craniofacial tumours correlating the angiographic result, the ease of surgery, and histology.

Materials and methods

After animal studies [4] we performed embolization using these microspheres in 56 patients (Table 1). Several catheter systems were utilized for embolization (3.6 F polyethylene catheter, 0.6 internal/1.0 external diameter Pursil catheter, Tracker 25 and 18) allowing us to study the feasibility and ease of use of the microspheres in these systems.

Of 56, 18 patients underwent postembolization operation (12 tumours, 6 facial AVMs), permiting detailed histological study of the pathological specimen. For these operated patients we compared the efficiency of the two ranges of microsphere size (Table 2).

The embolization material used was acrylic polymer microspheres that were calibrated by successive passages through carefully calibrated screen sieves, giving a narrow range of microsphere size. The size distribution was monitored by microscopic granuloscopy (Fig. 1 B). We obtained a range of microspheres between 100–1200 µm in diameter, which we divided into successive sizes of 200, 400, 600, and 950 µm ± 50 (type A). We compared embolization results of these carefully calibrated size ranges to a single size range of 500 µm ± 300 (type B) (Fig. 2). For all the patients the efficiency of microsphere embolization was evaluated by three criteria: (1) complete or partial angiographic devascularization on embolization and control angiograms; (2) operative criteria including feasibility of resection, ease of resection and operative blood loss; (3) histological consequences such as presence of and amount of tissue necrosis and the number of microspheres seen on histological slices of the operative specimen.

Table 1. Patients treated with microspheres

Pathology		Number	Correlation: angiography, surgery, histology
Tumours	Meningioma	3	3
	Nasopharyngeal fibroma	4	4
	Spinal metastases (renal carcinoma)	1	1
	Infratemporal fossa fibrosarcoma	1	1
	Hemangioblastoma	2	1
	Glomus tumour	1	1
	Temporoauricular sarcoma	1	1
	Neurofibroma	1	0
Facial AVMs	Lips	4	3
	Nose	1	1
	Eyelid	1	1
	Scalp	2	1
Spinal cord AVMs		19	0
Cerebral AVMs		13	0
Osler-Rendu		2	0
	Total	56	18

AVM, Arteriovenous malformation

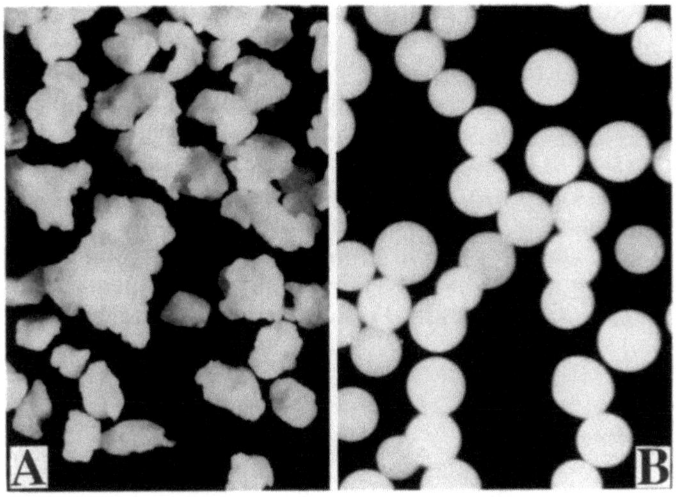

Fig. 1. **A** Irregularly shaped polyhedral particles of polyvinyl alcohol: size range distribution is large. **B** Carefully calibrated microspheres: size range distribution is more homogeneous

Results

In all 56 patients treated, embolization was possible and angiographic devascularization easily obtained and perfectly controlled. This was especially the case in treatment of spinal cord and cerebral AVMs with the narrow range of microsphere size. In no case was there aggregation of particles in the catheter, or involuntary proximal vessel occlusion.

For all 18 patients with either tumours or AVMs in which we compared the two size ranges, final angiographic results showed complete or satisfactory devascularization. In all cases, surgery was easy and without blood loss problems. Histological analysis of the operative specimens of the tumors embolised with the type A microspheres showed that the microspheres were present in all cases and more often, in large numbers (4/5), with associated tissue necrosis (4/5). On the other hand, the type B embolized tumours rarely had histological evidence of microspheres (4/7), and there was either slight or no tissue necrosis (5/7). In all the embolized and operated facial AVMs, there were numerous microspheres demonstrated histologically, without evidence of necrosis. There was sometimes (5/18), minimal inflammatory reaction in the embolized area.

Discussion

Spherical embolization materials were shown to be more efficient compared to PVA by Wright et al. [1]. Partial dog spleen embolization was more homogeneous and distal with dextran microspheres. Our clinical study utilises for the first time calibrated hydrophilic nonabsorbable microspheres [4].

In tumour embolization, angiographic devascularization and operative haemostatic goals are achieved regardless of the size range of particles used, or the level of arterial occlusion (proximal or distal). However, the possibility of obtaining tissue necrosis may, in certain cases, help in tumour removal. Nearly constant tissue necrosis is obtained with the small, narrow size range (200 μm ± 50) and is probably secondary to a very distal arterial network occlusion. The necrosis is directly related to the use of the very precisely calibrated narrow size range, allowing one to choose the correct diameter depending on the angioarchitecture of the lesion. A meningioma embolized with 200 ± 50 μm microspheres developed extensive necrosis and peritumoral oedema, causing significant mass effect and neurological deficit, which were completely reversible. This illustrates that tumours are more or less sensitive to embolization. Thus, in order to prevent this possible problem, we have modified our technique, and currently embolize intracranial lesion over several sessions, starting with the small size range microspheres.

In all cases of facial AVM, regardless of the size range used, histological examination showed numerous microspheres. Even though we used the more narrowly calibrated microspheres in only one case, we had the impression that we could better control the site of vascular

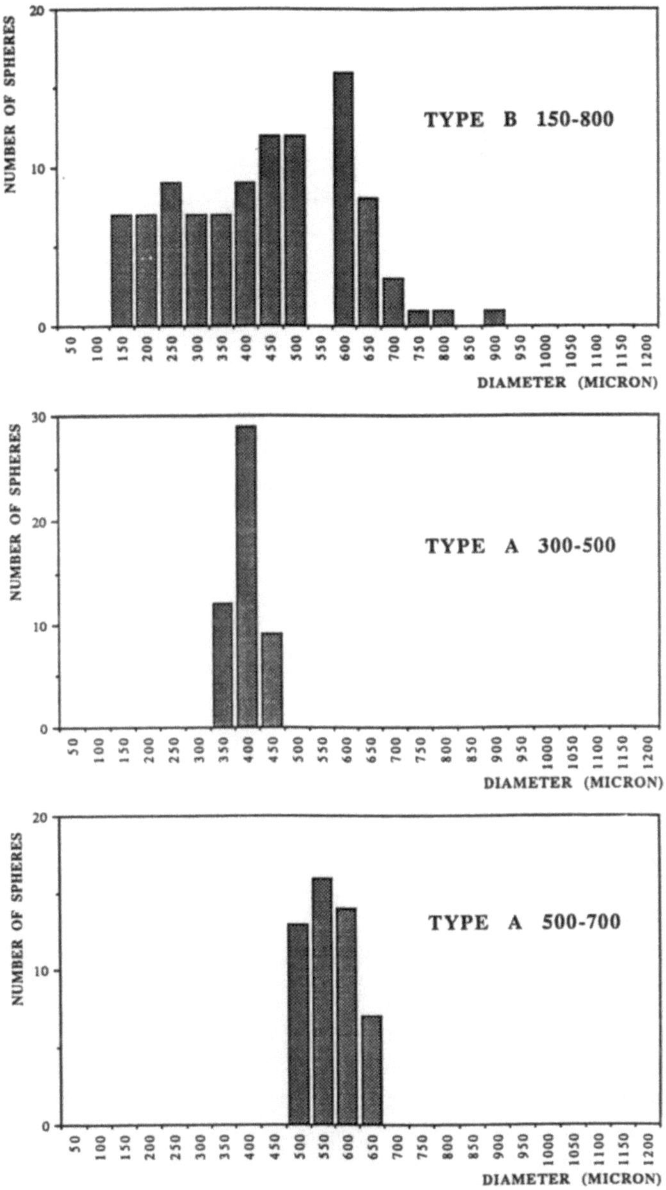

Fig. 2. Narrow and large size ranges of microspheres

Table 2. Angiography-surgery-histology correlation

Pathology	Large range	Narrow range
12 Tumours	7	5
Satisfactory devascularization	7/7	5/5
Operative benefit	7/7	5/5
Histology		
– Number of microspheres		
20–30	3/7	4/5
0– 3	4/7	1/5
– Necrosis		
+ + +	2/7	4/5
+ /0	5/7	1/5
6 Facial AVMs	5	1
Satisfactory devascularization	5/5	1/1
Operative benefit	5/5	1/1
Histology		
– Number of microspheres		
20–30	5/5	1/1
0– 3	0/5	0/1
– Necrosis		
+ + +	0/5	0/1
+ /0	5/5	1/1

occlusion by tailoring the microsphere size to the size of the vascular shunt. In this case, as opposed to cerebral and spinal cord AVMs which generally have larger shunts in the range of 500–700 μm, we used 200 ± 50 μm microspheres.

Conclusion

The endovascular size of occlusion must be defined by a careful angioarchitectural study of the lesion. It is thus necessary to be able to use multiple and precise calibre emboli adapted to the desired occlusion site. This is possible with use of the precisely calibrated narrow size range microspheres.

In conclusion, microspheres allow simple, complete, and rapid devascularization, without aggregate formation in the vessels or the catheters. In tumour embolization one can control the exact location of vascular occlusion. In AVMs, one can target the vascular shunt alone. Embolization helps the surgeon when performed preoperatively. Histological evidence confirms 100% mechanical occlusion, good tolerance, without tissue effects.

References

1. Wright KC, Anderson JH, Gianturco C, Wallace S, Chuang VP (1982) Partial splenic embolisation using polyvinyl alcohol foam, dextran, polystyrene, or silicone. Radiology 142: 351–354
2. Dion JE, Rankin RN, Vinuela F, Fox AJ, Wallace AC, Mervart M (1986) Dextran microsphere embolization: experimental and clinical experience with radiologic-pathologic correlation. Radiology 160: 717–721
3. Repa I, Moradian GP, Dehner LP, Tadavarthy SM, Hunter DW, Castaneda-Zuniga WR, Wright GB, Katkov H, Johnson P, Chrenka B, Amplatz K (1989) Mortalities associated with use of a commercial suspension of polyvinyl alcohol. Radiology 170: 395–399
4. Laurent A, Wassef M, Drouet L, Pignaud G, Merland JJ (1989) Etude histologique de plusieurs matériaux d'embolisation et d'un nouveau type de matériel sphérique et adhésif. Innov Tech Biol Med 10: 357–366

Dr. R. Beaujeux
Neuroradiologie
Hôpital Lariboisière
2 Rue A Paré
F-75010 Paris, France

Neuroradiology (1991) 33 [Suppl]: 565–566

Neuro radiology

© Springer-Verlag 1991

Gadolinium-DTPA-enhanced MRI of intracranial inflammatory diseases

K. Tsuchiya, K. Makita, S. Furui, and E. Takenaka

Department of Radiology, National Defense Medical College, Tokorozawa, Saitama, Japan

Summary. In 11 patients with intracranial inflammatory disease, we retrospectively evaluated gadolinium (Gd)-DTPA enhancement in MRI. The lesions included brain abscess ($n = 3$), subdural empyema ($n = 1$), epidural empyema ($n = 2$), meningitis ($n = 7$), and granuloma ($n = 1$). Brain abscess, subdural empyema, and epidural empyema were readily differentiated from the abscess fluid and surrounding oedema, since the capsule revealed enhancement. Abnormal meningeal enhancement, which was not always noted on enhanced CT scans, was demonstrated in all cases of meningitis. MRI with Gd-DTPA is of great value in the diagnosis of these disorders.

Key words: Magnetic resonance imaging – Gadolinium-DTPA – Brain abscess – Meningitis

The MRI appearance of intracranial infectious diseases has been described [1–7]. However, gadolinium (Gd)-DTPA enhancement in these diseases has not been thoroughly investigated [2, 6, 7]; the purpose of this study was to assess its value.

Patients and methods

MRI and CT studies were reviewed in 11 patients with intracranial infectious diseases. There were 9 male and 2 female patients, aged 0.3–68 years. The lesions included brain abscess ($n = 3$, bacterial), subdural empyema ($n = 1$, bacterial), epidural empyema ($n = 2$, bacterial), meningitis ($n = 7$, bacterial 5, fungal 1, and viral 1), and granuloma ($n = 1$, fungal). Two patients had two or three lesions. The diagnosis was proved both surgically and microbiologically in 5 patients with abscess and/or empyema. In other patients, it was based on the clinical presentation and laboratory cerebrospinal fluid findings. MRI was performed at 1.5 T to obtain pre-contrast spin-echo T1-weighted and T2-weighted images and post-contrast (0.1 mmol/kg Gd-DTPA) T1-weighted images. In all the patients, CT was performed with i.v. contrast material 0–14 days before or after the MRI study.

Results

In the 5 cases of brain abscess, subdural empyema, and/or epidural empyema, the capsule displayed significant enhancement on post-contrast MR images (Figs. 1, 2a). The enhancement was greater than that on enhanced CT

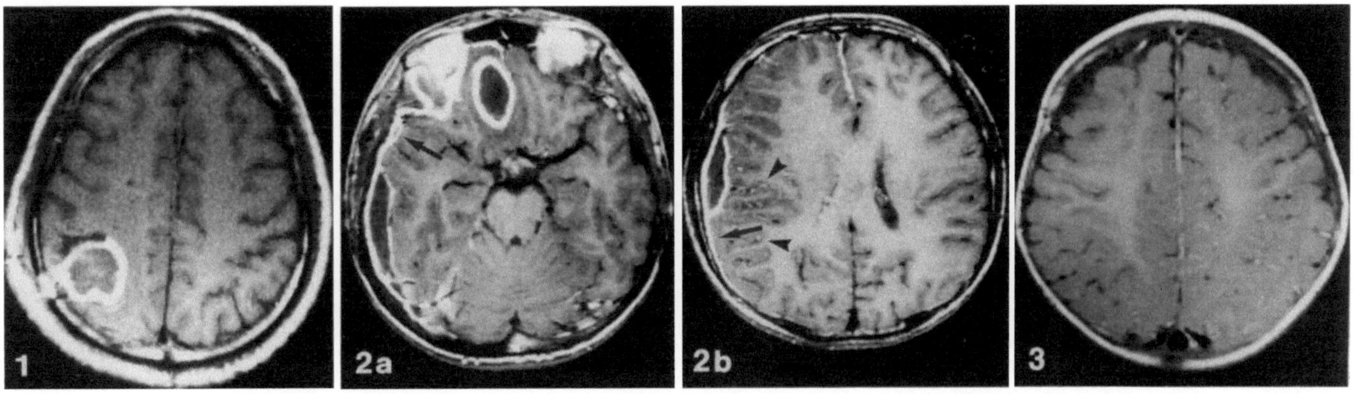

Fig. 1. Brain abscess (54-year-old man). Gadolinium (Gd)-DTPA-enhanced T1-weighted image (SE 500/38) demonstrates a ring-enhancing lesion in the right parietal lobe. Hypointensity anterior to the abscess is due to attempted drainage. The causative organism was salmonella

Fig. 2 a, b. Brain abscess, subdural empyema, and meningitis (13-year-old boy). Gd-DTPA-enhanced T1-weighted images (SE 500/30) reveal an abscess in the right frontal lobe and a right frontotemporal subdural empyema. Note abnormal meningeal enhancement due to meningitis (*arrowheads* in **b**) and thickening of the dura mater (*arrows* in **a, b**). Streptococcus was the causative organism

Fig. 3. Viral meningitis (4-month-old boy). Abnormal meningeal enhancement is noted in the left frontal and parietal lobes and in a part of the right parietal lobe on this Gd-DTPA-enhanced T1-weighted image (SE 500/30). The causative virus was not successfully identified scans. On precontrast MR images, the capsule was not clearly differentiated from the abscess fluid and surrounding oedema. In the 7 patients with meningitis, Gd-DTPA-enhanced images demonstrated abnormal meningeal enhancement with predominant involvement of the convexity surface (Figs. 2b, 3). Precontrast MR images showed no abnormality in all of the cases and enhanced CT was negative in 4. In the patient with cryptococcosis, tiny granulomas in the cerebral cortex were depicted only on Gd-DTPA-enhanced MR images.

Discussion

Brain abscess has been differentiated from focal cerebritis mainly on the basis of findings on enhanced CT [8]. In brain abscess, enhanced CT scans reveal ring-like, regular, and rather thin enhancement. On MRI, cerebritis, abscess fluid, and surrounding oedema are usually demonstrated as areas with prolongation of both T1 and T2. The abscess capsule is known to show T2 shortening due to free radicals produced by macrophages [6]. In our experience, however, the capsule is not clearly defined on T2-weighted images. The capsule demonstrates contrast enhancement with Gd-DTPA as shown in our clinical series as well as in a canine model reported previously [9]. This enhancement clearly differentiates the capsule, abscess fluid, and surrounding oedema and is of value in the diagnosis and subsequent management of brain abscess. The delineation of extra-axial empyemas is likewise facilitated on Gd-DTPA-enhanced MR images.

Our results indicate that Gd-DTPA-enhanced MRI is more sensitive than enhanced CT in defining the inflammatory process of the meninges. This is mainly due to greater contrast enhancement on MRI with Gd-DTPA than on enhanced CT. Especially in the convexity region, the absence of bone artefact also contributes to the high sensitivity of Gd-DTPA-enhanced MRI. In addition, previous investigation has indicated that MRI is more effective than CT in detecting complications of meningitis (e.g. ischaemia, abscess [7, 10]). Thus, MRI promises to be valuable in monitoring patients with meningitis.

In conclusion, from our limited series, we believe that MRI with Gd-DTPA plays an important role in the diagnosis of intracranial inflammatory disease.

References

1. Zimmerman RA, Bilaniuk LT, Sze G (1987) Intracranial infection. In: Brant-Zawadzki M, Norman D (eds) Magnetic resonance imaging of the central nervous system. Raven Press, New York, pp 235–257
2. Davidson HD, Steiner RE (1985) Magnetic resonance imaging in infections of the central nervous system. AJNR 6: 499–504
3. Schroth G, Kretzschmar K, Gawehn J, Voigt K (1987) Advantages of magnetic resonance imaging in the diagnosis of cerebral infections. Neuroradiology 29: 120–126
4. Sze G, Zimmerman RD (1988) The magnetic resonance imaging of infections and inflammatory diseases. Radiol Clin North Am 26: 839–859
5. Weingarten K, Zimmerman RD, Becker RD, Heier LA, Haimes AB, Deck MDF (1989) Subdural and epidural empyemas: MR imaging. AJNR 10: 81–87
6. Haimes AB, Zimmerman RD, Morgello S, Weingarten K, Becker RD, Jennis R, Deck MDF (1989) MR imaging of brain abscess. AJNR 10: 279–291
7. Chang KH, Han MH, Roh JK, Kim IO, Han MC, Kim CH (1990) Gd-DTPA-enhanced MR imaging of the brain in patients with meningitis: comparison with CT. AJNR 11: 69–76
8. Enzman DR, Britt RH, Yeager AS (1979) Experimental brain abscess evolution: computed tomography and neuropathologic correlation. Radiology 133: 113–122
9. Runge VM, Clanton JA, Price AC, Herzer WA, Allen JH, Partain CL, James AE Jr (1985) Evaluation of contrast-enhanced MR imaging in a brain-abscess model. AJNR 6: 139–147
10. Mathews VP, Kuharik MA, Edwards MK, D'Amour PG, Azzarelli BA, Dressen RG (1989) Gd-DTPA-enhanced MR imaging of experimental bacterial meningitis: evaluation and comparison with CT. AJNR 9: 1045–1050

Dr. K. Tsuchiya
Department of Radiology
National Defense Medical College
3-2, Namiki
Tokorozawa, Saitama, 359, Japan

Neuroradiology (1991) 33 [Suppl]: 567–568

Neuro radiology
© Springer-Verlag 1991

Neurological complications of AIDS: radiologic-pathologic correlation with special emphasis on the need for early biopsy

K. York Chynn[1], P. Kancherla[2], C. Sian[2], J. Edwards[1], C. Hilfer[1], H. P. Gaetz[2], and J. Scholes[2]

Departments of [1] Radiology and [2] Pathology, St. Luke's-Roosevelt Hospital Center and Columbia University, College of Physicans and Surgeons, New York, USA

Summary. Four cases were selected from a review of 73 autopsied cases with acquired immunodeficiency syndrome to emphasize the need for early biopsy. Their ages ranged from 23 to 63 years.

Key words: Aspergillosis – Acquired immune deficiency syndrome – Brain diseases – Cytomegalovirus infection – Lymphoma – Toxoplasmosis

In September 1987 an Acquired Immunodeficiency Syndrome (AIDS) Center Program was established at St. Luke's-Roosevelt Hospital Center, New York City. From January 1979 to December 1989, a total of 2621 newly diagnosed patients with AIDS were treated. In 1989 alone there were 897 in-patients with CDC-confirmed AIDS requiring 1409 Admissions. The clinical records, pathological report and roentgenological findings in 73 autopsied patients with AIDS were reviewed. Four cases were selected to emphasize the need for early biopsy.

Case reports

Case 1. A 50-year-old bisexual male was first admitted with focal seizure. Toxoplasmosis IgG titer was strongly positive. CT revealed an enhancing lesion in the right parietal area (Fig. 1a) which responded well to antitoxoplasmosis therapy. He was readmitted 3 months later with fever, and weakness of 10 days' duration. Repeat CT revealed an enhancing lesion in the left caudate nucleus which did not respond to antitoxoplasmosis treatment (Fig. 1b). The patient expired 24 days after admission. At autopsy, an irregular 3 × 3 cm lesion was noted in the left caudate nucleus area with a collapsed left frontal horn. This lesion proved microscopically to be an immunoblastic lymphoma.

Case 2. A 32-year-old intravenous (i. v.) drug and alcohol abuser was admitted with marked wasting, dysphagia and depression. CT showed two adjacent ring-enhancing lesions in the gray matter and corticomedullary junction (Fig. 2). The patient was treated empirically with antitoxoplasmosis therapy with some improvement clinically. However, 7 weeks later, repeat CT revealed no regression of lesions. In the meantime, serology was negative for *Toxoplasma* antibodies. Biopsy and culture of the left parietal area confirmed an *Aspergillus fumigatus* abscess. He expired 4 months after admission. The *A. fumigatus* abscess of the left parietal lobe was confirmed at autopsy. The source of the abscess was not found (especially on lung sectioning).

Case 3. A 37-year-old man with AIDS complained of nausea, vomiting and ataxia of a few days duration. Cranial CT revealed severe enhancement of the ependymal lining of both lateral ventricles consistent with ependymitis (Fig. 3). There was also some increased enhancement of the right choroid plexus. Cytomegalovirus (CMV) infection was suspected. The cerebrospinal fluid grew pneumococcus and i. v. penicillin was started. His condition continued to deteriorate and he expired 12 days after admission. At autopsy a high-grade diffuse large cell immunoblastic lymphoma (immunoblastic sarcoma) was seen to involve the choroid plexus, right and left basal ganglia, mamillary bodies, hippocampus and cerebellum. Involvement of the choroid plexus and basal ganglia was massive with diffuse infiltration into periventricular and Virchow-Robin spaces.

Case 4. A 32-year-old male with AIDS complained of left lower extremity weakness, increasing lateral divergence of the right eye and ataxia for 6 weeks. He had developed CMV retinitis a year previously, which resulted in loss of vision of the right eye. CT of the brain revealed a 1-cm nodular enhancement in the left high parietal region and two smaller enhancing lesions on the right side. MRI revealed high signal intensity lesions in the left parietal region, right parasagittal region and midbrain (Fig. 4a, b). All toxoplasmosis titers and cultures were negative. The patient expired about 3 weeks after admission. Postmortem examination revealed diffuse 0.2–1.0 cm lesions bilaterally involving both gray and white matter, brain stem and spinal cord. Extensive necrosis was present microscopically. Smudge cells consistent with CMV inclusions were seen surrounding these lesions. DNA hybridization was positive for CMV.

Discussion

The radiological findings in AIDS patients with toxoplasmosis [1], primary lymphoma [2], CMV infection [3, 4] and aspergillosis [5] have been well documented in the literature. Our selected cases, however, emphasize the significant atypical features which warrant sufficient attention.

Based on the radiological-pathological correlation of 73 autopsied cases we have seen in the last 5 years we can conclude that:

1. Primary lymphoma in AIDS patients may present unusual radiological findings such as: (a) intracerebral hemorrhage, (b) ventriculitis, and (c) poor or nearly no enhancement on contrast CT.
2. Radiological differentiation between toxoplasmosis and abscesses due to other organisms (e.g., aspergillus, Mycobacterium tuberculosis) and CMV encephalitis is sometimes not possible.
3. Concomitant or subsequent infection by more than one organism may occur. Lymphoma may coexist with toxoplasmosis.
4. MRI is more sensitive than CT in detecting lesions, but is no more specific.

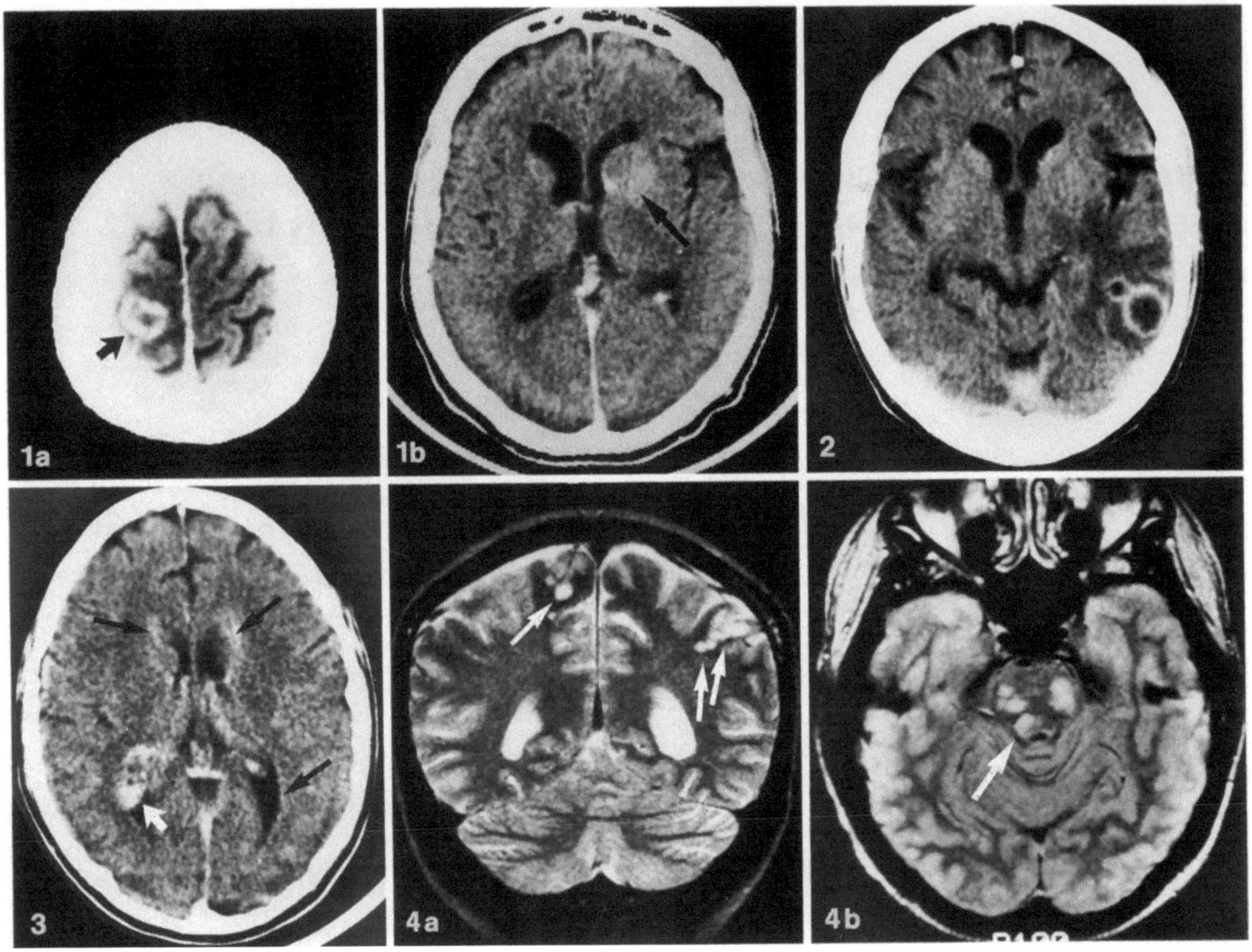

Fig. 1a, b. Case 1. **a** CT showing a ring-enhancing lesion in the right parietal region *(arrow)* which disappeared after antitoxoplasmosis therapy. **b** CT 3 months later, showing an enhancing lesion in the left caudate nucleus *(arrow)* which on autopsy proved to be immunoblastic lymphoma

Fig. 2. Case 2. CT showing two adjacent ring-enhancing lesions in the gray matter and corticomedullary junction of the left temporoparietal region which proved to be *Aspergillus fumigatus* abscesses

Fig. 3. Case 3. CT showing marked enhancement of the ependymal lining of both lateral ventricles *(arrows)* and an enhancing mass in the right choroid plexus *(white arrow)*. Although ependymitis is most commonly seen in cytomegalovirus (CMV) infection, we have observed it also in lymphoma and toxoplasmosis

Fig. 4a, b. Case 4. Multifocal CMV encephalitis with unusual radiological findings. **a** MRI coronal section, spin echo. TR 2500 TE 80 ms. High-intensity lesions demonstrated in the left parietal and the right parasagittal regions *(arrows)*. **b** MRI axial section, spin echo. TR 2500 TE 30 ms. High-intensity lesions in both cerebral peduncles and the right dorsal midbrain *(arrow)* with involvement of the medial longitudinal fasciculus, correlating with a right intranuclear ophthalmoplegia

Conclusion

Early stereotactic biopsy may detect treatable conditions and must be seriously considered when clinical response is poor.

Acknowledgements. We wish to thank Michael H. Grieco, M.D., Mary O'Mahony, M.P.H. and Steven Roffman, Ph.D. for providing the statistic information regarding the SLRHC AIDS center.

References

1. Navia BA, Petro CK, Jonathan WM, Cho E-S, Jordan BD, Price RW (1986) Cerebral toxoplasmosis complicating the acquired immune deficiency syndrome: clinical and neuropathological findings in 27 patients. Ann Neurol 19: 224–238
2. Lee Y-Y, Bruner JM, Van Tassel P, Libshitz HI (1986) Primary central nervous system lymphoma: CT and pathologic correlation. AJNR 7: 599–604
3. Post MJD, Hensley GT, Moskowitz, LB, Fischl M (1986) Cytomegalic inclusion virus encephalitis in patients with AIDS: CT, clinical and pathologic correlation. AJR 146: 1229–1234
4. Fuller GN, Guilloff RJ, Scaravilli F, Harcourt-Webster JN (1989) Combined HIV-CMV encephalitis presenting with brainstem signs. J Neurol Neurosurg Psychiatry 52: 975–979
5. Beal MF, O'Carrol CP, Kleinman GM, Grossman RI (1982) Aspergillosis of the nervous system. Neurology 32: 473–479

Dr. K. York Chynn
Department of Radiology
St. Luke's Hospital Center
Amsterdam Ave at 114th St.
New York, NY 10025, USA

Neuroradiology (1991) 33 [Suppl]: 569–570

Neuro
radiology
© Springer-Verlag 1991

Intracranial tuberculoma in AIDS: neuroradiological findings

J. M. Mercader[1,2], J. Perich[1], J. Berenguer[2], T. Pujol[2], and C. Cardenal[2]

[1] Centro Radiológico Computarizado, Barcelona, Spain
[2] Department of Radiology, Hospital Clínico, Barcelona, Spain

Summary. Tuberculous infection is common in the AIDS population in our country. During a 5-year period, 400 patients with AIDS were treated at our institution. Intracranial tuberculoma was demonstrated in 4 patients (1%). Diagnosis was by histological studies or therapeutic response. CT scans showed ring lesions with hypodense centre and ring enhancement. MIR studies showed lesions with prolongation of the T1 relaxation time; on T2-weighted sequences, a hypointense centre with hyperintense surrounding oedema was observed. Control MRI with gadolinium (Gd)-DTPA was performed in 1 patient, showing ring enhancement. Tuberculomas should be included in the differential diagnosis of intracranial space-occupying lesions in AIDS populations. Early diagnosis and prompt medical treatment are essential in reducing morbidity, as in our series.

Key words: Acquired immunodeficiency syndrome – Intracranial tuberculoma – Computed tomography – Magnetic resonance imaging

Disseminated tuberculosis is a common disease in AIDS patients in our country, although central nervous system involvement is rare. The aim of this study was to review the CT and MRI appearances of intracranial tuberculomas in our AIDS patients.

Case reports

During a 5-year period, 400 patients with AIDS were investigated at our institution. Brain tuberculoma was demonstrated in 4 patients (1%). Three were intravenous drug abusers and 1 was homosexual. Histological confirmation was available in 1 patient. In the remaining 3 patients the diagnosis was made on the basis of response to antituberculous therapy. CT was performed in all patients and MRI in only 2. Four other patients had tuberculous meningitis without brain mass lesions.

The CT appearance of brain tuberculoma was similar in all patients. Unenhanced CT showed ring lesions with peripheral oedema. After intravenous contrast medium an enhancing ring was observed. A hypodense triangular lesion without contrast enhancement was also seen in 1 patient, probably due to focal cerebritis. Three patients showed single lesions and one had two lesions. The locations of the tuberculomas were: cerebellar hemisphere (Fig. 1 a), brain stem (Fig. 2 a), capsulo-thalamic, frontal, and frontoparietal (Fig. 3).

MRI studies showed lesions with prolongation of the T1 relaxation time. On T2-weighted sequences a central zone of hypointensity surrounded by hyperintense oedema was observed (Figs. 1 b, 2 b). Follow-up gadolinium (Gd)-DTPA MRI examination was performed in 1 patient during antituberculous therapy and ring enhancement was observed on T1-weighted images (Fig. 2 c).

Discussion

Central nervous system lesions in patients with AIDS have been well described [1–4]. Tuberculous involvement is uncommon but not exceptional in our country. Neuromeningeal tuberculosis results from haematogenous spread from an extracerebral focus. The clinical spectrum may include meningitis, tuberculoma, or tuberculous abscess [4, 5].

On plain CT, brain tuberculomas are usually iso- or hyperdense lesions, and a hypodense central zone may be observed [6, 7]. After contrast injection, ring enhancement is commonly seen, but nodular or heterogeneous enhancement have also been described [7]. Central calcification or enhancement surrounded by ring enhancement have been described [8, 9], but we have not observed a "target sign" in our patients.

MRI usually shows lesions with long T1 relaxation time. The central caseous zone appears hypointense on T2-weighted sequences, surrounded by diffuse hyperintensity representing oedema [6, 10, 11]. Occasionally, an iso- or hypointense capsule may be observed [10, 11]. The centre of the tuberculoma may become hyperintense due to fluid collection [10, 11]. After Gd-DTPA injection, ring enhancement may be seen on T1-weighted sequences, as occurred in 1 of our patients.

Although rare, tuberculoma should be included in the differential diagnosis of intracranial space-occupying lesions in AIDS patients. Early diagnosis and prompt medical treatment are essential in reducing morbidity [5, 6, 11]. AIDS patients with tuberculous infection usually show good response to antituberculous therapy, as in our series.

References

1. Levy RM, Bredesen DE, Rosenblum ML (1985) Neuroradiological manifestations of the acquired immunodeficiency syndrome (AIDS): experience at UCSF and review of the literature. J Neurosurg 62: 475–495
2. Levy RM, Rosenbloom S, Perrat LV (1986) Neuroradiologic findings in AIDS; a review of 200 cases. AJR 147: 977–983

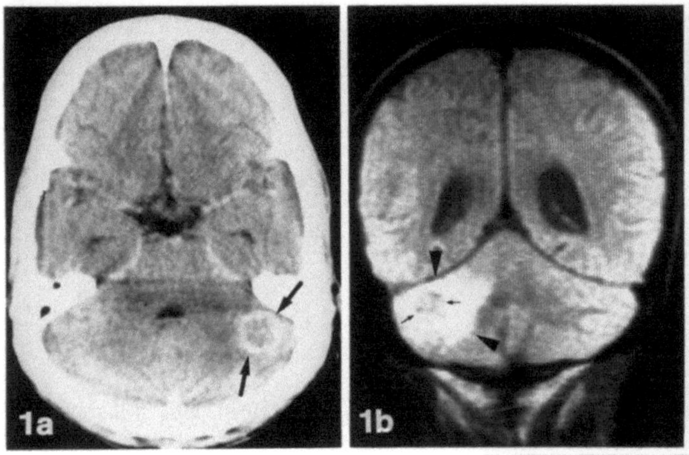

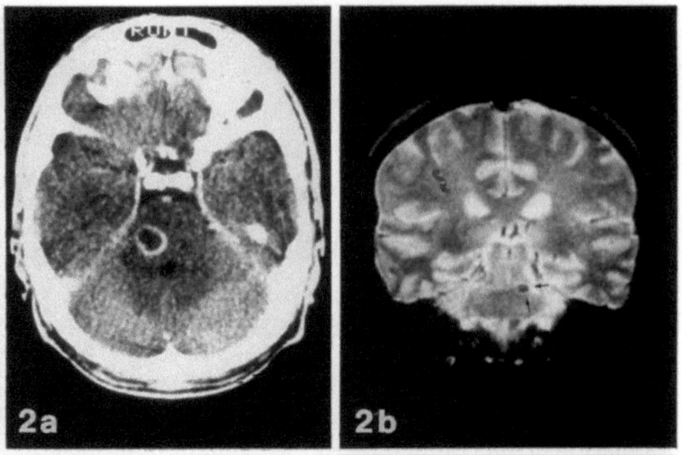

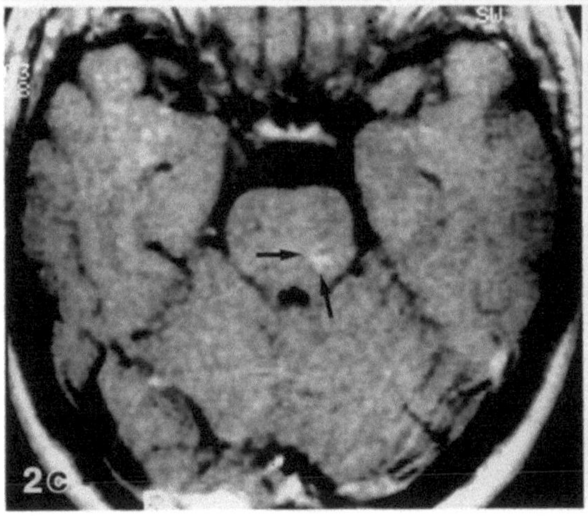

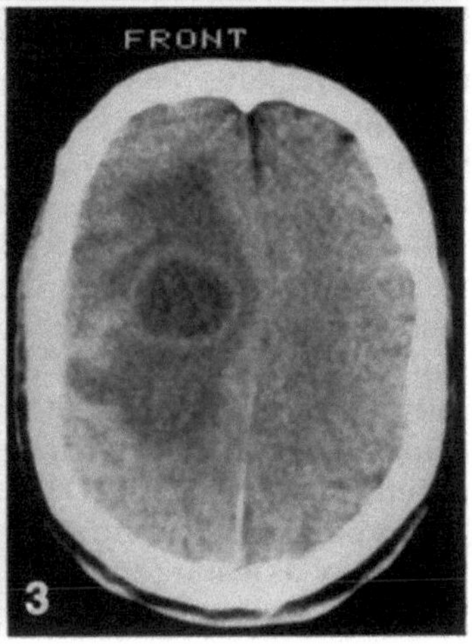

Fig. 1 a, b. Cerebellar tuberculoma. **a** Ring-enhancing lesion on post-contrast CT *(arrows)*. **b** Coronal MRI (2000/60) shows an iso- and hypointense lesion *(arrows)* with hyperintense peripheral edema *(arrowheads)*

Fig. 2 a–c. Brain-stem tuberculoma. **a** A hypointense lesion with ring enhancement is observed on postcontrast CT scan. **b** After antituberculous therapy, coronal MRI (2000/90) shows a hypointense lesion with peripheral hyperintensity *(arrows)*. **c** Gadolinium-DTPA-enhanced MRI (600/27) demonstrates ring enhancement *(arrows)*

Fig. 3. Unenhanced CT shows a ring lesion with a hypodense centre and peripheral oedema. Marked ring enhancement was observed on postcontrast CT (not shown)

3. Post MJD, Kursunoglu SJ, Hensley GT, Chan JC, Moskowitz LB, Hoffman TA (1985) Cranial CT in acquired immunodeficiency syndrome: spectrum of diseases and optimal contrast enhancement technique. AJR 145: 929–940
4. Olsen WL, Cohen W (1988) Neuroradiology of AIDS. In: Federle MP, Megibow AJ, Naidich DP (eds) Radiology of AIDS. Raven Press, New York pp 21–46
5. Bishburg E, Sunderam G, Reichman LB, Kapila R (1986) Central nervous system tuberculosis with the acquired immunodeficiency syndrome and its related complex. Ann Intern Med 105: 210–213
6. Talamás O, Del Brutto OH, García Ramos G (1989) Brain-stem tuberculoma. An analysis of 11 patients. Arch Neurol 46: 529–535
7. Whelan MA, Stern J (1981) Intracranial tuberculoma. Radiology 138: 75–81
8. Welchman JM (1979) Computerized tomography of intracranial tuberculomata. Clin Radiol 30: 567–573
9. Dyck A van (1988) CT of intracranial tuberculomas with specific reference to the "target sign". Neuroradiology 30: 329–336
10. Gupta RK, Jena A, Sharma A, Guha DK, Khusku S, Gupta AK (1988) MR imaging of intracranial tuberculomas. J Comput Assist Tomogr 12: 280–285
11. Salgado P, Del Brutto OH, Talamás O, Zenteno MA, Rodríguez Carbajal J (1989) Intracranial tuberculoma: MR imaging. Neuroradiology 31: 299–302

J. M. Mercader
Centro Radiológico Computarizado
Tavern 82
08006 Barcelona, Spain

Neuroradiology (1991) 33 [Suppl]: 571–572

Neuro-radiology
© Springer-Verlag 1991

Granulomas of the brain

N. K. Mishra, R. K. Goulatia, and A. Khosla

Department of Neuroradiology, Neurosciences Centre, All India Institute of Medical Sciences, New Delhi, India

Summary. Infective granulomas account for 15% of all space-occupying lesions of the brain. Tuberculomas are the most frequent granulomas (75%) followed by cysticercus granulomas (20%) and other granulomas (5%). CT scan in these patients provides an accurate method of diagnosis in these cases in conjunction with clinical details and response to medical therapy, in most instances. MRI provides additional information and could be useful if available in all cases.

Key words: Granuloma – Tuberculoma – Cysticercosis – Computed tomography – Brain

Inflammatory granulomas constitute approximately 15% of all intracranial space-occupying lesions [1, 2]. CT scans and case records of 200 such cases, seen at the AIIMS, New Delhi between January 1987 and December 1989 were analysed to assess the morphological characteristics of granulomas of different aetiologies on CT and in a few cases on MRI.

Patients and methods

Patients included in this study presented with symptoms and signs of raised intracranial pressure (ICP) (60%), focal neurological deficits (55%) and seizures (43%). The other presenting symptoms and signs are detailed in Table 1. The patients' age ranged from 1 year to 83 years and there were 104 male and 96 female patients in this group.

Results

Tuberculous granulomas were the most frequent (75%). Surgical excision and histopathological correlation was available in 17% of tuberculomas. In the rest diagnosis was arrived at by correlating clinical features, CT morphology and response to antituberculous therapy [3, 4]. CT scans showed either single or multiple enhancing "ring" lesions with isodense centre (Fig. 1), nodular (disc) lesions or bizzare irregularly enhancing large mass lesions, particularly in the posterior fossa, with varying grades of perilesional oedema and mass effect (Table 2). Evidence of meningitis with exudates in cistern, hydrocephalus, gyral enhancement was also seen in 18% cases [5–7]. Granulomas developed during the course of antituberculous therapy for tuberculous meningitis in 7% cases [8]. A calcified dot in the centre of a ring lesion, the "target" sign, was seen in 12 patients (8%) in the age group below 15 years [1, 9]. The majority of these lesions were single (74%) and the rest (26%) multiple. Sixteen patients had lesions in the brain stem [10, 11]. On antituberculous therapy, these lesions showed regression of perilesional oedema and reduction in size of the nodular or ring lesions within 8 weeks. In 16% cases resolution was delayed up to 9 months. As a final outcome, these lesions became calcified over a period of 12–18 months. Surgical excision in 17% cases was necessitated by worsening clinical condition. Excluded from this series were those patients who had solitary ring lesions on CT after seizures, which disappeared on anticonvulsant therapy alone. MRI performed in 5 cases with ring lesions showed a hypointense ring lesion with hyperintense core, surrounded by oedema on T2-weighted images. In

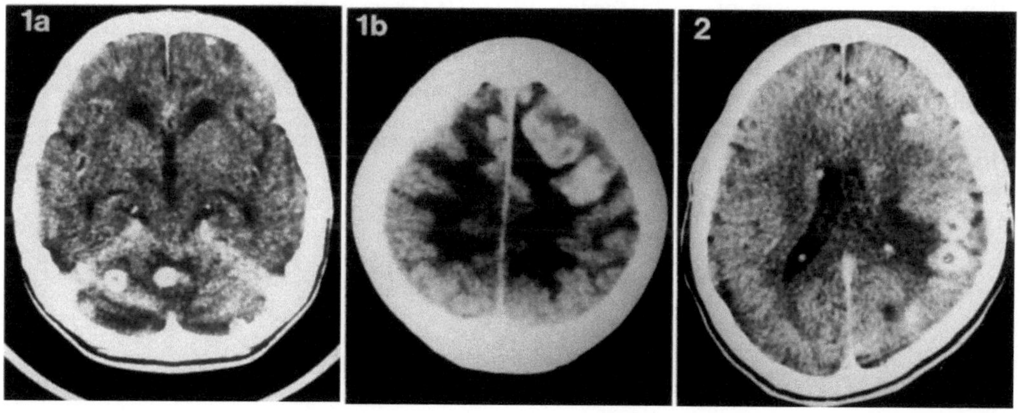

Fig. 1 a, b. Multiple supratentorial and infratentorial ring lesions

Fig. 2. Enhancing ring lesions with perifocal oedema and associated "cystic" and calcific lesions

Table 1. Granulomas of the brain: clinical features

1. Raised intracranial pressure	120–60%
2. Focal neurological deficits	110–55%
3. Seizure disorders	86–43%
4. Cerebellar signs	35–17.5%
5. Fever	54–27%
6. Meningitis	36–18%
7. Tuberculous focus elsewhere	18– 9%
8. Evidence of chronic sinus disease	8– 4%
9. Subcutaneous nodules of cysticercus	12– 6%

Table 2. Tuberculomas: CT morphology

	No. of cases = 150
1. Enhancing ring lesions with perifocal oedema	120–80%
2. Enhancing nodules with perifocal oedema	24–16%
3. Large irregular mass with rim enhancement and oedema	6– 4%
4. "Target" sign	12– 8%
5. Meningitis with exudates in cisterns	10– 7%
6. Multiple lesions	39–26%
7. Shift of midline structures	9– 6%

Table 3. Cysticercus granulomas: CT morphology

	No. of cases = 40
1. Multiple enhancing ring lesions with perifocal oedema	40–100%
2. Compressed ventricles and cisterns	24– 60%
3. Associated cystic lesions	36– 90%
4. Associated calcific lesions	32– 80%
5. Solitary "ring" lesions	4– 10%
6. Satisfactory response to medical therapy	30– 75%

2 cases with target sign, a central hypointense dot representing calcification was seen [12].

Cysticercosis is endemic in our country and 40 cases were analysed in this series [13]. Cysticercus granulomas account for up to 2.5% of intracranial space-occupying lesions and are also reported from many parts of the world [14]. Besides seizures, raised ICP and focal neurological deficits, 1 case presented with stroke. Subcutaneous cysticercus nodules were found in 12 cases (30%). CT scans in these cases showed enhancing ring lesions (Fig. 2) with hypodense core, surrounded by oedema with other calcific or purely cystic lesions (Table 3), few with calcified scolex [15]. Solitary ring lesions were seen in only 4 cases in this group. Excluded from this group were cases of purely cystic or calcified lesions and intraventricular cysts. Medical therapy with praziquantel or albendazole was favourable in 75% cases. MRI available in 6 cases showed hypointense rings with hyperintense core in T2-weighted images. Scolices were visualised in 2 cases on MRI.

Fungal granulomas were fewer and only 10 cases of proven fungal granulomas were analysed. None of these patients were immunocompromised. In 2 cases a history of chronic sinus disease was obtained. CT scan in these cases showed large enhancing masses, adjacent to diseased sinus, some with areas of hypodensity within the mass. Diagnosis was made on biopsy or surgical excision.

Conclusions

CT morphology in conjunction with clinical details and response to medical therapy is diagnostic in the majority of these granulomas. CT provides an excellent means of monitoring these cases at periodic intervals and obviates the need for surgical intervention, particularly for lesions in eloquent areas. MRI provides additional information and could be useful if used more frequently.

References

1. Bhargava S, Tandon PN (1980) Intracranial tuberculomas: a CT study. Br J Radiol 53: 935–945
2. Dastur HM (1975) Tuberculoma. In: Vinken PJ, Bruyn GW (eds) Handbook of clinical neurology, vol 35. North-Holland, Amsterdam, pp 413–426
3. Whelan MA, Stern J (1981) Intracranial tuberculoma. Radiology 138: 75–81
4. Vengsarkar US, Pisipaty RP, Parekh B (1986) Intracranial tuberculoma and the CT scan. J Neurosurg 64: 568–574
5. Draouat S, Abdenabi B, Ghanem M (1987) Computed tomography of cerebral tuberculoma. J Comput Assist Tomogr 11: 594–599
6. Welchman JM (1979) Computerised tomography of intracranial tuberculomata. Clin Radiol 30: 567–578
7. Bhatia R, Tandon P, Mishra NK (1986) Inflammatory lesions of the basal ganglia and thalamus: review of twenty-one cases. Neurosurgery 19: 983–988
8. Borah NC, Maheshwari MC, Mishra NK, Goulatia RK (1984) Appearance of tuberculoma during the course of TB meningitis. J Neurol 231: 269–270
9. VanDyk A (1988) CT of intracranial tuberculomas with specific reference to Target sign. Neuroradiology 30: 329–335
10. Mahanta A, Kalra L, Maheshwari MC, Mishra NK (1982) Brain stem tuberculoma. J Neurol 227: 249–253
11. Talamas O, Del Brutto OH, Garcia-Ramos G (1989) Brain stem tuberculoma: an analysis of 11 patients. Arch Neurol 46: 529–535
12. Gupta RK, Jena A, Sharma (1988) MR imaging of intracranial tuberculomas. J Comput Assist Tomogr 12: 280–286
13. Bhargava S (1983) Radiology including computed tomography of parasitic diseases of the CNS. Neurosurg Rev 6: 129–137
14. McCormick GF, Zee GS, Heiden J (1982) Cysticercosis cerebri: review of 127 cases. Arch Neurol 39: 534–539
15. Tandon PN (1983) Cerebral cysticercosis. Neurosurg Rev 6: 119–127

Dr. N. K. Mishra
Associate Professor
Department of Neuroradiology
Neurosciences Centre
A. I. I. M. S.
New Delhi-110029, India

Neuroradiology (1991) 33 [Suppl]: 573–574

Neuro radiology

© Springer-Verlag 1991

CT in subdural empyema

N. Khandelwal[1], N. Malik[1], A. Pathak[2], B. S. Sharma[2], V. K. Kak[2], and S. Suri

Departments of [1] Radiodiagnosis and [2] Neurosurgery, Postgraduate Institute of Medical Education and Research, Chandigarh, India

Summary. Forty-nine cases of subdural empyema were treated surgically between 1977 and 1990. Contrast-enhanced CT was obtained in 34 patients. It clearly showed the presence, location and extent of the collection in all cases. Diffuse collections, adjacent parenchymal involvement and delay in treatment were associated with a poor prognosis. Early accurate diagnosis and timely aggressive intervention helped to improve prognosis.

Key words: Empyema – Abscess – Subdural – Computed tomography

Subdural empyema (SDE) is an uncommon extra-axial bacterial infection accounting for approximately 13%–33% of all intracranial infections [1]. The majority of empyemas occur following acute sinusitis or otitis media and are associated with a fulminating clinical course. Less often, an empyema may occur following trauma or surgery and follow a prolonged, indolent course. The overall mortality has been reported to be as high as 30%–50% [2]. CT is highly reliable in the early diagnosis and precise anatomical localisation of SDE. It also demonstrates associated parenchymal involvement, e.g. oedema, infarction or abscess formation. In this study, CT studies of 34 patients with surgically proven SDE have been reviewed and correlated with clinicopathological data.

Patients and methods

Between 1977 and 1990, 49 cases of subdural empyema were treated at our institute. Thirty-four patients underwent contrast-enhanced CT. Plain CT was obtained in 10 patients and serial CT studies were carried out on 17 patients. There were 25 males and 9 females, whose ages ranged from 10 months to 80 years; they included 15 children, of whom 2 were infants.

Results

The presenting clinical features were fever (20 cases), headache (18), altered sensorium (18) and seizures (15). Examination revealed papilloedema (20 cases), hemiparesis (11), meningism (11) and cranial nerve palsies (2). The commonest aetiological factor was otitis media, in 12 cases, followed by trauma (8 cases) and surgery (4 cases). The cause could not be ascertained in 10 patients. Bacteriological examination of the pus yielded *Staphylococcus aureus* (8 cases), *Escherichia coli* (4), *Proteus mirabilis* (4) and multiple organisms, including anaerobes (6 cases). The pus was sterile on culture in 12 cases, presumably due to prior administration of antibiotics.

The CT diagnosis was established on criteria described in the literature [3]. Location and extent of SDE as established on CT are given in Table 1. Associated parenchymal involvement was seen in 10 cases, in the form of a brain abscess in 8 and infarction in 2 (Fig. 1). The collection was very small and close to bone in 4 cases, and could have escaped detection (Fig. 2). In 3 cases, initial CT revealed only a mild midline shift or cerebral oedema, the SDE being revealed on further CT studies after 2–3 days. A brain abscess was subsequently detected in 2 cases on postoperative CT. A unilocular, localised collection, without parenchymal abnormality, responded well to needle aspiration and antibiotics (Fig. 3). Multilocular, diffuse, parafalcine or posterior fossa SDE required burrhole evacuation, craniotomy or craniectomy. Re-exploration was required in 4 cases where serial CT demonstrated a large residual collection or a brain abscess. The overall mortality in the present series was 23.5%.

Discussion

SDE occurs most commonly following otorhinological infections. Subdural infections occur by way of retrograde thrombophlebitis via bridging emissary veins [3, 4]. Progression of thrombophlebitis to involve the cortical veins and dural sinuses leads to oedema and ischaemia of adjacent cortex. Without prompt treatment, an irreversible dural sinus and venous thrombosis ensues leading to secondary parenchymal infection and infarction.

Table 1. Location of subdural empyemas

Supratentorial			30
Convexity (diffuse)		24	
Bilateral	8		
Unilateral	16		
Parafalcine	14		
Convexity (focal)		6	
Frontoparietal	4		
Parietal	1		
Temporal	1		
Infratentorial			3
Combined			1

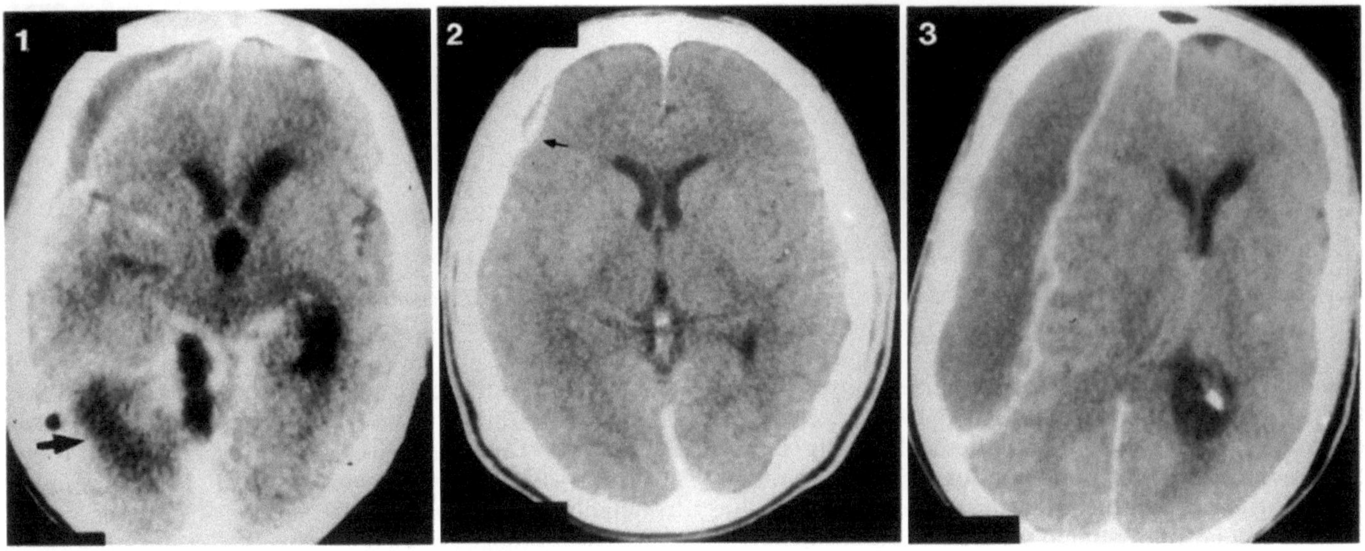

Fig. 1. Contrast-enhanced CT showing left frontal and loculated posterior interhemispheric collections. Note the parenchymal involvement (infarction) *(arrow)*

Fig. 2. Contrast-enhanced CT showing small hemispheric collection close to bone, which could be overlooked

Fig. 3. Contrast-enhanced CT showing huge unilocular hemispheric collection with intense irregular membrane enhancement

An aggressive surgical approach is the absolute requirement for successful treatment of this condition. In post-traumatic or postoperative cases, a well-formed limiting membrane develops, producing a localised infection with an indolent clinical course [5]. No obvious aetiological factor could be demonstrated clinically or radiologically in about 30% of cases in the present series. Clinically silent sinus or ear diseases may be demonstrated on CT, indicating a need for careful review of the basal sections [6].

The CT findings can be subtle early in the course of the disease. A small pocket of pus close to the bony vault, mild interhemispheric collections, lack of enhancement of the membrane and poor quality CT images are some of the factors which can lead to a negative study [3]. Minimal midline shift or cerebral oedema may be the only clues to the diagnosis. In such cases serial CT can demonstrate the location and extent of the collection, provided a high index of clinical suspicion is maintained.

The high mortality and morbidity associated with this condition are in part due to failure to recognise this entity, delay in treatment, inadequate surgical drainage and lack of wide-spread appreciation of management policies [7]. The changes of survival improve only if the disease is recognised before the onset of deterioration of consciousness or appearance of neurological signs or seizures. SDE should be suspected in cases of meningitis with a suspected extracerebral source of infection having focal neurological signs. Contrast-enhanced CT is obligatory even before performing lumbar puncture [8].

References

1. Danziger A, Price H, Schechter MM (1980) An analysis of 113 intracranial infections. Neuroradiology 19: 31–34
2. Smith HP, Hendrick EB (1983) Subdural empyema and epidural abscess in children. J Neurosurg 58: 392–397
3. Zimmermann RD, Leeds NE, Danziger A (1984) Subdural empyema: CT findings. Radiology 150: 417–422
4. Weingarten K, Zimmermann RD, Becker RD, Heier LA, Haimes AB, Deck MDF (1989) Subdural and epidural empyemas-MR imaging. AJR 152: 615–621
5. Post EM, Modesti LM (1981) Subacute postoperative subdural empyema. J Neurosurg 55: 761–765
6. Hodges J, Anslow P, Gillett G (1986) Subdural empyema-continuing diagnostic problem in the CT scan era. Q J Med 228: 387–393
7. Pathak A, Sharma BS, Mathuriya SN, Khosla VK, Khandelwal N, Kak VK (1990) Controversies in the management of subdural empyema – a study of 41 cases with review of literature. Acta Neurochir (Wien) 102: 25–32
8. Farkas AG, Marks JC (1986) Subdural empyema. An important diagnosis not to miss. Br Med J 293: 118–119

Dr. N. Khandelwal
Department of Radiodiagnosis
P. G. I. M. E. R.
Chandigarh-160012, India

Neuroradiology (1991) 33 [Suppl]: 575–577

Neuro
radiology
© Springer-Verlag 1991

Neuroacanthocytosis: correlation of clinical and neuroimaging abnormalities

J. E. Dervin[1], B. K. Kendall[1], and R. J. Hardie[2]

[1] Lysholm Radiological Department, [2] Department of Neurology, The National Hospital for Nervous Diseases, Queen Square, London, UK

Summary. The neuroimaging abnormalities in 11 patients with neuroacanthocytosis have been reviewed. In 4 of 6 patients studied by MRI, increased signal was returned from the corpus striatum and in 1 of the remaining cases increased pallidal signal was seen. Caudate nucleus atrophy was seen in just under three-quarters of cases. In 1 case studied by MRI at high field strength, low signal was seen in the posterior putamina on a heavily T2-weighted sequence, probably reflecting increased striatal iron. The imaging findings in neuroacanthocytosis appear to be very similar to Huntingdon's disease, but unlike Huntingdon's disease there appears to be no clear relationship between the degree of caudate nucleus atrophy and severity of clinical abnormalities.

Key words: Neuroacanthocytosis – Computed tomography – Magnetic resonance imaging

Neuroacanthocytosis is a specific degenerative neurological condition associated with the presence of abnormal erythrocytes, bearing spiky projections (*acantha,* thorn, Greek) in the peripheral blood smear. Creatinine kinase is usually elevated and lipoproteins are normal. A wide spectrum of clinical features can be encountered in this condition, dominated by movement disorders including chorea, tics, dystonia and parkinsonism; epileptic seizures, muscle wasting and emotional and cognitive changes also occur.

In five published cases, where necropsy has been performed, marked neuronal loss and gliosis were seen affecting the caudate, to a lesser extent the putamen and in two cases the pallidum; the cerebral cortex appears to be spared [1]. In a recent case at the National Hospital the pathological features of neuronal loss and gliosis were found in the pars reticulata; these findings have only previously been reported to involve the corpus striatum and pallidum.

Previous reports on the neuroimaging findings in neuroacanthocytosis have been limited; the largest series reported the CT findings in five patients [2]; the largest MRI series consisted of three patients [3].

Patients and methods

The neuroimaging findings in 11 patients with neuroacanthocytosis have been reviewed; 6 cases had MRI (5 at 0.26 T, 1 at 1.5 T); 3 of these patients had CT also; the remaining 5 cases had CT only. Peripheral blood samples were screened for acanthocytes in each pa-

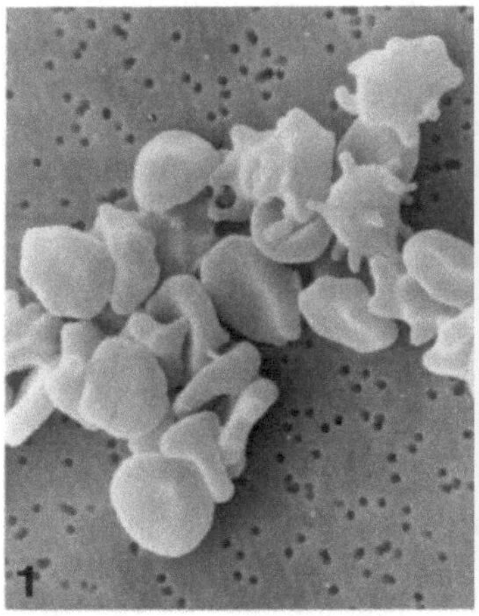
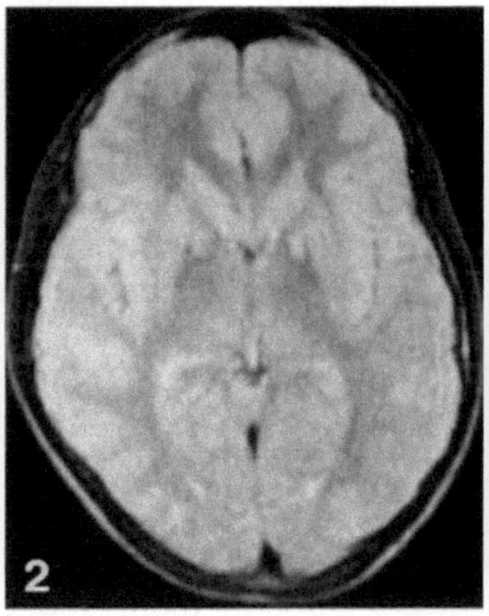
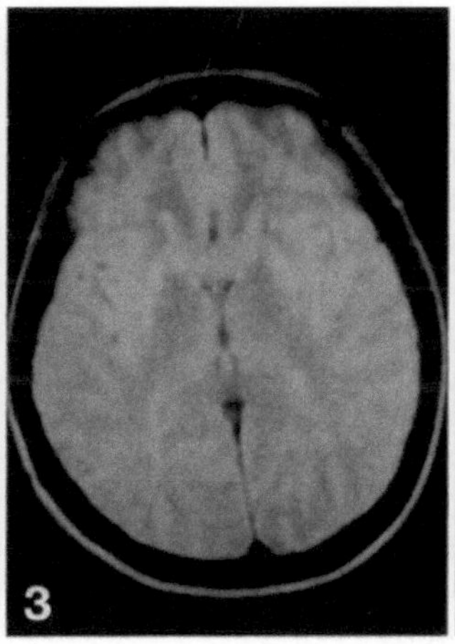
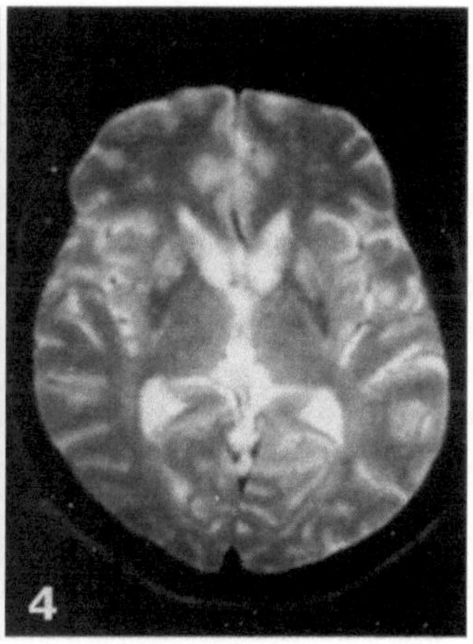

Fig. 1. Scanning electron microscopy (magnification × 4000) of peripheral blood smear showing several acanthocytes

Fig. 2. T2-weighted image obtained at 0.26 T shows increased signal in the globus pallidus bilaterally. SE 2000/80

Fig. 3. T2-weighted image obtained at 0.26 T shows increased striatal signal. SE 2000/80

Fig. 4. Heavily T2-weighted image obtained at 1.5 T. Mixed striatal signal is present with low signal in the posterior putamina

Table 1. Neuroimaging and clinical abnormalities

Patient	JD	KM	EC	CE	MH	SF	DB	KS	BL	FB	AB
Sex	M	F	M	M	F	F	F	M	F	F	F
MRI signal abnormalities	↑Pu ↑PV	↑Pu ↑PV	↑PV ↑CR ↑CS	↑GP	↑Pu	↑↓ Pu ↑ CS ↑ SC	–	–	–	–	–
Bicaudate diameter (mm) Normal < 15 mm	24	25	29	13	19	30	20	22	9	25	8
Location of CT low attenuation lesions	0	–	PV CR CS	0	–	–	0	0	CS SC	0	0
Cerebral atrophy	0	+	+	0	0	0	0	+	+	0	0
% Acanthocytes Normal < 3%	5	10	10	10	10	20	10	50	25	25	15
CPK (mU/ml) Normal < 195	692	401	47	103	860	410	213	261	840	–	109
Movement disorders	D	CDPT	CDPT	D	CDT	CPDT	CDT	CP	CT	CPT	DPT
Dementia	+	+	+	+	+	0	+	+	+	+	+
Seizures	0	0	0	0	+	0	+	+	+	0	0
EMG denervation	0	0	0	0	0	+	0	+	+	+	0
Age of onset (years)	33	40	62	8	22	24	28	44	21	44	12
Age at last examination	36	49	67	18	25	38	36	51	27	47	24

↑ (↓), Increased (decreased) signal intensity on T2-weighted sequences; Pu, putamen; GP, globus pallidus; PV, periventricular; CR, corona radiata; CS, centrum semiovale; SC, subcortical; C, chorea; D, dystonia; P, parkinsonism; T, tics; CPK, serum creatinine phosphokinase; 0, absent; +, present; –, not done

tient; for the purposes of this study an acanthocyte was defined as a dense, slightly contracted red cell which had a number of irregularly spaced thorny surface projections, often with terminal bulbs (Fig. 1). Other crenated forms such as ethinocytes were not counted as true acanthocytes. We regarded an acanthocyte count of over 3% as significant.

Results

Table 1 shows the neuroimaging and clinical abnormalities in all patients.

Discussion

In the two previous largest series which reported neuroimaging abnormalities in neuroacanthocytosis caudate nucleus atrophy was reported in all patients [2, 3], but in our series caudate nucleus atrophy was present in 8 cases (73%). We could not establish any relationship between the degree of caudate nucleus atrophy and the severity of clinical, erythrocyte or biochemical abnormalities, though it seems less common in younger patients. In 4 of the 6 patients studied by MRI increased signal was returned from the putamina and caudate nucleus (Fig. 1). All of these cases had atrophy of the caudate nucleus.

In 1 case, a 16-year-old boy (CE) there was no atrophy of the caudate head and CT appeared normal; MRI, however, revealed high signal foci in the globus pallidus bilaterally on a moderately T2-weighted sequence obtained at 0.26 T (Fig. 2); unlike most of our patients where chorea was a prominent feature the most striking movement disorder in this case was dystonia. In another case with similar clinical picture (JD), the radiological findings fell into the more general pattern with caudate nucleus atrophy and abnormal striatal signal (Fig. 3). An interesting observation was the presence of low signal in the posterior aspect of the putamina in the single case studied at high field strength (1.5 T), on a heavily T2-weighted sequence (Fig. 4). A similar observation has previously been reported; the most likely explanation for such T2 shortening is increased striatal iron, though this is not a recognised biochemical or histological feature of neuroacanthocytosis. The significance of increased iron in these extrapyramidal nuclei is uncertain, but it may be related to changes in regional metabolism. It is interesting to note that a recent biochemical investigation of neuroacanthocytosis revealed altered norepinephrine and dopamine levels in the striatum and globus pallidus [4]; iron is known to participate in the enzymatic synthesis of these amines.

Conclusions

The imaging findings in neuroacanthocytosis appear to be very similar to Huntingdon's disease, but unlike Huntingdon's disease there is no clear relationship between the degree of caudate nucleus atrophy and severity of clinical abnormalities. MRI may be useful in revealing abnormalities when CT is normal particularly when striatal changes are less prominent and caudate nucleus atrophy is absent. Further study of this condition with MRI at high field strength should elucidate the possible iron deposition.

References

1. Hardie RJ (1990) Neuroacanthocytosis: a clinical, haematological and pathological study in 19 cases. Brain (in press)
2. Serra S, Xerra A, Scribano E, Medurri M, Di Perri R (1987) Computerised tomography in amyotrophic choreo-acanthocytosis. Neuroradiology 29: 480–482
3. Rutledge JN, Hilal SK, Silver AJ, Detendi R, Fahn S (1987) Study of movement disorders and brain iron by MR. AJNR 8: 397–411
4. Yebebes JG de, Brin MF, Mena MA, De Felipe C, del Rio RM, Bazan E, Martinez A, Fahn S, Del Rio J, Vazquez A, Varela de Seijas E (1988) Neurochemical findings in neuroacanthocytosis. Mov Disord 3: 300–312

J. E. Dervin
Lysholm Radiological Department
The National Hospital for Nervous Diseases
Queen Square
London, UK

Neuroradiology (1991) 33 [Suppl]: 578–579

Neuro radiology
© Springer-Verlag 1991

Neurocysticercosis: comparison of CT scan and MRI

Study of 35 cases

S. B. Desai, V. C. Shah, D. J. Javri, and P. Rao

Breach Candy Hospital and Research Centre, Bombay, India

Summary. Thirty-five patients with intracranial cysticercosis were studied with CT and MRI prior to and after cysticidal therapy. MRI detected many more lesions than CT. Pre- and post-contrast CT could demonstrate only 15–65% of lesions identified on MRI. The morphology of cysticercus lesions was better and easily appreciated on MRI. Cerebrospinal fluid-equivalent cystic lesions containing mural nodules (pea in pod appearance) on T1-weighted images were pathognomonic of live cysticerci. MRI was superior in detecting dying cysticerci, but inferior to CT in identifying small calcified dead cysticerci.

Key words: Infection – Cysticercosis – Computed tomography – Magnetic resonance imaging – Pea in pod appearance

Cysticercosis is one of the most common parasitic diseases to affect the brain. The incidence of brain involvement is as high as 60–92% in cysticercosis. Cysticercosis is a parasitic infection endemic in parts of Asia, the Indian subcontinent, Africa and Latin America [1].

Humans serve as the intermediate hosts of *Taenia solium*, the pork tapeworm.

Cysticercosis is known to occur in pork eaters [2]. However, we have observed a rather paradoxical situation in India. Large numbers of our neurocysticercosis patients have been totally vegetarian. The mode of infection seems to be via infested vegetables.

Patients and methods

Thirty-five patients with neurocysticercosis were studied over a period of 1 year and detailed clinical assessment and routine investigations were done in all the cases. The criteria for diagnosis of neurocysticercosis are: (a) serum and cerebrospinal fluid (CSF) antibody titre; (b) biopsy of subcutaneous cyst; (c) CT; (d) pathognomonic MRI findings.

CT scans were obtained on a CT Somatom DR3, GE 9800, Toshiba TCT 80 and Hitachi CT scanner.

MRI was performed on a Siemens Magnetom superconducting magnet operating at 1.0 T. Multiple-slice spin-echo images were obtained at a short repetition time (TR) of 0.5–0.75 s and a longer TR of 2.5–3.0 s. Echo delay time (TE) was 17, 23 and 90 ms. Multiplanar imaging (axial, coronal and sagittal) with a slice thickness of 5.00–8.00 mm, an interslice gap of 0.8–1.6 mm and a matrix of 256×256 or 128×256 was used.

MR scans were obtained within 1–15 days following CT scans. In the majority of cases MRI was performed within 24–48 h of CT.

The lesion count was obtained per 25 cm^2 of brain area at various levels in the supratentorial region and the average value was calculated.

Results

Forty-one parallel CT and MRI studies were obtained in 35 patients. In a few cases the studies were carried out following therapy with either praziquantal or albendozole. The male to female ratio was 2.2:1. The majority of patients (82.8%) were in the second to fourth decade of life.

Our patients fell into four groups, based on CT and MRI findings. Group I (19 patients) had lesions in all stages. Group 2 (6 patients) had predominantly a very high number of live cysts (cyst burden). Group 3 (6 patients) had predominantly dying cysts. Group 4 (4 patients) showed predominantly dead cysts.

The patients in group 1 and 3 presented with seizures without focal deficit [3]. The patients in group 2 presented with dementia and raised intracranial pressure. Patients in group 4 usually had a long-standing history of seizures and had already received at least one course of anti-larval therapy.

Discussion

The cyst morphology had different CT and MRI appearances depending on the stage of evolution [4–6].

The live cysts on CT scan appeared as CSF equivalent density oval or circular lesions with or without identifiable hyperdense scolex within. There was no surrounding oedema or contrast enhancement [6]. On MRI, the live cysts revealed 5- to 20-mm-diameter round lesions of CSF equivalent intensity on both T1- and T2-weighted images [4]. An eccentric nodule of iso-intense scolex was well identified in almost all the cysts, producing a classical "pea-in-pod" appearance.

The dying cysts revealed ring/disc enhancing lesions on CT scans with surrounding oedema [6–8]. On MRI, the cyst fluid revealed intensity more than that of CSF on T1-weighted images and appreciable hyper-intensity on the T2-weighted images with significant surrounding oedema in all the cases. The scolex and cyst differentiation was not well identified. Dead cysticerci revealed punctate calcifications without surrounding oedema or contrast enhance-

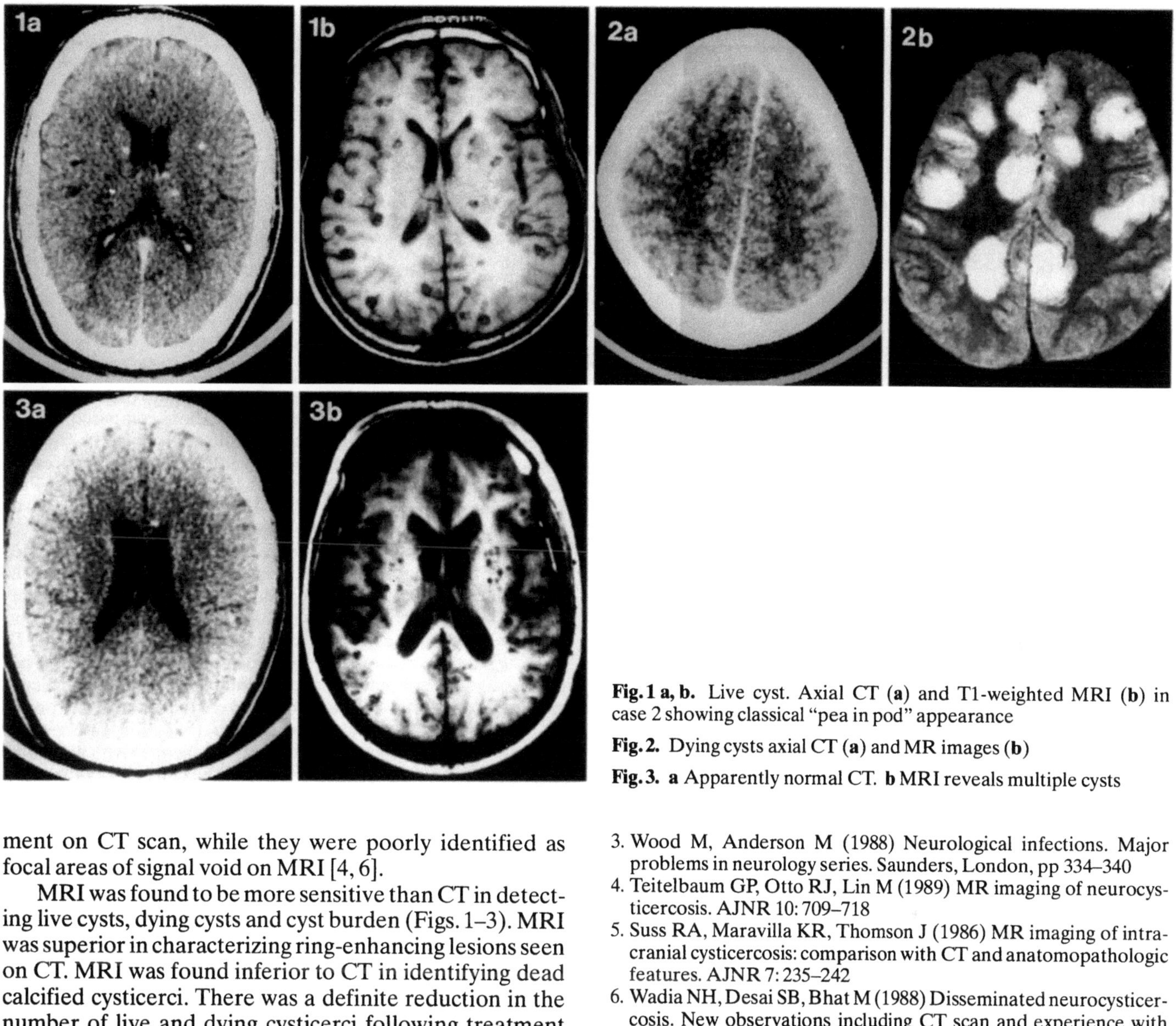

Fig. 1 a, b. Live cyst. Axial CT (**a**) and T1-weighted MRI (**b**) in case 2 showing classical "pea in pod" appearance

Fig. 2. Dying cysts axial CT (**a**) and MR images (**b**)

Fig. 3. **a** Apparently normal CT. **b** MRI reveals multiple cysts

ment on CT scan, while they were poorly identified as focal areas of signal void on MRI [4, 6].

MRI was found to be more sensitive than CT in detecting live cysts, dying cysts and cyst burden (Figs. 1–3). MRI was superior in characterizing ring-enhancing lesions seen on CT. MRI was found inferior to CT in identifying dead calcified cysticerci. There was a definite reduction in the number of live and dying cysticerci following treatment with albendozole. Our five patients who had symptomatic raised intracranial pressure had a very large number of live cysts (12.2–19.8/25 cm^2). This may give the possible quantitative correlation of cyst burden and pressure symptoms and may lead to therapeutic relevance in selecting the patients for cysticidal therapy.

References

1. McCormic GF, Zec CS, Heiden J (1982) Cysticercosis cerebri: review of 127 cases. Arch Neurol 39: 534–539
2. Sotelo J, Torres B, Rubio-Donnadiev F (1985) Praziquantel in the treatment of NCC. Neurology 35: 752–755
3. Wood M, Anderson M (1988) Neurological infections. Major problems in neurology series. Saunders, London, pp 334–340
4. Teitelbaum GP, Otto RJ, Lin M (1989) MR imaging of neurocysticercosis. AJNR 10: 709–718
5. Suss RA, Maravilla KR, Thomson J (1986) MR imaging of intracranial cysticercosis: comparison with CT and anatomopathologic features. AJNR 7: 235–242
6. Wadia NH, Desai SB, Bhat M (1988) Disseminated neurocysticercosis. New observations including CT scan and experience with treatment by praziquantel. Brain 111: 597–614
7. Handler LC, Mervis B (1983) Cerebral cysticercosis with reference to the natural history of parenchymal lesions. AJNR 4: 709–712
8. Cardenas Y, Gardenas J (1962) Cysticercosis of the central nervous system II. Pathologic and radiologic findings. J Neurosurg 19: 635–640

Dr. Viral Shah
MRI Center
Breach Candy Hospital
60 B Bhulabhai Desai Rd
Bombay 400-026, India

Neuroradiology (1991) 33 [Suppl]: 580–581

Neuro
radiology
© Springer-Verlag 1991

Changes in T1 and T2 on repeated MR brain scans in a cohort of HIV-positive patients

D. Kean[1], A. Blane[1], A. Chiswick[2], G. Goodwin[3], J.J.K. Best[1], and R. Brettle[2]

Departments of [1] Medical Radiology, [2] Infectious Diseases and [3] Psychiatry, University of Edinburgh, Edinburgh, UK

Summary. In an effort to detect changes in T1 and T2 values in a cohort of HIV patients, repeated MR brain scans were performed. These showed very little change in T1 or T2 and this small study illustrates the problems which will be encountered in any large study of this type.

Key words: Magnetic resonance imaging – Human immunodeficiency virus – Brain – White matter – Caudate nucleus

It has been demonstrated that magnetic resonance imaging (MRI) can detect white matter abnormalities, by virtue of increases in T1 and T2 values, in patients suffering from multiple sclerosis before focal lesions, i.e. plaques, are apparent [1]. It is also now well recognised that patients with HIV infection are liable to CNS complications such as encephalopathy and dementia and it is hoped that MRI may be able to monitor the onset and progression of this brain disease.

Patients and methods

In an effort to detect preclinical central nervous system changes in subjects infected with human immunodeficiency virus (HIV), MRI was performed on 64 HIV-positive patients. The cohort was composed of 10 homosexual males and the other 54 had been infected by blood transmission (32 males, 22 females; mean age 34 years). Thirty-eight patients were re-examined 1 year after their initial scan and the MR measurements of both examinations compared. All patients were staged according to the classification of the Centres for Disease Control, US Department of Health and Human Services [2]. An SR/IR interleaved sequence (TR 1 s, 200 ms) and a Carr-Purcell-Meiboom-Gill (TR 1.5 s, TE 32–128 ms) sequence were used to image the entire brain and from these transverse 12-mm-thick sections T1 and T2 measurements were obtained. The imaging device was a 0.08 T vertical field resistive system whose precision and accuracy measurements have been reported previously [3]. The more important measurement in this type of sequential study is precision which is approximately 3% using this imaging device. T1 and T2 measurements were obtained from the corona radiata of each hemisphere using an irregular region of interest facility (Fig. 1). Separate measurements were also obtained from the anterior and posterior portions of this white matter volume (Fig. 2). Measurements were also obtained from deep grey matter structures with particular reference to the caudate nucleus. Out of the patients who were reexamined, 25 remained in the same clinical stage, 10 had deteriorated by one stage and 3 had deteriorated by two stages.

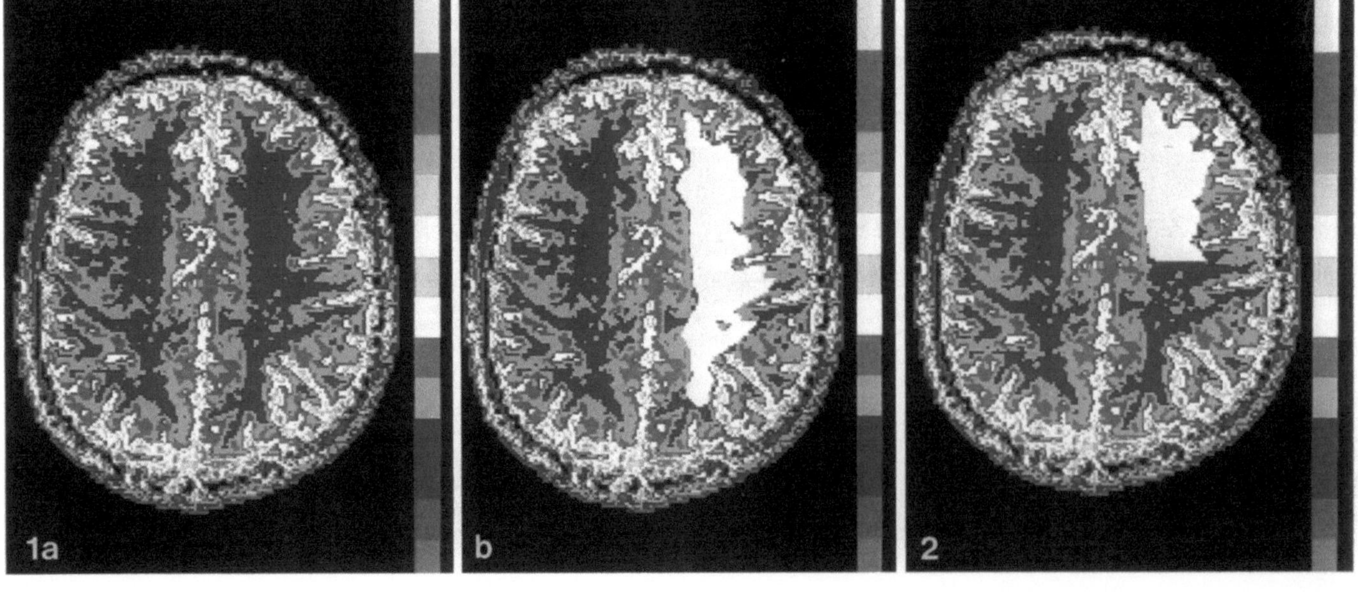

Fig. 1. **a** Normal calculated T1 map with no irregular areas described. **b** Transverse calculated T1 map showing, in white, an irregular area of interest drawn around the corona radiata

Fig. 2. Transverse calculated T1 map with only the anterior white matter described

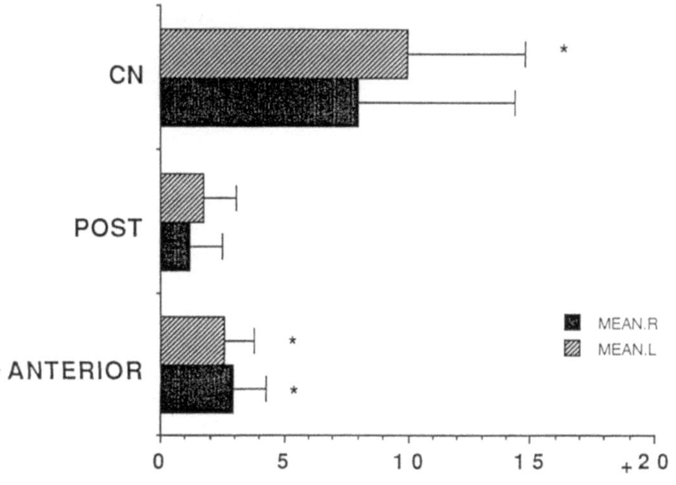

Fig. 3. Interval T1 changes barely reaching significance in anterior and posterior white matter areas and a larger change in the region of the head of the caudate.* $P = 0.045$

Results

There was no significant interval change either in T1 or T2 values obtained from the entire area of the corona radiata or when the anterior and posterior portions were measured individually. Measurements from deep grey matter, in particular the caudate nucleus, suggested that there was a slight increase in T1 values between examinations and some of these differences reached statistically significant levels (Fig. 3).

Discussion

It has been shown that there is no demonstrable change in white matter T1 or T2 values in a cohort of HIV subjects on sequential MRI. There may be changes in the caudate nucleus, but these changes are small and are susceptible to partial volume and registration errors. The magnitude of these changes, however, is in keeping with other physiological measurements in HIV subjects, such as serial auditory event related potentials which have been shown to deteriorate slightly on serial testing [4].

It appears, therefore, that this study will require longer term follow-up in a large cohort of subjects. It is also apparent that meticulous attention must be paid to the significant problems of registration and the methods of acquiring and extracting the numerical data before embarking on this study.

References

1. Ormerod I, Johnson G, MacManus D, du Boulay EPGH, McDonald WI (1986) Relaxation times of apparently normal cerebral white matter in multiple sclerosis. Acta Radiol [Suppl] 369: 382–384
2. Smith MA, Kean D, Best JJK, Douglas RHB, MacDonald HL (1984) Specification measurements of an NMR imager. Proceedings of the 3rd International Symposium on Magnetic Resonance in Medicine. Society for Magnetic Resonance in Medicine, New York, p 692
3. Centres for Disease Control, US Department of Health and Human Services (1986) Classification system for human T-lymphotrophic virus type 111/lymphadenopathy-associated virus infections Ann Intern Med 105: 234–237
4. Goodwin GM, Chiswick A, Egan V, St. Clair D, France AJ, Gray J, Jones ME, Welsby P, Brettle RP (1989) Neuropsychological testing and auditory event related potentials in the clinical examination of HIV seropositive drug misusers. In: Thompson P, Page ML (eds) Neuropsychiatric aspects of AIDS. Duphar, pp 30-39

Dr. D. Kean
Department of Medical Radiology
University of Edinburgh
Edinburgh, UK

Neuroradiology (1991) 33 [Suppl]: 582–583

Neuro-radiology
© Springer-Verlag 1991

CT of cranial nerve involvement in external ear disease

R. L. Guy, E. Wylie, S. A. Hickey, and K. A. Tonge

Departments of Radiology and Ear, Nose and Throat Surgery, St. Thomas'Hospital, London, UK

Summary. In malignant external otitis (MEO), the infection may spread from the external auditory meatus (EAM) along several routes: directly into the adjacent mastoid bone, anteriorly into the parotid gland and temporo-mandibular joint and inferiorly into the soft tissues of the infratemporal fossa. Within the infratemporal fossa the seventh and ninth to twelfth nerves may be involved just after they leave their exit foramina. In benign conditions of the external ear such as keratosis obturans, choleasteatoma and chronic otitis externa there may be a conductive deafness due to obstruction of the EAM but spread does not occur beyond the EAM and there are no cranial nerve palsies. Malignant conditions such as squamous cell carcinoma of the external ear may spread in a similar manner to MEO with resulting cranial nerve palsies. We have illustrated the typical patterns of spread and cranial nerve involvement in these different diseases.

Key words: Computed tomography – Malignant external otitis – Ear, neoplasms – Keratosis obturans – Otitis

Malignant external otitis (MEO) is a severe infection of the external auditory meatus (EAM) occuring predominantly in diabetics and usually caused by *Pseudomonas aeruginosa* [1]. It readily spreads to adjacent bone and along soft tissue planes with involvement of the lower cranial nerves and potentially fatal consequences. This pat-

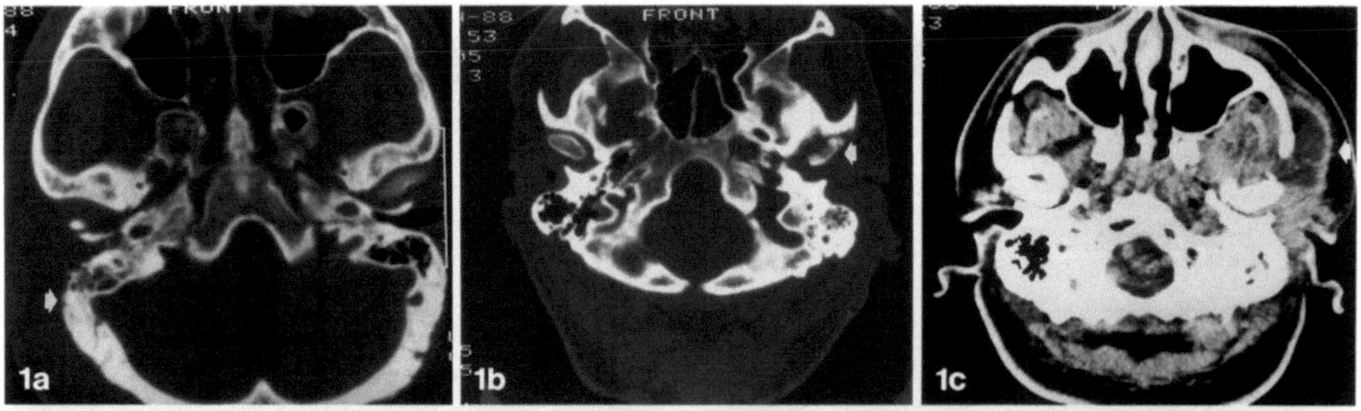

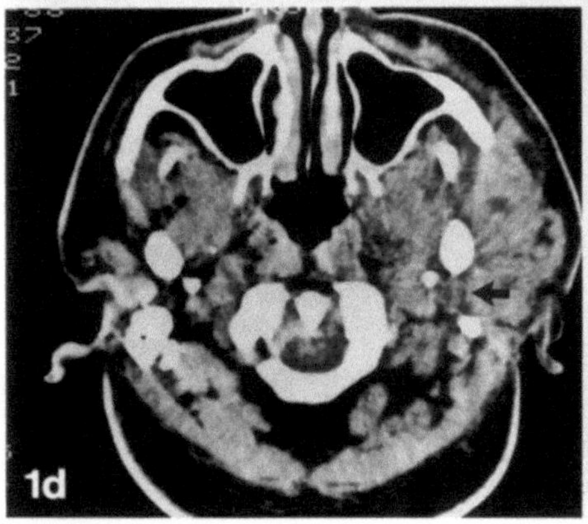

Fig. 1 a–d. Malignant external otitis (reproduced with the kind permission of *Clinical Radiology*). **a** Axial CT. There is erosion of the cortex of the right mastoid process *(arrow)* and clouding of the mastoid air cells. **b** Axial CT. There is erosion of the left temporomandibular joint *(arrow)*. **c** Axial CT. Soft tissue fills and surrounds the left external auditory meatus (EAM) with a low-density non-enhancing abscess in the masseter muscle *(arrow)*. **d** Axial CT. The soft tissue mass extends into the left infratemporal fossa, obliterating the subtemporal triangle *(arrow)*.

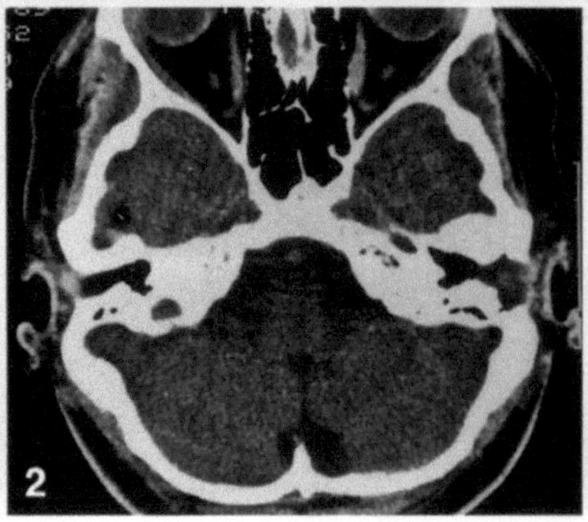

Fig. 2. Keratosis obturans. Axial CT. Soft tissue fills and remodels the left EAM

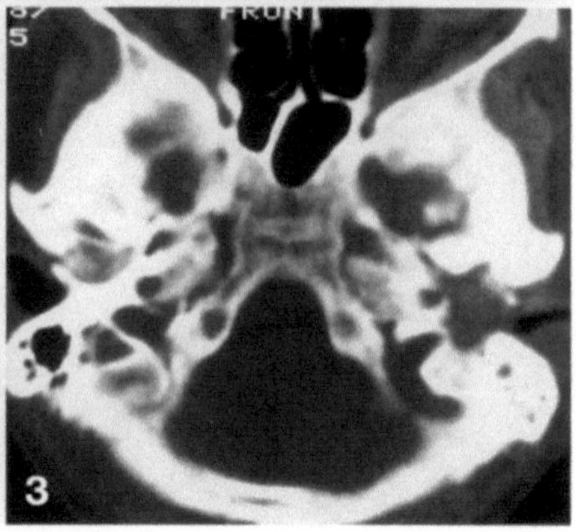

Fig. 3. Squamous cell carcinoma of the external ear. Axial CT. The soft tissue mass extends inferiorly from the left EAM

tern of spread and cranial nerve involvement has been compared with that in other benign and malignant conditions of the external ear.

Materials and methods

The CT studies of patients with external ear disease presenting to our department over a 2-year period were retrospectively reviewed.

Results and discussion

Soft tissue abnormalities of the external ear have been reviewed by Chakeres et al. [2]. CT is of particular value in occlusive conditions of the external ear because direct examination by otoscopy cannot reveal the extent of spread of disease.

There were four diabetic patients with MEO, three of whom had facial nerve palsies. All four patients had a soft tissue mass spreading out from the EAM with direct spread into the mastoid bone (Fig. 1a) and secondary involvement of the middle ear cavity. In all patients there was spread of the inflammatory process anteriorly with erosion of the temporomandibular joint (Fig. 1b), or abscess formation within the parotid gland or masseter muscle (Fig. 1c). In the three patients with seventh nerve palsies there was spread to the soft tissues of the infratemporal fossa. In particular there was obliteration of the fat planes delineating the subtemporal triangle between the styloid process, retromandibular vein and the mastoid process (Fig. 1d) where the facial nerve runs.

None of the patients with benign conditions of the external ear had cranial nerve palsies, although a conductive deafness was commonly due to occlusion of the external ear by soft tissue. In keratosis obturans there was soft tissue (desquamated keratin) filling and remodelling but not eroding the EAM (Fig. 2). In chronic otitis externa there was soft tissue thickening leading to occlusion of the EAM. Some associated mastoiditis was the only further spread of disease. Similarly, in external ear cholesteatoma, the only spread of the disease was to the mastoid process.

In squamous cell carcinoma of the external ear there was a soft tissue mass spreading out from the EAM with erosion of the mastoid bone. In addition there was spread anteriorly to the parotid gland and inferiorly to the infratemporal fossa with a facial nerve palsy (Fig. 3). This pattern of spread closely resembles that in MEO.

In our series, of the wide range of conditions causing stenosis of the EAM, only MEO and squamous cell carcinoma of the external ear were associated with cranial nerve palsies.

References

1. Chandler JR (1968) Malignant external otitis. Laryngoscope 78:1257–1294
2. Chakeres DW, Kapila A, LaMasters D (1985) Soft-tissue abnormalities of the external auditory canal: subject review of CT findings. Radiology 156:105–109

Dr. K. A. Tonge
Department of Radiology,
St. Thomas' Hospital,
Lambeth Palace Road,
London SE1 7EH, UK

Neuroradiology (1991) 33 [Suppl]: 584–585

Neuro
radiology
© Springer-Verlag 1991

MR demonstration of meningeal enhancement with gadolinium-DTPA

Y. Sakamoto, J. Shinzato, K. Yoshizumi, Y. Yamashita, Y. Korogi, H. Bussaka, and M. Takahashi

Department of Radiology, Kumamoto University School of Medicine, Kumamoto, Japan

Summary. Meningeal enhancement has been studied with gadolinium (Gd)-DTPA enhanced MRI in 12 normal and 24 abnormal cases. Pial enhancement was observed in meningeal carcinomatosis, while postoperative patients and sinus thrombosis never showed pial enhancement. Postoperative patients showed gradually decreasing dural enhancement over several months. These findings were useful differentiation of meningeal enhancement by Gd-DTPA MRI.

Key words: Magnetic resonance imaging – Meningeal enhancement – Postoperative state – Gadolinium-DTPA – Meningeal carcinomatosis

Gadolinium (Gd)-DTPA-enhancement of MRI can delineate meningeal pathology to better advantage, especially meningeal carcinomatosis and meningitis [1–3]. Meningeal enhancement is also recognised in some other conditions after Gd-DTPA injection, including the postoperative state and sinus thrombosis.

This report discusses (1) the degree of normal meningeal enhancement; (2) sequential changes of meningeal enhancement in the postoperative state; (3) differentiation of pathologies by meningeal enhancement patterns.

Materials and methods

The case material consisted of 12 patients considered to have no meningeal disease, and 24 who showed abnormal meningeal enhancement, including 14 postoperative studies, 8 meningeal carcinomatoses, 3 meningitides and 1 dural sinus thrombosis.

MRI was obtained by a 1.5 T superconductive unit (Siemens Magnetom) with a 256 × 256 matrix and one acquisition. Gd-DTPA (0.1 mmol/kg) was administrated at a rate of approximately 10 ml/min. Postcontrast T1-weighted spin echo images (TR/600 ms, TE/ ms) were obtained between 5–20 min after Gd-DTPA injection. Precontrast T1-weighted images were also obtained in a similar manner.

Correlation of the intervals after operation with the degree of meningeal enhancement was studied in the postoperative cases. Nine cases after surgery were followed sequentially for the changes of meningeal enhancement. The degree of meningeal enhancement was classified as: I, no meningeal enhancement; II, thin, vague and discontinuous meningeal enhancement; III, clear meningeal enhancement; IV, intensive enhancement with thickened meninges.

Results

Dural enhancement was often seen in the normal cases, but was vague and not consistant. The tentorium showed enhancement most frequently (70%) (Table 1).

In postoperative cases, intensive meningeal enhancement was shown within short intervals of the operation. The cases with longer intervals after surgery showed decreased meningeal enhancement (Table 2). The follow-up of 9 postoperative cases revealed decreasing meningeal enhancement (Table 3).

Table 1. Meningeal enhancement in 12 normal patients

	Dura mater				Pia mater
	Tentorium	Posterior fossa	Convexity	Cerebral falx	
I	•••	•••••• ••••	•••••• •	•••••• ••	•••••• ••••••
II	•••••• •		•••••	••••	
III					
IV					

Table 2. Degree of meningeal enhancement after surgery (14 cases)

	< 2 weeks	< 1 month	< 3 months	< 6 months	< 1 year
I				•	•
II		•	••••	•••	••
III	••	•	•••••	•	
IV	•••	••			•[a]

[a] In this case, the superior sagittal sinus was occluded at surgery

Table 3. Meningeal enhancement in the postoperative state

	Interval after operation					
	< 2 weeks	< 1 month	< 2 months	< 3 months	< 6 months	< 1 year
Case 1			III	II	II	
2		II			I	
3		III				II
4	III		II			
5	III					I
6			III	II		
7	IV		III		II	
8	IV		III	II		
9	IV		III		II	

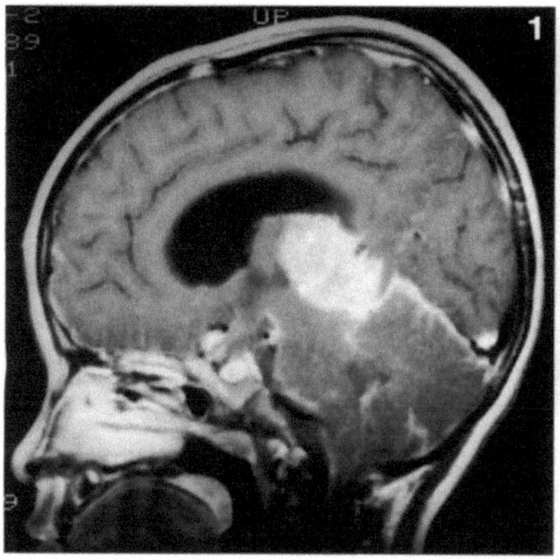

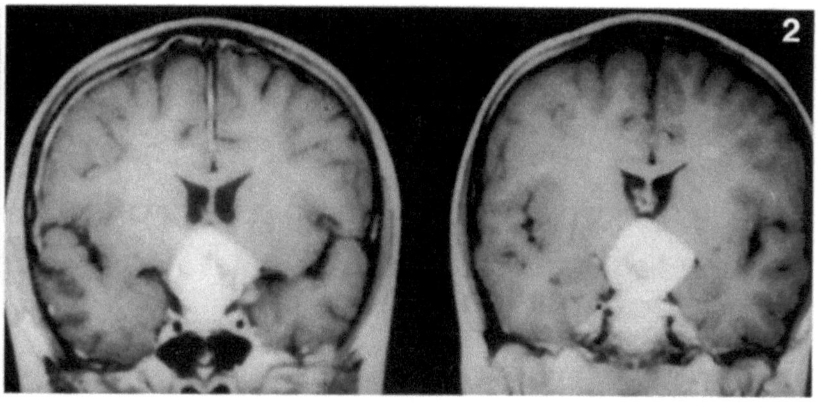

Fig. 1. A 2-year-old male with pineal germinoma. The pia mater on the surface of the brain stem and cerebellum, and the dura mater of the tentorium show marked meningeal enhancement

Fig. 2. A 45-year-old male after craniectomy. Dural enhancement is seen 1 month after operation *(left)*, and no pial enhancement is seen. At 3 months after operation *(right)* the dural enhancement is decreasing.

Table 4. Comparison of meningeal enhancement in various disease entities

Enhancement \ Pathology			Postoperative change	Meningeal carcinomatosis	Infectious meningitis	Dural sinus thrombosis
Pial enhancement			0/14	8/8	2/3	0/1
Dural enhancement	Degree of enhancement	IV	2/14	0/8	1/3	1/1
		III	6/14	1/8	0/3	0/1
		II	6/14	2/8	1/3	0/1
		Total	14/14	3/8	2/3	1/1
	Contralateral extension		4/14	0/3	1/2	1/1
	Transtentorial extension		1/14	1/3	1/2	0/1

The enhancement of the pia mater was shown only in the cases of meningitis and meningeal carcinomatosis (Fig. 1 and Table 4). Postoperative patients (Fig. 2) and sinus thrombosis never showed enhancement of the pia mater. This was useful for differentiation of these lesions.

Discussion

Good depiction of meningeal pathology in Gd-DTPA-enhanced MRI has two prerequisites. The first is an increase in signal after administration of Gd-DTPA, and the second that there are no adjacent structures which obscure meningeal enhancement. Unlike MRI, CT has the defect that meningeal enhancement is obscured by bony structures. Transient enhancement in the postoperative state is explained by meningal irritation, which is caused by the presence of blood in the subarachnoid space [1]. Decreased circulation in the meninges due to craniectomy can also be the cause of meningeal enhancement, while subdural effusion can be another cause. The same condition may be shown in the case of dural sinus thrombosis. Cases of the postoperative state can be followed for intervals of several months and decreasing meningeal enhancement contributes to the differential diagnosis.

All 8 cases of meningeal carcinomatosis showed pial enhancement, which was never seen in the cases of the postoperative state. This is an important finding for the differentiation of these conditions.

References

1. Sze G, Soletsky S, Bronen R, Krol G (1989) MR imaging of the cranial meninges with emphasis on contrast enhancement and meningeal carcinomatosis. AJNR 10: 965–975
2. Chang KH, Han MH, Roh JK, Kim IO, Han MC, Kim CW (1990) Gd-DTPA-enhanced MR imaging of the brain in patients with meningitis: comparisons with CT. AJNR 11: 69–76
3. Lee YY, Tien RD, Bruner JM, De Pena CA, Tassel PV (1989) Loculated intracranial leptomeningeal metastases: CT and MR characteristics. AJNR 10: 1171–1179

Dr. Y. Sakamoto
Department of Radiology
Kumamoto University School of Medicine
Kumamoto, Japan

Neuroradiology (1991) 33 [Suppl]: 586–588

Neuro-radiology
© Springer-Verlag 1991

Cryomicrotome analysis of the cavernous sinus and its adjacent structures for MR interpretation

Y. Korogi[1], M. Takahashi[1], F. Viñuela[2], J. R. Bentson[2], R. B. Lufkin[2], and W. N. Hanafee[2]

[1] Department of Radiology, Kumamoto University School of Medicine, Kumamoto, Japan
[2] Department of Radiological Sciences, UCLA School of Medicine, Los Angeles, California, USA

Summary. Whole-organ cryomicrotome sections from three cadavers were obtained to analyze MR appearance of various small structures of the cavernous sinus. MR images from five healthy volunteers and from 37 patients with an abnormal cavernous sinus were compared with cryomicrotome sections. The minute anatomy of the normal structures on MRI, including cranial nerves, small vessels and dural reflections, was best analyzed on the basis of cryomicrotome sections. MR images of normal structures and diseased states were also better explained.

Key words: Magnetic resonance imaging – Cavernous sinus – Cryomicrotome section

MRI now provides anatomical and pathological information about the normal structures and various abnormalities within the cavernous sinus [1–3]. This report discusses the MR appearance of the cavernous sinus in the light of cryomicrotome findings.

Materials and methods

Axial cryomicrotome sections of the sellar and parasellar regions of three fresh frozen cadaver heads were evaluated. The cryomicrotome freezing and sectioning techniques have previously been described [4]. T1- and T2-weighted spin echo (SE) images in five healthy volunteers, and in 15 patients with no known intracranial lesions were compared with cryomicrotome findings to establish the normal appearance of the cavernous sinus on MRI. Thirty-seven patients with abnormal cavernous sinuses were also examined.

The volunteers and patients were studied with a 1.5-T Siemens Magnetom system. In volunteers, technical factors of coronal and axial T1-weighted SE images were TR 600/TE 15 with 4–8 excitations, 128 × 256 matrix, 15 cm field of view, and 3 mm-thick sections. In patients, technical factors of T1-weighted SE images were TR 600/TE 15 with 1–2 excitations, 256 × 256 matrix, 30 cm field of view, and 3–5 mm thick section.

Results and discussion

The anatomy of the cavernous sinus is complex and has been reviewed recently [5–8]. The important landmarks of the cavernous sinus are cranial nerves, internal carotid artery, Meckel's cave and lateral and medial walls. Cranial nerve III was found to be located most superiorly in the cavernous sinus and to traverse the lateral wall before entering the superior orbital fissure (Fig. 1a). On the more inferior sections, cranial nerve IV, which was quite slender, was identified (Fig. 1b). It pierced the dura posterolateral to the third nerve and then, inferolateral to this nerve, traversed the lateral wall. The first division of the trigeminal nerve (V1) was entirely within the cavernous sinus, whereas the second and third divisions extended outside the cavernous sinus immediately beyond their origins (Fig. 1c). The sixth nerve lay so close to V1 that it was not possible to identify each nerve separately on MRI (Fig. 1c). These cranial nerves had some adjacent connective tissue (Fig. 1c). In the lower part of the cavernous sinus there was a prominent and consistently identified venous space, just below which cranial nerve V2 extended through the foramen rotundum anteriorly.

The cavernous sinus was located between the two layers of the dura mater, the periosteal layer forming the floor and most of the medial wall of the cavernous sinus, and the meningeal layer (dura propria) forming the roof, lateral wall, and the upper part of the medial wall [7]. A thick lateral wall and a thin dural membrane between the lateral margin of the pituitary gland and the cavernous sinus were identified (Fig. 1). Also noted was cavernous connective tissue lateral to the medial wall (Fig. 1b). Meckel's cave was identified as an oval or triangular dural pocket which was positioned just lateral to the posterior part of the cavernous sinus and contained the trigeminal nerve and cerebrospinal fluid (Fig. 1).

The signal intensity of normal and abnormal cavernous venous spaces was very variable in respect to the nerves and pituitary gland on MR images (Fig. 2). There have been a few reports which described the MR appearance of the normal and abnormal cavernous sinus [1–3]. Some authors stated that MR could demonstrate the cranial nerves even in T1-weighted SE images without contrast injection [1]. However, we found it impossible to differentiate venous spaces from the cranial nerves and connective tissue on pre- and postenhancement T1-weighted images. Gradient echo images proved to be an effective method of identifying structures within the cavernous sinus [3].

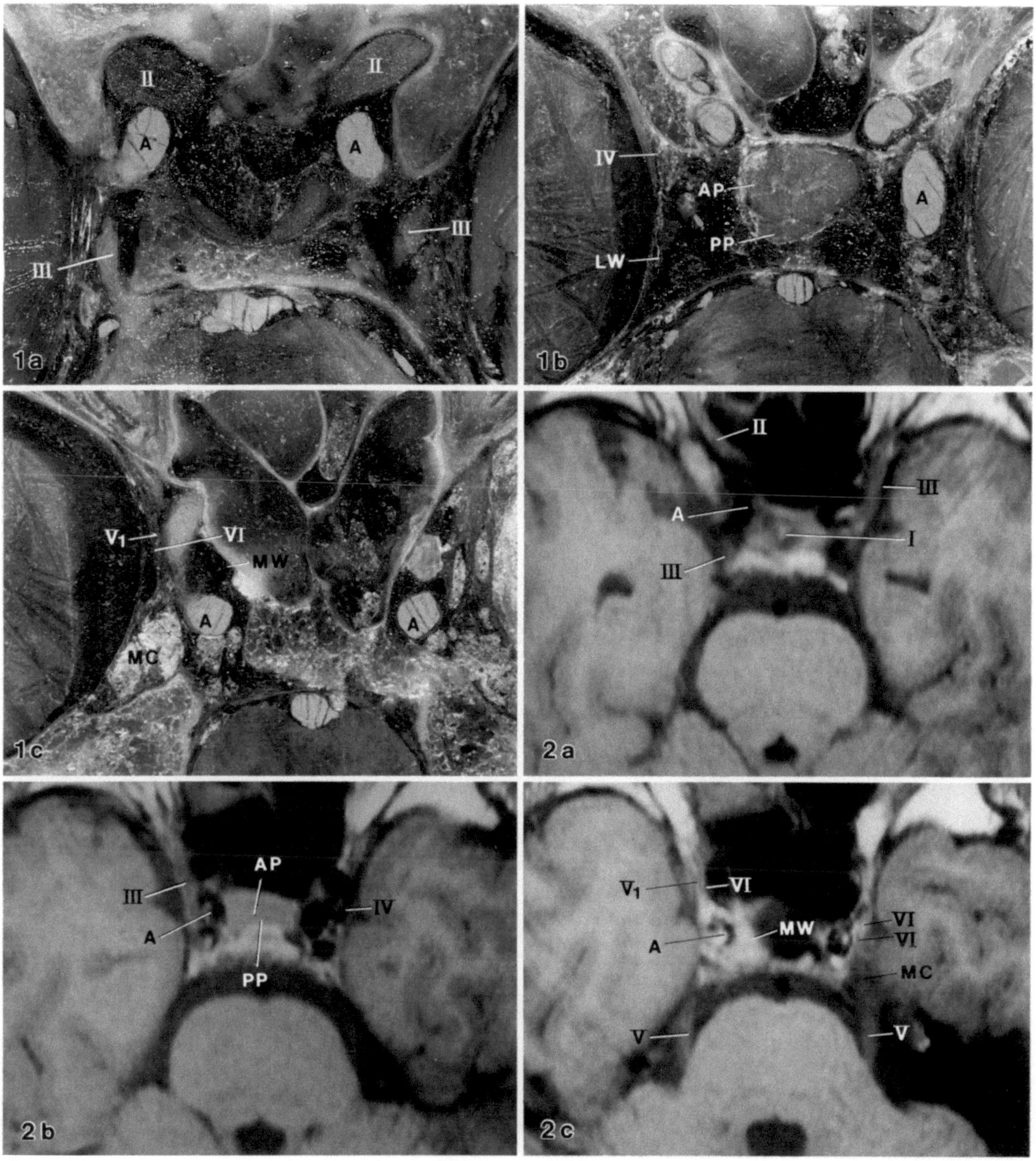

Figs. 1 and 2. Progressively more inferior cryomicrotome sections **(Fig. 1a–c)** and corresponding axial T1-weighted spin echo images **(Fig. 2a–c)** of cavernous sinus area. *II,* optic nerve; *III,* oculomotor nerve; *VI,* trochlear nerve; *V1,* ophthalmic division of trigeminal nerve; *V2,* maxillary division of trigeminal nerve; *IV,* abducens nerve; *MC,* Meckel's cave; *LW,* lateral wall of cavernous sinus; *MW,* medial wall of cavernous sinus; *A,* internal carotid artery; *I,* infundibulum; *AP,* anterior lobe of pituitary gland; *PP,* posterior lobe of pituitary gland

References

1. Daniels DL, Pech P, Mark L, Pojunas K, Williams AL, Haughton VM (1985) Magnetic resonance imaging of the cavernous sinus. AJR 144: 1009–1014
2. Hirsch WL Jr, Hryshko FG, Sekhar LN, Brunberg J, Kanal E, Latchaw RE, Curtin H (1988) Comparison of MR imaging, CT, and angiography in the evaluation of the enlarged cavernous sinus. AJNR 9: 907–915
3. Daniels DL, Czervionke LF, Bonneville JF, CattinF, Pech P, Mark L, Williams AL, Haughton VM (1988) MR imaging of the cavernous sinus: value of spin echo and gradient recalled echo images. AJNR 9:947–952
4. Rauschning W, Bergstrom K, Pech P (1983) Correlative cranio-spinal anatomy studies by computed tomography and cryomicrotomy. J Comput Assist Tomogr 7:9–13
5. Harris F, Rhoton AL Jr (1976) Anatomy of the cavernous sinus: microsurgical study J Neurosurg 45: 169–180
6. Umansky F, Nathan H (1982) The lateral wall of the cavernous sinus. J Neurosurg 56: 228–234
7. Taptas JN (1982) The so-called cavernous sinus: a review of the controversy and its implications for neurosurgeons. Neurosurgery 11: 712–717
8. Sekhar LN, Burgess J, Akin O (1987) Anatomical study of the cavernous sinus emphasizing operative approaches and related vascular and neural reconstruction.Neurosurgery 21: 806–816

Dr. Y. Korogi
Department of Radiology
Kumamoto University School of Medicine
Kumamoto, Japan

Neuroradiology (1991) 33 [Suppl]: 589–591

Neuro-radiology
© Springer-Verlag 1991

Hippocampal proton relaxometry in dementia

S. J. Karlik, D. H. Lee, and A. J. Fox

Department of Diagnostic Radiology, University Hospital, University of Western Ontario, London, Ontario, Canada

Summary. MRI was performed on 31 individuals with clinical diagnosis of senile dementia of the Alzheimer type and 52 age-matched controls to determine whether anatomically specific T1 and T2 relaxometry could detect differences related to dementia. Patient movement, technical and calibration factors decreased the usable cases to 26 controls and 13 dements. Increased T2 values in the hippocampal H2 field were observed in both hemispheres in the demented subjects ($p < 0.001$). No statistical differences were observed for six regions of temporal lobe, and other tissues including muscle, subcutaneous and clival fat. T1 and T2 values were prolonged for white matter lesions compared with uninvolved deep white matter. No correlation was observed between the increase in T2 value and the extended scale of dementia. Statistically significant prolongation of T2 relaxation times in the hippocampus may indicate intrinsic changes, but the overlap of measurements with controls makes the use of this technique nondiagnostic.

Key words: T1 – T2 – Hippocampus – Alzheimer's disease – dementia

The neuropathology of Alzheimer's disease shows a consistent and severe loss of hippocampal and entorhinal neurons. Because neuropathology describes changes seen at autopsy, specific identification of regional neural degeneration during disease is difficult beyond measures of atrophy in neuroimaging techniques. Quantitive MRI might prove useful for identifying specific anatomical or functional changes in select brain regions, such as the hippocampus, during the course of Alzheimer's disease [1–4]. These alterations could then be related to behavioural changes associated with degeneration in the neural substrate.

The MRI signal intensity depends on physical and chemical characteristics of the tissues under investigation. Relaxation times and intensity measurements in MRI can be of value in aiding the effectiveness of a clinical diagnosis [5]. To date, most studies have indicated that relaxation time changes are sensitive but not specific, a comment made frequently about the technique of MRI. It is also important to consider that some pathological processes may have several components, each of which affect relaxation times in different ways. Thus it is possible that combinations of events can yield normal tissue determinations in both MRI and relaxometric measurements [6]. In addition to intrinsic changes, there are many extrinsic factors which must be considered and controlled when performing proton relaxometry in vivo [7].

The purpose of this study was to examine the in vivo T1 and T2 relaxation times from a series of anatomically defined loci in the brain and, more specifically, in the hippocampus, to determine whether relaxometric measurements were sensitive to degeneration of the underlying neuronsal substrate.

Materials and methods

One hundred and two quantitive MRI scans were performed on volunteers from the U. W. O. Dementia Study on a GE Signa 1.5 Scanner. There were 31 patients with clinically confirmed senile dementia of the Alzheimer type (mean age, 70.29) and 52 age-matched (mean age, 70.97) controls. Pathological confirmation of these clinical diagnosis has not been possible as only 2 have come to autopsy. After the patient had the sagittal localizer and series of axial scans, a coronal series using TR2000; TE20/40/60/80, and either TR1000; TE20 and 500/20 or 600/20 were used for 3 mm slices through the hippocampus and temporal lobes. At 256 matrix, these studies took longer than conventional axial views used for radiological assessments and motion artefact was a problem. Some motion artefact is tolerable in axial images for interpretative techniques but produces significant errors in relaxometry. Three-millimetre slices, used to minimize volume averaging, were the thinnest available on the imager and a 100% gap was used in order to prevent interslice cross-talk. Three adjacent slices, which had the hippocampus and temporal lobes in view, were used for relaxometric analysis using the manufacturer's software. Figure 1 illustrates a coronal MRI with cursor positions for

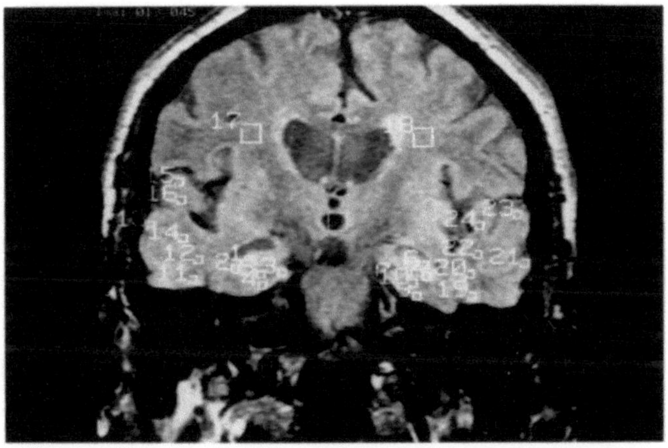

Fig. 1. Anatomical positions used to determine the relaxometric measurements. Cursor positions indicate 24 anatomical locations in the hippocampus temporal lobe and deep white matter bilaterally.

Table 1. Hippocampal relaxation times T1, T2 (mean ± SD)

	Control ($n = 26$) R	Dement ($n = 13$) R	Control L	Dement L
H2 field, grey	1258 ± 231 67 ± 6	1386 ± 244 74 ± 9**	1337 ± 271 67 ± 5	1498 ± 342 73 ± 7**
H1-subiculum, grey	1388 ± 268 66 ± 4	1318 ± 290 66 ± 9	1385 ± 157 66 ± 3	1263 ± 211* 66 ± 4
Presubiculum, grey	1339 ± 224 65 ± 4	1388 ± 326 66 ± 7	1398 ± 229 67 ± 4	1326 ± 311 67 ± 7
Parahippocampal gyrus, grey	1457 ± 232 63 ± 4	1453 ± 291 63 ± 3	1559 ± 282 64 ± 3	1502 ± 296 65 ± 3
Parahippocampal gyrus, white	1048 ± 256 60 ± 4	1126 ± 275 61 ± 4	997 ± 204 61 ± 3	1090 ± 192 65 ± 5

*$P < 0.05$; **$P < 0.001$

Table 2. Tissue relaxation times T1,T2 (mean ± SD)

	Control ($n = 26$)	Dement ($n = 13$)
Sucutanous fat ($n = 6$)	411 ± 59 48 ± 3	434 ± 51 48 ± 2
Clival fat	437 ± 81 52 ± 4	438 ± 62 52 ± 4
Muscle	1322 ± 380 34 ± 6	1322 ± 148 34 ± 3
White matter lesion	1312 ± 360 75 ± 12	1620 ± 361 87 ± 12
Deep white matter, frontal (all comparisons not significant)	746 ± 57 61 ± 3	737 ± 56 60 ± 3

bilateral areas: hippocampus ($n = 5$), temporal lobe($n = 6$), and deep white matter.

Results

Many cases had to be removed from the analysis due to a variety of problems resulting from technical factors and the patients. Motion artefact was a significant problem due to instability of the patients. Secondly, flow motion compensation was not used in acquiring the data for these relaxometric measurements and frequently pulsation artifacts from cerebral blood vessels caused "zippers" which interfered with specific measurements in hippocampus or temporal lobes. Thirdly, the manufacturer of the equipment changed the software midway during the study and a significant increase in T2 relaxation times resulted. The manufacturer's optimization of sequences provided additional signal/noise in long TE spin echo images. This improved the latter images and consequently resulted in prolonged T2 relaxation times when compared to the previous sequence. All the relaxometry data from patients scanned before this time were excluded. Finally, comprehensive phantom studies by ourselves and others [8] have indicated that relaxation times of a uniform phantom change as a function of slice location as well as location within a slice. Therefore, the data used for this analysis were from comparative slice locations referenced to the magnet isocentre and head imaging coil.

Tables 1 and 2 indicate the results from relaxometric determinations on 26 controls and 13 demented subjects. The T2 value in the H2 field in the hippocampus was significantly increased on both the right and left hemispheres of the demented subjects ($P < 0.001$). There was also a small increase in parahippocampal gyrus white matter in the dements on the left hemisphere side. There was no statistically significant difference between any measurement of controls and dements, for the six regions of temporal lobe grey and white matter (data not shown), or deep white matter which was not involved with lesions. There was no statistical difference between the readings for subcutaneous fat in six locations, or for clival fat or muscle in the identical slices used in determination of hippocampal relaxation times. As expected, the T1 and T2 values of white matter lesions for both groups were significantly prolonged when compared with uninvolved deep white matter (Table 2).

Discussion

After careful control for a number of confounding factors, it has been determined that the hippocampal H2 field in the demented cases shows a prolongation in T2. When T2 values were plotted as a function of the extended scale of dementia (ESD) (Fig. 2), a wide distribution was observed. This psychological test was performed on all volunteers and showed a wide range of ESD scores for the demented subjects and a trend towards prolonged relaxation times can be seen. There was a wide distribution of relaxation times in controls, which are clustered near an ESD score of 250 (normal score). No correlation between T2 relaxation times with this psychological test has been observed.

We conclude that T2 of hippocampal H2 field is significantly prolonged in demented subjects. Although significant, this prolongation overlaps widely in distribution with the control subjects. It is possible that T2 relaxation times in the H2 field may indicate some changes occurring in that tissue but the widespread distribution of these measurements in controls makes the use of this technique nondiagnostic. Secondly, as expected, white matter lesions show specific increase in T1 and T2 when compared with uninvolved deep white matter. Finally, relaxometric

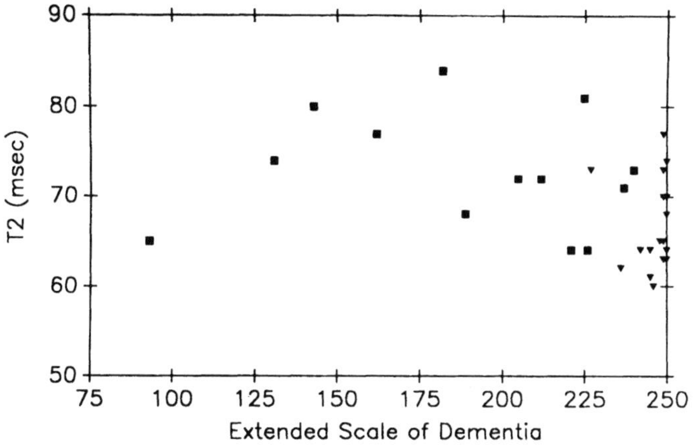

Fig. 2. Proton T2 relaxation times plotted as a function test for intellectual impairment

measurements of all other brain regions and adjacent tissues show remarkable constancy and afford internal controls.

References

1. Naidich TP, Daniels DL, Haughton VN, Pech P, Williams A, Pojunas K, Palacios E (1987) Hippocampal formation and related structures of the limic lobe: anatomic-MR correlation. Radiology 162: 755–761
2. Chawluk JB, Calcano-Perez JA, Zimmermann RA, Alavi A, Hurtig HI, Jamieson DG, Fazekas F, Reivich M (1988) Cortical signal abnormalities in Alzheimer's disease demonstrated by magnetic resonance imaging. Ann Neurol 24: 158–159
3. Kesslak JP, Nalcioglu C, Cotman CW (1989) Magnetic resonance imaging of the hippocampal – entorhinal circuitry in Alzheimer's disease. Soc Neurosci 15: 414–435
4. DeLeon MJ, George AE, Stylocpoulos LA, Smith G, Miller DC (1989) Early marker for Alzheimer's disease: the atrophic hippocampus. Lancet II: 672–673
5. Crooks LE, Hylton NM, Ortendahl DA, Posin JP, Kaufman L (1987) The value of relaxation times and density measurements in clinical MRI. Invest Radiol 22: 158–169 para 6. Karlik SJ, Strejan G, Gilbert JJ, Noseworthy JH (1986) NMR studies in experimental allergic encephalomyelitis (EAE): normalization of T1 and T2 with parenchymal cellular infiltration. Neurology 36: 1112–1114
7. Johnson G, Ormerod IEC, Barnes D, Tofts PS, MacManus D (1987) Accuracy and precision in the measurements of relaxation times from nuclear magnetic resonance images. Br J Radiol 60: 143–153

Dr. S. J. Karlik
Department of Diagnostic Radiology
University Hospital
University of Western Ontario
P. O. Box 5339
London, Ontario N6A 5A5, Canada

Neuroradiology (1991) 33 [Suppl]: 592–593

Neuro radiology
© Springer-Verlag 1991

Detection of pathological intracranial calcification by MRI

W. Schörner[1], D. Kunz[1], H. Henkes[1], J. C. Böck[1], B. Sander[1], and D. Schmidt[2]

Departments of [1] Radiology and [2] Neurology, University Clinic Rudolf Virchow/Charlottenburg, Free University, Berlin, Federal Republic of Germany

Summary. A total of 141 patients with CT-confirmed pathological intracranial calcification (PIC) were studied retrospectively with respect to their detectability by MRI using different pulse sequences. While 90% of calcified lesions were detected by MRI as pathological tissue changes, only 62% were recognised as being calcified. The detectability of PIC in MRI depended on the size and density of the calcification, on the surrounding tissue and the pulse sequence. Conventional T2-weighted SE images had the highest sensitivity in the detection of calcification. Conventional SE images did not reach CT sensitivity in the detection of PIC.

Key words: Brain, calcification – Brain, magnetic resonance imaging – Brain, calcinosis

MRI is recognised as the most sensitive imaging technique for the detection of parenchymal brain lesions [1–8]. The limited detectability of pathological intracranial calcification (PIC) is considered to be the major diagnostic drawback of MRI [1–6].

The purpose of this study was to determine the parameters that influence the detectability of PIC based on clinical MRI examinations.

Patients and methods

In 127 patients with 141 CT-confirmed PIC spin-echo (SE) sequences were used for T1-(SE 400/30), proton-density-(SE 1600/30) and T2-weighted images (SE 1600/70) on a 0.5 T scanner (Magnetom, Siemens, Erlangen, FRG).

All images were studied with respect to the detectability of PIC. Calcification was assumed in circumscribed areas of reduced signal intensity.

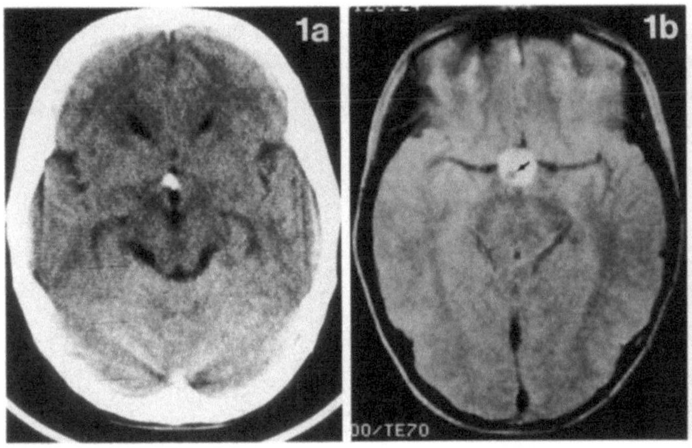

Fig. 1 a, b. Definite demonstration of calcification by MRI. Correlating to CT **(a)**, definite suprasellar calcification shown by MRI as profoundly reduced signal intensity *(arrow)* within a hyperintense tumour (T2-weighted image: SE 2000/70) **(b)** (14-year-old male, craniopharyngioma, histologically confirmed)

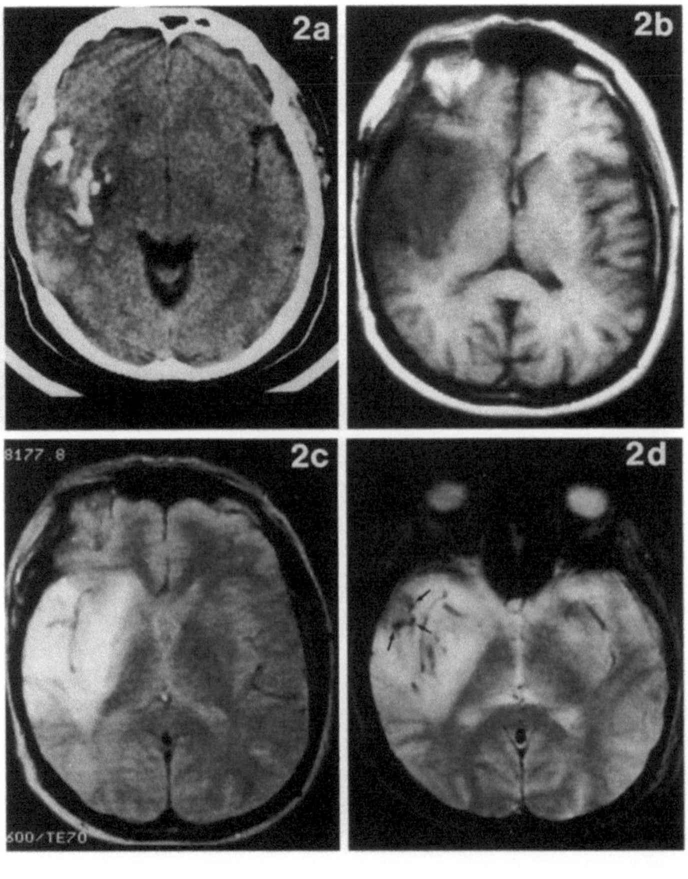

Fig. 2 a–d Detection of calcification by MRI according to the pulse sequence used. CT **(a)** shows multiple areas of calcification within a tumour of the right temporal lobe. While the T1-weighted image (GE 315/14 – the use of a GE instead of an SE sequence is of no relevance in this context) **(b)** shows no evidence of calcification due to hypointensity of tumour tissue, T2-weighted SE image (SE 1600/70), **(c)** shows an area of reduced signal within the hyperintense tumour tissue that did not correlate with the calcification on CT. T2-weighted image (GE 800/20 20°) **(d)** reveals an area of signal void *(arrows)* corresponding to calcification on CT (48-year-old male, oligodendroglioma, histologically confirmed)

Results

In 127 of 141 calcified lesions (90%) a pathological finding (not necessarily interpreted as calcification) was seen on MRI.

Of 141 calcified lesions, 87 (62%) were considered to be calcified after study of the MRI: these included 44 of 66 neoplasms, 23 of 34 vascular malformations, 7 of 15 inflammatory lesions and 13 of 26 cases of "isolated" calcification (e.g. Fahr's disease).

There was a significantly higher MRI detectability of large (>2 mm) PIC and PIC with high CT attenuation values (<100 Hu in CT) compared to small (<2mm) PICs and PIC with low CT attenuation values (<100 Hu in CT). In large PIC pathologically increased signal intensity of surrounding tissue improved PIC recognition (Fig. 1). In general, PIC was significantly more often demonstrated using T2-weighted images than using T1- or proton-density-weighted images ($P < 0.001$).

Discussion

In MRI signal intensity is determined by nuclear spin density, relaxation times T1 and T2, and proton motion [2,7]. When protons are associated with solids, T1 becomes long and T2 exceedingly short, leading to signal void [4, 5, 8]. Even though calcification has the characteristics of solids, its MRI intensity is usually higher than expected in most sequences [3–6].

In the present study, MRI demonstrated a pathological finding in 116 of 119 (97%) neoplastic, inflammatory and vascular lesions. We wish to emphasise that this did not result in unequivocal identification of all calcification. Most calcified intracranial lesions consist of pathological soft tissue and a circumscribed calcification. Therefore, the calcified lesion may be detected due to surrounding pathological soft tissue, but the calcification itself may be missed (Fig. 2) In our subpopulation "isolated" calcification in which by definition the calcification is not surrounded by any pathological soft tissue, MRI shows relatively little sensitivity (11/22) in the detection of calcification.

The calcification itself was detected in only 87 of 141 (62%) cases by MRI. In a prospective evaluation Oot et al. [4] recognised only 3 of 20 calcified lesions, whereas Holland et al. [3] considered 45% uncalcified lesions falsely as being calcified.

In accordance with other authors, we found that the detectability of PIC in MRI depends on size and CT attenuation [3–5]. Large PIC and PIC with high CT attenuation is significantly more often detected by MRI than small PIC and PIC with low CT attenuation. We confirm the phantom studies and clinical findings of Tsuruda and Bradley [5] and Oot et al. [4] that calcification is best detected when surrounded by hyperintense tissue (in T2-weighted images). In general conventional T2-weighted SE images showed the highest sensitivity for detection of calcification.

First initial results indicate that calcification detectability is considerably improved using a T2-weighted gradient-echo sequence [6] (Fig. 2).

References

1. Bradley WG Jr, Waluch V, Yadley RA, Wycoff RR (1984) Comparison of CT and MR in 400 patients with suspected disease of the brain and cervical spine cord. Radiology 152: 695–702
2. Brant-Zawadzki M (1988) MR imaging of the brain. Radiology 166: 1–10
3. Holland BA, Kucharcyzk W, Brant-Zawadzki M, Norman D, Haas DK, Harper PS (1985) MR imaging of calcified intracranial lesions. Radiology 157: 353–356
4. Oot RF, New PFJ, Pile-Spellman J, Rosen BR, Shoukimas GM, Davis KR (1986) The detection of intracranial calcifications by MR. Am J Neuroradiol 7: 801–809
5. Tsuruda JS, Bradley WG (1987) MR detection of intracranial calcification: a phantom study. Am J Neuroradiol 8: 1049–1055
6. Atlas SW, Grossmann RI, Hackney DB, Gomori JM, Campagna N, Goldberg HI, Bilaniuk LT, Zimmerman RA (1988) Calcified intracranial lesions: detection with gradient-echo-acquisition rapid MR imaging. Am J Neuroradiol 150: 1383–1389
7. Wehrli FW (1988) Principles of magnetic resonance. In: Stark DD, Bradley WG (eds) Magnetic resonance imaging. Mosby, St. Louis, pp 3–23
8. Higer HP, Bielke G (1986): Gewebecharakterisierung mit T1, T2 und Protonendichte: Traum und Wirklichkeit. Fortschr Röntgenstr 144: 597–605

Dr. W. Schörner
Department of Radiology
University Clinic Rudolf Virchow Charlottenburg
1000 Berlin, Federal Republic of Germany

Neuroradiology (1991) 33 [Suppl]: 594–595

Neuro radiology
© Springer-Verlag 1991

Follow-up MR in Wernicke's encephalopathy

M. Gallucci, A. Bozzao, A. Splendiani, A. Cifani, and R. Passariello

Department of Radiology, University of L'Aquila, L'Aquila, Italy

Summary. Very typical hyperintense areas surrounding the third ventricle and the aqueduct were identified in the acute phase of the disease in seven patients with Wernicke's encephalopathy, while clinical diagnosis was correct in only four of the patients (57%). After a period of 6–12 months, there was disappearance or reduction of the previously mentioned hyperintensities in all cases, with dilatation of the third ventricle and aqueduct.

Key words: Wernicke's encephalopathy – Alcoholism – Magnetic resonance imaging – Brain – Degenerative diseases

Wernicke's encephalopathy (WE) results from a nutritional deficiency of thiamine and is observed mainly, but not exclusively, in alcoholics [1–8].

The clinical diagnosis is often difficult and CT findings are neither constant nor specific [9]. We report seven cases of WE in which typical mesencephalic and diencephalic lesions have been documented by MRI in the acute and chronic phase of the disease.

Patients and methods

Seven patients, five males and two females (age 22–47 years), all alcoholics, were studied. They presented sudden palsy of the sixth cranial nerves (two cases), third cranial nerves (three cases), internuclear ophthalmoplegia (one case), vertical nystagmus (one case), always associated with bad general clinical conditions, ataxia of gait in six cases and stupor in five. The above-mentioned neurological symptoms had started within 72 h before our examination. The clinical diagnosis was of WE in only four cases, while in the others different diseases were suspected: brain-stem tumour in two cases (metastatic in one of them), demyelinating or vascular disease in the other.

MRI was performed by means of Ansaldo Esatom/MR 5000 equipment, operating at a 0.5 T magnetic field, obtaining spinecho (SE) sequences 1800/50–150, and 7 and 5 mm thickness, in transverse and coronal planes. Sagittal SE 350/30 scans, 5 mm thickness, were also obtained. Three patients also underwent CT examination. Six to 12 months later the patients were re-examined. At that time they all were in good general condition and the neurological evaluation showed normal ocular motility. The same equipment and techniques were employed.

Results

In the acute phase of the disease CT showed a non-enhancing hypodense area around the aqueduct in only one patient (Fig. 1a), while in all subjects T2-weighted sequences revealed very typical hyperintensity in the brain stem, around the aqueduct and surrounding the third ventricle (Figs. 1b, 2a). In one patient hyperintense tracks were evident in the mesencephalon along the course of the third nerve (Fig. 3a). The lesions described were analogous to the pathological changes described in postmortem studies. These findings, together with the history of chronic alcohol abuse and the clinical picture, led us to confirm the diagnosis of WE in the cases in which it was suspected, and to change the clinical impression in the others.

There was a moderate macrocytic anaemia and platelet reduction, with hyposideraemia, in four patients. Therefore, medical intramuscular therapy was prescribed with 590 mg thiamine and 30 mg folate therapy daily.

Follow-up MRI revealed marked reduction of the abnormalities previously demonstrated and third ventricle enlargement with aqueductal dilatation. The tissue degeneration suggested by the above-described hyperintensities had developed into tissue atrophy (Figs. 1c, 2b). CT became negative in the only case in which the brain-stem lesion was evident.

Discussion

Nowadays diagnosis of WE is based on the clinical findings by which Wernicke himself indentified this encephalopathy: ophthalmoplegia, ataxia and confusion [10].

However, postmortem studies demonstrated that the real incidence of WE is higher than clinically diagnosed, since typical lesions have been found in up to 2.2% of consecutive autopsies [5, 6]. Our work underlines that MRI can offer more satisfactory criteria for the identification of WE, since typical changes were present both in the acute and chronic phase in mesencephalo-diencephalic regions.

A previous report by us [11] has already described the capability of MRI to identify findings similar to those reported in postmortem studies. In one of the new cases, we were also able to identify a closer relationship with the clinical picture. This patient showed bilateral third nerve palsies which corresponded, in the acute phase, to very selective hyperintense stripes along the intramesencephalic roots of both third cranial nerves (Fig. 3).

The hyperintense areas are nonspecific, but could represent foci of oedema and demyelination, as being which Ghez [12] described the earliest in WE. Their disappearence and the presence of a thin hyperintense rim surrounding a dilated third ventricle and aqueduct suggested that tissue degeneration, followed by fibrillary astrocy-

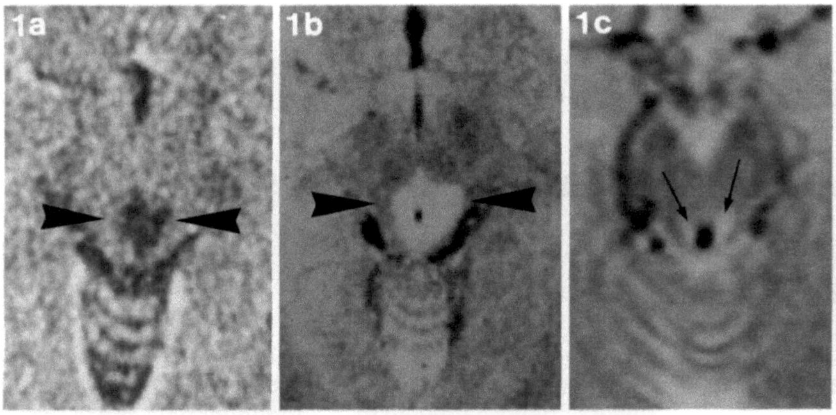

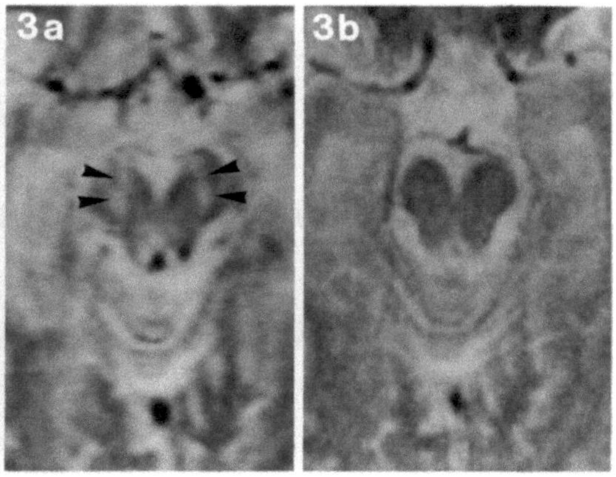

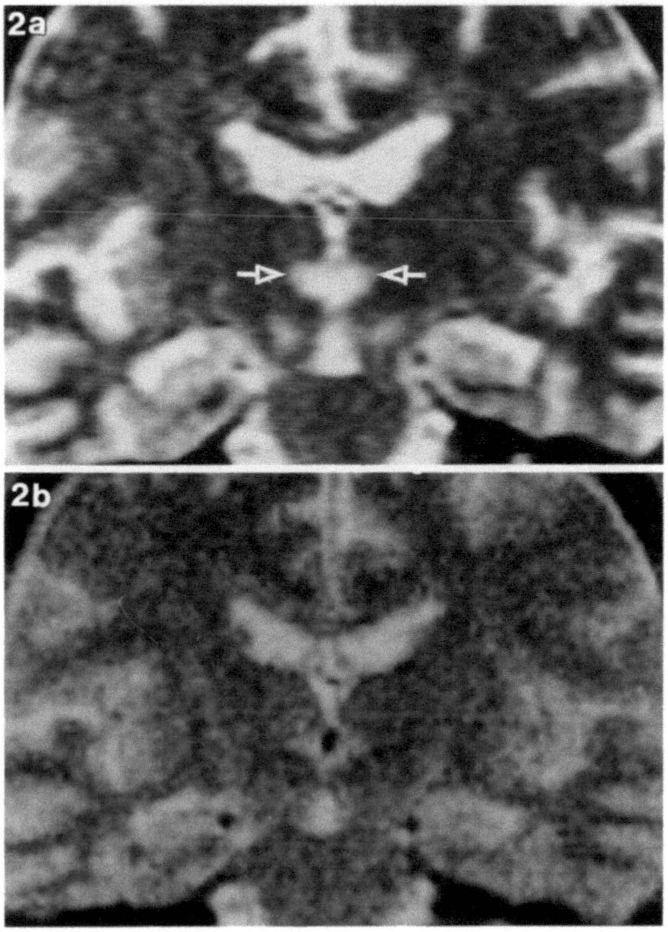

Fig. 1. **a** CT scan shows the presence of a non-enhancing lesion surrounding the aqueduct *(arrows)*. **b** The same lesion is hyperintense in T2-weighted SE sequence *(arrows)*. **c** On Follow-up evaluation the lesion is not detectable, the aqueduct is dilated and surrounded by a thin hyperintense rim *(arrows)*

Fig. 2. **a** Coronal T2-weighted SE sequence shows the presence of hyperintense areas around the third ventricle *(arrows)* **b** The lesions are reduced on follow-up examination; the third ventricle is dilated

Fig. 3. Hyperintense rims on T2-weighted axial scans along the course of the third nerve roots **(a)**, which disappeared on follow-up examination **(b)**

tosis had occurred, as reported in postmortem studies on chronic WE [1, 12, 13].

MRI is the most sensitive tool in identifying specific patterns in WE. MRI enabled us diagnose WE in all seven cases, while CT identified nonspecific lesions in 33% (1/3) and the clinical diagnosis was correct in 57% (4/7).

References

1. Gamper E (1928) Zur Frage der Polio-encephalitis haemorragica des chronischen Alkoholiker: anatomische Befunde beim alkoholischen Korsakow und ihre Beziehungen zum klinischen Bild. Dtsch Z Nervenheilkd 102: 122–129
2. Witt ED (1985) Neuroanatomical consequences of thiamine deficiency: a comparative analysis. Alcohol Alcohol 2: 201–221
3. Victor M, Adams RD (1981) On the etiology of alcoholic neurologic disease, with special reference to the role of nutrition. Am J clin Nutr 9: 379–397
4. Thompson AD, Ryle PR, Shaw GK (1983) Ethanol, thiamine and brain damage. Alcohol Alcohol 1: 27–43
5. Adams RD, Victor M (1985) Principles of neurology. McGraw-Hill, New York
6. Harper C (1978) Wernicke's encephalopathy: a more common disease than realised. A neuropathological study of 51 cases. J Neurol Neurosurg Psychiatry 42: 226–231
7. Lopez RI, Collins GH (1968). Wernicke's encephalopathy. A complication of chronic hemodialysis. Arch Neurol 18: 248–259
8. Nixon PF (1984) Is there a genetic component to the pathogenesis of the Wernicke-Korsakoff syndrome? Alcohol Alcohol 3: 219–221
9. Mc Dowell JR, Le Blanc HJ (1984) Computed tomography finding in Wernicke-Korsakoff syndrome. Arch Neurol 41: 435–454
10. Wernicke C (1881) Lehrbuch der Gehirnkrankheiten für Aerzte und Studenten, vol 2, Fischer, Berlin, pp 229–242
11. Galucci M, Bozzao A, Splendiani A, Masciocchi C, Passariello R (1990) MR demonstration of Wernicke's encephalopathy. AJNR 11 (in press)
12. Ghez C (1969) Vestibular paresis: a clinical feature of Wernicke disease. J Neurol Neurosurg Psychiatry 178: 134–139
13. Victor M, Adams RD, Collins GH (1971) The Wernicke-Korsakoff syndrome: a clinical and pathological study of 245 patients, 82 with post-mortem examinations. Davis, Philadelphia

Dr. Massimo Gallucci
Department of Radiology
Universita' dell'Aquila
Osp. S. M. Di Collemaggio
I-67100 L'Aquila, Italy

Neuroradiology (1991) 33 [Suppl]: 596–597

Neuro-radiology
© Springer-Verlag 1991

Primary cerebellar and spino-cerebellar ataxia: an MRI study

G. B. Bradac[1], A. Riva[1], L. Orsi[2], P. Mortara[2], and S. Duca[1]

Departments of [1] Neuroradiology and [2] Neurology, University of Turin, Turin, Italy

Summary. Fifty-eight patients with primary cerebellar and spino-cerebellar ataxia were studied with MRI. Macroscopic changes and areas of abnormal signal can be seen. These are not specific findings but the frequency of the lesions and their associations are different in the various groups of patients. In our experience MRI proved to be an excellent method of investigating these patients.

Key words: Primary cerebellar ataxia – Friedreich's ataxia

Three types of primary hereditary ataxia have been described on the basis of anatomicopathological features [1]: (a) Friedreich's disease, mainly characterized by degeneration of spinocerebellar tracts and posterior columns; (b) cerebellar atrophy, involving the cerebellum and inferior olives; (c) pontocerebellar atrophy, in which the pons and frequently other nervous structures are affected. The hereditary character was present in many patients but in others it could not be demonstrated. After the first descriptions many similar cases have been reported showing the great variability of the disease and the insufficiency of the above-mentioned classification. Today primary ataxias are classified on the grounds of clinical and genetic [2, 3] aspects, including mode of inheritance, age at onset and progression of the disease. Recently MRI has proved to be useful in studying these lesions in vivo [4–6].

Patients and methods

We examined 58 patients. There were cases of primary cerebellar ataxia (17 dominant, 10 recessive and 19 sporadic). Twelve cases were diagnosed as Friedreich's ataxia (FA). MRI was performed using 0.5 T equipment (Ansaldo-Esatom). T1/T2 (short/long echo)-weighted images in the axial, sagittal and in some cases coronal planes were obtained in one or two sessions. Slice thickness was 5–7 mm.

Results

Cerebellar atrophy (CA) was present in all cases of the dominant, sporadic and recessive groups. Severe CA was present in 70% of the dominant, 60% of the sporadic and 50% of the recessive cases.

Pontine atrophy (PA) was found in the dominant and sporadic groups (31%). In the dominant type the frequency of severe atrophy was significant (Fig. 1).

Spinal cord atrophy (SPA) occurred in 10 cases (21%). Seven patients belonged to the dominant type and in these SPA was associated with atrophy of the pons and was probably a consequence of it. The other 3 cases were of the sporadic group in which the pons appeared normal, similarly to most cases of FA.

In the supratentorial area severe cortical atrophy was present in 35% of the cases. This was more frequent in the recessive and in the sporadic group.

In 21 of 33 patients in all groups with the exception of FA, a technically correct study using T2-weighted images was obtained. In these cases hyperintense areas were recognizable in the caudal part of the pons, probably corresponding to degeneration of the raphe and of pontine transverse fibres (Fig. 2). This was commonly visible in cases of severe atrophy of the pons and in a few others without recognizable macroscopic changes. In addition, 14 cases displayed an abnormal signal at the level of the inferior olives and olivo-cerebellar fibres (Fig. 3). These findings were clearly predominant in the dominant type. No signal abnormalities were found in the basal ganglia or in the white matter.

Considering the cases of FA, CA was always present but it was never severe. SPA, which was demonstrable in every patient, was not associated with PA, with the exception of 3 cases where mild atrophy was recognizable (Fig. 4). Finally, cortical atrophy occurred but was rarely severe. As regards MRI findings and clinical aspects, we found that there was no significant correlation between the degree of CA and the age of onset, duration of the disease and the severity of ataxia. There was, however, always severe ataxia in those cases in which severe atrophy of the cerebellum and pons occurred together.

Discussion

We did not find any specific features typical of any group. However, there was a certain difference in the frequency of the lesions and in the combination of these. The dominant type was frequently characterized by a severe CA associated with severe pons atrophy. In a lot of these cases degeneration of the pontine transverse fibres as well as the olives was visible. In many cases atrophy of spinal cord was also present. In many of the recessive cases, CA was associated with severe atrophy of the cerebral cortex. SPA was the typical

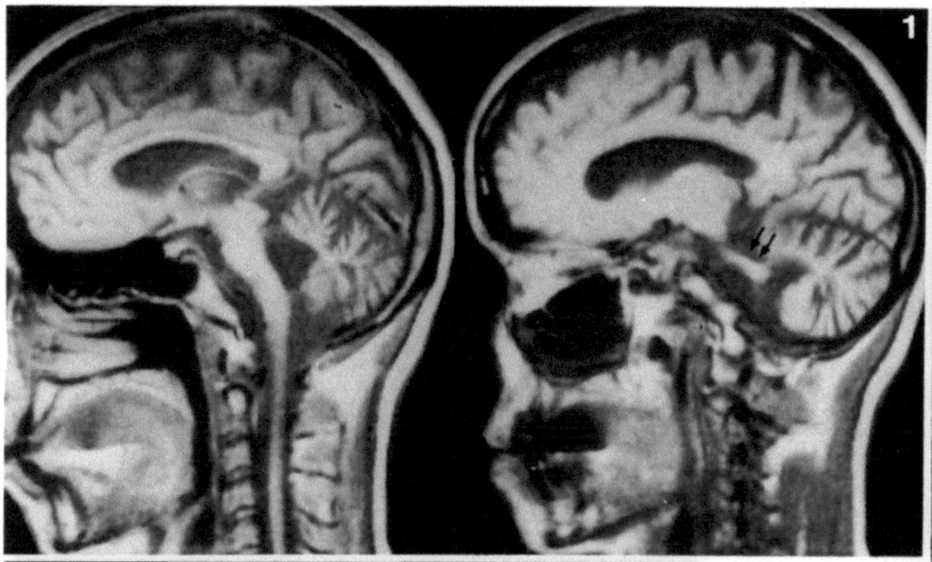

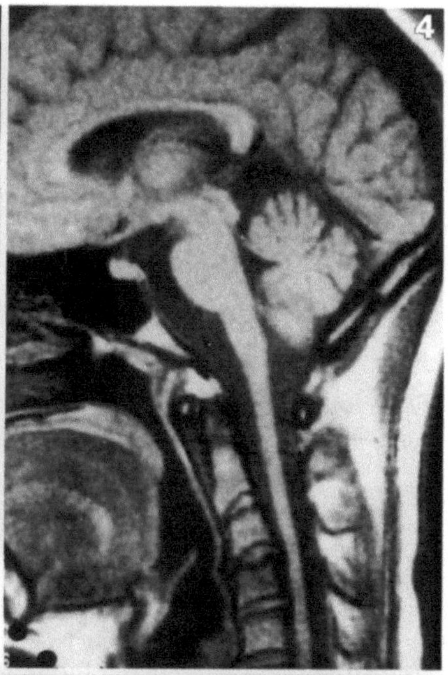

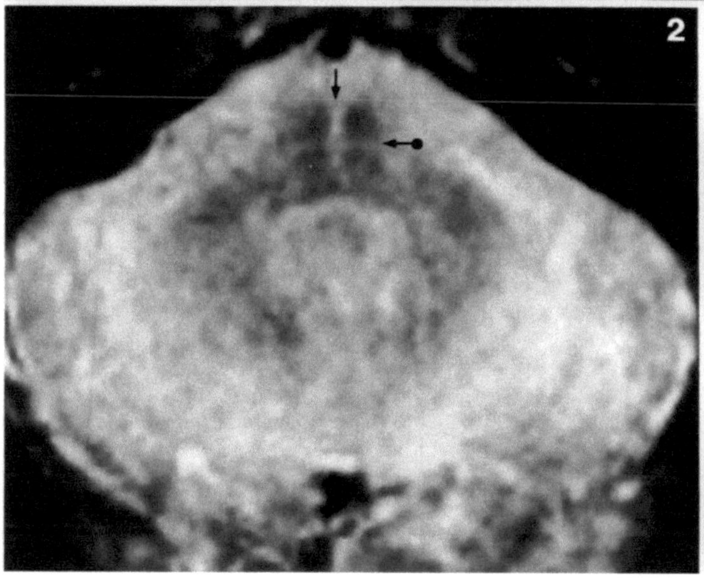

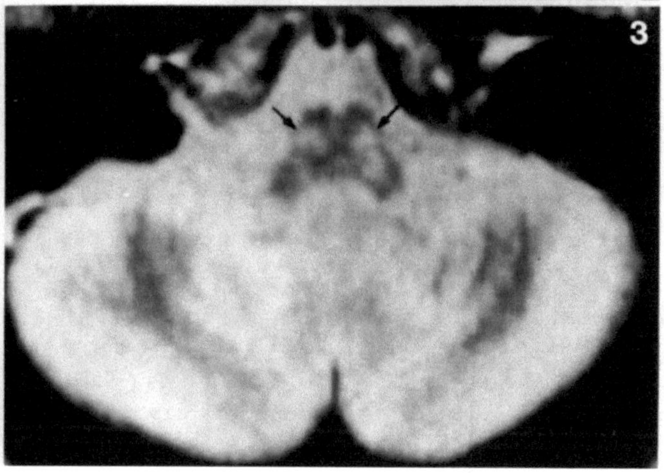

Fig. 1. A 37-year-old woman. Dominant. Severe atrophy of cerebellum, pons and middle cerebellar peduncles (→). There is also atrophy of the spinal cord and cerebral cortex

Fig. 2. A 42-year-old woman. Dominant. Severe atrophy of the pons. On this T2-weighted image there are areas of hyperintensity corresponding to degeneration of the raphe (→) and transverse pontine fibres (•→), while the pyramidal tracts *(black)* are normal

Fig. 3. A 35-year-old woman. Sporadic. Section at the level of inferior olives which appear highly hyperintense (→) on this T2-weighted image. The abnormal signal extends dorsally involving the olivo-cerebellar fibres

Fig. 4. A 30-year-old man. Friedreich's ataxia. Spinal cord atrophy, while the brain stem appears normal. Mild atrophy of the vermis and cerebral cortex

sign in FA, in which the brain stem was commonly normal. In the sporadic group each of the above described aspects was found. There was not always a good correlation between MRI findings and clinical symptoms.

References

1. Oppenheimer DR (1977) Diseases of basal ganglia, cerebellum and motor neurons. In: Blackwood W, Corsellis JAN (eds) Greenfield's neuropathology. Arnold Edinburgh, pp 608–651
2. Barbeau A, Sadibelouiz M, Sadibelouiz A, Roy M, (1984) A clinical classification of hereditary ataxias. Can J Neurol Sci 11: 501
3. Harding AE (1983) Classification of the hereditary ataxias and paraplegias. Lancet I: 1151
4. Bradac GB, Riva A, Mortara P. Orsi L, Riccio A (1989) Primary progressive cerebellar ataxia. Neuroradiology 31: 16
5. Savoiardo M, Strada L, Girotti F, Zimmerman RA, Grisoli M, Testa D, Petrillo R (1990) Olivopontocerebellar atrophy: MR diagnosis and relationship to multisystem atrophy. Radiology 174: 693
6. Wessel K, Schroth G, Diener MN, Müller-Farell W, Dichgans J (1989) Significance of MRI-confirmed atrophy of the cranial spinal cord in Friedreich's Ataxia. Eur Arch Psychiatry Neurol Sci 238: 225

Prof. G. B. Bradac
Neuroradiologica
Univ. Ospedale Molinette
Via Cherasco 15
I-10126, Turin, Italy

Neuroradiology (1991) 33 [Suppl]: 598–600

Neuro
radiology
© Springer-Verlag 1991

MRI in Wilson's disease of the brain

A. Mironov

Department of Neuroradiology, Kantonsspital, Aarau, Switzerland

Summary. Repeated MRI investigations of the skull with a 1.5 T instrument were carried out in three patients with biochemically and clinically diagnosed Wilson's disease. A pronounced decrease in the signal on T2 weighting was observed in all patients in the basal ganglia and brain stem nuclei which normally accumulate iron. There were also areas with an increased signal on T2 weighting in the regions without physiological iron deposits. In the region of the putamen, the caudate nucleus and the substantia nigra, striking target configurations were detected with marginal increase of the signal in T2 weighting. To our knowledge, similar target configurations have not yet been observed in the region of iron accumulating structures in Wilson's disease.

Key words: Wilson's disease – High field magnetic resonance imaging – Paramagnetic substances

Wilson's disease is an autosomal recessive disorder of copper metabolism characterised by abnormal retention of copper in the tissues, low serum copper and reduced or absent caeruloplasmin. Brain accumulation of copper begins later than that in the liver. Pathological changes in the brain include necrotising degeneration without inflammation but with variable glial response.

Numerous articles have dealt with CT findings in the brain including atrophy, either diffuse or focal, in the brain stem or basal ganglia. Areas of hypodensity in the lentiform nuclei, brain stem, cerebellar nuclei and cerebral hemisphere white matter are also frequently present [1–4]. Low-field MR images in the brain also reveal abnormalities in these areas with symmetrical or asymmetrical foci of increased signal intensity on T2-weighted images [5–8].

At high field strengths, decreased signal in the putamen on T2-weighted images has been reported in Wilson's disease [9] and probably reflects the T2 effect of the copper deposited due to a derangement in metabolism.

Patients, methods and results

Over a period of 2 years, we have carried out repeated MRI investigations (Gyroscan 1.5 T, 10 mT/m) in three patients with biochemical and clinical diagnosis of hepatolenticular degeneration or Wilson's disease. Spin echo sequences with T1 and T2 weighting were used.

With T1-weighting, slight to moderate atrophic changes of the cortex, basal ganglia, midbrain, pons and cerebellum were detected in all patients. Unilateral lacunae in the peripheral regions of the putamen adjacent to the external capsule were present in patients 2 and 3.

With T2-weighting, a severe decrease of the signal intensity was found in the putamen and substantia nigra, below that observed in globus pallidus, in patients 1 and 2. In patient 3, there was similar signal attenuation in the putamen and the caudate nucleus on the left. These coincided with a pronounced bilateral physiological signal reduction in the globus pallidus (Figs. 1, 2)

In addition, there were mainly symmetrical areas of increased signal in the mesencephalic tegmentum, the pontine tegmentum and periaqueductally with T2-weighting. Increased signal, not always symmetrical, but pronounced, occurred around the periphery of the putamen, the substantia nigra and the caudate nucleus (patient 1 and 2). The marked decrease in the signal of these nuclei with simultaneous marginal increase of the signal gave rise to a striking target configuration. Discrete macular signal elevations were also detected in the inner parts of the putamen, the caudate nucleus and the thalamus (patients 2 and 3). In patient 3, there were asymmetrical areas of high signal in the white matter of the corona radiata and the centrum semiovale on both sides.

In repeat investigations after penicillamine treatment, significant regression of the previously shown pathological changes was not detected.

Discussion

The terminal stage of cerebral Wilson's disease is characterised by a spongiform state, sealed off by cavitations with irreversible damage to the neurons. The basal ganglia, thalamus, midbrain nuclei, pontine and suprapontine structures and cerebellar nuclei have been described as predilection sites. An abnormal deposition of copper in the putamen was detected in postmortem investigations of the brain of patients with hepatolenticular degeneration [10].

Although paramagnetic copper plays an important role as a trace metal in brain metabolism, no predilection sites for physiological accumulation of this metal in healthy brain structures are known [11]. On the other hand, physiological and age-dependent accumulation of iron in the basal ganglia and the brain stem nuclei occurs. Owing to the local inhomogeneity of the accumulated paramagnetic iron, spin dephasing is caused in the magnetic field with subsequent decrease in signal of the iron-accumulating nuclei. The effect is more sensitive at higher field intensities and results in a decrease of the signal on T2 weighting [12, 13].

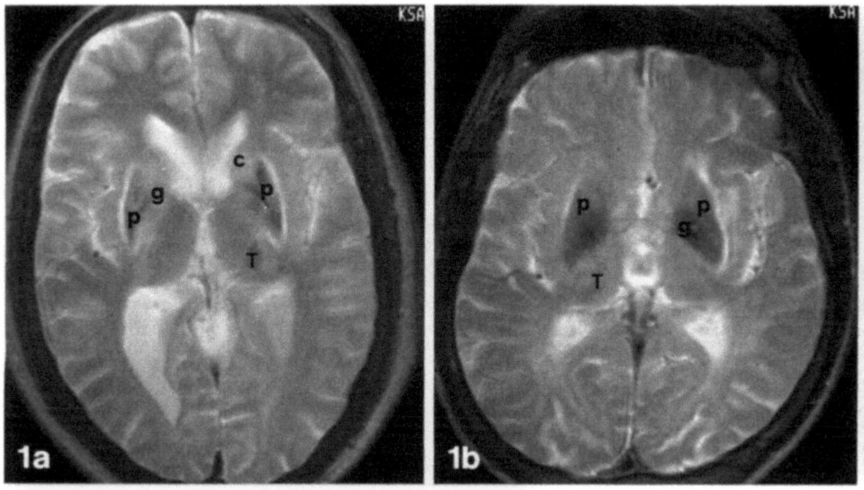

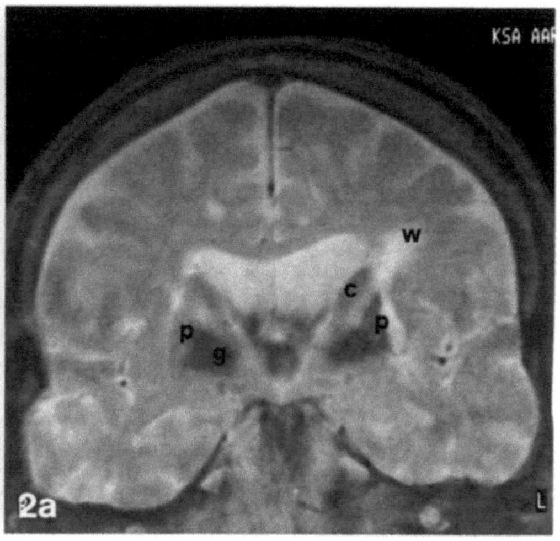

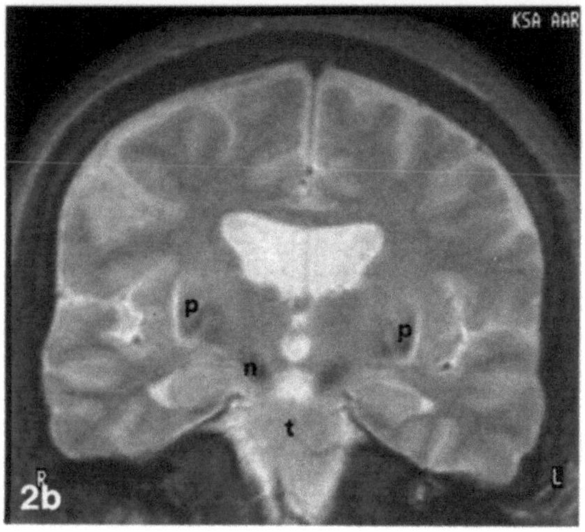

Fig. 1 a, b. Patient 2: **a** Axial and **b** coronal SE 2100/80 ms images display abnormally decreased signal intensity in the putamen *(p)* and substantia nigra *(n)* relative to globus pallidus *(g)*. Signal elevations occur in the caudate nucleus *(c)*, the thalamus *(T)* and the pontine tegmentum *(t)*. The marginal increase of the signal in the putamen *(p)* and the substantia nigra *(n)* gives rise to a target configuration

Fig. 2 a, b. Patient 3: **a** Axial and **b** Coronal SE 2100/80 ms images shows decreased signal and atrophy in the putamen *(p)* and the caudate nucleus *(c)* on the left coincidental with a pronounced signal reduction in the globus pallidus *(g)*. Asymmetrical signal elevations occur in the white matter *(w)* of corona radiata and the thalamus *(T)*. Also noted are marginal increases of the signal in the caudate nucleus *(c)*, the putamen *(p)* and the globus pallidus *(g)*, which suggest target configuration

The very severe decrease of the visual signal in the putamen, the substantia nigra and the caudate nucleus in our patients can be explained by the combination of the paramagnetic effects of abnormally accumulated copper with physiological iron accumulations already present in these nuclei. However, the mechanism and the predilection to copper accumulation remain unclear. The abnormal copper accumulation which has arisen for unclarified reasons is thus to be regarded as an early stage of the disease. In support of this chronology, we found only a circumscribed area of pronounced fall in the signal in the putamen in patient 1, probably attributable to the only slight accumulation of copper under regular therapy and monitoring.

With progression of the neuronal damage, a spongiform state develops with variable glial response, probably in a centripetal direction. This results in striking target configurations in the putamen, the caudate nucleus and the substantia nigra with peripheral signal elevation (status spongiosus) and central decrease in the signal (local inhomogeneity in magnetic susceptibility due to iron and copper). With further progression of the spongiform state, an increase of the signal also occurs even in the inner parts of the target configurations. As far as we know, the target configurations in cerebral Wilson's disease have not been observed previously.

Conclusions

The precise cause of the neuronal damage is not entirely evident, since the increased deposition of copper occurs in tissues which already contain abundant copper. In this context, the interpretation of the initial signal elevation on T2 weighting outside the areas with phyisological iron accumulations is ambivalent. On the one hand, the deposition of copper in these brain regions might not be detectable when there is no summation with the effect of iron, accumulated beforehand. Under these circumstances the spongiform state already caused is manifest as a signal elevation on T2 weighting. On the other hand, secondary neuronal damage might also occur without direct local accumulation of copper in these regions. Further study of the local metabolism of copper in the brain is required.

Without discussing the precise mechanisms hypothetically here, we believe that a deposition of copper at the beginning of the pathomorphological process exclusively in the iron-accumulating nuclei (mainly the putamen) and at a later time also in the structures not accumulating iron would appear to be plausible.

The striking target configuration of the putamen, the caudate nucleus and the substantia nigra might be directly proportional to the severity of brain damage.

References

1. Harik S, Post MJD (1981) Computed tomography in Wilson disease. Neurology 31: 107–110
2. Kendall BE, Pollock SS, Bass NM, Valentine AR (1981) Wilson's disease: Clinical correlation with cranial computed tomography. Neuroradiology 22: 1–5
3. Takano K, Kuroiwa Y, Shimada Y, Mannen T, Toyokura Y (1983) CT manifestation of cerebral white matter lesion in Wilson's disease.
4. Williams FJ, Walshe JM (1981) Wilson's disease: an analysis of the cranial computerized tomographic appearances found in 60 patients and the changes in response to treatment with chelating agents. Brain 104: 735–752
5. Aisen AM, Martel W, Gabrielsen T, Glazer G, Brewer G, Young AB, Hill G (1985) Wilson's disease of the brain: MR-imaging. Radiology 157: 137–141
6. Dörnemann H, Petsch R, Braitinger S (1987) MRI bei Morbus Wilson. Fortschr Röntgenstr 147: 570–571
7. Lawler GA, Pennock JM, Steiner RE, Jenkins WJ, Sherlock S, Young IR (1983) Nuclear megnetic resonance (NMR) imaging in Wilson's disease. J Comput Assist Tomogr 7: 1–8
8. Lukes SA, Aminoff MJ, Crooks L, Kaufman L, Mills C, Newton TH (1983) Nuclear magnetic resonance imaging in movement disorders. Ann Neurol 13: 690–691
9. I .utledge JN, Hilal SK, Silver AJ, Defendini R, Fahn S (1987) S udy of movement disorders and brain iron by MR. AJNR 8: 3)7–411
10. C uming JM (1948) The copper and iron content of brain and liver ii the normal and in hepato-lenticular degeneration. Brain 71: 4 10–415
11. I rayer B, Burger P, Hurwitz B, Dawson D, Cain J (1987) Re- c uced signal intensity on MR images of thalamus and putamen in r ıultiple sclerosis: increased iron content?
12. I)rayer B, Burger P, Darwin R, Riederer S, Herfkens R, Johnson (iA (1986) Magnetic resonance imaging of brain iron. AJNR 7: : 73–380
13. (iomori JM, Grossman RI, Goldberg HI, Zimmerman RA, Bila- ıink LT (1985) Intracranial hematomas: imaging bei high-field ΛR. Radiology 157: 87–93

Dr. A. Mironov
Ne ıroradiologie
Di: gnostische Radiologie
Ka ıtonsspital
CF -5001 Aarau, Switzerland

Neuroradiology (1991) 33 [Suppl]: 601–603

Neuro-radiology
© Springer-Verlag 1991

Intracranial calcified deposits are part of the diagnostic spectrum of neurofibromatosis type 2

L. Mayfrank[1], M. Moyadjer[1], and B. Wullich[2]

[1] Department of Neurosurgery, [2] Institute of Human Genetics and Anthropology, University of Freiburg, Freiburg, Federal Republic of Germany

Summary. Eleven consecutive patients with neurofibromatosis type 2 (NF-2) were investigated. CT revealed non-neoplastic intracranial calcified deposits in the choroid plexus, cerebellar cortex and on the surface of the cerebral cortex in seven of these patients. These abnormalities are most likely caused by calcium deposits in hamartomatous lesions. They are considered as part of the diagnostic spectrum of NF-2.

Key words: Neurofibromatosis – Intracranial calcification-Phacomatosis – Intracranial tumours – Computed tomography

Neurofibromatosis type 2 (NF-2) is a rare autosomal dominant inherited disorder characterized by the occurrence of neoplastic and malformative lesions. Multiple intracranial and spinal tumours, most frequently bilateral acoustic neuromas, neuromas of other cranial and spinal nerves and meningiomas, are the most common manifestation of the disease [1, 2]. This article reports on the incidence, location and significance of non-tumoral intracranial calcified deposits in NF-2.

Patients and methods

Eleven consecutive, unrelated patients with NF-2 (6 male, 5 female) were examined clinically and radiographically. The age of manifestation of the disorder ranged from 14 to 41 years (mean 22.5 years). All patients had multiple intracranial and spinal neuromas and/or meningiomas. Bilateral acoustic neuromas were found in 8 patients, all of whom additionally had intracranial meningiomas. Three further patients had one acoustic neuroma along with multiple other intracranial or spinal tumours (meningiomas or neuromas). The clinical features have been described in more detail elsewhere [3].

All patients underwent both plain and contrast-enhanced CT examinations. Five-millimetre slices were obtained in the axial plane and complemented as necessary by thin slices, reconstructions in the coronal or sagittal planes, or by bone view. Follow-up studies were performed with intervals ranging from 1 to 5 years (mean 3.0 years).

Results

CT revealed non-tumoral, intracranial calcified deposits in 7 out of the 11 patients. There was no abnormal enhancement or neoplastic mass lesion in corresponding locations. During the follow-up period no increase of the calcified deposits was observed.

In 6 cases abnormal calcification along the entire choroid plexus of either one or both lateral ventricles was observed, extending from the region of the foramen of Monro to the temporal horn (Fig. 1). In 4 patients the choroid plexus of the third ventricle was also calcified.

Areas with multiple nodular calcified lesions located in the folia of the cerebellar hemispheres were demonstrated in 4 patients (Figs. 1, 2). In 2 cases a craniotomy near the superficially located cerebellar calcification was performed in order to remove an acoustic neuroma, and no meningioma or cerebellar tumour was found in the region of the calcified deposits.

A nodular calcification in the region of the left lateral fissure was observed in 1 case (Fig. 3). It appeared to be located in or over the insular cortex. In 1 further patient multiple fine punctuate calcified lesions of less than 0.5 cm in diameter were observed on the surface of both cerebral hemispheres.

Discussion

This study demonstrates a high incidence of non-neoplastic intracranial calcified deposits in a series of 11 consecutive patients with clinically proven NF-2. Our results as well as a review of previously published cases [4–9] indicate that abnormal choroid plexus calcification is the most typical form of calcification in NF-2. Cerebellar or subependymal calcification, or calcified deposits on the supratentorial brain surface were observed less frequently (Table 1). We are not aware of any pathological study analysing the nature of non-tumoral calcified lesions in NF-2, but it is likely that they are caused by calcium deposits in hamartomatous lesions.

Major clinical manifestations in NF-2 patients are almost exclusively secondary to intracranial and spinal neoplastic lesions causing neurological symptoms. Non-neo-

Table 1. Summary of 19 reported neurofibromatosis type 2 patients with abnormal intracranial calcified deposits detected by CT [3–9]

Location of calcified deposits	Choroid plexus	Cerebellar cortex	Subependymal	Cerebral cortex
No. of cases	11	6	3	2

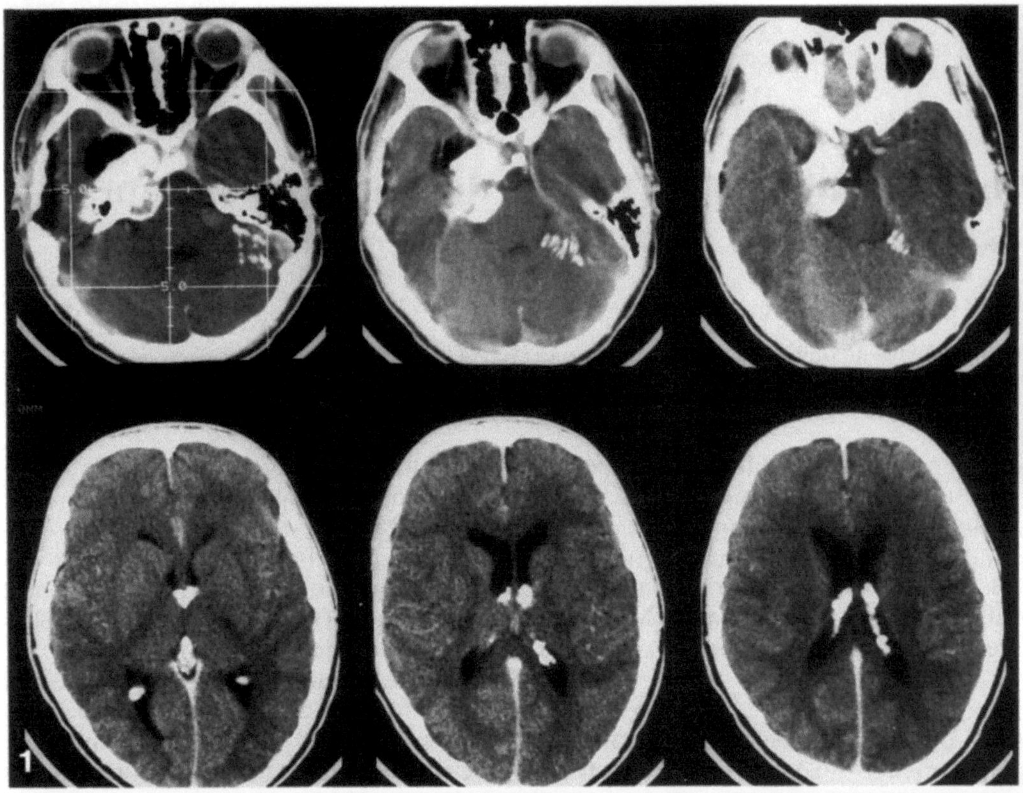
1

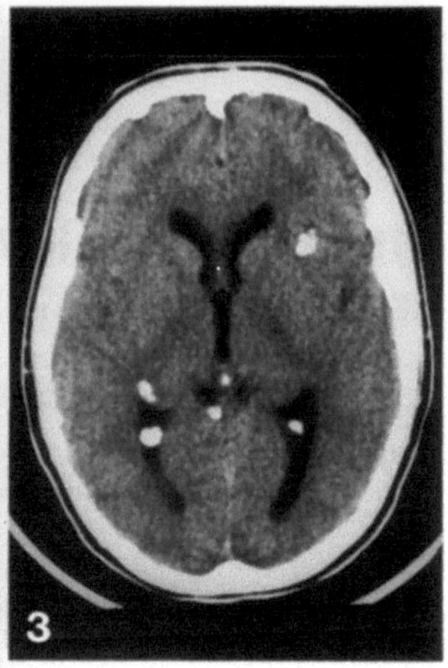
3

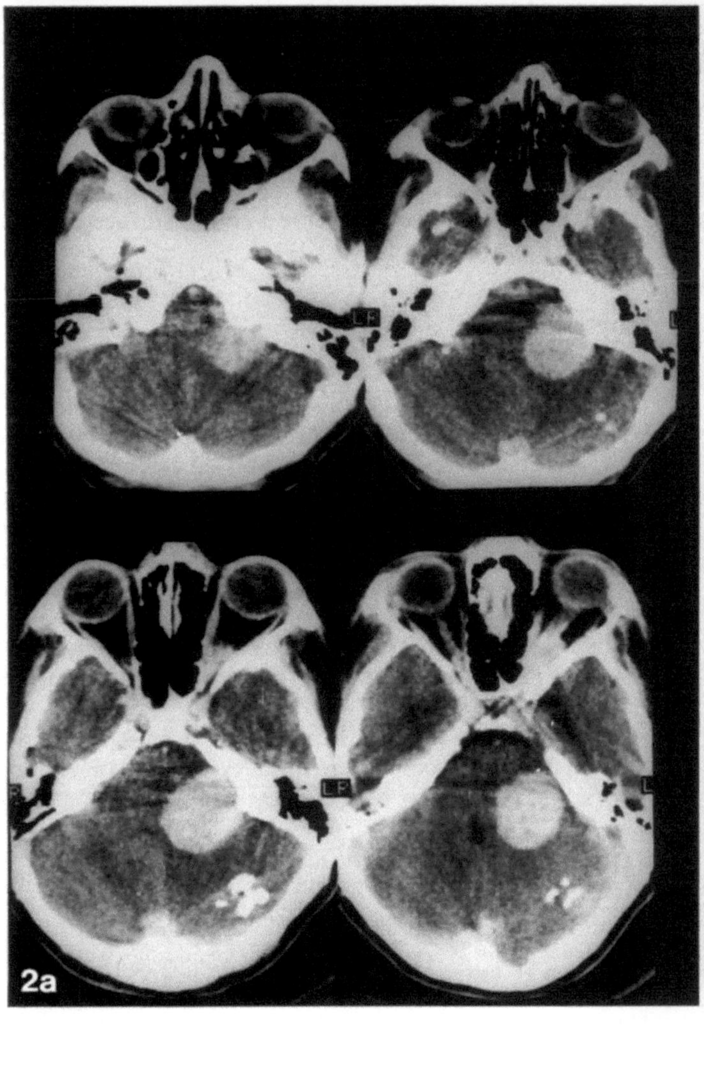
2a

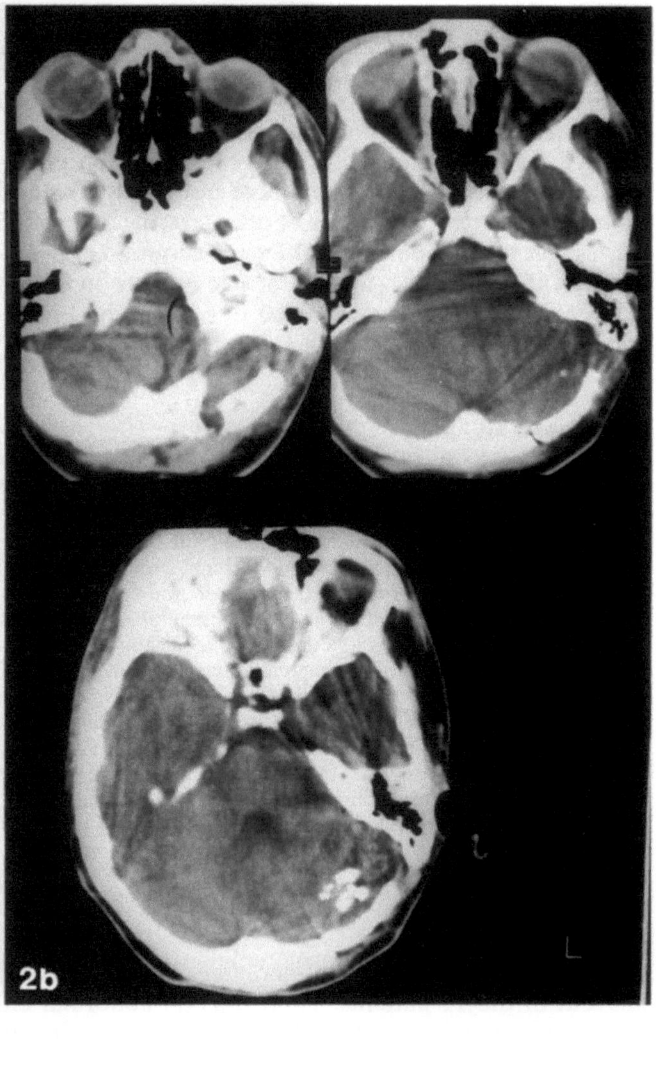
2b

Fig. 1. Contrast-enhanced CT. Calcification in the left cerebellar hemisphere and calcification of the choroid plexus. No change after contrast medium. Acoustic neuroma on the left side and partially resected meningioma of the right petrosal bone. A suboccipital craniotomy was performed on the left side for resection of the acoustic neuroma; no cerebellar or meningeal tumour in the region of the cerebellar calcification was found

Fig. 2. **a** Contrast-enhanced CT. Calcified deposits in the left cerebellar hemisphere. Bilateral acoustic neuromas. Non-enhanced CT after resection of the acoustic neuroma on the left side (**b**): The calcified cerebellar lesion has the same appearance as with contrast medium. Intraoperatively, no cerebellar tumour or meningioma were found

Fig. 3. CT before injection of contrast medium. Nodular calcification in or over the left insular cortex. No change after contrast medium

---

plastic abnormalities involving the central nervous system [10], skin, and eyes [11] also occur in NF-2. Some of these developmental lesions such as posterior capsular lens opacities or café-au-lait spots are of clinical interest, as they may precede the onset of symptoms of intracranial tumours, allowing early identification of family members with the gene. Recently, intracranial non-tumoural calcification was observed in 4 asymptomatic members of a family with NF-2, 3 of whom later developed tumours [12]. Thus, the demonstration of non-neoplastic calcification may help to establish a diagnosis of NF-2 before other stigmata of the disease become manifest.

References

1. Martuza RLK, Eldridge R (1988) Neurofibromatosis 2 (bilateral acoustic neurofibromatosis). N Engl J Med 318: 684–688
2. Kanter WR, Eldridge R, Fabricant R, Allen JC, Koerber T (1980) Central neurofibromatosis with bilateral acoustic neurinoma: genetic, clinical and biochemical distinctions from peripheral neurofibromatosis. Neurology 30: 851–859
3. Mayfrank L, Mohadjer M, Wullich B (1990) Intracranial calcified deposits in neurofibromatosis type 2. Neuroradiology 32:33–37
4. Modic MT, Weinstein MA, Rothner AD, Erenberg G, Duchesneau PM, Kaufmann B (1980) Calcification of the choroid plexus visualized by computed tomography. Radiology 15: 369–372
5. Vouge M, Pasquini U, Salvolini U (1980) CT findings of atypical forms of phakomatosis. Neuroradiology 20: 88–101
6. Gardeur D, Palmieri A, Mashaly R (1983) Cranial computed tomography in the phakomatoses. Neuroradiology 25: 293–304
7. Boruta P, Nadvornik P, Vrtelova N (1984) CT diagnosis of central neurofibromatosis. Medicamundi 29: 118–119
8. Arts WFM, Van Dongen KJ (1986) Intracranial calcified deposits in neurofibromatosis. J Neurol Neurosurg Psychiatry 49: 1317–1320
9. Van Tassel P, Yeakley JW, Lee KF (1987) Cerebellar calcification in central neurofibromatosis: CT in two cases. AJNR 8: 913–915
10. Rubinstein LJ (1986) The malformative central nervous system lesions in the central and peripheral forms of neurofibromatosis. Ann NY Acad Sci 486: 14–29
11. Kaiser-Kupfer MI, Freidlin V, Datiles MB, Edwards PA, Sherman JL, Parry D, McCain LM, Eldridge R (1989) The association of posterior lens opacities with bilateral acoustic neuromas in patients with neurofibromatosis type 2. Arch Ophtalmol 107: 541–544
12. Wertelecki W, Rouleau GA, Superneau DW, Forehand LW, Williams JP, Haines JL, Gusella JF (1988) Neurofibromatosis 2: clinical and DNA linkage studies of a large kindred. N Engl J Med 319: 278–283

Dr. Lothar Mayfrank
Department of Neurosurgery
Medical Faculty of the RWTH
Pauwelstrasse 30,
W-5100 Aachen, Federal Republic of Germany

Neuroradiology (1991) 33 [Suppl]: 604–606

Neuro radiology
© Springer-Verlag 1991

Measurement of caudate nucleus and putamen atrophy in patients with Huntington's disease

D. K. Kido[1], I. Shoulson[2], J. V. Manzione[1], and P. P. Harnish[1]

Departments of [1]Radiology and [2]Neurology, University of Rochester Medical Center, Rochester, New York, USA

Summary. Direct linear measurements of caudate nucleus widths are more accurate than indirect measurements (bicaudate distance) in detecting early atrophic changes using MRI in patients with Huntington's disease (HD). At 95% confidence level, caudate nucleus widths of 8 mm or less were found to be abnormal, while those 9 mm or larger were normal. Caudate nuclei widths were more sensitive than similar measurements of the putamen or of bicaudate-skull ratios as correlates of functional changes in patients with early HD.

Key words: Caudate nucleus – Putamen – Huntington's disease

Huntington's disease (HD) is an inherited central nervous system (CNS) disorder that results in motor and intellectual decline. Postmortem studies demonstrate extensive neural loss in the caudate nucleus, putamen, and globus pallidus, and more variable, less extensive loss in other regions of the basal ganglia and in the cerebral cortex and cerebellum [1, 2].

Caudate nucleus atrophy can be assessed indirectly using CT or MRI by determining the shortest transverse distance between the heads of the caudate nuclei (bicaudate distance) [3, 4]. Ratios between the bicaudate distance (CC) and the distance between the outer tables of the skull (OT) have been correlated with the motor and cognitive changes of HD [5, 6]. It is unknown whether direct measurements of the caudate nuclei and putamen offer any advantages over indirect measurements in correlating atrophy of these structures with early clinical features of HD. We, therefore, compared these three types of measurement in HD patients and age-matched control subjects.

Methods

Sixteen HD patients and 14 controls were included in this study. HD was diagnosed by the presence of movement disorders with confirmatory family history [mean age of HD patients = 41 ± 14 years; 11 females, 5 males]. A total functional capacity (TFC) score was assessed for each patient [7]. Based on this measure, 5 patients with HD were judged to be in stage I (TFC = 11–13), 7 in stage II (TFC = 7–10), and 4 in stage III (TFC = 3–6). Control subjects consisted of 14 patients who were suspected of having acoustic neuromas and who had normal MRI (mean age = 44 ± 10 years; 8 females, 6 males).

MRI was performed on a 1.5-T imager. Axial images were obtained using a spin echo sequence (TR 2000/TE 30, 60; slice thickness 5 mm; skip 1/2; 2 excitations; 256 × 256). All measurements of the caudate nucleus and putamen were made directly from images of the first echo and were accurate to 1 mm.

The width of the right and left caudate nuclei was measured directly by selecting the axial slice where they appeared largest (Fig. 1). Indirect bicaudate measurements were also made, and the distance between the outer tables of the skull at the level of the caudate nuclei was estimated by drawing a line between the inner surfaces of the subcutaneous fat on each side of the skull, in order to calculate a CC/OT ratio (Fig. 2).

The right and left putaminal widths were measured separately by drawing a horizontal line from the inner border of the putamen to its outer border (Fig. 1). The putamina were measured on the slice just superior to the anterior commissure at a level roughly through their middles. All MRI measurements were made independently of TFC clinical assessments.

Results

Both the indirect bicaudate (CC) and direct (caudate) measurements distinguished HD patients from controls (Table 1). Of the 16 HD patients, 15 had at least one caudate nucleus that was 8 mm or smaller, while all controls had caudate nuclei of 9 mm or larger (Fig. 3). Therefore, with 95% confidence, controls can be expected to have caudate nuclei that measure 9 mm or larger.

Direct measurements of the putamen revealed that 15 of the 16 HD patients had at least one putamen that was 9 mm or smaller, while all controls had putamina that were 10 mm or larger (Fig. 4). Controls can be expected to have

Table 1. Caudate nucleus and putamen measurements in Huntington's disease (HD) and controls (mm)[a]

	HD ($n = 16$)	Controls ($n = 14$)	
Caudate nucleus	6.8 ± 1.8	10.2 ± 0.6	$P = 0.000001$
Putamen	7.0 ± 2.3	11.9 ± 0.9	$P = 0.0000001$
CC	22.0 ± 4.7	10.7 ± 1.2	$P = 0.00000003$
OT	122.6 ± 5.9	121.6 ± 6.5	$P = 0.65$ (NS)
CT/OT	0.18 ± 0.04	0.09 ± 0.01	$P = 0.0000002$

[a] CC, Bicaudate distance; OT, distance between the outer tables of the skull

Mean measurements (± SD) in controls and patients, comparisons were made with the Student's *t*-test

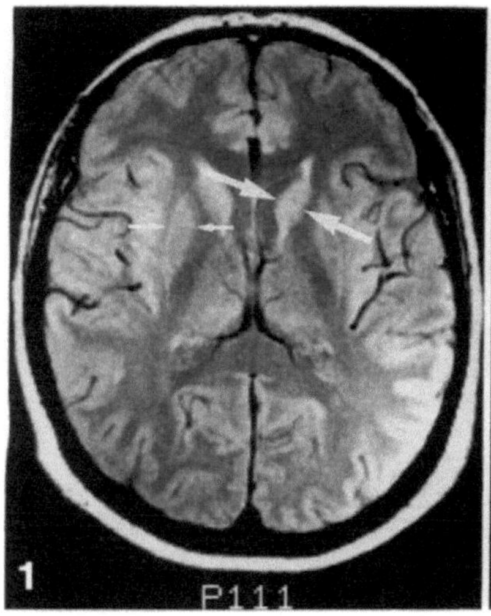

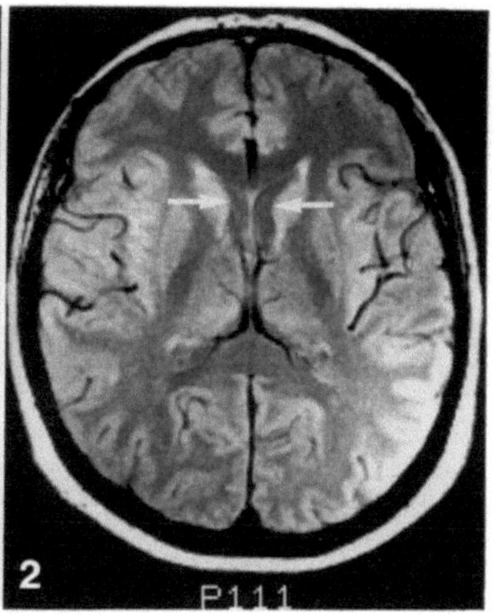

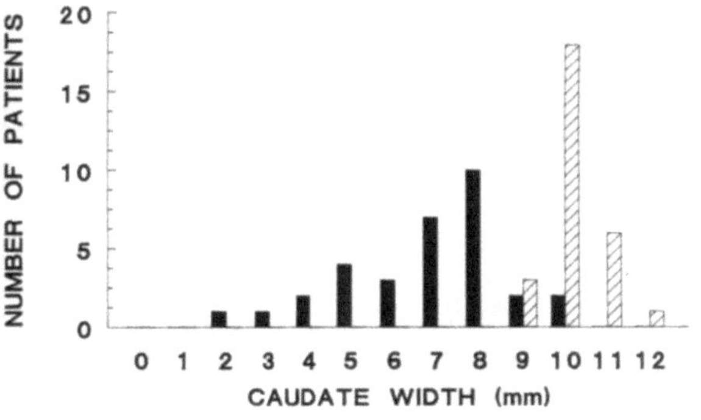

3

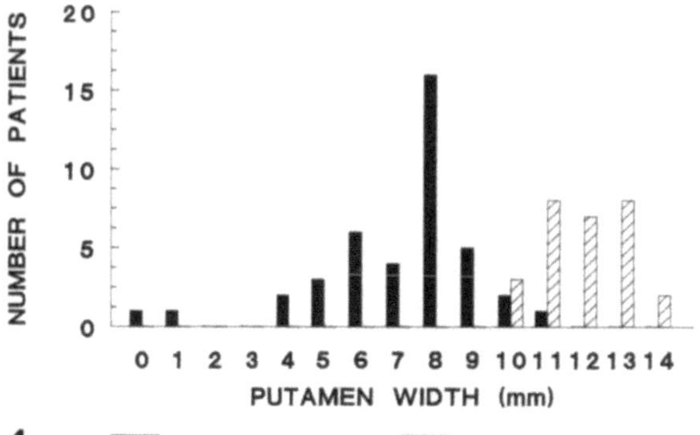

4

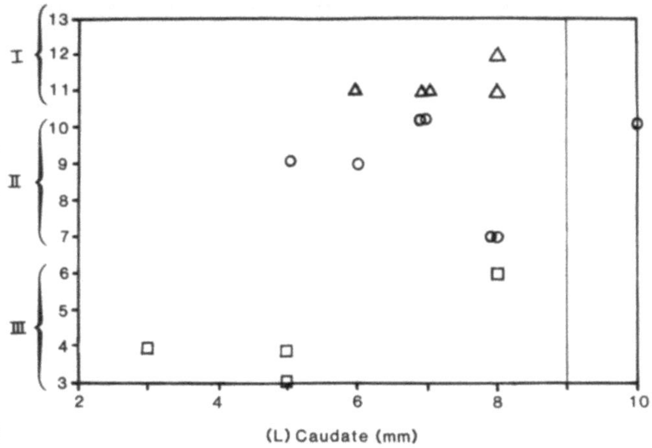

5

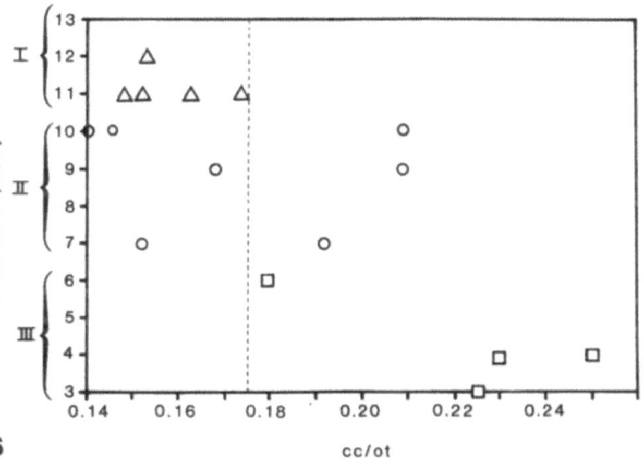

6

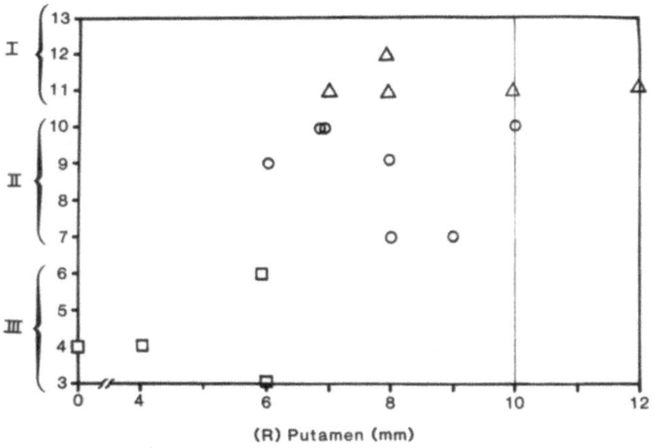

7

Fig. 1. Direct measurement of maximum left caudate nucleus width (between *large arrows*) and right putamen width (between *small arrows*) in millimeters; TR/TE 2000/30

Fig. 2. Indirect bicaudate measurements (between *arrows*); TR/TE 2000/30

Fig. 3. Caudate nucleus widths in patients with Huntington's disease (HD) and controls

Fig. 4. Putaminal widths in patients with HD and controls

Fig. 5. Relationship between direct caudate nucleus measurements and total functional capacity in patients with HD. The controls can be expected to have caudate nucleus widths to the right of the vertical line at 9 mm (95% confidence). Note the one circle to the right of the vertical line; △, stage I; ○, stage II; □, stage III

Fig. 6. Relationship between indirect caudate nucleus measurement (CC/OT) and total functional capacity in patients with HD. The controls can be expected to be to the left of the vertical line near 0.18 (95% confidence). Note that 9 triangles and circles are to the left of the line; △, stage I; ○, stage II; □, stage III

Fig. 7. Relationship between direct putamen measurements and total functional capacity in patients with HD. The controls can be expected to be to the right of the vertical line at 10 mm (95% confidence); △, stage I; ○, stage II; □, stage III putamina that measure 10 mm or larger (95% confidence).

Indirect and direct measurements of the caudate nuclei and putamen were compared with the independently determined TFC scores in HD patients (Figs. 5–7). Direct measurements of the caudate nucleus were better enabled detection of HD patients in stage I and II than the direct measurements of the putamen, which in turn were more accurate than the indirect CC/OT measurements. All three measurements enabled detection of all individuals with stage III HD.

Discussion

Direct caudate nucleus measurements in patients with early suspected HD are a more sensitive indication of atrophy than indirect bicaudate measurements because they are subject to less variation. Knowing that caudate nuclei 9 mm or more in width are normal with 95% confidence may be helpful in diagnosing borderline atrophy. A review of clinical radiology reports for our 16 HD patients revealed that 2 of the 16 studies were misinterpreted as normal. They would have been read as abnormal if direct caudate nucleus measurements had been taken. The fact that the caudate nucleus does not change in signal intensity or texture as it atrophies may contribute to the difficulty in determining borderline atrophy.

Acknowledgement. This work was supported in part by USPHS grant NS 17978.

References

1. Lange H, Thörner G, Hopf A, Schröder KF (1976) Morphometric studies of the neuropathological changes in choreatic diseases. J Neurol Sci 28: 401–425
2. Bruyn GW, Bots GTAM, Dom R (1979) Huntington's chorea: current neuropathological status. Adv Neurol 23: 83–93
3. Barr AN, Heinze WJ, Dobben GD, Valvassori GE, Sugar O (1978) Bicaudate index in CT of Huntington's disease and cerebral atrophy. Neurology 28: 1196–1200
4. Stober T, Wussow W, Schimrigk K (1984) Bicaudate diameter – the most specific and simple CT parameter in the diagnosis of Huntington's disease. Neuroradiology 26: 25–28
5. Shoulson I, Goldblatt D, Plumb S, Harder M, Kido D, Miller C, Behr J, Kennedy J, Caine E, Banford K, Kurlan R (1986) Motor correlates of early Huntington's Disease. Neurology 36: 341
6. Banford K, Caine E, Kido D, Hungerford M, Kennedy J, Behr J, Goldblatt D, Miller C, Kurlan R, Shoulson I (1986) Neuropsychological impairment in early HD: functional and CT correlates. Neurology 36: 102–103
7. Shoulson I, Fahn S (1979) Huntington's disease: clinical care and evaluation. Neurology 29: 1–3

Dr Daniel K. Kido
Department of Radiology
P.O. Box 648
University of Rochester Medical Center
Rochester, NY 14642, USA

Neuroradiology (1991) 33 [Suppl]: 607–608

Neuro radiology
© Springer-Verlag 1991

Decreasing gray/white matter contrast: an aging phenomenon

L. A. Heier, A. Orenstein, L. Schwartz, R. D. Zimmerman, and M. D. F. Deck

Cornell University Medical Center, New York, USA

Summary. The loss of gray/white matter differentiation on MR images of elderly people has been incidentally noted, but never verified of quantified. We have found that this is a reproducible and statistically significant occurence. Both hypertension and non-specific white matter disease are associated with it.

Key words: Brain – Aging

Materials and methods

The pathological basis and clinical implications of the loss of gray/white matter differentiation are unknown. Spin echo TR 2000/TE 40- and 80-ms images demonstrate the loss of contrast between gray and white matter with aging.

MRI (1.5 T) and charts of 165 randomly selected neurology outpatients were retrospectively reviewed. The intensities of the gray and white matter were each qualitatively matched to the display gray scale provided by the software on each image. This scale consisted of 16 contrast steps (Fig. 1). The number of contrast steps that separated the gray and white matter were recorded in two different corticomedullary locations on both the balanced (2000/40) and T2-weighted images (2000/80) in the frontal and parietal lobes at the level of the atria of the lateral ventricles. Thus, four measures of gray/white matter contrast were obtained. These are subsequently referred to as: (1) LVPD, which is the contrast measure of the parietal lobe at the level of the lateral ventricle on the proton density or balanced images; (2) FLPD, which is the contrast measure at the level of frontal lobe on the proton density or balanced images; (3) LVT2, which is the contrast measure of the parietal lobe at the level of the lateral ventricle on the T2-weighted images; (4) FLT2, which is the contrast measure at the level of the frontal lobe on the T2-weighted images. Each of these contrast measures was correlated with age and other clinical and radiographic parameters usually found with aging. These included hypertension, dementia, nonspecific white matter disease and large perivascular spaces. The amount of nonspecific white matter disease was graded on a scale of 0–3. The contrast scores of each of the four contrast measures ranges from 0 to 6 with 6 representing the highest degree of contrast between gray and white matter.

An attempt was made to measure the width of the gray matter, but this was unsuccessful as the edge between gray and white matter was too indistinct in older patients.

Spearman rank correlation coefficients were performed between each of the four contrast measures and both age and grade of nonspecific white matter disease. The comparison of contrast scores for the remaining categorical variables was made using the Mann-Whitney-Wilcoxon rank test (sex, large perivascular spaces, hypertension, dementia).

Results

Spearman rank correlation coefficients for each of the four contrast measures were found to correlate negatively with age and grade of white matter disease. Gray white contrast decreased with age (Fig. 2) and the degree of white matter disease. Each of the contrast measures was moderately to strongly negatively correlated with age. The correlation coefficients ranged from –0.60 to –0.71 where each P value was less than 0.0001. Contrast measures were also negatively correlated with the grade of white matter disease, although not quite as strongly as with age. Here the correlation coefficients ranged from –0.36 to –0.42 where again all P values were less than 0.0001 (Table 1).

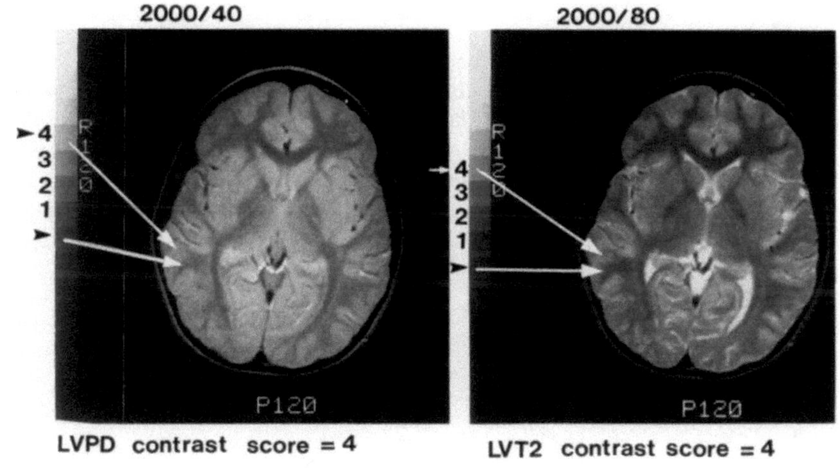

Fig. 1. SE TR 2000–40 and 80 ms axial images at the level of the atria of the lateral ventricles. The intensity of both the gray and white matter on each image is matched to the accompanying photographic gray scale. In each case four contrast steps separate the intensity of the gray and white matter giving a contrast score of 4

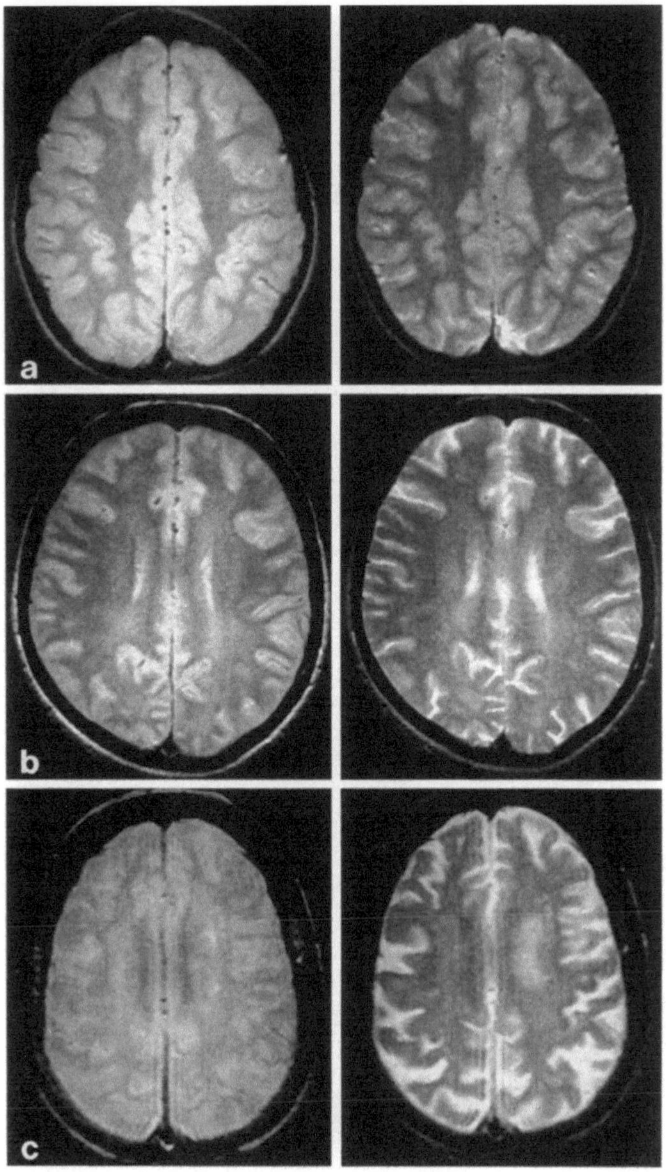

Fig. 2. a SE TR 2000–40 and 80 ms axial images of a 9-year-old female. **b** SE TR 2000–40 and 80 ms axial images of a 40-year-old female. **c** SE TR 2000–40 and 80 ms axial images of a 91-year-old female.

Table 1. Spearman rank correlation coefficients

Gray/white contrast measure	Age	White matter disease
LVPD	–0.60	0.42
FLPD	–0.61	0.40
LVT2	–0.71	0.39
FLT2	–0.67	0.36

LVPD, Parietal lobe at lateral ventricle on proton density or balanced images; FLPD, frontal lobe on proton density or balanced images; LVT2, parietal lobe at lateral ventricle on T2-weighted images; FLT2, frontal lobe on T2-weighted images

Table 2.

Contrast measure	–	Sex *P* value
LVPD		0.4578
FLPD		0.4992
LVT2		0.3413
FLT2		0.7344

Table 3.

Contrast measure	–	Virchow-Robin spaces *P* value
LVPD		0.2566
FLPD		0.6069
LVT2		0.3282
FLT2		0.7436

Table 4.

Contrast measure	–	Demential *P* value
LVPD		0.2165
FLPD		0.0886
LVT2		0.1767
FLT2		0.0789

Table 5.

Contrast measure	–	Hypertension *P* value
LVPD		0.0036
FLPD		0.0012
LVT2		0.0001
FLT2		0.0032

The Mann-Whitney-Wilcoxon rank test indicates that there are no differences in the contrast measures with respect to sex, large Virchow-Robin spaces or dementia. Tables 2–4 illustrate that none of the *P* values is significant. However, there were significant differences in contrast when the patient had a history of hypertension. Note that in Table 5 all the *P* values are less than 0.005.

Discussion

The loss of gray white matter differentiation with aging is a reproducible and statistically significant occurrence. Both hypertension and nonspecific white matter disease are significantly associated with it. It is speculated that with aging the gray matter loses water and becomes less hyperintense on balanced and T2-weighted images while the white matter gains water and becomes increasingly hyperintense resulting in the loss of contrast. Work is in progress to determine whether such a shift in water content between gray and white matter can be documented with MR spectroscopy.

Dr. Linda A. Heier
525 E 68th Street
New York, NY 10021, USA

Neuroradiology (1991) 33 [Suppl]: 609–611

Neuro radiology
© Springer-Verlag 1991

MRI and PET of CNS delayed radiation injury in an animal model

R. L. DeLaPaz[1], E. Lo[2], K. A. Frankel[2], M. H. Phillips[2], and J. I. Fabrikant[2]

[1] Department of Radiology, Stanford University Medical Center, Stanford, California, USA
[2] Lawrence Berkeley Laboratory, Berkeley, California, USA

Summary. Delayed CNS radiation injury was studied with magnetic resonance imaging (MRI) and positron emission tomography (PET) in the rabbit brain using 225 keV X-rays (60 Gy) and 230 MeV/u Bragg peak helium ions (15 and 30 Gy) to the left hemisphere. MRI at 2.5 months after X-irradiation showed increased signal on T2-weighted images and T1-weighted gadolinium(Gd)-DTPA contrast enhancement indicating increased tissue water content and blood-brain barrier (BBB) breakdown. Regional cerebral blood flow (rCBF) was reduced in the irradiated hemisphere. The 15 Gy helium irradiated cases showed no alterations on imaging studies. The 30 Gy cases showed alterations at 9–11 months including high signal on T2-weighted MR images and enhancement on T1-weighted Gd-DTPA MR images, primarily in the central white matter tracts and thalamus. These regions also showed reduced glucose utilization, measured by [18]FDG PET, and breakdown of the BBB, identified by [82]Rb PET. Histopathology showed white matter demyelination and edema corresponding to high signal changes on T2-weighted MRI and cystic necrosis with gliosis and dilated blood vessels in the thalamus, corresponding to Gd-DTPA contrast enhancement and [82]Rb PET. Cerebrovascular effects with BBB breakdown and tissue edema or necrosis may be a final common pathway for both "early delayed" CNS injury from high dose X-ray exposure and "late delayed" injury from heavy charged particle (helium) irradiation.

Key words: Brain, radiation injury – Blood-brain barrier – Cerebral blood flow – Magnetic resonance imaging – Positron emission tomography

---

Delayed reaction to radiation injury in the brain presents a serious potential complication in radiotherapy of intracranial disorders [1]. This study was undertaken to investigate the magnetic resonance imaging (MRI) and positron emission tomography (PET) changes with regional cerebral blood flow (rCBF) and histopathologic correlates following experimental, single dose radiation exposure.

Materials and methods

A total of 19 New Zealand White male rabbits (6–9 months old, 2.5 kg) were studied in one control group ($n = 4$) and three experimental groups each receiving a single dose of hemibrain irradiation: (1) 60 Gy 225 keV X-rays ($n = 5$; (2) 15 Gy 230 MeV Bragg peak helium (helium) ion ($n = 6$); or (3) 30 Gy 230 MeV/u Bragg peak helium ion ($n = 4$).

MRI studies were performed on a GE 1.5 T system using T1-weighted (SE 600/25, pre- and post-gadolinium (Gd)-DTPA, 1.0 mmol/kg IV) and T2-weighted (SE 2500/25, 50, 75, 100) images with a 15-cm RF coil, 12 cm field of vision (FOV), 256 × 256 matrix and 3-mm or 5-mm-thick slice (1 mm gap). MRI studies were obtained at 2-week intervals from irradiation through 2.5 months in group 1 (X-ray) animals and from 8 to 15 months after irradiation in groups 3 and 4 (helium ion) animals.

PET studies were performed on the helium-irradiated animals using the Donner 600 crystal imager with in-plane resolution of 2 mm and slice thickness of 4 mm. Fluorodeoxyglucose PET (7–8 mCi [18]FDG) studies were performed to examine cellular glucose uptake. [18]FDG freely crosses the BBB and is taken up and trapped by actively metabolizing neurons and glia [2]. Rubidium PET (24 mCi [82]Rb) studies were also conducted, to assess BBB integrity. [82]Rb is rapidly cleared from the brain vasculature so localization of tracer within the brain on PET indicates disruption of the BBB and accumulation of tracer in the brain parenchyma [3].

Measurements of rCBF were performed with radioactive cobalt ([57]Co) labelled styrene-divinyl resin microspheres (NEN-TRAC, Dupont) 15 µm in diameter, in the X-irradiated animals (2 at 1 month and 3 at 2.5 months post-irradiation), using standard techniques [4].

Histopathological analysis was conducted on 40-µm-thick brain slices from the helium-irradiated animals, corresponding to MRI and PET slice locations, using the hematoxylin and eosin stain for general morphology and Luxol fast blue for defining areas of demyelination.

Results

The MR images of rabbits in the 60 Gy 225 keV X-ray group demonstrated on abnormalities until approximately 2.5 months after irradiation. Gd-DTPA enhanced T1-weighted MR images at 2.5 months showed areas of contrast enhancement in the irradiated hemisphere, indicating the presence of focal disruption of the BBB, primarily in the white matter of the corona radiata and parts of the adjacent cortical gray matter, hippocampus and fimbria (Fig. 1).

There was no macroscopic evidence of tissue necrosis visible upon dissection of the X-irradiated brains for microsphere rCBF studies. Neurological deficits were not seen except for slight head tilt toward the irradiated hemisphere (left) in one animal. Control animal rCBF measurements were in the range fo 140–190 ml/100 g per minute in cortical regions, 80–90 ml/100 g per minute in the hippocampus, 110–150 ml/100 g per minute in the tha-

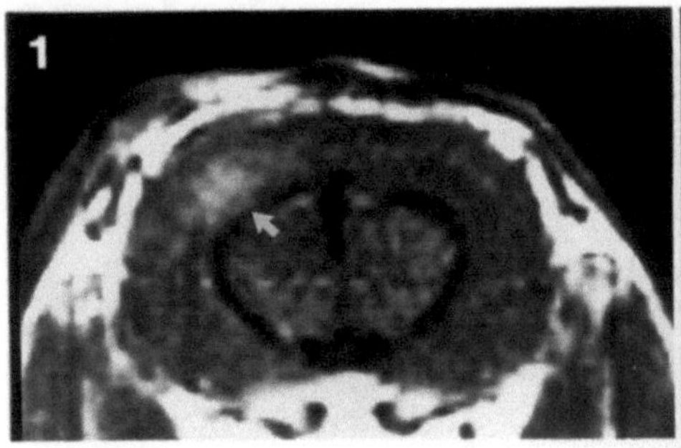

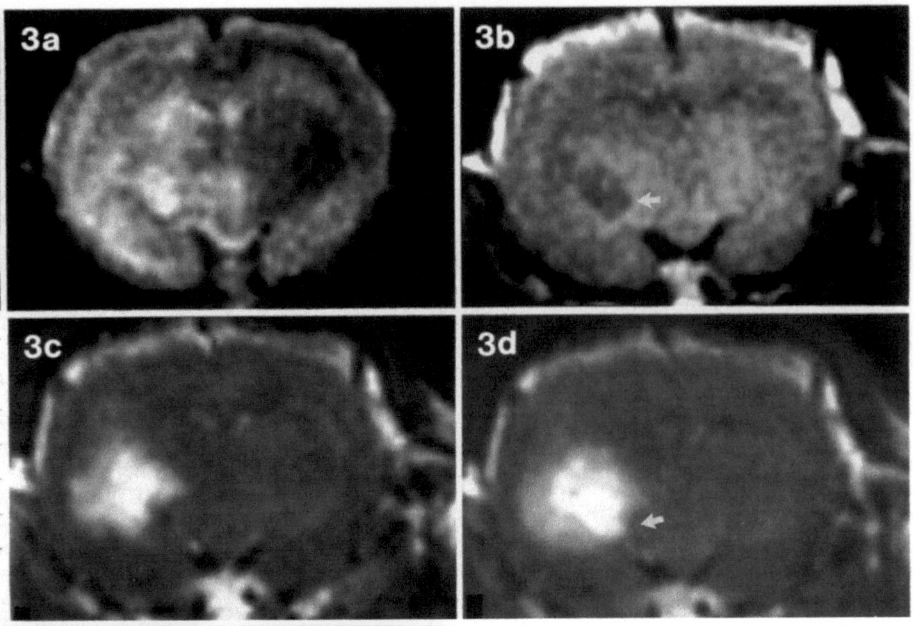

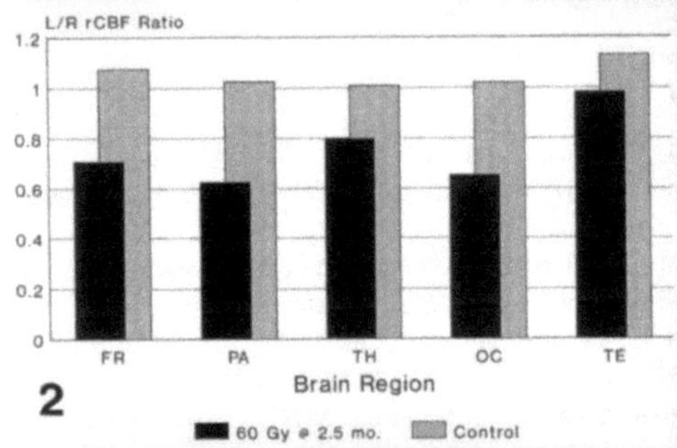

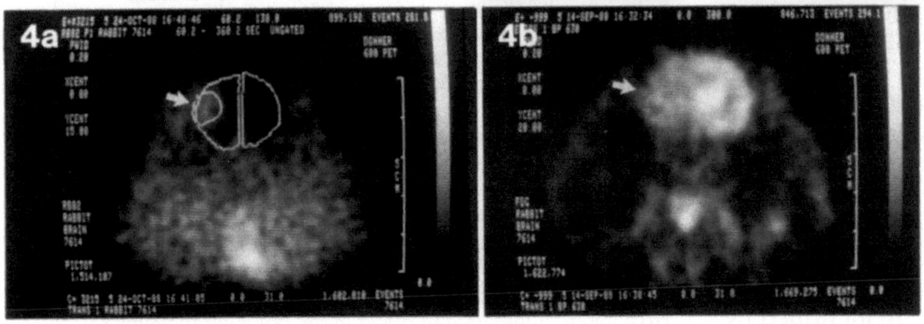

Fig. 1. Coronal Gd-DTPA-enhanced T1-weighted MR image of rabbit brain at 2.5 months after left hemibrain irradiation (60 Gy 225 keV X-rays) shows blood-brain barrier (BBB) breakdown, indicated by enhancement (high signal, *arrow*), in the corona radiata, hippocampus, fimbria and inner margins of cortical gray matter

Fig. 2. Radiation induced alterations in the left/right (irradiated/unirradiated) regional cerebral blood flow (rCBF) ratios at 2.5 months after treatment (60 Gy 225 keV X-rays). Statistically signficant ($P < 0.05$) reductions were seen in the frontal *(FR)*, parietal *(PA)*, thalamic *(TH)* and occipital *(OC)* regions but not in the temporal lobe *(TE)*

Fig. 3. a Coronal T2-weighted MR image of rabbit brain at 9 months following left hemibrain irradiation (30 Gy 230 MeV/u helium ions) shows extensive abnormal high signal in the irradiated hemisphere, primarily in corona radiata white matter, internal capsule, fimbria and thalamic regions. **b** The T1-weighted MR image shows abnormal low signal in a smaller area of the central irradiated volume, most pronounced in the lateral thalamus *(arrow)*. **c, d** Gd-DTPA T1-weighted MR images show enhancement, indicating BBB breakdown, in the perithalamic white matter and lateral thalamus (with delayed "fill-in" after 28 min, *arrow* in **d**) corresponding to the most prominent signal abnormalities on T2-and T1-weighted images and to cystic necrosis on histopathology

Fig. 4. a Coronal [82]Rb PET scan of the animal in Fig. 3 shows accumulation of tracer *(arrow)*, indicating BBB breakdown, which corresponds to Gd-DTPA enhancement on T1-weighted MRI. **b** The coronal [18]FDG PET scan shows extensive reduction in glucose utilization throughout the irradiated hemiphere *(arrow)* including cortex, basal ganglia and thalamus

lamus and striatum and 90–110 ml/100 g per minute in cerebellar hemispheres. Left/right rCBF ratios in controls were 0.9–1.1 in all structures (Fig. 2) and no significant differences were seen at 1 month post-irradiation. At 2.5 months, there were significant absolute decreases in rCBF in the irradiated hemisphere and in regional left/right ratios, compared to controls (Fig. 2). Changes were most prominent in cortical regions and thalamus with lesser changes in the hippocampus and no differences in the cerebellum.

The 15 Gy helium-irradiated cases showed no alterations on imaging studies out to 15 months post-irradiation. The 30 Gy helium cases showed alterations beginning at 9–11 months post-irradiation. None of the helium-irradiated rabbits developed neurologic deficits or feeding disorders. T2-weighted MR images showed abnormal high signal in the irradiated hemisphere, primarily in the white matter of the corona radiata, internal capusule, fimbria and thalamic regions (Fig. 3). T1-weighted images showed corresponding low signal changes over a smaller area in the central portion of the irradiated volume. Gd-DTPA T1-weighted images showed enhancement in the perithalamic white matter and lateral thalamus (with delayed "fill-in") corresponding to the signal abnormalities on T2- and T1-weighted images (Fig. 3).

The irradiated hemisphere also showed reduced glucose utilization throughout the cortical regions and deep nuclei, measured by [18]FDG PET (Fig. 4). Breakdown of the BBB, identified by [82]Rb PET, corresponded closely to the regions of Gd-DTPA enhancement on T1-weighted MR images (Fig. 4).

Histopathology in the 30 Gy helium animals showed demyelination and edema in the outer white matter tracts of the corona radiata without necrosis or signficant neuronal loss in cortical gray matter of the irradiated hemisphere. The white matter changes corresponded to regions of abnormal high signal on T2-weighted MR images and lay outside the areas of T1-weighted GdDTPA enhancement and [82]Rb PET activity. The deep white matter and peripheral thalamic areas showed cystic necrosis and vacuolation with widespread loss of neuronal and normal glial elements, chaotic proliferation of reactive astrocytes and lipid-laden microglia, and dilated blood vessels. These changes corresponded closely to high signal abnormalities on T2-weighted MRI and areas of BBB breakdown indicated by T1-weighted Gd-DTPA enhancement and tracer accumulation on [82]Rb PET.

Discussion

The rabbit brain appears to be a useful model for investigating the complex changes of delayed radiation injury with multiple imaging modalities and laboratory methods. A close correspondence was seen between abnormal high signal on T2-weighted images and histologic signs of tissue edema. The additional presence of BBB breakdown, indicated by T1-weighted MRI Gd-DTPA enhancement or [82]Rb PET, corresponded to more severe cystic necrosis. Metabolic suppression on [18]FDG PET and reduced microsphere rCBF also occurred in these regions but, as measures of more subtle tissue injury, were also seen in normal regions on MRI, [82]Rb PET and histology. The "early delayed" changes seen in the 60 Gy X-irradiated animals (reduced rCBF, tissue edema and BBB breakdown) suggest that cerebrovascular injury was an important component of the CNS radiation damage. The "late delayed" changes in the 30 Gy helium-irradiated animals occurred approximately 6–8 months after the X-ray-treated animals and also appeared to involve cerebrovascular injury. The deep regions of frank necrosis with dilated blood vessels, corresponding to high tissue water content (indicated by high signal on T2-weighted MRI) and BBB breakdown (indicated by Gd-DTPA and [82]Rb accumulation) suggest that vascular endothelial injury may be the primary mechanism of tissue injury. The data presented here support the hypothesis that cerebrovascular injury may be a "final common pathway" for CNS delayed radiation injury with radiation sources of widely different dose and relative biological effectiveness. However, primary tissue injury, especially to the oligodendroglial cell population, cannot be excluded as an alternate or co-mechanism for brain injury [5]. Metabolic suppression may be explained either by vascular injury causing reduced delivery of subtrates or direct cellular metabolic injury and deafferentation producing reduced metabolic demand [6]. Further work is needed to more precisely identify the specific mechanism.

References

1. Marks MP, DeLaPaz RL, Fabrikant JI, Frankel KA, Phillips MH, Levy RP, Enzmann DR (1988) Intracranial vascular malformations: imaging of charged particle radiosurgery, part 2. Complications. Radiology 168: 457–462
2. Di Chiro G, DeLaPaz RL, Brooks RA (1982) Glucose utilization of cerebral gliomas measured by (18F)-fluorodeoxyglucose and positron Emission tomography. Neurology 32: 1323–1329
3. Yen CK, Budinger TF (1981) Evaluation of blood-brain barrier permeability changes in rhesus monkey and man using 82Rb positron emission tomography. J Comput Assist Tomogr 5: 792–799
4. Heymann MA, Payne BD, Hoffman JI, Rudolph AM (1977) Blood flow measurements with radionuclide labelled particles. Prog Cardiovasc Dis 20: 55–79
5. Van der Kogel AJ (1986) Radiation-induced damage in the central nervous system: an interpretation of target cell responses. Br J Cancer 53 [Suppl 7]: 207–217
6. DeLaPaz RL, Patronas NJ, Brooks RA (1983) Positron emission tomographic study of suppression of gray-matter glucose utilization by brain tumors. Am J Neuroradiol 4: 826–829

Dr. Robert DeLaPaz
Neuroradiology Department of Radiology
Room S072
Stanford University Medical Center
Stanford, CA 94305, USA

Neuroradiology (1991) 33 [Suppl]: 612–613

Neuro radiology
© Springer-Verlag 1991

Subacute sclerosing panencephalitis: CT findings in acute and chronic cases

T. Kryst-Widźgowska[1], W. Sobczyk[2], J. Kulczycki[2], and P. Kozłowski[1]

[1] Department of Neuroradiology and [2] Clinic for Neurology Diseases, Institute of Psychiatry and Neurology, Warsaw, Poland

Summary. The accuracy of CT in the follow-up of subacute sclerosing panencephalitis (SSPE) was assessed in 31 patients aged 8–26 years. SSPE was diagnosed by the clinical symptoms, raised measles antibody titres in serum and EEG abnormalities. Patients were grouped into clinical stages according to Jabbour's classification. The CT examinations were carried out from 2 months to 6 years from the onset of the disease. Most significant findings on CT were hypodense areas in posterior parietal regions, generalised atrophy of the cerebral cortex and dilatation of the lateral and third ventricles.

Key words: Subacute sclerosing panencephalitis – White matter disease – Slow virus infection

Subacute sclerosing panencephalitis (SSPE) represents a slow virus disease related to the paramyxovirus group, with immunological, morphological and clinical features. SSPE is known to have worldwide distribution at a frequency of 0.5–1 million inhabitants per year and is a late complication of measles occurring 6–8 years after infection, affecting children between age of 7 and 9 and leading to progressive impairment of brain functions and to death.

Jabbour et al. [1] made the following clinical classification. In stage I patients have intellectual decline and behavioural changes. In stage II there is progressive intellectual deterioration, myoclonic seizures, ataxia and choreiform movements; some patients have ocular signs, e. g. cortical blindness, chorioretinitis and maculitis. In stage III, patients display less myoclonic movement, but diffuse rigidity. Stage IV includes coma, brain stem deficit and cachexia.

Clinical course was classified as follows: acute, death before 3 months; subacute, duration of 1–3 years; chronic, 4–8 years. On the basis of their observations and the treatment given in 125 cases, Sobczyk and Kulczycki [2] proposed classification of the clinical course as follows: acute, if the child reaches the third stage within 6 months from onset; subacute, when the patient reaches the third stage between 6 and 24 months of onset; chronic, if stage II is established during 2 years of observation. Clinical course is usually subacute. The disease is diagnosed by elevated titres of measles antibody in both the serum and cerebrospinal fluid (CSF) and by EEG with characteristic synchronous periodic high-voltage complexes. Diagnosis is founded on clinical, biochemical and EEG findings.

Patients and methods

Thirty-one patients aged 8–26 years were observed; there were 20 boys and 11 girls. Diagnosis was based on the history of measles, characteristic clinical symptoms, raised measles antibody titres in CSF and serum, Radermecker periodic complexes in EEG and CT. CT was performed in all patients, and we recorded white matter density, cortical atrophy and enlargement of the lateral ventricles by the Evans coefficient. CT was carried out between 2 months and 81 months from the onset, without contrast enhancement and without anaesthesia because there was sometimes only time for one slice.

Results

Eighteen children in stage II and I/II had the most dynamic changes on CT, because in this group hypodensity in the white matter, dilatation of the lateral ventricles and cortical atrophy are dominant (Fig. 1 a, b). Pathological scans were found in nearly all patients in this stage. In stage II/III and III less pathological CT scans were found. Dilatation of the lateral ventricles was detected in more than half of the group, but we found hypodensity in the white matter less frequently (Fig. 2 a, b). In the acute course of disease CT showed an abnormality in only one case. In the children with a subacute course of SSPE lateral ventricular dilatation was dominant. The chronic course in SSPE patients coincided with lateral ventricular dilatation and cortical atrophy in all cases (Fig. 3 a). In all cases of the chronic course group the Evans coefficient was more than 0.30, and dilatation of the lateral ventricles was marked (Fig. 3 b).

Discussion

The cerebral cortex and white matter of both hemispheres and brain stem are involved in SSPE. The cerebellum is usually spared. CT studies of SSPE patients have been published by a few authors, but in no study were enough patients investigated for the correlation of stage and course of the SSPE to be statistically significant [3, 4]. Radelicka et al. [5] analysed material comprising 26 CT studies in 8 cases and found cerebral oedema in stage II.

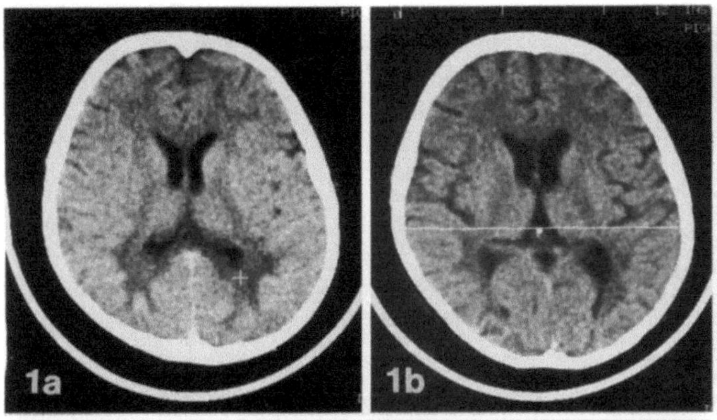

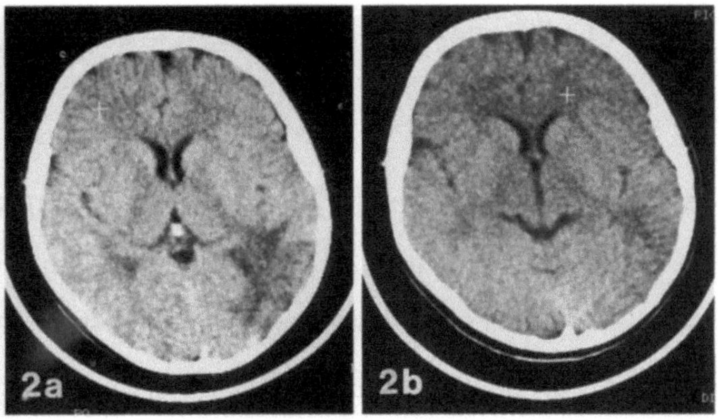

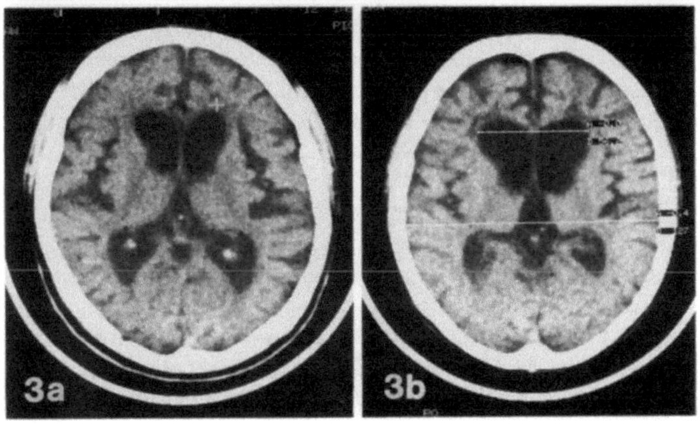

Fig. 1 a, b. Low-density areas are seen in the periventricular white matter of both hemispheres. Second examination after 6 months revealed slight but evident dilatation of the lateral ventricles and mild cortical atrophy. Clinical stage II, subacute clinical course

Fig. 2 a, b. Older sister of case presented in Fig. 1 a and b. Diffuse hypodensity areas in the periventricular localization and in the cortex of the parietal lobe in the left hemisphere. Second CT after 6 months revealed less prominent abnormalities. Clinical stage II/III. Subacute clinical course

Fig. 3 a. Patient 26 years old: 7 years observation and treatment. Dilated lateral ventricles and advanced cortical atrophy. Clinical stage II. Chronic clinical course

Fig. 3 b. Subacute sclerosing panencephalitis in a 15-year-old girl: 4 years observation. Advanced cortical atrophy and marked enlargement of the lateral and third ventricles. Clinical stage II/III. Chronic clinical course

In the series of Defianti et al. [6], CT was carried out in 14 patients (a total of 25 studies). They found mostly normal results in stages I and II, areas of white matter hypodensity, dilatation of the ventricles and cortical atrophy becoming more evident in stage III. Achram and Haddad [7] presented scans of 22 patients, some with Urografin i. v. enhancement but no significant change was observed after enhancement. They pointed out that CT findings are dependent on duration of disease and progressed over time. They did not find any abnormalities in stage I. Taly et al. [8] performed CT in 32 patients and besides typical changes found less well-known features: brain-stem atrophy without cerebral atrophy, focal areas of white matter hypodensity, and areas of hyperdensity.

CT appears to be a sensitive method to disclose advanced pathological changes in the periventricular white matter. In our series low-density changes in the white matter were recorded mostly during stage II, in all patients with a chronic course of SSPE with more than 24 months of observation. In conclusion, it seems to be a point for discussion and further observation whether dilatation of the lateral ventricles is secondary to white matter pathology and is significant in advanced cases, probably due to shrinkage of the periventricular white matter. Perivascular changes observed in morphological studies, e. g. perivascular cuffing of inflammatory cells may account for CT changes in advanced disease. A question for discussion is whether on neuropathological examination neurons may exhibit Alzheimer neurofibrillary degeneration and/or neuronal degeneration of the Symchowitz type, which is very rare and usually found only in aged patients [9].

References

1. Jabbour JT, Garcia JH, Lemmi H, Dagland J, Dulans PA, Sever JL (1969) Subacute sclerosing panencephalitis: a multidisciplinary study of eight cases. JAMA 207: 2248–2254
2. Sobczyk W, Kulczycki J (1981) Remarks on the antiviral treatment in the SSPE. Neurol Neurochir Pol 2: 143
3. Kingsley DP, Kendall BE (1981) Demyelinating and neurodegenerative disease in childhood. J Neuroradiol 8: 243–255
4. Pedersen H, Wulff CH (1982) Computed tomographic findings of early subacute sclerosing panencephalitis. Neuroradiology 23: 31–32
5. Radelicka H, Karkowska B, Michałowicz R (1984) Computed tomography in subacute sclerosing panencephalitis. Pol Przegl Radiol 48: 61–64
6. Defanti CA, Franza A, D'Angelo A, Breschi F (1986) SSPE: clinical, EEG and neuroradiological findings in a series of 69 cases. In: Subacute sclerosing panencephalitis. A reappraisal. Excerpta Medica, Amsterdam, pp 121–131
7. Achram M, Haddad FS (1986) CT scan abnormalities in subacute sclerosing panencephalitis. In: Subacute sclerosing panencephalitis. A reappraisal. Excerpta Medica, Amsterdam, pp 159–168
8. Taly AB, Arunodaya GR, Jayakumar PN, Nagaraja D, Araya BYT, Ravi V, Shetty KT, Shankar SK (1989) Computed tomography in SSPE. Third International Symposium on Subacute Sclerosing Panencephalitis. Vellore, India
9. Kulczycki J (1986) Subacute sclerosing panencephalitis. Discussion. In: Subacute sclerosing panencephalitis. A reappraisal. Excerpta Medica, Amsterdam, p 131

Dr. Teresa Kryst
Tomografia Komputerowa
Instytut Psychiatrii I Neurologii
Al. Sobieskiego 1/9
02-957 Warsaw, Poland

Neuroradiology (1991) 33 [Suppl]: 614–615

Neuroradiology
© Springer-Verlag 1991

Wilson's disease: CT and ultrasound

T. Kryst-Widźgowska[1], P. Kozłowski[1], M. Szleper[2], and A. Członkowska[2]

[1] Department of Neuroradiology and [2] Clinic for Neurovascular Diseases, Psychiatry and Neurology Institute, Warsaw, Poland

Summary. Seventy-one patients aged from 16 to 70 years with a diagnosis based on clinical and biochemical findings underwent CT of the head and abdomen and ultrasonography of the abdomen. Most frequently, cerebral and cerebellar cortical atrophy was noted; more rarely hypodensity in the basal ganglia was found. CT disclosed splenomegaly and a low density liver in 60% of the patients, cirrhosis of the liver in 12%. Ultrasonography showed parenchymal nodularity of the liver and enlargement of the spleen.

Key words: Hepatolenticular degeneration – Wilson's disease

Wilson's disease – hepatolenticular degeneration – results from abnormal deposits of copper in the liver and in the brain because of abnormal synthesis of ceruloplasmin; its inheritance is consistent with an autosomal recessive trait. Clinical manifestations are extrapyramidal and cerebellar signs; the Kayser-Fleischer corneal ring is pathognomonic. A decreased level of ceruloplasmin in the serum, instability of copper in the blood and high levels in the urine are characteristic laboratory findings of impaired copper metabolism. Clinical symptoms and signs develop in the second decade of life. We present the characteristic features of brain damage with special attention to the posterior fossa.

Patients and methods

Seventy-one patients with an established diagnosis of Wilson's disease, including the presymptomatic stage, were studied. There were 41 males and 30 females aged between 16 and 70 years. CT of the head and abdomen was carried out between 1 week and 36 years of observation. All patients had CT of the head without contrast enhancement. Brain CT abnormalities were recorded as follows: cortical atrophy, lateral ventricular enlargement, hypodensity in the basal ganglia, brain stem atrophy and atrophy of the cerebellar folia. In CT of the abdomen, the attenuation coefficients, size, shape of the liver and spleen were studied. Echogenicity of the liver was assessed in ultrasound examinations. The patients were divided into two groups according to duration of treatment and the time from diagnosis.

Results

The patients were divided into two groups: 20 patients observed and treated for less than 2 years, and 51 patients with follow-up ranging from 2 to 36 years. In both groups, on brain CT lateral ventricular enlargement and cortical diffuse atrophy dominated. Atrophy of the cerebellar folia was predominant in the second group and reached 41% (Fig. 1). Overall, reduced density of the basal ganglia and brain stem atrophy were found in 20–25% (Fig. 2a, b). Normal brain CT was found in 17.5%.

CT of the abdomen revealed diffuse reduction in density of the liver to + 18 to + 45 HU, with irregular areas of lower density in 50% of the patients. Cirrhotic shrunken livers, with irregular borders and humped surface and 60 to 70 HU attenuation coefficient were found in 12% patients (Fig. 3). In 1 case CT revealed advanced cirrhosis with ascites. A spleen larger than 110 mm was found in 50–54% of the patients. The attenuation coefficients of the spleen varied from 45 to 55 HU. In ultrasound examinations of the abdomen granulomatous parenchyma was found in 30% of the patients (Fig. 4): Enlargement of the spleen respectively in 54% and 50% as in the CT. No abnormalities in CT of the abdomen were found in 40% of the patients overall.

Discussion

Hepatolenticular degeneration has borne the name Wilson's disease since the original publication concerning its aetiology and pathology [1]. In that article the author stressed early lesions of the basal ganglia; he believed that liver involvement was less important. A direct relationship between excess copper deposits in the brain and liver was proved by Cumings in 1948 [2] and led to the development of appropriate therapy. The excess copper in the liver, central nervous system, eyes, kidneys and other organs leads to symptoms after 6 years of age; 50% of homozygotes have symptoms by 15 years of age [3]. Symptoms vary, as a result of liver and basal ganglia involvement.

CT has revealed structural changes in the brain and in the liver [4]. In the study of Williams and Walshe [5], CT appearances of the brain, and correlation with clinical findings and response to treatment were discussed. The authors stressed early symptoms related to the liver and spleen; ventricular dilatation occurred in 73%, cortical atrophy in 63%, basal ganglia hypodensity in 45% and posterior fossa atrophy in 10%. In our 71 patients CT of the brain revealed basal ganglia hypodensity less frequently: in 20%–23%. However, compared to that series,

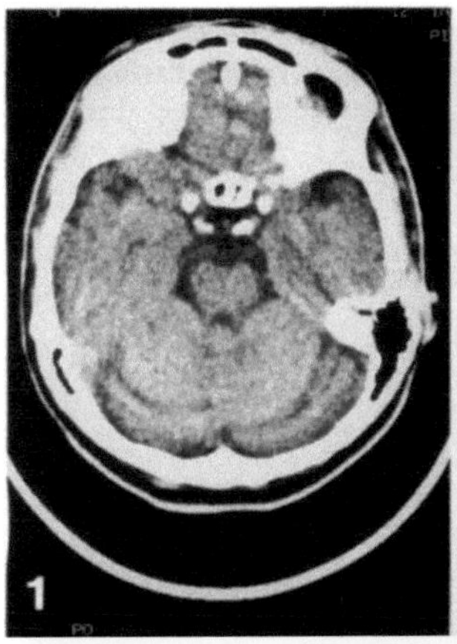

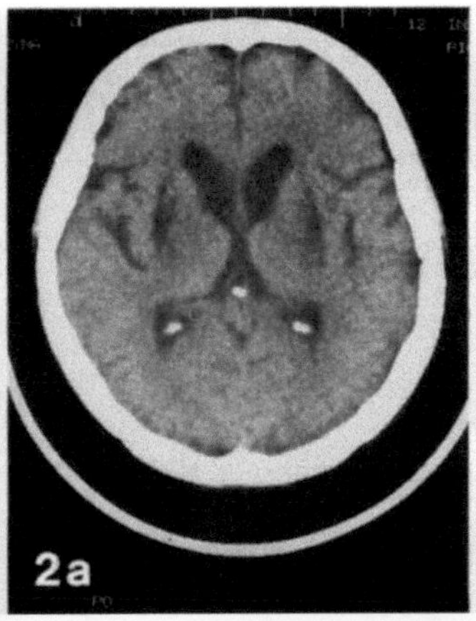

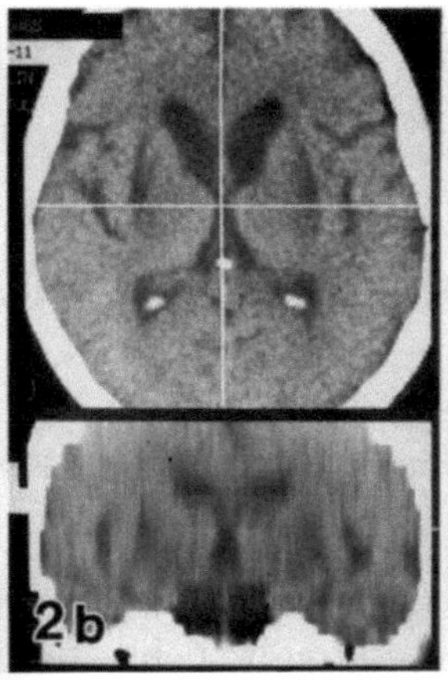

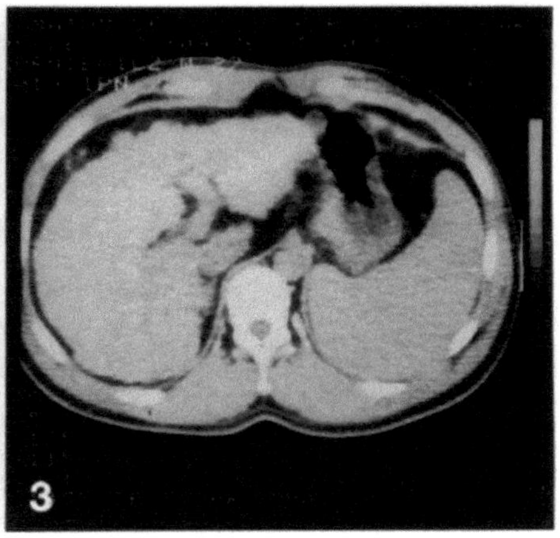

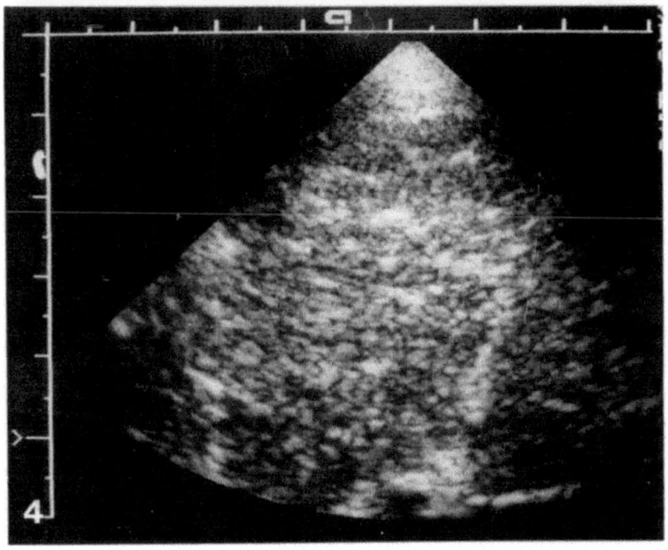

Fig. 1. Female 28 years old, presenting cerebellar symptoms. There is cerebellar and brain-stem atrophy. Five years observation and treatment

Fig. 2 a, b. There is bilateral hypodensity in the basal ganglia; as well as cortical atrophy and lateral ventricular dilatation. Female 32 years old with extrapyramidal and cerebellar signs. Two years observation

Fig. 3. A 27-year-old male with extrapyramidal symptoms. CT of the abdomen: there is a cirrhotic liver with irregular outline and splenomegaly

Fig. 4. Ultrasound of the liver. There is hyperechogenicity of nodular parenchyma. Liver CT of this patients is presented in Fig. 3

more patients in our material in the group with long duration had cerebellar folia atrophy (41%).

In the abdomen, structural changes in the liver were studied objectively with regard to density measurement and splenomegaly. The most consistent defect appears to be a varying degree low density, cirrhosis and splenomegaly. Ultrasound is more useful in demonstrating nodular liver regeneration. It would appear reasonable to monitor the patients by ultrasound and CT of the abdomen.

References

1. Wilson SA Kinnier (1912) Progressive lenticular degeneration. A familial nervous disease associated with cirrhosis of the liver. Brain 34: 295–309
2. Cumings JN (1948) The copper and iron content of brain and liver in the normal and in hepatolenticular degeneration. Brain 71: 410–415
3. Edmondson HA, Peters RL (1985) Liver, chapter 27. In: Anderson's pathology. Mosby, St. Louis, pp 1164–1166
4. Nelson RF, Guzman DA, Grahovac Z, Howse DCN (1979) Computerized cranial tomography in Wilson disease. Neurology 29: 866–868
5. Williams FJB, Walshe JM (1981) Wilson's disease. An analysis of the cranial computerized tomographic appearances found in 60 patients and the changes in response to treatment with chelating agents. Brain 104: 735–752

Dr. Teresa Kryst
Psychiatry and Neurology Institute
Tomografia Komputerowa
Al. Sobieskiego 1/9
02-957 Warsaw, Poland

Neuroradiology (1991) 33 [Suppl]: 616–617

Neuro-radiology
© Springer-Verlag 1991

Head injuries: 3 years' experience with ultralow field MRI

A. Janousek

Department of Traumatology, Lorenz Böhler Trauma Centre, Vienna, Austria

Summary. Patients with head injuries were investigated in the Lorenz Böhler Trauma Centre with ultralow field MRI. Acute extra- and intracerebral haematomas were identified and differentiated as well as brain contusions. This paper describes the typical signal intensities of intracerebral contusion and haematomas on T1- and T2-weighted images.

Key words: Cerebral trauma – Acute intracranial haematoma – Cerebral contusion

Almost all authors prefer CT to MRI for noninvasive diagnosis of acute intracranial haematoma (AIH) and cerebral contusion. Bradley and Schmidt [1] noted shortening of T1 and T2 in AIH. Gomori and Grossman [2] believe that a so-called hyperacute haematoma will be hypointense on T1-weighted images (T1-WI) and hyperintense on T2-weighted images (T2-WI). Our group was able to show that it is possible to detect early haematomas with ultralow field MRI (ULF-MRI) [3] and that it is a valuable tool in the diagnosis of acute craniocerebral trauma. Sipponen et al. [4] showed that acute haematoma is better seen on ULF-MR and that diagnostic difficulties increase with field strength.

Fig. 1. T2-weighted image (T2-WI) demonstrates hyperintensive contusion 3 days post-trauma

Fig. 2. T1-WI shows hypointensive contusion 3 days post-trauma

Fig. 3. After gadolinium(Gd)-DTPA the T1-WI demonstrates slight contrast enhancement

Fig. 4. The precontrast T1-WI 11 days later still shows low signal of the contusion

Fig. 5. The post Gd-DTPA scan demonstrates significant increase of the signal

Fig. 6. T2-WI shows a haematoma iso- and a little hypointense 3 days post-trauma

Fig. 7. Significant hyperintensity of the acute haematoma on the T1-WI

Fig. 8. At 0.5 T field-strength the T1-WI shows an almost isointense haematoma on the same day

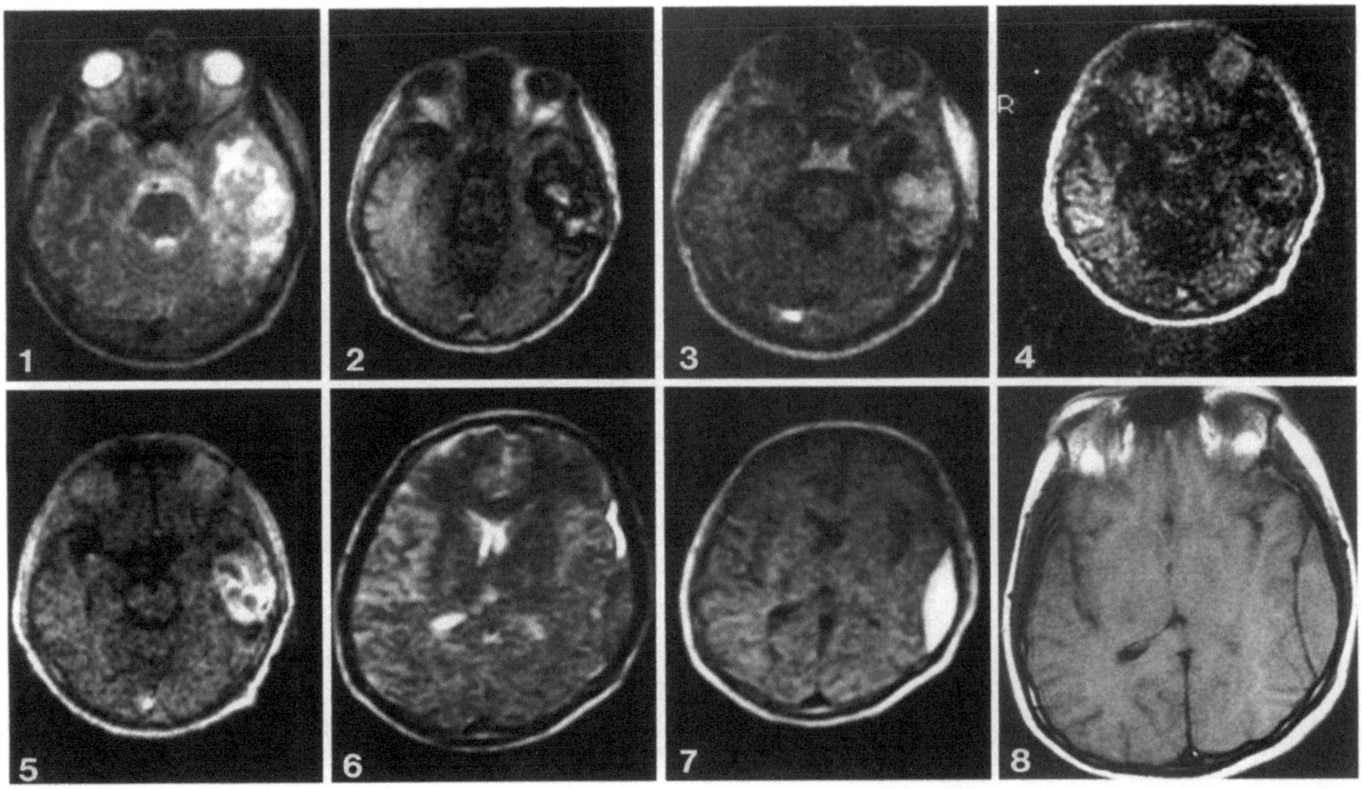

Materials and methods

In the Lorenz Böhler Trauma Centre we have been using ULF-MRI (Acutscan, Instrumentarium) since June 1987. The system has a field strength of 0.02 T. More than 600 examinations have been performed in patients with head injuries. A close-coupled head coil was used on all patients. Those who were under intensive care were intubated and ventilated during the examination. The time range of the examination was from about 90 min up to 3 years post-trauma. The standard study included a sagittal scout view and axial T2-WI with spin echo 2000/150 and T1-WI with inversion recovery 1000 (250)/40. When necessary, additional coronal images were obtained. Gadolinium(Gd)-DTPA enhanced images were obtained in some patients with brain contusion. The routine unenhanced investigation took about 25 min and included T1- and T2-WI.

Results

Contusion

Most brain contusions show only a slight change of signal in the first post-trauma image. Signal contrast may increase in the first 3 days. Contusions show increased signal intensity on T2-WI and are hypointense on T1-WI. After Gd-DTPA there was only slight contrast enhancement on T1-WI (Figs. 1–3). Contusions still show low signal 2 weeks post-trauma, but at this stage there is enhancement after Gd-DTPA (Figs. 4, 5).

Haematoma

About 2 h post-trauma haematomas are significantly hyperintense on T1-WI and almost isointense on T2-WI. This also applies 3 days post-trauma, at which time T1-WI from 0.5 T MRI show no significant increase in signal intensity (Figs. 6–8).

Discussion

We agree with other authors that imaging of (hyper)acute haematomas is difficult with high, mid and low field MRI. Our good results show that ULF-MRI is an excellent non-invasive tool for assessment of head injury. "Hyperacute" haematomas can be clearly identified by their characteristic high signal on T1-WI. It has been demonstrated that 0.5 T MRI shows no significant increase in signal intensity on T1-WI in similar cases. Brain contusion can be clearly identified and shows low signal on T1-WI. In the first 3 days there is only slight enhancement after Gd-DTPA; enhancement is at a maximum 2–3 weeks post-trauma. We interpret this as a defect in the blood-brain barrier.

Acknowledgement. I would like to thank to Dr. Andreas Neuhold from the Radiological Department of the Hospital Rudolfinerhaus, Vienna for the 0.5 T MR image.

References

1. Bradley WG, Schmidt PG (1985) Effect of methemoglobin formation on the MR appearance of subarachnoidal hemorrhage. Radiology 156: 99–103
2. Gomori JM, Grossman RI (1987) Head and neck hemorrhage. Magnetic Resonance Annual, pp 71–112
3. Janousek A, Leixnering M, Schreinlechner UP, Poigenfürst J (1988) Akute intracranielle Blutung: Frühzeitige Darstellung durch Magnetresonanz. Fortschr Röntgenstr 148: 589–590
4. Sipponen JT, Sepponen RE, Tanttu JI, Sivula A (1985) Intracranial haematomas studied by MR imaging at 0.17 and 0.02 T. J Comput Assist Tomogr 9: 698–704

Dr. A. Janousek
Lorenz Böhler Trauma Centre
Donaueschingenstrasse 13
A-1200 Vienna, Austria

Neuroradiology (1991) 33 [Suppl]: 618–620

Neuroradiology
© Springer-Verlag 1991

MRI in cerebral palsy: correlation between clinical and MR findings

M. H. Lipper[1], D. P. Chason[1], W. S. Cail[1], R. D. Ferguson[1], T. S. Park[2], and L. H. Phillips[3]

Departments of [1] Radiology, [2] Neurosurgery and
[3] Neurology, University of Virginia Health Sciences Center, Charlottesville, Virginia, USA

Summary. Fifty-one patients with spastic cerebral palsy referred for selective dorsal rhizotomy were studied by MRI to determine the degree of cerebral damage and predict surgical outcome. A close relationship was established between cerebral lesions such as periventricular leukomalacia, corpus callosum degeneration, porencephaly, atrophy and cortical infarction, and clinical severity of spasticity.

Key words: Spastic cerebral palsy – Periventricular leukomalacia – Corpus callosum degeneration – Magnetic resonance imaging

In devising an effective treatment for patients with spastic cerebral palsy such as selective dorsal rhizotomy, it is important that the degree, location and extent of cerebral damage as a result of perinatal anoxia be accurately determined in order to decide on suitability for this treatment and to predict outcome. MRI has proved to be the most accurate method to date for evaluating the lesions resulting from such cerebral damage.

Materials and methods

A standardized MR protocol consisting of T1-weighted sagittal and coronal and T2-weighted axial or coronal sequences was used to study 51 patients with spastic cerebral palsy referred for surgical treatment by selective dorsal rhizotomy to reduce spasm. The age range was between 2 and 13 years and there were 33 males and 18 females in the study. Thirty-four suffered from spastic diplegia, 8 had spastic triplegia and 9 spastic quadriplegia. MR findings such as periventricular leukomalacia (PVLM), degeneration of the corpus callosum (CCD), porencephaly, atrophy and cortical infarction were noted, and graded as mild, moderate or severe. These findings were compared with the severity of spasticity and gait disturbance which were classified as minimal, mild, moderate or severe.

Results

PVLM was present in 47 patients (92%) and appeared as: (1) white matter volume loss in the periventricular region and centrum semiovale seen as ventricular dilatation and white matter thinning; (2) cavitated infarcts in the immediate periventricular white matter – well defined regions of low signal intensity on T1-weighted images; (3) confluent areas of increased signal intensity on T2-weighted sequences in the periventricular white matter extending outwards to the gray-white matter junction, due to gliosis and demyelination.

Wallerian CCD, marked thinning or complete absence of segments of the corpus callosum, was detected in 43 (84%). These findings were further analyzed according to the degree of clinical severity in Tables 1 and 2. In addition, 10 Patients (20%) showed focal thinning of the gray matter with adjacent enlargement of the subarachnoid

Table 1. Incidence of periventricular leukomalacia (PVLM) in spastic cerebral palsy

			MR findings (%)			
Clinical severity			Normal	Mild PVLM	Moderate PVLM	Severe PVLM
Minimal	11/51	(21.5%)	37	45	9	9
Mild	22/51	(43%)	0	60	36	4
Moderate	7/51	(14%)	0	14	57	29
Severe	11/51	(21.5%)	0	0	45	55

Table 2. Incidence of corpus callosum degeneration (CCD) in spastic cerebral palsy

			MR findings (%)			
Clinical severity			Normal	Mild CCD	Moderate CCD	Severe CCD
Minimal	11/51	(21.5%)	73	18	0	9
Mild	22/51	(43%)	0	82	14	4
Moderate	7/51	(14%)	0	42	29	29
Severe	11/51	(21.5%)	0	9	9	82

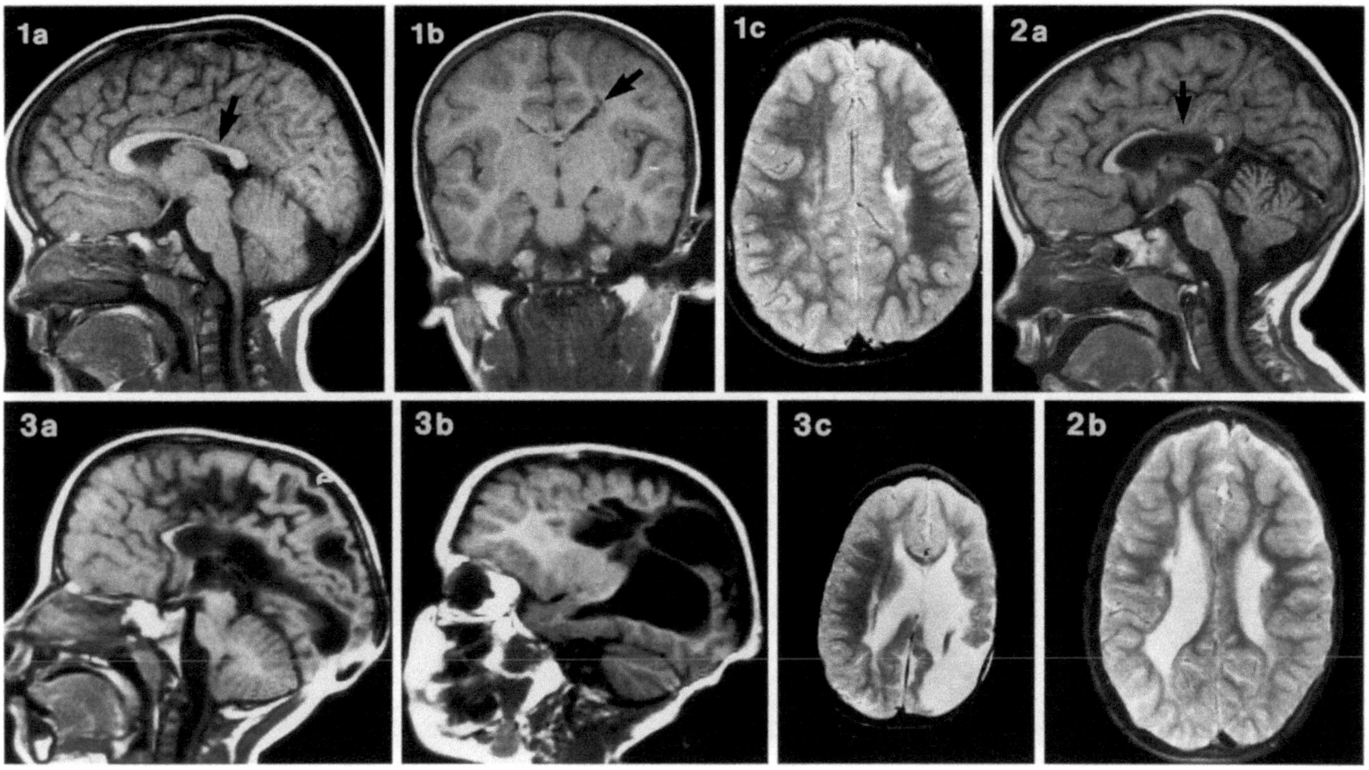

Fig. 1 a–c. Four-year-old male with mild spasticity. **a** Sagittal T1-weighted MR study (TR = 500 ms, TE = 17 ms), shows mild corpus callosum degeneration (CCD) *(arrow)*. **b** Coronal T1-weighted image (TR = 500 ms, TE = 17 ms), demonstrates a left periventricular cavitated infarct *(arrow)*. **c** Axial T2-weighted image (TR = 2500 ms, TE = 90 ms), shows a small left periventricular increased signal intensity consistent with periventricular leukomalacia (PVLM)

Fig. 2 a, b. Two-year-old male with moderate spasticity. **a** Sagittal T1-weighted image (TR = 500 ms, TE = 17 ms), with moderate CCD *(arrow)*. **b** T2-weighted coronal image (TR = 2500 ms, TE = 90 ms) shows severe white matter loss and PVLM

Fig. 3 a–c. Two-year-old female with severe spasticity. **a, b** Sagittal T1-weighted images (TR = 500 ms, TE = 17 ms), show severe CCD involving the entire corpus callosum, atrophy, cortical infarction and porencephaly. **c** Axial T2-weighted image (TR = 2500, TE = 90 ms) demonstrates bilateral volume loss, PVLM and left occipital cortical infarction and porencephaly

space and loss of distinction between gray and white matter consistent with cortical infarction.

Discussion

MRI is the most effective modality for the study of the extent and distribution of central nervous system lesions in cerebral palsy. PVLM and other lesions resulting from hypoxic-ischemic brain injury have been extensively described [1–6]. Because MRI accurately ascertains damage to the pyramidal system in the cerebral hemispheres, the information obtained could influence the choice of therapy [7]. As it is often difficult to clinically separate paresis from spasticity in these patients, the presence of infarction of the motor cortex suggests that paresis is present. One should, therefore, avoid surgical procedures which may weaken muscular strength. However, where spasticity predominates, selective dorsal rhizotomy may lead to considerable improvement in function.

Another interesting feature seen was the relationship between anatomical sites of cerebral lesions and Wallerian CCD. When the corpus callosum is divided into the five segments, one consisting of the genu, three separate segments in the body and one in the splenium [8], a close correlation can be made between the locations of the cerebral lesions and the distribution of Wallerian CCD, presumably due to the topographical organization of fibers coursing through the corpus callosum.

From this study it appears that a direct relationship exists between the severity of clinical findings and the incidence and severity of MRI changes in cerebral palsy, the worse the clinical status, the more severe the changes of PVLM and CCD. Furthermore, a distinct relationship was demonstrated between regions of the brain affected by PVLM and segmental Wallerian CCD. These findings as well as the presence of cortical infarction are useful in predicting the results of selective dorsal rhizotomy.

References

1. Baker L, Stevenson DK, Enzmann DR (1988) End-stage periventricular leukomalacia: MR evaluation. Radiology 168: 809–815
2. De Vries LS, Dubowitz LMS, Pennock JM, Bydder GM (1989) Extensive cystic leucomalacia: correlation of cranial ultrasound,

magnetic resonance imaging and clinical findings in sequential studies. Clin Radiol 40: 158–166
3. Flodmark O, Lupton B, Li D, Stimac GK, Roland EH, Hill A, Whitfield MF, Norman MG (1989) MR imaging of periventricular leukomalacia in childhood. AJNR 10: 111–118
4. Johnson MA, Pennock JM, Bydder GM, Dubowitz LMS, Thomas DJ, Young IR (1987) Serial MR imaging in neonatal cerebral injury. AJNR 8: 83–92
5. McArdle CB, Richardson CJ, Hayden CK, Nicholas DA, Amparo GE (1987) Abnormalities of the neonatal brain: MR imaging. II. Hypoxic-ischemic brain injury. Radiology 163: 395–403
6. Wilson DA, Steiner RE (1986) Periventricular leukomalacia: evaluation with MR imaging. Radiology 160: 507–511
7. Par : TS, Phillips LH, Torner JC (1989) Magnetic resonance imagi g in selective dorsal rhizotomy for spastic cerebral palsy. In: Neı rosurgery: state of the art reviews, vol. 4. Hanley and Belfus, Phi adelphia, pp 485–495
8. Del .acoste MC, Kirkpatrick JB, Ross ED (1985) Topography of the human corpus callosum. J. Neuropathol Exp Neurol 44: 578–591

Dr. M H. Lipper
Depa tment of Radiology, Box 170
Univ rsity of Virginia Health Sciences Center
Charl ottesville, Virginia 22908, USA

Neuroradiology (1991) 33 [Suppl]: 621–623

Neuroradiology
© Springer-Verlag 1991

Cortical blood flow reduction in capsular/putaminal aphasia syndromes shown by ^{123}I-amphetamine single-photon emission tomography

Y. Tsuda[1], M. Kitadai[1], K. Satoh[1], K. Nagatsuka[1], Y. Ayada[1], Y. Ohnishi[1], S. Kawasaki[2], and H. Matsuo[1]

[1] Second Department of Internal Medicine, and [2] Department of Radiology, Kagawa Medical School, Kagawa, Japan

Summary. Tomographic regional cerebral blood flow was measured by ^{123}I-amphetamine SPECT in three patients, who presented with motor or total aphasia showing capsular/putaminal infarctions on CT and MRI. The tomographic blood flow of the left frontoparietal cortex was decreased in all three cases and this persisted up to day 36 after onset in one case despite rapid resolution of the aphasia. An interruption of a neural connection between frontoparietal cortex and subcortical lesions, i.e. diaschisis, is regarded as a cause of cortical hypoperfusion in capsular/putaminal aphasia syndromes.

Key words: Capsular/putaminal aphasia syndromes – Cortical hypoperfusion – Diaschisis – ^{123}I-amphetamine single-photon emission tomography – Regional cerebral blood flow

The capsular/putaminal aphasia syndromes [1] are caused by lacunar infarctions in the lateral lenticulostriate artery territories of the dominant hemisphere [2]. We studied cortical blood flow (CBF) changes in patients with capsular/putaminal aphasia syndromes.

Subjects and methods

Tomographic CBF was measured by ^{123}I-amphetamine (IMP) SPECT using a single-head rotating gamma camera (GCA-90B, Toshiba, Japan) equipped with a high-resolution, low-energy collimator (FWHM = 4.5 mm), in three patients, who presented with motor aphasia and showed capsular or putaminal infarctions on CT and 1.5 T-MRI (Gyro-scan S15, Philips). The IMP SPECT images were obtained 30 min and 4 h p.i. of 111 mBq IMP. Images were reconstructed by a filtered back-projection method.

Results

A 58-year-old man (case 1, Fig. 1) presenting solely motor aphasia without hemiparesis showed a small infarct in the anterior limb of the left internal capsule on CT and MRI.

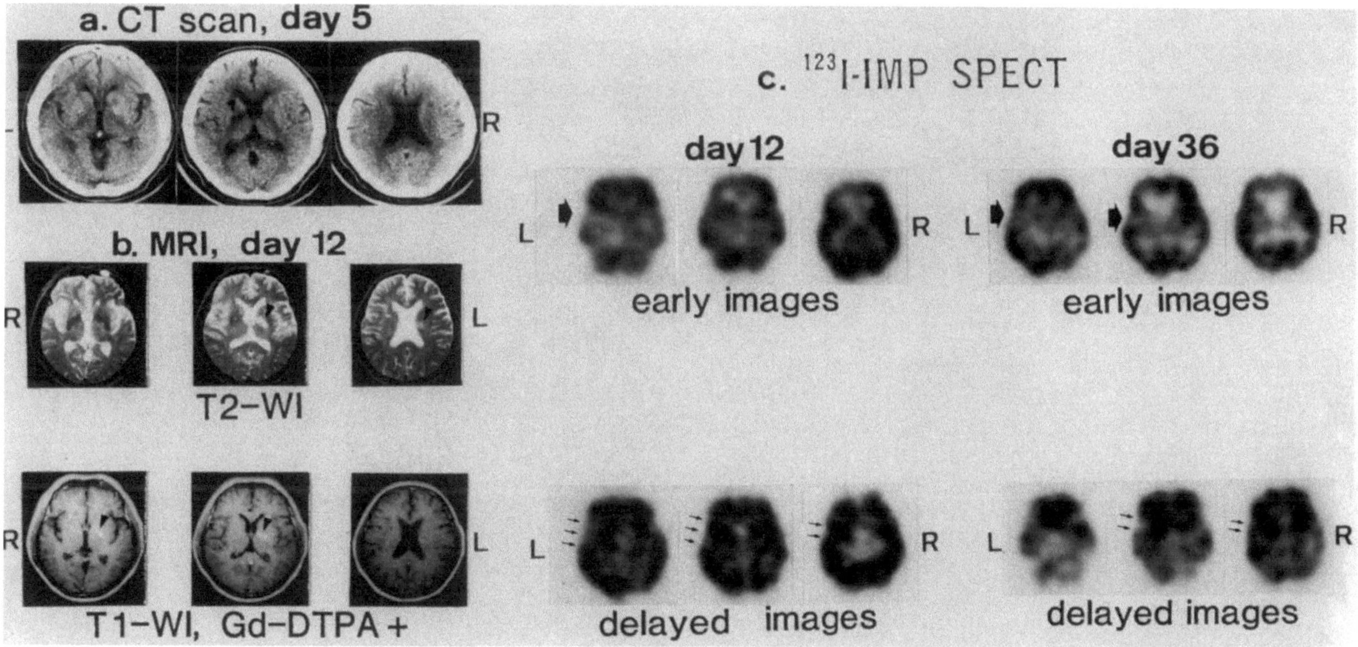

Fig. 1 a–c. A 58-year-old man (case 1) who presented with motor aphasia without hemiparesis: **a** CT; **b** MRI; **c** ^{123}I-amphetamine (IMP) SPECT

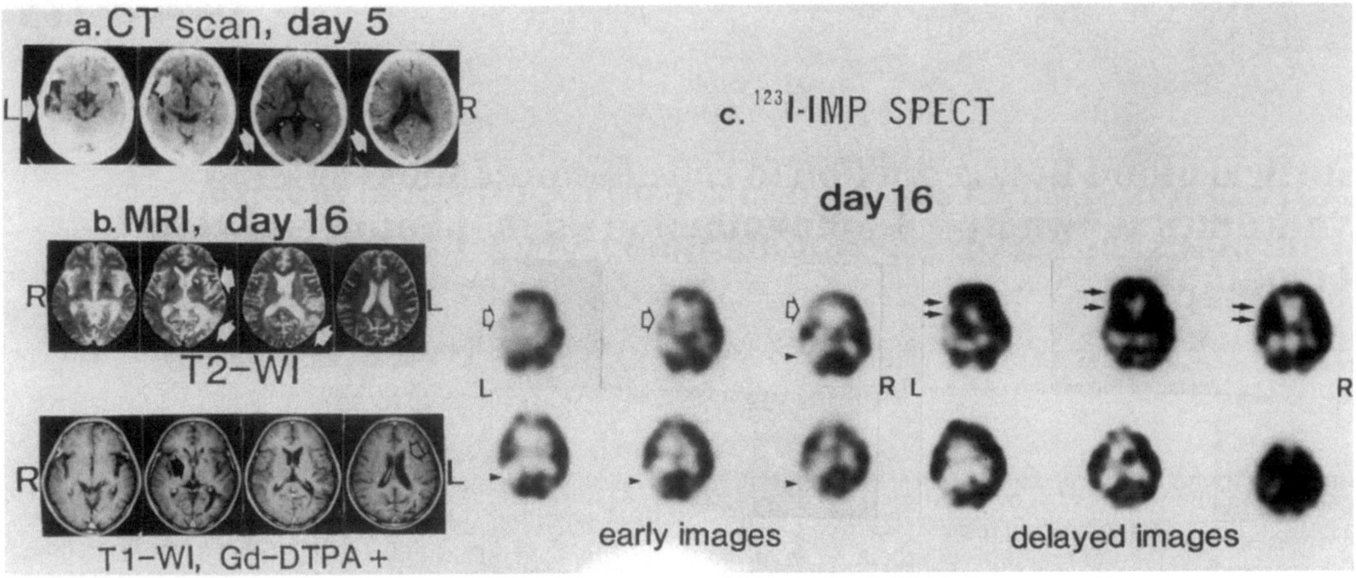

Fig. 2 a–c. A 58-year-old man (case 2) who presented with right hypesthesia and motor aphasia: **a** CT; **b** MRI; **c** ^{123}I-IMP SPECT

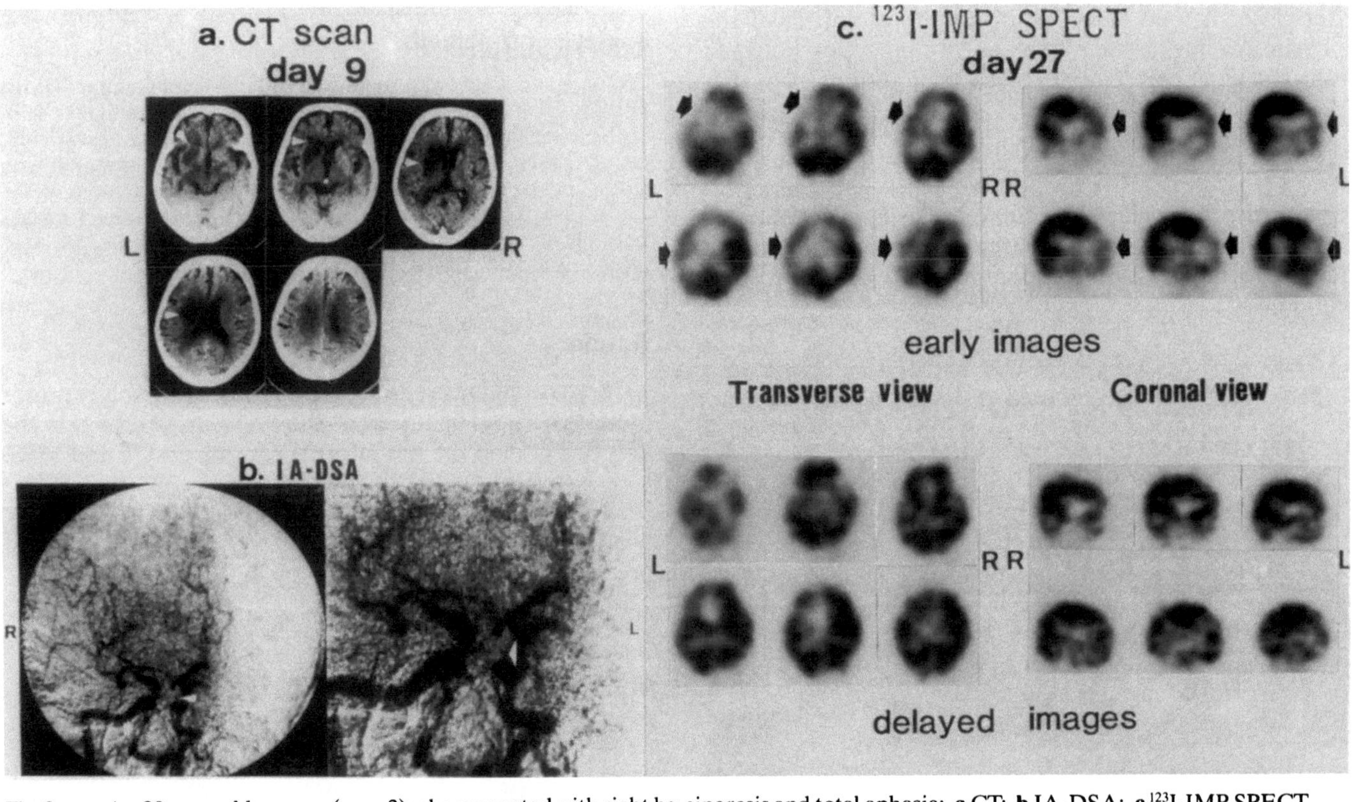

Fig. 3 a–c. An 80-year-old women (case 3) who presented with right hemiparesis and total aphasia: **a** CT; **b** IA-DSA; **c** ^{123}I-IMP SPECT

The motor aphasia of the patient disappeared within a short time of its onset. The CBF 12 days from onset was decreased in the left frontoparietal cortex and a partial redistribution phenomenon was observed in the delayed images by the IMP SPECT. The hypoperfusion and redistribution phenomenon persisted up to 36 days after onset despite an improvement of symptoms of aphasia. The other patient, a 58-year-old man (case 2, Fig. 2) presenting with right hypoaesthesia with motor aphasia showed an occlusion of the left carotid siphon with collaterals from the anterior communicating artery, while infarcts were observed in the left putamen and the watershed areas between the left middle and posterior cerebral arteries on CT and MRI. The CBF measured by IMP SPECT showed a global decrease in the areas of left frontal and parietotemporal cortex. The delayed images showed a redistribution phenomenon in the anterior parietal cortex. Another patient, an 80-year-old women, case 3, Fig. 3) presenting with a right hemiparesis with motor and sensory aphasia showed a left putaminal hypodense lesion on CT. Left carotid siphon occlusion was shown by intra-arterial digital subtraction angiography (IA-DSA). Global decreases of blood flow in the left cerebral cortex were observed in the early images, while redistribution phenomena were not observed in the delayed images of this patient.

Discussion

Aphasic patients with predominantly subcortical lesions in the internal capsule and putamen are defined as capsular/putaminal aphasia syndromes [1], which may be caused by lacunar infarction in the lateral lenticulostriate artery territories of the dominant hemisphere [2]. The lesions, seen in our three cases with aphasia are in accordance with these reports. On the other hand, striatocapsular infarction is reported with significant proximal carotid artery lesions as well as obstructive lesions at the bifurcation of the internal carotid artery [3]. Cases 2 and 3 in our study had proximal lesions of carotid siphon occlusion, which agree with the previous report [3]. Such proximal lesions might cause infarction in the lenticulostriate artery territories resulting in capsular/ putaminal aphasia syndromes. A prospective study of subcortical stroke cases showed rapid and complete improvements of aphasia symptoms within the first 6–8 weeks after onset [4], which is in accordance with our findings in cases 1 and 2. Cerebral blood flow studies in cases with subcortical aphasia showed cortical hypoperfusion evaluated with the two-dimensional ^{133}Xe intracarotid CBF [5] or with the tomographic CBF by HIPDM SPECT [6]. Such a finding of cortical hypoperfusion in capsular/putaminal aphasia syndromes is interpreted as the interruption of neural connection between the frontoparietal cortex of language processing and subcortical capsular/putaminal lesions, i. e. diaschisis [6].

References

1. Naeser MA, Alexander MP, Helm-Estabrooks N, Levine HL, Laughlin SA, Geschwind N (1982) Aphasia with predominantly subcortical lesion sites. Description of three capsular/putaminal aphasia syndromes. Arch Neurol 39: 2–14
2. Damasio AR, Damasio H, Rizzo M, Varney N, Gersh F (1982) Aphasia with nonhemorrhagic lesions in the basal ganglia and internal capsule. Arch Neurol 39: 15–20
3. Bladin PF, Berkovic SF (1984) Striatocapsular infarction: large infarcts in the lenticulostriate arterial territory. Neurology 34: 1423–1430
4. Fromm D, Holland AL, Swidell CS, Reinmuth OM (1985) Various consequences of subcortical stroke. Prospective study of 16 consecutive cases. Arch Neurol 42: 943–950
5. Skyhoj Olsen T, Bruhn P, Oeberg GE (1986) Cortical hypoperfusion as a possible cause of 'subcortical aphasia'. Brain 109: 393–410
6. Perani D, Vallar G, Cappa S, Messa C, Fazio F (1987) Aphasia and neglect after subcortical stroke. A clinical/cerebral perfusion correlation study. Brain 110: 1211–1229

Assist. Prof. Dr. Yoshiyasu Tsuda
Second Department of Internal Medicine
Kagawa Medical School
1750-1, Ikenobe, Miki-cho
Kagawa 761-07, Japan

Neuroradiology (1991) 33 [Suppl]: 624–626

Neuro
radiology
© Springer-Verlag 1991

Tomographic changes of regional cerebral blood flow treated by infusions of high-dose glycerol in acute cerebral embolism

Y. Tsuda[1], Y. Ayada[1], M. Kitadai[1], K. Satoh[1], Y. Sakamoto[1], Y. Ohnishi[1], K. Nagatsuka[1], M. Tanabe[2], and H. Matsuo

[1] Second Department of Internal Medicine and [2] Department of Radiology, Kagawa Medical School, Kagawa, Japan

Summary. Ten patients with acute cerebral embolism were treated with 10% glycerol infusion. The infusion of glycerol was continued for 2–3 weeks and increased maximally to 1600 ml/day. Regional cerebral blood flow (rCBF) was measured in six of ten patients by ^{123}I-amphetamine (IMP) SPECT. Two patients died of ischaemia of a whole hemisphere resulting in progressive herniation; one patient died from pneumonia. The other seven patients were helped despite ischaemia in the whole territory of a middle cerebral artery or in the midbrain. In most of these cases, delayed IMP SPECT images showed a partial redistribution phenomenon which might suggest a good prognosis. In the chronic stage, ischaemia is more clearly demonstrated than in the acute stage with the early images, particularly in the affected hemisphere, while in the delayed images a redistribution phenomenon was observed only in the unaffected hemisphere. This indicates paradoxically that redistribution of rCBF from hyperaemic to ischaemic zones might have existed in the acute stage of cerebral embolism.

Key words: Cerebral embolism – ^{123}I-amphetamine single-photon emission tomography – High-dose glycerol infusion – Regional cerebral blood flow

The cause of early death after cerebral embolism is brain oedema resulting in tentorial herniation. Glycerol has been reported to reduce intracranial pressure and early oedema formation [1–3], which is beneficial. With high-dose infusions of glycerol for more than 2 weeks, we evaluated tomographic regional cerebral blood flow (rCBF) and prognosis in patients with cerebral embolism accompanied by tentorial herniation.

Subjects and methods

Ten patients with acute cerebral embolism of cardiac origin (mean age 69 years) were treated with a 10% glycerol infusion within 6 h after onset. All the patients had atrial fibrillation at onset. The intravenous infusion of 10% glycerol, with 5% fructose added for the prevention of haemolysis (Glyceol, Chugai Pharmaceutical, Japan), was started as early as possible after onset. The initial infusion dose was 600–800 ml/day and was increased maximally to 1600 ml/day. The infusion was continued for 2–3 weeks, and CTwas carried out on days 1, 3, and 7 after onset. Tomographic rCBF images were obtained in six of ten cases by ^{123}I-amphetamine (IMP) SPECT using a rotating gamma camera (GCA-90B, Toshiba, Japan) equipped with a high-resolution, low-energy collimator (FWHM = 4.5 mm), as early (30 min p.i.) and delayed (4 h p.i.) images after i.v. injection of 111 mBq IMP sampled over 20–30 min with 64 images of 4 k matrix by a 360 ° rotation of the camera, respectively. Image reconstruction was by a filtered back projection method.

Results

Two patients (cases 1, 2) showing ischaemia of a whole hemisphere of the brain on CT died within a week, of progressive herniation. An 89-year-old woman (case 3) died of pneumonia 3 weeks after a second episode of embolism in the contralateral hemisphere, while the other seven im-

Table 1. Summary of patients and clinical prognosis

Case	Age (years)	Sex	Lesion	AF	VHD	HT	Prognosis
1.	65	F	total hemisphere (lt)	+	AR	–	Dead
2.	79	F	total hemisphere(lt)	+	–	+	Dead
3.	89	F	total MCA (rt-lt)	+	MR	–	Dead
4.	69	F	total MCA (rt)	+	MS	–	Fair
5.	46	F	total MCA (rt)	+	–	+	Good
6.	72	F	total MCA (rt)	+	–	–	Good
7.	74	M	total MCA (lt)	+	AR	+	Fair
8.	67	M	total MCA (lt)	sinus $\rightleftharpoons$ AF	–	–	Good
9.	59	F	partial MCA (rt)	sinus $\rightleftharpoons$ AF	–	–	Good
10.	67	F	midbrain (rt)	+	–	+	Fair

AF, Atrial fibrillation; VHD, valvular heart disease; HT, hypertension; MCA, middle cerebral artery territory; MS, mitral stenosis; MR, mitral regurgitation; AR, aortic regurgitation

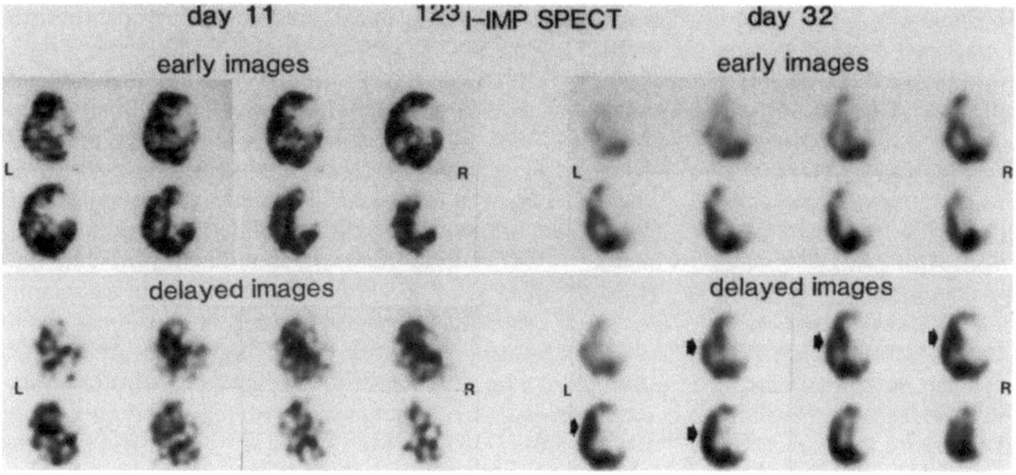

Fig. 1. Changes in early and delayed ^{123}I-amphetamine (IMP) SPECT images in a patient with acute cerebral embolism (case 5)

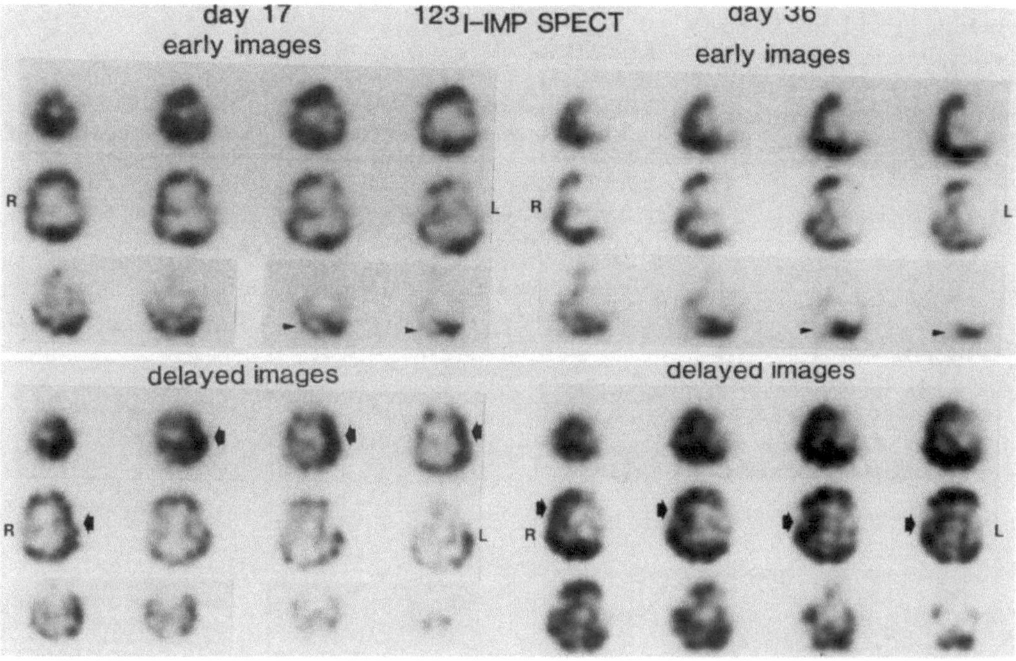

Fig. 2. Changes in early and delayed ^{123}I-IMP SPECT images in a patient with acute cerebral embolism (case 8)

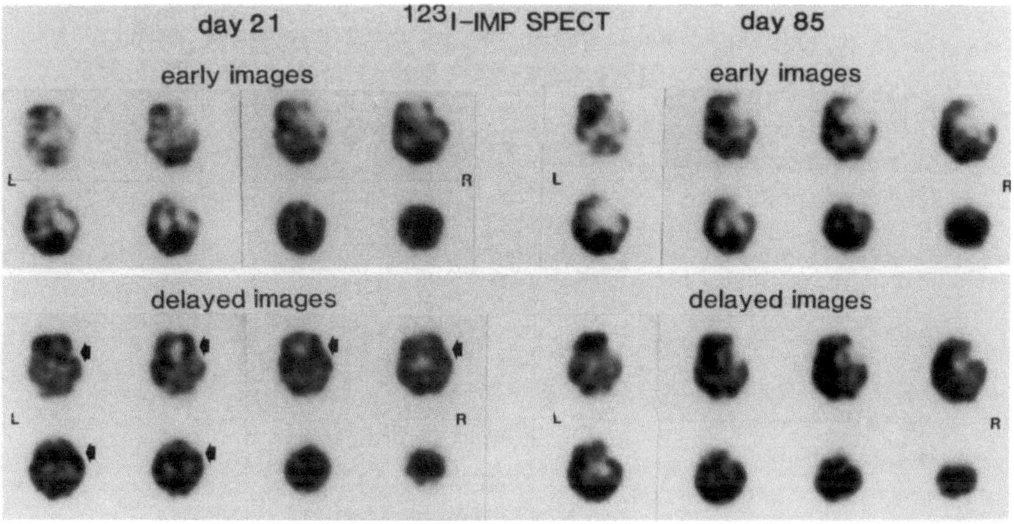

Fig. 3. Changes in early and delayed ^{123}I-IMP SPECT images in a patient with acute cerebral embolism (case 9)

proved despite global or partial ischaemia in the middle cerebral artery (MCA) territory in six cases (cases 4–8 and 9, respectively) and in the midbrain in one case (case 10). The prognosis is summarised in Table 1. In most of these cases, delayed IMP SPECT images during acute and chronic stages showed a partial redistribution phenomenon which might suggest a good prognosis. Figures 1–3 show early and delayed ^{123}I-IMP SPECT images in three cases after acute cerebral embolism with good prognosis (cases 5, 8, 9). Crossed cerebellar diaschisis was observed in case 8 in the early images on both days 17 and 36, as shown in Fig. 2. In the acute stage, the redistribution phenomenon was observed in the delayed images of cases 8 and 9 (Figs. 2, 3). In the chronic stage, ischaemia was more clearly shown in the early images of cases 5 and 8, particularly in the affected hemisphere, while the redistribution phenomenon in the unaffected hemisphere was observed in the delayed images as shown in Figs. 1 and 2. Such a redistribution in the unaffected hemisphere in the chronic stage was not observed in case 9 (Fig. 3), perhaps because the brain was less severely damaged in this case. Furthermore, haemolysis, or the rebound phenomenon was not observed after administration of glycerol, to which 5% fructose was added in many cases.

Discussion

The reduction of cerebral oedema by infusions of glycerol might improve cerebral circulation. The double-blind randomised trial of intravenous glycerol in acute stroke by Bayer et al. [1] showed a beneficial effect of the treatment by an analysis of the survival rates as compared with control patients without glycerol infusion. Cerebral embolism limited to the MCA territory might be helped by high-dose glycerol infusion and patients' outcome was better if the partial redistribution phenomenon had been observed in the delayed ^{123}I-IMP SPECT images in the acute and chronic stages. In the chronic stage in cases 5 and 8, more evident ischaemia in the early images and the redistribution phenomenon in the unaffected hemisphere in the delayed ^{123}I-IMP SPECT images, paradoxically indicate that redistribution of rCBF from hyperaemic to ischaemic zones [3] might have been shown by the early images in the acute stage after infusions of high-dose glycerol in cases with total MCA embolism. The redistribution phenomenon in a chronic stage in the unaffected hemisphere was not observed in a patient with partial MCA embolism (case 9), possibly due to less severely damaged brain.

References

1. Bayer AJ, Pathy MSJ, Newcombe R (1987) Double-blind randomised trial of intravenous glycerol in acute stroke. Lancet I: 405–408
2. Frank MSB, Nahata MC, Hilty MD (1981) Glycerol: a review of its pharmacology, pharmacokinetics, adverse reactions and clinical use. Pharmacotherapy 1: 147–160
3. Ott EO, Mathew NT, Meyer JS (1974) Redistribution of regional cerebral blood flow after glycerol infusion in acute cerebral infarction. Neurology 24: 1117–1126

Assist. Prof. Dr. Yoshiyasu Tsuda
Second Department of Internal Medicine
Kagawa Medical School
1750-1 Ikenobe, Miki-cho
Kagawa 761-07, Japan

Neuroradiology (1991) 33 [Suppl]: 627–628

Neuro-radiology
© Springer-Verlag 1991

Improvement of cortical blood flow and neurological deficits after extracranial-intracranial bypass in a patient with haemodynamically significant carotid lesions

Y. Tsuda[1], F. Okuda[1], K. Yamada[3], T. Hayakawa[3], Y. Ayada[1], M. Kitadai[1], K. Satoh[1], M. Ohkawa[2], and H. Matsuo[1]

[1] Second Department of Internal Medicine and [2] Department of Radiology, Kagawa Medical School, Kagawa, Japan
[3] Department of Neurosurgery, Osaka University Medical School, Osaka Japan

Summary. A 58-year-old man presented right hand hypaesthesia and dysarthria with memory disturbances and disorientation. CT and MRI showed small lesions on the left, while carotid angiography showed left carotid siphon occlusion and a stenosis of the proximal left anterior cerebral artery, with collaterals via the anterior communicating artery. ^{123}I-IMP SPECT images showed extensive hypoperfusion in the left anterior parietal cortex. From the haemodynamic point of view, bypass surgery was considered. After surgery, right hand hypaesthesia disappeared and speech became normal, with improved orientation and memory. Postoperative angiography showed good filling of the left middle cerebral artery from the bypass. Flow distributions showed good recovery in the left cerebral cortex. The extracranial-intracranial bypass improved neurological deficits and cortical blood flow in a patient with haemodynamically significant carotid lesions.

Key words: Carotid artery disease – Extracranial-intracranial arterial bypass – ^{123}I-IMP emission tomography – Magnetic resonance imaging – Regional cerebral blood flow

Whether bypass surgery might enhance cerebral circulation or not is still controversial [1–3] although its prophylactic effect was questioned by a cooperative study [4]. We studied a patient with haemodynamically significant

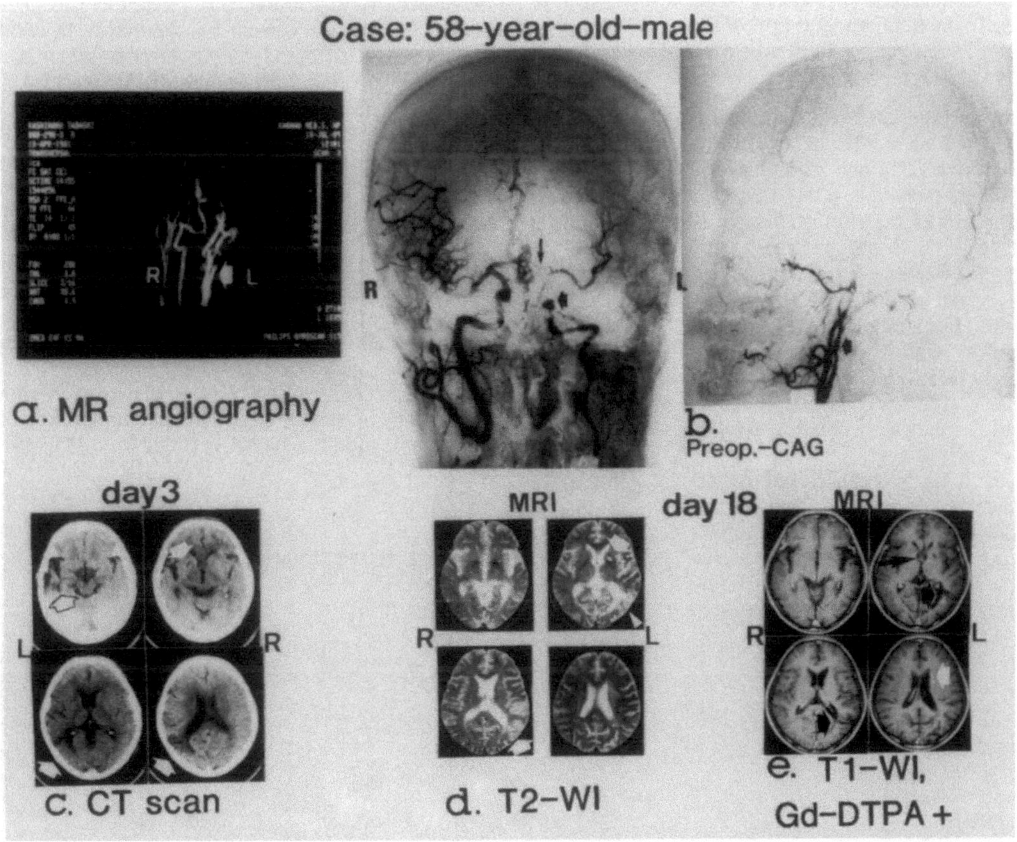

Fig. 1. Preoperative findings in **a** MR angiography, **b** carotid angiography, **c** CT, **d** T2-weighted MR images and **e** T1-weighted MR images enhanced by gadolinium-DTPA

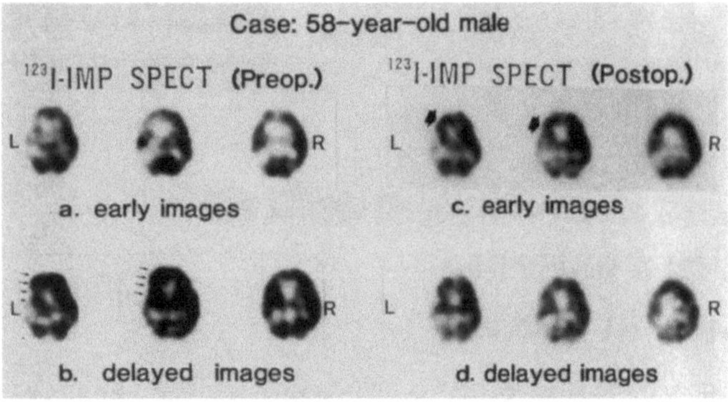

Fig. 2. Pre- *(left side)* and postoperative *(right side)* findings in the early **(a, c)** and delayed **(b, d)** images of ^{123}I IMP SPECT

carotid lesions who showed improvement of cortical flow and neurological deficits after the bypass.

Case report

A 58-year-old man had two episodes of transient ischaemic attack (TIA) in 3 years, showing right hemiparesis, right hand hypaesthesia, and dysarthria, which continued for 7 and 12 h, respectively. Two months prior to investigation, he experienced a transient episode of right hand tremor with motor aphasia. Subsequently, he showed memory disturbances and disorientation, which were noticed by his wife. At admission, he complained of right hand hypaesthesia and dysarthria, with memory disturbance, disorientation and dyscalculia.

Diagnostic evaluations. The patient was examined by CT, 1.5 T-MRI (Gyroscan S15, Philips), carotid angiography including MR angiography, and early (30 min p.i.) and delayed (4 h p.i.) ^{123}I *N*-isopropyl-*p*-iodoamphetamine (IMP) emission tomography (SPECT) using a rotating gamma camera (GCA-90B, Toshiba, Japan) equipped with a HRLE collimator (FWHM = 4.5 mm) sampled for 20–30 min after i.v. injection of 111 mBq IMP.

Preoperative study. MR angiography showed left carotid occlusion (shown by a white arrow in Fig. 1a), which was confirmed by carotid angiography (Fig. 1b) (shown by small arrows), showing a stenosis of the proximal left anterior cerebral artery (shown by a large arrow), with collaterals from the anterior communicating artery. CT and T2-weighted MR images showed small lesions in the left putamen, temporal subcortex, and temporo-occipital watershed area (shown by white arrows and arrowhead in Fig. 1c, d). In addition, T1-weighted images showed a small lesion enhanced by gadolinium-DTPA in the left periventricular region (shown by white arrow in Fig. 1e), suggesting recent infarction. The early IMP SPECT images showed hypoperfusion in the left anterior parietal cortex (Fig. 2a), while the delayed images showed redistribution (shown by small arrows in Fig. 2b) in the hypoperfused areas of early images.

From the haemodynamic point of view, it was considered that an extracranial-intracranial (EC-IC) arterial bypass was indicated, because the brain damage on CT and MRI was minimal, while collaterals via the anterior communicating artery were marginal due to severe stenosis of the proximal left anterior cerebral artery. In addition, a hypoperfused area in the early images, as well as redistribution in the delayed ones, were observed by ^{123}I IMP SPECT. The haemodynamic instability in this patient was considered to be correctable.

After successful bypass surgery, right hand hypaesthesia disappeared and speech became normal. His orientation improved, and he could calculate well.

Postoperative study. Postoperative cerebral angiography showed good filling into the left middle cerebral artery from the external carotid artery. CT and T2-weighted MR images showed small lesions in the left putamen, temporal subcortex and temporo-occipital watershed area, in addition to a left periventricular lesion. IMP SPECT showed a good recovery of blood flow in the left anterior parietal cortex (shown by arrows in Fig. 2c) without showing significant redistribution, postoperatively (Fig. 2d).

Discussion

The improvement of rCBF after EC-IC bypass has been reported in some studies to date [1–3]. However, the necessity for bypass surgery is still unclear in most cases, and its prophylactic efficacy has been questioned by a cooperative study [4]. In a rare case with haemodynamic instability showing TIAs with blood pressure changes reported by Baron et al. [1], EC-IC bypass might have been absolutely indicated as suggested by the pre- and postoperative studies or rCBF and cerebral oxygen metabolism. In our study, bypass surgery at least improved neurological deficits and three-dimensional cortical blood flow in a case with haemodynamically significant carotid lesions

References

1. Baron JC, Bousser MG, Rey A, Guillard A, Comar D, Castaigne P (1981) Reversal of focal "misery-perfusion syndrome" by extra-intracranial arterial bypass in hemodynamic cerebral ischemia. A case study with ^{15}O positron emission tomography. Stroke 12: 454–459
2. Tsuda Y, Kimura K, Iwata Y, Hayakawa T, Etani H, Fukunaga R, Yoneda S, Abe H (1984) Improvement of cerebral blood flow and or CO_2 reactivity after superficial temoral artery-middle cerebral artery bypass in patients with transient ischemic attacks and watershed-zone infarctions. Surg Neurol 22: 595–604
3. Vorstrup S, Lassen NA, Henriksen L, Haase J, Lindewald H, Boysen G, Paulson OB (1985) CBF before and after extracranial-intracranial bypass surgery in patients with ischemic cerebrovascular disease studied with ^{133}Xe-inhalation tomography. Stroke 16: 616–625
4. The EC/IC Bypass Study Group (1985) Failure of extracranial-intracranial arterial bypass to reduce the risk of ischemic stroke. Results of an international randomized trial. N Engl J Med 313: 1191–1200

Dr. Yoshiyasu Tsuda
Second Department of Internal Medicine
Kagawa Medical School
1750-1 Ikenobe, Miki-cho
Kagawa 761-07, Japan

SCIENTIFIC EXHIBITS

Neuroradiology (1991) 33 [Suppl]: 630–631

Neuro-radiology
© Springer-Verlag 1991

Cray-2 supercomputer image enhancement in neuroradiology

M. J. Kuhn[1], D. P. Lawrance[2], F. A. Reda III[1], and F. A. Wrestler[2]

[1] Southern Illinois University School of Medicine, St. John's Hospital, Springfield, Illinois, USA
[2] National Center of Supercomputing Applications, The Beckman Institute, University of Illinois, Urbana-Champaign, Illinois, USA

Summary. Because of its large central memory and high speed, a Cray-2 supercomputer was used to rapidly and simultaneously process entire neuroradiological image datasets. Test MRI sets consisting of quadruple spin echo images of the head, cervical spine and lumbar spine obtained on a General Electric 1.5 T imager were used. Principal component images were first computed and analyzed. A pseudocoloring technique was then applied for combining information from multiple images into a single composite. We found improved distinction between grey and white matter structures, improved visualization of intracranial vasculature and a decrease in the amount of imaging data that needed to be stored and transferred. We conclude that singular forms of neuroradiologic image enhancement are possible with appropriate image processing applications in supercomputer environments.

Key words: Image enhancement – Computer-assisted image processing – Computer simulation – Computer literacy

Scientific visualization is the presentation of numerical data as pictures; that is, the ability to "see the data". We have been involved in a collaborative effort of radiologists, computer programmers, and other support personnel, all contributing to the utilization of a Cray-2 supercomputer in neuroradiologic applications of scientific visualization.

Routine acquisition of neuroimaging data sets (CT, MRI) requires a substantial amount of computer and communications resources. Among the resources can be those for subsequent reprocessing. A number of computer environments are now evolving which are attractive for biomedical image processing including high-performance workstations, highly parallel computers, multiprocessors, and vector processors such as the Cray-2 [1]. The attractiveness of the Cray-2 is its large central memory store, its high clock speed, and its ability to operate on data vectors and to pipeline operations. These characteristics are useful in image processing because the same operators are often applied to the large number of pixels and voxels present in medical images.

Important constraining factors in digital radiography include limitations in image storage and transfer capability for both display and postprocessing [2]. If the information present in multislice image data could be compressed in some manner without significant loss of information, perhaps by compositing images, then image transfer and local storage requirements could be relaxed. Our work towards this end has primarily centered upon principal component image analysis, a model intensively used in the analysis of Landsar remote sensing images of Earth resources [3]. This is one technique by which redundant information present in sets of images can be removed, resulting in a set of intermediary images. These can yet again be visually combined using pseudocoloring, resulting in "data-dense" color images.

Materials and methods

Multislice quadruple spin echo sequences of the head, cervical, and lumbar spine were obtained on a 1.5 T General Electric Signa MRI imager. SE sequences of TR 2000 ms and TE 30, 60, 90, and 120 ms were used. Four principal component images were created for each slice (Fig. 1), computed from their corresponding covariance matrices, carried out on a Cray-2 supercomputer running UNICOS and using a general-purpose image processing program, Viewit, developed at the National Center for Supercomputing Applications [4].

Because the fourth principal component axis primarily corresponds to average tissue T2 decay rate, it discriminates grey and white matter to great advantage. Unlike T2-weighted images obtained using long TRs and TEs, the utilization of information from multiple echoes permits signal averaging which suppresses background noise at slight expense of T2 weighting. The third and second principal component images correspond to signal compartments unrelated to the first principal axis. The second component is particularly sensitive to partial volume and flow-void effects, preferentially enhancing intracranial vessels. The first principal component consists of mostly uncorrelated noise and was discarded. The principal component images were then computer-colored in shades of green, blue and red and superimposed (Fig. 2). The resulting superimposed image demonstrates more information than any individual principal component image or original unaltered spin echo image. Brain, fascia and muscle appear pink; dura mater, blue; bone marrow, red; and bone, white.

Discussion

The principal component images obtained are useful in their own right since they enhance certain structures of anatomic importance such as blood vessels and brain parenchyma. The colorization process magnifies these benefits in several ways. First, changes in hue are more detectable than changes in grey. Second, a wider dynamic

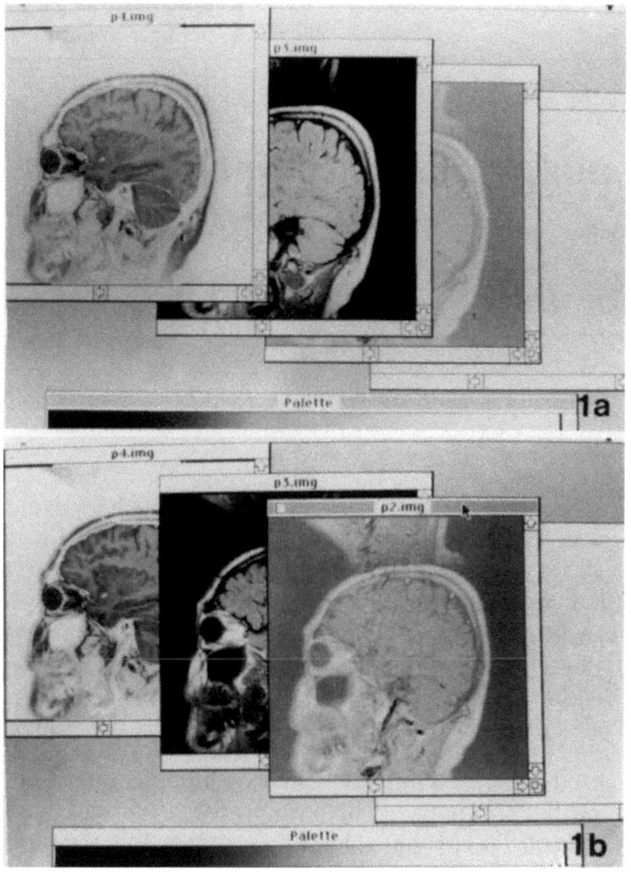

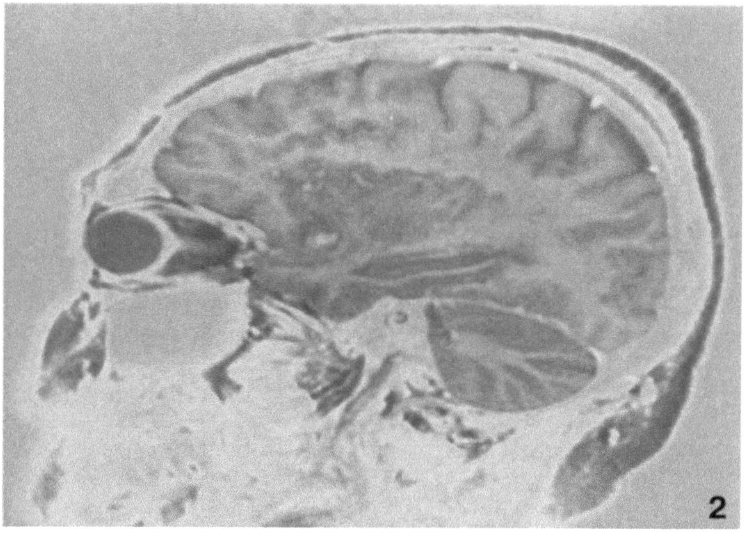

Fig. 1 a, b. The useful principal component images contained for each slice. The fourth **(a)** and second **(b)** principal component images are illustrated

Fig. 2. Superimposition of the colorized principal component images provides the greatest amount of data in a single image

range can be displayed using color than monochrome. Third, since the information density of the fourth principal component image is greater than that of any single preprocessed image, it might be possible to transmit all relevant clinical information by discarding data contained in the final principal component, thereby decreasing data transmission and storage requirements.

Supercomputers like the Cray-2, allowing intensive computation with short turnaround upon large medical image datasets, are extremely useful tools for investigating quickly novel techniques of image visualization and coding. This is significant because academic access to general-purpose supercomputers has dramatically improved over the past five years. General familiarity with useful computational methods of image processing will help to select hardware, software, and network features which should be optimized in a production diagnostic imaging system.

References

1. Smarr L (1988) The computational science revolution: technology, methodology, and sociology. In: Wilhelmsen RB (ed) High speed computing. University of Illinois Press, Urbana, pp 12–33
2. Cox GC, Templeton AW, Dwyer SJ (1986) Digital image management: networking, display and archiving. Radiol Clin North Am 24: 37–54
3. Richards JA (1986) Remote sensing digital image analysis. Springer, Berlin Heidelberg New York, pp 127–147
4. Potter C (1989) Viewit users' manual. National Center for Supercomputing Applications, Urbana Ill

Dr. Matthew J. Kuhn
Department of Radiology
St. John's Hospital
800 East Carpenter Street
Springfield, IL 62769, USA

Neuroradiology (1991) 33 [Suppl]: 632–633

Neuroradiology

© Springer-Verlag 1991

MRI in non-refractory temporal lobe epilepsy: hippocampal sclerosis and other temporal lesions

S. Iwasaki[1], T. Taoka[1], H. Nakagawa[1], K. Kichikawa[1], A. Fukusumi[1], H. Ohishi[1], H. Uchida[1], and Y. Kuru[2]

[1] Department of Radiology, Nara Medical University, Kashihara-shi, Nara, Japan
[2] Department of Radiology, Juntendo University Medical School, Bunkyo-ku, Tokyo, Japan

Summary. The MR images obtained from the coronal plane perpendicular to the hippocampus at 1.0/1.5 T in 18 patients with non-refractory temporal lobe epilepsy were closely examined to detect evidence of hippocampal sclerosis and other temporal lobe lesions. Hippocampal sclerosis was revealed by either brightness in the central region of the hippocampus or by smallness in 12 patients. Other temporal lobe lesions were found in 11 patients. Six patients had lesions in both the hippocampus and ipsilateral temporal lobe. These results are nearly identical to the findings of pathological examination in refractory epilepsy. Thus, MRI can be very useful even in non-refractory temporal lobe epilepsy.

Key words: Epilepsy – Temporal lobe epilepsy – Magnetic resonance imaging – Hippocampus – Ammon's horn sclerosis

The pathological changes seen in the hippocampus of epileptic patients have long been recognized as Ammon's horn sclerosis [1, 2]. However, the hippocampus is a small structure, and earlier diagnostic imaging, such as pneumoencephalography performed in conjunction with tomography, could only barely delineate its outline [3]. In the present study, we used MRI, which can depict the minute structure of the brain in any directional plane [4, 5], to examine the morphology of the hippocampus in cases of temporal lobe epilepsy with the coronal plane perpendicular to the hippocampus.

Subjects and methods

Eighteen patients with temporal lobe epilepsy, in whom clinical control was considered achievable with antiepileptic agents, were studied.

A superconducting MR imager operating at 1.5 T (Picker) or 1.0 T (Shimadzu) was used. All patients were investigated with perpendicular slices through the hippocampus. The slice thickness was 3–7 mm and gapless. For T1-weighted images, a spin echo sequence with TE of 20 ms and TR of 400 ms (two-dimensional Fourier transform) or TE of 18 ms and TR of 200 ms (three-dimensional Fourier transform), or inversion recovery with TI of 150 or 600 ms and TR of 2000–2300 ms was used. For T2-weighted images, a spin echo sequence with TE of 100 ms and TR of 2000 ms used.

Results

Extrahippocampal foci within the temporal lobe were found in 11 of the 18 cases (61.1%) (Table 1). Of these foci, the 2 cases of small brain damage, a neuroma, a case of MELAS (mitochondrial myopathy, encephalopathy, lactic acidosis, and strokelike episodes), an arachnoid cyst and a meningioma could be diagnosed by CT. Shrinkage of the hippocampus was found in 11 cases. In 10 of these and the one with normal-sized hippocampus, the central portion of the hippocampus showed hyperintensity on T2-weighted images. Thus, evidence of hippocampal sclerosis, either shrinkage or hyperintensity, was found in all 12 cases (66.7%) (Table 1, Fig. 1). A focus within the temporal lobe coexisting with sclerosis of the hippocampus was found in 6 cases (33.3%), with the lesions seen on the same side (Table 1, Fig. 2).

Discussion

Ammon's horn sclerosis is said to be chiefly a reduction of the volume of Sommer's sector, which corresponds to the outer portion of the hippocampus [1, 2]. However, in the

Table 1. MRI results in patients with temporal lobe epilepsy

Case no.	Age	Lesions		Hippocampus	
				Shrinkage	Hyperintensity in T2-weighted images
1	7	–		R	R
2	11	MELAS	(L)	L	L
3	19	Neuroma	(L)	–	–
4	21	–		R	R
5	23	–		R	R
6	24	Brain damage	(L)	L	L
7	25	–		R	R
8	28	–		–	–
9	32	–		L	L
10	33	Astrocytoma	(L)	–	–
11	34	Brain damage	(L)	–	–
12	41	Astrocytoma	(L)	–	L
13	41	Venous malformation	(L)	–	–
14	43	Gliosis	(R)	R	R
15	46	–		R	R
16	50	Cavernoma	(R)	–	–
17	59	Arachnoid cyst	(R)	R	R
18	75	Meningioma	(R)	R	–

R, Right side; L, left side

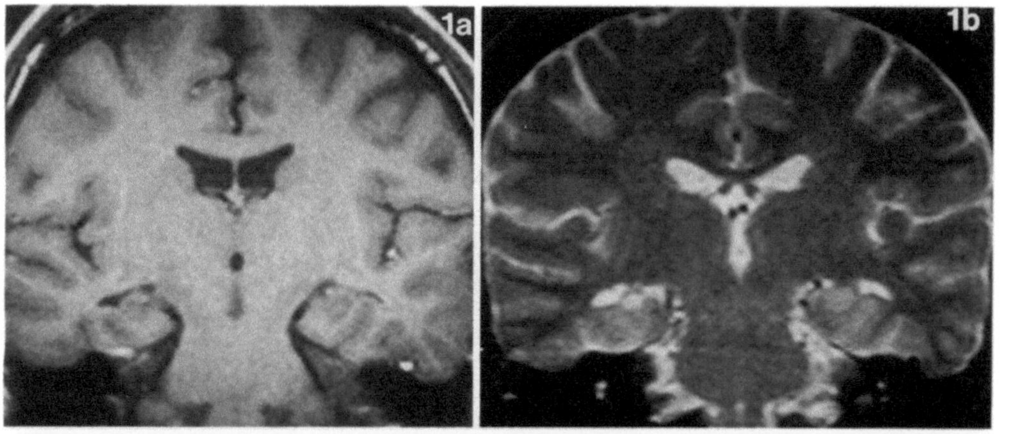

Fig. 1 a, b. Case 4. A 21-year-old man. No extrahippocampal focus is found. **a** An SE 400/20, 5-mm-thick image through the red nucleus shows an enlarged lateral cleft of the right inferior horn. **b** An SE 2000/100, 5-mm-thick image through the red nucleus shows an area of hyperintensity within the shrunken right hippocampus

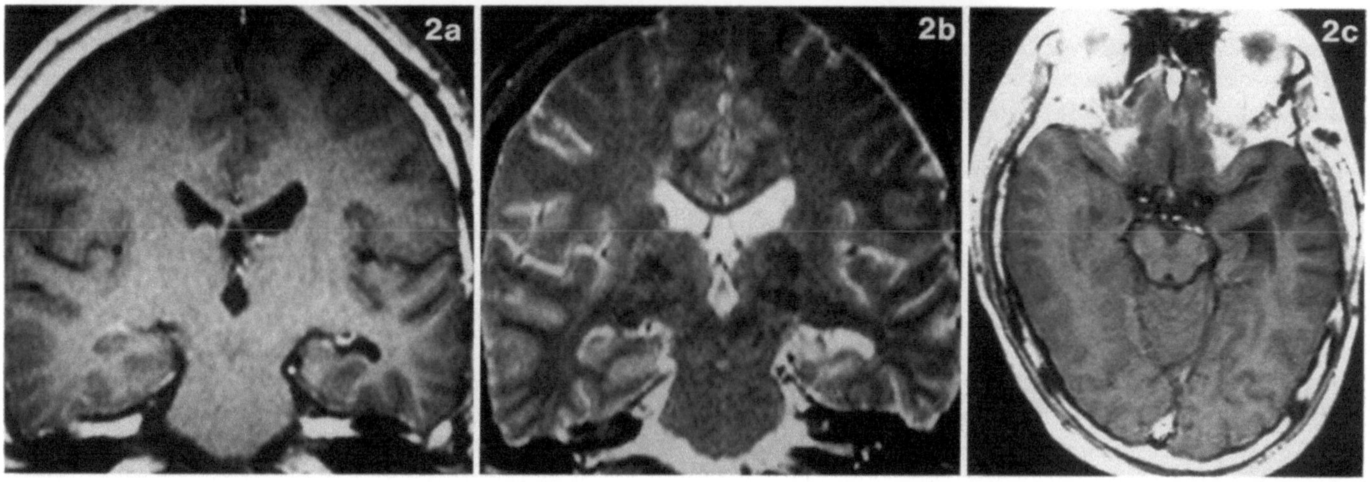

Fig. 2 a–c. Case 6. A 24-year-old man with a history of depressed fracture of the left temporal bone. **a** An SE 400/20, 6-mm-thick image through the tegmentum shows shrinkage of the left hippocampus. **b** An SE 2000/100, 5-mm-thick image through the same level as above shows hyperintensity within the left hippocampus. **c** The brain damage is visible in the left middle temporal gyrus

present cases, in which abnormalities were found in the hippocampus, the entire hippocampus except for the alveus, or the central portion of the hippocampus, showed hyperintensity on T2-weighted images. This suggests the strong possibility of demonstrating abnormalities not only of Sommer's sector but of the end-folium as well.

Bruton [1] performed a histopathological study of the temporal lobe in 249 cases of intractable temporal lobe epilepsy subjected to operation, and reported foci in the temporal lobe in 183 cases (73.5%), of which 122 (49%) were Ammon's horn sclerosis. Although the number of cases in the present series is too small to permit a statistical comparison, a similar tendency was seen even in temporal lobe epilepsy considered clinically controllable. The results of operation for temporal lobe epilepsy due to Ammon's horn sclerosis are considered excellent [1], and it is thought that the ability to diagnose Ammon's horn sclerosis accurately by imaging of the hippocampus is important.

Sclerosis of the hippocampus and foci in the temporal lobe can be demonstrated by MRI, suggesting that morphological confirmation comparable to histopathological examination can be obtained to elucidate pathological changes of epilepsy.

References

1. Bruton CJ (1988) The neuropathology of temporal lobe epilepsy. Oxford University Press, New York
2. Meldrum BS, Corsellis JAN (1984) Epilepsy. In: Hume Adams J, Corsellis JAN, Duchen LW (eds) Greenfield's neuropathology, 4th edn. Arnold, London, pp 921–950
3. Kuru Y (1976) Pneumoencephalography of today. Shinkei Kenkyu No Shinpo 20: 659–668
4. Naidich TP, Daniels DL, Haughton VM, Williams A, Pojunas K, Palacios E (1987) Hippocampal formation and related structures of the limbic lobe: anatomic-MR correlation. Radiology 162: 747–754
5. Triulzi F, Franceschi M, Fazio F, Del Maschio A (1988) Nonrefractory temporal lobe epilepsy: 1.5 T MR Imaging. Radiology 166: 181–185

Dr. Satoru Iwasaki
Department of Radiology, Nara Medical University
840, Kashihara-shi
Nara, 634 Japan

Neuroradiology (1991) 33 [Suppl]: 634–635

Neuro
radiology
© Springer-Verlag 1991

Three-dimensional visualization and models of brain tumour, skull, and spine derived from CT data

K. Heimberger[1], N. Pfafflmeyer[1], P. Solar[4], P. Samec[2], P. Vierlinger[5], and E. Schindler[3]

Department of Neuroradiology of [1] Neurological University Clinics and [2] City Hospital Rosenhugel,
[3] University Clinic of Neurosurgery, and [4] Department of Dentistry, Vienna University Clinics, Vienna, Austria
[5] Medizinelektronik Laboratory, Kiel, Federal Republic of Germany

Summary. Conventional methods like CT and MRI have been providing only two-dimensional reformattings of three-dimensional (3D) neuroanatomical and neuropathological structures. Endoplan is a new hard- and software containing system, interactively creating a genuine 3D reproduction, e.g. of a brain tumour as a model or as a computer-generated monitor view for cinematographic viewing, turning around a vertical axis. The system is based on an HP 300 computer and the MEK processing system. The contours of the object to be visualized three-dimensionally are defined by selecting density values from the object border's Hounsfield numbers on CT. The models of two brain tumours, one skull tumour, and a segment of the lumbar spine are demonstrated. 3D visualization and modelling can be used for topical and functional neurological diagnosis, neurological surgery and preparation for radiation therapy.

Key words: Brain tumour – Skull – Spine – Three-dimensional visualization

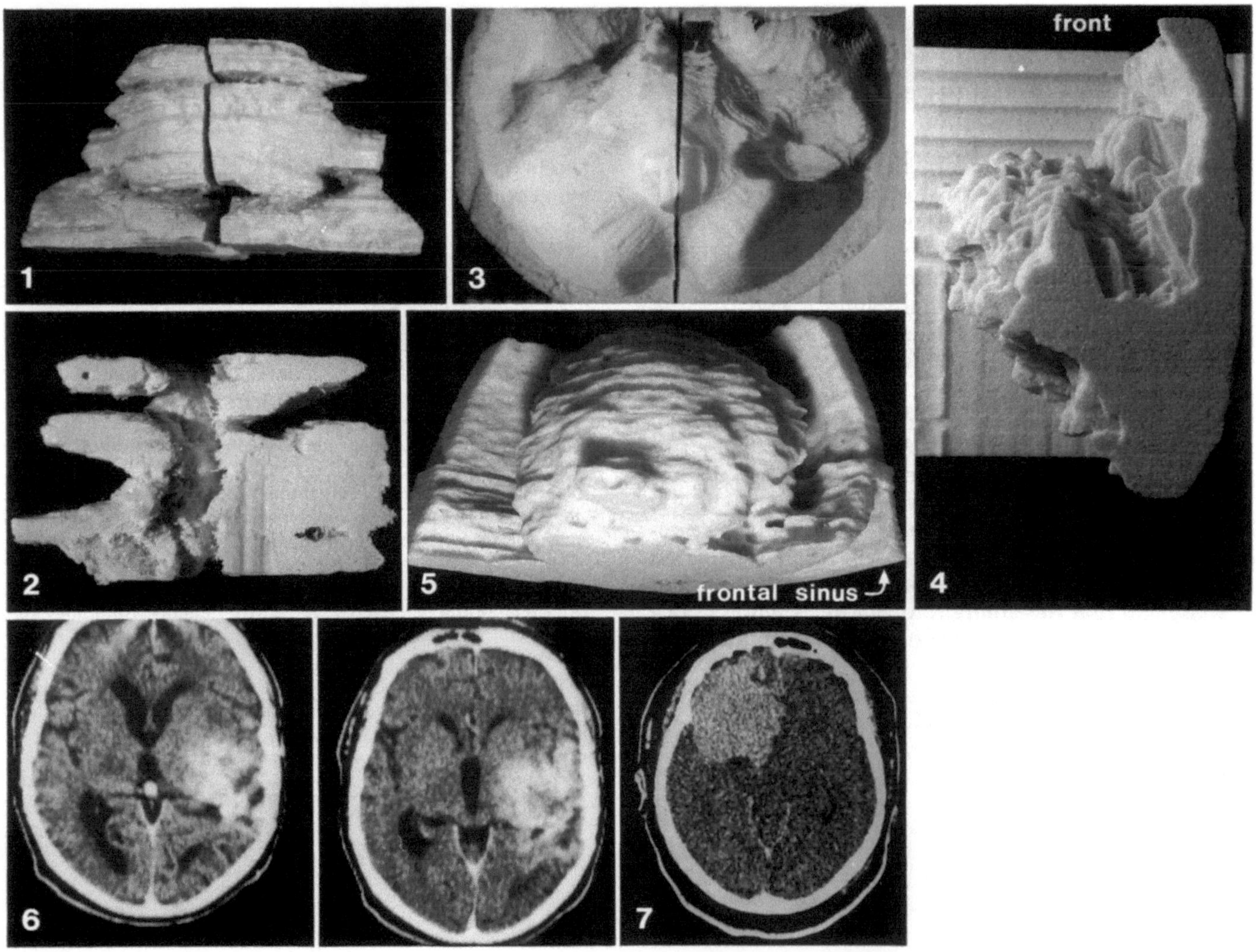

CT examinations were conducted on a Siemens Somatom 2N and DR (slice thickness and table advancement up to 2 mm). CT data are transferred to an HP 300 computer, where the object's contours are processed for reformatting. Sequences of pseudo-3D views for numerous projections of the object on a monitor are generated and serve as basis for a synthetic videofilm. There is the possibility for manual correction of automatically defined countours. Moreover, contours can be differently shaded and lit with different colours from different angles. Transferred and processed computer data control the movements of a cutter around four to five axes to fabricate the model [1]. The first models built were made of polystyrol (Figs. 1–3). Now, foamed polyurethane is preferred for better detail generation by the milling machine (Figs. 4, 5).

CT data from four patients were transferred to the Endoplan system for 3D reformatting: a 75-year-old female patient with an osteoma of the right petrous pyramid (Fig. 3); a 57-year-old male with a glioblastoma in the right temporoparietal region (Figs. 4, 6); an 82-year-old female with bilateral ischialgia (Figs. 1, 2); a 59-year-old male patient with a giant left frontal meningioma (Figs. 5, 7).

Results

After processing CT data and interpolation of anatomical structures between slices, models were cut by a computer-controlled milling machine. Photo prints were taken from the models. The glioblastoma patient and the meningioma patient had received i. v. contrast medium for facilitation of contour finding (Figs. 4–7). Automatic contour definition of the osteoma (Fig. 3) was exact and did not have to be corrected manually. The low CT density of intervertebral disc appears as air-gap in the model (Figs. 1, 2). Hounsfield numbers that are lower than the ones used at contour definition are usually presented as air gaps (intervertebral foramina, spinal canal, surrounding soft tissue – Fig. 2).

Fig. 1. Split model. Segmental part of the lumbar spine of an 82-year-old female with bilateral ischialgia. Anterior view. Lumbar disc spaces pictured as height reduced air gaps

Fig. 2. Same model as in Fig. 1; view of the median sagittal cut surface and the lining of the spinal canal with the possibility of measuring the diameters thereof

Fig. 3. Model of the skull base of a 75-year-old female patient. Osteoma of the right pyramid; top view

Fig. 4. Model of a right temporo-parietally situated glioblastoma which seems to adhere (but in reality is only in close proximity) to the internal table of the skull. The original CT from which this model was derived, is shown in Fig. 6

Fig. 5. Model of a giant left frontal meningioma. Oblique view from below right

Fig. 6. Original contrast enhanced CT from which the model of Fig. 4 was derived by aligning the contour along the contrast-enhanced region

Fig. 7. Original contrast enhanced CT from a series of which the model in Fig. 5 was derived

Discussion

CT data can be visualized three-dimensionally in 3 ways: in a synthetic video film with clockwise and counter-clockwise rotation around a vertical axis; in models; as photo prints of models. The models can be taken a part into several parts, revealing internal surfaces (e. g. osseous border of the spinal canal, Fig. 2). The clinical relevance of CT dataderived polyurethane models in the neurosciences is manifold: neuropathological/morphological relevance in measuring the extent of cranial lesions three-dimensionally [2], measuring therapy-induced volumetric changes, measuring the extent of cranial deformities [3]; neurosurgical relevance/operative simulation [4, 5]; neurophysiological relevance with possible overlapping of functional imaging like SPECT, magnetoencephalography (MEG) and consecutive recognition of diseased brain [6].

References

1. Brix F, Lambrecht T (1987) Individuelle Schädelherstellung auf der Grundlage computertomographischer Informationen. Fortschr Kiefer Ges Chir 32: 74–77
2. Stimac GK, Sundsten JW, Prothero JS, Prothero JW, Gerlach R, Sorbonne R (1988) 3D contour surfacing of the skull, face and brain from CT and MR images and from anatomic sections. AJR 151: 807–810
3. Vannier MW, Hildebolt CF, Marsh JL, Pilgram TK, McAlister WH, Shackelford GD, Offut CJ, Knapp RH (1989) Craniosynostoses: diagnostic value of 3D CT reconstruction. Radiology 173: 669–673
4. Chalif DJ, Dufresne CR, Ransohoff J, McCarthy JA (1988) 3D CT reconstructions of intracranial meningiomas. Neurosurgery 23: 570–575
5. Jackson IT, Bite U (1986) 3D CT scanning and major surgical reconstruction of the head and neck. Mayo Clin Proc 61: 546–555
6. Pietrzyk U, Herholz K, Heiss WD (1990) 3D alignment of functional and morphological tomograms. J Comput Assist Tomogr 14: 51–59

Dr. K. Heimberger
Department of Neuroradiology
Vienna University Clinics
Lazarettgasse 14
A-1090 Vienna, Austria

Neuroradiology (1991) 33 [Suppl]: 636–637

Neuroradiology
© Springer-Verlag 1991

Low-friction high-torque guide wire: a new way for superselective catheterization

K. Goto

Department of Interventional Neuroradiology, The Center for Central Nervous Diseases, Iizuka Hospital, Iizuka, Japan

Summary. A new plastic guide wire featuring a low-friction surface, high torque control and increased pushability whilst still maintaining floppiness of the distal end was developed for the sake of safer and quicker placement of microcatheters deep into the feeding arteries of various intracranial, spinal and craniofacial vascular lesions. The effectiveness of this guide wire was proven by our experience in using it 135 times in 65 cases.

Key words: Guide wire – Embolization – Arteriovenous malformation – cerebral arteriovenous fistula-dural – aneurysm-cerebral.

I report the development of a new guide wire for safer and quicker placement of microcatheters deep into various intracranial, spinal and craniofacial vascular lesions.

Materials and methods

The guide wire reported is a 0.016 inch, hydrophilic, polymer-coated guide wire (0.016 Radifocus, Terumo Europe, Leuven, Belgium). Its design and inner structure are shown in Fig. 1. The stiffness of the proximal part of this guide wire is 4 times that of the previous guide wire of the same design, which was 0.014 inch [1], thus generating more pushability.

Floppiness of the tip. A butting test was carried out by pressing the tip of the guide wire held at 30 mm from the distal tip end. The resulting load on this guide wire was $^1/_2$ to $^1/_6$ of that on four other widely used guide wires.

Low-friction surface. The hydrophilic polymer used for coating this guide wire has molecular chains on its surface. When wet, the polymer takes in water molecules between these chains, thus providing low-friction. The maximum sliding resistance which this guide wire met as it advanced through the microcatheter was $^1/_5$ to $^1/_2$ that of the others.

Torque control. Because the core is made of a superelastic alloy, this guide wire has high torque control. It is less likely that the tip of the guide wire will suffer permanent damage during use, allowing smooth insertion and removal.

Thrombogenicity. Due to hydrophilic polymer coating, thrombogenicity of this guide wire is markedly lower than that of Teflon-coated coiled-wires [2].

Vascular model. A vascular model (Fig. 2) was used to determine the optimal floppiness and angle of the tip of this guide wire. This model was also useful for practice in the use of the guide wire.

Case materials. Analyses were made of our experiences of the use of this guide wire 135 times in 65 cases of intracranial, spinal and craniofacial vascular lesions.

Case report

A 54-year-old male with an arteriovenous malformation in the left parietal lobe is reported. Angiography revealed marked elongation and increased tortuosity of the feeding arteries, which were given off from anterior and middle cerebral arteries (Fig. 3 a). The main feeding arteries were superselectively catheterized one by one with the help of this guide wire (Fig. 3 b). Embolization was done using 0.7–1.0 ml ethylene vinyl alcohol copolymer after confirming negative amylobarbital testing. Control angiography revealed a minimal residuum of the nidus, which was successfully resected without necessitating blood transfusion (Fig. 3 c).

Results

The visibility of the tip of the guide wire was excellent on every occasion. Smoothness in insertion and removal was also excellent every time. Torque control was excellent in 119 and good in 15 procedures. The guide wire failed to work in only 1 case. The average time needed to place the tip of the catheter into the optimal point for embolization was 10 min.

The following complications were encountered: perforation of the vessel wall (twice), angiospasm (3 times).

Permanent adhesion of tip of guide wire during use: none. Difficulty in insertion and removal during use: none.

Discussion

As the effectiveness of this guide wire was proven in the initial 10 cases, in whom the coil-type guide wire failed to work due to severe tortuosity of the vessels, we have been using this plastic guide wire only. The only complication was intimal damage associated with spasm of vessels caused by the tip of the guide wire, experienced 3 times in the initial cases, while manoeuvring the guide wire to pass sharp kinks in vessels.

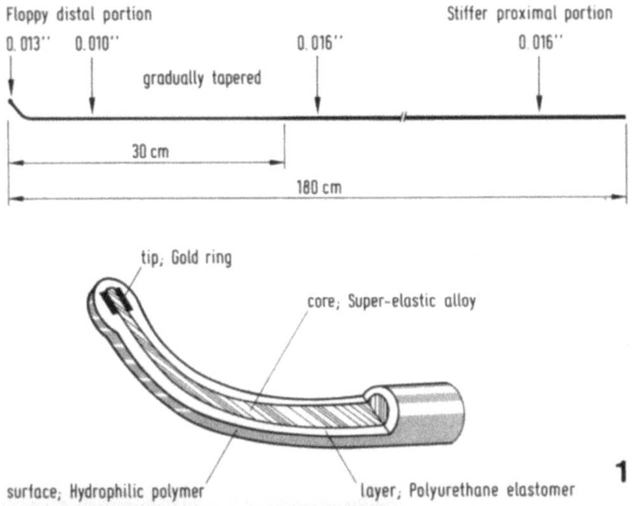

1

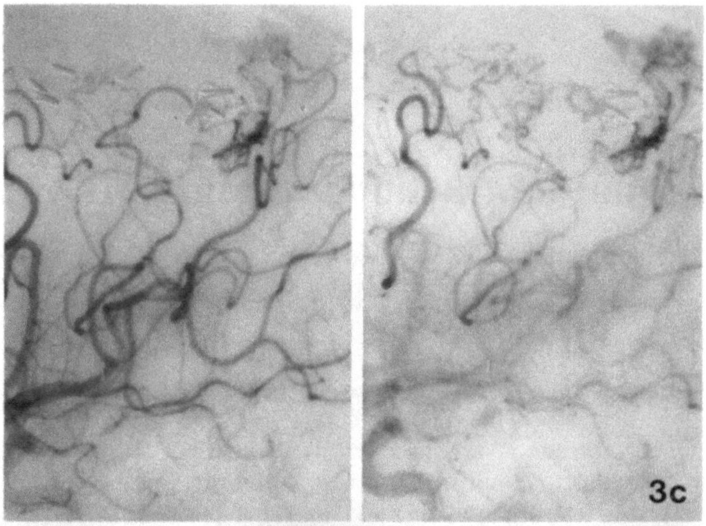

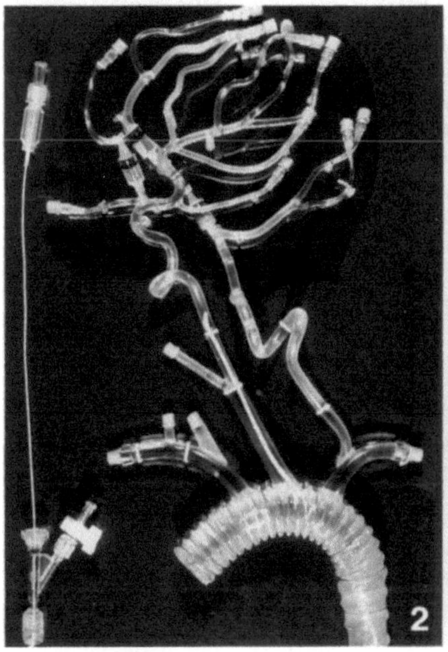

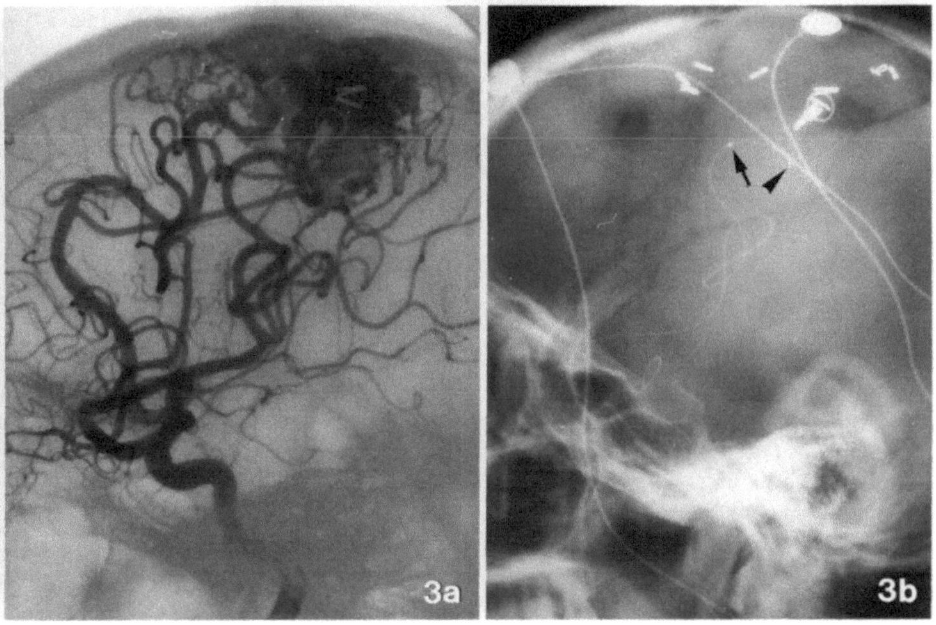

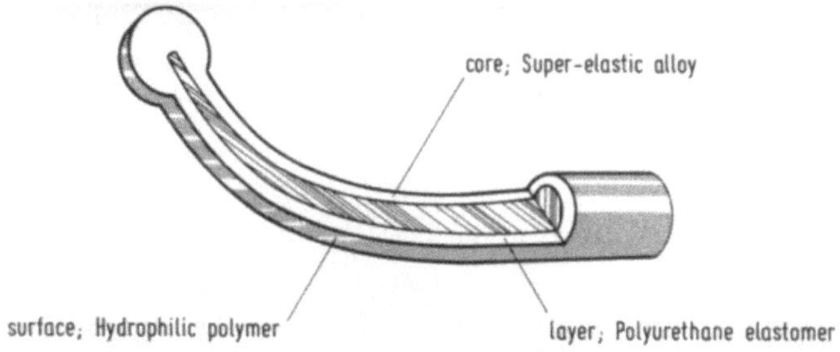

4

Fig. 1. Design and inner structure of 0.016 inch hydrophilic polymer-coated guide wire

Fig. 2. Vascular model of human cerebral arteries and aorta

Fig. 3. **a** Main feeders from anterior and middle cerebral arteries are very tortuous. **b** Selective cannulation into the central artery. *Arrow,* Tip of the guide wire; *arrowhead,* tip of the catheter. **c** Control angiography showing minimal residual nidus (stereo)

Fig. 4. Inner structure of the latest model of the hydrophilic polymer-coated guide wire

More recent advances have involved removing the gold ring to make the very tip more supple and placement of a small hydrophilic polymer-coated ball in order to prevent perforation of a vessel wall (Fig. 4). The radio-opacity of the tip was maintained by a platinum-containing layer of the ball.

References

1. Goto K (1988) Cerebral and cranial artery navigation without using a leak balloon – a new combination of a low-friction high torque guide wire and a thin supple catheter. AJNR 9: 1988
2. Pinto RS, Robbins E, Seidenwurm D (1989) Thrombogenicity of teflon versus copolymer-coated guide wires: evaluation with scanning electron microscopy. AJNR 10: 407–410

Dr. K. Goto
Department of Interventional Neuroradiology
The Center for Central Nervous Diseases
Iizuka Hospital
3-83 Yoshio-machi
Iizuka 820, Japan

Neuroradiology (1991) 33 [Suppl]: 638–639

Neuro-radiology
© Springer-Verlag 1991

Digital subtraction myelography of the cervical spine

P. H. Hoogland and H. W. Bodewes

Department of Radiology, Westeinde Hospital, The Hague, The Netherlands

Summary. In a consecutive series of 35 patients with clinical signs of a cervical radicular syndrome, real-time digital subtraction was used in the evaluation of intraspinal pulsations and results were compared with conventional myelography. Results were comparable; however, additional information was obtained by digital subtraction. Absence or reduction of root movement correlated with root deformities on conventional myelography. In 1 patient reduction of root movement in otherwise normal conventional myelography correlated with the clinically entrapped root, which was surgically confirmed.

Key words: Cervical myelography – Digital subtraction – Root pulsations – Radiculopathy – Spinal stenosis

Cervical myelography is still a frequently used examination method in patients presenting with cervical radiculopathy. It yields a good impression of the cervical roots and is in general a sensitive method for detecting the level of the radiculopathy [1].

Application of digital subtraction to cervical myelography allows the detection of flow of contrast medium intrathecally and demonstrates cerebrospinal fluid (CSF) and root pulsations, features hardly mentioned in literature and only in fluoroscopy [2, 3].

Patients and methods

Thirty-five patients with clinical signs of cervical radiculopathy were studied and we compared the results of conventional myelography (CM) and cervical myelography using digital subtraction. Cervical myelography was performed after intrathecal introduction of 10 ml contrast medium (Omnipaque 300) via a lateral C1–2 puncture. Digital subtraction was performed during intrathecal contrast injection and followed by plain films. The examinations were performed on a Siemens Angiotron (image frequency 50–60/s, matrix 512 × 512, spatial resolution 2.1 line pairs/mm). CM and digital subtraction myelography (DSM) were reviewed for cervical root deformities and spinal canal stenosis; DSM was additionally reviewed for its dynamic qualities. Movement of roots and CSF pulsations were both examined.

Results

The foremost advantage of DSM is a clear visualisation of the dynamic phenomena in the cervical spine. Three separate movements can be distinguished: pulsations of cord

Fig. 1. **a** Normal conventional myelography of patient with right-sided radiculopathy. **b** Digital subtraction of same patient. No subtraction artefact of fixed root

Fig. 2. **a** Conventional myelography of patient with left-sided radiculopathy. Root deformities on both sides at two levels. **b** Same patient. Digital subtraction shows root deformities (→) and spinal stenosis (→)

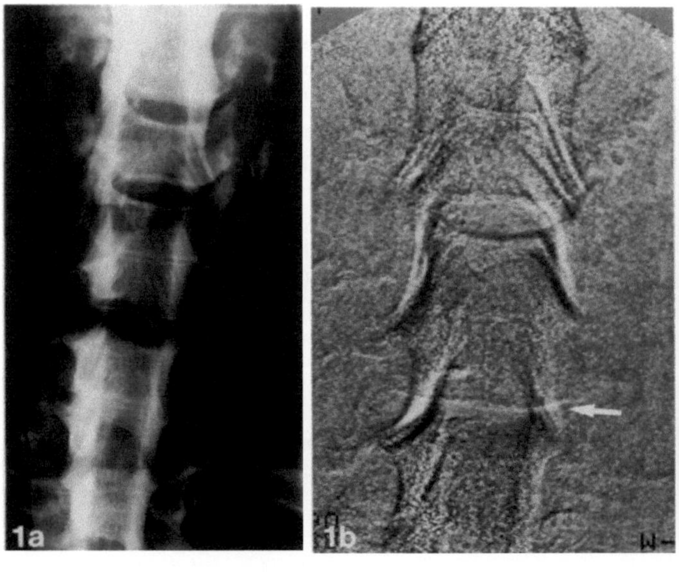

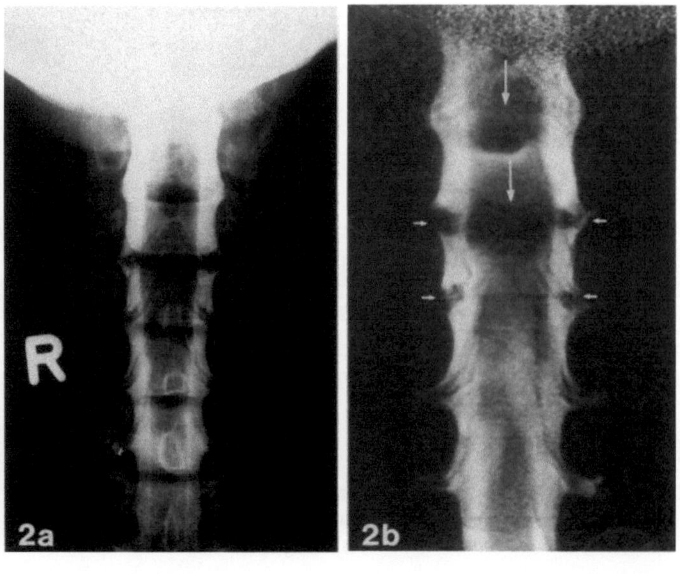

and roots, pulse waves in CSF (both related to the cardiac cycle) and a third movement that is less clearly detectable, synchronous with respiration and related to central venous pressure changes.

Consequently we were able to detect normal cord and root movements and normal CSF pulse waves as well. In 13 of 35 patients with a normal CM, digital subtraction permitted the detection of normal cord and root movements; CSF flow was readily demonstrated using real-time subtraction during contrast injection. Twenty-seven roots in 19 patients showed root deformities on CM and showed reduced or absent movement on the dynamic study of the same roots. Neurosurgical exploration of 12 roots in 10 patients yielded in 4 patients a herniated disc and in 8 patients osteophytes caused the deformities. In 2 patients with normal CM, DSM showed decreased movement of the clinically related root in comparison to contralateral, upper and lower roots. One of these 2 patients was operated upon, and a severely embedded and fixed root was found (Fig. 1). After intervention there was an uneventful recovery. In 8 patients decreased CSF pulsations at 14 levels correlated clearly with severe spinal stenosis found on CM (Fig. 2); however, 9 patients with a less severe stenosis on CM showed normal CSF pulsations.

Discussion

In cervical myelography additional information can be gained by digital subtraction. Diminished or absent root movement correlates with root deformities [2]. We were able to distinguish two separate phenomena in the cervical spine, which are both related to and synchronous with the cardiac cycle. In our opinion the first phenomenon, movement of cord and attached roots, is related to the direct systolic expansion of the brain, causing a downward shift of the cord and attached roots. The second phenomenon is a pulse wave in the CSF, particularly clearly observed during contrast injection. This CSF pulse wave is generated by conductance of intracranial and intraspinal arterial expansion to the CSF [3]. Absent or diminished root movement, while surrounding roots show normal movements and in otherwise normal myelography, in our opinion, can be a strong indication of pathology of this root. Decreased CSF pulsations at a particular level can indicate severe spinal stenosis. Besides better visualisation of separate roots [4], DSM can yield additional information; in particular, it permits a dynamic view in the analysis of root compression.

References

1. Modic MT, Masaryk TJ, Mulopulos GP, Bundschuh C, Han JS, Bohlman H (1986) Cervical radiculopathy: prospective evaluation with surface coil MR Imaging, CT with metrizamide and metrizamide myelography. Radiology 161: 753–759
2. Fox AJ, Lin JP, Pinto RS, Kricheff II (1975) Myelographic cervical nerve root deformities. Radiology 116: 355–361
3. Lane B, Kricheff II (1974) Cerebrospinal fluid pulsations at myelography: a videodensometric study. Radiology 110: 579–587
4. Voigt K, Vogl G (1988) Radikulographie in digitaler Subtraktionstechnik. Radiologe 28: 507–510

Dr. P. H. Hoogland
Department of Radiology
Westeinde Hospital
Lijnbaan 32
2512 VA The Hague
The Netherlands

Neuroradiology (1991) 33 [Suppl]: 640–641

Neuro radiology
© Springer-Verlag 1991

Dynamic imaging of cerebrospinal fluid leaks: localisation of fistulae by digital subtraction cisternography

D. MacVicar, J. V. Byrne, C. E. Ingram, and F. Sullivan

Department of Neuroradiology, Atkinson Morley's Hospital, London SW20, UK

Summary. Precise anatomical localisation of the site of cerebrospinal fluid (CSF) leakage is a notoriously difficult problem. Staining of nasal pledgets by dyes or radionuclides introduced into the subarachnoid space by lumbar puncture has proved a useful method of confirming CSF leakage, but has largely been replaced by computed tomographic positive contrast cisternography (CTC). However, since CT is essentially a static technique, visualisation of contrast within a fistulous track is usually fortuitous. We have performed fluoroscopy during intrathecal injection of radiographic contrast prior to CT and used digital subtraction of the video signal to visualise fistulae directly in patients with CSF leaks. Digital subtraction cisternography provides valuable information with no significant additional morbidity.

Key words: Cerebrospinal fluid fistula – Cisternography – Computed tomography – Digital subtraction

Computed tomographic cisternography (CTC) is generally accepted as the technique of choice in the investigation of patients with cerebrospinal fluid (CSF) leaks [1–3]. Iodinated contrast medium is injected intrathecally by lumbar puncture and high-resolution CT of the skull base and sinuses is performed. While a leak can frequently be confirmed by the presence of contrast medium in the sinuses, the site of the fistula must often be inferred from the pattern of their contamination. A method has recently been described which may directly demonstrate leaks by continuous fluoroscopy during the injection of contrast medium and subsequent digital subtraction of the recorded video signal [4]. We report our method of digital subtraction cisternography (DSC) and experience in ten patients.

Patients and methods

Ten patients were studied by DSC followed by CTC. Six had posttraumatic rhinorrhoea, four were postsurgical and all had current or recent leaks. No specific premedication is used. The patient is positioned prone on a screening table with the head immobilised in a movable craniostat with the clivus horizontal. Lateral cervical puncture with a 22-gauge spinal needle is performed and iohexol 240 injected with continuous lateral fluoroscopy until contrast medium reaches the rostral limit of the anterior cranial fossa floor. The video signal is recorded for subsequent digital subtraction (IDIS mobile unit, Quantel).

The patient is transferred in the prone position for direct coronal CT and then turned supine for axial images.

Results

Fistulae were directly visualised by DSC in eight patients and in seven patients the sites of leakage were confirmed at surgery. The technique facilitated interpretation of CTC in all positive studies and in two patients provided information which could not be deduced from CTC alone. Patients' details and the imaging/surgical findings are summarised in Table 1.

Discussion

In order to justify using DSC the technique must provide diagnostic information superior to that of CTC alone. Our results show that direct visualisation of fistulae can be achieved in the majority (8/10) of examinations, whereas direct visualisation was possible by CTC in only three patients.

Furthermore, interpretation of CTC was easier when data from the combined technique were evaluated together. For example, in case 1, CTC showed a defect in the pituitary fossa floor and contrast medium in sphenoid and ethmoid sinuses. This study alone could have been misinterpreted as ethmoidal contamination secondary to the sellar fistula. However, DSC clearly showed two fistulae, the second being through the floor of the anterior cranial fossa directly into the ethmoid air cells.

DSC was particularly helpful in studying patients with large fistulae. Contrast medium leaked rapidly through the fistula. In these patients, most of whom developed CSF rhinorrhea after surgery to the skull base, the fistula could be clearly demonstrated by DSC, whereas contrast medium was widely distributed and interpretation of CTC alone was difficult.

The technique thus provided additional information without the introduction of a second invasive procedure. Although transient headache was experienced during the procedure, no serious side-effects were observed and the increase in radiation dose was considered clinically justifiable.

Table 1. Summary of digital subtraction cisternography (DSC), computed tomographic cisternography (CTC) and surgical findings in ten patients investigated for cerebrospinal fluid (CSF) rhinorrhoea

Case	Age/sex	Previous surgery	DSC findings			CTC findings			Surgical findings
			CSF leak	Fistula visualised	Site	CSF leak	Fistula visualised	Site	
Post-traumatic rhinorrhoea									
1	47/M	Anterior fossa repair	Yes	Yes (2 sites)	Cribriform sella	Yes	Yes (1 site)	Sella	Yes
2	62/F	Anterior fossa repair	Yes	Yes	Frontal sinus	Yes	No	Frontal sinus	Yes
3	42/M	Anterior fossa repair	No	–	–	No	–	Petrous	Yes
4	51/M	None	Yes	Yes	Petrous	Yes	Yes	Petrous	Yes
5	39/F	None	Yes	Yes	Cribriform	Yes	Yes	Cribriform	Yes
6	57/F	None	Yes	Yes	Cribriform	Yes	No	Cribriform	No
Postoperative rhinorrhoea									
7	40/M	Transphenoidal hypophysectomy	No	No	–	Yes	No	Staining of nasal pleglets	No
8	64/M	Orbital clearance and cranioplasty	Yes	Yes	Cranioplasty	Yes	No	Orbit and frontal sinus	Yes
9	67/M	Orbital clearance and ethmoidectomy	Yes	Yes	Optic nerve sheath	Yes	No	Orbit	Yes
10	39/M	Resection of infra-temporal tumour	Yes	Yes	Middle fossa floor	Yes	No	Operative cavity and antrum	Yes

The combined technique is therefore recommended for the investigation of patients with recurrent and postoperative rhinorrhoea and when CTC alone fails to identify the fistula.

References

1. Manelfe C, Guiraud B, Tremoulet M (1977) Diagnosis of CSF rhinorrhea by computerised cisternography using metrizamide. Lancet II: 1073
2. Naidich TP, Moram CJ (1980) Precise anatomic localisation of atraumatic sphenoethmoidal cerebrospinal fluid rhinorrhea by metrizamide CT cisternography. J Neurosurg 53: 222–228
3. Chow JM, Goodman D, Mafee MF (1989) Evaluation of CSF rhinorrhea by computerised tomography with metrizamide. Otolaryngol Head Neck Surg 100: 99–105
4. Takahashi T, Mutsuga N, Aoki T, Handa T, Tanoi C, Yoshida J, Kobayashi T (1988) Localisation of dural fistulas using metrizamide digital subtraction fluoroscopic cisternography. J Neurosurg 68: 721–725

Dr. D. MacVicar
Department of Neuroradiology
Atkinson Morley's Hospital
Copse Hill
London SW20, UK

Neuroradiology (1991) 33 [Suppl]: 642–644

Neuroradiology

© Springer-Verlag 1991

Trigeminal neuralgia: indication for MRI?

D. Wimberger[2], J. Kramer[2], L. Prayer[2], R. Stiglbauer[2], and H. Imhof[2]

Departments of [1] Neurology, [2] Radiodiagnosis, MRI Institute, University of Vienna, Vienna, Austria

Summary. Forty-one patients with trigeminal symptoms affecting at least two divisions and variable involvement of other cranial nerves were examined with MRI. In 32 cases (78%) pathological findings occurred; 9 examinations (22%) were normal. Among 25 histologically verified cases only 1 was misdiagnosed. Thus accuracy and specificity suggest the use of MRI as a primary diagnostic tool in patients with this clinical picture.

Key words: Magnetic resonance imaging – Trigeminal nerve – Gasserian ganglion

About 25% of clinical trigeminal lesions involve the Gasserian ganglion or the preganglionic segment [1]. Other cranial nerves, arterial vessels and the cavernous sinus have close anatomical relationships to the trigeminal nerve in this region [2]. Most of these structures can be identified on thin-slice MR images.

Patients and methods

In 41 patients (16 men, 25 women), aged from 19 to 85 years (mean 33.3 years), the selection criteria were: symptoms from at least two trigeminal divisions and variable involvement of other cranial nerves. MRI was performed using a 1.5 T superconducting system and, T1-weighted (TR 700 ms/TE 15 ms) and T2-weighted (TR 2500 ms/TE 15.70 ms) axial and coronal images obtained, slice thickness 3 mm without intersection gap, with administration of 0.1 mmol gadolinium-DTPA/kg body weight.

Results

MR diagnoses are listed in Table 1; tumours are detailed in Table 2. Histological verification was obtained in 25 cases: 24 MR diagnoses were correct, 1 wrong: an epidermoid was mistaken for an arachnoid cyst because it gave signals identical to those of cerebrospinal fluid (CSF). Sixteen cases were not verified.

Discussion

The high percentage (78%) of pathological MRI findings results from our selection criteria. The variety of aetiologies is caused by the different anatomical structures of the region examined. Nerves, vessels, meninges and bones may be the origin of pathological processes [3].

Tumours originating from nerve sheaths (5 meningiomas, 3 neurinomas) were the most frequent neoplastic lesions (Fig. 1). This has also been observed by other authors [1, 4]. Pituitary adenomas are known to involve the cavernous sinus frequently [5]. Nevertheless the incidence of clinical cavernous syndromes, consisting of eye muscle palsies and trigeminal pain, in pituitary adenomas has not been reported up to now. Our 5 cases with pituitary adenomas presented clinical complaints due to cavernous syndromes. Nerve sheath tumours and pituitary adenomas could be differentiated from each other by imaging criteria concerning origin, signal characteristics and enhancement [3, 4]. With 1 exception, rare neoplasms did not have similar imaging features to the tumours mentioned above. Only a lymphoma imitated signals and enhancement of a neuroma (Fig. 2). De Pena et al. [6] observed a similar case. Meningeal involvement was seen in 3 patients with primary facial tumours. Supported by histological findings, Woodruff et al. [7] proposed that the mechanism of propagation in these cases is perineural extension. MRI provides information about

Table 1. MR diagnoses in patients with trigeminal neuralgia

MR diagnoses	Number of patients	(n = 41)
Neoplasm	$n = 17^a$	
Vascular structure	$n = 5$	
Cyst	$n = 4$	Pathological:
Meningiosis	$n = 3$	32 cases (78%)
Scar	$n = 2$	
Demyelinisation	$n = 1$	
No lesion found	$n = 9$	Normal: 9 cases (22%)

[a] Patient with Recklinghausen's disease had neuromas on both sides

Table 2. Types of tumour

Tumour	Number of patients	(n = 17)
Pituitary adenoma	$n = 5$	
Meningioma	$n = 5$	
Neuroma	$n = 2^a$	(Fig. 1)
Lymphoma	$n = 1$	(Fig. 2)
Chondroma	$n = 1$	
Chordoma	$n = 1$	
Teratoma	$n = 1$	
Histiocytosis X	$n = 1$	

[a] Patient with Recklinghausen's disease had neurinomas on both sides

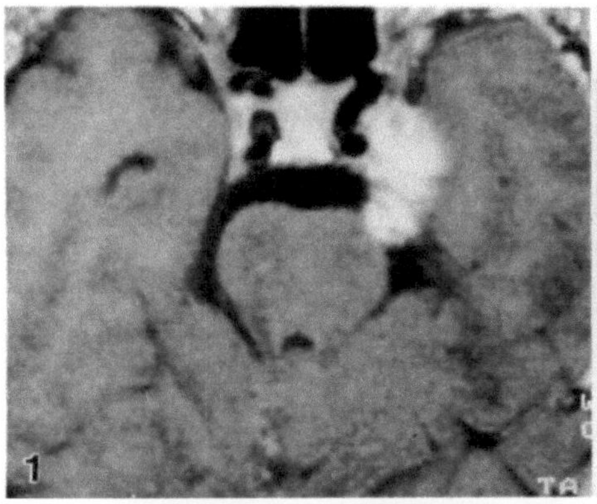

Fig. 1. A 50-year-old male patient with increasing trigeminal neuralgia on the left side of several months duration and including all three divisions. T1-weighted enhanced axial image. Trigeminal neuroma, originating from the Gasserian ganglion, with marked contrast enhancement

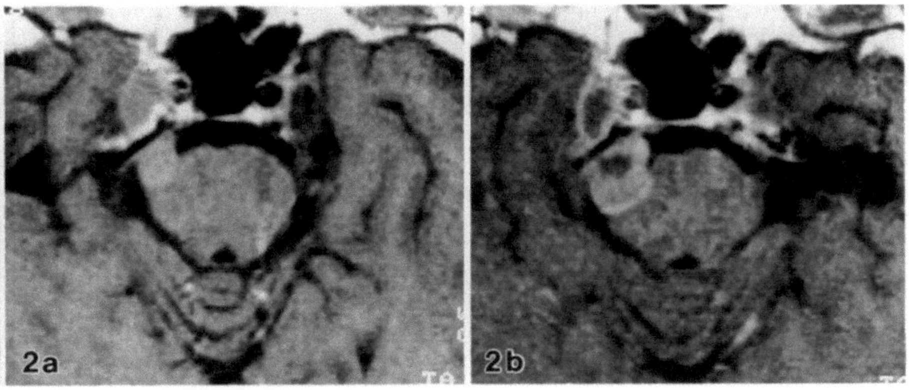

Fig. 2 a, b. A 68-year-old male patient with known extra-CNS lymphoma, sudden onset of a paratrigeminal syndrome on the right side. T1-weighted enhanced axial images. **a** Lymphomatous involvement of the right Gasserian ganglion and preganglionic segment, which is thickened and enhances with contrast medium. **b** After 3 weeks of radiation therapy and intrathecal methotrexate administration: central necrosis and extension of the lesion, remaining marginal contrast enhancement

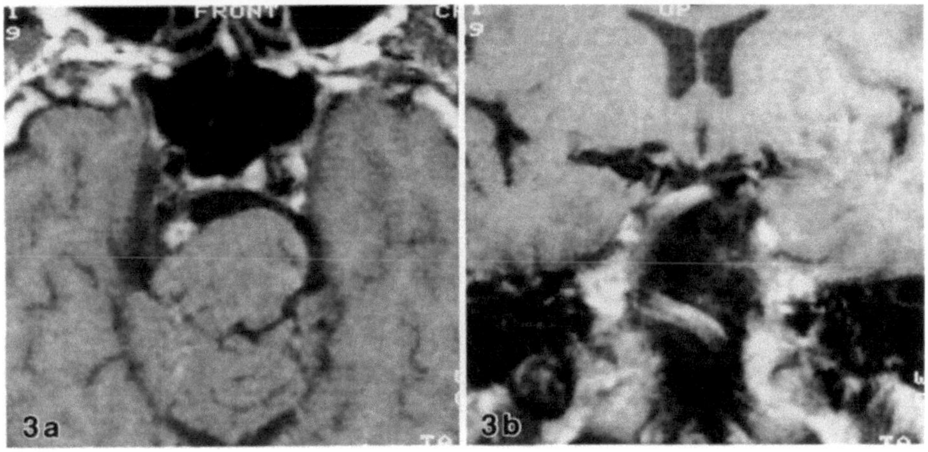

Fig. 3 a, b. A 59-year-old male patient with trigeminal neuralgia in the second and third divisions of the right side refractory to therapy. **a** T1-weighted axial image. Hyperintense cross-section of a vessel, compressing and displacing the root entry zone of the right trigeminal nerve. **b** T1-weighted coronal image. Widened and tortuous basilar artery with signs of slow flow

the exact extent of meningeal involvement, which is of interest for tumour staging.

Vascular compression was recognized as one of the major factors in the genesis of trigeminal neuralgia even before MRI was available [8, 9]. MRI clearly shows the anatomical relationships between vessel and nerve, and thus proves the vascular contact causing the clinical symptoms (Fig. 3) [10].

Mucocoeles can easily be identified on MRI because of their hyperintense T1-weighted signal, related to the protein content. Epidermoids can give CSF isointense signals in spite of their cholesterol content. Thus they may be misdiagnosed as arachnoid cysts [4].

Among the unverified cases there were 4 patients with multiple sclerosis and 1 patient with lupus erythematosus whose MRI was normal. In these cases the existence of lesions had to be assumed because of the history and the convincing clinical signs. In our opinion demyelinating or inflammatory lesions affecting the preganglionic segment may be overlooked by MRI because of the isointense surrounding CSF. The only demyelinating lesion we identified affected the root entry zone and extended to the pons.

Conclusion

The accuracy of MRI in identifying lesions affecting the Gasserian ganglion or the preganglionic segment (78% pathological findings) suggests that MRI should be the diagnostic tool of choice to examine patients with trigeminal complaints concerning at least two divisions. High specifity (only 1 case was misinterpreted) underlines this suggestion.

Acknowledgement. Supported in part by the Ludwig-Boltzmann-Institute of Radiophysical Tumour Diagnosis.

References

1. Hutchins LG, Hamsberger HR, Hardin CW, Dillon WP, Smoker WRK, Osborn AG (1989) The radiologic assessment of trigeminal neuropathy. AJNR 10: 1031–1038
2. Yasui T, Hakuba A, Soo Han K, Nishimura S (1989) Trigeminal neurinomas: operative approach in eight cases. J Neurosurg 71: 506–511
3. Kapila A, Chakeres DW, Blanco E (1984) The meckel cave: computed tomography study. Radiology 152: 425–433
4. Yuh WTC, Wright DC, Barloon TJ, Schultz DH, Yutaka S, Cervantes CA (1988) MR imaging of primary tumors of trigeminal nerve and meckel's cave. AJNR 9: 665–670
5. Scotti G, Chin-Yin Y, Dillon WP, Norman D, Colombo N, Newton TH, De Groot J, Wilson CB (1988) MR imaging of cavernous sinus involvement by pituitary adenomas. AJNR 9: 657–664
6. De Pena CA, Ya-Yen L, Van Tassel B (1989) Lymphomatous involvement of the trigeminal nerve and meckel cave: CT and MR appearance. AJNR 10: 15–17

7. Woodruff WW, Yeates AE, McLendon AE (1986) Perineural tumor extension to the cavernous sinus from superficial facial carcinoma: CT manifestations. Radiology 161: 395–399
8. De Lange EE, Vielvoye GJ, Voormolen JHC (1986) Arterial compression of the fifth cranial nerve causing trigeminal neuralgia: angiographic findings. Radiology 158: 721–727
9. Chung JW, Chang KH, Han MH, Kim BH, Song CS (1988) Computed tomography of cavernous sinus diseases. Neuroradiology 30: 319–328
10. Tash RT, Sze G, Leslie DR (1989) Trigeminal neuralgia: MR imaging features. Radiology 172: 767–770

Dr. Daniela Wimberger
Department of Neurology
University of Vienna
Lazarettgasse 14
A-1090 Vienna, Austria

Neuroradiology (1991) 33 [Suppl]: 645–646

Neuro radiology
© Springer-Verlag 1991

Computer aid in the interpretation of CT images of the head*

D. Teather[1], B. A. Teather[1], K. M. Wills[1], D. Plummer[2], and G. H. du Boulay[3]

[1] Medical Systems Research Centre, Leicester Polytechnic, Leicester, UK
[2] Department of Medical Physics, University College Hospital, London, UK [3] Institute of Neurology, Queen Square, London, UK

Summary. This paper describes the authors' experience in designing and constructing a statistically based computer advisor for CT. The modular PC system gives rapid access to statistical information, expert knowledge, textual explanations and reference diagrams and may offer considerable training benefits in radiology.

Key words: Expert system – Statistical diagnosis – Cerebral disease

CT advisor system

A prototype comptuer system (BRAINS) to aid in the interpretation of CT images for the diagnosis of cerebral disease, archiving of disease-related information and training in image interpretation has been developed by the authors [1, 2]. The BRAINS system represents one result of a long-term collaborative research program involving statisticians, computer scientists and radiologists [3–5] at the three institutions.

The system prompts the user to describe "abnormalities" visible on CT images. On the basis of the scan description, advice may be requested on diagnosis and the likely effect on diagnosis of "enhancement" of some tissues by injection of contrast medium. The description is entered by means of menus that form a tree-like structure. "HELP" is available in the form of textual explanations for all questions and options. A reference set of diagrams and images has been established to illustrate the various signs which may appear in the images. If diagnostic advice is sought, the system is able to indicate those signs which have provided evidence for the disease predicted, together with any that significantly conflict. The full system has been implemented on the Independent Display Console (IC) produced by International General Electric and additionally on a variety of PCs. The PC implementation currently displays reference diagrams but not images.

BRAINS: system design

In designing the system we have sought to provide more than a simple diagnostic advisor programmed to relate only to the case in hand. The statistical, textual, reference image/diagram databases may be accessed independently; thus the system may detail background and comparative information to the practising clinical radiologist and provide an accessible source of information for training.

Diagnostic advice provided by the system is statistically based and given in terms of 28 disease categories [3, 5]. The model used to provide disease predictions has been derived by extensive data analysis of 1500 cases with confirmed diagnoses and the acquisition of medical knowledge regarding which features might differentiate certain disease processes. The necessity of utilising hard statistical data in the calibration of subjective clinical judgements has been noted in both this and other applications [5, 6].

The need for an efficient means of interaction with the radiologist, requiring only minimal typing skills, led us to design a simple menu-based interface with a standard format for all dialogue screens [2]. The availability of an extensive range of HELP facilities provides an interface that is suitable for users with differing levels of computing and radiological expertise. Ease in use and in initial learning were paramount considerations in menu design and layout.

The system comprises a number of distinct modules of programme code allowing easy and rapid revision of the computer software [1, 7]. All textual information (menus, HELP etc.) is stored on computer file and may be edited to accommodate local variations in terminology without the necessity of reprogramming. The system could readily be translated into other national languages. The statistical data and model used to provide advice are also represented in text files to permit fine tuning of the advisor.

We have sought wherever possible to increase flexibility by separation of program code from the data and information that are manipulated. This design strategy will, for example, allow us to investigate alternative user interfaces [7].

BRAINS: evaluation results

A prototype system was first made available at the National Hospital for Nervous Diseases, for preliminary testing and evaluation in 1986. Subsequently, in 1987, the system underwent a major upgrade and was transferred to an "external" (i.e. previously unassociated) site for a rigo-

* This work was funded in part by grants from International General Electric, the Department of Health (STD) and the Polytechnic Central Funding Council

rous evaluation of acceptability and utility [7]. This external evaluation study involved eight radiologists of differing experience and two radiographers describing the plain CT studies of up to 20 cases.

The response of external users to the system was mixed. Many were unfamiliar with the concept of formal description of images which underlies the BRAINS system. It is essential that new users are made aware of the concepts underlying the system and the importance of accessing HELP facilities to clarify the use of different descriptors.

In general, users were slow to gain confidence in interacting with the system. We had underestimated the extent to which training would be required. It became apparent that users benefited greatly from person-to-person training with regular feedback and discussion. Such feedback greatly improved user confidence and performance in obtaining accurate descriptions.

Users reported positively on the educational benefit of the structured approach required to describe images. The training potential of the system was recognised by all users and this led us to develop a stand-alone PC system giving access to statistical data, help text, diagrams, diagnostic and enhancement advice.

The accuracy and reliability of the diagnostic advice is comparable to that of a trained neuroradiologist in the commoner cerebral diseases for which CT is performed. Interpretive performance from images of rare conditions will continue to improve as the archived database grows. Current work will provide helpful distinctions between gliomas of different grades of malignancy.

The PC implementation requires a 640K micro with 20 Mb hard disk and VGA monitor. The total disc space requirement for the program code, data/text files and diagrams is approximately 3.5 Mb. Response time is very acceptable, even on microcomputers of limited power.

The modular nature of the system also allows us to make subsets of the system available on small laptops and to provide a "shell" for the implementation of advisor systems for other imaging modalities.

The development of modular systems giving rapid access to statistical information, expert knowledge, textual explanations and reference diagrams and image sets could offer considerable benefits in radiology, particularly in training.

References

1. Teather D, Morton BA, du Boulay GH, Wills KM, Plummer D, Innocent PR (1985) Computer assistance for CT scan interpretation and cerebral disease diagnosis. Stat Med 4: 311–315
2. Plummer D, Teather D, Morton BA, Wills KM, du Boulay GH (1985) The development and assessment of a computer aid for use in the diagnosis of cerebral disease. Proceedings of the 9th International Conference on information processing in medical imaging, Washington DC, pp 310–324
3. Wills KM, du Boulay GH, Teather D (1981) Initial findings in the computer aided diagnosis of cerebral tumours using CT scan results. Br J Radiol 54: 948–952
4. Morton BA, Teather D, du Boulay GH (1984) Statistical modelling and diagnostic aids. Med Decis Making 4: 339–348
5. du Boulay GH, Teather D, Morton BA, Wills KM, Innocent PR, Plummer D (1987) BRAINS – a computer advisor system to aid in CT scan interpretation and cerebral disease diagnosis. Neuroradiology 29: 196–199
6. Leaper DJ, Horrocks JC, Staniland JR, Dombal FT de (1972) Computer assisted diagnosis of abdominal pain using estimates provided by clinicians. Br Med J 4: 350–354
7. Teather D, Teather BA, Wills KM, du Boulay GH, Plummer D, Isherwood I, Gholkar A (1988) Evaluation of computer advisor in the interpretation of CT images of the head. Neuroradiology 30: 511–517

Prof. D. Teather
Medical Systems Research Unit
School of Computing and Mathematical Sciences
Leicester Polytechnic
P. O. Box 143
Leicester, UK

Neuroradiology (1991) 33 [Suppl]: 647–648

Neuro radiology

© Springer-Verlag 1991

The value of CT-discography in the diagnosis and management of lumbar disc herniation

K. F. Lee[1,5], Y. S. Kim[3], T. K. Smith[2], N. H. Lebwohl[6], J. H. Suh[4], Y. E. Lee[7], and R. DeYoung[2]

Departments of [1] Radiology and [2] Orthopedic Surgery, The University of Texas Health Science Center, Houston, Texas, USA
Departments of [3] Neurosurgery and [4] Radiology, Yonsei University Medical Center, Seoul, Korea
Departments of [5] Radiology, [6] Orthopedic Surgery, and [7] Family Practice, University of Miami School of Medicine, Miami, Florida, USA

Summary. A comparison of the findings on surgical exploration of 105 lumbar discs revealed CT-discography to be more accurate than CT, MRI, myelography, or CT-myelography in the diagnosis of herniated nucleus pulposus (HNP). On the basis of our experience with CT-discography we recommend that this procedure be performed when the diagnosis of HNP is uncertain, or when significant discrepancy between clinical findings and imaging exists, inasmuch as direct visualization of the nucleus pulposus with radial tear or fissure can be best demonstrated on CT-discography. Nineteen patients demonstrated unilateral or incomplete filling of the nucleus pulposus due to compartmentalization (bipartite or tripartite nucleus pulposus) which was readily opacified using a longer inner needle. We believe this accounts in part for the results of our chymopapain treatments, which are better than those of previous reports. The authors caution that intrathecal passage of contrast medium is an absolute contraindication to chymopapain injection.

Key words: CT-discography – Herniated nucleus pulposus – Magnetic resonance imaging – CT-myelography – Discectomy

We have performed CT, MRI, myelography, CT-myelography (myelo-CT) and CT-discography on 69 patients who subsequently underwent 105 discectomies. In this paper we evaluate the comparative accuracy of each imaging modality for disc herniation (HNP).

Materials and methods

This series consists of 43 men (62.3%) and 26 women (37.7%), their mean age being 57.2 years. The indications for disc surgery included: low back pain, radicular pain, objective neurological deficit, positive straight-leg-raising test, and failure of conservative treatment for 1 month or longer, in addition to positive imaging tests (CT, MRI, myelography, myelo-CT, and CT-discography). High resolution imaging techniques employed were CT (GE-9800) with 1.5-mm slice thickness and multiplanar reformatted images and MRI (1.5 T Signa, GE) with 3-mm slice thickness in addition to lumbar myelography using a 22 gauge needle with intrathecal injection of 14 ml iohexol (Omnipaque) in a concentration of 180 mg I/ml. Each of the five radiological studies was read without knowledge of the results or clinical information. HNP were divided into bulging, protrusion, extrusion and sequestration.

Results

The diagnostic yields of the five imaging modalities in the 105 disc explorations are shown in Table 1. The bulging disc was adequately demonstrated by all five modalities except 1 overlooked on CT, but since there are only 3 cases in this category statistical analysis is difficult. CT-myelography demonstrated a high degree of accuracy, equal to that of MRI (92.4%). CT-discography showed the highest accuracy in all types of HNP, namely disc bulging, protrusion, extrusion, and sequestration (94.3%).

The pain response at the time of discography was 89.5% (94/105).

Table 1. Diagnostic yields of various imaging modalities on lumbar disc herniation (105 disc explorations)

Type of HNP	Disc no.	CT	Myelography	Myelo-CT	MRI	Disco-CT
Bulging	3	2 (66.7)	3 (100.0)	3 (100.0)	3 (100.0)	3 (100.0)
Protrusion	21	17 (80.9)	18 (85.7)	19 (90.5)	18 (85.7)	10 (90.5)
Extrusion	59	50 (84.7)	48 (81.3)	55 (93.2)	55 (93.2)	56 (94.9)
Sequestration	23	17 (73.9)	16 (69.5)	20 (87.0)	21 (91.3)	21 (91.3)
	105	86 (81.9)	85 (80.9)	97 (92.4)	97 (92.4)	99 (94.3)

HNP, Herniated nucleus pulposus

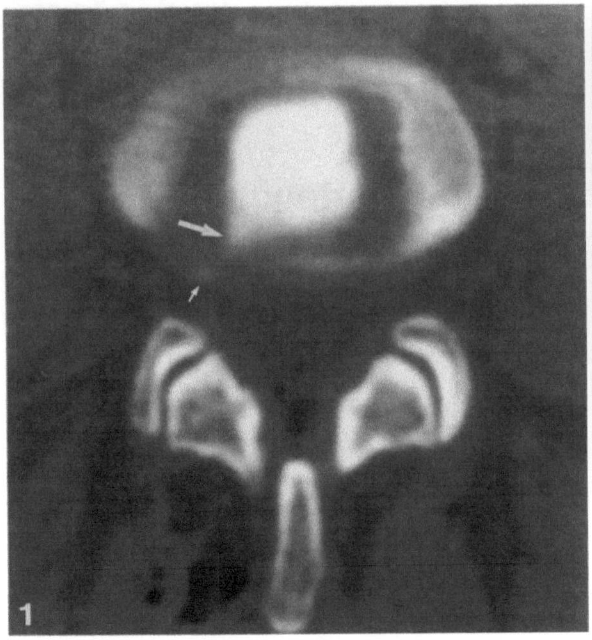

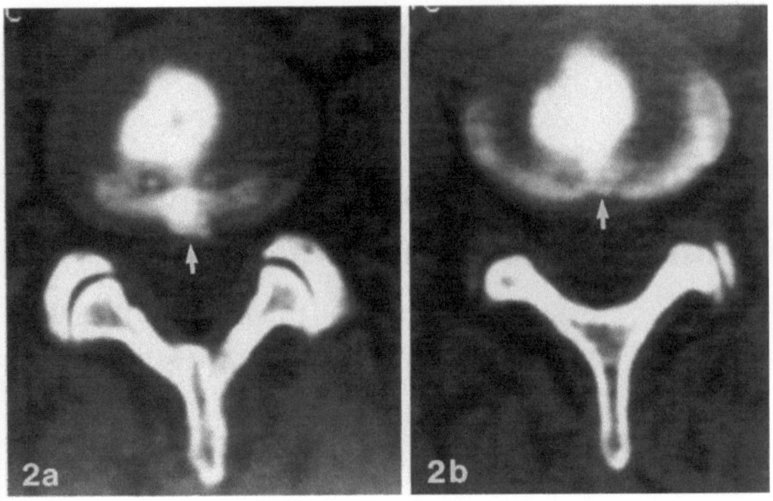

Fig. 1. A small laterally extruded disc *(small arrow)*, associated with a radial tear of the annulus *(large arrow)* is noted on CT-discogram

Fig. 2 a, b. Two CT-discographic images (1.5 mm thickness); **a** demonstrates the protruded disc better than **b** *(arrow)*

Discussion

No topic in radiology has caused more controversy than discography [1, 2]. Discography, has however, recently gained support with the publication of the North American Spine Society "position statement" favoring its use [3]. With a specially designed coaxial needle set (3.5 in. long 18-gauge outer needle and 6–7 in. long 22-gauge inner needle), one can place the tip of the needle more accurately and safely without damaging the perineural structures, including the exiting nerve. Nonionic isotonic contrast medium has been used for the disc distention test in order to avoid a pain response from irritant conventional contrast media. Poor pain response was noted when the nucleus pulposus was not well filled, especially when the HNP was calcified or ossified. So-called "sequestrated" discs could be opacified during discography while other diagnostic modalities failed to distinguish migrated extruded discs from true sequestrated discs in 9 instances. A small, laterally extruded disc was detected only by CT-discography (Fig. 1). Unless thin section (1.5 mm) CT were performed, a small central HNP might have been overlooked (Fig. 2). Although MRI is at least as reliable as CT-discography in the identification of herniated and degenerate disc [4, 5], it does not provide the ability to distinguish painful from asymptomatic levels. In addition, because of its higher resolution, CT has been shown to be more accurate for detection of small annular tears [6]. MRI abnormalities can be found in more than 20% of lumbar spine examinations in asymptomatic individuals [7]. The significance of the pain response, rather than the radiographic appearance, is well demonstrated in the study by Collhoun et al. [8].

Nineteen patients (15.2%) demonstrated compartmentalization of the nucleus pulposus (bipartite or tripartite septation) which was readily opacified with the use of a longer (7 in.) inner needle. We believe this accounts in part for the results (92%) of chemonucleolysis in our hands, as compared with previous reports [9, 10].

References

1. Holt EP Jr (1968) The question of lumbar discography. J Bone Joint Surg [Am] 50: 720–726
2. Simmons JW, Aprill CN, Dwyer AP, Brodsky AE (1988) Clin Orthop 237: 120–124
3. Executive Committee of the North American Spine Society (1988) Position statement on discography. Spine 13: 1343
4. Linson MA, Crowe CH (1990) Comparison of magnetic resonance imaging and lumbar discography in the diagnosis of disc degeneration. Clin Orthop 250: 160–163
5. Gibson MJ, Buckley J, Mawhinney R (1986) Magnetic resonance imaging and discography in the diagnosis of disc degeneration. A comparison study of 50 discs. J Bone Joint Surg [Br] 68: 369–373
6. Zucherman J, Derby R, Hsu K (1988) Normal magnetic resonance imaging with abnormal discography. Spine 13: 1355–1359
7. Boden SD, Davis DO, Dina TS (1990) Abnormal magnetic resonance scans of the lumbar spine in asymptomatic subjects. J Bone Joint Surg [Am] 72: 403–409
8. Collhoun E, McCall IW, Williams L (1988) Provocative discography as a guide to planning operations on the spine. J Bone Joint Surg [Br] 70: 267–271
9. Lee KF, Jones SC, Smith TK (1985) The role of CT-discography in the diagnosis of equivocal lumbar disc herniation and chemonucleolysis. Neuroradiology 27: 379
10. Lee KF, Kim YS, Smith TK, Suh JH, DeYoung R (1990) Improved results with CT-discography-guided chemonucleolysis. (in press)

Dr. K. F. Lee
Department of Radiology
The University of Texas Health Science Center
Houston, Texas, USA

Neuroradiology (1991) 33 [Suppl]: 649–650

Neuroradiology

© Springer-Verlag 1991

Using a personal computer data base to track patient profiles in neuroradiology

M. J. Kuhn and W. M. Choat

Department of Radiology, Southern Illinois University School of Medicine, St. John's Hospital, Springfield, IL, USA

Summary. The objective of this project was to facilitate the computerized storage of patient information for neuroradiologic research, educational and clinical purposes. Using Macintosh personal computers at radiologic interpretation stations, a template for entering patient information was created for neuroradiology. This information may at any time be retrieved, sorted, combined, or printed. The neuroradiologist then may easily find individual patients or sets of patients with specific diagnoses or findings or sort and combine an almost limitless assortment of other patient information. Rapid retrieval for research, educational conferences and clinical purposes is easily achieved.

Key words: Computer literacy – Computer simulation – Computer data base – Computer-assisted education

Much of the practice of medicine today is dominated by information processing: recording, retrieving and communicating data [1]. Automation and computerization of a radiologic work station offers many distinct advantages [2]. These include improved organization, increased efficiency and accuracy and the ability to track particular patients or diagnostic groups of patients through time.

Clinically, it is often necessary to follow patients through different stages of their neuroradiologic workup while having a clear understanding of previous examinations and their results. For teaching purposes it is important to be able to find examples of various diagnoses [3]. Conference preparation usually involves recalling recently studied patients. Research needs include the ability to store data securely on a subset of patients, adaptable to diagnostic trends, to determine frequencies of common and unusual diagnoses and to compare findings associated with different diagnoses, to identify and understand new relationships. These functions are readily achieved with this computer program.

Materials and methods

Apple Macintosh SE computers, a laser printer, and ACIUS' 4th dimension data base programs were purchased and strategies for developing the system were developed by a neuroradiologist (M.J.K.) and computer programmer (W.M.C.). A template for tracking patient information was developed, as described below.

The patient's name, date of birth, and medical record number are entered (Table 1) by a standard keyboard or "mouse". Specific information about the radiologic examination may then be entered, including date and type of examination, neuroradiologist, clinical history, diagnosis, findings, referring physician, pathological findings,

Table 1. The three data input screens

SIU Radiology Profile for Smythe, John

Medical Record #	Birth Date	Date of Exam
101456	2/10/61	3/25/90

Radiologist: Kuhn
Type of Exam: MRI

Diagnosis Sub-Speciality: Neuro

Glioblastoma multiforme, butterfly type

[Next Page]
[Accept] [Cancel]

SIU Radiology Profile for Smythe, John

History Referring M.D.: Mack

Seizure this morning. No prior symptoms other than occasional headaches for past few months.

Findings

Large enhancing mass in splenium of corpus callosum extending into both parietal lobes. Mass effect on the adjacent lateral ventricles is seen. No associated calcification of hemorrhage.

[Previous Page] [Next Page]
[Accept] [Cancel]

SIU Radiology Profile for Smythe, John

Pathology Proven? ○ Yes ○ No

Comments

Show at neuroradiology/neurosurgery Grand Rounds on April 19, 1990

Follow-up Date: 6/19/90

[Previous Page]
[Accept] [Cancel]

Table 2. A printed report. This is the "full page report". Other reports are smaller and list less patient information but allow many patients to be listed per page

Patient Profile for Smythe, John

Medical Record Number	Birth Date	
101456	2/10/61	
Radiologist	Referring MD	
Kuhn	Mack	
Exam Date	Exam Type	Sub Specialty
3/25/90	MRI	Neuro

History
Seizure this morning. No prior symptoms other than occasional headaches for past few months.

Diagnosis
Glioblastoma multiforme, butterfly type

Findings
Large enhancing mass in splenium of corpus callosum extending into both parietal lobes. Mass effect on the adjacent lateral ventricles is seen. No associated calcification or hemorrhage.

Comments
Show at neuroradiology/neurosurgery Grand Rounds on April 19, 1990

Follow-Up Date 6/19/90 Pathology Proven? Yes

and any comments. Lists of standard data entries were created and assigned to the particular fields. The person entering the data may select a word or phrase from the displayed list and then add other information as necessary.

Information stored may be viewed at the computer terminal or printed (Table 2) via Apple Talk to the nearby laser printer. Patients may be located by name, diagnosis, findings, date or type of examination, referring physician, clinical history, or comments. In addition the patients may be sorted or combined using multiple criteria.

Results

The data base is currently being used avidly by the neuroradiology division of the Southern Illinois University School of Medicine. The implementation of this data base into our research has decreased the amount of time spent searching for interesting or important cases and made possible more reliable searching techniques. New methods for determining numbers of patients with certain diagnoses, findings and patterns have been achieved. Listing and keeping track of patients in various research study groups are greatly simplified. Follow-up with referring neurologists and neurosurgeons is much more efficient and complete. Pathologic findings are permanently stored with radiologic data for future examination.

Discussion

Due to what is generally accepted as exceptional user-friendliness, Macintosh computers are used in radiology departments for many purposes [4]. Radiologists have always tried to keep track of interesting cases [5] and in this project we have used the Macintosh to great advantage in pursuing this goal. This method is both simple and highly effective. We believe that the relatively small investment required (less than US $ 5,000.00) is cost effective in our practice. Furthermore, the Macintosh computer and laser printer serve admirably in other functions such as word processing and electronic mail communication.

References

1. Barnett O (1990) Computers in medicine. JAMA 263: 2631–2633
2. Arenson RL (1986) Office Automation. Radiol Clin North Am 24: 87–95
3. Pieme TE (1988) Computer-assisted learning and evaluation in medicine. JAMA 260: 367–372
4. Greenes (1986) Computer-aided diagnostic strategy selection. Radiol Clin North Am 24: 105–120
5. Arenson RL (1986) Teaching with computers. Radiol Clin North Am 24: 97–103

Dr. Matthew J. Kuhn
Department of Radiology
St. John's Hospital
800 East Carpenter Street
Springfield, Illinois 62769, USA

Neuroradiology (1991) 33 [Suppl]: 651–652

Neuro radiology
© Springer-Verlag 1991

A new personal-computer-based image transfer system: impact on patient management

J. A. Spencer[1], P. L. Anslow[1], A. J. Molyneux[1], C. S. Barker[1], and D. Dobson[2]

[1] Section of Neuroradiology, The Radcliffe Infirmary, Oxford, UK
[2] Electronic Imaging Ltd., Oxford, UK

Summary. We describe the use of a new personal-computer-based image transfer and storage system in a regional neuroradiology department. The impact on patient management was analysed prospectively for 149 consecutive CT studies transferred by the system. Sixty-eight were of acute neurosurgical cases and a significant change in management resulted in 55 (81%). Seventy-three were sent for a neuroradiological opinion with a significant change in diagnosis or management occurring in 38 cases (52%). Overall 62% of images were transferred during normal working hours. The systems affords prompt specialist advice to clinicians and general radiologists in district hospitals. During the study the savings made by preventing interhospital transfer of head-injured patients for whom urgent neurosurgical care was inappropriate exceeded the costs of the system.

Key words: Image transfer – Computed tomography – Head injury

Transmission of CT images by telephone from district hospitals to their regional neurosurgical centre was introduced in 1984. The "Imtran" system used a video camera to capture images from a CT monitor screen at the "sender" hospital. The system did not gain wide acceptance but did demonstrate its potential [1]. A new system of image transfer by telephone, "Image Link", has been developed in Oxford. Based on an IBM-compatible personal computer, it is able to capture images directly and virtually instantaneously from the video output of all currently available CT systems. Its potential for transfer of high-quality CT images has allowed the provision of specialist radiological advice to these hospitals. The quality of the images transferred has also improved the confidence with which neurosurgical colleagues can offer advice to referring clinicians.

We analysed prospectively the impact of the system on patient management in a regional neuroradiology centre and six district hospitals equipped with "Image Link".

Patients and methods

A total of 149 consecutive CT studies transferred to and from our hospital by "Image Link" was analysed prospectively. The age of the patients ranged from 1 month to 83 years. The diagnoses made by referring clinicians and radiologists and the management plan for each patient prior to image transfer were compared with the scan diagnoses made by a consultant neuroradiologist and the revised management of the patient after neuroradiological and/or neurosurgical advice. The images were transferred predominantly for emergency neurosurgical advice and specialist radiological opinion although a number of useful accessory functions emerged (Table 1).

The "Image Link" system (Electronic Imaging Ltd., Oxford) comprises an IBM "AT"-compatible 16-bit computer with 1 MByte of RAM and a 40 MByte hard disk linked to two video monitors, one for control of text and one for display of images (256 grey scale). Additional purpose designed printed circuit boards are incorporated into the computer for acquisition and display of images. The direct and virtually instantaneous capture of the video output saves time compared with systems using video cameras such as "Imtran". The images are captured at the CT window and level settings chosen by the referring hospital and these cannot be manipulated by the receiver hospital. A complete file of the patient's details and images is stored in the system's hard disk at the "sender" hospital. Images are transferred using an error correcting modem over standard public telephone lines. Each image takes approximately 20 s to transfer (range 16–24 s). There is no discernible loss in image quality during transfer. Once received the images are also stored at the receiving hospital and may be scrolled through individually as in a normal CT examination or be displayed in groups of 4 or 16 images.

The system uses software providing pull-down menus for image capture, storage, transfer and display and will auto-dial and connect with the second system. After capturing the images – no more than a couple of minutes for most studies – the user does not have to oversee the transfer once the system has connected with the receiver hospital.

Results

Of the 149 studies transferred, 68 were of acute neurosurgical referrals with a request for transfer to the Oxford neurosurgical unit. Prior to the installation of "Image Link" it had been standard practice to transfer the patient urgently for CT and neurosurgical evaluation in Oxford. In 55 cases (81%) a significant change in management re-

Table 1. Categories of 149 CT studies transferred by "Image Link" over 4 months

Category	Number	Altering management (%)
Neurosurgical emergency	68	81
Neurosurgical follow-up	6	50
Radiological second opinion	50	56
Radiological primary opinion	23	43
Scanner breakdown	1	100
Postal delay[a]	1	100

[a] A patient referred urgently to neurosurgery outpatients arrived without his CT films; these were sent by "Image Link"

Table 2. Details of cases referred for radiological opinion (73 patients)

Secondary opinions		50
For neuroradiological advice	46	
Sent for advice to CT Body Centre	4	
Outcome		
Diagnosis confirmed		22
Normal	4	
Abnormal	18	
Altered diagnosis or treatment		28
Define abnormality	12	
Angiography advised	4	
Additional/different diagnosis	3	
Additional/different images advised	3	
Biopsy advised	2	
Interval operation advised	2	
Urgent operation	1	
Urgent angiography	1	
Primary opinions		23
Outcome		
Diagnosis confirmed		13
Normal	7	
Abnormal	6	
Altered diagnosis or treatment		10
Different diagnosis	4	
Biopsy	2	
Safety for lumbar puncture determined	2	
Suitability for anticoagulation decided	1	
Operation avoided	1	

sulted. Twenty-nine patients (43%) were not transferred because no neurosurgically treatable lesion was seen and in 25 interval transfer was planned. Six patients were scanned during convalescence at their district hospitals after treatment in Oxford.

Radiological advice was sought on 73 studies. Fifty were for second opinions, 46 sent by general radiologists for the attention of a consultant neuroradiologist. Four abdomino-pelvic studies of patients in the Radcliffe infirmary were sent to our Regional CT Body Scanning Centre for second opinions. In addition 23 studies were sent to the home of a neuroradiologist for advice on studies done out of hours at the Radcliffe Infirmary on current in-patients and emergency admissions. Overall in 38 of the 73 cases (52%) a significant change in diagnosis or management resulted following the advice of a consultant neuroradiologist. Details of these studies are given in Table 2. Of the 149 studies sent over a 4-month period, only 55 (38%) were sent outside normal scanning hours, reflecting extensive daytime use of the system.

Discussion

"Image Link" provides assistance for radiologists and clinicians and has a major impact on patient management. The great value of the system in the management of neurosurgical referrals was expected and is broadly similar to that found in centres which have used the "Imtran" system [1]. Interhospital transfer of comatose head-injured patients is dangerous [2] and should be avoided if at all possible. We believe that the high definition of images received via "Image Link" will further improve the confidence and quality of neurosurgical advice. The savings from ambulance journeys prevented in the study period alone exceeded the costs of the system (£ 7000 approximately). Morbidity and mortality from intracranial haematoma can be reduced from early detection by CT [3]. With the increased availability of CT scanners in district hospitals this diagnosis can be made prior to patient transfer. The impact of "Image Link" on neurosurgical referral and its implications for admission policy and bed use in a neurosurgical centre have been analysed elsewhere [4]. The high quality of the images received following transfer by "Image Link" and the ease of use of the system led to increasing numbers of referrals for radiological opinion during the study: 73 of 149 scans (49%) overall. Limited use of the "Imtran" system for this purpose was partly because of poor-quality imaging, and lack of confidence in the system (Griffiths, personal communication). Our experience with "Image Link" is quite the reverse.

Educational and training opportunities arose from use of the system. Trainees in the receiving centre, exposed to an increased number of acute and problem studies, and general radiologists in the referring hospitals benefited. Some of the latter voiced particular anxieties about head CT. Of the 22 second opinion scans in which the neuroradiologist confirmed the diagnosis, in 18 this was to increase confidence of diagnosis. Advice was also given on aspects of scan technique and imaging protocol. The system has helped to forge links between our unit and its referring district hospitals.

More than 40 "Image Link" systems have been installed in the United Kingdom; centres throughout the country are linked in one network. It seems likely that in time all hospitals will be linked by systems similar to "Image Link". With expansion of teleradiology the radiology departments in each hospital will be linked with viewing stations in their own hospitals, e.g. outpatient clinics. With digital systems for plain film radiography in the wings [5], systems such as "Image Link" will be able to "capture" their output and exploit their potential in the "filmless department" [6].

Acknowledgements. We would like to thank our neurosurgical colleagues for their help during the study and the many radiologists who sent increasing numbers of CT studies.

References

1. Griffith HB (1986) The IMTRAN revolution – telephone transmission of x-rays and scans. Bristol Med Chir J 101: 29–37
2. Gentleman D, Jennett B (1981) Hazards of inter-hospital transfer of comatose head-injured patients. Lancet II: 853–855
3. Teasdale G, Galbraith S, Murray L (1982) Management of traumatic intracranial haematoma. Br Med J 285: 1695–1697
4. Lee T, Latham J, Kerr RSC, Kaar G, Teddy PJT, Dobson D, Anslow P (1990) A new CT image transfer system: how does this affect the management of referrals to a regional neurosurgical service? Lancet (in press)
5. Hansell D (1990) Digital chest radiography: current status. Clin Radiol 41: 229–231
6. Craig JOMC (1988) The filmless department. Br J Hosp Med 40: 97–101

Dr. J. A. Spencer
Section of Neuroradiology
The Radcliffe Infirmary
Oxford OX2 6HE, UK

Neuroradiology (1991) 33 [Suppl]: 653–655

Neuro-radiology
© Springer-Verlag 1991

CT and MRI features of acute toxic encephalopathies

S. Batnitzky[1], R. Sherlock[2], J. H. McMillan[1], J. D. R. Miller[2], S. J. Rosenthal[1], and D. L. Nelson[1]

[1] Department of Diagnostic Radiology, University of Kansas Medical Center, Kansas City, USA
[2] The University of Alberta Hospitals, Edmonton, Alberta, Canada

Summary. A variety of toxins can cause degenerative brain lesions, both by chronic use of small amounts or by acute exposures from industrial accidents or suicide attempts. The most common neurotoxins encountered clinically are carbon monoxide, methanol, and ethylene glycol. CT and MRI play an important role in the assessment of the comatose patient. These imaging studies may suggest the cause of the coma in many instances. Immediate and appropriate therapy may be life saving.

Key words: Carbon monoxide – Ethylene glycol – Methanol – Encephalopathy

Material

Thirty-four patients who were hospitalized following ingestion of or exposure to various toxins were examined with cranial CT. Seven of these patients also had cranial MRI. Twenty-two patients were examined within 24 h after admission. Ten patients were examined 4–10 days after admission and delayed studies at 1 and 4 months were obtained in 2 patients. With the exception of 3 cases of carbon monoxide poisoning, all CT studies were performed without the use of intravenous contrast material. The MRI examinations utilized T1- and T2-weighted spin echo techniques. No contrast material was used. The ages of these patients ranged from 16 to 72 years. In 26 patients methanol was the offending toxin. In 6 patients carbon monoxide was the toxin and in 2 patients ethylene glycol was the causative agent. The majority of methanol and ethylene glycol intoxication occurred in alcoholics but several cases were the result of suicide attempts. In the case of carbon monoxide, 3 cases were due to accidental inhalation and 3 cases were the result of attempted suicide.

Results and discussion

The extreme toxicity of these agents makes rapid recognition and immediate treatment vital. Overall there were 14 deaths (13 from methanol and 1 from ethylene glycol). Five patients from the methanol group, 1 from the ethylene glycol group and 4 from the carbon monoxide group were left with profound neurological disturbances. Appropriate therapy and supportive measures may be life-saving if initiated rapidly [1]. Some of these toxins have a propensity for selective bilateral and symmetric involvement of the basal ganglia as well as the white matter. CT and MRI can demonstrate the extent and morphologic distribution of the brain changes in toxic encephalopathies and may suggest the cause in many instances. CT and MRI are also useful for determining the prognosis. In some instances it is difficult to categorize the areas of toxic involvement because of frequent additional brain damage from ensuing complications such as hypotension, anoxia and resuscitation efforts. This occurred in 4 patients in the methanol group.

Carbon monoxide

The affinity of hemoglobin for carbon monoxide is approximately 200–300 times its affinity for oxygen [2]. Exposure to even low concentrations of carbon monoxide can result in clinically significant reduction in the oxygen carrying capacity of the blood. Carbon monoxide poisoning preferentially involves the globus pallidus and white matter [2–5].

On CT, symmetric bilateral lesions can be seen in the globus pallidus (Fig. 1). Contrast enhancement in the region of these lesions may be seen 1–4 weeks following exposure to carbon monoxide [2, 3]. Symmetric ill- or well-defined lucent areas in the periventricular white matter are also common findings. On MRI, the globus pallidus and white matter lesions produce areas of increased signal intensity on T2-weighted images [5] (Figs. 2, 3). The severity of the white matter involvement provides the best clue to the prognosis [4]. The white matter changes may resolve (Fig. 3) or progress to varying degrees of permanent necrosis. Involvement of the globus pallidus is of no prognostic significance [4].

Bilateral symmetric globus pallidal necrosis is not specific for acute carbon monoxide poisoning. These changes may also be seen in hypoglycemia, barbiturate, hydrogen sulfide and cyanide intoxication [3].

Methanol and ethylene glycol

The sources of methanol and ethylene glycol are widespread with a multiplicity of uses. Methanol is found in industrial solvents, duplicating fluid, windshield wiper fluid, rubbing alcohol, bootleg or denatured alcohol, witch hazel, cologne and paint thinners. Ethylene glycol is found in detergents, paints, lacquers, polishes, cosmetics, deicers and antifreeze.

Characteristically, methanol and ethylene glycol intoxication are associated with metabolic acidosis with a large anion gap [6, 7]. Both methanol and ethylene glycol per se are nontoxic [6–8]. The CNS symptoms are due to

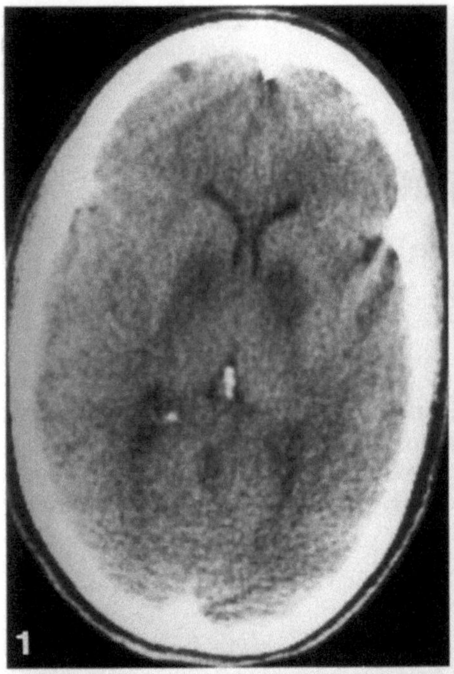

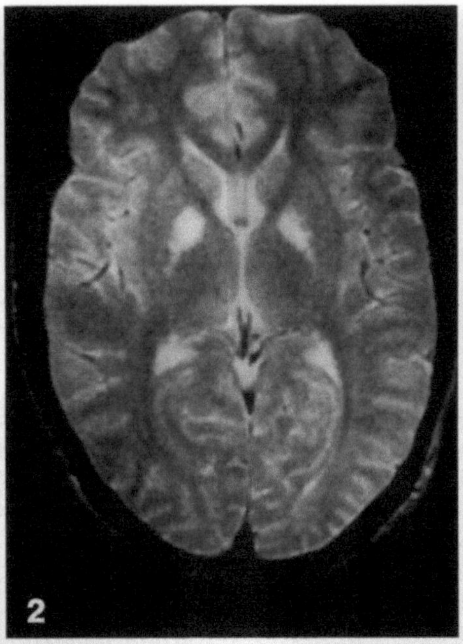

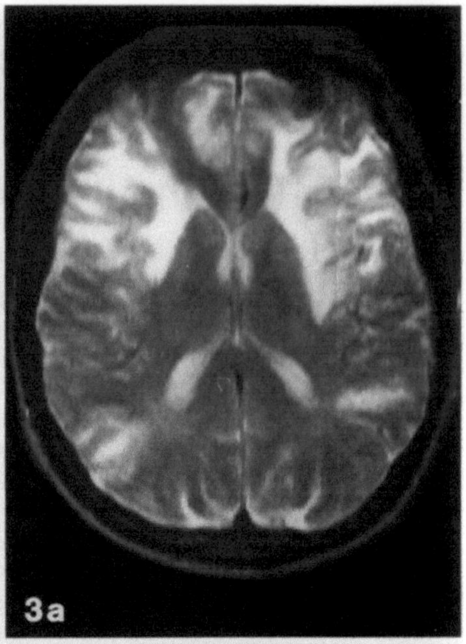

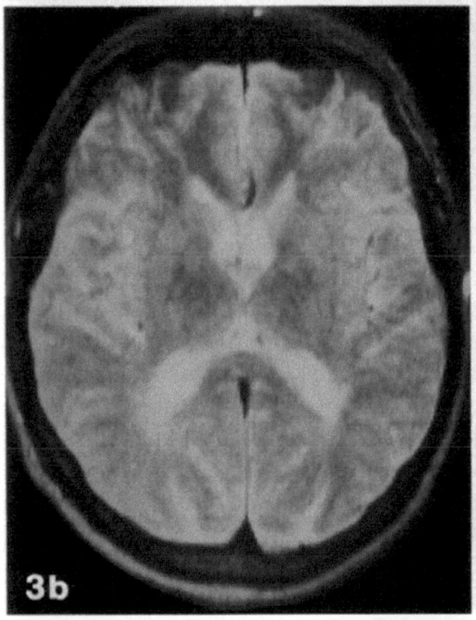

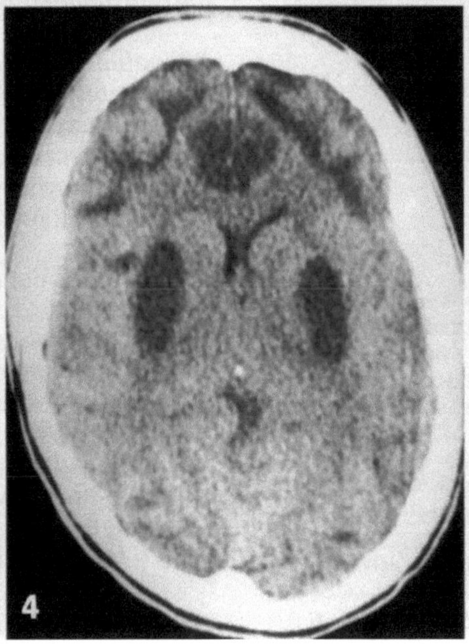

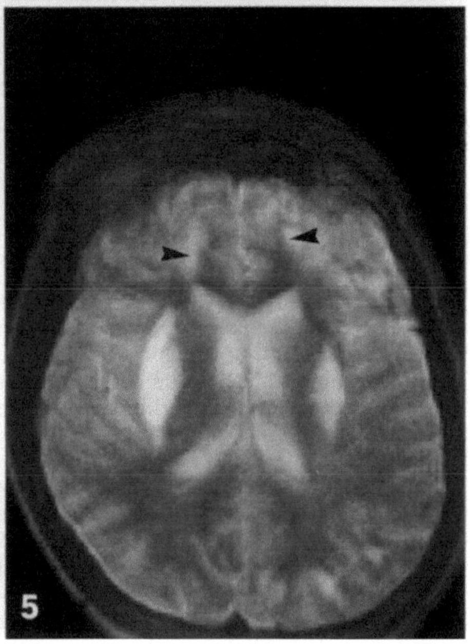

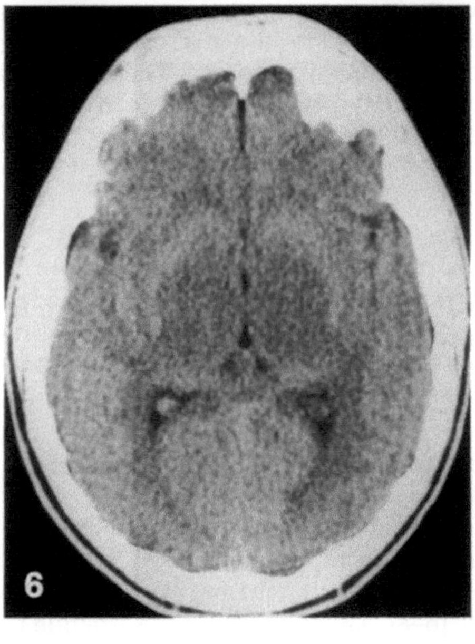

Fig. 1. Non-contrast CT in 27-year-old female who attempted suicide by inhaling carbon monoxide fumes demonstrates symmetric bilateral lucencies in the globus pallidus

Fig. 2. T2-weighted MRI in 25-year-old male with carbon monoxide intoxication demonstrates increased signal intensity in the globus pallidus bilaterally

Fig. 3 a, b. A 72-year-old male had accidental exposure to carbon monoxide while working on his car in a closed garage. **a** T2-weighted MR image demonstrates symmetric bilateral areas of increased signal intensity in the frontal white matter. The lateral ventricles are compressed and small. **b** Following hyperbaric oxygen therapy, the patient was discharged from hospital with no neurologic deficit. T2-weighted MR image taken 3 months later demonstrates resolution of the previously demonstrated abnormalities. Note the interval increase in ventricular size, which is still within normal limits for the patient's age

Fig. 4. Non-contrast CT in 23-year-old male with methanol intoxication demonstrates symmetric bilateral lucencies in the putamen. Bilateral symmetric frontal lucencies are also noted

Fig. 5. T2-weighted MR image in 45-year-old male with methanol intoxication demonstrates bilateral high signal intensity areas in the putamen and frontal lobes *(arrowheads)*

Fig. 6. Non-contrast CT in 16-year-old male with ethylene glycol intoxication demonstrates symmetric bilateral areas of decreased attenuation in the region of the thalamus the direct toxic effects of their metabolites and the associated severe metabolic acidosis [6–8].

Methanol intoxication has a propensity for symmetric bilateral, involvement of the putamen and the fronto-central white matter [1] (Figs. 4, 5). On CT, these areas have low attenuation values (Fig. 4). On MRI, these areas exhibit high signal on T2-weighted images (Fig. 5).

In the methanol group, 8 patients had normal CT and MRI scans. Treatment was initiated immediately because of a history or strong suspicion of methanol ingestion. All of these patients did well clinically with no residual ill effects.

Twenty-four of the 26 patients had admission methanol levels but in almost all cases there was usually a delay of a few hours from the time of ingestion. The methanol levels did not correspond to the clinical condition or CT appearance. However, there was clear correlation between the CT findings and the severity of the clinical symptoms. This has also been noted previously [1]. The presence of hemorrhage in the involved areas is a bad prognostic sign [1]. Putaminal, parenchymal or intraventricular hemorrhage was present in 6 patients who either died or were left with profound neurological deficits.

In ethylene glycol intoxication, areas of necrosis in the thalami, basal ganglia, pons, corpora quadrigemina and basal portions of the temporal lobes may be seen [9]. These are of low density on CT (Fig. 6) and have increased signal intensity on T2-weighted MR images. Diffuse cerebral edema with and without petechial hemorrhages may also be seen.

References

1. Aquilonius SM, Bergstrom K, Enoksson P, Hedstrand U, Lundberg PO, Mostrom U, Olsson Y (1980) Cerebral computed tomography in methanol intoxication. J Comput Assist Tomogr 4: 425–428
2. Nardizzi LR (1979) Computerized tomographic correlate of carbon monoxide poisoning. Arch Neurol 36: 38–39
3. Kim KS, Weinberg PE, Suh JH, Ho SU (1980) Acute carbon monoxide poisoning: computed tomography of the brain. AJNR 1: 399–402
4. Miura T, Mitomo M, Kawai R, Harada K (1985) CT of the brain in acute carbon monoxide intoxication: characteristic features and prognosis. AJNR 6: 739–742
5. Horowitz Al, Kaplan R, Sarpel G (1987) Carbon monoxide toxicity: MR imaging of the brain. Radiology 162: 787–788
6. Parry MF, Wallach R (1974) Ethylene glycol poisoning. Am J Med 57: 143–150
7. Scully RE, Galdabini JJ, McNeely BU (1979) Case records of the Massachusetts General Hospital. N Engl J Med 301: 650–657
8. McLean DR, Jcobs H, Mielke BW (1980) Methanol poisoning: a clinical and pathological study. Ann Neurol 8: 161–167
9. Maier W (1983) Cerebral computed tomography of ethylene glycol intoxication. Neuroradiology 24: 175–177

Dr. S. Batnitzky
Department of Diagnostic Radiology
University of Kansas Medical Center
Kansas City, KS 66103, USA

Neuroradiology (1991) 33 [Suppl]: 656–658

Neuro radiology
© Springer-Verlag 1991

MRI of Herpes simplex encephalitis

S. Batnitzky, H. I. Price, J. H. McMillan, S. J. Rosenthal, and L. H. Wetzel

Department of Diagnostic Radiology, University of Kansas Medical Center, Kansas City, Kansas, USA

Summary. Diagnosis of Herpes simplex encephalitis (HSE) is often delayed by nonspecific and poorly localizing neurological findings. Early diagnosis and treatment are critical for a favorable outcome. MRI, CT and radionuclide brain scan imaging, all sensitive noninvasive tests, were compared for diagnosis of HSE. MRI proved to be the most sensitive.

Key words: Herpes simplex virus – Encephalitis – Temporal lobe

Six patients with Herpes simplex encephalitis (HSE) whose ages ranged from 57 to 67 years were imaged using CT and MRI on the day of admission. Four CT studies were performed before and after intravenous contrast medium. In two cases noncontrast CT was obtained. MRI was performed using T1- and T2-weighted spin echo techniques. Radionuclide brain imaging (RNI) using ^{99m}Tc DTPA was performed in three patients on the day of admission or the following day. Follow-up MRI and CT was obtained in all patients. The diagnosis of HSE was verified by isolation of the virus (HSV) in two patients and by serological confirmation in the remaining patients.

Results

The initial imaging studies were performed 4–12 days after the onset of symptoms. Comparison of CT, MRI and RNI demonstrated that MRI was superior in sensitivity and speed of diagnosis. MRI was positive in all patients. CT was initially abnormal in only half but became positive in the others on follow-up. No contrast enhancement was seen on inital CT. In two of three patients in whom both CT and MRI were abnormal, the initial RNI was also abnormal. RNI was normal in one patient.

MRI demonstrated a far greater extent of involvement than CT or RNI. The temporal lobe was the dominant area of involvement in all patients. Involvement was unilateral in four cases (Fig. 1) and bilateral in two (Fig. 2), in whom CT and RNI demonstrated only unilateral disease. In two patients the orbitofrontal region was also involved (Fig. 3).

Discussion

HSV consists of two strains [1,2]: the oral strain (type 1) produces fulminant, necrotizing encephalitis in adults and children; the genital strain (type 2) is responsible for infection in neonates. In type 1 HSE the virus preferentially attacks the temporofrontal areas. The basis for this localization is not well understood. The mortality of untreated adult HSE is 70 % in 1 month and may approach 90 % at 6 months [1,3,4]. The mortality and morbidity of HSE may be reduced by antiviral therapy [1,5]. Early institution of therapy and, therefore, early diagnosis are essential. Diagnosis is often delayed by nonspecific and poorly localizing neurological findings and the lack of a specific noninvasive test. RNI, CT and MRI are all sensitive noninvasive imaging techniques which have been used to diagnose HSE [1,3,5–9]. The findings are not specific, but in patients clinically suspected of having HSE, these imaging studies can suggest a specific etiology. Bilateral temporal lobe abnormalities are almost pathognomonic for HSE (Fig. 2). Similarly an abnormality on both sides of the Sylvian fissure, the "transsylvian sign," is highly suggestive [5,8,9]. This latter finding was present in three of our cases on both CT and MRI (Figs. 1, 2). Sparing of the lenticular nucleus is characteristic [6].

CT and RNI within 4–5 days of the onset of symptoms are often normal [3,6,8,9]. RNI abnormalities have been observed as early as the 2nd–4th day after onset of neurological symptoms [7]. Contrast enhancement on CT is rarely detected until the 2nd week [9]. Although our series is small, our results suggest that MRI is the most sensitive noninvasive technique in early diagnosis. Abnormalities on MRI may be obvious days before CT changes, due to the high sensitivity of the T2-weighted spin-echo technique to increased brain water content. MRI demonstrates decreased signal on T1-weighted images (Fig. 1) and a pronounced increased signal on T2-weighted images (Figs. 1b, 2, 3). The abnormality shown on MRI is far more extensive than on concomitant CT and RNI.

MRI is superior to CT in the temporal lobe [9]. The middle cranial fossa is often obscured on CT by artifacts from the petrous and sphenoid bones, which do not occur with MRI. The basal, medial and lateral aspects of the temporal lobe are exquisitely imaged on coronal MRI (Fig. 3). The medial and basal gyri are spared in vascular occlusive lesions due to collateral blood supply [9]. Neoplastic involvement of the temporal lobe also tends to spare the medial and basal gyri, which areas are involved in HSE.

One of the pathological hallmarks of HSE is hemorrhage, seldom evident on imaging, as in most instances these are scattered microhemorrhages [5,9]. Only 11 were reported to have hemorrhage associated with the lesion on the initial imaging examination [5].

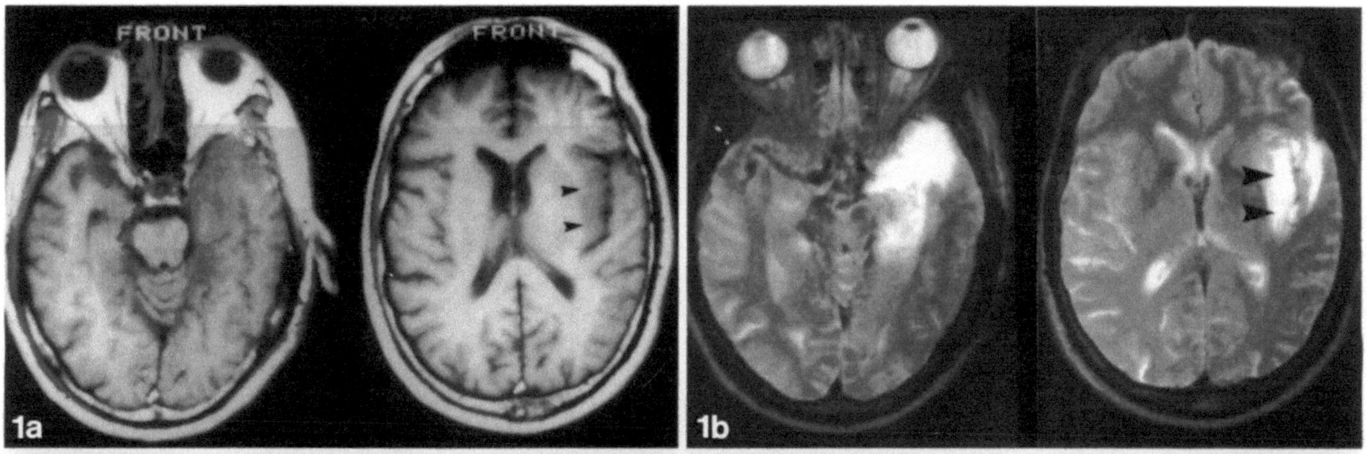

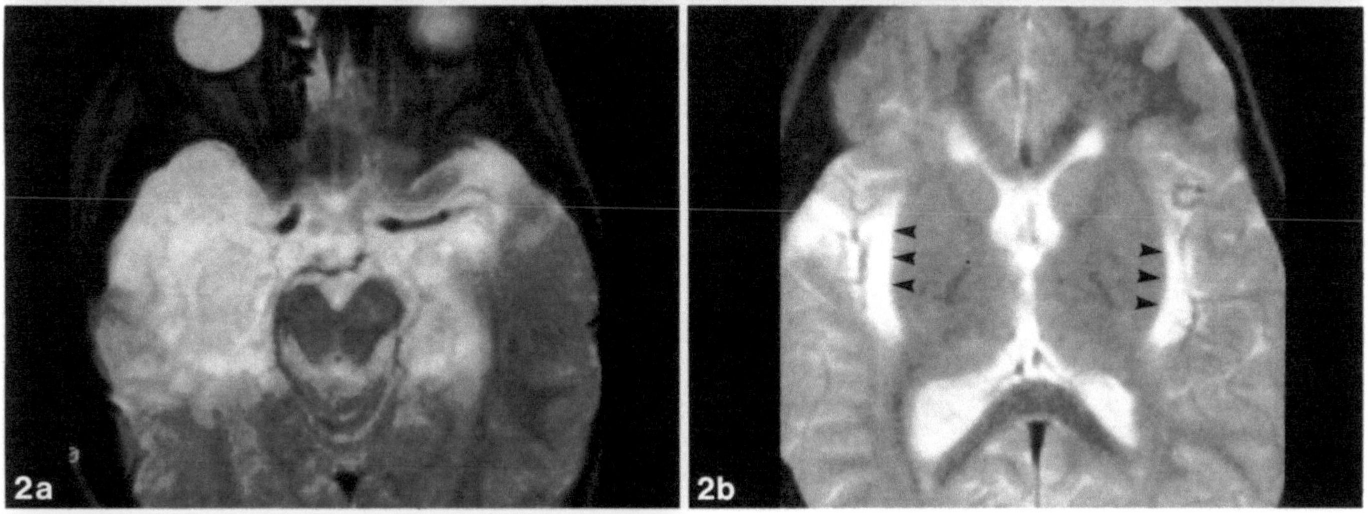

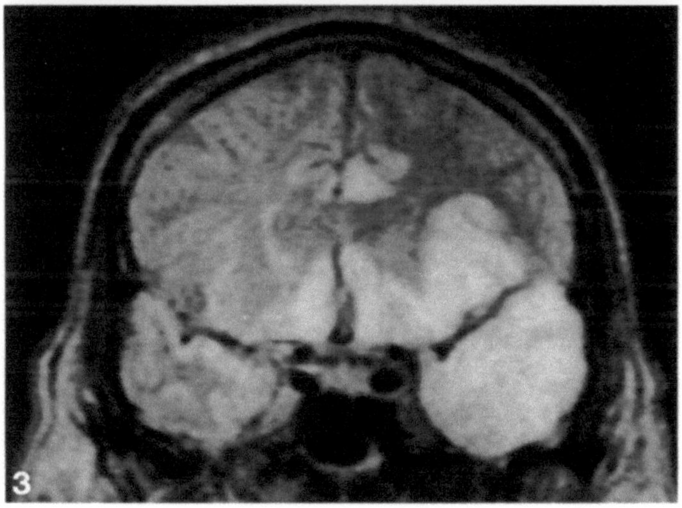

Fig. 1a, b. A 67-year-old male with left temporal Herpes simplex encephalitis (HSE). **a** T1-weighted MR images demonstrate decreased signal intensity in the left temporal lobe. There is decreased signal intensity in the insular area *(arrowheads)*, the "transsylvian sign", highly suggestive of HSE. Note sparing of the lenticular nucleus. **b** T2-weighted MR images demonstrate increased signal intensity in the left temporal lobe. The insular involvement is indicated by the *arrowheads*. CT and radionuclide brain scans did not demonstrate the same extent and degree of involvement as MRI

Fig. 2a, b. A 5-year-old girl with bilateral HSE. **a** T2-weighted MR image demonstrates increased signal intensity in both temporal lobes, right than left. **b** On a slightly more craniad T2-weighted MR image the right and left insular areas *(arrowheads)* are also involved

Fig. 3. Coronal T2-weighted MRI in a 54-year-old male with HSE demonstrates increased signal intensity in the entire left temporal lobe. There is involvement of both frontal lobes, greater on the left

Conclusions

MRI is the most sensitive noninvasive test for early diagnosis of HSE.

References

1. Griffith JF. Chien LT (1983) Herpes simplex virus encephalitis: diagnostic and treatment considerations. Med Clin North Am 67: 991–1008
2. Batnitzky S, Robinson RG, Wetzel LH, Lai CW, Halleran WJ III, McMillan JH (1986) Imaging studies in neonatal herpes simplex encephalitis. Acta Radiol (Stockh) [Suppl] 369: 197–199
3. Davis JM, Davis KR, Kleinman GM, Kirchner HS, Taveras J (1978) Computed tomography of herpes simplex encephalitis with clinico-pathological correlation. Radiology 129: 409–417
4. Morawetz RB, Whitley RJ, Murphy DM (1983) Experience with brain biopsy for suspected herpes encephalitis: a review of forty consecutive cases. Neurosurgery 12: 654–657

5. Neils EW, Lukin R, Tomsick TA, Tew JM (1987) Magnetic resonance imaging and computed tomography scanning of herpes simplex encephalitis. J Neurosurg 67: 592–594
6. Zimmerman RD, Russell EJ, Leeds NE, Kaufman D (1980) CT in the early diagnosis of herpes simplex encephalitis. AJR 143: 61–66
7. Karlin CA, Robinson RG, Hinthorn DR, Liu C (1978) Radionuclide imaging in herpes simplex. Radiology 126: 181–184
8. Enzmann DR, Ranson B, Norman D, Talberth E (1978) Computed tomography of herpes simplex encephalitis. Radiology 129: 419–425
9. Schroth G, Gawehn J, Thron A, Vallbracht A, Voight K (1987) Early diagnosis of herpes simplex encephalitis by MRI. Neurology 37: 179–183

Dr. S. Batnitzky
Department of Diagnostic Radiology
University of Kansas Medical Center
Kansas City
KS 66103, USA

Neuroradiology (1991) 33 [Suppl]: 659–660

Neuro-radiology
© Springer-Verlag 1991

Congestive cardiac manifestations from cerebrocranial arteriovenous shunts

Endovascular treatment in children

R. García Monaco, D. de Victor, H. Alvarez, and P. Lasjaunias

Department of Neuroradiology, Hôpital Bicêtre, Kremlin Bicêtre Cédex, France

Summary. Since 1984 the authors have been involved in the management of 30 children presenting with congestive cardiac manifestations secondary to cerebrocranial arteriovenous shunts. Medical treatment and follow-up or endovascular therapy were initially indicated depending on the age of the patients and the severity of the cardiac manifestations. The cardiac symptoms resolved (73%) or were improved (18%) in the patients treated by embolisation. The technique, challenges, indications and contraindications of endovascular therapy are discussed.

Key words: Embolisation – Neonate – Heart failure – Arteriovenous malformation

Cerebrocranial arteriovenous shunts (AVS) are infrequent causes of congestive cardiac failure (CCF). Cardiac manifestations vary from severe heart failure to asymptomatic cardiomegaly; all grades are possible. We report our experience of embolisation in CCF of cranial origin and discuss the best timing of intervention according to the clinical tolerance of the symptoms.

Patients and methods

The age at diagnosis was: 0–1 month in 19 cases, 1–12 months in 7 and 1–15 years in 4. In 23 (77%) of the patients the CCF was the main complaint, 13 having severe heart failure. In the remaining 7 (23%) macrocephaly or hydrocephalus were the prominent manifestations, a mild cardiac overload being discovered by complementary studies. The most frequent disease involved was vein of Galen aneurysmal malformation (VGAM) (22 patients). Dural or brain arteriovenous malformations (AVMs) or capillary haemangiomas were present in the remaining patients.

Embolisation was performed in 22 cases (5 neonates, 11 infants and 6 children). Another 2 patients are awaiting the appropriate time for embolisation. In 4 cases endovascular treatment was not indicated because of severe brain damage or inaccessible feeding vessels. Two other patients were lost to follow-up.

Embolisation was always performed by the femoral approach, by the Seldinger technique. IBCA or NBCA were used to embolise all AVMs or fistulae, whereas capillary haemangiomas were embolised with particles.

Results

In the embolised group CCF resolved in 16 (73%) of patients and in 4 (18%) there was significant clinical improvement. Two (9%) patients died, due to ineffective embolisation in a 3 kg baby with a VGAM and major

Table 1. Decision tree in the neonatal period

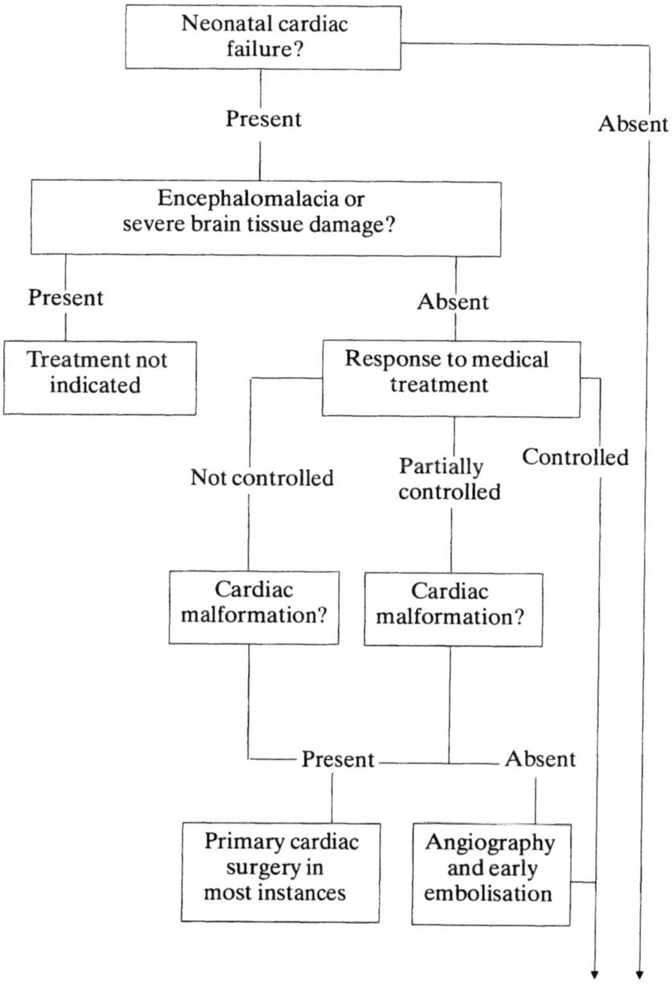

Table 2. Decision tree in infancy

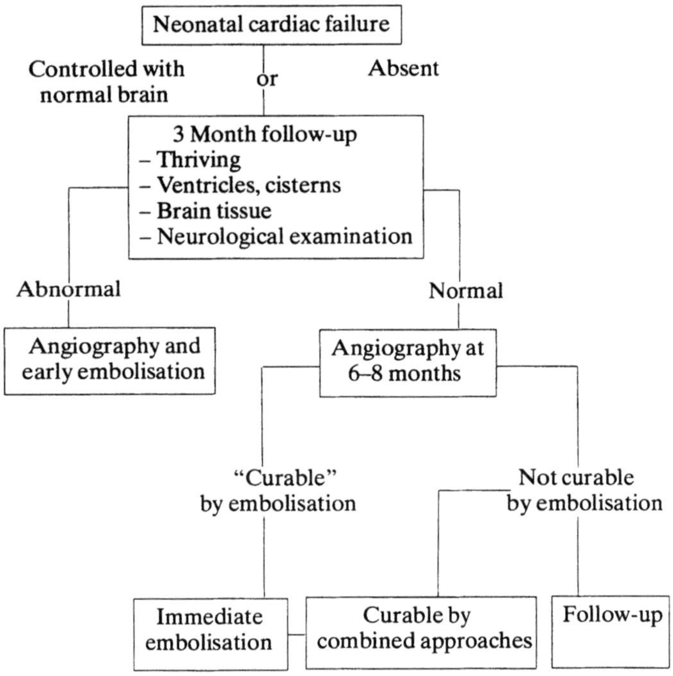

haemodynamic disorders during and after the procedure in a newborn with a brain AVM. In the non-embolised group, 2 infants are doing well and waiting for embolisation. The 4 patients rejected for embolisation have died. The overall mortality was 20%. Only 1 case of transient morbidity was seen after embolisation: skin necrosis after treatment of a capillary haemangioma that resolved spontaneously some months later.

Discussion

Severe CCF associated with intracranial vascular malformations occurs in the neonatal period. The older the child, the lower the chances of cardiac manifestations and the less severe they will be. In CCF with giant capillary haemangiomas of the face symptoms start with the proliferation phase of the lesion at 4–12 months of age.

The prognosis of newborns or infants with severe CCF of cranial origin has been classically considered very poor [1], with a mortality rate between 63% and 90% even with medical or surgical treatment [2]. This poor outcome has significantly improved since introduction of endovascular techniques [3, 4], with an overall mortality of 20% in our series.

Arterial embolisation presents some distinctive features when performed in newborns and infants [5]. The contrast medium and the small size of the femoral arteries constitute limiting factors. Femoral patency after intervention is essential to allow staged embolisation (if needed) and future normal growth of the lower limbs. The goal of arterial embolisation in newborns with severe failure is to decrease the flow of the cranial AVS. Eventually, the volume and pressure overload to the right atrium will be reduced, allowing stabilisation of cardiac function. Complete anatomical cure of the cerebral lesions is not mandatory at this stage. In view of the technical challenges, we think that embolisation is not needed in a newborn whose heart failure responds to medical treatment. In such a case we suggest periodic clinical follow up, and MRI examinations to survey neurological development. Occurrence of a warning sign or symptom will prompt embolisation. If not, pretherapeutic angiography is proposed at 6–8 months of age to determine the possibility of endovascular therapy. In these cases we think there is no indication for a "diagnostic" angiogram earlier in life, since CT and MRI provide all the necessary information. We believe that severe brain damage, shown by CT or MRI in a newborn, represents a contraindication to endovascular therapy, since neurological prognosis is ominous even with anatomical cure of the vascular lesion.

Conclusion

The traditional poor prognosis of congestive heart failure due to an intracranial lesion in early childhood must be revised. Management of these patients by the endovascular team will help to select the most appropriate form of treatment for the cardiac symptoms. Endovascular techniques can rapidly control, improve or cure most of these lesions and their symptoms with a reasonable chance of normal development. Morbidity and mortality are low if embolisation is properly indicated and scheduled, following a strict protocol (Tables 1, 2).

References

1. Pellegrino PA, Milanesi O, Saia OS, Carollo C (1987) Congestive heart failure secondary to cerebral arterio-venous fistula. Childs Nerv Syst 3: 141–144
2. Johnston IH, Whittle IR, Besser M, Morgan MK (1987) Vein of Galen malformation: diagnosis and management. Neurosurgery 20: 747–758
3. Lasjaunias P, Rodesch G, Terbrugge K, Pruvost P, Victor D de, Comoy J, Landrieu P (1988) Vein of Galen aneurysmal malformations. Report of 36 cases managed between 1982 and 1988. Acta Neurochir (Wien) 99: 26–37
4. Berenstein A, Lasjaunias P (1990) Endovascular treatment of brain, spinal cord and spinal lesions: surgical neuro-angiography, vol. 4. Springer, Berlin Heidelberg New York (in press)
5. García Monaco R, Alvarez H, Lasjaunias P (1990) Utilisation du minitorqueur dans les malformations artério-veineuses cérébrales du nouveau-né et du nourrisson. Rev Im Med 2: 263–264

Dr. P. Lasjaunias
Neuroradiologie Vasculaire
Hôpital Bicêtre
78 rue du Général-Leclerc
F-94275 Le Kremlin-Bicêtre Cedex, France

MIX
Papier aus verantwortungsvollen Quellen
Paper from responsible sources
FSC® C105338

If you have any concerns about our products,
you can contact us on
ProductSafety@springernature.com

In case Publisher is established outside the EU,
the EU authorized representative is:
Springer Nature Customer Service Center GmbH
Europaplatz 3, 69115 Heidelberg, Germany

Printed by Libri Plureos GmbH
in Hamburg, Germany